DISEA... DISORDERS

H A N D B O O K

DISEASES AND DISORDERS
DISORDERS
H A N D B O O K

Springhouse Corporation
Springhouse, Pennsylvania

STAFF FOR THIS VOLUME

CLINICAL STAFF

Clinical Director
Barbara McVan, RN

Clinical Editors
Mary Chapman Gyetvan, RN, BSEd
Judith A. Schilling McCann, RN, BSN

PUBLICATION STAFF

Executive Director, Editorial
Stanley Loeb

Executive Director, Creative Services
Jean Robinson

Design
John Hubbard (art director), Stephanie Peters (associate art director), Lorraine Carbo

Editing
Regina Daley Ford (project manager), Roberta Kangilaski

Copy Editing
David Moreau (manager), Edith McMahon (supervisor), Nick Anastasio, Keith de Pinho, Diane Labus, Doris Weinstock, Debra Young

Art Production
Robert Perry (manager), Anna Brindisi, Christopher Buckley, Loretta Caruso, Donald Knauss, Christina McKinley, Mark Marcin, Robert Wieder

Typography
David Kosten (manager), Diane Paluba (assistant manager), Nancy Wirs, Brenda Mayer, Brent Rinedoller, Joyce Rossi Biletz, Alicia Dempsey

Manufacturing
Deborah Meiris (manager), T.A. Landis

Project Coordination
Aline S. Miller (supervisor), Maureen Carmichael

Library of Congress Cataloging-in-Publication Data
Diseases and disorders handbook.

Bibliography: p.
Includes index.
1. Diseases—Handbooks, manuals, etc. 2. Internal medicine—Handbooks, manuals, etc. I. Springhouse Corporation. [DNLM: 1. Disease—handbooks. 2. Medicine—handbooks. WB 39 D611]
RC55.D56 1988 616 87-33568
ISBN 0-87434-157-4 (flex)
ISBN 0-87434-087-X (paper)

CONTENTS

ADVISORY BOARD, CONTRIBUTORS, AND CONSULTANTS

ADVISORY BOARD

Lillian S. Brunner, RN, MSN, ScD, FAAN, Nurse/Author, Brunner Associates, Inc., Berwyn, Pa.

Donald C. Cannon, MD, PhD, Resident in Internal Medicine, University of Kansas, School of Medicine, Wichita

Luther Christman, RN, PhD, Dean, Rush College of Nursing; Vice-President, Nursing Affairs, Rush–Presbyterian–St. Luke's Medical Center, Chicago

Kathleen A. Dracup, RN, DNSc, FAAN, Associate Professor, School of Nursing, University of California at Los Angeles

Stanley J. Dudrick, MD, FACS, Professor, Department of Surgery, and Director, Nutritional Support Services, University of Texas Medical School at Houston; St. Luke's Episcopal Hospital, Houston

Halbert E. Fillinger, MD, Assistant Medical Examiner, Philadelphia County

M. Josephine Flaherty, RN, PhD, Principal Nursing Officer, Department of National Health and Welfare, Ottawa

Joyce LeFever Kee, RN, MSN, Associate Professor, College of Nursing, University of Delaware, Newark

Dennis E. Leavelle, MD, Associate Professor, Mayo Medical Laboratories, Mayo Clinic, Rochester, Minn.

Roger M. Morrell, MD, PhD, FACP, Professor, Neurology and Immunology/Microbiology, Wayne State University, School of Medicine, Detroit; Chief, Neurology Service, Veterans Administration Medical Center, Allen Park, Mich.; Diplomate, American Board of Psychiatry and Neurology

Ara G. Paul, PhD, Dean, College of Pharmacy, University of Michigan, Ann Arbor

Rose Pinneo, RN, MS, Associate Professor of Nursing and Clinician II, University of Rochester, N.Y.

Thomas E. Rubbert, BSL, LLB, JD, Attorney-at-Law, Pasadena, Calif.

Maryanne Schreiber, RN, BA, Product Manager, Patient Monitoring, Hewlett-Packard Co., Waltham (Mass.) Division

Frances J. Storlie, RN, PhD, ANP, Director, Personal Health Services, Southwest Washington Health District, Vancouver

Claire L. Watson, RN, Clinical Documentation Associate, IVAC Corp., San Diego

CONTRIBUTORS

Virginia P. Arcangelo, RN, MSN, Instructor, Helene Fuld School of Nursing, Camden, N.J.

Charold L. Baer, RN, PhD, Professor, Department of Adult Health and Illness, The Oregon Health Sciences University School of Nursing, Portland

Katherine G. Baker, RN, MN, Clinical Specialist, UCLA Center for Health Sciences

Ardelina Albano Baldonado, RN, PhD, Assistant Dean and Director, Undergraduate Program, The Marcella Niehoff School of Nursing, Loyola University of Chicago

Cynthia Ashe Beebe, RN, Clinical Gynecologic Oncology Nurse, University of Virginia Medical Center, Charlottesville

Judy Beniak, RN, MPH, Program Director, Continuing Nursing Education, University of Minnesota, Minneapolis

Jo Anne Bennett, RN, MA, CNA, Adjunct Instructor, Lienhard School of Nursing, Pace University, Pleasantville, N.Y.

Patricia M. Bennett, RN, BSN, Unit Teacher, Urology Service, Massachusetts General Hospital, Boston

Margaret Hamilton Birney, RN, MSN, Lecturer, College of Nursing, Wayne State University, Detroit

Nora Lynn Bollinger, RN, MSN, Oncology Clinical Nurse Specialist, Walter Reed Army Medical Center, Washington, D.C.

Heather Boyd-Monk, RN, BSN, Assistant Director for Nursing Education Programs, Wills Eye Hospital, Philadelphia

Hirotaka Katsumata Bralley, RN, BSN, CRNA, Certified Registered Nurse Anesthetist, Cookeville (Tenn.) General Hospital

Barbara Gross Braverman, RN, MSN, CS, Psychiatric Clinical Nurse Specialist, Medical College of Pennsylvania, Philadelphia

Phyllis Bitner Brehm, RN, Medical Oncology Coordinator, Medical College of Pennsylvania, Philadelphia

Christine S. Breu, RN, MN, Research Associate, University of California, Los Angeles

Lillian S. Brunner, MSN, ScD, LittD, FAAN, Nurse/Author, Brunner Associates, Inc., Berwyn, Pa.

Joanne D'Agostino Bryanos, RN, MSN, Former Clinical Nurse Leader, Massachusetts General Hospital, Boston

Lizabeth A. Burke, RN, BSN, CPNP, Nurse Clinician, Children's Hospital of Philadelphia

Judith Suter Burkholder, RN, MSN, Clinical Director, Ambulatory Services, Yale–New Haven (Conn.) Hospital

Barbara J. Burns, RN, BSN, Medical Surgical Instructor, St. Elizabeth Hospital School of Nursing, Utica, N.Y.

Barbara R. Burroughs, RN, MSN, Home Infusion Clinical Nurse Specialist, nmc Homecare, Theranutrix, Delran, N.J.

Priscilla A. Butts, RN, MSN, Lecturer, School of Nursing, University of Pennsylvania, Philadelphia

Mary P. Cadogan, RN, MN, Former Instructor, Community Health Nursing, Yale University School of Nursing, New Haven, Conn.; Former Family Nurse Practitioner, Hill Health Center, New Haven

Linda Pelczynski Cagle, RN, MSN, Vice-President, Dynamedics Inc., St. Louis

G. Carpenter, MD, Associate Professor, Pediatrics, Thomas Jefferson University, Philadelphia

Barbara Walsh Clark, RN, MSN, Former Associate Professor of Nursing, Bucks County Community College, Newtown, Pa.

Constance C. Cooper, RN, Supervisor, Gastroenterology Services, Allegheny General Hospital, Pittsburgh

Susan Corbett, RN, Dermatology Nurse, Skin and Cancer Hospital and Mycosis Fungoides Center of Temple University Hospital, Philadelphia

Pam Cross, BSN, MS, Major, Army Nurse Corps; Clinical Head Nurse; Acute Care Psychiatric Ward, Eisenhower Army Medical Center, Fort Gordon, Ga.

Joanne Patzek DaCunha, RN, BS, Clinical Editor, Springhouse Corp., Springhouse, Pa.

T. Forcht Dagi, MD, FACS, Assistant Professor, Surgery and Anatomy, Georgetown University Hospital, Washington, D.C.

Mary Lou Damiano, RN, BA, ADN, Program Coordinator, Mountain States Regional Hemophilia Center, University of Arizona Health Sciences Center, Tucson

Helen Kline Davis, RN, MSN, Staff Nurse, Labor and Delivery, Thomas Jefferson University Hospital, Philadelphia

Fleda Dean, RN, BSN, AB, Staff Nurse, Yale–New Haven (Conn.) Hospital

Andrea L. Devoti, RN, MSN, CNRN, Nursing Supervisor, The Bryn Mawr (Pa.) Hospital

Stella R. Doherty, RN, MSN, Nursing Services Consultant for Tuberculosis, Commonwealth of Pennsylvania, Pennsylvania Department of Health, Division of Acute Infectious Disease Control, Harrisburg

Judy Donlen, RNC, MSN, Assistant Director of Nursing, Children's Hospital of Philadelphia

Gail D'Onofrio, RN, MS, Critical Care Specialist, Boston

Kathleen Dracup, RN, DNSc, CCRN, FAAN, Associate Professor, UCLA School of Nursing

Diane Dressler, RN, MSN, CCRN, Clinical Nurse Specialist, Midwest Heart Surgery Institute, Milwaukee

Colleen Jane Dunwoody, RN, BA, Clinical Instructor, Nursing Inservice Education, Presbyterian–University Hospital, Pittsburgh

Kathleen Joyce, MSN, Supervisory Clinical Nurse, Nephrology, National Institutes of Health, Clinical Center, Bethesda, Md.

Joyce LeFever Kee, RN, MSN, Associate Professor, College of Nursing, University of Delaware, Newark

Margaret A. Keen, RN, MSN, CNM, Associate Director/Midwifery Service, Kennedy Memorial Hospital–University Medical Center, Turnersville, N.J.

Karen Mabry Kennedy, RN, BSN, Formerly on Staff, Emergency Room, Winter Park (Fla.) Memorial Hospital

Ruth S. Kitson, RN, BAA(N), MBA, Director of Nursing, Critical Care, Toronto Western Hospital

Deborah J. LaCamera, RN, BSN, Nurse Epidemiologist, National Institutes of Health, Clinical Center, Bethesda, Md.

Mary Ann Lafferty-Della Valle, PhD, Research Associate, Department of Human Genetics, School of Medicine, and Lecturer, School of Nursing, University of Pennsylvania, Philadelphia

Cheryl Ann Gross Lane, RN, Former Oncology Nurse Specialist, Bowman Gray School of Medicine of Wake Forest University, Winston-Salem, N.C.

Linda Lass-Schuhmacher, RN, MEd, Adjunct Faculty, Department of Sociology, Suffolk University, Boston

Deborah J. Leisifer, RN, CCRN, Head Nurse, Medical/Surgical Intensive Care, Saint Francis Medical Center, Pittsburgh

Blanche M. Lenard, RN, Nurse Epidemiologist, Crozer-Chester Medical Center, Chester, Pa.

Dorrett N. Linton, RN, AD, Occupational Health Nurse, Rohm and Haas Company, Philadelphia

Patricia A. Lockhart-Pretti, RN, MS, Clinical Nurse Specialist in Neurology/Neurosurgery/Neuro-Rehabilitation, University Hospital, Boston

Pamela Peters Long, RN, BSN, Oncology Program Administrator and Clinical Coordinator, South Fulton Hospital, East Point, Ga.

Kenneth J. Mamot, RN, BS, Infection Control Consultant, The Genesee Hospital, Rochester, N.Y.

Joan Kern Manny, RN, Clinical Nurse, National Institutes of Health, Bethesda, Md.

Shirley Heaton Marshburn, RN, BSN, Assistant Director of Nursing, Hamad General Hospital Corporation, Doha Qatar, Arabian Gulf

Linda L. Martin, RN, MSN, Pulmonary Clinical Nurse Specialist, University of Virginia Medical Center, Charlottesville

Celestine B. Mason, RN, BSN, MA, Associate Professor, Pacific Lutheran University, Tacoma, Wash.

Donna McCarthy, RN, PhD, Post Doctoral Fellow, School of Nursing, University of Rochester (N.Y.)

Mary R. McCole, RN, BSN, Nurse Manager–Critical Care, Albert Einstein, Northern Division, Philadelphia

Edwina A. McConnell, RN, MS, Independent Nurse Consultant; Staff Nurse, Madison (Wis.) General Hospital

Joan P. McNamara, RN, I.V. Nurse Therapist, Abington (Pa.) Memorial Hospital

Vivian Meehan, RN, BA, Nurse Clinician for Eating Disorders Program, Highland Park (Ill.) Hospital; President and Founder, National Association for Anorexia Nervosa and Associated Disorders, Highland Park

Rita V. Miller, RN, BA, Former Nurse Manager, Presbyterian–University of Pennsylvania Medical Center, Philadelphia

M. Leslie Mitman, RN, BSN, Former Staff Nurse, Thomas Jefferson University Hospital, Philadelphia

Marilee Warner Mohr, RN, MSN, Supervisor, Women and Children Division, The Bryn Mawr (Pa.) Hospital

Anna P. Moore, RN, BSN, MS, Assistant Professor, Coordinator of Psychiatric Mental Health Nursing, Petersburg (Va.) General Hospital School of Nursing

Brenda M. Nevidjon, RN, MSN, Cancer Program Manager, Providence Medical Center, Seattle

Elaine H. Niggemann, RN, MD, Fellow, Division of Cardiology, Southwestern Medical School, Dallas

John J. O'Shea, Jr., MD, Chief Medical Staff Fellow, Clinical Immunology Section, Laboratory of Clinical Investigation, National Institute of Allergy and Infectious Diseases, National Institutes of Health, Bethesda, Md.

Mary Beth Lyman Pais, RN, BSN, MNEd, Head Nurse, Orthopaedics and Arthritis Rehabilitation, Presbyterian–University Hospital, Pittsburgh

A. June Partyka, RN, ET, Rehabilitation Nurse Coordinator, St. Francis Medical Center, Trenton, N.J.

Christene Perkins, RN, MN, Chairperson, Department of Nursing, Kettering (Ohio) College of Medical Arts

Adele W. Pike, RN, MSN, Clinical Nurse, National Institutes of Health, Clinical Center, Bethesda, Md.

Patricia Hogan Pincus, RN, MS, Technical Associate, University of Rochester (N.Y.) Medical Center; Infection Control Consultant, Hill Haven Nursing Home and Health Related Facility, Webster, N.Y.

Rosemary Carol Polomano, RN, MSN, CS, Oncology Clinical Specialist, Hospital of the University of Pennsylvania, Philadelphia

Katherine S. Puls, RN, MS, CNM, Nurse Midwife in Private Practice, Women's Alternative Health Care of Barrington (Ill.), Ltd.

Jo-Ellen Quinlan, RN, MSN, Gastrointestinal Nurse Clinician, Children's Hospital, Boston

Roger L. Ready, RN, CNA, Nurse Endoscopist, Mayo Clinic, Rochester, Minn.

Hazel V. Rice, RN, BS, MS, EdS, Associate Chairman, Southern College of SDA, Orlando, Fla.

Marilyn A. Roderick, RN, BSN, MD, Physician, General Practice, Redwood City, Calif.

Lisa Sehrt Rodriguez, RN, BSN, Staff Development Coordinator, Alton Ochsner Medical Foundation Hospital, New Orleans

Mary E. Ropka, RN, MS, Doctoral Student, University of Virginia, Charlottesville

Pamela M. Rowe, RN, BSN, MEd, Assistant Director of Nursing Education, Dartmouth-Hitchcock Medical Center, Hanover, N.H.

Sherrill Jantzi Rudy, RN, BSN, Pediatric Dermatology, Children's Hospital of Pittsburgh

Sarah A. Ryan, RN, Nurse Epidemiologist, Crozer-Chester Medical Center, Chester, Pa.

Linda Patti Sarna, RN, MN, Assistant Clinical Professor, UCLA School of Nursing

Karen Moore Schaefer, RN, MSN, Assistant Professor in Nursing, Cedar Crest College, Allentown, Pa.

Sandra Schuler, RN, MSN, Assistant Professor of Nursing, Montgomery College, Takoma Park, Md.

Marilyn R. Shahan, RN, MS, Nurse Epidemiologist, Denver Department of Health and Hospitals, Disease Control Service

Susan Budassi Sheehy, RN, MSN, CEN, Assistant Director/Trauma Service, St. Joseph Hospital, Tacoma, Wash.; Associate Clinical Professor, University of Washington School of Nursing, Seattle

Charlotte Shields, RN, BSN, Outreach Nurse Coordinator, Comprehensive Pediatric Rheumatology Center, Children's Hospital National Medical Center, Washington, D.C.

Jean A. Shook, RN, MS, CS, Psychiatric Clinical Nurse Specialist, Medical College of Pennsylvania, Philadelphia

Frances "Billie" Sills, RN, MSN, ARNP, Assistant Administrator, Nursing, The Institute for Rehabilitation and Research, Houston

Christine McNamee Smith, RN, BSN, Nurse Clinician, Thomas Jefferson University Hospital, Philadelphia

Janis B. Smith, RN, MSN, Nurse Consultant in Parent-Child Nursing, Pediatric Intensive Care, and Pediatric Cardiology and Cardiac Surgery, Wilmington, Del.

Sandra J. Somma, RN, BSN, Head Nurse, Department of Dermatology, Yale–New Haven (Conn.) Hospital

Brenda M. Splitz, RN, MSN, ANP, Adult Clinical Specialist; Clinical Coordinator, Nurse Practitioner Program; and Adjunct Faculty for Health Care Sciences, George Washington University Hospital, Washington, D.C.

Charlene Wandel Stanich, RN, MN, Associate Vice-President, Medical Nursing, Presbyterian–University Hospital, Pittsburgh

June L. Stark, RN, BSN, CCRN, Critical Care Instructor, Renal Nurse Consultant, New England Medical Center, Boston

Janice G. Stewart, RN, MSN, Manager of Nursing Support Resources, Thomas Jefferson University Hospital, Philadelphia

Frances J. Storlie, RN, PhD, CANP, Director, Personal Health Services, Southwest Washington Health District, Vancouver

Nancy S. Storz, RD, EdD, Adjunct Assistant Professor, University of Pennsylvania School of Nursing, Philadelphia

Mona R. Sutnick, RD, EdD, Nutrition Consultant, Sutnick Associates, Philadelphia; Lecturer in Community and Preventive Medicine, Medical College of Pennsylvania, Philadelphia

Basia Belza Tack, RN, MSN, ANP, Nursing Consultant, Mountain View, Calif.

Janet D'Agostino Taylor, RN, MSN, Program Director, Comprehensive Pulmonary Care Program, St. Elizabeth's Hospital, Brighton, Mass.

Maureen K. Toal, RN, BSN, Staff Nurse, Critical Care Unit, Sacred Heart Medical Center, Chester, Pa.

Sharon McBride Valente, RN, MN, CS, FAAN, Adjunct Assistant Professor, University of Southern California, Department of Nursing, Los Angeles; Clinical Specialist in Mental Health in Private Practice, Los Angeles

Susan VanDeVelde-Coke, RN, MA, MBA, Director of Nursing, Health Sciences Centre, Winnipeg, Manitoba

Mary Mishler Vogal, RN, MSN, CHN, Course Coordinator and Instructor, Helene Fuld School of Nursing, Camden, N.J.

Peggy L. Wagner, RN, MSN, CCRN, Cardiovascular Clinical Nurse Specialist, St. Michael Hospital, Milwaukee

Madeline Wake, RN, MSN, Administrator, Continuing Education in Nursing, Marquette University, Milwaukee

Connie A. Walleck, RN, MS, CNRN, Clinical Nurse Supervisor/Clinical Nurse Specialist, Neuro Trauma Center, Maryland Institute of Emergency Medical Services Systems, Baltimore

Joanne Schlosser Ware, RN, CCRN, Head Nurse, Progressive Care Unit, Martin Memorial Hospital, Stuart, Fla.

Joseph B. Warren, RN, BSN, Territory Manager/Neurosurgical Nurse Consultant, Kinetic Concepts, San Antonio, Tex.

Juanita Watson, RN, MSN, Director, Department of Continuing Education, Saint Agnes Medical Center, Philadelphia

Rosalyn Jones Watts, RN, EdD, Associate Professor of Nursing, University of Pennsylvania, Philadelphia

Terri E. Weaver, RN, MSN, CS, Pulmonary Clinical Nurse Specialist, Hospital of the University of Pennsylvania, Philadelphia; Clinical Instructor, University of Pennsylvania School of Nursing, Philadelphia

Erma L. Webb, RN, MS, Assistant Professor, Southern College of SDA, Orlando, Fla.

Joanne F. White, RN, MNEd, Associate Dean, School of Nursing, Duquesne University, Pittsburgh

Barbara A. Wojtklewicz, RNC, BSN, Former Adult Nurse Practitioner, Martha Eliot Health Center/Children's Hospital Medical Center, Jamaica Plain, Mass.

Hilary A. Wood, RN, SCM, Director, Cancer Treatment Center, Bethesda Hospital, Inc., Cincinnati

Gayle L. Ziegler, RN, MSN, Senior Research Assistant, University of Pittsburgh School of Medicine

Mary R. Zimmerman, RN, BSN, MS, Director of Nursing, Madison (Wis.) General Hospital

CONSULTANTS

Victoria J. Allen, RN, BSN, Clinical Nurse, National Institutes of Health, Clinical Center, Bethesda, Md.

John P. Atkinson, MD, Head, Division of Rheumatology, and Investigator, Howard Hughes Medical Institute, St. Louis; Professor of Microbiology and Immunology, Washington University School of Medicine, St. Louis

Edmund Martin Barbour, MD, Assistant Clinical Professor of Medicine, Wayne State University, Detroit

Garrett E. Bergman, MD, FAAP, Associate Professor of Pediatrics, Medical College of Pennsylvania, Philadelphia

Barbara Gross Braverman, RN, MSN, CS, Psychiatric Clinical Nurse Specialist, Medical College of Pennsylvania, Philadelphia

Lawrence W. Brown, MD, FAAP, FAAN, Associate Professor of Pediatrics and Neurology, Medical College of Pennsylvania, Philadelphia

A. Bruce Campbell, MD, PhD, Hematologist and Oncologist, Scripps Memorial Hospital, La Jolla, Calif.

G. Carpenter, MD, Associate Professor of Pediatrics, Thomas Jefferson University, Philadelphia

Linda L. Martin, RN, MSN, Pulmonary Clinical Nurse Specialist, University of Virginia Medical Center, Charlottesville

Margaret E. Miller, RN, MSN, Head and Neck Nurse Coordinator, Illinois Masonic Medical Center, Chicago

Terri Murrell, RN, MSN, Cardiovascular Clinical Nurse Specialist, Scripps Clinic, La Jolla, Calif.

John J. O'Shea, Jr., MD, Chief Medical Staff Fellow, Clinical Immunology Section, Laboratory of Clinical Investigation, National Institute of Allergy and Infectious Diseases, National Institutes of Health, Bethesda, Md.

Linda C. Pachucki, RN, MS, Diabetes Educator, Mount Sinai Medical Center, Milwaukee

Teresa A. Pellino, RN, MS, Director, Division of Education, National Association of Orthopaedic Nurses, Pitman, N.J.; Lecturer, University of Wisconsin, Madison

Frances W. Quinless, RN, PhD, Assistant Professor, Rutgers University College of Nursing, Newark, N.J.

Daniel W. Rahn, MD, Clinical Assistant Professor of Medicine, Yale University School of Medicine, New Haven, Conn.

Barbara Riegel, RN, MN, CS, Cardiovascular Clinical Nurse Specialist, Scripps Clinic and Research Foundation, San Diego

Janice R.J. Salyers, BS, RRT, Assistant Director, Respiratory Care, Duke University Medical Center, Durham, N.C.

Grannum R. Sant, MD, Assistant Professor of Urology, Tufts University School of Medicine, Boston

Joseph A. Scarola, MD, Staff Rheumatologist, Abington (Pa.) Memorial Hospital

Eric Z. Silfen, MD, Staff Physician, Emergency Department, and Clinical Instructor, Departments of Medicine and Emergency Medicine, Georgetown University Hospital, Washington, D.C.

Bryan P. Simmons, MD, Medical Director, Infection Control, Methodist Hospitals of Memphis

Janis B. Smith, RN, MSN, Nurse Consultant in Parent-Child Nursing, Pediatric Intensive Care, and Pediatric Cardiology and Cardiac Surgery, Wilmington, Del.

Brenda M. Splitz, RN, MSN, ANP, Adult Clinical Specialist; Clinical Coordinator, Nurse Practitioner Program; and Adjunct Faculty for Health Care Sciences, George Washington University Hospital, Washington, D.C.

Paul C. Summerell, RN, BSN, Assistant Head Nurse, Medical Intensive Care Unit, Duke University Medical Center, Durham, N.C.

Basia Belza Tack, RN, MSN, ANP, Nursing Consultant, Mountain View, Calif.

Richard W. Tureck, MD, Assistant Professor of Obstetrics and Gynecology, and Coordinator, In Vitro Fertilization/ Embryro Transfer Program, University of Pennsylvania School of Medicine, Philadelphia

A. Eugene Washington, MD, MSc, Assistant to the Director, Division of Sexually Transmitted Diseases, Centers for Disease Control, Atlanta

John K. Wiley, MD, FACS, Associate Clinical Professor of Neurosurgery, Wright State University School of Medicine, Dayton, Ohio

FOREWORD

In no other profession is maintaining excellence as critically important as it is in medicine. Proper patient management cannot be achieved without such dedication and the willingness to integrate individual efforts, expertise, and services with professional colleagues.

Keeping up with medical advances is increasingly difficult. At the same time medical technology is advancing, new financial constraints on health care providers are imposing stringent time and staffing pressures. To deliver quality patient care under these circumstances, medical professionals need a knowledge base that's accurate, easily accessible, and comprehensive.

Diseases and Disorders Handbook offers a dependable source of such information. The scope and organization of this unique handbook provide completely updated information on more than 480 disease processes in a comprehensive and coordinated, yet concise and ready manner. It includes, for example, the latest available information on acquired immunodeficiency syndrome (AIDS) and Alzheimer's disease (primary degenerative dementia), as well as *Chlamydia* infection. Students, trainees, and practitioners in all areas and at all levels of the health care profession will appreciate how current clinical information and relevant aspects of treatment are summarized in each entry.

The handbook is organized alphabetically, which makes locating a specific disease fast and simple.

Each entry begins with a *Description* that introduces the topic. Information may include a concise definition of the disorder, relevant pathophysiology, statistics, and prognosis.

A list of *Causes* follows. *Mode of transmission* and *Risk factors* are included when appropriate. A *Signs and symptoms* section lists the disease's expected clinical effects, and a *Diagnostic tests* section summarizes various clinical findings and special tests that suggest, confirm, or support the presence of the disease. The *Treatment* section describes commonly accepted forms of therapy, including surgery, and summarizes any ominous changes that signal onset of rapid, life-threatening deterioration in the patient's condition. The section on *Clinical implications* lists relevant information concerning customary care in the hospital and at home. Finally, a *Complications* section may be included. This section lists possible medical and psychological problems that may occur as a result of the disease.

When appropriate, each entry also includes helpful information on patient teaching, rehabilitation, and prevention. Teaching and prevention tips are often further emphasized in sidebars. Other carefully selected set-off pieces isolate and emphasize useful supplementary information.

I'm delighted to have the opportunity to introduce this most valuable addition to your professional library. I am confident that it will help you provide the best possible care for your patients.

—STANLEY J. DUDRICK, MD, FACS
Professor of Surgery
The University of Texas Medical
School at Houston/Hermann Hospital/
St. Luke's Episcopal Hospital
Houston

Abdominal aortic aneurysm

Description

Abdominal aneurysm, an abnormal dilation in the arterial wall, generally occurs in the aorta between the renal arteries and iliac branches. More than 50% of all patients with untreated abdominal aneurysms die, primarily from aneurysmal rupture, within 2 years of diagnosis. More than 85% die within 5 years.

Causes

• Arteriosclerosis (by far the most common)
• Cystic medial necrosis
• Trauma
• Syphilis
• Other infections

Signs and symptoms

Nonimminent rupture
—Asymptomatic pulsating mass in the periumbilical area
—Systolic bruit over the aorta
—Possible tenderness on deep palpation

Imminent rupture
Lumbar pain that radiates to the flank and groin from pressure on lumbar nerves

Rupture into peritoneal cavity
—Severe, persistent abdominal and back pain, mimicking renal or ureteral colic
—Signs of hemorrhage. These signs, such as weakness, sweating, tachycar-

dia, and hypotension, may be subtle due to retroperitoneal bleeding.

Diagnostic tests

Several tests can confirm suspected abdominal aneurysm.
• Serial ultrasonography allows determination of aneurysm size, shape, and location.
• Anteroposterior and lateral X-rays of the abdomen can detect aortic calcification, which outlines the mass, in at least 75% of patients.
• Aortography shows the condition of vessels proximal and distal to the aneurysm and the extent of the aneurysm but may underestimate aneurysm diameter, because it visualizes only the flow channel and not the surrounding clot.

Treatment

Usually, abdominal aneurysm requires resection of the aneurysm and replacement of the damaged aortic section with a Dacron graft. If an aneurysm is small and asymptomatic, surgery may be delayed; however, small aneurysms may rupture. Regular physical examination and ultrasound checks are necessary to detect enlargement, which may forewarn rupture. Large aneurysms or those that produce symptoms involve a significant risk of rupture and necessitate immediate repair. In patients with poor distal runoff, external grafting may be done.

Clinical implications

Abdominal aneurysm requires meticulous preoperative and postoperative care, psychological support, and comprehensive patient teaching. Following diagnosis, if rupture is not imminent, elective surgery allows time for additional preoperative tests to evaluate the patient's clinical status.

• Monitor vital signs, and type and cross match blood.

• As ordered, obtain kidney function tests (BUN, creatinine, electrolytes), blood samples (CBC with differential), EKG and cardiac evaluation, baseline pulmonary function tests, and blood gases.

• Be alert for signs of rupture, which may be immediately fatal. Watch closely for any signs of acute blood loss (decreasing blood pressure; increasing pulse and respiratory rate; cool, clammy skin; restlessness; and decreased sensorium).

• If rupture occurs, the first priority is to get the patient to surgery *immediately*. Medical antishock trousers may be used during transport. Surgery allows direct compression of the aorta to control hemorrhage. Large amounts of blood may be needed during the resuscitative period to replace blood loss. Renal failure due to ischemia is a major postoperative complication, possibly requiring hemodialysis.

• Before elective surgery, weigh the patient, insert an indwelling (Foley) catheter and I.V. line, and assist with insertion of an arterial line and pulmonary artery catheter to monitor fluid and hemodynamic balance. Give prophylactic antibiotics, as ordered.

• Explain the surgical procedure and the expected postoperative care in the ICU for patients undergoing complex abdominal surgery (I.V. lines, endotracheal and nasogastric intubation, mechanical ventilation).

• After surgery, in the ICU, closely monitor vital signs, intake and hourly output, neurologic status (level of consciousness, pupil size, sensation in arms and legs), and blood gases. Assess lung sounds and the depth, rate, and character of respirations at least every hour.

• Watch for signs of bleeding (increased pulse rate and respirations, hypotension), which may occur retroperitoneally from the graft site. Check abdominal dressings for excessive bleeding or drainage. Be alert for temperature elevations and other signs of infection. After nasogastric intubation for intestinal decompression, irrigate the tube frequently to ensure patency. Record the amount and type of drainage.

• Suction the endotracheal tube often. If the patient can breathe unassisted and has good lung sounds and adequate blood gases, tidal volume, and vital capacity 24 hours after surgery, he will be extubated and will require oxygen by mask. Weigh the patient daily to evaluate fluid balance.

• Help the patient walk as soon as he can (generally the 2nd day after surgery).

• Provide psychological support for the patient and family. Help ease their fears about the ICU, the threat of impending rupture, and surgery by providing appropriate explanations and answering all questions.

Abdominal injuries, blunt and penetrating

Description
Blunt and penetrating abdominal injuries may damage major blood vessels and internal organs. Their most immediate life-threatening consequences are hemorrhage and hypovolemic shock; later threats include infection. Prognosis depends on the extent of injury and the organs damaged but is generally improved by prompt diagnosis and surgical repair.

Causes
Blunt abdominal injuries
—Motor vehicle accidents
—Falls from heights
—Athletic injuries

Penetrating abdominal injuries
—Stab wounds
—Gunshot wounds

Signs and symptoms

Symptoms vary with the degree of injury and the organs damaged.

Blunt abdominal injuries
—Severe pain may radiate beyond the abdomen to the shoulders
—Bruises, abrasions, contusions
—Distention
—Tenderness
—Possible abdominal splinting or rigidity, nausea and vomiting, pallor, cyanosis, tachycardia, dyspnea

Penetrating abdominal injuries
—Obvious wounds (bullets often produce both entrance and exit wounds)
—Blood loss
—Pain, tenderness
—Possible pallor, cyanosis, tachycardia, dyspnea, hypotension

Diagnostic tests

Tests vary with the patient's condition but may include the following.
• Chest X-rays, preferably done with the patient upright, show free air.
• Abdominal films
• Examination of the stool and stomach aspirate for blood
• Several blood studies are generally performed. Decreased hematocrit and hemoglobin levels point to blood loss. Coagulation studies evaluate hemostasis. White blood cell count is usually elevated but does not necessarily point to infection; typing and cross matching precede blood transfusion.
• Arterial blood gas analysis evaluates respiratory status.
• Serum amylase levels often may be elevated in pancreatic injury.
• SGOT and SGPT levels increase with tissue injury and cell death.
• Intravenous pyelography and cystourethrography detect renal and urinary tract damage.
• Radioisotope scanning and ultrasound examination detect liver, kidney, or spleen injury.
• Angiography detects specific injuries, especially to the kidneys.
• Peritoneal lavage, with insertion of a lavage catheter, is performed to check for blood, urine, pus, ascitic fluid, bile, and chyle (a milky fluid absorbed by the intestinal lymph vessels during digestion).
• Computed tomography scan detects abdominal, head, or other injuries.
• Exploratory laparotomy detects specific injuries when other clinical evidence is incomplete.
• Other laboratory studies rule out associated injuries.

Treatment

Emergency treatment of abdominal injuries controls hemorrhage and prevents hypovolemic shock by the infusion of I.V. fluids and blood components. After stabilization, most abdominal injuries require surgical repair. Analgesics and antibiotics increase patient comfort and prevent infection. Most patients require hospitalization; if they are asymptomatic, they may require observation for only 6 to 24 hours.

Clinical implications

Emergency care in patients with abdominal injuries supports vital functions by maintaining airway patency, breathing, and circulation. At admission, immediately evaluate respiratory and circulatory status and, if possible, obtain a history of the trauma.
• To maintain airway patency and breathing, intubate the patient and provide mechanical ventilation, as necessary; otherwise, provide supplemental oxygen.
• Using a large-bore needle, start one or more I.V. lines for monitoring and rapid fluid infusion, using a normal saline solution. Then, draw a blood sample for laboratory studies. Also, insert a nasogastric tube and, if necessary, an indwelling (Foley) catheter; monitor stomach aspirate and urine for blood.

• Obtain vital signs for baseline data; continue to monitor every 15 minutes.
• Apply a sterile dressing to open wounds. Splint a suspected pelvic injury on arrival by tying the patient's legs together with a pillow between them. Move such a patient as little as possible.
• Give analgesics, as ordered. Usually, narcotics are not recommended, but if the pain is severe, give narcotics in small I.V. doses.
• Give tetanus prophylaxis and prophylactic I.V. antibiotics, as ordered.
• Prepare the patient for surgery. Get a consent form signed by the patient or a responsible relative. Remove dentures. Type and cross match blood.
• If the injury was caused by a motor vehicle accident, find out if the police were notified, and if not, notify them. If the patient suffered a gunshot or stab wound, notify the police, place all his clothes in a bag, and retain them for the police. Document the number and sites of the wounds. Contact the patient's family and offer them reassurance.

Complications
In both blunt and penetrating injuries, massive blood loss may cause hypovolemic shock. In general, damage to solid abdominal organs (liver, spleen, pancreas, kidneys) causes hemorrhage; damage to hollow organs (stomach, intestine, gallbladder, bladder) causes rupture and release of the organs' contents (including bacteria) into the abdomen, which in turn produces inflammation.

Abortion, spontaneous

Description
Spontaneous abortion is the expulsion of the products of conception from the uterus before fetal viability (fetal weight of less than 17½ oz [500 g] and gestation of less than 20 weeks). At least 75% of spontaneous abortions

(miscarriages) occur during the first trimester. (See *Types of Spontaneous Abortion*, p. 5.)

Causes
Fetal factors
These are the usual causes between 9 and 12 weeks of gestation.
—Defective embryologic development
—Faulty implantation of the fertilized ovum
—Failure of the endometrium to accept the fertilized ovum
Placental factors
These are the usual causes at approximately 14 weeks of gestation.
—Premature separation of the normally implanted placenta
—Abnormal placental implantation
—Abnormal platelet function
Maternal factors
These are the usual causes between 11 and 19 weeks of gestation.
—Infection
—Severe malnutrition
—Abnormalities of the reproductive organs (especially an incompetent cervix)
—Endocrine problems, such as thyroid dysfunction or lowered estriol secretion
—Trauma, including any type of surgery that necessitates manipulation of the pelvic organs
—Blood group incompatibility and Rh isoimmunization (still under investigation as a possible cause)
—Drug ingestion

Signs and symptoms
Prodromal symptoms of spontaneous abortion may include a pink discharge for several days or a scant brown discharge for several weeks before onset of cramps and increased vaginal bleeding. For a few hours, the cramps intensify and occur more frequently; then the cervix dilates for expulsion of uterine contents. If the entire contents are expelled, cramps and bleed-

Types of Spontaneous Abortion

• *Threatened abortion:* Bloody vaginal discharge occurs during the first half of pregnancy. Approximately 20% of pregnant women have vaginal spotting or actual bleeding early in pregnancy; of these, about 50% abort.
• *Inevitable abortion:* Membranes rupture and the cervix dilates. As labor continues, the uterus expels the products of conception.
• *Incomplete abortion:* Uterus retains part or all of the placenta. Before the 10th week of gestation, the fetus and placenta usually are expelled together; after the 10th week, separately. Because part of the placenta may adhere to the uterine wall, bleeding continues. Hemorrhage is possible because the uterus does not contract and seal the large vessels that feed the placenta.
• *Complete abortion:* Uterus passes all the products of conception. Minimal bleeding usually accompanies complete abortion because the uterus contracts and compresses the maternal blood vessels that fed the placenta.
• *Missed abortion:* Uterus retains the products of conception for 2 months or more after the death of the fetus. Uterine growth ceases; uterine size may even seem to decrease. Prolonged retention of the dead products of conception may cause coagulation defects, such as disseminated intravascular coagulation (DIC).
• *Habitual abortion:* Spontaneous loss of three or more consecutive pregnancies constitutes habitual abortion.
• *Septic abortion:* Infection accompanies abortion. This may occur with spontaneous abortion but usually results from an illegal abortion.

ing subside. However, if any contents remain, cramps and bleeding continue.

Diagnostic tests
• Human chorionic gonadotropin (HCG) in the blood or urine confirms pregnancy; decreased HCG levels suggest spontaneous abortion.
• Pelvic examination determines the size of the uterus and whether this size is consistent with the length of the pregnancy.
• Tissue cytology indicates evidence of products of conception.
• Hemoglobin and hematocrit levels are decreased due to blood loss.

Treatment
An accurate evaluation of uterine contents is necessary before planning treatment. The progression of spontaneous abortion cannot be prevented, except in those cases caused by an incompetent cervix. Hospitalization is necessary to control severe hemor-

rhage. Severe bleeding requires transfusion with packed RBCs or whole blood. Initially, I.V. administration of oxytocin stimulates uterine contractions. If remnants remain in the uterus, dilatation and curettage (D & C) or dilatation and evacuation (D & E) should be performed.

After an abortion, an Rh-negative female with a negative indirect Coombs' test should receive Rh₀ (D) immune globulin (human) to prevent future Rh isoimmunization.

Clinical implications
Before possible abortion
—Explain all procedures thoroughly.
—Do not allow the patient bathroom privileges, because she may expel uterine contents without knowing it.
—After she uses the bedpan, inspect the contents carefully for intrauterine material.
After abortion
—Note the amount, color, and odor of vaginal bleeding. Save all the pads the

patient uses, for evaluation.
—Administer analgesics and oxytocin, as ordered.
—Give good perineal care.
—Obtain vital signs every 4 hours for 24 hours.
—Monitor urinary output.
—Provide emotional support and counseling during the grieving process. Encourage the patient and her partner to express their feelings. Some couples may want to talk to a member of the clergy or, depending on their religion, may wish to have the fetus baptized.

Before patient discharge
—Tell the patient to expect vaginal bleeding or spotting. Instruct her to report immediately bleeding that lasts longer than 8 to 10 days or excessive, bright-red blood.
—Advise the patient to watch for signs of infection, such as a temperature higher than 100° F. (37.8° C.) and foul-smelling vaginal discharge.
—Encourage the gradual increase of daily activities to include whatever tasks the patient feels comfortable doing (cooking, sewing, cleaning, for example), as long as these activities do not increase vaginal bleeding or cause fatigue. Most patients return to work within 1 to 4 weeks.
—Urge 2 to 3 weeks' abstinence from intercourse, and encourage use of a contraceptive when intercourse is resumed.
—Instruct the patient to avoid using tampons for 2 to 4 weeks.
—Tell the patient to see her physician in 2 to 4 weeks for a follow-up examination.
—To minimize the risk of future spontaneous abortions, emphasize to the pregnant woman the importance of good nutrition and the need to exclude alcohol, cigarettes, and drugs. Most clinicians recommend that the couple wait two or three normal menstrual cycles after a spontaneous abortion has occurred before attempting conception.
—If the patient has a history of habitual spontaneous abortions, suggest that she and her partner have thorough examinations. For the woman, this includes premenstrual endometrial biopsy, a hormone assessment (estrogen, progesterone, and thyroid, follicle-stimulating, and luteinizing hormones), and hysterosalpingography and laparoscopy to detect anatomic abnormalities. Genetic counseling may also be indicated.

Abruptio placentae
(Placental abruption)

Description
In abruptio placentae, the placenta separates from the uterine wall prematurely, usually after the 20th week of gestation, producing hemorrhage. Bleeding is external or marginal (in 80% of patients) if a peripheral portion of the placenta separates from the uterine wall. Bleeding is internal or concealed (in the remaining 20%) if the central portion of the placenta becomes detached, in which case the still-intact peripheral portions trap the blood. Abruptio placentae occurs most often in multigravidas—usually in women over age 35—and is a common cause of bleeding during the second half of pregnancy. Conclusive diagnosis, when heavy maternal bleeding is present, generally necessitates termination of pregnancy. Fetal prognosis depends on gestational age and amount of blood lost; maternal prognosis is good if hemorrhage can be controlled.

Causes
Unknown

Risk factors
• Trauma, such as a direct blow to the uterus
• Placental site bleeding from a needle puncture during amniocentesis
• Chronic hypertension, which raises

pressure on the maternal side of the placenta
• Acute toxemia
• Pressure on the vena cava from an enlarged uterus

Signs and symptoms

Mild abruptio placentae
Separation is marginal; onset is gradual.
—Mild to moderate bleeding
—Vague lower abdominal discomfort
—Mild to moderate abdominal tenderness and uterine irritability
—Strong and regular fetal heart sounds

Moderate abruptio placentae
About 50% of the placenta separates; onset is gradual or abrupt.
—Continuous abdominal pain
—Moderate dark-red vaginal bleeding
—A very tender uterus that remains firm between contractions
—Barely audible or irregular and bradycardic fetal heart tones
—Possible signs of shock
—Labor (typically within 2 hours) that proceeds rapidly

Severe abruptio placentae
Nearly 70% of the placenta separates; onset is typically abrupt.
—Agonizing, unremitting uterine pain (often described as tearing or knifelike)
—Boardlike, tender uterus
—Moderate vaginal bleeding
—Rapidly progressive manifestations of shock
—Absence of fetal heart tones

Diagnostic tests
• Ultrasonography rules out placenta previa.
• Hemoglobin and platelet counts are decreased.
• Assays for fibrin split products, performed periodically, aid in monitoring the progression of abruptio placentae and detect the development of disseminated intravascular coagulation.

Treatment
Treatment of abruptio placentae is designed to assess, control, and restore the amount of blood lost; to deliver a viable infant; and to prevent coagulation disorders. Immediate measures for the patient with abruptio placentae include starting I.V. infusion (via large-bore catheter) of appropriate fluids (lactated Ringer's solution) to combat hypovolemia; drawing blood for hemoglobin and hematocrit determination and for typing and cross matching; initiating external electronic fetal monitoring; monitoring maternal blood pressure, pulse rate, and respirations; and assessing the amount of vaginal bleeding.

After determination of the severity of abruption and appropriate fluid and blood replacement, prompt delivery of the fetus by cesarean section is necessary if the fetus is alive but in distress. If the fetus is not in distress, monitoring continues; delivery is usually performed at the earliest sign of fetal distress. Because fetal blood may be lost through the placenta, a pediatric team should be on hand at delivery to immediately assess and treat the newborn for shock, blood loss, and hypoxia. If placental separation is severe and there are no signs of fetal life, vaginal delivery may be performed unless uncontrolled hemorrhage or other complications contraindicate it.

Clinical implications
• Check maternal blood pressure, pulse rate, respirations, central venous pressure, intake and output, and amount of vaginal bleeding every 10 to 15 minutes. Monitor fetal heart tones electronically.
• Prepare the patient and family for cesarean section. Thoroughly explain postpartum care, so the patient and family know what to expect.
• If vaginal delivery is elected, provide emotional support during labor. Because of fetal prematurity, the mother may not receive analgesics during labor and may experience intense pain. Reassure the patient

through labor, and keep her informed of fetal condition.

• Tactfully introduce the possibility of neonatal death. Tell the patient that survival depends primarily on gestational age, blood loss, and associated hypertensive disorders. Assure her that frequent monitoring and prompt management greatly reduce risk of mortality for the infant.

Complications
• Hemorrhage and shock
• Renal failure
• Disseminated intravascular coagulation (DIC)
• Maternal and fetal death

Achilles tendon contracture

Description
Achilles tendon contracture is a shortening of the Achilles tendon (tendo calcaneus or heel cord).

Causes
• Congenital structural anomaly
• Muscular reaction to chronic poor posture, especially in women who wear high-heeled shoes or joggers who land on the balls of their feet instead of their heels
• Paralytic conditions of the legs, such as poliomyelitis or cerebral palsy

Signs and symptoms
• Sharp, spasmodic pain during dorsiflexion of the foot characterizes reflexive Achilles tendon contracture.
• In footdrop (fixed equinus), contracture of the flexor foot muscle prevents placing the heel on the ground.

Diagnostic tests
A simple test confirms Achilles tendon contracture: while the patient keeps his knee flexed, the examiner places the foot in dorsiflexion; gradual knee extension forces the foot into plantar flexion.

Treatment
Conservative treatment aims to correct Achilles tendon contracture by raising the inside heel of the shoe, in reflexive contracture; gradually lowering the heels of shoes (sudden lowering can aggravate the problem), and stretching exercises, if the cause is high heels; or using support braces or casting to prevent footdrop, in a paralyzed patient. Alternative therapy includes using wedged plaster casts or stretching the tendon by manipulation. Analgesics may be given to relieve pain.

With fixed footdrop, treatment may include surgery (Z-tenotomy), but this procedure may weaken the tendon. Z-tenotomy allows further stretching by cutting the tendon. After surgery, a short leg cast maintains the foot in 90-degree dorsiflexion for 6 weeks. Some surgeons allow partial weight-bearing on a walking cast after 2 weeks.

Clinical implications
After surgery to lengthen the Achilles tendon:
• Elevate the casted foot to decrease venous pressure and edema. Raise the foot of the bed or support the patient's foot with pillows.
• Record the neurovascular status of the toes (temperature, color, sensation, capillary refill time, toe mobility) every hour for the first 24 hours, then every 4 hours. If you detect any changes, increase the elevation of the patient's legs, and notify the surgeon immediately.
• Prepare the patient for ambulation by having him dangle his foot over the side of the bed for short periods (5 to 15 minutes) before he gets out of bed, allowing for gradual increase of venous pressure. Assist the patient in walking, as ordered (usually within 24 hours of surgery), using crutches and a non-weight-bearing or touch-down gait.
• Protect the patient's skin with moleskin or by "petaling" the edges of the cast. Before discharge, teach the patient how to care for the cast, and ad-

vise him to elevate his foot regularly when sitting or whenever the foot throbs or becomes edematous. Also, make sure the patient understands how much exercise and walking are recommended after discharge.

• To prevent Achilles tendon contracture in paralyzed patients, apply support braces, universal splints, casts, or high-topped sneakers. Make sure that bed linens do not keep paralyzed feet in plantar flexion. For other patients, teach good foot care, and urge them to seek immediate medical care for foot problems. Warn women against wearing high heels constantly, and suggest regular foot (dorsiflexion) exercises.

Acne vulgaris

Description

An inflammatory disease of the sebaceous follicles, acne vulgaris affects adolescents primarily, but lesions can appear as early as age 8. Although acne strikes boys more often and more severely, in girls its onset usually is earlier and its duration tends to be longer, sometimes into adulthood. Prognosis is good with treatment.

Causes

Research now centers on hormonal dysfunction and oversecretion of sebum as possible primary causes.

Risk factors

• Use of oral contraceptives
• Certain medications, including corticosteroids, adrenocorticotropic hormone, androgens, iodides, bromides, trimethadione, phenytoin, isoniazid, lithium, and halothane
• Cobalt irradiation
• Hyperalimentation therapy
• Exposure to heavy oils, greases, or tars
• Trauma or rubbing from tight clothing

• Cosmetics
• Emotional stress

Signs and symptoms

• The acne plug may appear as a closed comedo, or whitehead (if it does not protrude from the follicle and is covered by the epidermis).
• The acne plug may appear as an open comedo, or blackhead (if it does protrude and is not covered by the epidermis).
• There may be characteristic acne pustules, papules, or, in severe forms, acne cysts or abscesses.
• Chronic, recurring lesions produce acne scars.

Treatment

Common therapy for severe acne includes benzoyl peroxide, a powerful antibacterial, alone or in combination with tretinoin, a keratolytic (retinoic acid or topical vitamin A); both agents may irritate the skin. Topical antibiotics, such as tetracycline, erythromycin, and clindamycin, may prove helpful in reducing the effects of acne.

Systemic therapy consists primarily of antibiotics, usually tetracycline, to decrease bacterial growth until the patient is in remission; then a lower dosage is used for long-term maintenance. Tetracycline is contraindicated during pregnancy because it discolors the teeth of the fetus. Erythromycin is an alternative for these patients. Exacerbation of pustules or abscesses during either type of antibiotic therapy requires a culture to identify a possible secondary bacterial infection.

Oral isotretinoin (Accutane), a newer treatment, combats acne by inhibiting sebaceous gland function and keratinization. But because of severe adverse effects, the usual 16- to 20-week course of isotretinoin is limited to those patients with severe papulopustular or cystic acne who do not respond to conventional therapy. Women of childbearing age should not take isotretinoin unless they use contraceptives, because birth defects can occur.

Females with particularly stubborn acne may benefit from the administration of estrogens to inhibit androgen activity. However, this method of treatment is usually a last resort, since improvement rarely occurs before 2 to 4 months and exacerbations may follow its discontinuation.

Other treatments for acne vulgaris include intralesional corticosteroid injections, exposure to ultraviolet light (but never when a photosensitizing agent, such as tretinoin, is being used), cryotherapy, or surgery.

Clinical implications

For those with acne, the main focus of nursing care is patient teaching about the disorder and its treatment and prevention.

• Check the patient's drug history. Certain medications, such as oral contraceptives, may cause an acne flare-up.

• Try to identify predisposing factors that can be eliminated or modified, such as emotional stress.

• Explain the possible causes of acne to the patient and family. Make sure they understand that prescribed treatment is more likely to improve acne than are strict diet and fanatic scrubbing with soap and water. In fact, overzealous washing can worsen the lesions. Provide written instructions regarding treatment.

• Instruct the patient receiving tretinoin to apply it at least 30 minutes after washing the face and at least 1 hour before bedtime. Warn against using this medication around the eyes or lips. After treatments, the skin should look pink and dry. If it appears red or starts to peel, the preparation may have to be weakened or applied less often. Advise the patient to avoid exposure to sunlight or to use a sunscreening agent.

• If the prescribed regimen includes tretinoin and benzoyl peroxide, instruct the patient to avoid skin irritation by using one preparation in the morning and the other at night.

• Instruct the patient to take tetracycline on an empty stomach and not to take it along with antacids or milk since it interacts with their metallic ions and will be poorly absorbed.

• If the patient is taking isotretinoin, tell him to avoid vitamin A supplements, which can worsen any adverse effects. Also teach him how to deal with dryness of the skin and mucous membranes, which usually occurs during treatment.

• Inform the patient that acne takes a long time to clear; complete resolution may require years. Encourage him to continue local skin care even after acne clears. Explain the adverse effects of all medications.

• Pay special attention to the patient's perception of his physical appearance, and offer emotional support.

Acquired immunodeficiency syndrome (AIDS)

Description

AIDS is characterized by progressive weakening of cell-mediated (T cell) immunity, which makes the patient susceptible to opportunistic infections and unusual cancers. (See *Common Opportunistic Infections with AIDS*, pp. 12-13, and *Kaposi's Sarcoma*.) Diagnosis rests on careful correlation of the patient's history and clinical features rather than on laboratory criteria. The time between probable exposure to the virus and diagnosis averages 1 to 3 years. In children, incubation time appears to be shorter, with a mean of 8 months. More than 75% of AIDS victims die within 2 years of diagnosis. The term AIDS-related complex (ARC) is used to describe patients who manifest signs and symptoms suggestive of AIDS and have antibodies to the AIDS virus, but who have no opportunistic infections or neoplasms.

Kaposi's Sarcoma

Kaposi's sarcoma (KS) is a neoplasm characterized by purple or blue patches, plaques, or nodular skin lesions that spread widely in the AIDS patient. The lesions seldom drain or bleed. The most common sites for these lesions include the skin, oral mucosa, lymph nodes, GI tract, lungs, and visceral organs. Lesions of the GI tract are associated with diarrhea, nausea, loss of appetite, and weight loss. Lesions of the lungs are associated with congestion and difficult breathing. Lesions of the lymphatic system are associated with severe extremity and facial swelling and pain secondary to swelling.

The following treatments are used for KS:
• Skin lesions may be successfully removed by surgical incision with no further treatment indicated.
• Tumors that require further treatment are generally responsive to local irradiation.
• Chemotherapeutic agents are also used. These include doxorubicin, vinblastine, bleomycin, interferon, and interleukin-2.
• Many experimental protocols are being tested in the treatment of KS in AIDS. The physician should be asked about availability and more information.

Causes
A retrovirus called the human immunodeficiency virus (HIV) or AIDS-related virus (ARV)

Mode of transmission
• Direct inoculation alone via intimate sexual contact, especially associated with trauma to the rectal mucosa
• Transfusion of blood or blood products
• Contaminated needles
• Perinatal transmission from mother to fetus

Risk factors
• Multiple sexual contacts with homosexual and bisexual men
• Present or past abuse of intravenous drugs
• Hemophilia
• Transfusions of blood or blood products
• Heterosexual contact with someone who has AIDS or is at risk for it
• Prenatal and perinatal exposure to AIDS
• Breast-fed infants of mothers who have AIDS or are at risk for AIDS

Signs and symptoms
There is wide variation in the clinical course before an initial diagnosis of AIDS.
Nonspecific manifestations
These often precede complications.
—Fatigue
—Afternoon fevers
—Night sweats
—Weight loss
—Diarrhea
—Cough
Specific manifestations
Patients who have these signs and symptoms may be otherwise asymptomatic until abrupt onset of complications.
—Opportunistic infections (See *Common Opportunistic Infections with AIDS*, pp. 12-13.)
—Kaposi's sarcoma (See *Kaposi's Sarcoma*.)

Diagnostic tests
• The HIV antibody test detects the presence of antibodies to the virus responsible for AIDS. A positive result indicates previous exposure to the virus and means the individual may be contagious and capable of transmitting

Common Opportunistic Infections with A.I.D.S.

INFECTION	SIGNS AND SYMPTOMS	TREATMENT
Candida Albicans Infection *Candida albicans* is a fungus that causes one of the most common opportunistic infections associated with AIDS. *C. albicans* is commonly present in the mucous membranes of the mouth, throat, esophagus, or rectum.	The two most common signs and symptoms of oral and esophageal candidiasis are the presence of white, cottage cheese–like patches in the mouth and dysphagia (swallowing difficulty). Common symptoms of candidal proctitis are rectal pain, pruritus, and discharge.	For oral candidiasis, clotrimazole troches and nystatin oral suspension are used. For esophageal candidiasis, ketoconazole is administered. For candidal proctitis, clotrimazole cream is applied to the affected area. Treatment will generally continue for the entire course of illness because of the underlying immunodeficiency.
Cytomegalovirus (CMV) Infection CMV, one of the herpes viruses, may result in serious, widespread infection in AIDS patients. The most common sites for CMV infection include the lungs, adrenal glands, eyes, central nervous system, gastrointestinal tract, male genitourinary tract, and blood.	Unexplained fever, malaise, gastrointestinal ulcers, swollen lymph nodes, enlarged liver and spleen, and blurred vision are common signs and symptoms that may be related to CMV infection. Vision changes leading to blindness are not uncommon.	No effective therapy for CMV infection exists at this time. DHPG, an experimental drug, may help to slow the virus, particularly when eye infection is identified.
Cryptosporidium Enterocolitis *Cryptosporidium enterocolitis* is an intestinal infection caused by a protozoan (one-celled animal). The disease may be untreatable and very distressing in the person with AIDS. The causal organism is found primarily in the small bowel and rarely in other organs.	The two major symptoms of *C. enterocolitis* are cramping abdominal pain and chronic, profuse, watery diarrhea.	Therapy for *C. enterocolitis* has been largely ineffective. Spiramycin, an antibiotic with anti-*Toxoplasma* activity, has been helpful in some cases of severe diarrhea. Diphenoxylate hydrochloride with atropine or loperamide may also help. Kaolin and pectin mixtures may be taken for mild diarrhea.

Common Opportunistic Infections with A.I.D.S. *(continued)*

INFECTION	SIGNS AND SYMPTOMS	TREATMENT
Herpes Simplex Herpes simplex is a chronic infection caused by a herpes virus. It is often a reactivation of an earlier herpes infection.	The most common signs and symptoms of herpes simplex virus are red, blisterlike lesions occurring in oral, anal, and genital areas. Lesions may also be found on the esophageal and tracheobronchial mucosa in AIDS patients. The patient generally complains of pain, bleeding, or discharge.	Acyclovir ointment is used topically to adequately cover all lesions. The drug is given orally in capsule form. Treatment may have to continue indefinitely to prevent recurrence.
Herpes Zoster Herpes zoster, also known as shingles, is an acute infection caused by the chicken pox virus.	Herpes zoster is characterized by small clusters of painful, reddened papules (small, circumscribed, superficial skin elevations) that follow the route of inflamed nerves. It may be disseminated.	Herpes zoster is most often treated with acyclovir capsules until healed. Treatment may have to continue indefinitely to prevent recurrence. Intravenous acyclovir has been effective in treating disseminated herpes zoster lesions in some patients. Medications may be used to relieve pain associated with herpes zoster infection.

***Pneumocystis Carinii* Pneumonia (PCP)**
PCP is a protozoan infection found in the air sacs of the lungs. It is the most common lung infection found in patients with AIDS.
	The three most common signs and symptoms of PCP are fever, shortness of breath, and a dry, nonproductive cough.	PCP is treated with co-trimoxazole or pentamidine isethionate.
		    Oxygen therapy may be used continuously or as needed. An oxygen concentrator may be more cost-effective for long-term home intervention.
		    Oral morphine solution may be ordered to reduce respiratory rate and anxiety.
		
		(continued)

Common Opportunistic Infections with A.I.D.S. *(continued)*

INFECTION	SIGNS AND SYMPTOMS	TREATMENT
Mycobacterium Avium Intracellulare (MAI) Infection MAI infection is caused by bacteria commonly found in the environment. The bacteria rarely cause infection in the healthy individual. However, in the patient with AIDS, the bacteria may spread throughout the patient's blood, lymph nodes, bone marrow, liver, lungs, and gastrointestinal tract.	The four most common signs and symptoms of MAI infection are fever, diarrhea, weight loss, and debilitation. These signs and symptoms are often masked by or confused with those of other opportunistic infections.	Treatment involves a multidrug regimen, including isoniazid, ethambutol, and rifampin. Ansamycin and clofazimine are experimental drugs that may be added to this regimen. (This regimen has shown poor results, however.) Besides ansamycin and clofazimine, other experimental protocols to treat MAI infection may be available. Ask the physician about this.
Toxoplasmosis Toxoplasmosis, caused by a protozoan, results in acute or chronic brain infection in patients with AIDS. Toxoplasmosis occurs generally as a secondary opportunistic infection and less frequently as a primary infection.	Localized neurologic defects, such as seizures, memory loss, confusion, weakness, and lethargy, are common signs and symptoms of toxoplasmosis.	Pyrimethamine and sulfadiazine is the most common regimen used for toxoplasmosis.
Progressive Multifocal Leukoencephalopathy (PML) PML is a central nervous system disorder caused by a papovavirus that causes gradual brain degeneration.	Progressive dementia, memory loss, confusion, and weakness are the most common symptoms of PML. Other neurologic complications, such as seizures, may occur.	No treatments are currently available for PML. Supportive care is given to help manage symptoms.

the virus; it does not mean that the individual has or will get ARC or AIDS.

• T_4:T_8 ratio is characteristically decreased.

• T_4 lymphocytes are characteristically severely depleted.

• Skin testing with common antigens confirms impaired cell-mediated immunity.

Treatment

Currently no cure exists for AIDS. However, researchers continue to explore methods to arrest growth of HIV or to restore lost immune function.

• Although bone marrow transplant has failed to improve immune function, I.V. infusion of interleukin-2 and interferon has shown limited effectiveness.

• The experimental antiviral drug azidothymidine (AZT) has shown promise in impeding progress of HIV and is being made more widely available to AIDS patients.

• Other drug treatment for AIDS varies, depending on the AIDS-related disorder present. Although many of the causative infectious organisms are responsive to drugs, infection tends to recur when treatment is discontinued.

• The development of a vaccine to help combat AIDS is now under investigation by researchers. It will be many years before such a vaccine is available for general use.

Clinical implications

Although AIDS is not thought to be transmitted by casual contact, you should observe special precautions when caring for an AIDS patient. Wear gloves and a gown when handling blood, other body fluids, excretions, or potentially contaminated objects or surfaces. If such contact occurs, wash your hands immediately with soap and water. Of course, thorough handwashing is necessary before and after any contact with suspected and diagnosed AIDS patients. Generally, follow precautions appropriate for hepatitis B: properly labeling all specimens col-

---

Preventing A.I.D.S.

Measures to prevent the spread of AIDS include the following:

• Practicing protective sex or safe sex, or avoiding vaginal or anal intercourse with infected individuals

• Wearing a condom during vaginal or anal intercourse

• Following sexual practices in which no semen, vaginal fluid, or blood is exchanged (considered safer)

• Knowing a sexual partner and his or her habits

• Avoiding sex with prostitutes

• Preventing blood transmission by not sharing needles and syringes

• Avoiding use of recreational drugs. These can do serious harm to the patient with AIDS. Opiates, alcohol, and marijuana, which can act as immunosuppressants, may increase the patient's vulnerability to infection. Moreover, research suggests that, although inhaled nitrates do not play a role in the development of AIDS itself, they may increase the risk of Kaposi's sarcoma in homosexual men afflicted with AIDS.

• In women who are HIV-positive, avoiding pregnancy. Mother-to-infant transmission can occur during pregnancy or after pregnancy when breast-feeding.

In addition, individuals who test positive for HIV antibodies should not donate blood, body organs or tissues, or sperm. These individuals should also follow infection-control guidelines, as explained by the physician.

Teaching Topics in A.I.D.S.

- Explanation of normal immune response and how the AIDS virus affects it
- The current status of AIDS research
- Tests to support diagnosis and to confirm complications
- Treatment for any complications
- Activity and dietary modifications
- Symptoms of opportunistic infections and cancers
- Prevention of AIDS transmission, including safe sexual practices
- Measures to prevent infection
- Availability of support groups and other services

---

lected from the patient; placing soiled linen in a labeled, impervious bag; and disposing of needles (unsheathed) in a puncture-resistant container.

• Monitor the patient for fever, noting its pattern. Also assess for tender, swollen lymph nodes, and check laboratory values regularly. Be alert for signs of infection, such as skin breakdown, cough, sore throat, and diarrhea.

• Encourage daily oral rinsing with normal saline or bicarbonate solution. To relieve oral *Candida* infection or stomatitis, offer the patient hydrogen peroxide or Benadryl-Kaopectate solution (swish and spit). Avoid glycerin swabs, which dry mucous membranes.

• Record the patient's caloric intake. Total parenteral nutrition (TPN) may be necessary to maintain adequate caloric intake, but it provides a potential route for infection.

• If the patient develops Kaposi's sarcoma, monitor the progression of lesions. Provide meticulous skin care, especially in the debilitated patient.

• Recognize that diagnosis of AIDS is typically emotionally charged because of the social impact and discouraging prognosis of the disease. The patient may face the loss of his job and financial security as well as the support of his family and friends. Coping with an altered body image and the emotional burden of untimely death may also overwhelm the patient. Be as sup-

portive as possible. (Also see *Preventing AIDS*, p. 15, and *Teaching Topics in AIDS*.)

Actinomycosis

Description

Actinomycosis is an infection that produces granulomatous, suppurative lesions with abscesses. Common infection sites are the head, neck, thorax, and abdomen, but infection can spread to contiguous tissues, causing multiple draining sinuses. Less common sites include the bones, brain, liver, kidneys, and female reproductive organs. Actinomycosis is likely to infect people with dental disease. The causative organism occurs as part of the normal flora of the throat, tonsillar crypts, and mouth (particularly around carious teeth).

Causes

Traumatic introduction of the grampositive anaerobic bacillus *Actinomyces israelii* into body tissues

Signs and symptoms
Cervicofacial actinomycosis
—Painful, indurated swellings in the mouth or neck
—Fistulas that open onto the skin
—Appearance of sulfur granules (yellowish gray masses that are actually colonies of *A. israelii*) in the exudate

Pulmonary actinomycosis
—Fever
—Productive cough
—Possible hemoptysis
—Sinus formation through the chest wall
Gastrointestinal actinomycosis
—Abdominal pain
—Fever
—Possible palpable mass
—External sinus

Diagnostic tests
• Isolation of *A. israelii* in exudate or tissue confirms actinomycosis.
• Microscopic examination of sulfur granules helps identify the infection.
• Gram staining of excised tissue or exudate reveals branching gram-positive rods.
• Chest X-ray shows lesions in unusual locations, such as the shaft of a rib.

Treatment
High-dose I.V. penicillin or tetracycline therapy precedes surgical excision and drainage of abscesses in all forms of the disease and continues for 3 to 6 weeks. Following parenteral therapy, treatment with oral penicillin or tetracycline may continue for 1 to 6 months.

Clinical implications
• Dispose of all dressings in a sealed plastic bag.
• After surgery, provide proper aseptic wound management.
• Administer antibiotics, as ordered. Before giving the first dose, obtain an accurate patient history of allergies. Watch for hypersensitivity reactions, such as rash, fever, itching, and signs of anaphylaxis. If the patient has a history of any allergies, keep epinephrine 1:1,000 and resuscitative equipment available.
• Stress the importance of good oral hygiene and proper dental care.

Acute tubular necrosis
(Acute tubulointerstitial nephritis)

Description
Acute tubular necrosis (ATN) accounts for about 75% of all cases of acute renal failure and is the most common cause of acute renal failure in critically ill patients. ATN injures the tubular segment of the nephron, causing renal failure and uremic syndrome. Mortality ranges from 40% to 70%, depending on complications from underlying diseases. Nonoliguric forms of ATN have a better prognosis. (See *Pathophysiologic Mechanisms*, p. 18.)

Causes
Ischemic injury
—Circulatory collapse
—Severe hypotension
—Trauma
—Hemorrhage
—Dehydration
—Cardiogenic or septic shock
—Surgery
—Anesthetics
—Transfusion reactions
Nephrotoxic injury
—Ingestion of certain chemical agents
—Hypersensitivity reaction of the kidneys (See *Nephrotoxic Injury*, p. 19.)

Signs and symptoms
• Oliguria (or rarely anuria)
• Confusion, which may progress to uremic coma

Diagnostic tests
• Urinalysis reveals low specific gravity and sediment containing RBCs and casts.
• Urine osmolality is low (less than 400 mOsm/kg).
• Urine sodium level is high (40 to 60 mEq/liter).
• BUN and serum creatinine levels are elevated.
• Serum potassium is elevated.

Pathophysiologic Mechanisms

ATN may result from the following:
• Diseased tubular epithelium that allows leakage of glomerular filtrate across the membranes and reabsorption of filtrate into the blood
• Obstruction of urine flow by the collection of damaged cells, casts, RBCs, and other cellular debris within the tubular walls
• Ischemic injury to glomerular epithelial cells, resulting in cellular collapse and decreased glomerular capillary permeability
• Ischemic injury to vascular endothelium, eventually resulting in cellular swelling and obstruction

• EKG may show dysrhythmias (from electrolyte imbalances) and, with hyperkalemia, widening QRS segment, disappearing P waves, and tall, peaked T waves.

Treatment

Treatment for patients with ATN consists of vigorous supportive measures during the acute phase until normal renal function resumes.

Initial treatment may include administration of diuretics and infusion of a large volume of fluids to flush tubules of cellular casts and debris and to replace fluid loss. However, this treatment carries a risk of fluid overload. Long-term fluid management requires daily replacement of projected and calculated losses (including insensible loss).

Other appropriate measures to control complications include transfusion of packed RBCs for anemia and administration of antibiotics for infection. Hyperkalemia may require emergency I.V. administration of 50% glucose, regular insulin, and sodium bicarbonate. Sodium polystyrene sulfonate with sorbitol may be given P.O. or by enema to reduce extracellular potassium levels. Peritoneal dialysis or hemodialysis may be needed if the patient is catabolic.

Clinical Implications

• Maintain fluid balance. Watch for fluid overload, a common complication of therapy. Accurately record intake and output, including wound drainage, nasogastric output, and peritoneal dialysis and hemodialysis balances. Weigh the patient daily.
• Monitor hemoglobin and hematocrit, and administer blood products, as needed. Use fresh packed cells instead of whole blood to prevent fluid overload and congestive heart failure.
• Maintain electrolyte balance. Monitor laboratory results, and report imbalances. Enforce dietary restriction of foods containing sodium and potassium, such as bananas, orange juice, and baked potatoes. Check for potassium content in prescribed medications (for example, penicillin V potassium). Provide adequate calories and essential amino acids while restricting protein intake to maintain an anabolic state. Total parenteral nutrition may be indicated in the severely debilitated or catabolic patient.
• Use aseptic technique, particularly when handling catheters, since the debilitated patient is vulnerable to infection. Immediately report fever, chills, delayed wound healing, or flank pain if the patient has an indwelling (Foley) catheter in place.
• Watch for complications. If anemia worsens (pallor, weakness, lethargy with decreased hemoglobin), administer RBCs, as ordered. For acidosis, give sodium bicarbonate or assist with dialysis in severe cases, as ordered. Watch for signs of diminishing renal

Nephrotoxic Injury

Incidence of acute tubular necrosis (ATN) from ingestion or inhalation of toxic substances is rising. This exposure may occur in the hospital, to an already debilitated patient, from such toxic agents as antibiotics (aminoglycosides, for example) and contrast media. Other nephrotoxic agents include pesticides, fungicides, heavy metals (mercury, arsenic, lead, bismuth, uranium), and organic solvents containing carbon tetrachloride or ethylene glycol (cleaning fluids or industrial solvents). Ingestion of these substances may be accidental or intentional.

Nephrotoxic injury causes multiple symptoms similar to those of renal failure, particularly azotemia, anemia, acidosis, overhydration, and hypertension; and, less frequently, fever, skin rash, and eosinophilia.

Treatment consists of identifying the nephrotoxic substance, eliminating its use, and removing it from the body by any means available, such as hemodialysis in extreme cases. Treatment is supportive during the course of acute renal failure.

---

perfusion (hypotension, decreased urine output). Encourage coughing and deep breathing to prevent pulmonary complications.

• Perform passive range-of-motion exercises. Provide good skin care; apply lotion or bath oil for dry skin. Help the patient to walk as soon as possible, but guard against exhaustion.

• Provide reassurance and emotional support. Encourage the patient and family to express their fears. Fully explain each procedure; repeat the explanation each time the procedure is done. Help the patient and family set realistic goals according to individual prognosis.

• To prevent ATN, make sure all patients are well hydrated before surgery or after X-rays that use a contrast medium. Administer mannitol, as ordered, to high-risk patients before and during these procedures. Carefully monitor patients receiving blood transfusions to detect early signs of transfusion reaction (fever, rash, chills), and discontinue transfusion immediately if signs occur.

Complications
• Infection, the leading cause of death in ATN
• Congestive heart failure
• Uremic pericarditis
• Pulmonary edema
• Anemia
• Intractable vomiting
• Uremic lung

Adenoid hyperplasia
(Adenoid hypertrophy)

Description
A fairly common childhood condition, adenoid hyperplasia is enlargement of the lymphoid tissue of the nasopharynx.

Causes
The precise cause is unknown.

Risk factors
• Heredity
• Repeated infection
• Chronic nasal congestion
• Persistent allergy
• Inefficient nasal breathing

Signs and symptoms
Characteristic signs and symptoms
—Mouth breathing
—Snoring
—Frequent, prolonged nasal congestion

Other possible signs and symptoms
—Distinctive facial features, such as slightly elongated face, open mouth, highly arched palate, shortened upper lip, and a vacant expression
—Signs of nocturnal respiratory insufficiency, such as intercostal retractions and nasal flaring

Diagnostic tests
• Nasopharyngoscopy or rhinoscopy confirms adenoid hyperplasia by visualizing abnormal tissue mass.
• Lateral pharyngeal X-rays show obliteration of the nasopharyngeal air column.

Treatment
Adenoidectomy is the treatment of choice for adenoid hyperplasia and is commonly recommended for the patient with prolonged mouth breathing, nasal speech, adenoid facies, recurrent otitis media, constant nasopharyngitis, and nocturnal respiratory distress. This procedure usually eliminates recurrent nasal infections and ear complications and reverses any secondary hearing loss.

Clinical implications
Focus the care plan on sympathetic preoperative care and diligent postoperative monitoring.
Before surgery
• Describe the hospital routine and arrange for the patient and parents to tour relevant areas of the hospital.
• Explain adenoidectomy to the child, using illustrations, if necessary, and detail the recovery process. Reassure him that he will probably need to be hospitalized only 2 nights. If hospital protocol allows, encourage one parent to stay with the child and participate in his care.
After surgery
• Maintain a patent airway. Position the child on his side, with head down, to prevent aspiration of draining secretions.
• Frequently check the throat for bleeding. Be alert for vomiting of old,

partially digested blood ("coffee grounds"). Closely monitor vital signs, and report excessive bleeding, rise in pulse rate, drop in blood pressure, tachypnea, and restlessness.
• If no bleeding occurs, offer cracked ice or water when the patient is fully awake.
• Tell the parents that their child may have a nasal voice temporarily.

Complications
Adenoid hyperplasia can obstruct the eustachian tube and predispose to otitis media, which in turn can lead to fluctuating conductive hearing loss. Stasis of nasal secretions from adenoidal inflammation can lead to sinusitis. Pulmonary hypertension and cor pulmonale can result if nocturnal respiratory insufficiency occurs.

Adenovirus infection

Description
Adenoviruses cause acute self-limiting febrile infections, with inflammation of the respiratory or ocular mucous membranes, or both. All infections occur in epidemics. The incubation period is usually less than 1 week; acute illness lasts less than 5 days and can be followed by prolonged asymptomatic reinfection.

Causes
Adenovirus has 35 known serotypes.

Transmission
• Direct inoculation into the eye
• Fecal-oral transmission
• Inhalation of an infected droplet

Signs and symptoms
Clinical features vary. (See *Major Adenoviral Infections.*)

Diagnostic tests
• Isolation of the virus from respiratory or ocular secretions, or fecal smear provides definitive diagnosis

Major Adenoviral Infections

DISEASE	AGE-GROUP	CLINICAL FEATURES
Acute febrile respiratory illness	Children	Nonspecific cold-like symptoms, similar to other viral respiratory illness: fever, pharyngitis, tracheitis, bronchitis, pneumonitis
Acute respiratory disease	Adults (usually military recruits)	Malaise, fever, chills, headache, pharyngitis, hoarseness, dry cough
Viral pneumonia	Children and adults	Sudden onset of high fever, rapid infection of upper and lower respiratory tracts, skin rash, diarrhea, intestinal intussusception
Acute pharyngo-conjunctival fever	Children (particularly after swimming in pools or lakes)	Spiking fever lasting several days, headache, pharyngitis, conjunctivitis, rhinitis, cervical adenitis
Acute follicular conjunctivitis	Adults	Unilateral tearing and mucoid discharge; later, milder symptoms in other eye
Epidemic keratoconjunctivitis	Adults	Unilateral or bilateral ocular redness and edema, preorbital swelling, local discomfort, superficial opacity of the cornea without ulceration
Hemorrhagic cystitis	Children (boys)	Hematuria, dysuria, urinary frequency

during epidemics; however, typical symptoms alone can confirm diagnosis.
• Differential leukocyte count can show lymphocytosis in children.
• Chest X-ray may show pneumonitis in respiratory disease.

Treatment
Supportive treatment includes bed rest, antipyretics, and analgesics. Ocular infections may require corticosteroids and direct supervision by an ophthalmologist. Hospitalization is required in cases of pneumonia (in infants) to prevent death and in epidemic keratoconjunctivitis (EKC) to prevent blindness.

Clinical implications
During the acute illness, monitor respiratory status and intake and output. Give analgesics and antipyretics, as needed. Stress the need for bed rest.

To help minimize the incidence of adenoviral disease, instruct all patients in proper handwashing to reduce fecal-oral transmission. EKC can be prevented by sterilization of ophthalmic instruments, adequate chlorination of swimming pools, and avoidance of swimming pools during EKC epidemics.

Killed virus vaccine (not widely available) and a live oral virus vaccine can prevent adenoviral infection and are recommended for high-risk groups.

Adrenal hypofunction
(Addison's disease, adrenal insufficiency)

Description

Primary adrenal hypofunction (Addison's disease) occurs when more than 90% of the adrenal gland is destroyed. It is the most common form of adrenal insufficiency. Addison's disease is an autoimmune process in which circulating antibodies react specifically against the adrenal tissue. It is characterized by decreased mineralocorticoid, glucose, and androgen secretion. Adrenal hypofunction can also occur secondary to a disorder outside the gland, but aldosterone secretion frequently continues intact. With early diagnosis and adequate replacement therapy, prognosis for adrenal hypofunction is good.

Acute adrenal insufficiency, or adrenal crisis (addisonian crisis), is a medical emergency requiring immediate, vigorous treatment. It is a critical deficiency of mineralocorticoids and glucocorticoids, and generally follows acute stress, trauma, or surgery in patients who have chronic adrenal insufficiency.

Causes
Addison's disease
—Tuberculosis
—Bilateral adrenalectomy
—Hemorrhage into the adrenal gland
—Neoplasms
—Fungal infections
Secondary adrenal hypofunction
—Hypopituitarism
—Abrupt withdrawal of long-term corticosteroid therapy
—Removal of a nonendocrine, ACTH-secreting tumor
Adrenal crisis
This occurs when the body's stores of glucocorticoids are exhausted in a person with adrenal hypofunction caused by trauma, surgery, or other physiologic stresses.

Signs and symptoms
Addison's disease
—Weakness
—Fatigue
—Weight loss
—Nausea and vomiting
—Anorexia
—Chronic diarrhea
—Conspicuous bronze coloration of the skin, especially in the creases of the hand and over the metacarpophalangeal joints, elbows, and knees
—Darkening of scars and areas of vitiligo (absence of pigmentation)
—Increased pigmentation of the mucous membranes, especially the buccal mucosa
—Cardiovascular abnormalities, such as postural hypotension, decreased cardiac size and output, and a weak, irregular pulse
—Decreased tolerance for even minor stress
—Poor coordination
—Fasting hypoglycemia
—Craving for salty food
—Possible retardation of axillary and pubic hair growth in females, decreased libido, and, in severe cases, amenorrhea
Secondary adrenal hypofunction
Clinical effects similar to Addison's disease without hyperpigmentation, hypotension, and electrolyte abnormalities
Adrenal crisis
—Profound weakness and fatigue
—Severe nausea and vomiting
—Hypotension
—Dehydration
—Occasional high fever

Diagnostic tests
• 24-hour urine collection for 17-ketosteroids and 17-hydroxycorticoste-

roids establishes baseline urine steroid levels.

• Plasma cortisol levels are decreased.

• Serum potassium level is increased.

• Blood urea nitrogen (BUN) level is increased.

• Hematocrit, lymphocyte, and eosinophil counts are elevated.

• X-rays show a small heart and adrenal calcification.

• Special provocative tests necessary to determine if adrenal hypofunction is primary or secondary include metyrapone and ACTH stimulation tests.

Treatment

For all patients with primary or secondary adrenal hypofunction, corticosteroid replacement, usually with cortisone or hydrocortisone (both also have mineralocorticoid effect), is the primary treatment and must continue for life. Addison's disease may also necessitate desoxycorticosterone I.M., a pure mineralocorticoid, or fludrocortisone P.O., a synthetic drug that acts as a mineralocorticoid; both prevent dangerous dehydration and hypotension. Women with Addison's disease who have muscle weakness and decreased libido may benefit from testosterone injections but risk unfortunate masculinizing effects.

Teaching Topics in Adrenocortical Insufficiency

• An explanation of the type of disorder: primary or secondary

• Warning signs and prevention of adrenal crisis

• Serial diagnostic tests to evaluate hormone levels

• Dietary modifications, with special emphasis on sodium and glucose needs

• Activity restrictions and need for rest

• Hormone replacement therapy

Adrenal crisis requires prompt I.V. bolus administration of 100 mg hydrocortisone. Later, 50- to 100-mg doses are given I.M. or are diluted with dextrose in saline solution and given I.V. until the patient's condition stabilizes; up to 300 mg/day of hydrocortisone and 3 to 5 liters of I.V. saline solution may be required during the acute stage. With proper treatment, the crisis usually subsides quickly; blood pressure should stabilize, and water and sodium levels return to normal. After the crisis, maintenance doses of hydrocortisone preserve physiologic stability.

Clinical implications

Adrenal crisis

• Monitor vital signs carefully, especially for hypotension, volume depletion, and other signs of shock (decreased level of consciousness and urine output). Watch for hyperkalemia before treatment and for hypokalemia after treatment (from excessive mineralocorticoid effect).

• If the patient also has diabetes, check blood glucose levels periodically, since steroid replacement may necessitate adjustment of insulin dosage.

• Record weight and intake and output carefully, since the patient may have volume depletion. Until onset of mineralocorticoid effect, force fluids to replace excessive fluid loss.

Maintenance therapy

• Arrange for a diet that maintains sodium and potassium balances.

• If the patient is anorectic, suggest six small meals a day to increase calorie intake. Ask the dietitian to provide a diet high in protein and carbohydrates. Keep a late-morning snack available in case the patient becomes hypoglycemic.

• Observe the patient receiving steroids for cushingoid signs, such as fluid retention around the eyes and face. Watch for fluid and electrolyte imbalance, especially if the patient is receiving mineralocorticoids. Monitor weight and check blood pressure to assess body fluid status. Remember, steroids administered in the late afternoon or evening may cause central nervous system stimulation and insomnia in some patients. Check for petechiae, since the patient bruises easily.

• In women receiving testosterone injections, watch for and report facial hair growth and other signs of masculinization. A dosage adjustment may be necessary.

• If the patient receives glucocorticoids alone, observe for orthostatic hypotension or electrolyte abnormalities, which may indicate a need for mineralocorticoid therapy.

• Explain that lifelong steroid therapy is necessary. Advise him of symptoms of overdose and underdose. Tell him that dosage may need to be increased during times of stress (when he has a cold, for example). Warn that infection, injury, or profuse sweating in hot weather may precipitate adrenal crisis.

• Instruct the patient always to carry a medical identification card stating that he takes a steroid and giving the name of the drug and the dosage. Teach the patient how to give himself an injection of hydrocortisone. Tell him to keep available an emergency kit containing hydrocortisone in a prepared syringe for use in times of stress. Warn that any stress may necessitate additional cortisone to prevent a crisis. (See *Teaching Topics in Adrenocortical Insufficiency*, p. 23.)

Adrenogenital syndrome

Description
Adrenogenital syndrome is an endocrine disorder resulting from abnormal activity of the adrenal cortex. Less than normal amounts of cortisol and greater than normal amounts of androgen are produced. This syndrome may be inherited (congenital adrenal hyperplasia [CAH]) or acquired (adrenal virilism). (See *Acquired Adrenal Virilism*, for further information on this type. Also see *Hermaphroditism*, p. 26.)

CAH is the most prevalent adrenal disorder in infants and children; simple virilizing CAH and salt-losing CAH are the most common forms. In both forms, a deficiency of the enzyme 21-hydroxylase results in underproduction of cortisol. In salt-losing CAH, 21-hydroxylase is almost completely absent, causing a precipitous fall in plasma cortisol levels and aldosterone, which, in combination with the excessive production of salt-wasting compounds, precipitates acute adrenal crisis. This crisis may be fatal in infants.

Other rare CAH enzyme deficiencies lead to increased or decreased production of affected hormones. (Also see *Acquired Adrenal Virilism*.)

Causes
CAH is transmitted as an autosomal recessive trait.

Signs and symptoms
Simple virilizing CAH
—Tall childhood stature
—Short adult stature
In females, signs and symptoms also include the following.
—Ambiguous genitalia (enlarged clitoris, with urethral opening at base; some labioscrotal fusion) but normal genital tract and gonads
—Signs of progressive virilization, such as early appearance of pubic and axillary hair, deep voice, acne, and facial hair
—Failure to begin menstruation at puberty
In males, signs and symptoms also include the following.
—Accentuated prepubertal masculine characteristics, such as an enlarged phallus, with frequent erections and deepened voice
—Small testes at puberty
Salt-losing CAH
—Apathy

Acquired Adrenal Virilism

Acquired adrenal virilism results from virilizing adrenal tumors, carcinomas, or adenomas. This rare disorder is twice as common in females as it is in males. Although acquired adrenal virilism can develop at any age, its clinical effects vary with the patient's age at onset.

• *Prepubescent girls:* Pubic hair, clitoral enlargement; at puberty, no breast development, menses delayed or absent

• *Prepubescent boys:* Hirsutism, macrogenitosomia precox (excessive body development, with marked enlargement of genitalia). Occasionally, the penis and prostate equal those of an adult male in size; however, testicular maturation fails to occur.

• *Women (especially middle-aged):* Dark hair on legs, arms, chest, back, and face; pubic hair extending toward navel; oily skin, sometimes with acne; menstrual irregularities; muscular hypertrophy (masculine resemblance); male pattern balding; atrophy of breasts and uterus

• *Men:* No overt signs; discovery of tumor usually accidental

• *All patients:* Good muscular development; taller than average during childhood and adolescence; short stature as adults due to early closure of epiphyses

Diagnostic tests include the following.

• *Urinary total 17-ketosteroids (17-KS):* Greatly elevated, but levels vary daily; dexamethasone P.O. does not suppress 17-KS

• *Plasma levels of dehydroepiandrosterone (DHA):* Greatly elevated

• *Serum electrolytes:* Normal

• *X-ray of kidneys:* May show downward displacement of kidneys by tumor

Treatment requires surgical excision of tumor and metastases (if present), when possible, or radiation therapy and chemotherapy. Preoperative treatment may include glucocorticoids. With treatment, prognosis is very good in patients with slow-growing and nonrecurring tumors. Periodic follow-up urine testing (for increased 17-KS) to check for possible tumor recurrence is essential.

—Failure to eat
—Diarrhea

In females, signs and symptoms also include the following.

—More complete virilization than apparent in simple virilizing CAH
—Male external genitalia without testes

In males, signs and symptoms also include the following.

—No external genital abnormalities
—Adrenal crisis developing in the first week of life (may be fatal if not recognized)

Diagnostic tests

Several tests confirm the diagnosis of CAH.

• Urine 17-ketosteroids (17-KS) are elevated but can be suppressed by administering dexamethasone P.O.

• Urinary metabolites of hormones, particularly pregnanetriol, are elevated.

• Plasma 17-hydroxyprogesterone is elevated.

• Urine 17-hydroxycorticosteroids are normal or decreased.

• Hyperkalemia, hyponatremia, and hypochloremia in the presence of excessive urinary 17-KS and pregnanetriol and decreased urinary aldosterone confirm salt-losing CAH during first week of life.

Treatment

Simple virilizing CAH requires correction of the cortisol deficiency and inhibition of excessive pituitary ACTH production by daily administration of cortisone or hydrocortisone. Such treatment returns androgen production to normal levels. Measurement of urinary 17-KS determines the initial dose of cortisone or hydrocortisone; this dose is usually large and is given I.M. Later dosage is modified according to decreasing urinary 17-KS levels. Infants must continue to receive cortisone or hydrocortisone I.M. until age 18 months; after that, they may take it P.O.

The infant with salt-losing CAH in adrenal crisis requires immediate I.V. sodium chloride and glucose infusion to maintain fluid and electrolyte balance and to stabilize vital signs. If saline and glucose infusion does not control symptoms while diagnosis is being established, desoxycorticosterone I.M. and, occasionally, hydrocortisone I.V. are necessary. Later, main-tenance includes mineralocorticoid (desoxycorticosterone) and glucocorticoid (cortisone or hydrocortisone) replacement.

Sex chromatin and karyotype studies determine the genetic sex of patients with ambiguous external genitalia. Females with masculine external genitalia require reconstructive surgery, such as correction of the labial fusion and of the urogenital sinus. Such surgery is usually scheduled between ages 1 and 3, after the effect of cortisone therapy has been assessed.

Clinical implications

• Suspect CAH in infants hospitalized for failure to thrive, dehydration, or diarrhea, as well as in tall, sturdy-looking children with a record of numerous episodic illnesses.
• When caring for an infant with ad-

Hermaphroditism

True hermaphroditism (hermaphrodism, intersexuality) is a rare condition characterized by both ovarian and testicular tissues. External genitalia are usually ambiguous but may be completely male or female, and thus can mask hermaphroditism until puberty. The hermaphrodite almost always has a uterus (fertility is rare) and ambiguous gonads distributed:

• *bilaterally:* testis and ovary on both sides, ovatestes
• *unilaterally:* ovary or testis on one side; an ovatestis on the other side
• *asymmetrically or laterally:* an ovary and a testis on opposite sides.

Since the Y chromosome is needed to develop testicular tissue, hermaphroditism in infants with XX karyotypes is particularly perplexing but may possibly result from mosaicism (XX/XY, XX/XXY), hidden mosaicism, or hidden gene alterations. In patients with XX karyotype, ovaries are usually better developed than in those with XY karyotype. Fifty percent of hermaphrodites have 46,XX karyotype, 20% have 46,XY, and 30% are mosaics.

Although ambiguous external genitalia suggest hermaphroditism, chromosomal studies (particularly a buccal smear for Barr bodies, indicating an XX karyotype), a 24-hour urine specimen for 17-ketosteroids to rule out congenital adrenal hyperplasia, and gonadal biopsy are necessary to confirm it.

Sexual assignment, based on the anatomy of the external genitalia, and prognosis for most successful plastic reconstruction, should be made as early as possible to prevent physical and psychological consequences of delayed reassignment. During such surgery, inappropriate reproductive organs are removed to prevent incongruous secondary sex characteristics at puberty. Hormonal replacement may be necessary.

Nursing intervention emphasizes psychological support of the parents and reinforcement of their choice about sexual assignment.

renal crisis, keep the I.V. line patent, infuse fluids, and give steroids, as ordered. Monitor body weight, blood pressure, and serum electrolytes carefully, especially sodium and potassium levels. Watch for cyanosis, hypotension, tachycardia, tachypnea, and signs of shock. Keep external stress to a minimum.

• If the child is receiving maintenance therapy with steroid injections, rotate I.M. injection sites to prevent atrophy. Tell parents to do the same. Teach them the possible adverse effects (cushingoid symptoms) of long-term therapy. Explain that maintenance therapy with hydrocortisone, cortisone, or implanted desoxycorticosterone pellets is essential for life.

• Warn parents not to withdraw these drugs suddenly, since potentially fatal adrenal insufficiency will result. Instruct parents to report stress and infection, which require increased steroid dosages.

• Monitor the patient receiving desoxycorticosterone for edema, weakness, and hypertension. Be alert for significant weight gain and rapid changes in height, since normal growth is an important indicator of adequate therapy.

• Instruct the patient to wear a medical identification bracelet indicating that he is on prolonged steroid therapy and providing dosage information.

• Help parents of a female infant with male genitalia to understand that she is physiologically a female and that this abnormality can be surgically corrected. Arrange for counseling, if necessary.

Adult respiratory distress syndrome (ARDS)
(Shock, stiff, white, wet, or Da Nang lung)

Description
A form of pulmonary edema that causes acute respiratory failure, adult respiratory distress syndrome (ARDS) results from increased permeability of the alveolocapillary membrane. Fluid accumulates in the lung interstitium, alveolar spaces, and small airways, causing the lung to stiffen. Effective ventilation is thus impaired, prohibiting adequate oxygenation of pulmonary capillary blood. Severe ARDS can be fatal; however, patients who recover may have little or no permanent lung damage.

Causes
• Aspiration of gastric contents
• Sepsis (primarily gram-negative)
• Trauma (lung contusion, head injury, long-bone fracture with fat emboli)
• Oxygen toxicity
• Viral, bacterial, or fungal pneumonia
• Microemboli (fat or air emboli or disseminated intravascular coagulation [DIC])
• Drug overdose (barbiturates, glutethimide, narcotics)
• Blood transfusion
• Smoke or chemical inhalation (nitrous oxide, chlorine, ammonia)
• Hydrocarbon and paraquat ingestion
• Pancreatitis, uremia, or miliary tuberculosis (rare)
• Near-drowning

Signs and symptoms
• Rapid, shallow breathing
• Dyspnea
• Hypoxemia
• Intercostal and suprasternal retractions
• Rales and rhonchi
• Restlessness
• Apprehension
• Mental sluggishness
• Motor dysfunction
• Tachycardia

Diagnostic tests
• Arterial blood gases (ABGs) on room air show decreased PO_2 (less than 60 mm Hg) and PCO_2 (less than 35 mm Hg). The resulting pH usually reflects

respiratory alkalosis. As ARDS becomes more severe, ABGs show respiratory acidosis (increasing PCO_2 [more than 45 mm Hg]) and metabolic acidosis (decreasing HCO_3 [less than 22 mEq/liter]) and a decreasing PO_2 despite oxygen therapy.

• Pulmonary artery catheterization helps identify the cause of pulmonary edema by evaluating pulmonary capillary wedge pressure (PCWP); allows collection of pulmonary artery blood, which shows decreased oxygen saturation, reflecting tissue hypoxia; measures pulmonary artery pressure; and measures cardiac output by thermodilution techniques.

• Serial chest X-rays initially show bilateral infiltrates; in later stages, ground-glass appearance and eventually (as hypoxemia becomes irreversible) "whiteouts" of both lung fields.

• Sputum Gram stain culture and sensitivity and blood cultures detect infections.

• Toxicology screen detects drug ingestion.

• Serum amylase determination is performed if pancreatitis is a consideration.

Treatment

When possible, treatment is designed to correct the underlying cause of ARDS and to prevent progression and potentially fatal complications. Supportive medical care consists of administering humidified oxygen by a tight-fitting mask, which allows for use of continuous positive airway pressure (CPAP). Hypoxemia that does not respond adequately to these measures requires ventilatory support with intubation, volume ventilation, and positive end-expiratory pressure (PEEP). Other supportive measures include fluid restriction, diuretics, and correction of electrolyte and acid-base abnormalities.

When ARDS requires mechanical ventilation, sedatives, narcotics, or neuromuscular blocking agents such as tubocurarine or pancuronium bromide may be ordered to minimize restlessness (thereby reducing oxygen consumption and carbon dioxide production) and to facilitate ventilation. When ARDS results from fat emboli or chemical injuries to the lungs, a short course of high-dose steroids may help if given early. Treatment with sodium bicarbonate may be necessary to reverse severe metabolic acidosis, and use of fluids and vasopressors may be required to maintain blood pressure. Nonviral infections require antimicrobial drugs.

Clinical implications

ARDS requires careful monitoring and supportive care.

• Frequently assess the patient's respiratory status. Be alert for retractions on inspiration. Note rate, rhythm, and depth of respirations, and watch for dyspnea and the use of accessory muscles of respiration. On auscultation, listen for adventitious or diminished breath sounds. Check for clear, frothy sputum that may indicate pulmonary edema.

• Observe and document the hypoxemic patient's neurologic status (level of consciousness, mental sluggishness).

• Maintain a patent airway by suctioning, using sterile, nontraumatic technique. When necessary, instill normal saline solution to help liquefy tenacious secretions.

• Closely monitor heart rate and blood pressure. Watch for dysrhythmias that may result from hypoxemia, acid-base disturbances, or electrolyte imbalance. With pulmonary artery catheterization, know the desired PCWP level, check readings often, and watch for decreasing mixed venous oxygen saturation.

• Monitor serum electrolytes, and correct imbalances. Measure intake and output, and weigh patient daily.

• Check ventilator settings frequently, and empty condensation from tubing promptly to assure maximum oxygen delivery. Monitor ABG studies; check for metabolic and respiratory acidosis and PO_2 changes. The patient with severe hypoxemia may need controlled mechanical ventilation with positive airway pressure. Give sedatives, as needed, to reduce restlessness. Since PEEP may decrease cardiac output, check for hypotension, tachycardia, and decreased urine output. Suction only as needed so that PEEP is maintained. Reposition often and record any increase in secretions, temperature, or hypotension that may indicate a deteriorating condition.

• Monitor nutrition, maintain joint mobility, and prevent skin breakdown. Plan patient care to allow periods of uninterrupted sleep.

• Provide emotional support. Warn the patient who is recovering from ARDS that recovery will take some time and that he will feel weak for a while.

• Watch for and immediately report all respiratory changes in the patient who has suffered injuries that may adversely affect the lungs, especially during the 2- to 3-day period after the injury, when the patient may appear to be improving.

Complications
• Hypoxemia
• Respiratory acidosis

Alcoholism

Description
Alcoholism is a chronic disorder marked by uncontrolled intake of alcoholic beverages that interferes with physical or mental health, social and familial relationships, and occupational responsibilities. Alcoholism cuts across all social and economic groups, involves both sexes, and occurs at all stages of the life cycle, beginning as early as elementary school age. It has no known cure.

Causes
No definite cause of alcoholism has been clearly identified. However, various biologic, psychological, and sociocultural factors have been considered.

Signs and symptoms
Characteristic signs and symptoms
—Need for daily or episodic use of alcohol for adequate function
—Inability to discontinue or reduce alcohol intake
—Episodes of anesthesia or amnesia during intoxication
—Episodes of violence during intoxication
—Interference with social and familial relationships and occupational responsibilities
Other possible signs and symptoms
—Unexplained traumatic injuries
—Unexplained mood swings
—Unresponsiveness to sedatives
—Poor personal hygiene
—Secretive behavior (possibly an attempt to hide disease or alcohol supply)
—Consumption of alcohol in any form when deprived of usual supply
—Hostility when confronted with drinking problem (if patient has not yet recognized its existence)

Diagnostic tests
• Blood alcohol level documents recent alcohol ingestion. A level of 0.10% weight/volume (200 mg/dl) is generally accepted as the level of intoxication. It cannot confirm alcoholism, but by knowing how recently the patient has been drinking you can tell when to expect withdrawal symptoms.

• A complete serum electrolyte count may be necessary to identify electrolyte abnormalities. In severe hepatic disease, BUN level is increased and serum glucose level is decreased.

• Serum ammonia levels may be increased.

• Urine toxicology may help to determine if the alcoholic with alcohol withdrawal syndrome or another acute complication abuses other drugs as well.

• Hepatic function studies, revealing increased serum cholesterol, lactate dehydrogenase (LDH), SGOT, SGPT, and creatine phosphokinase levels, may point to hepatic damage.

• Elevated serum amylase and lipase levels point to acute pancreatitis.

• A hematologic workup can identify anemia, thrombocytopenia, increased prothrombin time, and increased partial thromboplastin time.

Symptoms of Alcohol Withdrawal

SYMPTOM	MILD	MODERATE	SEVERE
Motor impairment	Inner tremulousness with hand tremors	Visible tremors	Gross uncontrollable bodily shaking
Anxiety	Mild restlessness	Obvious motor restlessness and painful anxiety	Extreme restlessness and agitation with intense fearfulness
Sleep disturbance	Restless sleep or insomnia	Marked insomnia and nightmares	Total wakefulness
Appetite	Impaired appetite	Marked anorexia	Rejection of all food and fluid except alcohol common
GI symptoms	Nausea	Nausea and vomiting	Dry heaves and vomiting
Confusion	None	Variable	Marked confusion and disorientation
Hallucinations	None	Vague, transient visual and auditory hallucinations and illusions; commonly nocturnal; often with insight	Visual and occasional auditory hallucinations, usually of fearful or threatening content; misidentification of persons and frightening delusions related to hallucinatory experiences
Pulse rate	Tachycardia	Pulse, 100 to 120	Pulse, 120 to 140
Blood pressure	Normal or slightly elevated systolic	Usually elevated systolic	Elevated systolic and diastolic
Sweating	Slight	Obvious	Marked hyperhidrosis
Convulsions	None	Possible	Common

Treatment and clinical implications

Total abstinence is the only effective treatment. Supportive programs that offer detoxification, rehabilitation, and aftercare (including continued involvement in Alcoholics Anonymous [AA]) produce the best long-term results.

Treatment during acute withdrawal may include administration of I.V. glucose for hypoglycemia and forcing fluids containing thiamine and other B complex vitamins to correct nutritional deficiencies and help metabolize glucose. (See also *Symptoms of Alcohol Withdrawal.*)

When caring for a patient in alcohol withdrawal, carefully monitor mental status, heart rate, lung sounds, blood pressure, and temperature every ½ to 6 hours, depending on the severity of symptoms. Orient the patient to reality, since he may have hallucinations and may try to harm himself or others. If he is combative or disoriented, you may have to restrain him temporarily. Take seizure precautions. Administer drugs, as ordered, which may include antianxiety agents, anticonvulsants, or antidiarrheal or antiemetic agents. Participate in the plan of care for medical symptoms and complications. Observe for signs of depression or suicide. Also, encourage adequate nutrition.

Once the alcoholic is sober, treatment aims to help him stay sober. Educate the patient and his family about his illness. Encourage participation in a rehabilitation program. Warn him that he will be tempted to drink again and will not be able to control himself after the first drink. Therefore, he must abstain from alcohol *totally* for the rest of his life. Two forms of treatment may help him abstain: aversion therapy, if ordered, and supportive counseling. Unfortunately, neither is completely effective.

Aversion or deterrent therapy employs a daily oral dose of disulfiram. This drug interferes with alcohol metabolism and allows toxic levels of acetaldehyde to accumulate in the patient's blood, producing immediate and potentially fatal distress if the patient drinks alcohol up to 2 weeks after taking it. The reaction includes nausea, vomiting, facial flushing, headache, shortness of breath, red eyes, blurred vision, sweating, tachycardia, hypotension, and fainting. It may last from 30 minutes to 3 hours or longer. The patient needs close medical supervision during this time. Warn the patient taking disulfiram that even a small amount of alcohol will induce this adverse reaction and that the longer he takes the drug, the greater will be his sensitivity to alcohol. Because of this, he must avoid even medicinal sources of alcohol, such as mouthwash, cough syrups, liquid vitamins, or cold remedies. Paraldehyde, a sedative, is chemically similar to alcohol and may also provoke a disulfiram reaction.

Aversion therapy is contraindicated during pregnancy and in patients with diabetes, heart disease, severe hepatic disease, or any disorder in which such a reaction could be especially dangerous. Instruct patients taking this drug that they may continue this treatment for months or years and that they should remain under medical supervision.

Another form of deterrent therapy attempts to induce aversion by administering alcohol with an emetic. However, for long-term success with deterrent therapy, the sober alcoholic must learn to fill the place alcohol once occupied in his life with something constructive. Indeed, for patients with abnormal dependency needs or for those who also abuse other drugs, deterrent therapy with disulfiram may only substitute one drug dependency for another. It should be used prudently.

Supportive counseling or individual, group, or family psychotherapy may improve the alcoholic's ability to cope with stress, anxiety, and frustration and help him gain insight into the personal problems and conflicts that may have led him to alcohol abuse. Occasionally, a doctor may order a tranquilizer to relieve overwhelming anxiety during rehabilitation, but such drugs are dangerous because of their potential for transferring addiction and for inducing coma and death when combined with alcohol.

In AA, a self-help group with more than a million members worldwide, the alcoholic finds emotional support from others with similar problems. Offer to arrange a visit from an AA member.

Spouses of alcoholics can find encouragement in Al-Anon, another self-help group; children, in Alateen. Family involvement in rehabilitation can reduce family tensions. For alcoholics who have lost all contact with family and friends and who have a long history of unemployment, trouble with the law, or other problems associated with alcohol abuse, rehabilitation may involve job training, sheltered workshops, halfway houses, or other supervised facilities.

Providing comprehensive treatment for alcoholics can help them maintain sobriety and may limit family disruptions that could contribute to the development of alcoholism in offspring.

Complications
• Gastritis
• Acute pancreatitis
• Anemia
• Malnutrition and other nutritional deficiencies
• Hepatitis
• Cirrhosis (common)
• Cardiomyopathy
• Congestive heart failure
• Organic brain damage such as Wernicke-Korsakoff syndrome
• Traumatic injuries due to falls

Allergic purpura
(Henoch-Schönlein purpura, anaphylactoid purpura)

Description
Allergic purpura, a nonthrombocytopenic purpura, is an acute or chronic vascular inflammation affecting the skin, joints, and gastrointestinal and genitourinary tracts, in association with allergy symptoms. When allergic purpura primarily affects the gastrointestinal tract, with accompanying joint pain, it is called Henoch-Schönlein purpura or anaphylactoid purpura. However, the term allergic purpura applies to purpura associated with many other conditions, such as erythema nodosum.

Fully developed allergic purpura is persistent and debilitating. Allergic purpura affects males more often than females and is most prevalent in children from age 3 to 7.

An acute attack of allergic purpura can last for several weeks and is potentially fatal (usually from renal failure); however, most patients do recover. Prognosis is more favorable for children than adults.

Causes
• Most common: An autoimmune reaction directed against vascular walls, triggered by a bacterial infection (particularly streptococcal infection)
• Allergic reactions to some drugs and vaccines
• Allergic reactions to insect bites
• Allergic reactions to some foods, such as wheat, eggs, milk, chocolate

Signs and symptoms
Typically, upper respiratory infection occurs 1 to 3 weeks before the onset of symptoms.
Skin symptoms
—In adults, characteristically purple, macular, ecchymotic, of varying size; appearing in symmetric patterns on the arms and legs; accompanied by pruritus, paresthesia, and occasionally angioneurotic edema
—In children, urticarial and expanding, becoming hemorrhagic; appearing on the arms and legs in symmetrical patterns; possible scattered petechiae on the legs, buttocks, and perineum
Gastrointestinal symptoms
These are common in Henoch-Schön-

lein syndrome and may precede overt cutaneous signs of purpura.
—Transient or severe colic
—Tenesmus and constipation
—Vomiting
—GI bleeding
—Occult blood in stool
—Possible intussusception

Musculoskeletal symptoms
—Rheumatoid pains, usually in the legs and feet
—Periarticular effusions, usually in the legs and feet

Genitourinary symptoms
—Renal hemorrhages resulting in microscopic hematuria and renal function disturbances
—Bleeding from the mucosal surfaces of the ureters, bladder, or urethra

Other possible signs and symptoms
—Moderate and irregular fever
—Headache
—Anorexia
—Localized edema of the hands, feet, or scalp

Diagnostic tests

• Tourniquet test is positive.
• White blood cell count is elevated.
• Erythrocyte sedimentation rate is elevated.
• Coagulation and platelet function test are normal.
• Small bowel X-rays may reveal areas of transient edema.
• Tests for blood in the urine and stool are often positive.
• BUN and creatinine tests are increased and may indicate renal involvement.

Treatment

Treatment is generally symptomatic; for example, severe allergic purpura may require steroids to relieve edema and analgesics to relieve joint and abdominal pain. Some patients with chronic renal disease may benefit from immunosuppression with azathioprine, along with identification of the provocative allergen. *Accurate allergy history is essential.*

Clinical implications

• Encourage maintenance of an elimination diet to help identify specific allergenic foods to be eliminated from the patient's diet.
• Monitor skin lesions and level of pain. Provide analgesics, as needed.
• Watch carefully for complications: GI and genitourinary tract bleeding, edema, nausea, vomiting, headache, hypertension (with nephritis), abdominal rigidity and tenderness, and absence of stool (with intussusception).
• To prevent muscle atrophy in the bedridden patient, perform passive or active range-of-motion exercises.
• Provide emotional support and reassurance, especially if the patient is temporarily disfigured by florid skin lesions.
• After the acute stage, stress the need for the patient to *immediately* report *any* recurrence of symptoms (most common about 6 weeks after initial onset) and to return for follow-up urinalysis as scheduled.

Complications

• Chronic glomerulonephritis, especially following a streptococcal infection
• Renal failure
• GI and genitourinary tract bleeding
• Edema
• Nausea and/or vomiting
• Headache
• Hypertension (with nephritis)
• Abdominal rigidity and tenderness
• Absence of stool (with intussusception)

Allergic rhinitis

Description

Allergic rhinitis is a reaction to airborne (inhaled) allergens. Depending on the allergen, the resulting rhinitis and conjunctivitis may be seasonal (hay fever) or occur year-round (perennial allergic rhinitis). It is most prevalent in young children and adolescents, but can occur in all age-groups. Seasonal pollen allergy may exacerbate symptoms of perennial rhinitis.

Causes
Hay fever
—Wind-borne pollens such as tree pollens in spring, grass pollens in summer, and weed pollens in fall
—Mold (fungal spores) in summer and fall
Perennial allergic rhinitis
—House dust
—Feather pillows
—Mold
—Cigarette smoke
—Upholstery
—Animal dander

Signs and symptoms
Hay fever
—Paroxysmal sneezing
—Profuse watery rhinorrhea
—Nasal obstruction or congestion
—Pruritus of the nose and eyes
—Pale, cyanotic, edematous nasal mucosa
—Red and edematous eyelids and conjunctivae
—Excessive lacrimation
—Headache or sinus pain
—Dark circles under the eyes ("allergic shiners")
—Occasional itching in the throat, malaise, and fever
Perennial allergic rhinitis
—Chronic nasal obstruction often extending to eustachian tube obstruction, particularly in children
—Dark circles under the eyes ("allergic shiners")

Diagnostic tests
• Microscopic examination of sputum and nasal secretions reveals large numbers of eosinophils.
• Blood chemistry shows normal or elevated IgE.
• Skin testing can pinpoint the responsible allergens when paired with tested responses to environmental stimuli and interpreted in light of the patient's history.

Treatment and clinical implications
Treatment aims to control symptoms by eliminating the environmental antigen, if possible, and by drug therapy and immunotherapy. Antihistamines effectively block histamine effects but commonly produce anticholinergic adverse effects (sedation, dry mouth, nausea, dizziness, blurred vision, and nervousness). However, new antihistamines, such as terfenadine (Seldane), produce fewer adverse effects and are much less likely to cause sedation. Topical intranasal steroids produce local anti-inflammatory effects with minimal systemic adverse effects.

The most commonly used drugs are flunisolide (Nasalide) and beclomethasone (Beconase, Vancenase). Generally, these drugs are not effective for acute exacerbations; nasal decongestants and oral antihistamines may be needed instead. Advise the patient to use intranasal steroids regularly, as

---

Preventing Allergic Rhinitis

To reduce exposure to airborne allergens, follow these guidelines:
• Sleep with the windows closed.
• Avoid the countryside during pollination seasons.
• Use air-conditioning to filter allergens and keep down moisture and dust.
• Eliminate dust-collecting items, such as wool blankets, deep-pile carpets, and heavy drapes, from the home.
• Consider drastic changes in life-style, such as relocation to a pollen-free area either seasonally or year-round in severe and resistant cases.

prescribed, for optimal effectiveness.

Cromolyn sodium (Nasalcrom) may be helpful in preventing allergic rhinitis. However, this drug may take up to 4 weeks to produce a satisfactory effect and must be taken regularly during allergy season.

When caring for the patient with allergic rhinitis, monitor his compliance with prescribed treatment regimens and note any changes in symptom control or signs of drug misuse.

Long-term management includes immunotherapy, or desensitization with injections of extracted allergens, administered preseasonally, coseasonally, or perenially. Seasonal allergies require particularly close dosage regulation. Before such injections, assess the patient's symptom status. Afterward, watch for adverse reactions, including anaphylaxis and severe localized erythema. Keep epinephrine and emergency resuscitative equipment available. Observe the patient for 30 minutes after the injection. Tell him to call the physician if a delayed reaction occurs. (See also *Preventing Allergic Rhinitis*.)

Alport's syndrome

Description
Alport's syndrome is a nephritis that affects males more often and more severely than females. Men with hematuria and proteinuria often develop end-stage renal disease in their thirties or forties.

Streptococcal infection is not linked to Alport's syndrome, but respiratory infection often precipitates recurrent bouts of hematuria.

Causes
This syndrome is hereditary. It is transmitted as an X-linked, autosomal trait.

Signs and symptoms
• Most common: Recurrent gross or microscopic hematuria that typically appears during early childhood
• Next most common: Deafness
• Proteinuria
• Pyuria
• Red blood cell casts in urine
• Ocular symptoms such as cataracts and, less commonly, keratoconus, microspherophakia, myopia, retinitis pigmentosa, and nystagmus
• Hypertension (often associated with progressive renal failure)
• Possible flank pain or other abdominal symptoms

Diagnostic tests
• Renal biopsy confirms diagnosis.
• Urinalysis is performed on all family members to detect proteinuria, pyuria, red blood cell casts, and hematuria.
• Blood studies detect immunoglobulins and complement components.
• Audiometry testing identifies deafness.

Treatment and clinical implications
Effective treatment is supportive and symptomatic. It may include antibiotic therapy for associated respiratory or urinary tract infection; a hearing aid for hearing loss; eyeglasses or contact lenses to improve vision; antihypertensive therapy for associated hypertension; and dialysis or renal transplantation for end-stage renal failure.

Refer the patient and family for genetic counseling as appropriate.

Alzheimer's disease
(Primary degenerative dementia)

Description
Alzheimer's disease is a presenile dementia that accounts for over half of all dementias. The brain tissue of patients with primary degenerative dementia has three hallmark features: neurofibrillary tangles, neuritic

Organic Brain Syndrome

Although many behavioral disturbances are clearly linked to organic brain dysfunction, the clinical syndromes associated with this type of impairment are sometimes hard to detect because they are not determined solely by the affected area of the brain or even by the extent of tissue damage. Instead, the way in which the patient's personality interacts with the brain injury determines the specific clinical effects that develop. General symptoms often include impairment of orientation, memory, and intellectual and emotional function. These primary cognitive deficits help to distinguish organic brain syndromes from neurosis and depression.

Diagnosis of an organic brain syndrome depends on a detailed history of the onset of cognitive and behavioral disturbances; a complete neurologic assessment; and such tests as electroencephalograms, computed tomography scans, brain X-rays, cerebrospinal fluid analysis, and psychological studies. Organic brain syndromes are classified by etiology and specific clinical effects. Causes include infection, brain trauma, nutritional deficiency, cerebrovascular disease, degenerative disease, tumor, toxins, and metabolic or endocrine disorders.

Effective treatment requires correction of the underlying cause. Special considerations may include reality orientation, emotional support for the patient and family, providing a safe environment, mat therapy for an agitated or aggressive patient, and referral for psychological counseling.

plaques, and granulovascular degeneration. Because this is a primary progressive dementia, the prognosis for a patient with this disease is poor.

Causes

The cause of primary degenerative dementia is unknown. Several factors are thought to be implicated. These include neurochemical factors, such as deficiencies in the neurotransmitters acetylcholine, somatostatin, substance P, and norepinephrine; environmental factors, such as aluminum and manganese; viral factors, such as slow-growing central nervous system viruses; trauma; and genetic immunologic factors.

Signs and symptoms

Onset is insidious. Initial changes are almost imperceptible, but they gradually progress to serious problems.
Initial signs and symptoms
—Forgetfulness
—Recent memory loss
—Difficulty learning and remembering new information
—Deterioration in personal hygiene and appearance
—Inability to concentrate
Later signs and symptoms
—Difficulty with abstract thinking and activities that require judgment
—Progressive difficulty in communication
—Severe deterioration in memory, language, and motor function, resulting in coordination loss and an inability to speak or write
—Repetitive actions or perseveration (a key sign)
—Personality changes such as restlessness and irritability
—Nocturnal awakenings
—Disorientation
—Urinary or fecal incontinence (common in final stages)
—Possible twitching and seizures in late stages
—Susceptibility to infection (often the cause of death)

Diagnostic tests
• Psychometric testing and neurologic

examination can help establish the diagnosis.

• Positron emission transaxial tomography scan measures the metabolic activity of the cerebral cortex and may help confirm early diagnosis.

• Electroencephalogram and computed tomography scan may help diagnose later stages of Alzheimer's disease.

Treatment
Therapy consists of cerebral vasodilators, such as ergoloid mesylates (Hydergine), isoxsuprine (Vasodilan), and cyclandelate (Cyclospasmol), to enhance the brain's circulation; hyperbaric oxygen to increase oxygen supply to the brain; psychostimulators, such as methylphenidate (Ritalin), to enhance the patient's mood; and antidepressants if depression seems to exacerbate the patient's dementia. Most drug therapies currently being used are experimental. These include choline salts, lecithin, physostigmine, deanol, enkephalins, and naloxone, which may slow the disease process. Another approach to treatment includes avoiding antacids, use of aluminum cooking utensils, and aluminum-containing deodorants to help decrease aluminum intake.

Clinical implications
Overall care is focused on supporting the patient's abilities and compensating for those abilities he has lost.

• Establish an effective communication system with the patient and family to help them adjust to the patient's altered cognitive abilities.

• Offer emotional support to the patient and family. Teach them about the disease, and listen to their concerns.

• Protect the patient from injury by providing a safe, structured environment.

• Encourage the patient to exercise, as ordered, to help maintain mobility.

• Set up an appointment with a social services agency, which will help the family assess its financial status and handle legal matters such as power of attorney.

• Refer the family to support groups; they may find solace in knowing that others are going through the same devastating experience. To locate support groups in your area, contact your local Alzheimer's Disease and Related Disorders Association (ADRDA), or contact the national ADRDA. (See also *Organic Brain Syndrome*.)

Amebiasis
(Amebic dysentery)

Description
Amebiasis is an acute or chronic protozoal infection that produces varying degrees of illness. Extraintestinal amebiasis can induce hepatic abscess and infections of the lungs, pleural cavity, pericardium, peritoneum, and, rarely, the brain. It occurs worldwide but is most common in the tropics, subtropics, and other areas with poor sanitation and health practices. Prognosis is generally good, although complications increase mortality.

Causes
Entamoeba histolytica, which exists in two forms: a cyst that can survive outside the body and a trophozoite that cannot survive outside the body

Mode of transmission
Ingestion of feces, contaminated food, or contaminated water

Signs and symptoms
The clinical effects of amebiasis vary with the severity of the infestation. In some cases the patient is asymptomatic.

Acute amebic dysentery
—Sudden high fever of 104° to 105° F. (40° to 40.5° C.)
—Chills
—Abdominal cramping
—Profuse, bloody diarrhea with tenesmus

—Diffuse abdominal tenderness
Chronic amebic dysentery
—Intermittent diarrhea that lasts for 1 to 4 weeks and recurs several times a year
—Foul-smelling mucus- and blood-tinged diarrheal stools 4 to 8 times daily (in severe cases, up to 18 times daily)
—Mild fever
—Vague abdominal cramps
—Tenderness over the cecum and ascending colon
—Possible weight loss and hepatomegaly

Diagnostic tests
• Isolation of *E. histolytica* (cysts and trophozoites) in fresh feces or aspirates from abscesses, ulcers, or tissue confirms acute amebic dysentery.
• Indirect hemagglutination test yields positive results with current or previous infection.
• Complement fixation usually is positive only during active disease.
• Barium studies rule out nonamebic causes of diarrhea, such as polyps and cancer.
• Sigmoidoscopy detects rectosigmoid ulceration; a biopsy may be helpful.

Treatment and clinical implications
Drugs used to treat amebic dysentery include metronidazole, an amebicide at intestinal and extraintestinal sites; emetine hydrochloride, also an amebicide at intestinal and extraintestinal sites, including the liver and lungs; iodoquinol (diiodohydroxyquin), an effective amebicide for asymptomatic carriers; chloroquine, for liver abscesses, not intestinal infections; and tetracycline (in combination with emetine hydrochloride, metronidazole, or paromomycin), which supports the antiamebic effect by destroying intestinal bacteria on which the amoebae normally feed.

Tell patients with amebiasis to avoid drinking alcohol when taking metronidazole. The combination may cause nausea, vomiting, and headache.

Patients with amebiasis should not have preparatory enemas, since these may remove exudates and destroy the trophozoites, thus interfering with test results.

Complications
• Amebic granuloma (ameboma), often mistaken for cancer
• Intestinal stricture
• Hemorrhage
• Intussusception
• Perforation of intestine resulting in spread to liver and from there to lungs, pleural cavity, and, rarely, the brain
• Brain abscess (a rare complication, usually fatal)

Amputation, traumatic

Description
Traumatic amputation is the accidental loss of a body part, usually a finger, toe, arm, or leg. In complete amputation, the member is totally severed; in partial amputation, some soft-tissue connection remains. Prognosis has improved as a result of improved early emergency and critical care management, new surgical techniques, early rehabilitation, prosthesis fitting, and prosthesis design. New limb reimplantation techniques have been moderately successful, but incomplete nerve regeneration remains a major limiting factor.

Causes
Traumatic amputations usually result directly from accidents with factory, farm, or power tools or from motor vehicle accidents.

Treatment
Because the greatest immediate threat after traumatic amputation is blood loss and hypovolemic shock, emergency treatment consists of local measures to control bleeding, fluid

replacement with normal saline solution and colloids, and blood replacement, as needed. Reimplantation remains controversial, but it is becoming more common and successful because of advances in microsurgery. If reconstruction or reimplantation is possible, surgical intervention attempts to preserve usable joints. When arm or leg amputations are done, the surgeon creates a stump to be fitted with a prosthesis. A rigid dressing permits early prosthesis fitting and rehabilitation.

Clinical implications

Every traumatic amputee requires careful monitoring of vital signs. If amputation involves more than just a finger or toe, assessment of airway, breathing, and circulation is also required. Since profuse bleeding is likely, watch for signs of hypovolemic shock, and draw blood for hemoglobin, hematocrit, and typing and cross matching. In partial amputation, check for pulses distal to the amputation. After any traumatic amputation, assess for other traumatic injuries, as well.

During emergency treatment, monitor vital signs (especially in hypovolemic shock); cleanse the wound; and give tetanus prophylaxis, analgesics, and antibiotics, as ordered. After complete amputation, flush the amputated part with sterile saline solution, wrap it in a moist sterile towel or gauze, and put it in a plastic bag. Then place the bag in a container of ice. Flush the wound with sterile saline solution, apply a sterile pressure dressing, and elevate the limb. Notify the reimplantation team. After partial amputation, position the limb in normal alignment, and drape it with towels or dressings soaked in sterile normal saline solution.

Preoperative care includes thorough wound irrigation and debridement (using a local anesthetic). Postoperative dressing changes using sterile technique help prevent skin infection and ensure skin graft viability. Help the amputee cope with his altered body image. Reinforce exercises, and emphasize the need to prevent stump trauma.

Amyloidosis

Description

Amyloidosis is a rare, chronic disease resulting in the accumulation of an abnormal fibrillar scleroprotein (amyloid), which infiltrates body organs and soft tissues. Reticuloendothelial cell dysfunction and abnormal immunoglobulin synthesis occur in some types of amyloidosis. The disease is classified in two ways, based on histologic findings: perireticular type, which affects the inner coats of blood vessels, and pericollagen type, which affects the outer coats of blood vessels and also involves the parenchyma. Prognosis varies with type and with the site and extent of involvement. Amyloidosis sometimes results in permanent—usually even life-threatening—organ damage.

Causes

• Heredity, especially in persons of Portuguese ancestry
• May occur in conjunction with tuberculosis, chronic infection, rheumatoid arthritis, multiple myeloma, Hodgkin's disease, paraplegia, and brucellosis
• May accompany the aging process

Signs and symptoms

Amyloidosis produces dysfunction of the kidneys, heart, gastrointestinal (GI) tract, peripheral nerves, and, rarely, the liver. Any of the following symptoms may occur.
• Proteinuria leading to nephrotic syndrome and eventual renal failure
• Faint heart sounds
• Intractable congestive heart failure
• Stiffness and enlargement of the tongue, which hinders enunciation
• Malabsorption, which may become

chronic, leading to malnutrition and predisposing the patient to infection
• GI bleeding
• Infiltration of blood vessels along the GI tract
• Abdominal pain
• Constipation
• Diarrhea
• Peripheral neuropathy
• Rarely, liver enlargement, often with azotemia, anemia, albuminuria, and mild jaundice

Diagnostic tests
• Histologic examination of a tissue biopsy specimen using a polarizing or electron microscope is necessary to confirm the diagnosis. Rectal mucosa biopsy is preferable, since it is less hazardous than kidney or liver biopsy. Depending on the location of amyloid deposits, other biopsy sites include the gingiva, skin, and nerves.
• EKG shows low voltage and conduction or rhythm abnormalities resembling those of myocardial infarction in cardiac amyloidosis.
• Liver function studies are generally normal, except for slightly elevated serum alkaline phosphatase in hepatic amyloidosis.

Treatment
Treatment is mainly supportive but may include corticosteroids and other immunosuppressives to minimize inflammation. Transplantation may be useful for amyloidosis-induced renal failure. Patients with cardiac amyloidosis require conservative treatment; digitalis must be given with caution to prevent dangerous dysrhythmias. Malnutrition caused by malabsorption in end-stage GI involvement may require total parenteral nutrition.

Clinical implications
• Maintain nutrition and fluid balance; give analgesics to relieve intestinal pain; control constipation or diarrhea; and manage infection and fever.
• Provide good mouth care for the pa-

tient with tongue involvement. Refer him for speech therapy, if needed. Provide an alternative method of communication if he cannot talk.
• Assess airway patency when the tongue is involved, and prevent respiratory tract compromise by gentle and adequate suctioning, when indicated. Keep a tracheostomy tray at bedside.
• When long-term bed rest is necessary, properly position the patient, and turn him often to prevent decubitus ulcers. Perform range-of-motion exercises to prevent contractures.
• Provide psychological support. Exercise patience and understanding to help the patient cope with this chronic illness.

Amyotrophic lateral sclerosis
(Lou Gehrig's disease, ALS)

Description
Amyotrophic lateral sclerosis is the most common motor neuron disease of muscular atrophy. Other motor neuron diseases include progressive muscular atrophy and progressive bulbar palsy. (See also *Motor Neuron Disease.*) In inherited ALS (approximately 10% of cases), men and women are affected equally. In noninherited ALS, incidence is highest among persons whose occupations require strenuous physical labor. Generally, onset occurs between ages 40 and 70. ALS is fatal within 3 to 10 years after onset, usually because of aspiration pneumonia or respiratory failure.

Precipitating factors for acute deterioration include trauma, viral infections, and physical exhaustion. Disorders that must be differentiated from ALS include central nervous system syphilis, multiple sclerosis, spinal cord tumors, and syringomyelia.

Causes
• Autosomal dominant inheritance
• Nutritional deficiency of motor neu-

rons related to a disturbance in enzyme metabolism
• Metabolic interference in nucleic acid production by the nerve fibers
• Autoimmune disorders that affect immune complexes in the renal glomerulus and basement membrane

Signs and symptoms
• Atrophy and weakness, especially in the muscles of the forearms and the hands
• Impaired speech
• Difficulty chewing and swallowing
• Difficulty breathing
• Normal mental status
• Possible choking and excessive drooling

Diagnostic tests
• Electromyography and muscle biopsy help show nerve rather than muscle disease.
• Examination of cerebrospinal fluid reveals increased protein content in one third of patients.

Treatment
No effective treatment exists for ALS. Management aims to control symptoms and provide emotional, psychological, and physical support.

Clinical implications
This cruel, demeaning neurologic disease challenges the patient's and his care givers' ability to cope. Since mental status remains intact while progressive physical degeneration takes place, the patient acutely perceives every change. Care begins with a complete neurologic assessment, a baseline for future evaluations of disease progression.
• Implement a rehabilitation program designed to maintain independence as long as possible.
• Help the patient obtain equipment, such as a walker and a wheelchair. Arrange for a visiting nurse to oversee home care, to provide support, and to

---

Motor Neuron Disease

In its final stages, motor neuron disease affects both upper and lower motor neuron cells. However, the site of initial cell damage varies.
• *Progressive bulbar palsy:* Degeneration of upper motor neurons in the medulla oblongata
• *Progressive muscular atrophy:* Degeneration of lower motor neurons in the spinal cord
• *Amyotrophic lateral sclerosis:* Degeneration of upper motor neurons in the medulla oblongata and lower motor neurons in the spinal cord

---

teach the family about the illness.
• Depending on the patient's muscular capacity, assist with bathing, personal hygiene, and transfers from wheelchair to bed. Help establish a regular bowel and bladder routine.
• To help the patient handle increased accumulation of secretions and dysphagia, teach him to suction himself. He should have a suction machine handy at home to reduce fear of choking.
• To prevent skin breakdown, provide good skin care when the patient is bedridden. Turn him often, keep his skin clean and dry, and use sheepskins or pressure-relieving devices.
• If the patient has trouble swallowing, give him soft, solid foods and position him upright during meals. Gastrostomy and nasogastric tube feedings may be necessary if he can no longer swallow. Teach the patient (if he is still able to feed himself) or family how to administer gastrostomy feedings.
• Provide emotional support. Prepare the patient and family for his eventual death, and encourage the start of the grieving process. Patients with ALS

Teaching Topics in A.L.S.

• Explanation of how motor neuron degeneration affects muscles and motor function
• Preparation for electromyography, nerve conduction studies, and other tests to help distinguish ALS from other disorders
• The importance of exercise in maintaining strength in unaffected muscles
• Dietary changes, such as use of semisoft foods
• Techniques for nasogastric and gastrostomy tube feedings, if needed
• Palliative medications
• Techniques for respiratory support
• Alternative communication techniques
• Availability of information from the Muscular Dystrophy Association

---

may benefit from a hospice program. (See also *Teaching Topics in ALS*.)

Anal fissure

Description
Anal fissure is a laceration or crack in the lining of the anus that extends to the circular muscle. Posterior fissure, the most common, is equally prevalent in males and females. Anterior fissure, the rarer type, is 10 times more common in females. An anal fissure may be an acute or chronic condition. Prognosis is very good, especially with fissurectomy and good anal hygiene.

Causes
• Passage of large, hard stools that stretch the lining beyond its limits
• Strain on the perineum during childbirth (anterior fissure)
• Occasionally, proctitis, anal tuberculosis, or carcinoma
• Rarely, scar stenosis (anterior fissure)

Signs and symptoms
Acute anal fissure
—Tearing, cutting, or burning pain during or immediately after bowel movement
—Drops of blood seen on toilet paper or underclothes

—Painful anal sphincter spasms
—Pain and bleeding on digital examination
—Direct visualization of fistula upon eversion by gentle traction on perianal skin
Chronic anal fissure
—Scar tissue that hampers normal bowel evacuation
—Pain and bleeding on digital examination
—Direct visualization of fistula upon eversion by gentle traction on perianal skin

Diagnostic tests
Anoscopy shows the longitudinal tear and helps establish the diagnosis.

Treatment and clinical implications
Treatment varies according to severity of the tear. For superficial fissures without hemorrhoids, forcible digital dilatation of anal sphincters under local anesthesia stretches the lower portion of the anal sphincter. For complicated fissures, treatment includes surgical excision of tissue, adjacent skin, and mucosal tags, and division of internal sphincter muscle from external.
• Prepare the patient for rectal examination, and explain the necessity of the procedure.
• Provide hot sitz baths, warm soaks, and local anesthetic ointment to re-

lieve pain. A low-residue diet, adequate fluid intake, and stool softeners prevent straining during defecation.

• Control diarrhea with diphenoxylate or other antidiarrheals.

Anaphylaxis

Description

Anaphylaxis is an exaggerated hypersensitivity reaction to a previously encountered antigen. The response, which is mediated by antibodies of the IgE class of immunoglobulins, causes the release of histamine, kinin, and substances that affect smooth muscle. A severe reaction may precipitate vascular collapse, leading to systemic shock and, sometimes, death.

Causes

The source of anaphylactic reactions is ingestion of or other systemic exposure to sensitizing drugs or other substances, including the following.

• Penicillin (the most common cause)
• Serums
• Vaccines
• Allergen extracts
• Enzymes
• Hormones
• Antibiotics other than penicillin
• Sulfonamides
• Local anesthetics
• Salicylates
• Polysaccharides
• Diagnostic chemicals, including radiographic contrast media containing iodine
• Foods
• Sulfite-containing food additives
• Insect venom
• Rarely, ruptured hydatid cyst

Signs and symptoms

Anaphylactic reaction usually produces sudden physical distress within seconds or minutes after exposure to an allergen. (A delayed or persistent reaction may occur up to 24 hours later.) The severity of symptoms depends on the original sensitizing dose of antigen, the amount and distribution of antibodies, and the route of entry and size of the dose of antigen.

General initial symptoms
—Feeling of impending doom or fright
—Weakness
—Sweating
—Sneezing
—Shortness of breath
—Nasal pruritus
—Urticaria
—Angioedema

Cardiovascular symptoms
—Hypotension
—Shock
—Cardiac dysrhythmias, which may precipitate circulatory collapse if not treated

Respiratory symptoms
—Nasal mucosal edema
—Profuse watery rhinorrhea
—Itching
—Nasal congestion
—Sudden sneezing attacks
—Hoarseness, stridor, and dyspnea (early signs of acute respiratory failure)

Gastrointestinal and genitourinary symptoms
—Severe stomach cramps
—Nausea
—Diarrhea

Preventing Anaphylaxis

To prevent anaphylaxis, follow these guidelines:
• With food or drug allergy, avoid the offending food or drug in all its forms.
• With allergy to insect stings, avoid open fields and wooded areas during the insect season and carry an anaphylaxis kit (epinephrine, antihistamine, tourniquet) when outdoors.
• Wear a medical identification bracelet identifying the allergy or allergies.

—Urinary urgency
—Incontinence

Treatment

Anaphylaxis is always an emergency. It requires an *immediate* injection of epinephrine 1:1,000 aqueous solution, 0.1 to 0.5 ml, repeated every 5 to 20 minutes, as necessary. In the early stages of anaphylaxis, when the patient has not lost consciousness and is normotensive, give epinephrine I.M. or S.C., and help it move into circulation faster by massaging the site of injection. In severe reactions, when the patient has lost consciousness and is hypotensive, give epinephrine I.V.

Maintain airway patency. Observe for early signs of laryngeal edema (stridor, hoarseness, and dyspnea), which will probably necessitate endotracheal intubation or a tracheotomy and oxygen therapy. In case of cardiac arrest, begin cardiopulmonary resuscitation.

Watch for hypotension and shock, and maintain circulatory volume with volume expanders (plasma, plasma expanders, saline, and albumin), as needed. Stabilize blood pressure with the I.V. vasopressors norepinephrine and dopamine. Monitor blood pressure, central venous pressure, and urine output as a response index.

After the initial emergency, administer other medications as ordered: S.C. epinephrine, longer-acting epinephrine, corticosteroids, and diphenhydramine I.V. for long-term management; and aminophylline I.V. over 10 to 20 minutes for bronchospasm. (Caution: Rapid infusion of aminophylline may cause or aggravate severe hypotension.)

Clinical Implications

• To prevent anaphylaxis, teach the patient to avoid exposure to known allergens.

• If a patient must receive a drug to which he is allergic, prevent a severe reaction by making sure he receives careful desensitization with gradually increasing doses of the antigen or advance administration of steroids.

• Of course, a person with a known allergic history should receive a drug with a high anaphylactic potential only after cautious pre-testing for sensitivity. Closely monitor the patient during testing, and make sure you have resuscitative equipment and epinephrine ready.

• When any patient needs a drug with a high anaphylactic potential (particularly parenteral drugs), make sure he receives each dose under close medical observation.

• Closely monitor a patient undergoing diagnostic tests, such as intravenous pyelography, cardiac catheterization, and angiography, that use radiographic contrast media. (See also *Preventing Anaphylaxis,* p. 43.)

Ankylosing spondylitis
(Rheumatoid spondylitis, Marie-Strümpell disease)

Description

A chronic, usually progressive inflammatory disease, ankylosing spondylitis primarily affects the sacroiliac, apophyseal, and costovertebral joints and adjacent soft tissue. The disease progresses unpredictably and can go into remission, exacerbation, or arrest at any stage. Generally, it begins in the sacroiliac joints and gradually progresses to the lumbar, thoracic, and cervical regions of the spine. Deterioration of bone and cartilage can lead to fibrous tissue formation and eventual fusion of the spine or peripheral joints. Progressive disease is well-recognized in men, but diagnosis is often overlooked or missed in women, who tend to have more peripheral joint involvement.

Causes

• A familial tendency has been strongly suggested by recent evidence.

• Immunologic activity is suggested

by the presence of histocompatibility antigen HLA-B27 (in more than 90% of patients with this disease) and circulating immune complexes.

Signs and symptoms

The presence of symptoms other than back pain depends on the disease stage.
• Intermittent low back pain, usually most severe in the morning or after a period of inactivity
• Stiffness and limited motion of the lumbar spine
• Pain and limited expansion of the chest due to involvement of the costovertebral joints
• Peripheral arthritis involving shoulders, hips, and knees
• Kyphosis in advanced stages, caused by chronic stooping to relieve symptoms
• Hip deformity and associated limited range of motion
• Tenderness over sites of inflammation
• Mild fatigue, fever, anorexia, or weight loss
• Occasional iritis
• Aortic regurgitation and cardiomegaly
• Upper lobe pulmonary fibrosis (mimics tuberculosis)

Diagnostic tests

• Test for HLA-B27 histocompatibility antigen is positive.
• Characteristic X-rays, which confirm the diagnosis, reveal blurring of the bony margins of joints in the early stage, bilateral sacroiliac involvement, patchy sclerosis with superficial bony erosions, eventual squaring of vertebral bodies, and "bamboo" spine with complete ankylosis.
• Erythrocyte sedimentation rate may be slightly elevated.
• Alkaline phosphatase may be slightly elevated.
• Creatinine phosphokinase levels may be slightly elevated.
• A negative rheumatoid factor helps rule out rheumatoid arthritis, which produces similar symptoms.

Treatment

No treatment reliably stops progression of this disease. Management aims to delay further deformity by good posture, stretching and deep-breathing exercises, and, in some patients, braces and lightweight supports. Anti-inflammatory analgesics, such as aspirin, indomethacin, and sulindac, control pain and inflammation.

Severe hip involvement usually necessitates surgical hip replacement. Severe spinal involvement may require a spinal wedge osteotomy to separate and reposition the vertebrae. This surgery is performed only on selected patients because of the risk of spinal cord damage and the long convalescence involved.

Clinical implications

Ankylosing spondylitis can be an extremely painful and crippling disease. The main nursing responsibility is to promote patient comfort. When dealing with such a patient, keep in mind that limited range of motion makes simple tasks difficult. Offer support and reassurance. Contact the local Arthritis Foundation chapter for a support group.

Administer medications, as ordered. Apply local heat and provide massage to relieve pain. Assess mobility and degree of discomfort frequently. Teach and assist with daily exercises, as needed, to maintain strength and function. Stress the importance of maintaining good posture.

If treatment includes surgery, provide good postoperative nursing care. Since ankylosing spondylitis is a chronic, progressively crippling condition, a comprehensive treatment plan should also reflect counsel from a social worker, visiting nurse, and dietitian. To minimize deformities, advise the patient to:
• avoid any physical activity that places undue stress on the back, such as lifting heavy objects
• stand upright; sit upright in a high,

straight chair; and avoid leaning over a desk
• sleep in a prone position on a hard mattress and avoid using pillows under neck or knees
• avoid prolonged walking, standing, sitting, or driving
• perform regular stretching and deep-breathing exercises and swim regularly, if possible
• have height measured every 3 to 4 months to detect any tendency toward kyphosis
• seek vocational counseling if work requires standing or prolonged sitting at a desk.

Anorectal abscess and fistula

Description

Anorectal abscess is a localized collection of pus due to inflammation of the soft tissue near the rectum or anus. Such inflammation may produce an anal fistula—an abnormal opening in the anal skin—that may communicate with the rectum.

As the anorectal abscess produces more pus, a fistula may form in the soft tissue beneath the muscle fibers of the sphincters (especially the external sphincter), usually extending into the perianal skin. The internal (primary) opening of the abscess or fistula is usually near the anal glands and crypts; the external (secondary) opening, in the perianal skin. (See *Types of Anorectal Abscess.*)

Causes

• An abrasion or tear in the lining of the anal canal, rectum, or perianal skin, and subsequent infection by *Escherichia coli,* staphylococci, or streptococci as a result of trauma from objects such as enema tips or ingested eggshells or fish bones
• Systemic illness, such as ulcerative colitis or Crohn's disease

Signs and symptoms

Anorectal abscess
—Characteristic: Throbbing pain and tenderness at the abscess site
—Presence of a hard, painful lump that prevents comfortable sitting
Anorectal fistula
—Pruritic drainage, causing perianal irritation
—Pink, red, elevated, discharging sinus or ulcer on the skin near the anus
—Possible chills, fever, nausea, vomiting, and malaise depending on the

---

Types of Anorectal Abscess

• *Perianal abscess* (80% of patients): A red, tender, localized, oval swelling close to the anus. Sitting or coughing increases pain, and pus may drain from the abscess. Digital examination reveals no abnormalities.
• *Ischiorectal abscess* (15% of patients): Involves the entire perianal region on the affected side of the anus. It is tender but may not produce drainage. Digital examination reveals a tender induration bulging into the anal canal.
• *Submucous or high intermuscular abscess* (5% of patients): May produce a dull, aching pain in the rectum; tenderness; and, occasionally, induration. Digital examination reveals a smooth swelling of the upper part of the anal canal or lower rectum.
• *Pelvirectal abscess* (rare): Produces fever, malaise, and myalgia but no local anal or external rectal signs or pain. Digital examination reveals a tender mass high in the pelvis, perhaps extending into one of the ischiorectal fossae.

severity of infection
—A palpable indurated tract, a drop or two of pus, and a depression or ulcer in the midline anteriorly or at the dentate line posteriorly (may be found on digital examination)

Diagnostic tests
Sigmoidoscopy, barium studies, and colonoscopy may be done to rule out other conditions.

Treatment
Anorectal abscesses require surgical incision under caudal anesthesia to promote drainage. Fistulas require fistulotomy—removal of the fistula and associated granulation tissue—under caudal anesthesia. If the fistula tract is epithelialized, treatment requires fistulectomy—removal of the fistulous tract—followed by insertion of drains, which remain in place for 48 hours.

Clinical implications
• After incision to drain anorectal abscess, provide adequate medication for pain relief, as ordered.
• Examine the wound frequently to assess proper healing, which should progress from the inside out. Healing should be complete in 4 to 5 weeks for perianal fistulas and in 12 to 16 weeks for deeper wounds.
• Inform the patient that complete recovery takes time. Offer encouragement.
• Stress the importance of perianal cleanliness.
• Dispose of soiled dressings properly.
• Be alert for the first postoperative bowel movement. The patient may suppress the urge to defecate because of anticipated pain; the resulting constipation increases pressure at the wound site. Such a patient benefits from a stool-softening laxative such as psyllium (Hydrocil, Metamucil).

Anorexia nervosa

Description
Anorexia nervosa, probably a psychological disturbance, is characterized by self-imposed starvation and consequent emaciation, nutritional deficiency disorders, and atrophic changes. Gorging, vomiting, and purging may occur during starvation or after normal weight is restored. This disorder primarily affects adolescent females and young adults but is not uncommon among older women. Occasionally it also affects males. Anorexia nervosa usually develops in a patient whose weight is normal or who may be only 5 pounds (2.3 kg) overweight.

Prognosis varies but is improved if the diagnosis is made early or if the patient voluntarily seeks help and wants to overcome the disorder. Nevertheless, mortality ranges from 5% to 15%, the highest mortality associated with a psychological disturbance.

Causes
The cause is unknown. Researchers in neuroendocrinology are seeking a physiologic cause but have found nothing definite. Clearly, however, social attitudes that equate slimness with beauty play some role in provoking this disorder; family factors are also clearly implicated.

Signs and symptoms
Any of the following symptoms may be present.
• 25% or greater weight loss for no organic reason, coupled with a morbid dread of being fat and a compulsion to be thin (cardinal symptoms)
• Anger and ritualistic behavior
• Skeletal muscle atrophy
• Loss of fatty tissue
• Hypotension
• Constipation
• Dental caries
• Susceptibility to infection

- Blotchy or sallow skin
- Intolerance to cold
- Lanugo on the face and body
- Dryness or loss of scalp hair
- Amenorrhea
- Restless activity and vigor (despite undernourishment), such as exercising avidly without apparent fatigue
- Obsession with food or cooking but refusal to eat
- Distorted body image (belief that she is fat despite evidence to the contrary)
- Gorging followed by self-induced vomiting or self-administration of laxatives or diuretics
- Feelings of despair, hopelessness and worthlessness, guilt, anxiety, low self-esteem, or depression
- Blood pressure below 50 mm Hg, signaling circulatory collapse
- Cardiac dysrhythmias, which may lead to cardiac arrest

Diagnostic tests
Laboratory data are usually normal unless weight loss exceeds 30%. Initial laboratory tests include the following.
- Complete blood count
- Serum creatinine
- Blood urea nitrogen
- Serum uric acid
- Serum cholesterol
- Total serum protein
- Serum albumin
- Serum electrolytes (sodium, potassium, chloride, bicarbonate)
- Serum calcium
- SGOT and SGPT
- Fasting blood glucose
- Urinalysis
- Electrocardiogram

Treatment
Treatment aims to promote weight gain or control the patient's compulsive gorging and purging, and to correct the underlying dysfunction. Hospitalization in a medical or psychiatric unit may be required to improve the patient's precarious physical state. Hospitalization may be as brief as 2 weeks or may stretch from a few months to

2 years or longer. Treatment is difficult, and results are often discouraging. Fortunately, many clinical centers are now developing programs for managing eating disorders in both inpatients and outpatients.

Treatment approaches may include behavior modification (privileges are dependent on weight gain); curtailing activity for physical reasons (such as cardiac dysrhythmias); vitamin and mineral supplements; a reasonable diet, with or without liquid supplements; hyperalimentation (subclavian, peripheral, or enteral [enteral and peripheral routes carry less risk of infection]); and group, family, or individual psychotherapy.

All forms of psychotherapy, from psychoanalysis to hypnotherapy, have been used in treating anorexia nervosa, with varying success. To be successful, such therapy should address the patient's underlying problems of low self-esteem, guilt, and anxiety; feelings of hopelessness and helplessness; and depression. Most therapists consider task-centered approaches and therapeutic flexibility important requirements for success.

Clinical implications
- During hospitalization, regularly monitor vital signs and intake and output. Weigh the patient daily—before breakfast, if possible. However, since such a patient often fears being weighed, the routine for this may differ greatly.
- Frequently offer small portions of food or drinks, if the patient wants them. Often, nutritionally complete liquids are more acceptable, since they eliminate choices between foods—something the anorexic patient often finds difficult.
- If tube feedings or other special feeding measures become necessary, explain these measures completely to the patient and be ready to discuss her fears or reluctance; however, limit the discussion about food itself.
- Discuss the patient's need for food

with her matter-of-factly. Point out that improved nutrition can correct abnormal laboratory findings.
• If edema or bloating occurs after the patient has returned to normal eating behavior, reassure her that this phenomenon is temporary. She will probably find this condition frightening.
• Encourage the patient to recognize and assert her feelings freely. If she understands that she can be assertive, she may gradually learn that expressing her true feelings will not result in her losing control or love.
• Remember: The anorexic patient uses exercise, preoccupation with food, ritualism, manipulation, and lying as mechanisms that preserve the only control she feels she has in her life.
• Her family may need therapy to uncover and correct faulty interactions. Advise family members to avoid discussing food with her. Her weight may be monitored by someone acceptable to her, her family, and her therapist. You or the physician may refer the patient and her family to Anorexia Nervosa and Associated Disorders (ANAD), a national information and support organization.

Anxiety states
(Anxiety neuroses)

Description
Anxiety is a feeling of apprehension caused by a threat to a person or his values. Some describe it as an exaggerated feeling of impending doom, dread, or uneasiness. Unlike fear—a reaction to danger from a specific external source—anxiety is a reaction to an internal threat, such as an unacceptable impulse or a repressed thought that is below a conscious level. Occasional anxiety is a normal part of life. However, overwhelming anxiety can cause an anxiety state—uncontrollable, unreasonable anxiety that narrows perceptions and interferes

with normal functioning.

Anxiety states can be acute or chronic. An acute state, or panic disorder, often begins between ages 15 and 35. Studies show that families of patients with panic disorders have a high incidence of alcoholism and that these patients have increased mortality caused by suicide and heart disease, especially mitral valve prolapse.

Chronic anxiety that lasts for more than a month is called a generalized anxiety disorder and has an uncertain prognosis.

Causes
• Conflict, whether intrapsychic, sociopersonal, or interpersonal, promotes an anxiety state.
• Genetic predisposition is suggested by research that has proven that anxiety states run in families.

Signs and symptoms
Psychological or physiologic symptoms of anxiety states vary with the degree of anxiety.
Generalized anxiety disorder
Mild to moderate psychological and physical symptoms, which may include the following, last for a month or more, but no panic attacks occur.
—Restlessness
—Sleeplessness
—Appetite changes
—Irritability
—Repeated questioning
—Constant attention- or reassurance-seeking behavior
—Fatigue on awakening and worry about possible misfortunes
—Difficulty concentrating, causing unawareness of surroundings
—Orientation to the past, not the present or future
—Feeling apprehensive, helpless, angry, fearful, "keyed-up," tearful, withdrawn, or afraid of losing self-confidence or control
—Lack of initiative
—Criticism of himself and others
—Self-deprecation
—Diaphoresis

Recognizing a Panic Attack

A panic attack is a brief period of intense apprehension or fear; it may last from minutes to hours. A history of three or more panic attacks within 3 weeks that are unrelated to extreme physical exertion, life-threatening situations, or phobias confirms panic disorder.

During a panic attack, the patient will display four or more of these signs and symptoms:
- Chest pains
- Palpitations
- Dyspnea
- Choking or smothering feeling
- Vertigo, dizziness, or unsteadiness
- Feelings of faintness
- Depersonalization or feeling of unreality
- Tingling in the hands and feet
- Shaking or trembling
- Hot and cold flashes
- Diaphoresis
- Fear of going crazy, dying, or being out of control during a panic attack

Diagnostic tests
- Various laboratory tests rule out other organic causes of the patient's symptoms, such as hyperthyroidism, pheochromocytoma, coronary artery disease, paroxysmal tachycardia, and Meniere's disease.
- Psychological tests rule out other psychiatric disorders such as phobia, obsessive-compulsive disorders, depression, and acute schizophrenia.
- Routine laboratory tests should include a complete blood count with differential.

Treatment
A combination of organic and psychotherapeutic treatments may help a patient with an anxiety disorder. The benzodiazepine antianxiety drugs may relieve mild anxiety and improve the patient's ability to cope with stress. Tricyclic antidepressants or higher doses of benzodiazepines may relieve severe anxiety and panic attacks. These drugs can ease distress and facilitate psychotherapy or psychoanalysis.

Clinical implications
When caring for an anxious patient, your role is primarily supportive and protective. Your goal will be to help the patient develop effective coping mechanisms to manage his anxiety.
- If the patient must take antianxiety drugs or tricyclic antidepressants, administer medications, as ordered, and evaluate the patient's response.
- Stress the importance of taking the medications exactly as prescribed for maximum effectiveness.
- Warn the patient and his family that these drugs may cause adverse effects, such as drowsiness, fatigue, ataxia, blurred vision, slurred speech, tremors, and hypotension.
- Tell the patient to avoid simultaneous use of alcohol or any central nervous system depressants. He should also avoid driving and other hazardous tasks until he develops a tolerance for the drug's sedative effects.

—Dilated pupils
—Dry mouth
—Difficulty swallowing
—Frequent urination
—Dysuria
—Rapid respirations
—Flushing or pallor
—Diarrhea or constipation
—Nausea
—Vomiting
—Belching
—Sexual dysfunction
—Cold, clammy hands

Panic disorder
Acute anxiety causes a panic attack with severe signs and symptoms. (See *Recognizing a Panic Attack*.) After a panic attack, the patient may not remember what precipitated it and may feel depersonalized. Usually, chronic anxiety persists between attacks.

• Advise him to discontinue medications only with the physician's approval, because abrupt withdrawal could cause severe symptoms.

• If the patient has a panic attack, protect him during the attack. Show him how to take slow, deep breaths if he is hyperventilating. Carefully explain the physiologic reasons for these symptoms. Avoid making judgments or critical comments.

• When panic subsides, encourage the patient to face his anxiety, because avoidance only increases it. Help him recognize the symptoms of his anxiety and his coping mechanisms, such as depression, withdrawal, demanding or violent behavior, denial, and manipulation.

• Explore alternative behaviors; encourage him to take up activities that will distract him from his anxiety.

• Make referrals for psychiatric treatment, as needed, for such problems as chronic anxiety and disturbed coping mechanisms. Provide telephone numbers for hotlines, psychiatric emergency help, and other emergency agencies.

Aplastic anemia
(Hypoplastic anemia)

Description
Aplastic anemia is a deficiency of all of the formed elements of the blood, representing a failure of the cell-generating capacity of the bone marrow. It usually develops when damaged or destroyed stem cells inhibit RBC production. Less commonly, it develops when damaged bone marrow microvasculature creates an unfavorable environment for cell growth and maturation. Although often used interchangeably with other terms for bone marrow failure, aplastic anemia properly refers to pancytopenia resulting from the decreased functional capacity of a hypoplastic, fatty bone marrow. Two forms of idiopathic aplastic anemia have been identified: congenital hypoplastic anemia (anemia of Blackfan and Diamond), which develops between ages 2 months and 3 months; and Fanconi's syndrome, in which chromosomal abnormalities are usually associated with multiple congenital anomalies—such as dwarfism and hypoplasia of the kidneys and spleen. Mortality for aplastic anemia with severe pancytopenia is 80% to 90%. Death may result from bleeding or infection.

Causes
• Drugs
• Toxic agents, such as benzene and chloramphenicol
• Radiation
• Immunologic factors (suspected but unconfirmed)
• Severe disease, especially hepatitis
• Preleukemia and neoplastic infiltration of bone marrow
• Congenital abnormalities (a possible cause of idiopathic anemias)
• Induced change in the development of the fetus (suspected as a cause in the absence of a consistent familial or genetic history of aplastic anemia)

Signs and symptoms
Clinical features of aplastic anemia vary with the severity of pancytopenia, often develop insidiously, and may include the following signs and symptoms:
• Progressive weakness
• Fatigue
• Shortness of breath
• Headache
• Pallor
• Ultimately tachycardia and congestive heart failure
• Ecchymoses
• Petechiae
• Hemorrhage, especially from the mucous membranes (nose, gums, rectum, vagina) or into the retina or central nervous system
• Infection (fever, oral and rectal ulcers, sore throat) but without characteristic inflammation

Diagnostic tests

Confirmation of aplastic anemia requires a series of laboratory tests.

• RBCs are usually normochromic and normocytic (although macrocytosis [larger than normal erythrocytes] and anisocytosis [excessive variation in erythrocyte size] may exist), with a total count of 1,000,000/cu mm or less. Absolute reticulocyte count is very low.

• Serum iron level is elevated (unless bleeding occurs), but total iron-binding capacity is normal or slightly reduced. Hemosiderin is present, and tissue iron storage is visible microscopically.

• Platelet, neutrophil, and WBC counts fall.

• Coagulation tests (bleeding time), reflecting decreased platelet count, are abnormal.

• Bone marrow biopsies taken from several sites may yield a "dry tap" or show severely hypocellular or aplastic marrow, with a varying amount of fat, fibrous tissue, or gelatinous replacement; absence of tagged iron (since the iron is deposited in the liver rather than in bone marrow) and megakaryocytes; and depression of erythroid elements.

Treatment

Effective treatment must eliminate any identifiable cause and provide vigorous supportive measures, such as packed RBC, platelet, and experimental HLA-matched leukocyte transfusions. Even after elimination of the cause, recovery can take months. Bone marrow transplantation is the treatment of choice for anemia due to severe aplasia and for patients who need constant RBC transfusions.

Reverse isolation is necessary to prevent infection in patients with low leukocyte counts. The infection itself may require specific antibiotics; however, these are not given prophylactically because they tend to encourage resistant strains of organisms. Patients with low hemoglobin counts may need respiratory support with oxygen, in addition to blood transfusions.

Other appropriate forms of treatment include corticosteroids to stimulate erythroid production (successful in children, unsuccessful in adults), marrow-stimulating agents, such as androgens (which are controversial), and immunosuppressive agents (if the patient does not respond to other therapy).

Clinical implications

• If platelet count is low (less than 20,000/cu mm), prevent hemorrhage by avoiding I.M. injections, suggesting the use of an electric razor and a soft toothbrush, humidifying oxygen to prevent drying of mucous membranes (dry mucosa may bleed), and promoting regular bowel movements through the use of a stool softener and a proper diet to prevent constipation (which can cause rectal mucosal bleeding). Also, apply pressure to venipuncture sites until bleeding stops. Detect bleeding early by checking for blood in urine and stool and assessing skin for petechiae.

• Help prevent infection by washing your hands thoroughly before entering the patient's room, making sure the patient is receiving a nutritious diet (high in vitamins and proteins) to improve his resistance, and encouraging meticulous mouth and perianal care.

• Watch for life-threatening hemorrhage, infection, adverse effects of drug therapy, or blood transfusion reaction. Make sure routine throat, urine, and blood cultures are done regularly and correctly to check for infection. Teach the patient to recognize signs of infection, and tell him to report them immediately.

• If the patient has a low hemoglobin count, which causes fatigue, schedule frequent rest periods. Administer oxygen therapy, as needed. If blood transfusions are necessary, assess for a transfusion reaction by checking the patient's temperature and watching for the development of other signs, such

as rash, hives, itching, back pain, restlessness, and shaking chills.
• Reassure and support the patient and family by explaining the disease and its treatment, particularly if the patient has recurring acute episodes. Encourage the patient who does not require hospitalization to continue his normal life-style, with appropriate restrictions (such as regular rest periods), until remission occurs.
• To prevent aplastic anemia, monitor blood studies carefully in the patient receiving anemia-inducing drugs.
• Support efforts to educate the public about the hazards of toxic agents.

Appendicitis

Description
The most common major surgical disease, appendicitis is inflammation of the vermiform appendix due to an obstruction, which sets off an inflammatory process that can lead to infection, thrombosis, necrosis, and perforation. Since the advent of antibiotics, the incidence and the death rate of appendicitis have declined; if untreated, this disease is invariably fatal.

Causes
Appendicitis probably results from an obstruction of the intestinal lumen caused by the following.
• A fecal mass
• Stricture
• Barium ingestion
• Viral infection

Signs and symptoms
Initial symptoms
—Abdominal pain, generalized or localized in the right upper abdomen, eventually localizing in the right lower abdomen (McBurney's point)
—Anorexia
—Nausea
—Vomiting

—Boardlike abdominal rigidity
—Retractive respirations
—Increasingly severe abdominal spasms and rebound spasms. Rebound tenderness on the opposite side of the abdomen suggests peritoneal inflammation.
Later symptoms
—Constipation, although diarrhea is also possible
—Slight fever of 99° to 102° F. (37.2° to 38.9° C.)
—Tachycardia
—Sudden cessation of abdominal pain (indicates perforation or infarction of the appendix)

Diagnostic tests
The white blood cell (WBC) count is moderately elevated, with increased immature cells.

Treatment
Appendectomy is the only effective treatment. If peritonitis develops, treatment involves gastrointestinal intubation, parenteral replacement of fluids and electrolytes, and administration of antibiotics.

Clinical implications
If appendicitis is suspected, or during preparation for appendectomy, follow these guidelines:
• Administer I.V. fluids to prevent dehydration. *Never* administer cathartics or enemas, as they may rupture the appendix. Give the patient nothing by mouth, and administer analgesics judiciously, since they may mask symptoms.
• To lessen pain, place the patient in the Fowler position. (This is also helpful postoperatively.) *Never* apply heat to the lower right abdomen; this may cause the appendix to rupture.

After appendectomy, follow these guidelines.
• Monitor vital signs and intake and output. Give analgesics, as ordered.
• Encourage the patient to cough, deep breathe, and turn frequently to prevent pulmonary complications.

• Document bowel sounds, passing of flatus, or bowel movements—signs of the return of peristalsis. These signs in a patient whose nausea and abdominal rigidity have subsided indicate readiness to resume oral fluids.

• Watch closely for possible surgical complications. Continuing pain and fever may signal an abscess. The complaint that "something gave way" may mean wound dehiscence. If an abscess or peritonitis develops, incision and drainage may be necessary. Frequently assess the dressing for wound drainage.

• Assist the patient to ambulate as soon as possible after surgery—usually within 12 hours.

• If peritonitis complicated appendicitis, a nasogastric tube may be needed to decompress the stomach and reduce nausea and vomiting. If so, record drainage, and give good mouth and nose care.

Complications

If the appendix ruptures or perforates, the infected contents spill into the abdominal cavity, causing peritonitis, the most common and most perilous complication of appendicitis.

Arterial occlusive disease

Description

Arterial occlusive disease is the obstruction or narrowing of the lumen of the aorta and its major branches, causing an interruption of blood flow, usually to the legs and feet. This disorder may affect the carotid, vertebral, innominate, subclavian, mesenteric, and celiac arteries. Occlusions may be acute or chronic. This disease is a frequent complication of atherosclerosis.

Arterial occlusive disease is more common in males than in females. Prognosis depends on the location of the occlusion, the development of collateral circulation to counteract reduced blood flow, and, in acute disease, the time elapsed between occlusion and its removal.

Causes

• Emboli formation
• Thrombosis
• Trauma or fracture

Risk factors

• Smoking
• Aging
• Hypertension
• Hyperlipemia
• Diabetes
• Family history of vascular disorders, myocardial infarction, or cerebrovascular accident

Signs and symptoms

Signs and symptoms depend on the site of the arterial occlusion. (For further information, see *Arterial Occlusive Disease*.)

Diagnostic tests

Pertinent supportive diagnostic tests include the following.

• Arteriography demonstrates the type (thrombus or embolus), location, and degree of obstruction, and the collateral circulation. Arteriography is particularly useful in chronic disease or for evaluating candidates for reconstructive surgery.

• Doppler ultrasonography and plethysmography are noninvasive tests that, in acute disease, show decreased blood flow distal to the occlusion.

• Ophthalmodynamometry helps determine degree of obstruction in the internal carotid artery by comparing ophthalmic artery pressure with brachial artery pressure on the affected side. A difference greater than 20% suggests insufficiency.

• Electroencephalography and computed tomography may be necessary to rule out brain lesions.

Treatment

Generally, treatment of arterial occlusive disease depends on the cause, lo-

Arterial Occlusive Disease

SITE OF OCCLUSION	SIGNS AND SYMPTOMS
Carotid arterial system • Internal carotids • External carotids	Neurologic dysfunction: transient ischemic attacks (TIAs) due to reduced cerebral circulation produce unilateral sensory or motor dysfunction (transient monocular blindness, hemiparesis), possible aphasia or dysarthria, confusion, decreased mentation, and headache. These usually last 5 to 10 minutes but may persist up to 24 hours, and may herald a stroke. Absent or decreased pulsation with an auscultatory bruit over the affected vessels.
Vertebrobasilar system • Vertebral arteries • Basilar arteries	Neurologic dysfunction: TIAs of brain stem and cerebellum produce binocular visual disturbances, vertigo, dysarthria, and "drop attacks" (falling down without loss of consciousness). Less common than carotid TIA.
Innominate • Brachiocephalic artery	Neurologic dysfunction: signs and symptoms of vertebrobasilar occlusion. Indications of ischemia (claudication) of right arm; possible bruit over right side of neck.
Subclavian artery	Subclavian steal syndrome (characterized by the backflow of blood from the brain through the vertebral artery on the same side as the occlusion, into the subclavian artery distal to the occlusion); clinical effects of vertebrobasilar occlusion and exercise-induced arm claudication. Possible gangrene of the digits.
Mesenteric artery • Superior (most commonly affected) • Celiac axis • Inferior	Bowel ischemia, infarct necrosis, and gangrene; sudden, acute abdominal pain; nausea and vomiting; diarrhea; leukocytosis; and shock due to massive intraluminal fluid and plasma loss.
Aortic bifurcation (saddle block occlusion, an emergency associated with cardiac embolization)	Sensory and motor deficits (muscle weakness, numbness, paresthesias, paralysis), and signs of ischemia (sudden pain; cold, pale legs with decreased or absent peripheral pulses) in both legs.
Iliac artery (Leriche's syndrome)	Intermittent claudication of lower back, buttocks, and thighs, relieved by rest; absent or reduced femoral or distal pulses; possible bruit over femoral arteries; impotence in males.
Femoral and popliteal artery (associated with aneurysm formation)	Intermittent claudication of the calves on exertion; ischemic pain in feet; pretrophic pain (heralds necrosis and ulceration); leg pallor and coolness; blanching of feet on elevation; gangrene; no palpable pulses in ankles and feet.

cation, and size of the obstruction. For patients with mild chronic disease, treatment usually consists of supportive measures, elimination of smoking, hypertension control, and walking exercise. For patients with carotid artery occlusion, antiplatelet therapy may begin with dipyridamole and aspirin. For those with intermittent claudication caused by chronic arterial occlusive disease, pentoxifylline (Trenatal) may improve blood flow through the capillaries. This drug is particulary useful for patients who are not good candidates for surgery.

Acute arterial occlusive disease usually necessitates surgery to restore circulation to the affected area. Appropriate surgical procedures may include embolectomy, thromboendarterectomy, patch grafting, bypass grafting, and lumbar sympathectomy. Amputation becomes necessary with failure of arterial reconstructive surgery or with the development of complications.

Other appropriate therapy includes heparin to prevent emboli (for embolic occlusion) and bowel resection after restoration of blood flow (for mesenteric artery occlusion).

Clinical implications
• Provide comprehensive patient teaching, such as proper foot care. Explain all diagnostic tests and procedures. Advise the patient to stop smoking and to follow the prescribed medical regimen closely.

Preoperatively, during an acute episode, follow these guidelines:
• Assess the patient's circulatory status by checking for the most distal pulses and by inspecting his skin color and temperature.
• Provide pain relief, as needed.
• Administer heparin by continuous I.V. drip, as ordered.
• Wrap the patient's affected foot in soft cotton batting, and reposition it frequently to prevent pressure on any one area. Strictly avoid elevating or applying heat to the affected leg.

• Watch for signs of fluid and electrolyte imbalance, and monitor intake and output for signs of renal failure (urine output less than 30 ml/hour).
• If the patient has carotid, innominate, vertebral, or subclavian artery occlusion, monitor him for signs of cerebrovascular accident, such as numbness in an arm or leg and intermittent blindness.

Postoperatively, follow these guidelines.
• Monitor the patient's vital signs. Continuously assess his circulatory function by inspecting skin color and temperature and by checking for distal pulses. In charting, compare earlier assessments and observations. Watch closely for signs of hemorrhage (tachycardia, hypotension), and check dressings for excessive bleeding.
• In carotid, innominate, vertebral, or subclavian artery occlusion, assess neurologic status frequently for changes in level of consciousness or muscle strength and pupil size.
• In mesenteric artery occlusion, connect nasogastric tube to low intermittent suction. Monitor intake and output (low urine output may indicate damage to renal arteries during surgery). Check bowel sounds for return of peristalsis. Increasing abdominal distention and tenderness may indicate extension of bowel ischemia with resulting gangrene, necessitating further excision, or it may indicate peritonitis.
• In saddle block occlusion, check distal pulses for adequate circulation. Watch for signs of renal failure and mesenteric artery occlusion (severe abdominal pain), and for cardiac dysrhythmias, which may precipitate embolus formation.
• In iliac artery occlusion, monitor urine output for signs of renal failure from decreased perfusion to the kidneys, as a result of surgery. Provide meticulous catheter care.
• In both femoral and popliteal artery occlusion, assist with early ambulation, but do not allow the patient to sit for an extended period.

Teaching Topics in Arterial Occlusive Disease

• Major causes of reduced arterial blood flow—atherosclerosis and arteriosclerosis
• How intermittent claudication and arterial ulcers develop
• Preparation for arteriography, Doppler ultrasonography, blood clotting studies, and possibly serum lipid and lipoprotein measurements
• Relief of intermittent claudication with rest or by placing leg in a dependent position
• Regular exercise to prevent further occlusion and to develop collateral circulation
• Anticoagulant drugs—proper use and precautions
• Preventing infection and ulcers
• Caring for ulcers, including dressing changes
• Preparation for possible surgery—sympathectomy, endarterectomy, arterial bypass grafting, revascularization

---

• When caring for a patient who has undergone amputation, check the stump carefully for drainage. Elevate the stump, as ordered, and administer adequate analgesic medication. Since phantom limb pain is common, explain this phenomenon to the patient.

• When preparing the patient for discharge, instruct him to watch for signs of recurrence (pain, pallor, numbness, paralysis, absence of pulse) that can result from graft occlusion or occlusion at another site. Warn him against wearing constrictive clothing. (See also *Teaching Topics in Arterial Occlusive Disease*.)

Complications
• Gangrene
• Uncontrolled infection
• Intractable pain

Asbestosis

Description
Asbestosis is a form of pneumoconiosis characterized by diffuse interstitial fibrosis. It can develop as much as 15 to 20 years after regular exposure to asbestos has ended. Asbestos also causes pleural plaques and mesotheliomas of pleura and the peritoneum; a potent co-carcinogen, it aggravates the risk of lung cancer in cigarette smokers.

Causes
Asbestosis results from the inhalation of respirable asbestos fibers (50 microns or more in length, 0.5 microns or less in diameter), which assume a longitudinal orientation in the airway, move in the direction of airflow, and penetrate respiratory bronchioles and alveolar walls.

Risk factors
People who work in the following industries have a higher risk of developing asbestosis.
• Mining and milling of asbestos
• Construction (where asbestos is used in a prefabricated form)
• Fireproofing and textile industries
• Industries involving the production of paints, plastics, and brake and clutch linings

Asbestos-related diseases also develop in the following groups.
• Families of asbestos workers, as a result of exposure to fibrous dust shaken off the workers' clothing at home

• Individuals who are exposed to fibrous dust or waste piles from nearby asbestos plants

Signs and symptoms
• Dyspnea on exertion. This is usually the first symptom, typically occurring after 10 years' exposure, and increasing until it occurs even at rest.
• Dry, crackling rales at the lung bases
• Dry cough (may be productive in smokers)
• Chest pain, often pleuritic
• Recurrent respiratory infections
• Tachypnea
• Hypoxia

Diagnostic tests
• Sputum and lung tissue reveal ferruginous bodies and asbestos bodies, which are inhaled fibers that have become encased in a brown, proteinlike sheath rich in iron.
• Chest X-rays show fine, irregular, and linear diffuse infiltrates; extensive fibrosis results in a "honeycomb" or "ground-glass" appearance. X-rays may also show pleural thickening and pleural calcification, with bilateral obliteration of costophrenic angles and, in later stages, an enlarged heart with a classic "shaggy" heart border.
• Pulmonary function studies show the following.
—Vital capacity (VC), forced vital capacity (FVC), and total lung capacity (TLC): decreased
—Forced expiratory volume measured in 1 second (FEV_1): decreased or normal
—Defusing capacity for carbon monoxide (DL_{CO}): reduced when fibrosis destroys alveolar walls and thickens alveolar capillary membrane
• Arterial blood gas analysis shows the following.
—PO_2: decreased
—PCO_2: low due to hyperventilation

Treatment and clinical implications
The goal of treatment is to relieve respiratory symptoms and, in advanced disease, manage hypoxia and cor pulmonale. Respiratory symptoms may be relieved by chest physiotherapy techniques, such as controlled coughing and segmental bronchial drainage, with chest percussion and vibration. Aerosol therapy, inhaled mucolytics, and increased fluid intake (at least 3 liters/day) may also help relieve respiratory symptoms. Diuretics, digitalis preparations, and salt restriction may be indicated for patients with cor pulmonale. Hypoxia requires oxygen administration by cannula or mask (1 to 2 liters/minute), or by mechanical ventilation if arterial oxygen cannot be maintained above 40 mm Hg. Respiratory infections require prompt administration of antibiotics.
• Teach the patient to prevent infections by avoiding crowds and persons with infections and by receiving influenza and pneumococcal vaccines.
• Improve the patient's respiratory efficiency by encouraging physical reconditioning, energy conservation in daily activities, and relaxation techniques.

Complications
• Pulmonary hypertension
• Right ventricular hypertrophy
• Cor pulmonale
• Finger clubbing

Ascariasis
(Roundworm infection)

Description
Ascariasis is a roundworm infection that occurs in two phases: early pulmonary and prolonged intestinal. After ingestion, the worm ova hatch and release larvae, which penetrate the intestinal wall and reach the lungs through the bloodstream. After about 10 days in pulmonary capillaries and

alveoli, the larvae migrate to the bronchioles, bronchi, trachea, and epiglottis. There they are swallowed and return to the intestine to mature into worms.

Causes
Ascaris lumbricoides, a large roundworm resembling an earthworm

Mode of transmission
• It is transmitted to humans by ingestion of soil contaminated with human feces that harbor *A. lumbricoides* ova.
• Direct transmission occurs when contaminated soil is eaten.
• Indirect transmission occurs when poorly washed raw vegetables grown in contaminated soil are eaten.
• Ascariasis never passes directly from person to person.

Signs and symptoms
Mild infection
—Vague stomach discomfort
—Vomiting worms or passing worms in the stool
Severe infection
—Stomach pain
—Vomiting
—Restlessness
—Disturbed sleep
—Intestinal obstruction (in extreme cases)
—Pneumonitis and other symptoms that occur reflect the area invaded by larvae when they migrate via the lymphatic and the circulatory systems.

Diagnostic tests
• Complete blood count shows eosinophilia.
• X-rays show characteristic bronchovascular markings: infiltrates, patchy areas of pneumonitis, and widening of hilar shadows when migrating larvae invade the alveoli.

Treatment
Anti-ascaris drug therapy, the primary treatment, uses pyrantel or piperazine to temporarily paralyze the worms, permitting peristalsis to expel them.

Mebendazole is also used to block helminth nutrition. These drugs are up to 95% effective, even after a single dose. In multiple helminth infection, one of these drugs must be the first treatment; using some other anthelmintic first may stimulate *A. lumbricoides* perforation into other organs. No specific treatment exists for migratory infection, since anthelmintics affect only mature worms.

In intestinal obstruction, nasogastric suctioning controls vomiting. When suctioning can be discontinued, instill piperazine and clamp the tube. If vomiting does not occur, give a second dose of piperazine orally 24 hours later, as ordered. If this is ineffective, treatment probably requires surgery.

Clinical implications
• Although isolation is unnecessary, properly dispose of feces and soiled linen, and carefully wash your hands after patient contact.
• If the patient is receiving nasogastric suction, be sure to give him good mouth care.
• Teach the patient to prevent reinfection by washing hands thoroughly, especially before eating and after defecating, and by bathing and changing underwear and bed linens daily.
• Inform the patient of drug adverse effects. Tell him piperazine may cause stomach upset, dizziness, and urticaria. Remember, piperazine is contraindicated in convulsive disorders. Pyrantel produces red stools and vomitus and may cause stomach upset, headache, dizziness, and skin rash. Mebendazole may cause abdominal pain and diarrhea.

Aspergillosis

Description
Aspergillosis is a rare, opportunistic infection capable of causing inflammatory, granulomatous lesions on or in any organ. The fungus that causes

this disease is normally present in the mouth and sputum and only produces clinical infection in persons who become especially vulnerable to it. Such vulnerability can result from excessive or prolonged use of antibiotics and from glucocorticoids or other immunosuppressive therapy. It can also result from Hodgkin's disease, irradiation, leukemia, azotemia, alcoholism, sarcoidosis, organ transplant, bronchitis, bronchiectasis, tuberculosis, or some other cavitary lung disease.

Aspergillosis occurs in four major forms: aspergilloma, which produces a fungus ball in the lungs, called mycetoma; allergic aspergillosis, a hypersensitive asthmatic reaction to aspergilli antigens; aspergillosis endophthalmitis, an infection of the anterior and posterior chambers of the eye that can lead to blindness; and disseminated aspergillosis, a rare, acute, and usually fatal infection that produces septicemia, thrombosis, and infarction of virtually any organ, but especially the heart, lungs, brain, and kidneys.

Aspergillus may cause infection of the ear (otomycosis), cornea (mycotic keratitis), and prosthetic heart valves (endocarditis); pneumonia (especially in persons receiving immunosuppressants, such as cyclophosphamide); sinusitis; and brain abscesses. Its incubation period ranges from a few days to weeks. Prognosis varies with each form. Occasionally, aspergilloma causes fatal hemoptysis. Disseminated aspergillosis is almost always fatal.

Causes
Fungi of the genus *Aspergillus,* usually *A. fumigatus, A. flavus,* and *A. niger*

Mode of transmission
Aspergillus is found worldwide, often in fermenting compost piles and damp hay. It is transmitted through inhalation of fungal spores or, in aspergillosis endophthalmitis, the invasion of spores through a wound or other tissue injury. It is a common laboratory contaminant.

Signs and symptoms
Aspergilloma
—Asymptomatic in some cases
—Mimics tuberculosis in some cases. Productive cough, purulent or blood-tinged sputum, dyspnea, empyema, and lung abscess
Allergic aspergillosis
—Wheezing
—Dyspnea
—Cough with some sputum production
—Pleural pain
—Fever
Aspergillosis endophthalmitis
—Clouded vision
—Pain
—Reddened conjunctiva
—Purulent exudate from the anterior and posterior chambers of the eye
Disseminated aspergillosis
—Thrombosis
—Infarctions
—Typical signs of septicemia (chills, fever, hypotension, delirium)
—Azotemia
—Hematuria
—Urinary tract obstruction
—Headaches
—Seizures
—Bone pain and tenderness
—Soft tissue swelling
—Death (can occur rapidly after infection)

Diagnostic tests
Aspergilloma
Chest X-ray reveals a crescent-shaped radiolucency surrounding a circular mass, but this is not definitive for aspergillosis.
Allergic aspergillosis
Sputum examination shows eosinophils.
Aspergillosis endophthalmitis
A culture or exudate showing *Aspergillus* is diagnostic.
Disseminated aspergillosis
Culture and examination of affected

tissue can confirm the diagnosis, but this form is usually diagnosed at autopsy.

Treatment and clinical implications

Aspergillosis does not require isolation. Treatment of aspergilloma necessitates local excision of the lesion and supportive therapy, such as chest physiotherapy and coughing, to improve pulmonary function. Allergic aspergillosis requires desensitization and, possibly, steroids. Disseminated aspergillosis and aspergillosis endophthalmitis require a 2- to 3-week course of I.V. amphotericin B (as well as prompt cessation of immunosuppressant therapy) and possibly flucytosine. However, disseminated aspergillosis often resists amphotericin B therapy and rapidly progresses to death.

Asthma

Description

Asthma is a chronic reactive airway disorder that produces episodic, reversible airway obstruction via bronchospasms, increased mucus secretion, and mucosal edema. The disorder may result from external allergens (extrinsic asthma) or internal nonallergenic factors (intrinsic asthma). In many asthmatics, especially children, intrinsic and extrinsic asthma coexist. Although this common condition can strike at any age, half of all cases occur in children under age 10. Underlining the significance of hereditary predisposition, about one third of all asthmatics share the disease with at least one member of their immediate family, and three fourths of children with two asthmatic parents also have asthma.

Causes

Extrinsic asthma
—Pollen
—Animal dander
—House dust or mold
—Kapok or feather pillows
—Food additives containing sulfites
—Any other sensitizing substances

Intrinsic asthma
—Irritants
—Emotional stress
—Fatigue
—Endocrine changes
—Temperature and humidity changes
—Exposure to noxious fumes

Other causes
—Aspirin
—Various nonsteroidal anti-inflammatory drugs (such as indomethacin and mefenamic acid)
—Tartrazine, a yellow food dye
—Exercise
—Occupational exposure to various allergenic factors such as platinum

Sign and symptoms

Extrinsic asthma
This is usually accompanied by manifestations of atopy (Type I IgE-mediated allergy), such as eczema and allergic rhinitis.

Intrinsic asthma
Most cases are preceded by a severe respiratory infection, especially in adults.

Acute asthma attack
This begins dramatically, with simultaneous onset of severe multiple symptoms, or insidiously, with gradually increasing respiratory distress.
—Sudden dyspnea
—Wheezing
—Tightness in chest
—Cough productive of thick, clear, or yellow sputum
—Feeling of suffocation
—Inability to speak more than a few words without pausing for breath during a severe attack
—Tachypnea, though respiratory rate is frequently normal
—Audible wheezing
—Obvious use of accessory respiratory muscles
—Rapid pulse
—Profuse perspiration
—Hyperresonant lung fields

How to Treat Status Asthmaticus

Unless it is promptly and correctly treated, status asthmaticus may lead to fatal respiratory failure. The patient with increasingly severe asthma unresponsive to drug therapy is usually admitted to the intensive care unit for the following care.

- As ordered, give corticosteroids, epinephrine, and I.V. aminophylline.
- Frequently check arterial blood gas measurements to assess respiratory status, particularly after ventilator therapy or a change in oxygen concentration.
- Carefully administer oxygen (the patient will be hypoxemic), and, if necessary, assist in endotracheal intubation and mechanical ventilation (when he has an elevated PCO_2).
- Administer I.V. fluids according to the patient's clinical status and age. (Dehydration is likely because of inadequate fluid intake and increased insensible loss.)
- Help position the patient for frequent chest X-rays.

—Diminished breath sounds with wheezes and rhonchi
—Cyanosis, confusion, and lethargy. These indicate the onset of life-threatening status asthmaticus and respiratory failure.

Diagnostic tests

- Pulmonary function studies reveal signs of airway obstructive disease (decreased flow rates and forced expiratory volume in 1 second [FEV_1]), low-normal or decreased vital capacity, and increased total lung and residual capacity. However, pulmonary function studies may be normal between attacks. Typically, the patient has decreased PO_2 and PCO_2 levels. In severe asthma, PCO_2 may be normal or increased, indicating severe bronchial obstruction. In fact, FEV will probably be less than 25% of the predicted value. Initiating treatment tends to decrease PO_2, making frequent arterial blood gas analysis mandatory. Even when the asthmatic attack appears under control, the spirometric values (FEV and forced expiratory flow between 25% and 75% of vital capacity) remain abnormal. Residual volume remains abnormal for the longest period—up to 3 weeks after the attack.

- Complete blood count with differential shows increased eosinophil count.
- Chest X-ray shows possible hyperinflation, with areas of local atelectasis (mucus plugging).
- Skin testing for specific allergens may be necessary if no allergic history exists.
- Inhalation bronchial challenge testing evaluates the clinical significance of allergens identified by skin testing.

Treatment

The best treatment for asthma is prevention by identifying and avoiding precipitating factors such as allergens or irritants. Usually, such stimuli cannot be removed entirely. Desensitization to specific antigens may be helpful but is rarely totally effective or persistent.

Drug treatment for asthma usually includes some form of bronchodilator and is more effective when begun soon after onset of symptoms. Drugs used include rapid-acting epinephrine; epinephrine in oil, which is not recommended for infants; terbutaline; aminophylline; theophylline and theophylline-containing oral preparations; oral sympathomimetics; corticosteroids; and aerosolized sympathomimetics such as isoproterenol or albuterol. Arterial blood gases help determine the severity of an asthmatic attack and the patient's response to treatment. (Also see *How to Treat Status Asthmaticus.*)

Clinical implications

During an acute attack, follow these guidelines:

• First, maintain respiratory function and relieve bronchoconstriction, while allowing mucus plug expulsion.

• If the attack is induced by exercise, you may be able to control it by having the patient sit down, rest, and sip warm water. This helps slow breathing, promotes bronchodilation, and loosens secretions. (Before exercising, asthmatic children should use an oral bronchodilator for 30 to 60 minutes or an inhaled bronchodilator for 15 to 20 minutes. Cromolyn sodium can also be used to prevent exercise-induced bronchospasm; have the patient inhale one capsule no more than 1 hour before exercising.)

• Find out if the patient has a nebulizer and if he has used it. The asthmatic should have access to an isoproterenol or isoetharine nebulizer at all times. He should take no more than two or three whiffs every 4 hours, however. If he needs the nebulizer again in less than 4 hours, give it and call the physician for further instructions. (Overuse of a nebulizer can progressively weaken the patient's response until it has no effect at all. Extended overuse can even lead to cardiac arrest and death, but this is rare.)

• Loss of breath is terrifying, so reassure the patient that you will help him. Then, place him in a semi-Fowler position, encourage diaphragmatic breathing, and urge him to relax as much as possible.

• Consider status asthmaticus unrelieved by epinephrine a medical emergency.

• Administer humidified oxygen by nasal cannula at 2 liters/minute to ease difficulty in breathing and to increase arterial oxygen saturation. Later, adjust oxygen according to the patient's vital functions and arterial blood gas measurements.

• Administer drugs and I.V. fluids as ordered. Continue epinephrine, and administer aminophylline I.V. as a loading dose, followed by I.V. drip. (Caution: Elderly patients with hepatic or cardiac insufficiency or those taking erythromycin are predisposed to aminophylline toxicity.) Young patients and those who smoke or who are receiving barbiturates have increased aminophylline metabolism and require a larger dose. Simultaneously, a loading dose of corticosteroids can be given I.V. or I.M. Combat dehydration with I.V. fluids until the patient can tolerate oral fluids, which will help loosen secretions.

Preventing Recurrent Asthma Attacks

To prevent recurrent asthma attacks:

• Instruct the patient to breathe deeply, cough up secretions accumulated overnight, and allow time for medication to work. He can best loosen secretions by coughing correctly—inhaling fully and gently, then bending over with arms crossed over the abdomen before coughing—and by drinking 3 liters of liquid daily.

• Tell the patient and his family that the patient should avoid known allergens, irritating fumes of any kind, aerosol spray, smoke, and automobile exhaust.

• Refer the patient to community resources such as the American Lung Association and the Asthma and Allergy Foundation.

Teaching Topics in Asthma

- An explanation of how asthma triggers elicit bronchospasm, airway edema, and mucus production
- Complications such as status asthmaticus
- Identification of asthma triggers
- Preparation for arterial blood gas (ABG) analysis, pulmonary function tests, and other diagnostic studies
- Importance of diet and adequate hydration
- Drugs and their administration
- How to use an oral inhaler
- How to control an asthma attack
- Warning signs and prevention of respiratory infection
- Availability of support groups, such as the American Lung Association

---

During long-term care, follow these guidelines.

• Supervise the patient's drug regimen. Make sure he knows how to use aerosolized bronchodilator drugs properly. When the patient is using an aminophylline bronchodilator, monitor his blood levels, as oral absorption of aminophylline can be erratic. With long-term steroid therapy, watch for cushingoid adverse effects. Because of their respiratory depressant effect, sedatives and narcotics are not recommended. (Also see *Preventing Recurrent Asthma Attacks*, p. 63, and *Teaching Topics in Asthma*.)

Ataxia-telangiectasia

Description

Ataxia-telangiectasia is a disorder characterized by progressively severe ataxia (impaired ability to coordinate movement), telangiectasia (permanent dilation of groups of superficial capillaries and venules), and chronic, recurrent sinopulmonary infections that may reflect both humoral (B cell) and cell-mediated (T cell) immunodeficiencies. It has neurologic, endocrine, and vascular aspects. The earliest and most dominant signs of cerebellar ataxia usually appear within 2 years after birth, but may develop later. As-

sociated telangiectasia usually appear after ataxia and may not develop until age 9.

Approximately 80% of affected children develop recurrent or chronic respiratory infections because of IgA deficiency early in life, but some may be symptom-free for 10 years or more. These children are unusually vulnerable to lymphomas, particularly lymphosarcomas and lymphoreticular malignancies, and may also develop leukemia, adenocarcinoma, dysgerminoma, or medulloblastoma. They may fail to develop secondary sex characteristics during puberty and eventually may become mentally retarded. Rarely, a patient shows signs of progeria: premature graying, senile keratoses, and vitiligo.

The degree of immunodeficiency determines the rate of deterioration. Some patients die within several years; others survive until their thirties. Severe abnormalities cause rapid clinical deterioration and premature death due to overwhelming sinopulmonary infection or malignancy.

Signs and symptoms
Cerebellar ataxia
—Continual and involuntary jerky (choreoathetoid) movements
—Nystagmus
—Pseudoparkinsonism
—Motor restlessness

—Dystonias

—Unsteady gait, with forward leaning to maintain balance

—Decreased arm movements

—Purposeless tremors

Telangiectasia

—Lesion on the sclera (usually the first sign)

—Lesions on the bridge of the nose, the ear, or the antecubital or popliteal areas

Diagnostic tests

• Immunologic tests confirm early diagnosis.

• IgA is usually selectively absent (in 60% to 80%), or IgA and IgE are deficient.

• B cell count is normal, but antibody responses are diminished.

• Hassall's corpuscles are absent on examination of thymic tissue.

• Serum levels of oncofetal proteins are high.

• T cells are decreased.

• Computed tomography, magnetic resonance imaging, and pneumoencephalography demonstrate degenerative neurologic changes.

Treatment and clinical implications

No treatment is yet available to stop progression of ataxia-telangiectasia. However, prophylactic or early and aggressive therapy with broad-spectrum antibiotics is essential to prevent or control recurrent infections.

To help parents protect their child from infections, advise them to avoid crowds and persons who have infections, and teach them to recognize early signs of infection. Also teach physical therapy and postural drainage techniques if their child has chronic bronchial infections. As always, stress proper nutrition and adequate hydration.

Immune globulin infusion or injection can passively replace missing antibodies in an IgG-deficient patient and may also help prevent infection. (This treatment may not help an IgA-deficient patient, however.) The effectiveness of other forms of immunotherapy—such as fetal thymus transplant or histocompatible bone marrow transplant—is unproven.

Parents of a child with ataxia-telangiectasia may have questions about the vulnerability of future offspring and may need genetic counseling. They may also need psychological therapy to help them cope with their child's long-term illness and inevitable early death.

Atelectasis

Description

Atelectasis is incomplete expansion of lobules (clusters of alveoli) or lung segments, which may result in partial or complete lung collapse. This causes the loss of regions of the lung for gas exchange. Unoxygenated blood passes through these areas unchanged, thereby producing hypoxia. Atelectasis may be chronic or acute. It occurs to some degree in many patients undergoing upper abdominal or thoracic surgery. Prognosis depends on prompt removal of any airway obstruction, relief of hypoxia, and reexpansion of collapsed lobule(s) or lung(s).

Causes

• Bronchial occlusion by mucus plugs (a special problem in persons with chronic obstructive pulmonary disease)

• Bronchiectasis

• Cystic fibrosis

• Heavy smoking

• Occlusion by foreign bodies

• Bronchogenic carcinoma

• Inflammatory lung disease

• Idiopathic respiratory distress syndrome of the newborn (hyaline membrane disease)

• Oxygen toxicity

• Pulmonary edema

• Any condition that inhibits full lung expansion or makes deep breathing

painful, such as upper abdominal surgical incisions, rib fractures, tight dressings, or obesity
• Prolonged immobility
• Mechanical ventilation using constant small tidal volumes without intermittent deep breaths
• Central nervous system depression (as in drug overdose), which eliminates periodic sighing

Signs and symptoms

Clinical effects vary with the cause of collapse, the degree of hypoxia, and any underlying disease.
• Dyspnea. May be mild and subside without treatment if atelectasis involves only a small area of the lung; severe if massive collapse occurs
• Anxiety
• Cyanosis
• Diaphoresis
• Decreased breath sounds
• Dull sound on percussion if a large portion of the lung is collapsed
• Peripheral circulatory collapse
• Tachycardia
• Substernal or intercostal retraction
• Compensatory hyperinflation of unaffected areas of the lung
• Mediastinal shift to the affected side
• Elevation of the ipsilateral hemidiaphragm

Diagnostic tests

• Chest X-ray shows characteristic horizontal lines in the lower lung zones and, with segmental or lobar collapse, characteristic dense shadows often associated with hyperinflation of neighboring lung zones in widespread atelectasis. However, extensive areas of "microatelectasis" may exist without abnormalities on chest X-ray.
• Bronchoscopy may be included in diagnostic procedures to rule out an obstructing neoplasm or a foreign body if the cause is unknown.

Treatment

Treatment includes incentive spirometry, chest percussion, postural drainage, and frequent coughing and deep-breathing exercises. If these measures fail, bronchoscopy may be helpful in removing secretions. Humidity and bronchodilators can improve mucociliary clearance and dilate airways; they are sometimes used with a nebulizer.

Atelectasis secondary to an obstructing neoplasm may require surgery or radiation therapy Postoperative thoracic and abdominal surgery patients require analgesics to facilitate deep breathing, which minimizes the risk of atelectasis.

Clinical implications

• To prevent atelectasis, encourage postoperative and other high-risk patients to cough and deep breathe every 1 to 2 hours. To minimize pain during coughing exercises in postoperative patients, hold a pillow tightly over the incision; teach the patient this technique as well. *Gently* reposition these patients often and help them walk as soon as possible. Administer adequate analgesics to control pain.
• During mechanical ventilation, tidal volume should be maintained at 10 to 15 ml/kg of the patient's body weight to ensure adequate expansion of lungs. Use the sigh mechanism on the ventilator, if appropriate, to intermittently increase tidal volume at the rate of three to four sighs per hour.
• Use an incentive spirometer to encourage deep inspiration through positive reinforcement. Teach the patient how to use the spirometer, and encourage him to use it every 1 to 2 hours.
• Humidify inspired air and encourage adequate fluid intake to mobilize secretions. To promote loosening and clearance of secretions, use postural drainage and chest percussion.
• If the patient is intubated or uncooperative, provide suctioning, as needed. Use sedatives with discretion, since they depress respirations and the cough reflex and suppress sighing. But remember that the patient will not co-

operate with treatment if he is in pain.
- Assess breath sounds and ventilatory status frequently and report any changes immediately.
- Teach the patient about respiratory care, including postural drainage, coughing, and deep breathing.
- Encourage the patient to stop smoking, to lose weight, or both, as needed. Refer him to appropriate support groups for help.
- Provide reassurance and emotional support, since the patient will undoubtedly be frightened by his limited breathing capacity.

Atrial septal defect

Description
An atrial septal defect (ASD) is an opening between the left and right atria that allows shunting of blood between the chambers. Blood shunts from left to right because left atrial pressure normally is slightly higher than right atrial pressure. This pressure difference forces large amounts of blood through the defect. The result is right heart volume overload, affecting the right atrium, right ventricle, and pulmonary arteries. Eventually, the right atrium enlarges, and the right ventricle dilates to accommodate the increased blood volume.

Ostium secundum defect (most common) occurs in the region of the fossa ovalis and, occasionally, extends inferiorly, close to the vena cava. Sinus venosus defect occurs in the superior-posterior portion of the atrial septum, sometimes extending into the vena cava, and is almost always associated with abnormal drainage of pulmonary veins into the right atrium. Ostium primum, a defect of the primitive septum, occurs in the inferior portion of the septum primum and is usually associated with atrioventricular valve abnormalities (cleft mitral valve) and conduction defects.

Although ASD is usually a benign defect during infancy and childhood, delayed development of symptoms and complications makes it one of the most common congenital heart defects diagnosed in adults. Prognosis is excellent in asymptomatic persons, but poor in those with cyanosis caused by large, untreated defects.

Causes
The specific cause of this congenital abnormality is unknown.

Signs and symptoms
Childhood
—Often asymptomatic, especially in preschoolers
—Tired feeling after extreme exertion
—Possible growth retardation if large shunts are present
—Early to midsystolic murmur heard on auscultation at the second or third left intercostal space, superficial in quality
—Low-pitched diastolic murmur occurs in patients with large shunts, heard on auscultation at the lower left sternal border; becomes more pronounced on inspiration; may be difficult to hear
—Fixed, widely split S_2 heart sound and a systolic click or late systolic murmur at the apex
Adulthood
—Pronounced fatigability
—Dyspnea on exertion, frequently to the point of severe limitation (especially after age 40)
—An accentuated S_2 heart sound, a pulmonary ejection click, and an audible S_4 sound possible in older patients with large uncorrected defects and fixed pulmonary hypertension
—Clubbing
—Cyanosis
—Syncope (with severe pulmonary vascular disease)
—Hemoptysis (with severe pulmonary vascular disease)

Diagnostic tests
The following findings help confirm the diagnosis.

• Chest X-ray shows an enlarged right atrium and right ventricle, a prominent pulmonary artery, and increased pulmonary vascular markings.

• EKG may be normal but often shows right axis deviation, prolonged P-R interval, varying degrees of right bundle branch block, right ventricular hypertrophy, atrial fibrillation (particularly in severe cases after age 30), and, in ostium primum, left axis deviation.

• Echocardiography measures the extent of right ventricular enlargement and may locate the defect. (Other causes of right ventricular enlargement must be ruled out.)

• Cardiac catheterization confirms ASD by demonstrating that right atrial blood is more oxygenated than superior vena caval blood—indicating a left-to-right shunt—and determines the degree of shunting and pulmonary vascular disease. Dye injection shows ASD size and location, the location of pulmonary venous drainage, and atrioventricular valve competence.

Treatment and clinical implications

Since ASD seldom produces complications in infants and toddlers, surgery can be delayed until they reach preschool or early school age. A large defect may need immediate surgical closure with sutures or a patch graft. Although experimental, treatment for a small ASD may involve insertion of an umbrellalike patch using a cardiac catheter instead of open-heart surgery.

• Before cardiac catheterization, explain pre- and post-test procedures to the child and parents. If possible, use drawings or other visual aids to explain it to the child.

• As needed, teach the patient about antibiotic prophylaxis to prevent infective endocarditis.

• If surgery is scheduled, teach the child and parents about the ICU and introduce them to the staff. Show parents where they can wait during the operation. Explain postoperative procedures, tubes, dressings, and monitoring equipment.

• After surgery, closely monitor vital signs, central venous and intraarterial pressures, and intake and output. Watch for atrial dysrhythmias, which may remain uncorrected.

Complications

Complications, which rarely occur in children, include the following.

• Congestive heart failure
• Pulmonary hypertension
• Infective endocarditis
• Right ventricular hypertrophy

Basal cell epithelioma
(Basal cell carcinoma)

Description
Basal cell epithelioma is a slow-growing destructive skin tumor. Although its pathogenesis is uncertain, some experts now hypothesize that it originates when, under certain conditions, undifferentiated basal cells become carcinomatous instead of differentiating into sweat glands, sebum, and hair. Most of these tumors (94%) occur on parts of the body with abundant pilosebaceous follicles, especially on the face. Three types occur: noduloulcerative, superficial, and sclerosing (morphealike) basal cell epitheliomas. This carcinoma usually occurs in persons over age 40. It is more prevalent in blond, fair-skinned males, and is the most common malignant tumor affecting whites.

Causes
- Prolonged sun exposure (most common)
- Arsenic ingestion
- Radiation exposure
- Burns
- Vaccinations (rare)

Signs and symptoms
Noduloulcerative
These occur most often on the face, particularly on the forehead, eyelid margins, and nasolabial folds.
—Early-stage lesions: Small, smooth pinkish translucent papular lesions with telangiectatic vessels on the surface and occasionally pigmentation
—Late-stage lesions: enlarged, centers depressed, borders firm and elevated, eventually ulcerating and becoming locally invasive
—"Rodent ulcers": ulcerated tumors, which rarely metastasize. These occur if late-stage lesions are not treated. They can spread, if untreated, to vital areas and become infected or cause massive hemorrhage if they invade large blood vessels.
Superficial
These occur most often on chest and back.
—Oval or irregularly shaped, light-pigmented plaques with sharply defined, slightly elevated threadlike borders.
—Scaly, with small atrophic areas in the center that resemble psoriasis or eczema
—Usually chronic and noninvasive
Sclerosing
These occur on the head and neck.
—Waxy, sclerotic, yellow to white plaques without distinct borders
—Often resemble small patches of scleroderma

Diagnostic tests
Basal cell epitheliomas are diagnosed by clinical appearance and by the following tests.
- Incisional or excisional biopsy
- Histologic study

Treatment
Depending on the size, location, and depth of the lesion, treatment may include curettage and electrodesicca-

tion, chemotherapy, surgical excision, irradiation, or chemosurgery.

• Curettage and electrodesiccation offer good cosmetic results for small lesions.

• Topical 5-fluorouracil is often used for superficial lesions. This medication produces marked local irritation or inflammation in the involved tissue but no systemic effects.

• Microscopically controlled surgical excision carefully removes recurrent lesions until a tumor-free plane is achieved. After removal of large lesions, skin grafting may be required.

• Irradiation is used for elderly or debilitated patients who might not withstand surgery.

• Chemosurgery is often necessary for persistent or recurrent lesions. Chemosurgery consists of periodic applications of a fixative paste (such as zinc chloride) and subsequent removal of fixed pathologic tissue. Treatment continues until tumor removal is complete.

Clinical implications

• Instruct the patient to eat frequent small meals that are high in protein. Suggest eggnogs, "blenderized" foods, or liquid protein supplements if the lesion has invaded the oral cavity and caused eating problems.

• Tell the patient that to prevent disease recurrence, he needs to avoid excessive sun exposure and use a strong sunscreen or sunshade to protect his skin from damage by ultraviolet rays.

• Advise the patient to relieve local inflammation from topical 5-fluorouracil with cool compresses or with corticosteroid ointment.

• Instruct the patient with noduloulcerative basal cell epithelioma to wash his face gently when ulcerations and crusting occur. Scrubbing too vigorously may cause bleeding.

Bell's palsy

Description

Bell's palsy is a disease that blocks conduction of nerve impulses from the seventh cranial nerve (facial), which is responsible for motor innervation of the facial muscles. The conduction block is due to an inflammatory reaction around the nerve (usually at the internal auditory meatus). Onset is rapid. The disorder affects all age-groups, but it occurs most often in patients under age 60. In 80% to 90% of patients, it subsides spontaneously, with complete recovery in 1 to 8 weeks; however, recovery may be delayed in the elderly. If recovery is partial, contractures may develop on the paralyzed side of the face. Bell's palsy may recur on the same or opposite side of the face.

Causes

• Infection
• Hemorrhage
• Tumor
• Meningitis
• Local trauma

Signs and symptoms

• Unilateral facial weakness
• Occasionally, aching pain around the angle of the jaw or behind the ear
• Mouth droops, causing drooling on the affected side
• Distorted taste perception over the affected anterior portion of the tongue
• Smooth forehead
• Markedly impaired ability to close eye on weak side
• Incomplete eye closure and Bell's phenomenon (eye rolling upward as eye is closed)
• Excessive tearing when patient attempts to close affected eye
• Inability to raise the eyebrow, smile, show the teeth, or puff out the cheek

Diagnostic tests

Electromyography helps predict the level of expected recovery by distinguishing temporary conduction defects from a pathologic interruption of nerve fibers.

Treatment and clinical implications

Treatment consists of prednisone, an oral corticosteroid that reduces facial nerve edema and improves nerve conduction and blood flow. After the 14th day of prednisone therapy, electrotherapy may help prevent atrophy of facial muscles.

• During treatment with prednisone, watch for steroidal adverse effects.

• To reduce pain, apply moist heat to the affected side of the face, taking care not to burn the skin.

• To help maintain muscle tone, massage the patient's face with a gentle upward motion two to three times daily for 5 to 10 minutes, or have him massage his face himself. When he is ready for active exercises, teach him to exercise by grimacing in front of a mirror.

• Advise the patient to protect his eye by covering it with an eye patch, especially when outdoors. Tell him to keep warm and avoid exposure to dust and wind. When exposure is unavoidable, instruct him to cover his face.

• To prevent excessive weight loss, help the patient cope with difficulty in eating and drinking. Instruct him to chew on the unaffected side of his mouth. Provide a soft, nutritionally balanced diet, eliminating hot foods and fluids. Arrange for privacy at mealtimes to reduce embarrassment.

• Apply a facial sling to improve lip alignment. Also, give the patient frequent and complete mouth care, being particularly careful to remove residual food that collects between the cheeks and gums.

• Offer psychological support. Give reassurance that recovery is likely within 1 to 8 weeks.

Benign prostatic hypertrophy

Description

Although most men over age 50 have some prostatic enlargement, in benign prostatic hypertrophy or hyperplasia (BPH), the prostate gland enlarges sufficiently to compress the urethra and cause some overt urinary obstruction. BPH begins with changes in periurethral glandular tissue. As the prostate enlarges, it may extend into the bladder and obstruct urinary outflow by compressing or distorting the prostatic urethra. BPH may also cause formation of a pouch in the bladder that retains urine when the rest of the bladder empties. This retained urine may lead to calculus formation or cystitis. Depending on the size of the enlarged prostate, the age and health of the patient, and the extent of obstruction, BPH is treated symptomatically or surgically.

Causes

• Hormonal activity (suggested by recent evidence)
• Neoplasm
• Arteriosclerosis
• Inflammation
• Metabolic or nutritional disturbances

Signs and symptoms

Clinical features of BPH depend on the extent of prostatic enlargement and the lobes affected.

Early
—Reduced urinary stream caliber and force
—Difficulty starting micturition (straining)
—Feeling of incomplete voiding
—Occasional urinary retention

Later
—More frequent urination
—Nocturia
—Incontinence
—Possible hematuria

—Complete urinary obstruction may follow infection or ingestion of decongestants, tranquilizers, alcohol, antidepressants, or anticholinergics.

Other signs and symptoms
—Visible midline mass (distended bladder)
—Enlarged prostate, disclosed by rectal palpation
—Possible secondary anemia and renal insufficiency

Diagnostic tests

When symptoms are severe, cystourethroscopy is the definitive diagnostic measure, but this examination is performed only immediately before surgery, to help determine the best operative procedure. It can show prostate enlargement, bladder wall changes, and a raised bladder.
• Intravenous pyelography may indicate urinary tract obstruction, calculi or tumors, and filling and emptying defects in the bladder.
• Elevated BUN and creatinine levels suggest impaired renal function.
• Urinalysis and urine culture show hematuria, pyuria, and, when bacterial count is more than 100,000/mm³, urinary tract infection.

Treatment

Conservative therapy includes prostatic massages, sitz baths, short-term fluid restriction (to prevent bladder distention), and, if infection develops, antimicrobials. Regular sexual intercourse may help relieve prostatic congestion.

Surgery is the only effective therapy for relief of acute urinary retention, hydronephrosis, severe hematuria, and recurrent urinary tract infection or for palliative relief of intolerable symptoms. A transurethral resection may be performed if the prostate weighs less than 2 ounces (56.7 g). (Weight is approximated by digital examination.) In this procedure, a resectoscope removes tissue with a wire loop and electric current. For patients who are not good surgical risks, continuous drainage with an indwelling (Foley) catheter alleviates urinary retention.

Other appropriate procedures involve open surgical removal.
• Suprapubic (transvesical): Most common and especially useful when prostatic enlargement remains within the bladder
• Perineal: For a large gland in an older patient; usually results in impotence and incontinence
• Retropubic (extravesical): Allows direct visualization; potency and continence are usually maintained

Clinical implications

Prepare the patient for diagnostic tests and surgery, as appropriate. (See *Teaching Topics in BPH*.)
• Monitor and record the patient's vital signs, intake and output, and daily weight. Watch closely for signs of postobstructive diuresis (such as increased urine output and hypotension).
• Administer antibiotics, as ordered, for urinary tract infection, urethral instrumentation, and cystoscopy.
• If urinary retention is present, insert a Foley catheter (although this is usually difficult in a patient with BPH). If the catheter cannot be passed transurethrally, assist with suprapubic cystostomy (under local anesthetic). Watch for rapid bladder decompression.
• After prostate surgery, maintain patient comfort, and watch for and prevent postoperative complications. Observe for immediate dangers— shock and hemorrhage—of prostatic bleeding. Check the catheter frequently (every 15 minutes for the first 2 to 3 hours) for patency and urine color; check the dressings for bleeding.
• Postoperatively, many urologists insert a three-way catheter and establish continuous bladder irrigation. Keep the catheter open at a rate sufficient to maintain returns that are clear and light pink. Watch for fluid overload from absorption of the irrigating fluid into

Teaching Topics in B.P.H.

- An explanation of nonmalignant tissue overgrowth in the prostate
- Signs and symptoms of BPH
- The importance of treatment to prevent complications, such as bladder infection or rupture
- Preparation for physical examination of the prostate and for blood tests, urinalysis, and invasive diagnostic tests
- An explanation of radiation therapy, if appropriate
- An explanation of open prostatectomy or transurethral resection of the prostate
- At-home catheter care, if appropriate
- Referral for sexual counseling, if appropriate, to deal with postoperative infertility or, rarely, impotence

systemic circulation. If a regular catheter is used, observe it closely. If drainage stops because of clots, irrigate the catheter, as ordered, usually with 80 to 100 ml normal saline solution, while maintaining *strict* aseptic technique.

- Also watch for septic shock, the most serious complication of prostatic surgery. Immediately report severe chills, sudden fever, tachycardia, hypotension, or other signs of shock. Start rapid infusion of antibiotics I.V., as ordered. Watch for pulmonary embolus, heart failure, and renal shutdown. Monitor vital signs, central venous pressure, and arterial pressure continuously. The patient may need intensive supportive care in the intensive care unit.

- Administer belladonna and opium suppositories or other anticholinergics, as ordered, to relieve painful bladder spasms that often occur after transurethral resection.

- Take patient comfort measures after an open procedure: provide suppositories (except after perineal prostatectomy), analgesic medication to control incisional pain, and frequent dressing changes.

- Continue infusing I.V. fluids until the patient can drink sufficient fluids

(2 to 3 liters/day) to maintain adequate hydration.

- Administer stool softeners and laxatives, as ordered, to prevent straining. Do not check for fecal impaction, since a rectal examination may precipitate bleeding.

- After the catheter is removed, the patient may experience urinary frequency, dribbling, and occasional hematuria. Reassure him that he will gradually regain urinary control. Explain this to the patient's family so they can reinforce this reassurance.

- Reinforce prescribed limits on activity. Warn the patient against lifting, strenuous exercise, and long automobile rides, since these increase bleeding tendency. Also caution the patient to restrict sexual activity for at least several weeks after discharge.

- Instruct the patient to follow the prescribed oral antibiotic drug regimen, and tell him the indications for using gentle laxatives. Urge him to seek medical care immediately if he cannot void, if he passes bloody urine, or if he develops a fever.

Complications
- Infection
- Renal insufficiency
- Hemorrhage
- Shock

Berylliosis
(Beryllium poisoning, beryllium disease)

Description

Berylliosis, a form of pneumoconiosis, is a systemic granulomatous disorder with dominant pulmonary manifestations. It occurs in two forms: acute nonspecific pneumonitis and chronic noncaseating granulomatous disease with interstitial fibrosis, which may cause death from respiratory failure and cor pulmonale. The mechanism by which berylliosis exerts its toxic effect is unknown. The disease is generally associated with the milling and use of beryllium. Most patients with chronic interstitial disease become only slightly to moderately disabled by impaired lung function and other symptoms, but with each acute exacerbation the prognosis worsens.

Causes

- Inhalation of beryllium dusts, fumes, and mists
- Absorption through the skin

Risk factors

The following individuals are at risk for developing berylliosis.

- Beryllium alloy workers
- Ray tube makers
- Gas mantle workers
- Missile technicians
- Nuclear reactor workers
- Families of workers mentioned above, as a result of dust shaken off workers' clothing at home
- People living near plants where beryllium alloy is used

Signs and symptoms

Dermal absorption of beryllium
—Itchy rash, which usually subsides within 2 weeks after exposure
—"Beryllium ulcers" from accidental implantation of beryllium in the skin

Acute berylliosis
—Swelling and ulceration of nasal mucosa
—Progressive, dry cough
—Tightness in chest
—Substernal pain
—Tachycardia
—Signs of bronchitis

Chronic berylliosis
This develops 10 to 15 years after exposure in about 10% of patients with acute berylliosis.
—Increasing dyspnea
—Mild chest pain
—Dry, unproductive cough
—Tachypnea

Other signs and symptoms
—Hepatosplenomegaly
—Renal calculi
—Lymphadenopathy
—Anorexia
—Fatigue

Diagnostic tests

- Chest X-rays in acute berylliosis may be suggestive of pulmonary edema, showing acute miliary process or a patchy acinous filling, and diffuse infiltrates with prominent peribronchial markings. In chronic berylliosis, X-rays show reticulonodular infiltrates and hilar adenopathy and large coalescent infiltrates in both lungs.
- Pulmonary function studies show decreased vital capacity, forced vital capacity, residual volume/total lung capacity, defusing capacity for carbon monoxide, and decreased compliance as lungs stiffen from fibrosis.
- Arterial blood gas analysis shows decreased PO_2 and PCO_2.
- The in vitro lymphocyte transformation test diagnoses berylliosis and monitors workers for occupational exposure to beryllium.
- Positive beryllium patch test establishes only hypersensitivity to beryllium, not the presence of disease.
- Tissue biopsy and spectrographic analysis are positive for most exposed workers but not absolutely diagnostic.
- Urinalysis may show beryllium in urine, but this only indicates exposure.

Treatment and clinical implications

Beryllium ulcer requires excision or curettage. Acute berylliosis requires prompt corticosteroid therapy. Hypoxia may require oxygen administration by nasal cannula or mask (1 to 2 liters/minute). Severe respiratory failure requires mechanical ventilation if arterial oxygen cannot be maintained above 40 mm Hg.

Chronic berylliosis is usually treated with corticosteroids, although it is not certain that steroids alter disease progression. Lifelong maintenance therapy may be necessary.

Respiratory symptoms may be treated with bronchodilators, increased fluid intake (at least 3 liters/day), and chest physiotherapy techniques. Diuretics, digitalis preparations, and salt restriction may be useful in patients with cor pulmonale.

• Teach the patient to prevent infection by avoiding crowds and persons with infection and by receiving influenza and pneumococcal vaccines.

• Encourage the patient to practice physical reconditioning, energy conservation in daily activities, and relaxation techniques.

Complications
• Septal perforation
• Tracheitis
• Bronchitis
• Respiratory failure
• Pneumothorax
• Pulmonary hypertension
• Right ventricular hypertrophy
• Cor pulmonale

Bipolar affective disorder

Description
Bipolar affective disorder is marked by severe pathologic mood swings from euphoria to sadness, by spontaneous recoveries, and by a tendency to recur. The cyclic (bipolar) form consists of separate episodes of mania (elation) and depression; however, manic or depressive episodes can be predominant, or the two moods can be mixed. When depression is the predominant mood, the patient has the unipolar form of the disease. The manic form is more prevalent in young patients, and the depressive form in older ones. Bipolar disorder recurs in 80% of patients; as they grow older, the attacks of illness recur more frequently and last longer. This illness is associated with significant mortality; 20% of patients commit suicide, often just as depression lifts.

Causes
Causes are not clearly understood but are believed to be multiple and complex, and may involve hereditary, biologic, psychological, interpersonal, and social and cultural factors.

Risk factors
Although bipolar affective disorder often appears without identifiable predisposing factors, the following problems may precede the onset of bipolar illness.
• Early loss of a parent
• Parental depression
• Incest
• Abuse
• Bereavement
• Disruption of an important relationship
• Severe accidental injury

Signs and symptoms
The manic and the depressive phases of bipolar disorder produce characteristic mood swings and other behavioral and physical changes. Before the onset of overt symptoms, many patients with this illness have an energetic and outgoing personality with a history of wide mood swings.
Depressive phase
—Loss of self-esteem
—Overwhelming inertia
—Hopelessness
—Despondency
—Withdrawal

—Apathy
—Sadness
—Helplessness
—Increased fatigue, difficulty sleeping (falling asleep, staying asleep, or early-morning awakening)
—Tiredness on awakening; the patient usually feels worse in the morning.
—Anorexia, causing significant weight loss without dieting
—Psychomotor retardation, with slowed speech, movement, and thoughts, difficulty concentrating. Although usually not disoriented or intellectually impaired, the patient may offer slow, one-word answers in a monotonic voice.
—Multiple somatic complaints, such as constipation, fatigue, headache, chest pains, or heaviness in the limbs. The patient may worry excessively about having cancer or some other severe illness. In an elderly patient, such physical symptoms may be the only clues to his depression.
—Excessive and hypochondriacal concern about body changes
—Guilt and self-reproach over past events
—As depression deepens, possible feelings of worthlessness and belief that he is wicked and deserves to be punished

Acute manic phase
This phase is marked by recurrent, distinct episodes of persistently euphoric, expansive, or irritable mood. It must be associated with four of the following symptoms that persist for at least 1 week.
—Increase in social, occupational, or sexual activity with physical restlessness
—Unusual talkativeness or pressure to keep talking
—Flight of ideas or the subjective experience that thoughts are racing
—Inflated self-esteem, grandiosity
—Decreased need for sleep
—Distractibility, attention too easily drawn to trivial stimuli
—Excessive involvement in activities

that have a high potential for painful but unrecognized consequences (shopping sprees, reckless driving). The manic patient has little control over incessant pressure of ideas, speech, and activity; he ignores the need to eat, sleep, or relax.

Hypomania
This is more common than acute mania. It is not associated with flight of ideas, delusions, or absence of discretion and self-control.
—A classic triad of symptoms: Elated but unstable mood, pressure of speech, and increased motor activity
—Other signs and symptoms: Hyperactivity, easy distractibility, talkativeness, irritability, impatience, impulsiveness, and much energy.

Diagnostic tests
Psychological tests such as rating scales of increased or decreased activity, speech, or sleep may support the diagnosis, which rests primarily on observation and psychiatric history.

Treatment
Treatment for an acute manic or depressive episode may require brief hospitalization to provide drug therapy or electroconvulsive therapy (ECT).
• Monoamine oxidase (MAO) inhibitors such as phenelzine (Nardil) and tricyclic antidepressants such as imipramine (Tofranil) relieve depression without causing the amnesia or confusion that commonly follows ECT.
• In ECT, an electric current is passed through the temporal lobe to produce a controlled grand mal seizure. ECT is an effective treatment for persistent depression. It is less effective in the manic phase. However, it is the treatment of choice for middle-aged, agitated, and suicidal patients.
• Lithium therapy can dramatically relieve symptoms of mania and hypomania and may prevent recurrence of depression. In some patients, maintenance therapy with lithium has prevented recurrence of symptoms for decades. Lithium has a narrow ther-

apeutic range, so treatment must include close monitoring. Because therapeutic doses of lithium produce adverse effects in many patients, compliance may be a problem. In those who fail to respond to lithium, or to treat acute symptoms before onset of lithium effect, haloperidol (Haldol) may be effective. (Onset of lithium effect takes 7 to 10 days.)

Clinical implications

The depressed patient needs continual positive reinforcement to improve his self-esteem.

- Encourage him to talk or to write down his feelings if he is having trouble expressing them. Listen attentively and respectfully, and allow him time to formulate his thoughts if he seems sluggish.
- Provide a structured routine, including activities to boost confidence and promote interaction with others (for instance, group therapy), and keep reassuring him that depression will lift.
- To prevent possible self-injury or suicide, remove harmful objects from the patient's environment (glass, belts, rope, bobby pins), observe him closely, and strictly supervise his medications.
- Record all observations and conversations with the patient, since these records are valuable for evaluating his condition.
- Do not forget the patient's physical needs. If he is too depressed to take care of himself, help him.

In caring for the manic patient, follow these guidelines.

- Remember the manic patient's physical needs. Encourage him to eat; he may jump up and walk around the room after every mouthful but will sit down again if you remind him.
- Encourage short naps during the day, and assist with personal hygiene.
- Provide emotional support, maintain a calm environment, and set realistic goals for behavior.
- Provide diversional activities suited to a short attention span; firmly discourage him if he tries to overextend himself.
- When necessary, reorient the patient to reality, and tactfully divert conversations when they become intimately involved with other patients or staff members.
- Set limits in a calm, clear, and self-confident manner for the manic patient's demanding, hyperactive, manipulative, and acting-out behaviors. Setting limits tells the patient you will provide security and protection by refusing inappropriate and possibly harmful requests. Avoid leaving an opening for the patient to test or argue.
- Listen to requests attentively and with a neutral attitude, but avoid power struggles if a patient tries to put you on the spot for an immediate answer. Explain that you will consider the request seriously and will respond later.
- Collaborate with other staff members to provide consistent responses to the patient's manipulations or acting out.
- Watch for early signs of frustration (when the patient's anger escalates from verbal threats to hitting an object). Tell the patient firmly that threats and hitting are unacceptable and that these behaviors show he needs help to control his behavior. Then tell him that staff will help him move to a quiet area and will help him control his behavior so he will not hurt himself or others. Staff who have practiced as a team can work effectively to prevent acting-out behavior or to remove and confine a patient.
- Alert the staff team promptly when acting-out behavior escalates. It is safer to have help available before you need it than to try controlling an anxious or frightened patient by yourself.
- Once the incident is over and the patient is calm and in control, discuss his feelings with him and offer suggestions to prevent recurrence.

Bladder cancer

Description

Bladder tumors can develop on the surface of the bladder wall (papillomas, benign or malignant) or grow within the bladder wall (generally more virulent) and quickly invade underlying muscles. Almost all bladder tumors (90%) are transitional cell carcinomas, arising from the transitional epithelium of mucous membranes. They may result from malignant transformation of benign papillomas. Less common bladder tumors include adenocarcinomas, epidermoid carcinomas, squamous cell carcinomas, sarcomas, tumors in bladder diverticula, and carcinoma in situ.

Bladder tumors are most prevalent in people over age 50 and are more common in men than in women. The incidence of bladder tumors rises in densely populated industrial areas. Bladder cancer accounts for about 2% to 4% of all cancers.

Causes

Unknown

Risk factors

• Exposure to environmental carcinogens, such as 2-naphthylamine, benzidine, tobacco, nitrates, and coffee, is known to predispose to transitional cell tumors.
• Members of certain industrial groups such as rubber workers, cable workers, weavers, aniline dye workers, hairdressers, petroleum workers, spray painters, and leather finishers are at high risk for developing these tumors.
• Living in geographic areas where schistosomiasis is endemic (such as Egypt) increases the risk.
• The disease is associated with chronic bladder irritation and infection in people with kidney stones, indwelling (Foley) catheters, and chemical cystitis caused by cyclophosphamide.

Signs and symptoms

• Asymptomatic in early stages in approximately one fourth of patients
• Gross, painless, intermittent hematuria (often with clots in the urine) is commonly the first sign.
• Suprapubic pain after voiding occurs in patients with invasive lesions.
• Other clinical effects include bladder irritability, urinary frequency, nocturia, and dribbling.

Diagnostic tests

• Cystoscopy and biopsy confirm bladder cancer. They should be performed when hematuria first appears. When these procedures are performed under anesthesia, a bimanual examination is usually done to determine if the bladder is fixed to the pelvic wall.
• Intravenous pyelography can identify a large, early-stage tumor or an infiltrating tumor. It can also delineate functional problems in the upper urinary tract and can assess the degree of hydronephrosis.
• Urinalysis can detect ureteral obstruction or rigid deformity of the bladder wall.
• Pelvic arteriography can reveal tumor invasion into the bladder wall.
• Computed tomography demonstrates the thickness of the involved bladder wall and detects enlarged retroperitoneal lymph nodes.

Treatment

Superficial bladder tumors are removed through transurethral (cystoscope) resection and fulguration (electrical destruction). This procedure is adequate when the tumor has not invaded the muscle. However, additional tumors may develop, and the fulguration may have to be repeated every 3 months for years.

Tumors too large to be treated through a cystoscope require segmental bladder resection to remove a full-thickness section of the bladder. This procedure is feasible only if the tumor is not near the bladder neck or ureteral orifices. Bladder instillations of thiotepa after transurethral resections may also help control such tumors.

For infiltrating bladder tumor, radical cystectomy is the treatment of choice. The week before cystectomy, treatment may include 2,000 rads of external beam therapy to the bladder. The surgeon forms a urinary diversion, usually an ileal conduit. The patient must then wear an external pouch continuously. Other diversions include ureterostomy, nephrostomy, vesicostomy, ileal bladder, ileal loop, and sigmoid conduit.

Males are impotent following radical cystectomy and urethrectomy, because such resection damages the sympathetic and the parasympathetic nerves that control erection and ejaculation. At a later date, the patient may desire a penile implant, to make sexual intercourse (without ejaculation) possible.

Treatment for patients with advanced bladder cancer includes cystectomy to remove the tumor, radiation therapy, and systemic chemotherapy, such as cyclophosphamide, 5-fluorouracil, doxorubicin, and cisplatin. This combined treatment has sometimes been successful in arresting this disease.

Clinical implications
• Provide psychological support. Encourage the patient to have a positive outlook about the stoma.
• Before surgery, assist in selection of the stoma site by assessing the patient's abdomen in varying positions. The usual site is in the rectus muscle, to minimize the risk of subsequent herniation. Make sure that the selected stoma site is visible to the patient.
• After surgery, encourage the patient to look at the stoma. If he has difficulty doing this, leave the room for a few minutes while the stoma is exposed. Offer the patient a mirror to make viewing easier.
• To obtain a specimen for culture and sensitivity, catheterize the patient, using sterile technique.

• If the patient with surgically induced impotence was sexually active before surgery, elicit psychological support and understanding for the patient from his partner. Also, suggest alternative methods of sexual expression.
• Except for heavy lifting and contact sports, the patient with a urinary stoma may participate in various athletic and physical activities.
• When a patient with a urinary diversion is discharged, arrange for follow-up home care from a visiting nurse.
• Make a referral to an enterostomal therapist, if one is available.
• Teach the patient about his urinary stoma. Instruction usually begins 4 to 6 days after surgery. Encourage the patient's spouse or a friend or relative to attend the teaching sessions, and advise this person beforehand that a negative reaction to the stoma can impede the patient's adjustment.
• All individuals at high risk for bladder cancer should have periodic cytologic examinations and should know about the danger of significant exposure to irritants, toxins, and carcinogens. Many industries have taken measures to protect workers from possible exposure to aromatic amines, such as 2-naphthylamine and benzidine, and have reduced incidence of bladder cancer among their workers.
• For added information, refer ostomates to the American Cancer Society or to the United Ostomy Association.

Blastomycosis
(North American blastomycosis, Gilchrist's disease)

Description
Blastomycosis is a disease that usually infects the lungs and produces bronchopneumonia. Less frequently, this fungus may disseminate through the blood and cause osteomyelitis and CNS, skin, and genital disorders. The

incubation period may range from weeks to months. Untreated blastomycosis is slowly progressive and usually fatal; however, spontaneous remissions occasionally occur. With antifungal drug therapy and supportive treatment, the prognosis for patients with blastomycosis is good.

Causes
Blastomyces dermatitidis, a yeastlike fungus that normally inhabits the soil and is endemic to the southeastern United States

Mode of transmission
Probably inhaled by people who are in close contact with the soil

Signs and symptoms
Pulmonary blastomycosis
—Dry, hacking, or productive cough (occasionally hemoptysis)
—Pleuritic chest pain
—Fever
—Shaking
—Chills
—Night sweats
—Malaise
—Anorexia
—Weight loss
Cutaneous blastomycosis
Small, painless, nonpruritic, nondistinctive, raised, reddened macules or papules on exposed body parts
Other signs and symptoms
Occurrence of these signs and symptoms depends on fungal dissemination.
—Dissemination to the bone causes soft-tissue swelling, tenderness, and warmth over bony lesions, which generally occur in the thoracic, lumbar, and sacral regions; long bones of the legs; and, in children, the skull.
—Genital dissemination produces painful swelling of the testes, the epididymis, or the prostate; deep perineal pain; pyuria; and hematuria.
—CNS dissemination causes meningitis or cerebral abscesses and results in decreased level of consciousness, lethargy, and change in mood or affect.

Diagnostic tests
• Culture of *B. dermatitidis* from skin lesions, pus, sputum, or pulmonary secretions is required.
• Microscopic examination of tissue biopsy from the skin or the lungs, or of bronchial washings, sputum, or pus is required as the physician finds appropriate.
• Complement fixation testing is not conclusive, but a high titer in extrapulmonary disease is a poor prognostic sign.
• Immunodiffusion testing detects antibodies for the A and B antigen of blastomycosis.
• Chest X-ray is required if pulmonary blastomycosis is suspected. It may show pulmonary infiltrates.
• WBC count and erythrocyte sedimentation rate are increased.
• Serum globulin is slightly increased.
• Alkaline phosphatase is increased in bone lesions.

Treatment and clinical implications
All forms of blastomycosis respond to amphotericin B. Care is mainly supportive.
• In severe pulmonary blastomycosis, check for hemoptysis. If the patient is febrile, provide a cool room and give tepid sponge baths.
• If blastomycosis causes joint pain or swelling, elevate the joint and apply heat. In CNS infection, watch the patient carefully for decreasing level of consciousness and unequal pupillary response. In men with disseminated disease, watch for hematuria.
• Infuse I.V. amphotericin B slowly (too rapid infusion may cause circulatory collapse). During infusion, monitor vital signs (temperature may rise but should subside within 1 to 2 hours). Watch for decreased urine output, and monitor laboratory results for increased BUN, increased creatinine, and hypokalemia, which may indicate renal toxicity. Report any hearing loss, tinnitus, or dizziness immediately. To

relieve adverse effects of amphotericin B, give antiemetics and antipyretics, as ordered.

Blepharitis

Description

Blepharitis is a common inflammatory condition of the lash follicles and meibomian glands of the upper or lower eyelids. It often occurs in children and is often bilateral. It usually occurs as seborrheic (nonulcerative) blepharitis or as staphylococcal (ulcerative) blepharitis. Both types may coexist. Blepharitis tends to recur and become chronic. It can be controlled if treatment begins before onset of ocular involvement.

Causes

- Seborrhea of the scalp, eyebrows, and ears generally causes seborrheic blepharitis.
- *Staphylococcus aureus* infection causes ulcerative blepharitis.
- Pediculosis (from *Phthirus pubis* or *Pediculus humanus capitis*) of the brows and lashes, which irritates the lid margins.

Signs and symptoms

- Redness of the eyelid margins
- Itching of affected eye(s)
- Burning of affected eye(s)
- Foreign-body sensation
- Sticky, crusted eyelids on waking
- Unconscious rubbing of eyes
- Continual blinking
- Greasy scales (in seborrheic blepharitis)
- Flaky scales on lashes, loss of lashes, and ulcerated areas on lid margins (in ulcerative blepharitis)
- Nits on lashes (a sign of pediculosis)

Diagnostic tests

Culture of ulcerated lid margins shows *S. aureus* in ulcerative blepharitis.

Treatment

Early treatment is essential to prevent recurrence or complications. Treatment depends on the type of blepharitis.

- In seborrheic blepharitis, daily shampooing (using a mild shampoo on a damp applicator stick or a washcloth) removes scales from the lid margins. The scalp and eyebrows are shampooed frequently.
- In ulcerative blepharitis, sulfonamide eye ointment is applied or an appropriate antibiotic is given.
- In blepharitis caused by pediculosis, treatment requires removal of nits (with forceps) or application of ophthalmic physostigmine ointment as an insecticide. A film of ointment on the cornea may cause pupil constriction and possible headache, conjunctival irritation, and blurred vision.

Clinical implications

- Instruct the patient to remove scales from the lid margins daily with an applicator stick or a clean washcloth.
- Teach the patient the following method for applying warm compresses. First, run warm water into a clean bowl, and immerse a clean cloth in the water and wring it out. Then place the warm cloth against the closed eyelid (be careful not to burn the skin). Hold the compress in place until it cools. Continue this procedure for 15 minutes.
- If blepharitis results from pediculosis, check the patient's family and other contacts, and notify local health authorities.

Complications

In ulcerative blepharitis, chalazions and styes may develop.

Bone tumors, primary malignant
(Sarcomas of bone, bone cancer)

Description
Primary malignant bone tumors are rare, constituting less than 1% of all malignant tumors. Most bone tumors are secondary, caused by seeding from a primary site. Primary malignant bone tumors are more common in males, especially in children and adolescents, although some types do occur in persons between ages 35 and 60. They may originate in osseous or nonosseous tissue. Osseous bone tumors arise from the bony structure itself; they include osteogenic sarcoma (the most common), parosteal osteogenic sarcoma, chondrosarcoma, and malignant giant cell tumor. Together

Classifying Primary Malignant Bone Tumors

TYPE	CLINICAL FEATURES	TREATMENT
Osseous origin		
Osteogenic sarcoma	• Osteoid tumor present in specimen • Tumor arises from bone-forming osteoblast and bone-digesting osteoclast • Occurs most often in femur, but also tibia and humerus; occasionally, in fibula, ileum, vertebra, or mandible • Usually in males age 10 to 30	• Surgery (tumor resection, high thigh amputation, hemipelvectomy, interscapulothoracic surgery) • Radiation • Chemotherapy • Combination of above
Parosteal osteogenic sarcoma	• Develops on surface of bone instead of interior • Progresses slowly • Occurs most often in distal femur, but also in tibia, humerus, and ulna • Usually in females age 30 to 40	• Surgery (tumor resection, possible amputation, interscapulothoracic surgery, hemipelvectomy) • Chemotherapy • Combination of above
Chondrosarcoma	• Develops from cartilage • Painless; grows slowly, but is locally recurrent and invasive • Occurs most often in pelvis, proximal femur, ribs, and shoulder girdle • Usually in males age 30 to 50	• Hemipelvectomy, surgical resection (ribs) • Radiation (palliative) • Chemotherapy
Malignant giant cell tumor	• Arises from benign giant cell tumor • Found most often in long bones, especially in knee area • Usually in females age 18 to 50	• Curettage • Total excision • Radiation

Classifying Primary Malignant Bone Tumors *(continued)*

TYPE	CLINICAL FEATURES	TREATMENT
Nonosseous origin		
Ewing's sarcoma	• Originates in bone marrow and invades shafts of long and flat bones • Usually affects lower extremities, most often femur, innominate bones, ribs, tibia, humerus, vertebra, and fibula; may metastasize to lungs • Pain increasingly severe and persistent • Usually in males age 10 to 20 • Prognosis poor	• High-voltage radiation (tumor is very radiosensitive) • Chemotherapy to slow growth • Amputation only if no evidence of metastases
Fibrosarcoma	• Relatively rare • Originates in fibrous tissue of bone • Invades long or flat bones (femur, tibia, mandible) but also involves periosteum and overlying muscle • Usually in males age 30 to 40	• Amputation • Radiation • Chemotherapy • Bone grafts (with low-grade fibrosarcoma)
Chordoma	• Derived from embryonic remnants of notochord • Progresses slowly • Usually found at end of spinal column and in spheno-occipital, sacrococcygeal, and vertebral areas • Characterized by constipation and visual disturbances • Usually in males age 50 to 60	• Surgical resection (often resulting in neural defects) • Radiation (palliative or when surgery not applicable, as in occipital area)

they make up 60% of all malignant bone tumors. Nonosseous tumors arise from hematopoietic, vascular, and neural tissues; they include Ewing's sarcoma, fibrosarcoma, and chordoma. Osteogenic and Ewing's sarcomas are the most common bone tumors in childhood.

Causes

• Theories point to heredity, trauma, and excessive radiotherapy.
• Some evidence suggests that primary malignant bone tumors arise in areas of rapid growth, since children and young adults with such tumors seem to be much taller than average.

Signs and symptoms

• Bone pain is the most common indication. It is often more intense at night and is not usually associated with mobility. Pain is dull and usually localized, although it may be referred

from the hip or spine and result in weakness or a limp.
• Mass or tumor, which may be tender and may swell
• Pathologic fractures
• Cachexia, fever, and impaired mobility (may occur in late stages)
(See also *Classifying Primary Malignant Bone Tumors*, pp. 82-83.)

Diagnosis
• Biopsy (by incision or by aspiration) is essential for confirming primary malignant bone tumors.
• Bone X-rays and radioisotope bone and computed tomography scans show tumor size.
• Serum alkaline phosphatase is usually elevated in patients with sarcoma.

Treatment
Surgery (usually amputation) and radiation are the treatments of choice, sometimes combined with chemotherapy and immunotherapy. Sometimes radical surgery (such as hemipelvectomy or interscapulothoracic amputation) is necessary. However, surgical resection of the tumor (often with preoperative radiation *and* postoperative chemotherapy) has saved limbs from amputation. Chemotherapeutic drugs include doxorubicin, high-dose methotrexate with leucovorin rescue, vincristine, cyclophosphamide, cisplatin, bleomycin, dactinomycin, and melphalan. Adjuvant immunotherapy uses interferon or the transfer factor (a dialyzable extract of immune lymphocytes that transfers cell-mediated immunity).

Clinical implications
• Be sensitive to the enormous emotional strain caused by the threat of amputation. If amputation is inevitable, teach the patient how to readjust his body weight so he will be able to get in and out of bed and wheelchair. Teach exercises that will help him do this even before surgery.

• After surgery, check vital signs every hour for the first 4 hours, then every 2 hours for the next 4 hours, and then every 4 hours if the patient is stable. Tape a tourniquet to the bed in case of hemorrhage. Check the dressing periodically for oozing. Elevate the foot of the bed or the stump on a pillow for the first 24 hours. (Be careful not to leave the stump elevated for more than 48 hours, as this may led to contractures.)
• To ease the patient's anxiety, administer analgesics for pain before morning care. If necessary, brace the patient with pillows, keeping the affected part at rest.
• Since the patient may have thrombocytopenia, make sure he uses a soft toothbrush and an electric razor to avoid bleeding. Do not give I.M. injections or take rectal temperatures. Be careful not to bump the patient's arms or legs; his low platelet count causes bruising.
• Encourage fluids to prevent dehydration. Record intake and output accurately. After a hemipelvectomy, insert a nasogastric tube to prevent abdominal distention. Continue low gastric suction for 2 days after surgery or until the patient can tolerate a soft diet. Administer antibiotics to prevent infection of the rectum. Give transfusions, if necessary, and administer medication to control pain. Keep drains in place to facilitate wound drainage and prevent infection. Use an indwelling (Foley) catheter until the patient can void voluntarily.
• Watch for adverse reactions to radiation treatment: nausea, vomiting, and dryness of skin with excoriation.
• Encourage early rehabilitation. Start physical therapy 24 hours postoperatively. Pain is usually not severe after amputation. If it is, watch for a wound complication, such as hematoma, excessive stump edema, or infection.
• Be aware of the "phantom limb" syndrome. Tell the patient this sensation is normal after amputation and usually subsides.

• To avoid contractures and assure the best conditions for wound healing, warn the patient not to hang the stump over the edge of the bed; sit in a wheelchair with the stump flexed; place a pillow under his hip, knee, or back or between his thighs; lie with his knees flexed; rest an above-the-knee (AK) stump on the crutch handle; or abduct an AK stump.

• Wash the stump, massage it gently, and keep it dry until it heals. Make sure the bandage is firm and is worn day and night. Know how to reapply the bandage to shape the stump for a prosthesis.

• Help the patient select a prosthesis. The rehabilitation staff will make the final decision, but since most patients are totally uninformed about choosing a prosthesis, give some guidelines. Generally, children need relatively simple devices, while elderly patients may require prostheses that provide stability. Consider personal and family finances, too. Children outgrow prostheses; advise parents to select inexpensive ones.

• The same points are applicable for an interscapulothoracic amputee, but losing an arm causes a greater cosmetic problem.

• Try to instill a positive attitude toward recovery. Urge the patient to resume an independent life-style. Refer elderly patients to community health services, if necessary. Suggest tutoring for children to help them keep up with schoolwork.

Botulism

Description

Botulism, a life-threatening paralytic illness, is usually the result of ingesting inadequately cooked contaminated foods, especially those with low acid content, such as home-canned fruits and vegetables, sausages, and smoked or preserved fish or meat. Rarely, it is a result of wound infection with *Clostridium botulinum*. Recently, findings have shown that an infant's GI tract can become colonized with *C. botulinum* from some unknown source. The exotoxin is then produced within the infant's intestine.

Mortality from botulism is about 25%. Death is most often caused by respiratory failure during the first week of illness.

Causes

An exotoxin produced by the gram-positive, anaerobic bacillus *Clostridium botulinum*

Signs and symptoms

In adults
—Dry mouth
—Sore throat
—Weakness
—Vomiting
—Diarrhea
—Ptosis
—Diplopia
—Dysarthria
—Descending weakness or paralysis of muscles in the extremities or trunk
—Dyspnea from respiratory paralysis

In infants
—Constipation
—Feeble cry
—Depressed gag reflex
—Inability to suck
—Flaccid facial expression
—Ptosis
—Ophthalmoplegia
—Generalized muscle weakness
—Hypotonia
—Areflexia
—Striking loss of head control
—Respiratory arrest (likely)

Diagnostic tests

• Identification of the offending toxin in the patient's serum, stool, gastric content, or the suspected food confirms the diagnosis.

• An electromyogram (EMG) showing

diminished muscle action potential after a single supramaximal nerve stimulus is also diagnostic.

Treatment and clinical implications

Treatment consists of I.V. or I.M. administration of botulinum antitoxin (available through the Centers for Disease Control).

If you suspect ingestion of contaminated food, follow these guidelines:

• Obtain a careful history of the patient's food intake for the past several days. Check to see if other family members exhibit similar symptoms and share a common food history.

• Observe carefully for abnormal neurologic signs. If the patient returns home, tell his family to watch for signs of weakness, blurred vision, and slurred speech, and to return the patient to the hospital immediately if such signs appear.

• If ingestion has occurred within several hours, induce vomiting, begin gastric lavage, and give a high enema to purge any unabsorbed toxin from the bowel.

If clinical signs of botulism appear, follow these guidelines.

• Admit the patient to the ICU, and monitor cardiac and respiratory functions carefully.

• Administer botulinum antitoxin, as ordered, to neutralize any circulating toxin. Before giving antitoxin, obtain an accurate patient history of allergies, especially to horses, and perform a skin test. Afterward, watch for anaphylaxis or other hypersensitivity and for serum sickness. Keep epinephrine 1:1,000 (for S.C. administration) and emergency airway equipment available.

• Closely assess and accurately record neurologic function, including bilateral motor status (reflexes, ability to move arms and legs).

• Give I.V. fluids, as ordered. Turn the patient often, and encourage deep-breathing exercises. Isolation is not required.

• Because botulism is sometimes fatal, keep the patient and family informed regarding the course of the disease.

• Immediately report all cases of botulism to local public health authorities.

• To help prevent botulism encourage patients to observe proper techniques in processing and preserving foods. Warn them to avoid even *tasting* food from a bulging can or one with a peculiar odor and to sterilize by boiling any utensil that comes in contact with suspected food. Ingestion of even a small amount of food contaminated with botulism toxin can prove fatal.

Brain abscess
(Intracranial abscess)

Description

Brain abscess is a free or encapsulated collection of pus usually found in the temporal lobe, cerebellum, or frontal lobes. It can vary in size and may occur at single or multiple loci. Untreated brain abscess is usually fatal. With treatment, prognosis is only fair, and about 30% of patients develop focal seizures. Multiple metastatic abscesses secondary to systemic or other infections have the poorest prognosis.

Causes

• Brain abscess is usually secondary to another infection.

• Common infecting organisms include *Staphylococcus aureus, Streptococcus viridans,* and *Streptococcus hemolyticus.*

Risk factors

• Otitis media
• Sinusitis
• Dental abscess
• Mastoiditis
• Subdural empyema
• Bacterial endocarditis
• Bacteremia
• Pulmonary or pleural infection

• Pelvic, abdominal, and skin infections
• Cranial trauma
• Rarely, congenital heart disease

Signs and symptoms

General symptoms
—Signs of infection such as fever, pallor, and bradycardia are absent or appear late unless associated with a predisposing condition.
—Constant intractable headache, worsened by straining
—Nausea, vomiting
—Seizures
—Nystagmus
—Decreased vision
—Inequality of pupils
—Change in level of consciousness, varying from drowsiness to deep stupor

Focal symptoms
—Temporal lobe abscess: Auditory-receptive dysphasia, central facial weakness, hemiparesis
—Cerebellar abscess: Dizziness, coarse nystagmus, gaze weakness on lesion side, tremor, ataxia
—Frontal lobe abscess: Expressive dysphasia, hemiparesis with unilateral motor seizure, drowsiness, inattention, mental function impairment

Diagnostic tests
• Electroencephalography, computed tomography (CT) scan, and, occasionally, arteriography (which highlights abscess by a halo) help locate the site.
• Examination of cerebrospinal fluid can help confirm infection, but most doctors agree that lumbar puncture is usually too risky, because it can release increased intracranial pressure (ICP) and provoke cerebral herniation.
• Culture and sensitivity testing of drainage identify the causative organism.
• Skull X-rays, radioisotope scan, and, rarely, ventriculography may be done.

Treatment
Therapy consists of antibiotics to combat the underlying infection and surgical aspiration or drainage of the abscess. However, surgery is delayed until the abscess becomes encapsulated (CT scan helps determine this) and is contraindicated in patients with congenital heart disease or another debilitating cardiac condition. Administration of a penicillinase-resistant antibiotic, such as nafcillin or methicillin, for at least 2 to 3 weeks before surgery can reduce the risk of spreading infection. Other treatment during the acute phase is palliative and supportive, and includes mechanical ventilation, administration of I.V. fluids with diuretics (urea, mannitol), and glucocorticoids (dexamethasone) to combat increased ICP and cerebral edema. Anticonvulsants, such as phenytoin and phenobarbital, help prevent seizures.

Clinical implications
The patient with an acute brain abscess requires intensive monitoring.
• Frequently assess neurologic status.
• Record vital signs at least every 1 to 2 hours.
• Monitor fluid intake and output carefully, since fluid overload could contribute to cerebral edema.
• If surgery is necessary, explain the procedure to the patient and answer his questions.
• After surgery, continue frequent neurologic assessment. Monitor vital signs and intake and output.
• Watch for signs of meningitis (nuchal rigidity, headaches, chills, sweats), an ever-present threat.
• Be sure to change a damp dressing often, using aseptic technique and noting amount of drainage. To promote drainage and prevent reaccumulation of the abscess, position the patient on the operative side.
• If the patient remains stuporous or comatose for an extended period, give meticulous skin care to prevent decubitus ulcers, and position him to preserve function and prevent contractures.
• If the patient requires isolation be-

cause of postoperative drainage, make sure he and his family understand why.
• Initiate ambulation as soon as possible.

Brain tumors, malignant

Description
Malignant brain tumors (gliomas, meningiomas, and schwannomas) are common. They may occur at any age. In adults, incidence is generally highest between ages 40 and 60. In children, incidence is generally highest before age 1 and then again between ages 2 and 12. In children, brain tumors are one of the most common causes of death from cancer.

Causes
Unknown

Signs and symptoms
Generally, clinical features result from increased intracranial pressure (ICP); these features vary with the type of tumor, its location, and the degree of invasion. (See *Classifying Malignant Brain Tumors*.)

Diagnostic tests
• Biopsy identifies the histologic type and provides the definitive diagnosis.
• Skull X-rays, brain scan, computed tomography, magnetic resonance imaging, and cerebral angiography can locate the tumor.
• Lumbar puncture shows increased pressure and protein, decreased glucose, and occasionally, tumor cells in cerebrospinal fluid (CSF).

Treatment
Treatment includes removing a resectable tumor, reducing the size of a nonresectable tumor, relieving cerebral edema or ICP, relieving symptoms, and preventing further neurologic damage.

Mode of therapy depends on the tumor's histologic type, radiosensitivity, and anatomic location and may include surgery, radiation, chemotherapy, or decompression of increased ICP with diuretics, corticosteroids, or possibly ventriculoatrial or ventriculoperitoneal shunting of CSF.

Clinical implications
A patient with a brain tumor requires comprehensive neurologic assessment, teaching, and supportive care. During your first contact with the patient, perform a comprehensive assessment (including a complete neurologic evaluation) to provide baseline data and to help develop your care plan. Obtain a thorough health history concerning onset of symptoms. Assist the patient and his family in coping with the treatment, potential disabilities, and changes in life-style resulting from his tumor.

Throughout hospitalization, follow these guidelines:
• Carefully document seizure activity (occurrence, nature, duration).
• Maintain airway patency.
• Monitor patient safety.
• Administer anticonvulsants, as ordered.
• Check continuously for changes in neurologic status, and watch for increase in ICP.
• Watch for and immediately report sudden unilateral pupillary dilation with loss of light reflex. This ominous change indicates imminent transtentorial herniation.
• Monitor respiratory changes carefully. Abnormal respiratory rate and depth may point to increasing ICP or herniation of the cerebellar tonsils from expanding infratentorial mass.
• Monitor temperature carefully. Fever commonly follows hypothalamic anoxia but might also indicate meningitis. Use hypothermia blankets preoperatively and postoperatively to keep the patient's temperature down and minimize cerebral metabolic demands.
• Administer steroids and antacids, as ordered. Observe and report signs of

Classifying Malignant Brain Tumors

TUMOR	CLINICAL FEATURES
Meningioma • Most common nongliomatous brain tumor (15% of primary brain tumors) • Peak incidence among 50-year-olds; rare in children; more common in females (ratio 3:2) • Arises from the meninges • Common locations include parasagittal area, sphenoidal ridge, anterior part of the base of the skull, cerebellopontile angle, spinal canal • Benign, well-circumscribed, highly vascular tumors that compress underlying brain tissue by invading overlying skull	*General:* • Headache and vomiting • Seizures (in two thirds of patients) • Changes in mental activity • Similar to schwannomas *Localizing:* • Skull changes (bony bulge) over tumor • Sphenoidal ridge, indenting optic nerve: Unilateral visual changes and papilledema • Prefrontal parasagittal: Personality and behavioral changes • Motor cortex: Contralateral motor changes • Anterior fossa compressing both optic nerves and frontal lobes: Headache and bilateral vision loss • Pressure on cranial nerves causes varying symptoms
Schwannoma *(acoustic neurinoma, neurilemoma, cerebellopontile angle tumor)* • Accounts for approximately 10% of all intracranial tumors • Higher incidence in women • Onset of symptoms between ages 30 and 60 • Affects the craniospinal nerve sheath, usually cranial nerve VIII; also, V and VII, and to a lesser extent, VI and X on the same side as the tumor • Benign, but often classified as malignant because of its growth patterns; slow-growing—may be present for years before symptoms occur	*General:* • Unilateral hearing loss with or without tinnitus • Stiff neck and suboccipital discomfort • Secondary hydrocephalus • Ataxia and uncoordinated movements of one or both arms due to pressure on brain stem and cerebellum *Localizing:* • V: Early—facial hypoesthesia or paresthesia on side of hearing loss; unilateral loss of corneal reflex • VI: Diplopia or double vision • VII: Paresis progressing to paralysis (Bell's palsy) • X: Weakness of palate, tongue, and nerve muscles on same side as tumor
Medulloblastoma • Rare glioma • Incidence highest in children age 4 to 6 • Affects males more than females • Frequently metastasizes via CSF	*General:* • Increased ICP *Localizing:* • Brain stem and cerebrum: Papilledema, nystagmus, hearing loss, flashing lights, dizziness, ataxia, paresthesias of face, cranial nerve palsies (V, VI, VII, IX, X, primarily sensory), hemiparesis, suboccipital tenderness; compression of supratentorial area produces other general and focal symptoms

Classifying Malignant Brain Tumors *(continued)*

TUMOR	CLINICAL FEATURES
Glioblastoma multiforme *(spongioblastoma multiforme)* • Peak incidence between ages 50 and 60; twice as common in males; most common glioma • Unencapsulated, highly malignant; grows rapidly and infiltrates the brain extensively; may become enormous before diagnosed • Occurs most often in cerebral hemispheres, especially frontal and temporal lobes (rarely in brain stem and cerebellum) • Occupies more than one lobe of affected hemisphere; may spread to opposite hemisphere by corpus callosum; may metastasize into CSF, producing tumors in distant parts of the nervous system	*General:* • Increased ICP (nausea, vomiting, headache, papilledema) • Mental and behavioral changes • Altered vital signs (increased systolic pressure; widened pulse pressure, respiratory changes) • Speech and sensory disturbances • In children, irritability, projectile vomiting *Localizing:* • Midline: headache (bifrontal or bioccipital); worse in morning; intensified by coughing, straining, or sudden head movements • Temporal lobe: Psychomotor seizures • Central region: Focal seizures • Optic and oculomotor nerves: Visual defects • Frontal lobe: Abnormal reflexes, motor responses
Oligodendroglioma • Third most common glioma • Occurs in middle age; more common in women • Slow-growing	*General:* • Mental and behavioral changes • Decreased visual acuity and other visual disturbances • Increased ICP *Localizing:* • Temporal lobe: Hallucinations, psychomotor seizures • Central region: Seizures (confined to one muscle group or unilateral) • Midbrain or third ventricle: Pyramidal tract symptoms (dizziness, ataxia, paresthesias of the face) • Brain stem and cerebrum: Nystagmus, hearing loss, dizziness, ataxia, paresthesias of face, cranial nerve palsies, hemiparesis, suboccipital tenderness, loss of balance
Ependymoma • Rare glioma • Most common in children and young adults • Occurs most often in fourth and lateral ventricles	*General:* • Similar to oligodendroglioma • Increased ICP and obstructive hydrocephalus, depending on tumor size

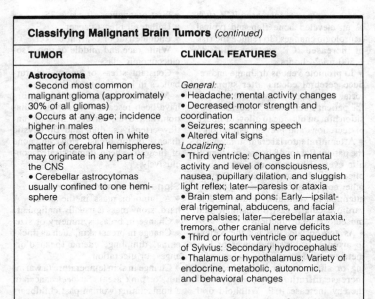

Classifying Malignant Brain Tumors *(continued)*

TUMOR	CLINICAL FEATURES
Astrocytoma • Second most common malignant glioma (approximately 30% of all gliomas) • Occurs at any age; incidence higher in males • Occurs most often in white matter of cerebral hemispheres; may originate in any part of the CNS • Cerebellar astrocytomas usually confined to one hemisphere	*General:* • Headache; mental activity changes • Decreased motor strength and coordination • Seizures; scanning speech • Altered vital signs *Localizing:* • Third ventricle: Changes in mental activity and level of consciousness, nausea, pupillary dilation, and sluggish light reflex; later—paresis or ataxia • Brain stem and pons: Early—ipsilateral trigeminal, abducens, and facial nerve palsies; later—cerebellar ataxia, tremors, other cranial nerve deficits • Third or fourth ventricle or aqueduct of Sylvius: Secondary hydrocephalus • Thalamus or hypothalamus: Variety of endocrine, metabolic, autonomic, and behavioral changes

Reprinted by permission of Elsevier Science Publishing Co., Inc., from *Cancer Nursing—A Holistic Multidisciplinary Approach*, 2nd ed., by Ardelina A. Baldonado and Dulcelina A. Stahl. (Garden City, N.Y.: Medical Examination Publishing Co., 1980)

stress ulcer: abdominal distention, pain, vomiting, and tarry stools.
• Restrict fluids to 1,500 ml/24 hours. Administer osmotic diuretics, such as mannitol or urea, as ordered. Carefully monitor fluid and electrolyte balance.
• Radiation therapy is usually delayed until after the surgical wound heals, but it can induce wound breakdown even then. Therefore, observe the wound carefully for infection and sinus formation. Because radiation may cause brain inflammation, monitor closely for signs of rising ICP.
• Since the nitrosoureas—carmustine (BCNU), lomustine (CCNU), and procarbazine—used as adjuncts to radiotherapy and surgery can possibly cause delayed bone marrow depression, tell the patient to watch for and immediately report any signs of infection or bleeding that appear within 4 weeks after the start of chemotherapy. Before chemotherapy, give prochlorperazine or another antiemetic, as ordered, to minimize nausea and vomiting.
• Teach the patient and his family early signs of recurrence. Urge compliance with therapy.
• Since brain tumors may cause residual neurologic deficits that handicap the patient physically or mentally, begin rehabilitation early. Encourage independence in daily activities. As necessary, provide aids for self-care and mobilization, such as bathroom rails for wheelchair patients. If the patient is aphasic, arrange for consultation with a speech pathologist.

Surgery requires additional nursing care.
• After craniotomy, continue to monitor general neurologic status and

watch for signs of increased ICP, such as an elevated bone flap and typical neurologic changes. To reduce the risk of increased ICP, restrict fluids to 1,500 ml/24 hours.

• To promote venous drainage and reduce cerebral edema after supratentorial craniotomy, elevate the head of the patient's bed about 30 degrees. Position him on his side to allow drainage of secretions and prevent aspiration.

• After infratentorial craniotomy, keep the patient flat for 48 hours, but logroll him every 2 hours to minimize complications of immobilization. Prevent other complications by paying careful attention to ventilatory status and to cardiovascular, gastrointestinal, and musculoskeletal functions.

• As appropriate, instruct the patient to avoid Valsalva's maneuver or isometric muscle contractions when moving or sitting up in bed. These can increase intrathoracic pressure and thereby increase ICP. Withhold oral fluids, which may provoke vomiting and consequently increase ICP.

Breast cancer

Description

Breast cancer is the second most common cancer affecting women and is second only to lung cancer as the cause of death in women age 35 to 54. It occurs in men, but rarely. The 5-year survival rate has improved from 53% in the 1940s to 65% in the 1970s. This is because of earlier diagnosis and the variety of treatment modes now available. The death rate, however, has not changed in the past 50 years.

Causes

Unknown

Risk factors

• Family history of breast cancer
• Long menstrual cycles
• Early onset of menses or late onset of menopause

• First pregnancy after age 35
• Unilateral breast cancer
• Endometrial or ovarian cancer
• White race and middle or upper socioeconomic class
• Constant stress or unusual disturbances in home or work life

Many other predisposing factors have been researched, such as radiation, hair dyes, estrogen therapy, antihypertensives, diet, and fibrocystic disease of the breast. However, none of these has been demonstrated conclusively.

Signs and symptoms

• A lump or mass in the breast. A hard, stony mass is usually malignant.
• Change in breast symmetry or size
• Change in breast skin, such as thickening, dimpling, edema (peau d'orange), or ulceration
• Change in skin temperature (a warm, hot, or pink area). Suspect cancer in a nonlactating woman past childbearing age until proven otherwise.
• Unusual drainage or discharge. Spontaneous discharge of any kind in a nonnursing, nonlactating woman warrants investigation; so does any discharge produced by breast manipulation (greenish black, white, creamy, serous, or bloody). If a nursing infant rejects one breast, this may suggest possible breast cancer.
• Change in the nipple, such as itching, burning, erosion, or retraction
• Pain is not usually a symptom of breast cancer unless the tumor is advanced, but it should be investigated.
• Bone metastasis, pathologic bone fractures, and hypercalcemia

Diagnostic tests

• Regular breast self-examination followed by immediate evaluation of any abnormality is the most reliable method of detection.
• Mammography, ultrasonography, thermography, and surgical biopsy are other diagnostic measures.
• Bone scan, computed tomography,

measurement of alkaline phosphatase levels, liver function studies, and liver biopsy can detect distant metastases.

• A hormonal receptor assay done on the tumor can determine if it is estrogen- or progesterone-dependent. This test is important in making therapy decisions.

Treatment
Much controversy exists over treatment of breast cancer; therapy should take into consideration the stage of the disease, the woman's age and menopausal status, and the disfiguring effects of the surgery. Treatment may include one or any combination of the following.

Surgery
Lumpectomy (excision of the tumor)

is the initial surgery; this procedure also aids in determining tumor cell type. It is often done on an outpatient basis and is the only surgery some patients require, especially those with a small tumor and no evidence of axillary node involvement. Radiation therapy is often combined with this surgery.

A two-stage procedure, in which the surgeon removes the lump, confirms that it is malignant, and discusses treatment options with the patient, is desirable because it allows the patient to participate in her treatment plan. Sometimes, if the tumor is diagnosed as clinically malignant, such planning can be done before surgery.

In lumpectomy and dissection of the axillary lymph nodes, the tumor and

---

Patient-Teaching Aid: Preventing Infection after Axillary Node Dissection or Radiation Therapy

Dear Patient:
Because edema makes tissue especially vulnerable to injury, take special care of the arm and hand on the surgical side.

Some don'ts
• Don't hold a cigarette in the affected hand.
• Don't use it to carry your purse or anything heavy.
• Don't wear a wristwatch or other jewelry on it.
• Don't cut or pick at cuticles or hangnails.
• Don't work near thorny plants or dig in the garden without heavy gloves.
• Don't reach into a hot oven with it.
• Don't permit injection into it.
• Don't permit blood to be drawn from it.
• Don't allow your blood pressure to be taken on it.

Some do's
• Do wear a loose rubber glove on this hand when washing dishes.
• Do wear a thimble when sewing.
• Do apply lanolin hand cream daily if your skin is dry.
• Do wear your Life Guard Medical Aid tag engraved with CAUTION OR PREVENT—LYMPHEDEMA ARM—NO TESTS—NO HYPOS.
• Do contact your doctor immediately if your arm gets red, feels warm, or is unusually hard or swollen.
• Do elevate your arm if it feels heavy.
• Do show this hand care sheet to your surgeon.

This patient-teaching aid may be reproduced by office copier for distribution to patients.
© 1988, Springhouse Corporation

Information courtesy of the Cleveland Clinic, Department of Physical Medicine and Rehabilitation.

the axillary lymph nodes are removed, leaving the breast intact. A simple mastectomy removes the breast but not the lymph nodes or pectoral muscles. Modified radical mastectomy removes the breast and the axillary lymph nodes. Radical mastectomy, the performance of which has declined, removes the breast, pectoralis major and minor, and the axillary lymph nodes.

Postmastectomy, reconstructive surgery can create a breast mound if the patient desires it and if she does not demonstrate evidence of advanced disease. Additional surgery to modify hormone production may include oophorectomy, adrenalectomy, and hypophysectomy. (With adrenalectomy or hypophysectomy, the patient is required to take daily cortisone supplements for the rest of her life.)

Chemotherapy

Various cytotoxic drug combinations are being used, either as adjuvant therapy (in patients with axillary lymph node involvement but no evidence of distant metastasis) or as primary therapy (when metastasis has occurred), based on a number of factors, including the patient's premenopausal or postmenopausal status.

Radiation therapy

Primary radiation therapy *after* tumor removal is effective for small tumors in early stages with no evidence of distant metastasis. It is also used to prevent or treat local recurrence.

Other methods

Breast cancer patients may also receive estrogen, progesterone, or androgen therapy; anti-androgen therapy with aminoglutethimide; or anti-estrogen therapy, specifically tamoxifen, a new drug with few adverse effects that inhibits DNA synthesis. Tamoxifen is used in postmenopausal women and is most effective against estrogen receptor positive tumors. The success of these newer drug therapies, along with growing evidence that breast cancer is a systemic, not local, disease, has led to a decline in ablative surgery.

Clinical implications

To provide good care for a breast cancer patient, begin with a history; assess the patient's feelings about her illness, and determine what she knows about it and what she expects. Preoperatively, be sure you know what kind of surgery the patient will have, so you can prepare her properly. If a mastectomy is scheduled, in addition to the usual preoperative preparation (skin preparation, nothing by mouth), provide the following information:

• Teach the patient how to deep breathe and cough to prevent pulmonary problems.

• Instruct her to rotate her ankles to help prevent thromboembolism.

• Tell her she can ease her pain by lying on the affected side or by placing a hand or pillow on the incision.

• Preoperatively, show her where the incision will be. Inform her that she will receive pain medication and that she need not fear addiction. Remember, adequate pain relief encourages coughing and turning and promotes general well-being. A small pillow under the arm anteriorly provides comfort.

• Tell her that she may move about and get out of bed as soon as possible (even as soon as the anesthesia wears off or the first evening after surgery).

• Explain to her that after mastectomy, an incisional drain or some type of suction (Hemovac) is used to remove accumulated serous or sanguineous fluid and to keep the tension off the suture line, promoting healing.

In postoperative care, follow these guidelines.

• Inspect the dressing anteriorly and posteriorly, and report excessive bleeding promptly.

• Measure and record the amount and color of drainage. It is bloody during the first 4 hours and then becomes serous.

• Monitor circulatory status (blood pressure, pulse, respirations, bleeding).

• Monitor intake and output for at least

Postoperative Arm and Hand Care

Hand exercises for the patient who is prone to lymphedema can begin on the day of surgery. Plan arm exercises with the physician, because he can anticipate potential problems with the suture line.

• Have the patient open her hand and close it tightly six to eight times every 3 hours while she is awake.

• Elevate the arm on the affected side on a pillow above the heart level.

• Encourage the patient to wash her face and comb her hair—an effective exercise.

• Measure and record the circumference of the patient's arm 2¼" (6 cm) from her elbow. Indicate the exact place you measured. By remeasuring a month after surgery and at intervals during and following radiation therapy, you will be able to determine whether lymphedema is present. The patient may complain that her arm is heavy—an early sign of lymphedema.

• When the patient is home, she can elevate her arm and hand by supporting it on the back of a chair or a couch.

---

48 hours after general anesthesia.

• Prevent lymphedema of the arm, which may be an early complication of any breast cancer treatment that involves lymph node dissection. (See *Preventing Infection After Axillary Node Dissection or Radiation Therapy*, p. 93, and *Postoperative Arm and Hand Care*.) Such prevention is very important, because lymphedema cannot be treated effectively.

• Inspect the incision. Encourage the patient and her partner to look at her incision as soon as feasible—perhaps when the first dressing is removed.

• Advise the patient to ask her physician about reconstructive surgery or to call the local or state medical society for the names of plastic and reconstructive surgeons who regularly perform surgery to create breast mounds. Such reconstruction may be planned prior to the mastectomy.

• Instruct the patient about breast prostheses. The American Cancer Society's Reach to Recovery group can provide instruction, emotional support, and a list of area stores that sell prostheses.

• Give psychological and emotional support. Many patients react to the fear of cancer and to disfigurement, and worry about loss of sexual func-

tion. Explain that breast surgery does not interfere with sexual function and that the patient may resume sexual activity as soon as she desires after surgery. She may experience "phantom breast syndrome" (a phenomenon in which a tingling or a pins-and-needles sensation is felt in the area of the amputated breast tissue) or depression following mastectomy. Listen to the patient's concerns, offer support, and refer her to an appropriate organization, such as the American Cancer Society's Reach to Recovery—which offers group support to help breast cancer patients in the hospital and at home.

Bronchiectasis

Description

A condition marked by chronic abnormal dilation of bronchi and destruction of bronchial walls, bronchiectasis can occur throughout the tracheobronchial tree or can be confined to one segment or lobe. However, it is usually bilateral and involves the basilar segments of the lower lobes. This disease has three forms: cylindrical (fusiform), varicose, and saccular (cystic). (See *Forms of Bronchial Dilation.*) It affects people of both sexes and all ages. Because of the availability of antibiotics to treat acute respiratory tract infections, the incidence of bronchiectasis has dramatically decreased in the past 20 years. Bronchiectasis is irreversible.

Causes

This disease results from conditions associated with repeated damage to bronchial walls and abnormal mucociliary clearance, which cause a breakdown of supporting tissue adjacent to airways. Such conditions include the following.

• Mucoviscidosis (cystic fibrosis of the pancreas)

• Immunologic disorder (agammaglobulinemia, for example)

• Recurrent, inadequately treated bacterial respiratory tract infections, such as tuberculosis

• Measles, pneumonia, pertussis, or influenza

• Obstruction (by a foreign body, tumor, or stenosis) in association with recurrent infection

• Inhalation of corrosive gas or repeated aspiration of gastric juices into the lungs

• Congenital anomalies (uncommon)

Signs and symptoms

• Initially, bronchiectasis may be asymptomatic.

• The classic symptom is a chronic cough that produces copious, foul-smelling, mucopurulent secretions, possibly totaling several cupfuls daily.

• Characteristic findings include coarse rales during inspiration over involved lobes or segments, occasional wheezes, dyspnea, weight loss, malaise, clubbing, recurrent fever, chills, and other signs of infection.

Diagnostic tests

• Chest X-rays show peribronchial thickening, areas of atelectasis, and scattered cystic changes.

• Bronchography, the most reliable diagnostic test, reveals the location and extent of the disease.

• Bronchoscopy helps identify the source of secretions or the site of bleeding in hemoptysis.

• Sputum culture and Gram stain identify predominant organisms.

• Blood count checks for possible anemia and leukocytosis.

• Pulmonary function studies detect decreased vital capacity, decreased expiratory flow, and hypoxemia. These tests also help determine the physiologic severity of the disease and the effects of therapy, and help evaluate patients for surgery.

Treatment

Treatment includes antibiotics, given P.O. or I.V., for 7 to 10 days or until sputum production decreases. Bronchodilators, with postural drainage and chest percussion, help remove secretions if the patient has bronchospasm and thick, tenacious sputum. Bronchoscopy may occasionally be used to aid mobilization of secretions. Hypoxemia requires oxygen therapy. Severe hemoptysis often requires lobectomy or segmental resection.

Clinical implications

Throughout this illness, provide supportive care and help the patient adjust to the permanent changes in life-style that irreversible lung damage necessitates. Thorough patient teaching is vital.

• Administer antibiotics, as ordered, and explain all diagnostic tests. Perform chest physiotherapy, including postural drainage and chest percussion designed for involved lobes several times a day. The best times to do this are early morning and just before bedtime. Instruct the patient to maintain each position for 10 minutes, then perform percussion and tell him to cough. Show family members how to do postural drainage and percussion. Also teach the patient coughing and deep-breathing techniques to promote good

Forms of Bronchial Dilation

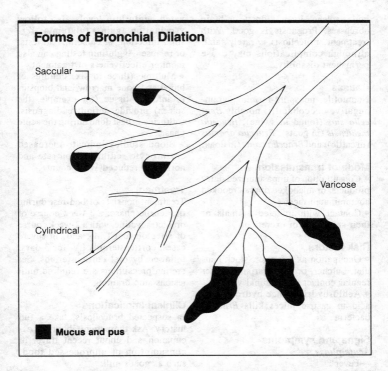

Saccular

Varicose

Cylindrical

■ Mucus and pus

ventilation and the removal of secretions.
• Advise the patient to stop smoking, since it stimulates secretions and irritates the airways. Refer the patient to a local self-help group.
• Provide a warm, quiet, comfortable environment, and urge the patient to rest as much as possible. Encourage balanced, high-protein meals to promote good health and tissue healing, and plenty of fluids to aid expectoration. Give frequent mouth care to remove foul-smelling sputum. Teach the patient to dispose of all secretions properly.
• Tell the patient to avoid air pollutants and people with upper respiratory tract infections. Instruct him to take medications (especially antibiotics) exactly as ordered.
• To help prevent this disease, vigor-

ously treat bacterial pneumonia and stress the need for immunization to prevent childhood diseases.

Complications
Advanced bronchiectasis may produce chronic malnutrition and amyloidosis, as well as right heart failure and cor pulmonale due to hypoxic pulmonary vasoconstriction.

Brucellosis
(Undulant fever, Malta fever)

Description
Brucellosis is an acute febrile illness transmitted to humans from animals. It is rarely found in the United States. Brucellosis causes fever, profuse sweating, anxiety, general aching, and

bone, spleen, liver, kidney, or brain abscesses. Prognosis is good. With treatment, brucellosis is rarely fatal, although complications may cause permanent disability.

Causes
Nonmotile, nonspore-forming, gram-negative coccobacilli, notably *Brucella suis* (found in swine), *Brucella melitensis* (in goats), *Brucella abortus* (in cattle), and *Brucella canis* (in dogs)

Mode of transmission
• Consumption of unpasteurized dairy products, or uncooked or undercooked contaminated meat
• Contact with infected animals or their secretions or excretions

Risk factors
• Occupation as a farmer, stock handler, butcher, or veterinarian or other regular contact with animal vectors
• Achlorhydria, since hydrochloric acid in gastric juices kills *Brucella* bacteria

Signs and symptoms
Acute phase
—Fever
—Chills
—Profuse sweating
—Fatigue
—Headache
—Backache
—Enlarged lymph nodes
—Hepatosplenomegaly
—Weight loss
Chronic phase
—Recurrent depression
—Sleep disturbances
—Fatigue
—Headache
—Sweating
—Sexual impotence
—Hepatosplenomegaly
—Enlarged lymph nodes

Diagnostic tests
• Agglutinin titers of 1:160 or more usually occur within 3 weeks of developing this disease. However, ele-

vated agglutinin levels also follow vaccination against tularemia, *Yersinia* infection, or cholera; skin tests; or relapse. Agglutinin testing can also monitor effectiveness of treatment.
• Multiple (three to six) cultures of blood and bone marrow, and biopsies of infected tissue (for example, the spleen) provide definitive diagnosis. Culturing is best done during the acute phase.
• Blood studies indicate increased erythrocyte sedimentation rate and normal or reduced WBC count.

Treatment
Treatment consists of bed rest during the febrile phase; a 3-week course of oral tetracycline, with a 2-week course of streptomycin I.M.; and, in severe cases, corticosteroids I.V. for 3 days, followed by oral corticosteroids. Secretion precautions are required until lesions stop draining.

Clinical implications
In suspected brucellosis, take a full history. Ask the patient about his occupation and about recent travel or consumption of unprocessed food, such as goat's milk.
• During the acute phase, monitor and record the patient's temperature every 4 hours. Be sure to use the same route (oral or rectal) every time. Ask the dietary department to provide between-meal milk shakes and other supplemental foods to counter weight loss. Watch for heart murmurs, muscle weakness, vision loss, and joint inflammation; all may point to complications.
• During the chronic phase, watch for depression and disturbed sleep patterns. Administer sedatives, as ordered, and plan care to allow adequate rest.
• Keep suppurative granulomas and abscesses dry. Double-bag and properly dispose of all secretions and soiled dressings. Give reassurance that this infection *is* curable.
• Before discharge, stress the impor-

tance of continuing medication for the prescribed duration. To prevent recurrence, advise patients to cook meat thoroughly and avoid using unpasteurized milk. Warn meat packers and other persons at risk of occupational exposure to wear rubber gloves and goggles.

Complications

- Abscess and granuloma formulation in subcutaneous tissues, lymph nodes, liver, spleen, and (in the chronic phase) in testes, ovaries, kidneys, and brain (meningitis and encephalitis)
- Osteomyelitis
- Orchitis
- Rarely, subacute bacterial endocarditis

Buerger's disease
(Thromboangiitis obliterans)

Description
Buerger's disease—an inflammatory, nonatheromatous occlusive condition—causes segmental lesions and subsequent thrombus formation in the small and medium arteries (and sometimes the veins), resulting in decreased blood flow to the feet and legs. This disorder may produce ulceration and eventually gangrene. Incidence is highest among men of Jewish ancestry, age 20 to 40, who smoke heavily.

Causes
Although the cause of Buerger's disease is unknown, a definite link exists to smoking, suggesting a hypersensitivity reaction to nicotine.

Signs and symptoms
- Intermittent claudication of the instep aggravated by exercise and relieved by rest
- During exposure to low temperature, the feet initially become cold, cyanotic, and numb; later, they redden, become hot, and tingle.
- Occasionally, Buerger's disease also affects the hands, possibly resulting in painful fingertip ulcerations.
- Other signs and symptoms may include impaired peripheral pulses, migratory superficial thrombophlebitis, and, in later stages, ulceration, muscle atrophy, and gangrene.

Diagnostic tests
- Doppler ultrasonography shows diminished circulation in the peripheral vessels.
- Plethysmography helps detect decreased circulation in the peripheral vessels.
- Arteriography locates lesions and rules out atherosclerosis.

Treatment and clinical implications
The primary goals of treatment are to relieve symptoms and prevent complications. Such therapy may include an exercise program that uses gravity to fill and drain the blood vessels or, in severe disease, a lumbar sympathectomy to increase blood supply to the skin. Amputation may be necessary for nonhealing ulcers, intractable pain, or gangrene.
- Strongly urge the patient to discontinue smoking permanently, to enhance the effectiveness of treatment. If necessary, refer him to a smoking cessation program.
- Warn the patient to avoid precipitating factors, such as emotional stress, exposure to extreme temperatures, and trauma.
- Teach proper foot care, especially the importance of wearing well-fitting shoes and cotton or wool socks. Show the patient how to inspect his feet daily for cuts, abrasions, and signs of skin breakdown, such as redness and soreness. Remind him to seek medical attention immediately after any trauma.
- If the patient has ulcers and gangrene, enforce bed rest and use a padded footboard or bed cradle to prevent pressure from bed linens. Protect the feet with soft padding. Wash them gently with a mild soap and tepid wa-

ter, rinse thoroughly, and pat dry with a soft towel.

• Provide emotional support. If necessary, refer the patient for psychological counseling to help him cope with restrictions imposed by this chronic disease. If he has undergone amputation, assess rehabilitative needs, especially regarding changes in body image. Refer him to physical therapists, occupational therapists, and social service agencies, as needed.

Bulimia

Description
Bulimia is marked by recurring episodes of eating binges followed by induced vomiting. Other essential features include an awareness that the binge-purge eating pattern is abnormal, a fear of inability to control eating binges, and depressed mood and self-deprecating thoughts after a binge-purge episode.

This disorder primarily affects females of young adult or adolescent age (generally slightly older than those with anorexia nervosa). Patients are commonly perceived by others as "perfect" students, mothers, or career women; an adolescent may be distinguished for participation in competitive activities, such as gymnastics, sports, or ballet. The weight loss in bulimia is rarely life-threatening. Bulimia is much less common, but tends to be more severe, in males.

Causes
The exact cause of bulimia is unknown, but various psychosocial factors are thought to contribute to its development. They include family disturbance or conflict, maladaptive learned behavior, struggle for control or self-identity, and cultural overemphasis on physical appearance. Recent psychiatric theory leans strongly toward considering bulimia a syndrome of depression.

Signs and symptoms
• Episodic binge eating that may occur as often as several times a day
• Induced vomiting (purging), which allows eating to continue until abdominal pain, sleep, or the presence of another person interrupts it
• Frequent weight fluctuations; weight usually stays within normal range through the use of diuretics, laxatives, vomiting, and exercise.
• Hyperactivity, peculiar eating habits or rituals, frequent weighing
• Distorted body image

Diagnostic tests
The typical bulimic eating pattern is rarely confused with any physical disorder. Laboratory tests may be needed to rule out hypokalemia and alkalosis associated with electrolyte imbalances or dehydration.

Treatment
The bulimic patient knows that her eating pattern is abnormal, but cannot control it. Therefore, treatment focuses on breaking the binge-purge cycle and helping the patient regain control over eating behavior. Treatment usually occurs in an outpatient setting. It includes behavior modification therapy, possibly in highly structured psychoeducational group meetings. Individual psychotherapy and family therapy, which address the eating disorder as a symptom of unresolved conflict, may also be used. Antidepressant drugs, such as imipramine, may be helpful because bulimia is often associated with depression. The patient may also benefit from participation in self-help groups such as Overeaters Anonymous.

Clinical implications
• Help the patient regain control over eating behavior by encouraging her to keep a daily record of everything she has eaten, to eat only at mealtimes and

only at the table, and to reduce her access to food by limiting choice or quantity.

• Help the patient develop more adaptive coping skills by encouraging her to recognize and verbalize feelings, by reinforcing realistic perceptions about weight and appearance, and by encouraging participation in the prescribed therapy program.

• Suggest to the patient and her family the American Anorexia/Bulimia Association, Inc., and Anorexia Nervosa and Associated Disorders (ANAD) as sources of additional information and community support.

Burns

Description
A major burn is a horrifying injury, necessitating painful treatment and a long period of rehabilitation. It is often fatal or permanently disfiguring and incapacitating (both emotionally and physically). In the United States, about 2 million persons annually suffer burns. Of these, 300,000 are burned seriously and over 6,000 are fatalities, making burns the nation's third greatest cause of accidental death.

Causes
Thermal burns (most common)
—Residential fires
—Motor vehicle accidents
—Playing with matches
—Improperly stored gasoline
—Space heater or electrical malfunctions
—Arson
—Improper handling of firecrackers
—Scalding accidents
—Kitchen accidents
—Parental abuse
Chemical burns
Contact with or ingestion, inhalation, or injection of acids, alkalis, or vesicants
Electrical burns
—Contact with faulty electrical wiring

or with high-voltage power lines
—Chewing of electric cords by young children
Friction or abrasion burns
Harsh rubbing of skin against a coarse surface
Sunburn
Excessive exposure to sunlight

Signs and symptoms
(See *Assessing Burns,* p. 102.)

Treatment and clinical implications
Immediate, aggressive burn treatment increases the patient's chance for survival. Later, supportive measures and strict aseptic technique can minimize infection. Because burns necessitate such comprehensive care, good nursing can make the difference between life and death.

If burns are minor, immerse the burned area in cool saline solution (55° F. [12.8° C.]) or apply cool compresses. Next, soak the wound in a mild antiseptic solution to cleanse it, and give pain medication, as ordered. Debride the devitalized tissue, taking care not to break any blisters. Cover the wound with an antimicrobial agent and a nonstick bulky dressing. Administer tetanus prophylaxis, as ordered. Provide aftercare instructions for the patient. Stress the importance of keeping the dressing dry and clean, elevating the burned extremity for the first 24 hours, taking analgesics as ordered, and returning for a wound check in 2 days.

In moderate and major burns, immediately assess the patient's airway, breathing, and circulation (ABC). Be especially alert for signs of smoke inhalation and pulmonary damage: singed nasal hairs, mucosal burns, voice changes, coughing, wheezing, soot in the mouth or nose, and darkened sputum. As ordered, assist with endotracheal intubation and administer 100% oxygen. With ABC assured, take a brief history of the burn. Draw blood samples for complete blood

Assessing Burns

One goal of assessment is to determine the *depth* of skin and tissue damage. A partial-thickness burn damages the epidermis and part of the dermis, while a full-thickness burn affects the epidermis, dermis, and subcutaneous tissue. However, a more traditional method gauges burn depth by degrees, although most burns are a combination of different degrees and thicknesses.

• *First degree*—Damage is limited to the epidermis, causing erythema and pain.

• *Second degree*—The epidermis and part of the dermis are damaged, producing blisters and mild-to-moderate edema and pain.

• *Third degree*—The epidermis and dermis are damaged. No blisters appear, but white, brown, or black leathery tissue and thrombosed vessels are visible.

• *Fourth degree*—Damage extends through deeply charred subcutaneous tissue to muscle and bone.

Another assessment goal is to estimate the *size* of a burn. This is usually expressed as the percentage of body surface area (BSA) covered by the burn. The Rule of Nines chart most commonly provides this estimate, although the Lund and Browder chart is more accurate, because it allows for BSA changes with age. A correlation of the burn's depth and size permits an estimate of its severity.

• *Major*—Third-degree burns on more than 10% of BSA; second-degree burns on more than 25% of adult BSA (more than 20% in children); burns of hands, face, feet, or genitalia; burns complicated by fractures or respiratory damage; electrical burns; all burns in poor-risk patients

• *Moderate*—Third-degree burns on 2% to 10% of BSA; second-degree burns on 15% to 25% of adult BSA (10% to 20% in children)

• *Minor*—Third-degree burns on less than 2% of BSA; second-degree burns on less than 15% of adult BSA (in children).

Here are other important factors in assessing burns:

• Location—Burns on the face, hands, feet, and genitalia are most serious, because of possible loss of function.

• Configuration—Circumferential burns can cause total occlusion of circulation in an extremity as a result of edema. Burns on the neck can produce airway obstruction, whereas burns on the chest can lead to restricted respiratory expansion.

• History of complicating medical problems—Note disorders that impair peripheral circulation, especially diabetes, peripheral vascular disease, and chronic alcohol abuse.

• Other injuries sustained at the time of the burn.

• Patient age—Victims under age 4 or over age 60 have a higher incidence of complications and, consequently, a higher mortality.

• Pulmonary injury can result from smoke inhalation.

count, electrolytes, glucose, blood urea nitrogen, creatinine, arterial blood gases, and typing and cross matching.

Control bleeding, and remove smoldering clothing (soak it first in saline solution if it is stuck to the patient's skin), rings, and other constricting items. Be sure to cover burns with a clean, dry, sterile bed sheet. (*Never* cover large burns with saline-soaked dressings, since they can drastically lower body temperature.)

Begin I.V. therapy immediately to prevent hypovolemic shock and maintain cardiac output. Use one of the following two formulas as a general guideline for the amount of fluid replacement the first 24 hours postburn. (Vary the specific infusions according to the patient's response, especially urinary output.)

• Baxter formula: 4 ml lactated Ringer's solution/kg/% BSA/24 hours. Give one half of the total amount over first 8 hours postburn and the remainder over next 16 hours.

• Brooke formula: Colloids (plasma, plasmanate, dextran) 0.5 ml/kg/% BSA + lactated Ringer's solution 1.5 ml/kg/% BSA + 2,000 ml dextrose in water for adults (less for children). Give one half of the total amount over the first 8 hours postburn and the remainder over the next 16 hours.

Closely monitor intake and output, and frequently check vital signs. Although it may make you nervous, do not be afraid to take the patient's blood pressure because of burned limbs.

In the hospital, a central venous pressure line and additional I.V. lines (using venous cutdown, if necessary), and an indwelling (Foley) catheter may be inserted. To combat fluid evaporation through the burn and the release of fluid into interstitial spaces (possibly resulting in hypovolemic shock), continue fluid therapy, as ordered.

Check vital signs every 15 minutes (the physician may insert an arterial line if blood pressure is unobtainable with a cuff). Send a urine specimen to the laboratory to check for myoglobinuria and hemoglobinuria.

Insert a nasogastric tube to decompress the stomach and avoid aspiration of stomach contents.

Electrical and chemical burns demand special attention. Tissue damage from electrical burns is difficult to assess, because internal destruction

---

Managing Burns with Skin Grafts

When a patient has a limited, well-defined burn, he may need a *temporary graft* to minimize fluid and protein loss from the burn surface, prevent infection, and reduce pain. Types of temporary grafts include the following:
• Allografts (homografts), which are usually cadaver skin
• Xenografts (heterografts), which are typically pigskin
• Biosynthetic grafts, which are a combination of collagen and synthetics
    To treat a full-thickness burn, a patient may need an *autograft*. This method uses the patient's own skin—usually a split-thickness graft—to replace the burned skin. For areas where appearance or joint movement is important, the autograft will be transplanted intact. In flat areas where appearance is less critical, the graft may be meshed (fenestrated) to cover up to three times its original size.
    When burns cover the entire body surface, a new method—the *test-tube skin graft*—may provide lifesaving treatment. In this method, a small full-thickness biopsy yields epidermal cells that are cultured into sheets and then grafted onto the burns. According to its developers, this smooth, supple test-tube skin represents a major advance in the treatment of extensive burns.

along the conduction pathway is usually greater than the surface burn would indicate. Electrical burns that ignite the patient's clothes may cause thermal burns as well. If the electric shock caused ventricular fibrillation and cardiac and respiratory arrest, begin cardiopulmonary resuscitation at once. Get an estimate of the voltage. (For more details, see "Electric Shock," p. 255.)

In a chemical burn, irrigate the wound with copious amounts of water or normal saline solution. Using a weak base ($NaHCO_3$) to neutralize hydrofluoric acid, hydrochloric acid, or sulfuric acid on skin or mucous membrane is controversial, particularly in the emergency phase, since the neutralizing agent can produce more heat and tissue damage.

If the chemical entered the patient's eyes, flush them with large amounts of water or saline solution for at least 30 minutes. In an alkali burn, irrigate until the pH of the cul-de-sacs returns to 7.0. Have the patient close his eyes, and cover them with a dry, sterile dressing. Note the type of chemical causing the burn and the presence of any noxious fumes. The patient will need an ophthalmologic examination.

Do not treat the burn wound itself in the emergency department if the patient is to be transferred to a specialized burn care unit within 4 hours after the burn. Instead, prepare the patient for transport by wrapping him in a sterile sheet and a blanket for warmth and elevating the burned extremity to decrease edema. Then, transport immediately. (For more information see *Managing Burns with Skin Grafts*, p. 103.)

C

Calcium imbalance

Description

Calcium plays an indispensable role in cell permeability, formation of bones and teeth, blood coagulation, transmission of nerve impulses, and normal muscle contraction. Nearly all (99%) of the body's calcium is found in the bones. The remaining 1% exists in ionized form in serum, and maintenance of that ionized calcium in the serum is critical to normal neurologic function. The parathyroid glands regulate ionized calcium and determine its resorption into bone, absorption from the gastrointestinal mucosa, and excretion in urine and feces. Severe calcium imbalance requires emergency treatment. A deficiency (hypocalcemia) can lead to tetany and convulsions. An excess (hypercalcemia) can lead to cardiac dysrhythmias.

Causes

Hypocalcemia

—Inadequate intake of calcium and vitamin D

—Hypoparathyroidism. Injury, disease, or surgery may decrease or eliminate secretion of parathyroid hormone (PTH), which is necessary for calcium absorption and normal serum calcium levels.

—Malabsorption or loss of calcium from the gastrointestinal tract may result from increased intestinal motility due to severe diarrhea or laxative abuse. Malabsorption of calcium can also result from inadequate levels of vitamin D or PTH, or from a reduction in gastric acidity, decreasing the solubility of calcium salts.

—Severe infections or burns, in which diseased and burned tissue traps calcium from the extracellular fluid

—Overcorrection of acidosis, resulting in alkalosis, which decreases ionized calcium and induces symptoms of hypocalcemia

—Pancreatic insufficiency, which may cause malabsorption of calcium and subsequent calcium loss in feces. In pancreatitis, participation of calcium ions in saponification contributes to calcium loss.

—Renal failure, resulting in excessive excretion of calcium secondary to increased retention of phosphate

—Hypomagnesemia, which causes decreased PTH secretion and blocks the peripheral action of that hormone

Hypercalcemia

—Hyperparathyroidism, which increases serum calcium levels by promoting calcium absorption from the intestine, resorption from bone, and reabsorption from the kidneys

—Hypervitaminosis D can promote increased absorption of calcium from the intestine.

—Tumors raise serum calcium levels by destroying bone or by releasing PTH or a PTH-like substance, osteoclast-activating factor, prostaglandins, and perhaps, a vitamin D-like sterol.

—Multiple fractures and prolonged immobilization release bone calcium and raise the serum calcium level.

—Multiple myeloma promotes loss of calcium from bone.
—Milk-alkali syndrome
—Sarcoidosis
—Hyperthyroidism
—Adrenal insufficiency
—Thiazide diuretics
—Loss of serum albumin secondary to renal disease

Signs and symptoms
Hypocalcemia
—Perioral paresthesia
—Twitching
—Carpopedal spasm
—Tetany
—Seizures
—Possible laryngospasm
—Possible dysrhythmias
—Chvostek's sign
—Trousseau's sign
(See *Chvostek's and Trousseau's Signs*, p. 107.)
Hypercalcemia
—Muscle weakness
—Decreased muscle tone
—Lethargy
—Anorexia
—Constipation
—Nausea
—Vomiting
—Depression or apathy
—Polydipsia
—Polyuria
—When severe, dysrhythmias, coma, cardiac arrest

Diagnostic tests
• A serum calcium level less than 4.5 mEq/liter confirms hypocalcemia.
• A serum calcium level above 5.5 mEq/liter confirms hypercalcemia. (Since approximately half of serum calcium is bound to albumin, however, changes in serum protein must be considered when interpreting serum calcium levels.)
• Sulkowitch's urine test shows increased calcium precipitation in hypercalcemia.
• EKG reveals lengthened QT interval, prolonged ST segment, and dysrhythmias in hypocalcemia; and

shortened QT interval and heart block in hypercalcemia.

Treatment
Treatment varies and requires correction of acute imbalance, followed by maintenance therapy and correction of the underlying cause. Mild hypocalcemia may require nothing more than dietary adjustment to allow adequate intake of calcium, vitamin D, and protein, possibly with oral calcium supplements. Acute hypocalcemia is an emergency that needs immediate correction by I.V. administration of calcium gluconate or calcium chloride. Chronic hypocalcemia also requires vitamin D supplements to facilitate gastrointestinal absorption of calcium.

Treatment of hypercalcemia primarily eliminates excess serum calcium through hydration with normal saline solution, which promotes calcium excretion in urine. Loop diuretics, such as ethacrynic acid and furosemide, also promote calcium excretion. (Thiazide diuretics are contraindicated in hypercalcemia, because they inhibit calcium excretion.) Corticosteroids, such as prednisone and hydrocortisone, are helpful in treating sarcoidosis, hypervitaminosis D, and certain tumors. Plicamycin can also lower serum calcium level and is especially effective against hypercalcemia secondary to certain tumors. Calcitonin may also be helpful in certain instances. Sodium phosphate solution administererd P.O. or by retention enema promotes deposition of calcium in bone and inhibits its absorption from the gastrointestinal tract.

Clinical implications
• Watch for hypocalcemia in patients receiving massive transfusions of citrated blood and in those with chronic diarrhea, severe infections, and insufficient dietary intake of calcium and protein (especially the elderly).
• Monitor serum calcium levels every 12 to 24 hours, and report a calcium

level less than 4.5 mEq/liter immediately. When giving calcium supplements, frequently check pH, since an alkalotic state that exceeds 7.45 pH inhibits calcium ionization. Check for Trousseau's and Chvostek's signs.

• Administer calcium gluconate by slow I.V. infusion in 5% dextrose in water (*never* in saline solution, which encourages renal calcium loss). Do not add calcium gluconate to I.V. solutions containing bicarbonate; it will precipitate. When administering calcium solutions, watch for anorexia, nausea, and vomiting—possible signs of overcorrection of hypercalcemia.

• If the patient is receiving calcium chloride, watch for abdominal discomfort.

• Monitor the patient closely for a possible drug interaction if he is receiving digitalis with large doses of oral calcium supplements. Watch for signs of digitalis toxicity (anorexia, nausea, vomiting, yellow vision, cardiac dysrhythmias). Administer oral calcium supplements 1 to 1½ hours after meals or with milk.

• Provide a quiet, stress-free environment for the patient with tetany. Observe seizure precautions for patients with severe hypocalcemia, which may lead to convulsions.

• To prevent hypocalcemia, advise all patients—especially the elderly—to eat foods rich in calcium, vitamin D, and protein, such as fortified milk and cheese. Explain how important calcium is for normal bone formation and blood coagulation. Also discourage chronic use of laxatives.

If the patient has hypercalcemia, follow these guidelines.

• Monitor serum calcium levels frequently. Watch for cardiac dysrhythmias if serum calcium level exceeds 5.7 mEq/liter. Increase fluid intake to dilute calcium in serum and urine and to prevent renal damage and dehydration. Watch for signs of congestive heart failure in patients receiving normal saline solution diuresis therapy.

• Administer loop diuretics (not thia-

Chvostek's and Trousseau's Signs

To check for Chvostek's sign, tap the facial nerve above the mandibular angle, adjacent to the earlobe. A facial muscle spasm that causes the patient's upper lip to twitch confirms tetany.

To check for Trousseau's sign, apply a blood pressure cuff to the patient's arm. A carpopedal spasm that causes thumb adduction and phalangeal extension confirms tetany.

---

zide diuretics), as ordered. Monitor intake and output, and check urine for renal calculi and acidity. Provide acid-ash drinks, such as cranberry or prune juice, since calcium salts are more soluble in acid than in alkali.

• Check EKG and vital signs frequently.

• Encourage ambulation as soon as possible. Handle the patient with chronic hypercalcemia *gently* to prevent pathologic fractures. If the patient is bedridden, reposition him frequently, and encourage range-of-motion exercises to promote circulation and prevent urinary stasis and calcium loss from bone.

• To prevent recurrence, suggest a low-calcium diet, with increased fluid intake.

Candidiasis
(Candidosis, moniliasis)

Description

Candidiasis is usually a mild, superficial fungal infection. Rarely, fungi enter the bloodstream and invade the kidneys, lungs, endocardium, brain, or other structures, causing serious infections. Such systemic infection is most prevalent among drug addicts and patients already hospitalized, particularly diabetic and immunosuppressed patients. Prognosis varies and depends on the patient's resistance.

Causes

• Most cases of *Candida* infection result from *Candida albicans* and *Candida tropicalis*.

• Other infective strains include *Candida parapsilosis* (cutaneous infection, endocarditis) and *Candida guillermondi* (endocarditis).

Risk factors

• Broad-spectrum antibiotic therapy (most common)
• Diabetes mellitus
• Carcinoma
• Immunosuppressive drug therapy
• Radiation therapy
• Aging
• Drug abuse
• I.V. therapy
• Hyperalimentation
• Urinary catheterization

Signs and symptoms

Superficial candidiasis

—Skin: Scaly, erythematous, papular rash, sometimes covered with exudate, appearing below the breast, between fingers, and at the axillae, groin, and umbilicus. In diaper rash, papules appear at the edges of the rash.

—Nails: Red, swollen, darkened nail bed; occasionally, purulent discharge and separation of a pruritic nail from the nail bed

—Oropharyngeal mucosa (thrush): Cream-colored or bluish white patches of exudate on the tongue, mouth, or pharynx that reveal bloody engorgement when scraped. These may swell, causing respiratory distress in infants. They are only occasionally painful but cause a burning sensation in the throats and mouths of adults.

—Esophageal mucosa: Dysphagia, retrosternal pain, regurgitation, and, occasionally, scales in the mouth and throat

—Vaginal mucosa: White or yellow discharge, with pruritus and local excoriation; white or gray raised patches on vaginal walls, with local inflammation; dyspareunia

Systemic candidiasis

—General: Chills; high, spiking fever; hypotension; prostration; and occasional rash

—Pulmonary: Hemoptysis, cough, fever

—Renal: Fever, flank pain, dysuria, hematuria, pyuria

—Brain: Headache, nuchal rigidity, seizures, focal neurologic deficits

—Endocardium: Systolic or diastolic murmur, fever, chest pain

—Eye: Endophthalmitis, blurred vision, orbital or periorbital pain, scotoma, and exudate

Diagnostic tests

• Gram stain of skin, vaginal scrapings, pus, or sputum gives evidence of *Candida* and diagnoses superficial candidiasis.

• Skin scrapings prepared in potassium hydroxide solution can also diagnose superficial infection.

• Blood or tissue culture specimen is needed to diagnose systemic infections.

Treatment

Treatment first aims to improve the underlying condition that predisposes the patient to candidiasis, such as controlling diabetes or discontinuing antibiotic therapy and catheterization, if possible. Nystatin is an effective antifungal for superficial candidiasis. Topical amphotericin B is effective for candidiasis of the skin and nails; so is gentian violet, which is also effective for thrush and vaginal infections but is rarely used because it stains the skin. Clotrimazole and miconazole are effective in mucous membrane and vaginal *Candida* infections. Ketoconazole is the treatment of choice for chronic candidiasis of the mucous membranes. Treatment for systemic infection consists of I.V. amphotericin B, flucyto-sine, or miconazole.

Clinical implications

• Instruct a patient using nystatin solution to swish it around his mouth for several minutes before swallowing. Swab nystatin on the oral mucosa of an infant with thrush. Provide a non-irritating mouthwash to loosen tenacious secretions and a soft toothbrush to avoid irritation. Relieve mouth discomfort with a topical anesthetic, such as lidocaine, at least 1 hour before meals. (It may suppress the gag reflex and cause aspiration.)
• Provide a soft diet for the patient with severe dysphagia. Tell the patient with mild dysphagia to chew food thoroughly.
• Use cornstarch or dry padding in intertriginous areas of obese patients to prevent irritation.
• Note dates of insertion of I.V. catheters, and replace them according to institutional policy, to prevent phlebitis.
• Assess the patient with candidiasis for underlying systemic causes, such as diabetes mellitus. If the patient is receiving amphotericin B for systemic candidiasis, he may have severe chills, fever, anorexia, nausea, and vomiting. Premedicate with aspirin, antihistamines, or antiemetics to help reduce adverse effects.
• Frequently check vital signs of patients with systemic infections. Provide appropriate supportive care. In patients with renal involvement, carefully monitor intake and output, and urine blood and protein.
• Daily check high-risk patients, especially those receiving antibiotics, for patchy areas, irritation, sore throat, bleeding of mouth or gums, or other signs of superinfection. Check for vaginal discharge; record color and amount.
• Encourage women in their third trimester of pregnancy to be examined for vaginal candidiasis to protect their infants from infection at birth.

Cardiac tamponade

Description

In cardiac tamponade, a rapid, unchecked rise in intrapericardial pressure impairs diastolic filling of the heart. The rise in pressure usually results from blood or fluid accumulation in the pericardial sac. If fluid accumulates rapidly, this condition is commonly fatal and requires emergency lifesaving measures. Slow accumulation and rise in pressure, as in pericardial effusion associated with malignancies, may not produce immediate symptoms, since the fibrous wall of the pericardial sac can gradually stretch to accommodate as much as 1 to 2 liters of fluid.

Causes

• Idiopathic (Dressler's syndrome)
• Effusion (in malignancy, bacterial infections, tuberculosis, and, rarely, acute rheumatic fever)
• Hemorrhage from trauma (such as gunshot or stab wounds of the chest, perforation by catheter, or cardiac surgery)
• Hemorrhage from nontraumatic causes (such as rupture of the heart or great vessels, or anticoagulant therapy in a patient with pericarditis)
• Acute myocardial infarction
• Uremia

Signs and symptoms

Classic
—Neck vein distention
—Reduced arterial blood pressure
—Muffled heart sounds on auscultation
—Pulsus paradoxus (an abnormal inspiratory drop in systemic blood pressure greater than 15 mm Hg)
Others
—Possible dyspnea
—Tachycardia
—Narrow pulse pressure
—Restlessness
—Hepatomegaly

Diagnostic tests

• Chest X-ray shows slightly widened mediastinum and cardiomegaly.

• EKG is rarely diagnostic of tamponade but is useful to rule out other cardiac disorders. It may reveal changes produced by acute pericarditis.

• Pulmonary artery catheterization detects increased right atrial pressure, right ventricular diastolic pressure, and central venous pressure.

• Echocardiography records pericardial effusion with signs of right ventricular and atrial compression.

Treatment

The goal of treatment is to relieve intrapericardial pressure and cardiac compression by removing accumulated blood or fluid. Pericardiocentesis (needle aspiration of the pericardial cavity) or surgical creation of an opening dramatically improves systemic arterial pressure and cardiac output with aspiration of as little as 25 ml of fluid. Such treatment necessitates continuous hemodynamic and EKG monitoring in the intensive care unit. Trial volume loading with temporary I.V. normal saline solution with albumin, and perhaps an inotropic drug, such as isoproterenol or dopamine, is necessary in the hypotensive patient to maintain cardiac output. Although these drugs normally improve myocardial function, they may further compromise an ischemic myocardium after myocardial infarction.

Depending on the cause of tamponade, additional treatment may include the following:

• In traumatic injury, blood transfusion or a thoracotomy to drain reaccumulating fluid or to repair bleeding sites

• In heparin-induced tamponade, the heparin antagonist protamine sulfate

• In warfarin-induced tamponade, vitamin K

Clinical implications

If the patient needs pericardiocentesis, follow these guidelines:

• Explain the procedure to the patient. Keep a pericardial aspiration needle attached to a 50-ml syringe by a three-way stopcock, an EKG machine, and an emergency cart with a defibrillator at the bedside. Make sure equipment is turned on and ready for immediate use. Position the patient at a 45- to 60-degree angle. Connect the precordial EKG lead to the hub of the aspiration needle with an alligator clamp and connecting wire, and assist with fluid aspiration. When the needle touches the myocardium, you will see an ST-segment elevation or premature ventricular contractions.

• Monitor blood pressure and central venous pressure (CVP) during and after pericardiocentesis. Infuse I.V. solutions, as ordered, to maintain blood pressure. Watch for a decrease in CVP and a concomitant rise in blood pressure, which indicate relief of cardiac compression.

• Watch for complications of pericardiocentesis, such as ventricular fibrillation, vagovagal arrest, or coronary artery or cardiac chamber puncture. Closely monitor EKG changes, blood pressure, pulse rate, level of consciousness, and urine output.

If the patient needs thoracotomy, follow these guidelines:

• Explain the procedure to the patient. Tell him what to expect postoperatively (chest tubes, drainage bottles, administration of oxygen). Teach him how to turn, deep-breathe, and cough.

• Give antibiotics, protamine sulfate, or vitamin K, as ordered.

• Postoperatively, monitor critical factors such as vital signs and arterial blood gases, and assess heart and breath sounds. Give pain medication, as ordered. Maintain the chest drainage system, and be alert for complications such as hemorrhage and dysrhythmias.

Cardiogenic shock

Description
Sometimes called pump failure, cardiogenic shock is a condition of diminished cardiac output that severely impairs tissue perfusion. It reflects severe left ventricular failure and occurs as a serious complication in nearly 15% of all patients hospitalized with acute myocardial infarction (MI). Cardiogenic shock typically affects patients whose area of infarction exceeds 40% of muscle mass. In such patients, mortality may exceed 85%. Most patients with cardiogenic shock die within 24 hours of onset. Prognosis for those who survive is extremely poor.

Causes
Cardiogenic shock can result from any condition that causes significant left ventricular dysfunction with reduced cardiac output, including the following:
• Myocardial infarction (most common)
• Myocardial ischemia
• Papillary muscle dysfunction
• End-stage cardiomyopathy

Signs and symptoms
• Cold, pale, clammy skin
• A drop in systolic blood pressure to 30 mm Hg below baseline, or a sustained reading below 80 mm Hg not attributable to medication
• Tachycardia
• Rapid, shallow respirations
• Oliguria (less than 20 ml urine/hour)
• Restlessness
• Mental confusion and obtundation
• Narrowing pulse pressure
• Cyanosis
• Gallop rhythm and faint heart sounds on auscultation
• A holosystolic murmur, if shock results from ventricular septum or papillary muscle rupture

Diagnostic tests
• Pulmonary artery pressure monitoring shows increased pulmonary artery pressure (PAP) and increased pulmonary capillary wedge pressure (PCWP), reflecting a rise in left ventricular end-diastolic pressure (preload) and increased resistance to left ventricular emptying (afterload) caused by ineffective pumping and increased peripheral vascular resistance. Thermodilution technique measures decreased cardiac index (less than 2.2 liters/minute).
• Invasive arterial pressure monitoring reveals hypotension from impaired ventricular ejection.
• Arterial blood gases may show metabolic acidosis and hypoxia.
• EKG may show evidence of acute MI, ischemia, or ventricular aneurysm.
• Elevated enzyme levels (creatine phosphokinase [CPK], lactate dehydrogenase [LDH], serum glutamic-oxaloacetic transaminase [SGOT], and serum glutamic-pyruvic transaminase [SGPT]) point to myocardial infarction or ischemia and suggest congestive heart failure or shock. CPK and LDH isoenzyme determinations may confirm acute myocardial infarction.

Treatment
Treatment aims to enhance cardiovascular status by increasing cardiac output, improving myocardial perfusion, and decreasing cardiac workload with various cardiovascular drugs and mechanical-assist techniques. Drug therapy may include dopamine I.V., a vasopressor that increases cardiac output, blood pressure, and renal blood flow; norepinephrine, a more potent vasoconstrictor; and nitroprusside I.V., a vasodilator that may be used with a vasopressor to further improve cardiac output by decreasing peripheral vascular resistance (afterload) and reducing left ventricular end-diastolic pressure (preload). However, the patient's blood pressure must be adequate to support nitroprusside therapy and must be monitored closely.

The intra-aortic balloon pump (IABP) is a mechanical-assist device that attempts to improve coronary artery perfusion and decrease cardiac workload. The inflatable balloon pump is surgically inserted through the femoral artery into the descending thoracic aorta. The balloon inflates during diastole to increase coronary artery perfusion pressure and deflates before systole (before the aortic valve opens) to reduce resistance to ejection (afterload) and therefore lessen cardiac workload. Improved ventricular ejection, which significantly improves cardiac output, and a subsequent vasodilation in the peripheral vasculature lead to lower preload volume.

When drug therapy and IABP insertion fail, treatment may require an experimental device—the ventricular assist pump or the artificial heart.

Clinical Implications

• At the first sign of cardiogenic shock, check the patient's blood pressure and heart rate. If the patient is hypotensive or is having difficulty breathing, make sure he has a patent I.V. line and a patent airway, and provide oxygen to promote tissue oxygenation. Notify the physician immediately.

• Monitor arterial blood gases to measure oxygenation and detect acidosis from poor tissue perfusion. Increase oxygen flow as indicated by blood gas measurements. Check complete blood count (CBC) and electrolytes.

• After diagnosis, monitor cardiac rhythm continuously. Assess skin color, temperature, and other vital signs often. Watch for a drop in systolic blood pressure to less than 80 mm Hg (usually compromising cardiac output further). Report hypotension immediately.

• An indwelling (Foley) catheter may be inserted to measure urine output. Notify the physician if output drops below 30 ml/hour.

• Using a pulmonary artery catheter, closely monitor PAP, PCWP, and, if equipment is available, cardiac output. A high PCWP indicates congestive heart failure and should be reported immediately.

• When a patient is on the IABP, reposition him often and perform passive range-of-motion exercises to prevent skin breakdown. However, do not flex the patient's "ballooned" leg at the hip, since this may displace or fracture the catheter. Assess pedal pulses and skin temperature and color to make sure circulation to the leg is adequate. Check the dressing on the insertion site frequently for bleeding, and change it according to institutional policy. Also, check the site for hematoma or signs of infection, and culture any drainage.

• After the patient has become hemodynamically stable, the frequency of balloon inflation is gradually reduced to wean him from the IABP. During weaning, watch for monitor changes, chest pain, and other signs of recurring cardiac ischemia and shock.

• Provide psychological support. Because the patient and family may be anxious about the intensive care unit and about the IABP and other tubes and devices, offer reassurance. To ease emotional stress, plan your care to allow the patient frequent rest periods, and provide for privacy.

Cardiomyopathy, dilated

Description

Dilated cardiomyopathy results from extensively damaged myocardial muscle fibers, although the exact causes are poorly understood. This disorder interferes with myocardial metabolism and grossly dilates the ventricles without proportional compensatory hypertrophy, causing the heart to take on a globular shape and to contract poorly during systole. Dilated cardiomyopathy leads to intractable congestive heart failure, dysrhythmias, and emboli. Since this disease is usually not diagnosed until it is in the advanced stages, prognosis is usually poor.

Causes
Primary
—Unknown
Secondary
The mechanism whereby the following conditions induce cardiac damage is unknown, and there is no evidence of a direct cause-and-effect relationship:
—Alcoholism
—Viral infections
—Muscle disorders such as myasthenia gravis and progressive muscular dystrophy
—Infiltrative disorders such as hemo-chromatosis and amyloidosis
—Sarcoidosis
—Endocrine disorders such as hyperthyroidism and pheochromocytoma
—Nutritional disorders such as thiamine deficiency and kwashiorkor (protein deficiency)
—Pregnancy, especially in multiparous women over age 30 with pre-eclampsia or malnutrition

Signs and symptoms
• Shortness of breath
• Orthopnea
• Dyspnea on exertion
• Paroxysmal nocturnal dyspnea
• Fatigue
• Irritating dry cough at night
• Edema

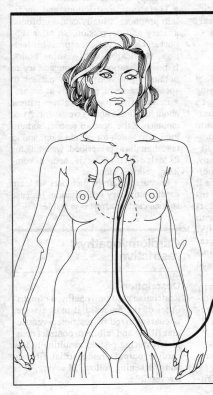

Intraaortic Balloon Pump

An effective method of reducing myocardial oxygen consumption, the intra-aortic balloon pump approximates the action of the heart in response to an EKG signal. It inflates during ventricular diastole, displacing blood proximally and increasing coronary artery perfusion. It deflates before systole, decreasing aortic pressure and resistance to ventricular flow. The end result is decreased ventricular workload.

- Liver engorgement
- Jugular venous distention
- Peripheral cyanosis
- Possible sinus tachycardia or atrial fibrillation
- Diffuse apical impulses
- Pansystolic murmur (mitral and tricuspid regurgitation secondary to cardiomegaly and weak papillary muscles)
- S_3 and S_4 gallop rhythms

Diagnostic tests
No single test confirms dilated cardiomyopathy.
- EKG and angiography rule out ischemic heart disease. EKG may also show biventricular hypertrophy, sinus tachycardia, atrial enlargement, and, in 20% of patients, atrial fibrillation.
- Chest X-ray demonstrates cardiomegaly (usually affecting all heart chambers), pulmonary congestion, or pleural effusion.

Treatment
In dilated cardiomyopathy, the goal of treatment is to correct the underlying causes and to improve the heart's pumping ability with digitalis, diuretics, oxygen, and a restricted-sodium diet. Therapy may also include prolonged bed rest, selective use of steroids, and, possibly, pericardiotomy, which is still investigational. Vasodilators reduce preload and afterload, thereby decreasing congestion and increasing cardiac output. Acute heart failure necessitates vasodilation with nitroprusside I.V. or nitroglycerin I.V. Long-term treatment may include prazosin, hydralazine, isosorbide dinitrate, and, if the patient is on prolonged bed rest, anticoagulants.

When these treatments fail, therapy may require a heart transplant for carefully selected patients. (Also see *Intra-aortic Balloon Pump*, p. 113.)

Clinical implications
In the patient with acute heart failure, follow these guidelines:
- Monitor for signs of progressive failure (decreased arterial pulses, increased neck vein distention) and compromised renal perfusion (oliguria, increased blood urea nitrogen [BUN] and serum creatinine levels, electrolyte imbalances). Weigh the patient daily.
- If the patient is receiving vasodilators, check blood pressure and heart rate frequently. If he becomes hypotensive, stop the infusion and place him supine, with legs elevated to increase venous return and to ensure cerebral blood flow.
- If the patient is receiving diuretics, monitor for signs of resolving congestion (decreased crackles and dyspnea) or too-vigorous diuresis. Check serum potassium for hypokalemia, especially if therapy includes digitalis.
- Therapeutic restrictions and uncertain prognosis usually cause profound anxiety and depression, so offer support and let the patient express his feelings. Be flexible with visiting hours. If hospitalization is prolonged, try to obtain permission for the patient to spend occasional weekends at home.
- Before discharge, teach the patient about his illness and its treatment. Also, emphasize the need to restrict sodium intake, to watch for weight gain, and to take digitalis as prescribed, watching for its toxic effects (anorexia, nausea, vomiting, yellow vision).
- Encourage family members to learn cardiopulmonary resuscitation, because sudden cardiac arrest is possible.

Cardiomyopathy, restrictive

Description
Restrictive cardiomyopathy, a rare disorder of the myocardial musculature, is characterized by restricted ventricular filling and failure to contract completely during systole, resulting in low cardiac output. Endocardial fibrosis and thickening follow. If severe, it is irreversible.

Causes
Primary restrictive cardiomyopathy
—Unknown
Restrictive cardiomyopathy syndrome
In amyloidosis, infiltration of amyloid into the intracellular spaces in the myocardium, endocardium, and subendocardium

Signs and symptoms
• Fatigue
• Dyspnea
• Orthopnea
• Chest pain
• Generalized edema
• Liver engorgement
• Peripheral cyanosis
• Pallor
• S_3 or S_4 gallop rhythms

Diagnostic tests
• In advanced stages of this disease, chest X-ray shows massive cardiomegaly, affecting all four chambers of the heart.
• Echocardiography rules out constrictive pericarditis as the cause of restricted filling by detecting increased left ventricular muscle mass and differences in end-diastolic pressures between the ventricles.
• EKG may show low-voltage complexes, hypertrophy, or atrioventricular conduction defects.
• Arterial pulsation reveals blunt carotid upstroke with small volume.
• Cardiac catheterization demonstrates increased left ventricular end-diastolic pressure and rules out constrictive pericarditis as the cause of restricted filling.

Treatment
Although no therapy currently exists for restricted ventricular filling, digitalis, diuretics, and a restricted-sodium diet ease symptoms of congestive heart failure.

Oral vasodilators—such as isosorbide dinitrate, prazosin, and hydralazine—may control intractable congestive heart failure. Anticoagulant therapy may be necessary to prevent thrombophlebitis in the patient on prolonged bed rest.

Clinical implications
• In the acute phase, monitor heart rate and rhythm, blood pressure, urine output, and pulmonary artery pressure readings to help guide treatment.
• Give psychological support. Provide appropriate diversionary activities for the patient restricted to prolonged bed rest. Since a poor prognosis may cause profound anxiety and depression, be especially supportive and understanding, and encourage the patient to express his fears. Refer him for psychosocial counseling, as necessary, for assistance in coping with his restricted life-style. Be flexible with visiting hours whenever possible.
• Before discharge, teach the patient to watch for and report signs of digoxin toxicity (anorexia, nausea, vomiting, yellow vision); to record and report weight gain; and, if sodium restriction is ordered, to avoid canned foods, pickles, smoked meats, and excessive use of table salt.

Carpal tunnel syndrome

Description
Carpal tunnel syndrome, the most common of the nerve entrapment syndromes, results from compression of the median nerve at the wrist, within the carpal tunnel (formed by the carpal bones and the transverse carpal ligament). The median nerve, along with blood vessels and flexor tendons, passes through this tunnel to the fingers and thumb. Compression neuropathy causes sensory and motor changes in the median distribution of the hand.

Carpal tunnel syndrome usually occurs in women between ages 30 and 60 and poses a serious occupational health problem. Assembly-line workers and packers and persons who repeatedly use poorly designed tools are most likely to develop this disorder.

Any strenuous use of the hands—sustained grasping, twisting, or flexing—aggravates this condition.

Causes

• Many conditions can cause the contents or structure of the carpal tunnel to swell and press the median nerve against the transverse carpal ligament. Such conditions include rheumatoid arthritis, flexor tenosynovitis (often associated with rheumatic disease), nerve compression, pregnancy, renal failure, menopause, diabetes mellitus, acromegaly, edema following Colles' fracture, hypothyroidism, amyloidosis, myxedema, benign tumors, tuberculosis, and other granulomatous diseases.

• Another source of damage to the median nerve is dislocation or acute sprain of the wrist.

Signs and symptoms

• Weakness, pain, burning, numbness, or tingling in one or both hands. This paresthesia affects the thumb, forefinger, middle finger, and half of the fourth finger.

• Inability to clench the hand into a fist

• Nail atrophy

• Dry, shiny skin

• Pain possibly spreading to the forearm and, in severe cases, as far as the shoulder

• Decreased sensation to light touch or pinpricks in the affected fingers

Diagnostic tests

• Tinel's sign (tingling over the median nerve on light percussion) is present.

• Positive response to Phalen's wrist-flexion test (holding the forearms vertically and allowing both hands to drop into complete flexion at the wrists for 1 minute) reproduces symptoms of carpal tunnel syndrome.

• A compression test supports the diagnosis: A blood pressure cuff inflated above systolic pressure on the forearm for 1 to 2 minutes provokes pain and paresthesia along the distribution of the median nerve.

• Electromyography detects a median nerve motor conduction delay of more than 5 milliseconds.

• Other laboratory tests may identify underlying disease.

Treatment

Conservative treatment should be tried first, including resting the hands by splinting the wrist in neutral extension for 1 to 2 weeks. If a definite link has been established between the patient's occupation and the development of carpal tunnel syndrome, he may have to seek other work. Effective treatment may also require correction of an underlying disorder. When conservative treatment fails, the only alternative is surgical decompression of the nerve by sectioning the entire transverse carpal tunnel ligament. Neurolysis (freeing of the nerve fibers) may also be necessary.

Clinical implications

• Administer mild analgesics, as needed. Encourage the patient to use his hands as much as possible; however, if the condition has impaired the dominant hand, you may have to help with eating and bathing.

• Teach the patient how to apply a splint. Tell him not to make it too tight. Show him how to remove the splint to perform gentle range-of-motion exercises, which should be done daily. Make sure the patient knows how to do these exercises before he is discharged.

• After surgery, monitor vital signs, and regularly check the color, sensation, and motion of the affected hand.

• Advise the patient who is about to be discharged to occasionally exercise his hands in warm water. If the arm is in a sling, tell him to remove the sling several times a day to do exercises for his elbow and shoulder.

• Suggest occupational counseling for the patient who has to change jobs because of carpal tunnel syndrome.

Cataract

Description

A common cause of vision loss, a cataract is a gradually developing opacity of the lens or lens capsule of the eye. Cataracts commonly occur bilaterally, with each progressing independently. Exceptions are traumatic cataracts, which are usually unilateral, and congenital cataracts, which may remain stationary. Cataracts are most prevalent in persons over age 70, as part of aging. Prognosis is generally good. Surgery improves vision in 95% of affected persons.

Causes

• Senile cataracts develop in the elderly, probably because of changes in the chemical state of lens proteins.

• Congenital cataracts occur in newborns as genetic defects or as a result of maternal rubella during the first trimester.

• Traumatic cataracts develop after a foreign body injures the lens with sufficient force to allow aqueous or vitreous humor to enter the lens capsule.

• Complicated cataracts occur secondary to uveitis, glaucoma, retinitis pigmentosa, or detached retina. They may also occur in the course of a systemic disease such as diabetes, hypoparathyroidism, or atopic dermatitis, and they can result from ionizing radiation or infrared rays.

• Toxic cataracts result from drug or chemical toxicity with ergot, dinitrophenol, naphthalene, and phenothiazines. They result from galactose in patients with galactosemia.

Signs and symptoms

• Painless, gradual blurring and loss of vision

• With progression, whitening of the pupil

• Other possible symptoms: Appearance of halos around lights, blinding glare from headlights at night, and glare and poor vision in bright sunlight

Diagnostic tests

• Shining a penlight on the pupil reveals the white area behind it (unnoticeable until the cataract is advanced) and suggests a cataract.

• Ophthalmoscopy or slit-lamp examination confirms the diagnosis by revealing a dark area in the normally homogeneous red reflex.

Treatment

Treatment consists of surgical extraction of the opaque lens and postoperative correction of visual deficits. The current trend is to perform the surgery as a 1-day procedure.

Surgical procedures include the following:

• Extracapsular cataract extraction, the most common procedure, removes the anterior lens capsule and cortex, leaving the posterior capsule intact. With this procedure, a posterior chamber intraocular lens (IOL) is implanted in place of the patient's own lens. (A posterior chamber IOL is the most common type now used in the United States.) This procedure is used for patients of all ages.

• Intracapsular cataract extraction removes the entire lens within the intact capsule by cryoextraction (the moist lens sticks to an extremely cold metal probe for easy and safe removal with gentle traction). Once the lens is removed, an IOL is implanted in either the pupil or the anterior chamber. If an IOL implant is not used, the visual deficit is corrected with contact lenses or aphakic glasses.

• Phacoemulsification fragments the lens with ultrasonic vibrations and aspirates the pieces. Occasionally, this is performed on patients under age 30.

• Discission and aspiration can still be used for children with soft cataracts, but this procedure has largely been replaced by the use of multifunction suction cutting instruments.

Possible complications of surgery

Teaching Topics in Cataracts

- An explanation of the disease
- Risk of progressive vision loss without surgery
- Surgical lens removal
- Preparation for intraocular lens implant or fitting for corrective contact lens or glasses
- Postoperative instructions, including activity restrictions, medication, and schedule for follow-up tests and examinations
- Eye drops and their administration
- Eye patch application, if necessary
- Eye shield application, if necessary

include loss of vitreous (during surgery), wound dehiscence (from loosening of sutures and flat anterior chamber or iris prolapse into the wound), hyphema, pupillary block glaucoma, retinal detachment, and infection.

A patient with an IOL implant may experience improved vision once the eye patch is removed; however, the IOL corrects distance vision only. The patient will also need either corrective reading glasses or a corrective contact lens, which will be fitted 4 to 8 weeks after surgery.

Where no IOL has been implanted, the patient may be given temporary aphakic cataract glasses; in about 4 to 8 weeks, he will be fitted with his own corrective glasses.

Some patients who have an extracapsular cataract extraction develop a secondary membrane in the posterior lens capsule (which has been left intact), resulting in decreased visual acuity. But this membrane can be removed by the Nd:YAG laser, which cuts an area out of the center of the membrane, thereby restoring vision. Laser therapy alone cannot be used to remove a cataract, however.

Clinical implications

After surgery to extract a cataract, follow these guidelines:
- Because the patient will be discharged after he recovers from anesthesia, remind him to return for a checkup the next day and warn him to avoid activities that increase intraocular pressure, such as straining.
- Urge the patient to protect the eye from accidental injury by wearing an eye shield (a plastic or metal shield with perforations) or glasses during the day, and an eye shield at night.
- Administer antibiotic ointment or drops to prevent infection and steroids to reduce inflammation, or combination steroid-antibiotic eye drops.
- Watch for the development of complications, such as iris prolapse, a sharp pain in the eye, or hyphema. Report them immediately.
- Before discharge, teach correct instillation of eye drops, and instruct the patient to notify the physician immediately if he experiences sharp eye pain. Caution him about activity restrictions, and advise him that it takes several weeks before he will receive his corrective reading glasses or lenses. (See *Teaching Topics in Cataracts*.)

Celiac disease
(Idiopathic steatorrhea, nontropical sprue, gluten enteropathy, celiac sprue)

Description

Celiac disease, a relatively uncommon disorder, is characterized by poor food absorption and intolerance of gluten, a protein in wheat, barley, rye, oats, and foods made from them. Such malabsorption in the small bowel results from atrophy of the villi and a decrease in the activity and amount of enzymes in the surface epithelium. It usually affects children, but may occur in adults. With elimination of gluten from the patient's diet, prognosis is good, but residual bowel changes may persist in adults.

Causes
This disorder probably results from environmental factors and a genetic predisposition, but the exact mechanism is unknown. Two theories prevail:
• The first suggests that the disease involves an abnormal immune response. (The presence of HLA-B8 antigen in such a person may be the primary determinant of celiac disease, according to recent studies.)
• The second theory proposes that an intramucosal enzyme defect produces an inability to digest gluten. Resulting tissue toxicity produces rapid cell turnover, increases epithelial lymphocytes, and damages surface epithelium of the small bowel.

Signs and symptoms
Gastrointestinal
Recurrent attacks of diarrhea, steatorrhea, abdominal distention from flatulence, stomach cramps, weakness, anorexia, or, occasionally, increased appetite without weight gain
Musculoskeletal
Tetany and bone pain, especially in the lower back, rib cage, and pelvis
Neurologic
Peripheral neuropathy, convulsions, or paresthesia
Dermatologic
Dry skin; eczema; generalized fine, sparse, prematurely gray hair; brittle nails; localized hyperpigmentation on the face, lips, or mucosa
Endocrine
Amenorrhea, hypometabolism
Psychosocial
Mood changes and irritability

Diagnostic tests
• Small-bowel biopsy shows histologic changes that confirm the diagnosis.
• A glucose tolerance test shows poor absorption of glucose.

• A D-xylose tolerance test shows low urine and blood levels of xylose (less than 3 grams over a 5-hour period); however, the presence of renal disease may cause a false-positive result.
• Serum carotene levels measure absorption. (The patient ingests carotene for several days before the test; since the body neither stores nor manufactures carotene, low serum levels indicate malabsorption.)
• Analyses of stool specimens (after a 72-hour stool collection) show excess fat.
• Barium X-rays of the small bowel show protracted barium passage. The barium shows up in a segmented, coarse, scattered, and clumped pattern; the jejunum shows generalized dilation.
• Hemoglobin, hematocrit, leukocyte, and platelet counts are low.
• Albumin, sodium, potassium, cholesterol, and phospholipid levels are decreased.
• Prothrombin time is reduced.

Treatment
Treatment requires elimination of gluten from the patient's diet for life. Even with this exclusion, full return to normal absorption and bowel histology may not occur for months or at all.

Supportive treatment may include supplemental iron, vitamin B_{12} and folic acid, reversal of electrolyte imbalance (by I.V. infusion, if necessary), I.V. fluid replacement for dehydration, corticosteroids (prednisone, hydrocortisone) to treat accompanying adrenal insufficiency, and vitamin K for hypoprothrombinemia.

Clinical implications
• Explain the necessity of a gluten-free diet to the patient (and to his parents, if the patient is a child). Advise elimination of wheat, barley, rye, oats, and foods made from them, such as breads and baked goods. Suggest substitution of corn or rice. Advise the

patient to consult a dietitian for a gluten-free diet that is high in protein but low in carbohydrates and fats. Depending on individual tolerance, the diet initially consists of proteins and gradually expands to include other foods. Assess the patient's acceptance and understanding of the disease, and encourage regular reevaluation.

• Observe nutritional status and progress by daily calorie counts and weight checks. Also, evaluate tolerance to new foods. In the early stages, offer small, frequent meals to counteract anorexia.

• Assess fluid status: record intake, urine output, and number of stools (may exceed 10 per day). Watch for signs of dehydration, such as dry skin and mucous membranes, and poor skin turgor.

• Check serum electrolyte levels. Watch for signs of hypokalemia (weakness, lethargy, rapid pulse, nausea, diarrhea) and hypocalcemia (impaired blood clotting, muscle twitching, tetany).

• Monitor prothrombin time, hemoglobin, and hematocrit. Protect the patient from bleeding and bruising. Administer vitamin K, iron, folic acid, and vitamin B_{12}, as ordered. Early in treatment, give hematinic supplements I.M., using a separate syringe for each. Use the Z-track method to give iron I.M. If the patient can tolerate oral iron, give it between meals, when absorption is best. Dilute oral iron preparations, and give them through a straw to prevent staining teeth.

• Protect patients with osteomalacia from injury by keeping the side rails up and assisting with ambulation, as necessary.

• Give steroids, as ordered, and assess regularly for cushingoid adverse effects, such as hirsutism and muscle weakness.

Complications
• Fluid and electrolyte imbalances
• Nonspecific ulcers in the small bowel, which may perforate or bleed (in adults)
• Rickets in children and compression fractures in adults from vitamin D deficiency
• Normochromic, hypochromic, or macrocytic anemia from poor absorption of folate, iron, and vitamin B_{12} and hypoprothrombinemia from jejunal loss of vitamin K
• Osteomalacia, osteoporosis
• Psoriasis, rosacea, dermatitis herpetiformis
• Adrenocortical insufficiency if malabsorption is severe

Cerebral aneurysm

Description
Cerebral aneurysm is a localized dilation of a cerebral artery that results from a weakness in the arterial wall. Cerebral aneurysms usually arise at an arterial junction in the circle of Willis, the circular anastomosis forming the major cerebral arteries at the base of the brain. (See *Most Common Sites of Cerebral Aneurysm.*) Cerebral aneurysms frequently rupture and cause subarachnoid hemorrhage. Sometimes bleeding also spills into brain tissue and subsequently forms a clot. This may result in potentially fatal increased intracranial pressure (ICP) and brain tissue damage.

Prognosis is guarded. Probably half of the patients suffering subarachnoid hemorrhages die immediately. With new and better treatment, prognosis is improving, however.

Causes
• Congenital defect
• Degenerative process
• Combination of both

Signs and symptoms
• Occasional premonitory symptoms include headache, nuchal rigidity, stiff back and legs, and intermittent nausea.
• Typical abrupt onset causes sudden

Most Common Sites of Cerebral Aneurysm

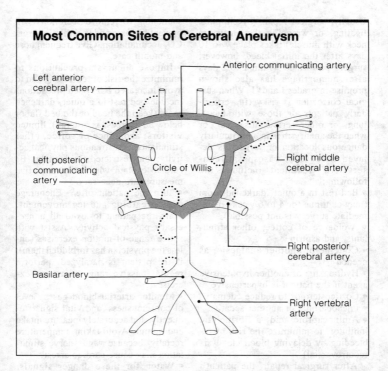

Left anterior cerebral artery

Anterior communicating artery

Left posterior communicating artery

Circle of Willis

Right middle cerebral artery

Basilar artery

Right posterior cerebral artery

Right vertebral artery

severe headache, nausea, vomiting, and possible altered level of consciousness.

• Meningeal irritation results in nuchal rigidity, back and leg pain, fever, restlessness, irritability, occasional seizures, and blurred vision.

• Bleeding into brain tissue causes hemiparesis, hemisensory defects, dysphagia, and visual defects.

• Possible oculomotor nerve compression causes diplopia, ptosis, dilated pupil, and inability to rotate the eye. (See *Grading Ruptured Cerebral Aneurysms*, p. 123.)

Diagnostic tests

• Angiography can confirm an unruptured cerebral aneurysm. Unfortunately, diagnosis of cerebral aneurysm usually follows its rupture.

• Lumbar puncture can detect blood in cerebrospinal fluid (CSF) and increased ICP.

• Skull X-ray may show calcification in the walls of a large aneurysm.

• EKG often shows flattened or depressed T waves.

• Computed tomography locates the clot and identifies hydrocephalus, areas of infarction, and extent of blood spillage within the cisterns around the brain.

• Other baseline laboratory studies include complete blood count, urinalysis, measurement of arterial blood gases, coagulation studies, serum osmolality, and electrolyte and glucose levels.

Treatment

Treatment aims to reduce the risk of rebleeding by repairing the aneurysm.

Usually, surgical repair (by clipping, ligating, or wrapping the aneurysm neck with muscle) takes place 7 to 10 days after the initial bleed; however, surgery performed within 1 to 2 days after hemorrhage has also shown promise in grades I and II. When surgical correction is risky (in very elderly patients or those with heart, lung, or other serious diseases), or when the aneurysm is in a particularly dangerous location or surgery is delayed because of vasospasm, conservative treatment includes the following:

• Bed rest in a quiet, darkened room (may continue for 4 to 6 weeks if immediate surgery is not possible)
• Avoidance of coffee, other stimulants, and aspirin
• Codeine or another analgesic, as needed
• Hydralazine or another hypotensive agent if the patient is hypertensive
• Corticosteroids to reduce edema
• Phenobarbital or another sedative
• Aminocaproic acid, a fibrinolytic inhibitor, to minimize the risk of rebleeding by delaying blood clot lysis (controversial)

After surgical repair, the patient's condition depends on the extent of damage from the initial bleed and the degree of success of treatment for resulting complications. Surgery cannot improve the patient's neurologic condition unless it removes a hematoma or reduces the compression effect.

Clinical implications

An accurate neurologic assessment, good patient care, patient and family teaching, and psychological support can speed recovery and reduce complications. Follow these guidelines:
• During initial treatment after hemorrhage, establish and maintain a patent airway, because the patient may need supplementary oxygen. Position the patient to promote pulmonary drainage and prevent upper airway obstruction. If he is intubated, preoxygenation with 100% oxygen before

suctioning to remove secretions will prevent hypoxia and vasodilation from CO_2 accumulation. Give frequent nose and mouth care.
• Impose aneurysm precautions to minimize the risk of rebleeding and to avoid increased ICP. Such precautions include bed rest in a quiet, darkened room (keep the head of the bed flat or below 30 degrees, as ordered); limited visitors; avoidance of coffee, other stimulants, and strenuous physical activity; and restricted fluid intake. Be sure to explain why these restrictive measures are necessary.
• Turn the patient often. Encourage deep breathing and leg movement. Warn the patient to avoid all unnecessary physical activity. Assist with active range-of-motion exercises (unless the physician has forbidden them); if the patient is paralyzed, perform regular passive range-of-motion exercises.
• Monitor arterial blood gases, level of consciousness, and vital signs frequently, and accurately measure intake and output. Avoid taking temperature rectally, because vagus nerve stimulation may cause cardiac arrest.
• Watch for these danger signals, which may indicate an enlarging aneurysm, rebleeding, intracranial clot, vasospasm, or other complications: decreased level of consciousness, unilateral enlarged pupil, onset or worsening of hemiparesis or motor deficit, increased blood pressure, slowed pulse, worsening of headache or sudden onset of a headache, renewed or worsened nuchal rigidity, renewed or persistent vomiting.
• Give fluids, as ordered, and monitor I.V. infusions to avoid increased ICP.
• If the patient has facial weakness, assist him during meals, placing food in the unaffected side of his mouth. If he cannot swallow, insert a nasogastric tube, as ordered, and give all tube feedings slowly. Prevent skin break-

Grading Ruptured Cerebral Aneurysms

The severity of symptoms varies considerably from patient to patient, depending on the site and amount of bleeding. To better describe their conditions, patients with ruptured cerebral aneurysms are grouped as follows:

• *Grade I: Minimal bleed.* Patient is alert with no neurologic deficit; he may have a slight headache and nuchal rigidity.
• *Grade II: Mild bleed.* Patient is alert, with a mild to severe headache, nuchal rigidity, and, possibly, third nerve palsy.
• *Grade III: Moderate bleed.* Patient is confused or drowsy, with nuchal rigidity and, possibly, a mild focal deficit.
• *Grade IV: Severe bleed.* Patient is stuporous, with nuchal rigidity and, possibly, mild to severe hemiparesis.
• *Grade V: Moribund (often fatal).* If nonfatal, patient is in deep coma or decerebrate.

down by taping the tube so it does not press against the nostril.
• If the patient can eat, provide a high-bulk diet (bran, salads, fruit) to prevent straining at stool, which can increase ICP. Get an order for a stool softener, such as docusate sodium, or a mild laxative; administer as ordered. *Do not* force fluids. Implement a bowel program based on previous habits. If the patient is receiving steroids, check the stool for blood.
• With third or facial nerve palsy, administer artificial tears to the affected eye, and tape the eye shut at night to prevent corneal damage.
• To minimize stress, give a sedative, as ordered. Watch for signs of oversedation, and report them immediately. If the patient is confused, raise the side rails to help protect him from injury. If possible, avoid using restraints, because these can cause agitation and increase ICP.
• Administer hydralazine or another hypotensive agent, as ordered. Carefully monitor blood pressure and report *any* significant change, but especially a rise in systolic pressure, immediately.
• Administer aminocaproic acid I.V. in 5% dextrose in water, P.O. or as ordered. Give it at least every 2 hours to maintain therapeutic blood levels.

(Renal insufficiency may require dosage adjustment.) Monitor the patient for adverse reactions, such as nausea and diarrhea (most common with oral administration) and phlebitis (most common with I.V. administration). Reduce deep vein thrombosis by applying antiembolism stockings.
• If the patient cannot speak, establish a simple means of communication, or use cards or a slate. Try to limit conversation to topics that will not further frustrate the patient. Encourage his family to speak to him in a normal tone, even if he does not seem to respond.
• Provide emotional support, and include the patient's family in his care as much as possible. Encourage family members to adopt a positive attitude, but discourage unrealistic goals.
• Before discharge, make a referral to a visiting nurse or a rehabilitation center when necessary.

Complications

Cerebral aneurysm poses three major threats: increased ICP, rebleeding, and vasospasm.
• Increased ICP may push the brain downward, impair brain stem func-

tion, and cut off blood supply to the part of the brain that supports vital functions, resulting in death.

• Generally, after the initial bleeding episode, a clot forms and seals the rupture, which reinforces the wall of the aneurysm for 7 to 10 days. However, after the seventh day, fibrinolysis begins to dissolve the clot and increases the risk of rebleeding, which produces signs and symptoms similar to those accompanying the initial hemorrhage. Rebleeds during the first 48 to 72 hours following initial hemorrhage are not uncommon. They contribute to the high mortality.

• Why vasospasm occurs is not clearly understood. Usually, it occurs in blood vessels adjacent to the aneurysm, but it may extend to major vessels of the brain, causing ischemia and altered brain function.

• Other complications include acute hydrocephalus (a result of abnormal accumulation of CSF within the cranial cavity because of CSF blockage by blood or adhesions) and pulmonary embolism (a possible adverse effect of therapy with aminocaproic acid or deep vein thrombosis).

Cerebral contusion

Description
Cerebral contusion is bruising of brain tissue as a result of a severe blow to the head. More serious than a concussion, contusion disrupts normal nerve functions in the bruised area and may cause loss of consciousness, cerebral hemorrhage or edema, and even death. (See *Hemorrhage, Hematoma, and Tentorial Herniation.*)

Cause
Trauma (acceleration-deceleration or coup-contrecoup injuries)

Signs and symptoms
• Loss of consciousness
• Scalp wounds
• Hemiparesis
• Decorticate or decerebrate posturing
• Labored breathing
• Unequal pupils
• Drowsiness, confusion, disorientation, agitation, or violence when conscious
• Temporary aphasia and unilateral numbness after regaining consciousness

Diagnostic tests
• Skull X-rays rule out fractures and may help to show a shift in brain tissue.
• Cerebral angiography outlines vasculature.
• Computed tomography shows ischemic or necrotic tissue and subdural, epidural, and intracerebral hematomas.

Treatment and clinical implications
• Establish a patent airway. As ordered, assist with a tracheotomy or endotracheal intubation (for an unconscious patient with no cervical spine fracture). Perform a neurologic examination, focusing on the level of consciousness, motor responses, and intracranial pressure (ICP).
• Start I.V. fluids with 5% dextrose in 0.45% normal saline solution. Hypotonic fluids are not indicated; they may aggravate cerebral edema. Mannitol I.V. may be given to reduce cerebral edema. Dexamethasone I.V. or I.M. will be given for several days to control cerebral edema.
• Type and cross match blood for a patient suspected of having intracerebral hemorrhage. A blood transfusion may be needed and possibly a craniotomy, to control bleeding and to aspirate blood.
• Insert an indwelling (Foley) cathe-

ter, as ordered. Monitor intake and output. With unconscious patients, insert a nasogastric tube to prevent aspiration.

• Enforce absolute bed rest. Observe for cerebrospinal fluid (CSF) leaks. Check bed sheets for a blood-tinged spot surrounded by a lighter ring (halo sign). If CSF leaks develop, raise the head of the bed 30 degrees. If you detect CSF leaks from the nose, place a gauze pad under the nostrils. Be sure to tell the patient not to blow his nose, but to wipe it instead. If CSF leaks from the ear, position the patient so that the ear drains naturally. Do not pack the ear or nose.

• Monitor vital signs and respirations regularly (usually every 15 minutes). Abnormal respirations could indicate a breakdown in the respiratory center in the brain stem and possible impending tentorial herniation—a neurologic emergency.

• Perform frequent neurologic checks. Assess for restlessness, level of consciousness, and orientation.

• After the patient is stabilized, clean and dress any superficial scalp wounds. (If the skin has been broken, tetanus prophylaxis may be in order.) Assist with suturing, if necessary.

Hemorrhage, Hematoma, and Tentorial Herniation

Among the most serious consequences of a head injury are hemorrhage, hematoma, and tentorial herniation. An epidural hemorrhage or hematoma results from a rapid accumulation of blood between the skull and the dura mater; a subdural hemorrhage or hematoma, from a slow accumulation of blood between the dura mater and the subarachnoid membrane. Intracerebral hemorrhage or hematoma occurs within the cerebrum itself. Tentorial herniation occurs when injured brain tissue swells and squeezes itself through the tentorial notch, constricting the brain stem.

Epidural hemorrhage or hematoma can cause immediate loss of consciousness, followed by a lucid interval lasting minutes to hours, which eventually gives way to a rapidly progressive decrease in the level of consciousness. Other effects are contralateral hemiparesis, progressively severe headache, ipsilateral pupillary dilation, and signs of increased ICP: decreasing pulse and respirations and increasing systolic blood pressure.

With a subacute or chronic subdural hemorrhage or hematoma, blood accumulates slowly, so symptoms may not occur until days after the injury. In an acute subdural hematoma, symptoms appear earlier because blood accumulates within 24 hours of the injury. Loss of consciousness occurs, often with weakness or paralysis. Intracerebral hemorrhage or hematoma usually causes nuchal rigidity, photophobia, nausea, vomiting, dizziness, convulsions, decreased respiratory rate, and progressive obtundation.

Tentorial herniation causes drowsiness, confusion, dilation of one or both pupils, hyperventilation, nuchal rigidity, bradycardia, and decorticate or decerebrate posturing. Irreversible brain damage or death can occur rapidly.

Intracranial hemorrhage may require a craniotomy, to locate and control bleeding and to aspirate blood. Epidural and subdural hematomas are usually drained by aspiration through burr holes in the skull. Increased ICP may be controlled with mannitol I.V., steroids, or diuretics, but emergency surgery is usually required.

Cerebral palsy

Description
The most common cause of crippling in children, cerebral palsy comprises a group of neuromuscular disorders resulting from prenatal, perinatal, or postnatal central nervous system (CNS) damage. Although nonprogressive, these disorders may become more obvious as an affected infant grows older.

Three major types of cerebral palsy occur—spastic, athetoid, and ataxic—sometimes in mixed forms. Motor impairment may be minimal (sometimes apparent only during physical activities such as running) or severely disabling. Associated defects, such as seizures, speech disorders, and mental retardation, are common. Early diagnosis is essential for effective treatment and requires careful clinical observation during infancy and precise neurologic assessment.

All infants should have a screening test for cerebral palsy as a regular part of their 6-month checkup. Prognosis varies. In mild impairment, proper treatment may make a near-normal life possible.

Causes
Conditions that result in cerebral anoxia, hemorrhage, or other damage are probably responsible for cerebral palsy.
Prenatal causes
—Maternal infection (especially rubella)
—Radiation
—Anoxia, toxemia
—Maternal diabetes
—Abnormal placental attachment
—Malnutrition
—Isoimmunization
Perinatal and birth difficulties
—Forceps delivery
—Breech presentation
—Placenta previa
—Abruptio placentae
—Depressed maternal vital signs from general or spinal anesthetic
—Prolapsed cord, with delay in delivery of head
—Premature birth
—Prolonged or unusually rapid labor
—Multiple birth (especially infants born last in a multiple birth)
Infection or trauma during infancy
—Kernicterus resulting from erythroblastosis fetalis
—Brain infection
—Head trauma
—Prolonged anoxia
—Brain tumor
—Cerebral circulatory anomalies, causing blood vessel rupture
—Systemic disease, resulting in cerebral thrombosis or embolus

Risk factors
• Low birth weight
• Low Apgar scores at 5 minutes
• Seizures
• Metabolic disturbances

Signs and symptoms
Spastic form (most common)
—Hyperactive deep tendon reflexes
—Increased stretch reflexes
—Rapid alternating muscle contraction and relaxation
—Muscle weakness
—Underdevelopment of affected limbs
—Muscle contraction in response to manipulation
—Tendency toward contractures
—Typical walking on toes with scissors gait (crossing one foot in front of the other)
Athetoid form
—Involuntary movements such as grimacing, wormlike writhing, dystonia, and sharp jerks. These impair voluntary movement and affect arms more than legs. They worsen during stress, decrease with relaxation, and disappear during sleep.
Ataxic form
—Disturbed balance

Recognizing Symptoms of Cerebral Palsy

Suspect cerebral palsy whenever an infant:
• has difficulty sucking or keeping the nipple or food in his mouth
• seldom moves voluntarily, or has arm or leg tremors with voluntary movement
• crosses his legs when lifted from behind rather than pulling them up or "bicycling" like a normal infant
• has legs that are hard to separate, making diaper changing difficult
• persistently uses only one hand or, as he gets older, uses his hands well but not his legs.

—Incoordination (especially of the arms)
—Hyperactive reflexes
—Nystagmus
—Muscle weakness
—Tremor
—Lack of leg movement during infancy
—Wide gait when beginning to walk
—Sudden or fine movements are almost impossible.

Combination
—Difficulty in eating, especially swallowing
—Retarded growth and development
—Frequent impaired speech
—Frequent dental problems
—Vision and hearing defects (common)
—Reading disabilities (common)
—Possible mental retardation
—Possible seizure disorders. (See also *Recognizing Symptoms of Cerebral Palsy.*)

Treatment
Cerebral palsy cannot be cured, but proper treatment can help affected children reach their full potential within the limits set by this disorder. Such treatment requires a comprehensive and cooperative effort involving physicians, nurses, teachers, psychologists, the child's family, and occupational, physical, and speech therapists. Home care is often possible. Treatment usually includes the following:
• Braces or splints and special appliances, such as adapted eating utensils and a low toilet seat with arms, to help these children perform activities independently
• An artificial urinary sphincter for the incontinent child who can use the hand controls
• Range-of-motion exercises to minimize contractures
• Orthopedic surgery to correct contractures
• Phenytoin, phenobarbital, or another anticonvulsant to control seizures
• Sometimes, muscle relaxants or neurosurgery to decrease spasticity

Children with milder forms of cerebral palsy should attend a regular school; severely afflicted children need special education classes.

Clinical implications
A child with cerebral palsy may be hospitalized for orthopedic surgery and for treatment of other complications. Follow these guidelines:
• Speak slowly and distinctly. Encourage the child to ask for things he wants. Listen patiently, and do not rush him.
• Plan an adequate diet to meet the child's high energy needs.
• During meals, maintain a quiet, unhurried atmosphere with as few distractions as possible. The child may need special utensils and a chair with a solid footrest. Teach him to place

food far back in his mouth to facilitate swallowing.

• Encourage the child to chew food thoroughly, drink through a straw, and suck on lollipops to develop the muscle control needed to minimize drooling.

• Allow the child to wash and dress independently, assisting only as needed. The child may need clothing modifications.

• Give all care in an unhurried manner; otherwise, muscle spasticity may increase.

• Encourage the child and his family to participate in the care plan so they can continue it at home.

• Care for associated hearing or visual disturbances, as necessary.

• Give frequent mouth care and dental care, as necessary.

• Reduce muscle spasms that increase postoperative pain by moving and turning the child carefully after surgery.

• After orthopedic surgery, give good cast care. Wash and dry the skin at the edge of the cast frequently, and rub it with alcohol. Reposition the child frequently, check for foul odor, and ventilate under the cast with a blow-dryer. Use a flashlight to check for skin breakdown beneath the cast. Help the child relax, perhaps by giving a warm bath, before reapplying a bivalved cast.

• Work with parents to set realistic goals, based on your understanding of normal growth and development.

• Assist in planning crafts and other activities.

• Stress the child's need to develop peer relationships; warn the parents against being overprotective.

• Identify and deal with family stress. Parents may feel unreasonable guilt about their child's handicap and may need psychological counseling.

• Make a referral to supportive community organizations. For more information, tell parents to contact the United Cerebral Palsy Association, Inc., or their local cerebral palsy agency.

Cerebrovascular accident
(Stroke)

Description

A cerebrovascular accident (CVA) is a sudden impairment of cerebral circulation in one or more of the blood vessels supplying the brain. CVA interrupts or diminishes oxygen supply and frequently causes serious damage or necrosis in brain tissues. The sooner circulation returns to normal after CVA, the better chances are for complete recovery.

CVAs are classified according to their course of progression. The least severe is the transient ischemic attack (TIA), or "little stroke," which results from a temporary interruption of blood flow. (See *Transient Ischemic Attack*.) A progressive stroke, or stroke-in-evolution (thrombus-in-evolution), begins with slight neurologic deficit and worsens in a day or two. In a complete stroke, neurologic deficits are maximal at onset.

CVA is the third most common cause of death in the United States today and the most common cause of neurologic disability. It strikes 500,000 people each year; half of them die as a result. About half of those who survive a CVA remain permanently disabled and experience a recurrence within weeks, months, or years.

Causes

• Thrombosis (most common)
• Embolism
• Hemorrhage

Risk factors

• History of TIAs
• Atherosclerosis
• Hypertension
• Dysrhythmias
• Rheumatic heart disease
• Diabetes mellitus
• Gout
• Postural hypotension
• Cardiac or myocardial enlargement

- High serum triglyceride levels
- Lack of exercise
- Use of oral contraceptives
- Cigarette smoking
- Family history of CVA

Signs and symptoms

Clinical features of CVA vary with the artery affected (and, consequently, the portion of the brain it supplies), the severity of damage, and the extent of collateral circulation that develops to help the brain compensate for decreased blood supply. If CVA occurs in the left hemisphere, it produces symptoms on the right side; if in the right hemisphere, symptoms are on the left side. However, a CVA that causes cranial nerve damage produces signs of cranial nerve dysfunction on the same side as the hemorrhage. Symptoms are usually classified according to the artery affected. (Symptoms can also be classified as premonitory, generalized, and focal.)

Middle cerebral artery

Aphasia, dysphasia, visual field cuts, or hemiparesis on affected side (more severe in the face and arm than in the leg)

Carotid artery

Weakness, paralysis, numbness, sensory changes, visual disturbances on affected side, altered level of consciousness, bruits, headaches, aphasia, or ptosis

Vertebrobasilar artery

Weakness on affected side, numbness around lips and mouth, visual field cuts, diplopia, poor coordination, dysphagia, slurred speech, dizziness, amnesia, or ataxia

Anterior cerebral artery

Confusion, weakness and numbness (especially in the leg) on affected side, incontinence, loss of coordination, impaired motor and sensory functions, or personality changes

Posterior cerebral arteries

Visual field cuts, sensory impairment, dyslexia, coma, cortical blindness; paralysis usually absent

Diagnostic tests

- Computed tomography (CT) shows evidence of thrombotic or hemor-

---

Transient Ischemic Attack

A TIA is a recurrent episode of neurologic deficit, lasting from seconds to hours, that clears within 12 to 24 hours. It is usually considered a warning sign of an impending thrombotic CVA. In fact, TIAs have been reported in 50% to 80% of patients who have had a cerebral infarction from such thrombosis. The age of onset varies. Incidence rises dramatically after age 50 and is highest among blacks and men.

In TIA, microemboli released from a thrombus probably temporarily interrupt blood flow, especially in the small distal branches of the arterial tree in the brain. Small spasms in those arterioles may impair blood flow and also precede TIA. Predisposing factors are the same as for thrombotic CVAs. The most distinctive characteristics of TIAs are the transient duration of neurologic deficits and complete return of normal function. The symptoms of TIA easily correlate with the location of the affected artery. These symptoms include double vision, speech deficits (slurring or thickness), unilateral blindness, staggering or uncoordinated gait, unilateral weakness or numbness, falling because of weakness in the legs, and dizziness.

During an active TIA, the aim of treatment is to prevent a completed stroke and consists of aspirin or anticoagulants to minimize the risk of thrombosis. After or between attacks, preventive treatment includes carotid endarterectomy or cerebral microvascular bypass.

Preventing CVA

Teach all patients (especially those at high risk) to follow these guidelines.
- Follow a low-cholesterol, low-salt diet.
- Maintain appropriate weight.
- Increase activity.
- Avoid smoking.
- Avoid prolonged bed rest.
- Minimize stress.
- Control diseases, such as diabetes or hypertension, if present.

rhagic stroke, tumor, or hydrocephalus.
- Brain scan shows ischemic areas but may not be positive for up to 2 weeks after CVA.
- Lumbar puncture may yield bloody cerebrospinal fluid in hemorrhagic stroke.
- Ophthalmoscopy may show signs of hypertension and atherosclerotic changes in retinal arteries.
- Angiography outlines blood vessels and pinpoints the site of occlusion or rupture.
- EEG may help to localize the area of damage.

Treatment

Surgery to improve cerebral circulation for patients with thrombotic or embolic CVA includes endarterectomy (removal of atherosclerotic plaques from inner arterial walls) or microvascular bypass (anastomosis of an extracranial vessel to an intracranial vessel).

Medications useful in CVA include the following:
- Anticonvulsants, such as phenytoin or phenobarbital, to treat or prevent seizures
- Stool softeners, such as docusate sodium, to prevent straining, which increases intracranial pressure (ICP)
- Corticosteroids, such as dexamethasone, to minimize associated cerebral edema

- Analgesics, such as codeine, to relieve headache that may follow hemorrhagic CVA

Usually, aspirin is contraindicated in hemorrhagic CVA because it increases bleeding tendencies, but it may be useful in preventing TIAs.

Clinical implications

- Maintain patent airway and oxygenation. Loosen constricting clothes. Watch for ballooning of the cheek with respiration. The side that balloons is the side affected by the stroke. If the patient is unconscious, he could aspirate saliva, so keep him in a lateral position to allow secretions to drain naturally, or suction secretions, as needed. Insert an artificial airway, and start mechanical ventilation or supplemental oxygen, if necessary.
- Check vital signs and neurologic status, record observations, and report any significant changes to the physician. Monitor blood pressure, level of consciousness, pupillary changes, motor function (voluntary and involuntary movements), sensory function, speech, skin color, temperature, signs of increased ICP, and nuchal rigidity or flaccidity.
- Remember, if CVA is impending, blood pressure rises suddenly, pulse is rapid and bounding, and the patient may complain of headache.
- Watch for signs of pulmonary emboli, such as chest pains, shortness of breath, dusky color, tachycardia, fever, and changed sensorium.
- If the patient is unresponsive, monitor arterial blood gases frequently and alert the physician to increased PCO_2 or decreased PO_2 levels.
- Maintain fluid and electrolyte balance. If the patient can take liquids P.O., offer them as often as fluid limitations permit. Administer I.V. fluids, as ordered. Never give too much too fast, because this can increase ICP. Offer the urinal or bedpan every 2 hours. If the patient is incontinent, he may need an indwelling (Foley) catheter, but this should be avoided, if pos-

sible, because of the risk of infection.

• Ensure adequate nutrition. Check for gag reflex before offering small oral feedings of semisolid foods. Place the food tray within the patient's visual field. If oral feedings are not possible, insert a nasogastric tube.

• Manage GI problems. Be alert for signs that the patient is straining at stool, because this increases ICP. Modify diet; administer stool softeners, as ordered; and give laxatives, if necessary. If the patient vomits (usually during the first few days), keep him positioned on his side to prevent aspiration.

• Give careful mouth care. Clean and irrigate the patient's mouth to remove food particles. Care for his dentures, as needed.

• Provide meticulous eye care. Remove secretions with a cotton ball and sterile normal saline solution. Instill eye drops, as ordered. Patch the patient's affected eye if he cannot close the lid.

• Position the patient, and align his extremities correctly. Use high-topped sneakers to prevent footdrop and contracture.

• Use eggcrate, flotation, or pulsating mattresses, or sheepskin to prevent decubitus ulcers.

• To prevent pneumonia, turn the patient at least every 2 hours.

• Elevate the affected hand to control dependent edema, and place it in a functional position.

• Assist the patient with exercise. Perform range-of-motion exercises for both the affected and unaffected sides. Teach and encourage the patient to use his unaffected side to exercise his affected side.

• Give medications, as ordered, and watch for and report adverse effects.

• Establish and maintain communication with the patient. If he is aphasic, set up a simple method of communicating basic needs. Then, remember to phrase your questions so he will be

Teaching Topics in CVA

• An explanation of the type of CVA: thrombotic, embolic, or hemorrhagic
• Preparation for diagnostic tests, such as a CT scan and cerebral angiography
• If necessary, an explanation of the type of surgery: craniotomy, carotid endarterectomy, or extracranial/intracranial bypass
• The importance of rehabilitation in minimizing neurologic deficits
• A balanced program of activity and rest
• Dietary adjustments, such as semisoft foods for dysphagia
• Assistive devices
• Communication tips for the patient and his family
• Home safety tips
• Risk factors in CVA
• Sources of additional information and support

able to answer using this system. Repeat yourself quietly and calmly. (Remember, he is not deaf!) Use gestures if necessary to help him understand. Even the unresponsive patient can hear, so do not say anything in his presence you would not want him to hear and remember.

• Provide psychological support. Set realistic short-term goals. Involve the patient's family in his care when possible, and explain his deficits and strengths.

• Begin your rehabilitation of the patient with CVA on admission. The amount of teaching you will have to do depends on the extent of neurologic deficit.

• Establish rapport with the patient. Spend time with him, and provide a means of communication. Simplify your language, asking yes-or-no questions whenever possible. Do not correct his speech or treat him like a child. Remember that building rapport may be difficult because of the mood changes that may result from brain damage or from being dependent.

• If necessary, teach the patient to comb his hair, dress, and wash. With the aid of a physical and an occupational therapist, obtain appliances, such as walking frames, hand bars by the toilet, and ramps, as needed. If speech therapy is indicated, encourage the patient to begin as soon as possible, and follow through with the speech pathologist's suggestions.

• To reinforce teaching, involve the patient's family in all aspects of rehabilitation. With their cooperation and support, devise a realistic discharge plan, and let them help decide when the patient can return home.

• Before discharge, warn the patient or his family to report any premonitory signs of CVA, such as severe headache, drowsiness, confusion, and dizziness. Emphasize the importance of regular follow-up visits.

• If aspirin has been prescribed to minimize the risk of embolic stroke, tell the patient to watch for possible GI bleeding related to ulcer formation. Make sure the patient realizes that he cannot substitute acetaminophen for aspirin. (See *Preventing CVA*, p. 130, and *Teaching Topics in CVA*, p. 131.)

Cervical cancer

Description

The third most common cancer of the female reproductive system, cervical cancer is classified as either preinvasive or invasive.

Preinvasive carcinoma ranges from minimal cervical dysplasia, in which the lower third of the epithelium contains abnormal cells, to carcinoma in situ, in which the full thickness of epithelium contains abnormally proliferating cells (also known as cervical intraepithelial neoplasia [CIN]). Preinvasive cancer is curable 75% to 90% of the time with early detection

and proper treatment. If untreated (and depending on the form in which it appears), it may progress to invasive cervical cancer.

In invasive carcinoma, cancer cells penetrate the basement membrane and can spread directly to contiguous pelvic structures or disseminate to distant sites by lymphatic routes. Invasive carcinoma of the uterine cervix is responsible for 8,000 deaths annually in the United States alone. Usually, invasive carcinoma occurs between ages 30 and 50; rarely, under age 20.

Causes
Unknown

Risk factors
• Intercourse at a young age
• Multiple sexual partners
• Multiple pregnancies
• Venereal infections

Signs and symptoms
Preinvasive cervical cancer is asymptomatic.
Early invasive
—Abnormal vaginal bleeding
—Persistent vaginal discharge
—Postcoital pain and bleeding
Advanced
—Pelvic pain
—Vaginal leakage of urine and feces from a fistula
—Anorexia
—Weight loss
—Fatigue

Diagnostic tests
• Cytologic examination (Pap smear) can detect cervical cancer before clinical evidence appears.
• Colposcopy can detect the presence and extent of preclinical lesions.
• Biopsy and histologic examination can confirm the diagnosis.
• Additional studies, such as lymphangiography, cystography, and scans, can detect metastasis.
(See *Staging Cervical Cancer*.)

Staging Cervical Cancer

Stage 0: Carcinoma in situ, intraepithelial carcinoma
Stage I: Carcinoma is strictly confined to the cervix (extension to the corpus should be disregarded)
Stage Ia: Microinvasive carcinoma (early stromal invasion)
Stage Ib: All other cases of Stage I. Occult cancer should be marked "occ."
Stage II: Carcinoma extends beyond the cervix but has not extended to the pelvic wall. The carcinoma involves the vagina, but not as far as the lower third.
Stage IIa: No obvious parametrial involvement
Stage IIb: Obvious parametrial involvement
Stage III: Carcinoma has extended to the pelvic wall. On rectal examination, there is no cancer-free space between the tumor and the pelvic wall. The tumor involves the lower third of the vagina. All cases with a hydronephrosis or nonfunctioning kidney are included, unless they are known to be due to other cause.
Stage IIIa: No extension to the pelvic wall
Stage IIIb: Extension to the pelvic wall and/or hydronephrosis or nonfunctioning kidney
Stage IV: Carcinoma has extended beyond the true pelvis or has clinically involved the mucosa of the bladder or rectum. A bullous edema as such does not permit a case to be allotted to Stage IV.
Stage IVa: Spread of the growth to adjacent organs
Stage IVb: Spread to distant organs

Reprinted from *Manual for Staging of Cancer* (Chicago: American Joint Committee for Cancer Staging and End Results Reporting, 1983). Used with permission.

Treatment

Appropriate treatment depends on accurate clinical staging. Preinvasive lesions may be treated with total excisional biopsy, cryosurgery, laser destruction, conization (and frequent Pap smear follow-up), or, rarely, hysterectomy. Therapy for invasive squamous cell carcinoma may include radical hysterectomy and radiation therapy (internal, external, or both).

Clinical implications

Management of cervical cancer requires skilled preoperative and postoperative care, comprehensive patient teaching, and emotional and psychological support.

• If you assist with a biopsy, drape and prepare the patient as for routine Pap smear and pelvic examination. Have a container of formaldehyde ready to preserve the specimen during transfer to the pathology laboratory. Explain to the patient that she may feel pressure, minor abdominal cramps, or a pinch from the punch forceps. Reassure her that pain will be minimal, because the cervix has few nerve endings.

• If you assist with cryosurgery, drape and prepare the patient as if for a routine Pap smear and pelvic examination. Explain that the procedure takes approximately 15 minutes, during which time the physician will use refrigerant to freeze the cervix. Warn the patient that she may experience abdominal cramps, headache, and sweating, but reassure her that she will feel little, if any, pain.

• If you assist with laser therapy, drape and prepare the patient as if for a routine Pap smear and pelvic examina-

Internal Radiation Safety Precautions

There are three cardinal safety rules in internal radiation therapy:
• *Time*. Wear a radiosensitive badge. Remember, your exposure increases with time, and the effects are cumulative. Therefore, carefully plan the time you spend with the patient to prevent overexposure. (However, do not rush procedures, ignore the patient's psychological needs, or give the impression that you cannot get out of the room fast enough.)
• *Distance*. Radiation loses its intensity with distance. Avoid standing at the foot of the patient's bed, where you are in line with the radiation.
• *Shield*. Lead shields reduce radiation exposure. Use them whenever possible.

In internal radiation therapy, remember that the patient is radioactive while the radiation source is in place, usually 48 to 72 hours.
• Pregnant women should not be assigned to care for these patients.
• Check the position of the source applicator every 4 hours. If it appears dislodged, notify the physician immediately. If it is completely dislodged, remove the patient from the bed; pick up the applicator with long forceps, place it on a lead-shielded transport cart, and notify the physician immediately.
• *Never* pick up the source with your bare hands. Notify the physician and radiation safety officer whenever there is an accident, and keep a lead-shielded transport cart on the unit as long as the patient has a source in place.

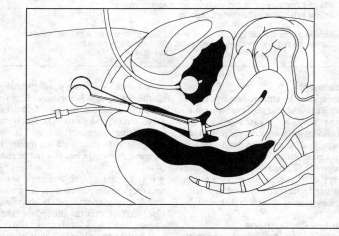

tion. Explain that the procedure takes approximately 30 minutes and may cause abdominal cramps.
• After excisional biopsy, cryosurgery, or laser therapy, tell the patient to expect a discharge or spotting for about 1 week. Advise her not to douche, use tampons, or engage in sexual intercourse during this time. Tell her to watch for and report signs of infection. Stress the need for a follow-up Pap smear and a pelvic examination within 3 to 4 months after these procedures and periodically thereafter.
• After surgery, monitor vital signs every 4 hours. Watch for and immediately report signs of complications, such as bleeding, abdominal disten-

tion, severe pain, wheezing, or other breathing difficulties. Administer analgesics, prophylactic antibiotics, and subcutaneous heparin, as ordered. Encourage deep breathing and coughing.

• Explain that external outpatient radiation therapy, when necessary, continues for about 4 to 6 weeks. The patient may be hospitalized for a 2- to 3-day course of internal radiation treatment (an intracavitary implant of radium, cesium, or some other radioactive material). Find out if the patient is to have internal or external therapy, or both. Usually, internal radiation therapy is the first procedure.

• Check to see if the radioactive source will be inserted while the patient is in the operating room (preloaded) or at the bedside (afterloaded). If the source is preloaded, the patient returns to her room "hot," and safety precautions begin immediately.

• Remember that safety precautions—time, distance, and shielding—begin as soon as the radioactive source is in place. Inform the patient that she will require a private room. (See *Internal Radiation Safety Precautions*.)

• Explain the preloaded internal radiation procedure, and answer the patient's questions. Internal radiation requires a 2- to 3-day hospital stay, a bowel preparation, a povidone-iodine vaginal douche, a clear liquid diet, and nothing by mouth the night before the implantation; it also requires an indwelling (Foley) catheter. Tell the patient that the procedure is performed in the operating room under a general anesthetic, during which time she is placed in the lithotomy position and a radium applicator is inserted. The radioactive source is implanted in the applicator by the physician.

• If the patient is to have afterloaded radiation therapy, explain that a member of the radiation team will implant the source after she is returned to her room from surgery.

• Encourage the patient to lie flat and limit movement while the source is in place. If she prefers, elevate the head of the bed slightly.

• Check vital signs every 4 hours; watch for skin reaction, vaginal bleeding, abdominal discomfort, or evidence of dehydration. Make sure the patient can reach everything she needs without stretching or straining. Assist her in range-of-motion arm exercises (leg exercises and other body movements could dislodge the source). If ordered, administer a tranquilizer to help the patient relax and remain still. Organize the time you spend with the patient to minimize your exposure to radiation.

• Inform visitors of safety precautions, and hang a sign listing these precautions on the patient's door.

• Teach the patient to watch for and report uncomfortable adverse effects. Since radiation therapy may increase susceptibility to infection by lowering the white blood cell count, warn the patient during therapy to avoid persons with obvious infections.

• Reassure the patient that this disease and its treatment should not radically alter her life-style or prohibit sexual intimacy.

Chalazion

Description

A chalazion is a granulomatous inflammation of a meibomian gland in the upper or lower eyelid. This common eye disorder is characterized by localized swelling and usually develops slowly over several weeks. A chalazion may become large enough to press on the eyeball, producing astigmatism; a large chalazion seldom subsides spontaneously. It is usually benign and chronic and can occur at any age. In some patients, it is likely to recur. Persistently recurrent chalazions, especially in an adult, necessitate biopsy to rule out meibomian cancer.

Cause

Obstruction of the meibomian (sebaceous) gland

Signs and symptoms

• A painless, hard lump that usually points toward the conjunctival side of the eyelid

• A red or red-yellow elevated area on the conjunctival surface

Treatment and clinical implications

• Initial treatment consists of application of warm compresses to open the lumen of the gland and, occasionally, instillation of sulfonamide eye drops. If such therapy fails, or if the chalazion presses on the eyeball or causes a severe cosmetic problem, incision and curettage under local anesthetic may be necessary. After such surgery, a pressure eye patch applied for 8 to 24 hours controls bleeding and swelling. After removal of the patch, treatment again consists of warm compresses applied for 10 to 15 minutes, two to four times daily, and antimicrobial eye drops or ointment to prevent secondary infection.

• Teach proper lid hygiene to the patient disposed to chalazions (water and mild baby shampoo applied with a cotton applicator).

• Instruct the patient how to properly apply warm compresses: Take special care to avoid burning the skin; always use a clean cloth; discard used compresses. Tell the patient to start applying warm compresses at the first sign of lid irritation to increase the blood supply and keep the lumen open.

Chancroid
(Soft chancre)

Description

Chancroid is a venereal disease characterized by painful genital ulcers and inguinal adenitis. This infection occurs worldwide but is particularly common in tropical countries. It affects males more often than females. Chancroidal lesions may heal spontaneously and usually respond well to treatment in the absence of secondary infections.

Causes

Hemophilus ducreyi, a short, nonmotile, gram-negative streptobacillus

Mode of transmission

Sexual contact

Risk factors

Poor personal hygiene in males, especially those who are uncircumcised

Signs and symptoms

• After a 3- to 5-day incubation period, a small papule appears at the site of entry, usually the groin or inner thigh; in the male, it may appear on the penis; in the female, on the vulva, vagina, or cervix. (Occasionally, this papule may erupt on the tongue, lip, breast, or navel.)

• The papule (more than one may appear) rapidly ulcerates, becoming painful, soft, and malodorous; bleeds easily; and produces pus. It is gray and shallow, with irregular edges, and measures up to 1″ (2.5 cm) in diameter.

• Within 2 to 3 weeks, inguinal adenitis develops, creating suppurated, inflamed nodes that may rupture into large ulcers or buboes.

• Headache and malaise occur.

• During the healing stage, phimosis may develop.

Diagnostic tests

• Gram stain smears of ulcer exudate or bubo aspirate are 50% reliable.

• Blood agar cultures are 75% reliable.

• Biopsy confirms diagnosis but is reserved for resistant cases or those in which malignancy is suspected.

• Dark-field examination and serologic testing rule out other venereal diseases (genital herpes, syphilis, lymphogranuloma venereum), which cause similar ulcers.

Treatment
Co-trimoxazole usually cures chancroid within 2 weeks. An alternative to sulfonamides, erythromycin may prevent detection of coexisting syphilis. Aspiration of fluid-filled nodes helps prevent infection from spreading.

Clinical implications
• Make sure the patient is not allergic to sulfonamides or any other prescribed drug before giving the initial dose.
• Instruct the patient not to apply creams, lotions, or oils on or near genitalia or on other lesion sites.
• Tell the patient to abstain from sexual contact until healing is complete (usually about 2 weeks after treatment begins) and to wash the genitalia daily with soap and water. Instruct uncircumcised males to retract the foreskin to thoroughly cleanse the glans penis.
• To prevent chancroid, advise patients to avoid sexual contact with infected persons, to use condoms during sexual activity, and to wash the genitalia with soap and water after sexual activity.

Chédiak-Higashi syndrome

Description
Chédiak-Higashi syndrome (CHS) is characterized by morphologic changes in granulocytes that impair their ability to respond to chemotaxis and to digest or "kill" invading organisms. The child with CHS has recurrent bacterial infections, most commonly caused by *Staphylococcus aureus* but also by streptococci and pneumococci. CHS also affects certain animals.

Causes
CHS is transmitted as an autosomal recessive trait. In many cases, it seems linked to consanguinity.

Signs and symptoms
• Infections in skin, subcutaneous tissue, and lungs with possible fever
• Possible hepatosplenomegaly
• Partial albinism involving ocular fundi, skin, and hair
• Photophobia
• Progressive motor and sensory neuropathy (may eventually cause debilitation and inability to walk or perform activities of daily living)

Diagnostic tests
• Peripheral smear detects characteristic morphologic changes in granulocytes.
• Functional studies confirm delayed chemotaxis of granulocytes and impaired intracellular digestion of organisms.

Treatment
When prevention of infection fails, the next best step is early detection and vigorous treatment of infection with antimicrobials and surgical drainage, if indicated. In a few patients, large doses of vitamin C (ascorbic acid) have helped enhance chemotaxis of abnormal granulocytes, although without associated clinical improvement.

Clinical implications
• Provide meticulous skin care to maintain skin integrity and prevent infection.
• Teach the patient and his family how to prevent and recognize infection, especially in areas of decreased sensation.
• After surgical drainage of infection, provide diligent wound care. Irrigate draining or open wounds and change sterile dressings frequently.
• Administer antimicrobials, as ordered, and monitor the patient for drug adverse effects. Also check the I.V. site frequently.

• Suggest sunglasses or a visor, or both, to minimize discomfort from photophobia. Also teach the patient how to avoid injury associated with decreased sensation or motor coordination.

• Offer emotional support to help the patient and his family cope with this difficult disorder and maintain as normal a life-style as possible.

Complications

Patients who survive recurrent bouts of infection commonly develop marked proliferation of granulocytes or lymphocytes, resembling lymphoreticular malignancy. These cells infiltrate the liver, spleen, and bone marrow, causing progressively severe hepatosplenomegaly, thrombocytopenia, neutropenia, and anemia. Eventually, this cellular proliferation is fatal.

Chest injuries, blunt

Description

Chest injuries account for one fourth of all trauma deaths in the United States. Many are blunt chest injuries, which include myocardial contusion and rib and sternal fractures that may be simple, multiple, displaced, or jagged. Such fractures may cause potentially fatal complications, such as hemothorax, pneumothorax, hemorrhagic shock, and diaphragmatic rupture.

Causes

• Motor vehicle accidents (most common)
• Sports injuries
• Blast injuries

Signs and symptoms
Rib fractures
—Tenderness, slight edema over the fracture site
—Pain that worsens with deep breathing and movement, causing shallow, splinted respirations

Sternal fractures
—Persistent chest pains, even at rest. (See *Complications of Blunt Chest Injuries*.)

Diagnostic tests

• Chest X-rays may confirm rib and sternal fractures, pneumothorax, flail chest, pulmonary contusions, lacerated or ruptured aorta, tension pneumothorax (mediastinal shift), diaphragmatic rupture, lung compression, or atelectasis with hemothorax.

• With cardiac damage, EKG changes may show right bundle branch block.

• Serial serum glutamic-oxaloacetic transaminase (SGOT), serum glutamic-pyruvic transaminase (SGPT), lactate dehydrogenase, creatine phosphokinase, and MB fraction are elevated.

• Retrograde aortography reveals aortic laceration or rupture.

• Contrast studies and liver and spleen scans detect diaphragmatic rupture.

• Other studies, such as echocardiography, computed tomography, and cardiac and lung scans, show the extent of injury.

Treatment and clinical implications

Blunt chest injuries call for immediate physical assessment, control of bleeding, maintenance of a patent airway, adequate ventilation, and fluid and electrolyte balance. In addition, follow these guidelines:

• Check pulses (including peripheral pulses) and level of consciousness. Evaluate color and temperature of skin, depth of respiration, use of accessory muscles, and length of inhalation compared to exhalation.

• Observe tracheal position. Look for distended jugular veins and paradoxical chest motion. Listen to heart and lung sounds carefully; gently palpate for subcutaneous emphysema (crepitation) or structural disintegrity of the ribs.

• Obtain a thorough history of the injury. Unless severe dyspnea is present, ask the patient to locate the pain, and

Complications of Blunt Chest Injuries

• *Pneumothorax* results if a fractured rib tears the pleura and punctures a lung. This usually produces severe dyspnea, cyanosis, agitation, extreme pain, and, when air escapes into chest tissue, subcutaneous emphysema.

• *Flail chest* may result from multiple rib fractures. A portion of the chest wall "caves in", which causes a loss of chest wall integrity and prevents adequate lung inflation. Bruised skin, extreme pain caused by rib fracture, disfigurement, paradoxical chest movements, and rapid, shallow respirations are all signs of flail chest, as are tachycardia, hypotension, respiratory acidosis, and cyanosis.

• *Tension pneumothorax* can result from flail chest. This is a condition in which air enters the chest but cannot be ejected during exhalation; life-threatening thoracic pressure buildup causes lung collapse and subsequent mediastinal shift. The cardinal symptoms of tension pneumothorax include tracheal deviation (away from the affected side), cyanosis, severe dyspnea, absent breath sounds (on the affected side), agitation, distended jugular veins, and shock.

• *Hemothorax* occurs when a rib lacerates lung tissue or an intercostal artery, causing blood to collect in the pleural cavity, thereby compressing the lung and limiting respiratory capacity. It can also result from rupture of large or small pulmonary vessels. Massive hemothorax is the most common cause of shock following chest trauma.

• *Pulmonary contusions* result in hemoptysis, hypoxia, dyspnea, and possible obstruction.

• *Myocardial contusions* produce tachycardia, dysrhythmia, conduction abnormalities, and ST-T segment changes.

• *Diaphragmatic rupture* (usually on the left side) causes severe respiratory distress. Unless treated early, abdominal viscera may herniate through the rupture into the thorax, compromising both circulation and the lungs' vital capacity.

Other complications include laceration or rupture of the aorta, which is nearly always immediately fatal; myocardial tears; cardiac tamponade; pulmonary artery tears; ventricular rupture; and bronchial, tracheal, or esophageal tears or rupture.

ask if he is having trouble breathing. Obtain an order for appropriate laboratory studies (arterial blood gas analysis, cardiac enzyme studies, complete blood count, typing and cross matching).

• For simple rib fractures, give mild analgesics, encourage bed rest, and apply heat. Do not strap or tape the chest.

• For more severe fractures, assist with administration of intercostal nerve blocks. (Obtain X-rays both before and after to rule out pneumothorax.) Intubate the patient in the event of excessive bleeding or hemopneumothorax. Chest tubes may be inserted, especially if bleeding is prolonged. To prevent atelectasis, turn the patient frequently, and encourage coughing and deep breathing.

• For pneumothorax, assist during placement of a large-bore needle into the second intercostal space—in the midclavicular line on the affected side or in the midaxillary line at the fourth intercostal space—to aspirate as much air as possible from the pleural cavity and to reexpand the lungs. When time permits, insert chest tubes attached to water-seal drainage and suction.

• For flail chest, place the patient in the semi-Fowler position. Wrap the affected area with an elastic bandage, or pad it with a thick dressing. Then, tape it with wide adhesive, to stabilize the chest wall. As temporary first aid, place sandbags on the affected side, or exert manual pressure over the flail segment on exhalation. Using an endotracheal tube, give oxygen at a high flow rate under positive pressure. Reposition the patient, suction frequently, give postural drainage, maintain acid-base balance, and provide controlled mechanical ventilation until paradoxical motion of the chest wall ceases. Observe for signs of tension pneumothorax. Start I.V. therapy, using lactated Ringer's or normal saline solution.

• For hemothorax, treat shock with I.V. infusions of lactated Ringer's or normal saline solution. Administer oxygen, and assist with insertion of chest tubes into the fifth or sixth intercostal space at the midaxillary line to remove blood. Monitor vital signs and blood loss. Watch for and immediately report falling blood pressure, rising pulse rate, and uncontrolled hemorrhage. All of these mandate thoracotomy to stop bleeding.

• For pulmonary contusions, give limited amounts of colloids (salt-poor albumin, whole blood, or plasma), as ordered, to replace volume and maintain oncotic pressure. Give analgesics, diuretics, and, if necessary, corticosteroids, as ordered (use of steroids is controversial). Monitor arterial blood gases to ensure adequate ventilation. Provide oxygen therapy, mechanical ventilation, and chest tube care, as needed.

• For suspected cardiac damage, close intensive care or telemetry may detect dysrhythmias and prevent cardiogenic shock. Impose bed rest in the semi-Fowler position (unless the patient requires shock position); as needed, administer oxygen, analgesics, and supportive drugs, such as digitalis, to control heart failure or supraventricular dysrhythmia. Watch for cardiac tamponade, which calls for pericardiocentesis. Essentially, provide the same care as for a patient who has suffered a myocardial infarction.

• For myocardial rupture, septal perforations, and other cardiac lacerations, immediate surgical repair is mandatory. Less severe ventricular wounds require a digital or balloon catheter; atrial wounds, a clamp or balloon catheter.

• For the few patients with aortic rupture or laceration who reach the hospital alive, immediate surgery is mandatory, using synthetic grafts or anastomosis to repair the damage. Give large volumes of I.V. fluids (lactated Ringer's or normal saline solution) and whole blood, along with oxygen at very high flow rates. Apply medical antishock trousers, and transport the patient promptly to the operating room.

• For tension pneumothorax, expect to assist with insertion of a spinal, or 14G to 16G, needle into the second intercostal space at the midclavicular line, to release pressure in the chest. After that, insert a chest tube to normalize pressure and reexpand the lung. Administer oxygen under positive pressure, along with I.V. fluids.

• For a diaphragmatic rupture, insert a nasogastric tube to temporarily decompress the stomach, and prepare the patient for surgical repair.

Chest wounds, penetrating

Description
Penetrating chest wounds, depending on their size, may cause varying degrees of damage to bones, soft tissue, blood vessels, and nerves. Mortality and morbidity from a chest wound depend on the size and severity of the wound. Gunshot wounds are usually more serious than stab wounds, both because they cause more severe lacerations and more rapid blood loss and because ricochet frequently damages large areas and multiple organs. With prompt, aggressive treatment, up to 90% of patients with penetrating chest wounds recover.

Causes
• Stab wounds from a knife or ice pick are the most common penetrating chest wounds; gunshot wounds are a close second.
• Explosions or firearms fired at close range are the usual source of large, gaping wounds.

Signs and symptoms
• Obvious chest wound
• Sucking sound, as the diaphragm contracts and air enters the chest cavity through the wound
• Varying levels of consciousness
• Severe pain, with splinted respirations
• Rapid, weak, thready pulse

Diagnostic tests
• Arterial blood gases assess respiratory status.
• Chest X-rays before and after chest tube placement evaluate injury and tube placement.
• Results of complete blood count show low hemoglobin and hematocrit, reflecting severe blood loss.

Treatment and clinical implications
Penetrating chest wounds require immediate support of respiration and circulation, prompt surgical repair of tissue injury, and appropriate measures to prevent complications. Follow these guidelines:
• Immediately assess airway, breathing, and circulation. Establish a patent airway, and support ventilation, as needed. Monitor pulses frequently for rate and quality.
• Place an occlusive dressing (such as petrolatum-impregnated gauze) over the sucking wound. Monitor for signs of tension pneumothorax (tracheal shift, respiratory distress, tachycardia, tachypnea, diminished or absent breath sounds on the affected side); if tension pneumothorax develops, temporarily remove the occlusive dressing to create a simple pneumothorax.

• Control blood loss (also remember to look *under* the patient to estimate loss), type and cross match blood, and replace blood and fluids, as necessary.
• Assist with chest X-ray and placement of chest tubes (using water-seal drainage) to reestablish intrathoracic pressure and to drain blood in hemothorax. A second X-ray will evaluate the position of tubes and their function.
• After the patient's condition has stabilized, surgery can repair the damage caused by the wound.
• Throughout treatment, monitor central venous pressure and blood pressure to detect hypovolemia, and assess vital signs. Provide analgesics as appropriate. Tetanus and antibiotic prophylaxis may be necessary.
• Reassure the patient, especially if he was the victim of a violent crime. Report the incident to the police in accordance with local laws. Help contact the patient's family, and offer them reassurance.

Complications
Penetrating chest wounds may also cause lung lacerations (bleeding and substantial air leakage through the chest tube), arterial lacerations (loss of more than 100 ml blood/hour through the chest tube), and hemothorax. Other effects may include dysrhythmias, cardiac tamponade, mediastinitis, subcutaneous emphysema, esophageal perforation, bronchopleural fistula, and tracheobronchial, abdominal, or diaphragmatic injuries.

Chlamydial infections

Description
Chlamydial infections—including urethritis in men, cervicitis in women, and lymphogranuloma venereum (LGV) in both—are linked to one organism: *Chlamydia trachomatis*. They are the most common sexually transmitted diseases in the United States.

However, because symptoms of many chlamydial infections do not appear until late in the course of the disease, sexual transmission of the organism often occurs unknowingly.

Trachoma inclusion conjunctivitis, a chlamydial infection that occurs rarely in the United States, is a leading cause of blindness in Third World countries.

Cause

C. trachomatis

Mode of transmission

Mucosal contact with an infected person

Signs and symptoms

Lymphogranuloma venereum (LGV)
—Primary lesion: painless vesicle or nonindurated ulcer, 2 to 3 mm in diameter (frequently unnoticed)
—Regional lymphadenopathy (after 1 to 4 weeks); inguinal lymph node swelling (2 weeks later)
—Systemic symptoms, such as myalgia, headache, fever, chills, backache, weight loss

Proctitis
—Diarrhea, tenesmus, pruritus, bloody or mucopurulent discharge, or diffuse or discrete ulceration in the rectosigmoid colon

Cervicitis
—Cervical erosion, mucopurulent discharge, pelvic pain, or dyspareunia

Endometritis or salpingitis
—Pain and tenderness of the abdomen, cervix, uterus, and lymph nodes; chills; fever; vaginal discharge; or dysuria

Urethral syndrome
—Dysuria, pyuria, or urinary frequency

Epididymitis
—Painful scrotal swelling, urethral discharge

Prostatitis
—Lower back pain, urinary frequency, dysuria, nocturia, urethral discharge, or painful ejaculation

Urethritis
—Dysuria, erythema and tenderness of the urethral meatus, urinary frequency, pruritus, or urethral discharge

Diagnostic tests

• A swab culture from the site of infection (urethra, cervix, rectum) usually establishes the diagnosis of urethritis, cervicitis, salpingitis, endometritis, or proctitis.
• Culture of aspirated blood, pus, or cerebrospinal fluid establishes the diagnosis of epididymitis, prostatitis, or LGV.
• Direct visualization of cell scrapings or exudate with Giemsa stain or fluorescein-conjugated monoclonal antibodies may be attempted if the site is accessible, but tissue cell cultures are more sensitive and specific.
• Serologic tests to determine previous exposure to *C. trachomatis* include complement fixation and microimmunofluorescence (Micro IF) tests. Although the enzyme-linked immunosorbent assay is as effective as the Micro IF test at detecting *C. trachomatis* antibody, its value is uncertain.

Treatment

Recommended treatment is tetracycline P.O. for 7 to 21 days, or erythromycin or sulfamethoxazole P.O. for at least 7 days. Patients with LGV require extended treatment. In pregnant women with chlamydial infections, erythromycin (stearate base) is the treatment of choice, because of the adverse effects of tetracycline and sulfonamides on fetal growth and development.

Clinical implications

• To prevent contracting a chlamydial infection, double-bag all soiled dressings and contaminated instruments, and wear gloves when handling contaminated material and giving patient care.

• Make sure the patient understands dosage requirements of prescribed medications. Stress the importance of completing the course of drug therapy even after symptoms subside.
• To prevent reinfection during treatment, urge abstinence from intercourse or encourage use of condoms.
• Urge the patient to inform sexual contacts of his infection so they can seek treatment. Report all cases to local public health authorities for follow-up on sexual contacts.
• Check newborns of infected mothers for signs of infection. Take specimens for culture from the infant's eyes, nasopharynx, and rectum. (Positive rectal cultures will peak by 5 to 6 weeks postpartum.)

Complications

Untreated, chlamydial infections can lead to such complications as acute epididymitis, salpingitis, pelvic inflammatory disease, and eventually sterility. In pregnant women, chlamydial infections are also associated with spontaneous abortion, premature delivery, and neonatal death, although a direct link with *C. trachomatis* has not been established.

Children born of infected mothers may contract trachoma inclusion conjunctivitis, otitis media, and pneumonia during passage through the birth canal.

Chloride imbalance

Description

Hypochloremia and hyperchloremia are, respectively, conditions of deficient or excessive serum levels of the anion chloride. A predominantly extracellular anion, chloride accounts for two thirds of all serum anions. Secreted by stomach mucosa as hydrochloric acid, it provides an acid medium conducive to digestion and activation of enzymes. Chloride also participates in maintaining acid-base and body water balances, influences the osmolality or tonicity of extracellular fluid, plays a role in the exchange of oxygen and carbon dioxide in red blood cells, and helps activate salivary amylase (which in turn activates the digestive process).

Causes

Hypochloremia

—Decreased chloride intake or absorption, as in low dietary sodium intake, sodium deficiency, potassium deficiency, or metabolic alkalosis; prolonged use of mercurial diuretics; or administration of dextrose I.V. without electrolytes
—Excessive chloride loss, resulting from prolonged diarrhea or diaphoresis; loss of hydrochloric acid in gastric secretions from vomiting, gastric suctioning, or gastric surgery

Hyperchloremia

—Excessive chloride intake or absorption (as in hyperingestion of ammonium chloride, or ureterointestinal anastomosis), allowing reabsorption of chloride by the bowel
—Hemoconcentration caused by dehydration
—Compensatory mechanisms for other metabolic abnormalities, as in metabolic acidosis, neurogenic hyperventilation caused by brain stem injury, and hyperparathyroidism

Signs and symptoms

Hypochloremia associated with hyponatremia
—Muscular weakness
—Twitching

Hypochloremia associated with loss of gastric secretions
—Muscle hypertonicity
—Tetany
—Shallow, depressed breathing

Hyperchloremia associated with hypernatremia and fluid volume excess
—Agitation

—Tachycardia
—Hypertension
—Pitting edema
—Dyspnea
Hyperchloremia associated with metabolic acidosis
—Deep, rapid breathing
—Weakness
—Diminished cognitive ability
—Coma

Diagnostic tests
• Serum chloride level < 98 mEq/liter confirms hypochloremia; supportive values with metabolic alkalosis include serum pH > 7.45 and serum CO_2 > 32 mEq/liter.
• Serum chloride level > 108 mEq/liter confirms hyperchloremia; with metabolic acidosis, serum pH is < 7.35 and serum CO_2 is < 22 mEq/liter.

Treatment
In either kind of chloride imbalance, treatment must correct the underlying disorder. The aims of treatment for hypochloremia are to correct the condition that causes excessive chloride loss and to give oral replacement, such as salty broth. When oral therapy is not possible or when emergency measures are necessary, treatment may include normal saline solution I.V. (if hypovolemia is present) or chloride-containing drugs such as ammonium chloride to increase serum chloride levels and potassium chloride for metabolic alkalosis.

For severe hyperchloremic acidosis, treatment consists of sodium bicarbonate I.V. to raise serum bicarbonate level and permit renal excretion of the chloride anion, because bicarbonate and chloride compete to combine with sodium. For mild hyperchloremia, lactated Ringer's solution is administered; it converts to bicarbonate in the liver, thus increasing base bicarbonate to correct acidosis.

Clinical implications
When managing the patient with hypochloremia, follow these guidelines:
• Monitor serum chloride levels frequently, particularly during I.V. therapy.
• Watch for signs of hyperchloremia or hypochloremia. Be alert for respiratory difficulty.
• To prevent hypochloremia, monitor laboratory results (serum electrolyte levels and arterial blood gases) and fluid intake and output of patients who are vulnerable to chloride imbalance, particularly those recovering from gastric surgery. Record and report excessive or continuous loss of gastric secretions. Also report prolonged infusion of dextrose in water without saline.

When managing the patient with hyperchloremia, follow these guidelines:
• Check serum electrolyte levels every 3 to 6 hours. If the patient is receiving high doses of sodium bicarbonate, watch for signs of overcorrection (metabolic alkalosis, respiratory depression) or lingering signs of hyperchloremia, which indicate inadequate treatment.
• To prevent hyperchloremia, check laboratory results for elevated serum chloride level or potassium imbalance if the patient is receiving I.V. solutions containing sodium chloride, and monitor fluid intake and output. Also, watch for signs of metabolic acidosis. When administering I.V. fluids containing lactated Ringer's solution, monitor flow rate according to the patient's age, physical condition, and bicarbonate level. Report any irregularities promptly.

Cholecystitis, cholelithiasis, and related disorders

Description
Diseases of the gallbladder and biliary tract are common and frequently pain-

---

Gallbladder and Biliary Tract Disorders

Cholelithiasis, stones or calculi in the gallbladder (gallstones), results from changes in bile components. It is the leading biliary tract disease, affects over 20 million Americans, and accounts for the third most common surgical procedure performed in the United States—cholecystectomy. Prognosis is usually good with treatment unless infection occurs, in which case prognosis depends on its severity and response to antibiotics.

Choledocholithiasis occurs when gallstones passed out of the gallbladder lodge in the common bile duct, causing partial or complete biliary obstruction. Prognosis is good unless infection develops.

Cholecystitis, acute or chronic inflammation of the gallbladder, is usually associated with a gallstone impacted in the cystic duct, causing painful distention of the gallbladder. The acute form is most common during middle age; the chronic form, among the elderly. Prognosis is good with treatment.

Cholangitis, infection of the bile duct, is frequently associated with choledocholithiasis and may follow percutaneous transhepatic cholangiography. Widespread inflammation may cause fibrosis and stenosis of the common bile duct. Prognosis for this rare condition is poor—stenosing or primary sclerosing cholangitis is almost always fatal.

Gallstone ileus involves small-bowel obstruction by a gallstone. Typically, the gallstone travels through a fistula between the gallbladder and small bowel and lodges at the ileocecal valve. This condition is most common in the elderly. Prognosis is good with surgery.

---

ful conditions that usually require surgery and may be life-threatening. They are often associated with deposition of calculi and inflammation. Generally, gallbladder and duct diseases occur in middle age. Between ages 20 and 50, they are six times more common in women, but incidence in men and women becomes equal after age 50. Incidence rises with each succeeding decade. (See *Gallbladder and Biliary Tract Disorders.*)

Causes
The exact cause of gallstone formation is unknown, but abnormal metabolism of cholesterol and bile salts is a likely cause.

Risk factors
Possible risk factors for gallstone formation include the following:
• High-calorie, high-cholesterol diet, associated with obesity
• Elevated estrogen levels from oral contraceptives, postmenopausal therapy, pregnancy, or multiparity
• Antilipemic clofibrate
• Diabetes mellitus, ileal disease, hemolytic disorders, liver disease, and pancreatitis

Signs and symptoms
Acute cholelithiasis, acute cholecystitis, choledocholithiasis
—Classic attack with severe midepigastric or right upper quadrant pain radiating to the back or referred to the right scapula, frequently following meals rich in fats
—Recurring fat intolerance
—Belching that leaves a sour taste in the mouth
—Flatulence
—Indigestion
—Diaphoresis
—Nausea
—Chills and low-grade fever
—Possible jaundice and clay-colored stools with common duct obstruction
Cholangitis
—Abdominal pain

—High fever and chills
—Possible jaundice and related itching
—Weakness, fatigue
Gallstone ileus
—Nausea and vomiting
—Abdominal distention
—Absent bowel sounds, if complete bowel obstruction
—Intermittent colicky pain over several days

Diagnostic tests

• Ultrasound examination reflects calculi in the gallbladder with 96% accuracy.
• Percutaneous transhepatic cholangiography, done under fluoroscopic control, distinguishes between gallbladder disease and cancer of the pancreatic head in patients with jaundice.
• Endoscopic retrograde cholangiopancreatography visualizes the biliary tree after endoscopic examination of the duodenum, cannulation of the common bile and pancreatic ducts, and injection of contrast medium.
• HIDA scan (technetium-labeled iminodiacetic acid, ^{99m}Tc HIDA) of the gallbladder detects obstruction of the cystic duct.
• Computed tomography, although not used routinely, helps distinguish between obstructive and nonobstructive jaundice.
• X-ray of the abdomen identifies calcified, but not cholesterol, calculi with 15% accuracy.
• Oral cholecystography shows calculi in the gallbladder and biliary duct obstruction.
• Intravenous cholangiography visualizes the ductal system (rarely used).
• Laboratory tests showing elevated icteric index, total bilirubin, urine bilirubin, and alkaline phosphatase support the diagnosis. White blood cell count is slightly elevated during a cholecystitis attack. Serum amylase distinguishes gallbladder disease from

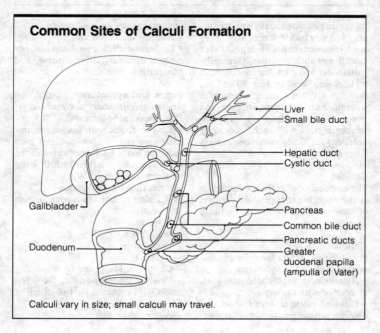

Common Sites of Calculi Formation

Liver
Small bile duct
Hepatic duct
Cystic duct
Gallbladder
Pancreas
Common bile duct
Pancreatic ducts
Greater duodenal papilla (ampulla of Vater)
Duodenum

Calculi vary in size; small calculi may travel.

pancreatitis.
• Serial enzyme tests and EKG should precede diagnostic tests if heart disease is suspected. (See *Common Sites of Calculi Formation*.)

Treatment
Surgery, usually elective, is the treatment of choice for gallbladder and duct disease. Surgery may include cholecystectomy, cholecystectomy with operative cholangiography, and possibly exploration of the common bile duct. Other treatment includes a low-fat diet to prevent attacks and vitamin K for itching, jaundice, and bleeding tendencies caused by vitamin K deficiency. Treatment during an acute attack may include insertion of a nasogastric tube and an I.V. line, and antibiotic administration.

A recently developed nonsurgical treatment for choledocholithiasis involves insertion of a flexible catheter, formed around a T tube, through a sinus tract into the common bile duct. Guided by fluoroscopy, the catheter is directed toward the stone. A Dormia basket is threaded through the catheter, opened, twirled to entrap the calculi, closed, and withdrawn.

Chenodiol, a newly available drug that dissolves radiolucent calculi, provides an alternative for patients who are poor surgical risks or who refuse surgery. However, use of chenodiol is limited by the need for prolonged treatment, the high incidence of adverse effects, and the frequency of calculi reformation after treatment is stopped.

Clinical implications
• Before surgery, teach the patient to deep-breathe, cough, expectorate, and perform leg exercises that are necessary after surgery. Also teach splinting, repositioning, and ambulation techniques. Explain the procedures that will be performed before, during, and after surgery, to help ease the patient's anxiety and ensure his cooperation.
• After surgery, monitor vital signs for signs of bleeding, infection, or atelectasis. Evaluate the incision site for bleeding. Serosanguineous and bile drainage is common during the first 24 to 48 hours if the patient has a wound drain such as a Jackson-Pratt or Penrose drain. If, after a choledochostomy, a T-tube drain is placed in the duct and attached to a drainage bag, make sure the drainage tube is not kinked. Also check that connecting tubing from the T tube is well secured to the patient to prevent dislodging. Measure and record drainage daily (200 to 300 ml is normal). Teach patients who will be discharged with a T tube how to empty it, change the dressing, and provide proper skin care.
• Monitor intake and output. Allow the patient nothing by mouth for 24 to 48 hours or until bowel sounds return and nausea and vomiting cease.
• Encourage deep-breathing and leg exercises every hour. The patient should ambulate in the evening or morning after surgery. Provide antiembolism stockings to support leg muscles and promote venous blood flow.
• Administer adequate medication to relieve pain, especially before such activities as deep breathing and ambulation, which increase pain.
• At discharge (usually 4 to 10 days after surgery), advise the patient against heavy lifting or straining for 6 weeks. Urge him to walk daily. Tell him that food restrictions are unnecessary unless he has an intolerance to a specific food or some underlying condition (diabetes, atherosclerosis, obesity).

Cholera
(Asiatic cholera, epidemic cholera)

Description
Cholera is an acute enterotoxin-mediated GI infection that produces profuse diarrhea, vomiting, massive fluid

and electrolyte loss, and possibly hypovolemic shock, metabolic acidosis, and death. Even with prompt diagnosis and treatment, cholera is fatal in up to 2% of children because of difficulty with fluid replacement; in adults, it is fatal in fewer than 1%. Untreated cholera may be fatal in as many as 50% of victims, however. Cholera infection confers only transient immunity.

Causes
Gram-negative, mobile, aerobic bacterium *Vibrio cholerae*

Mode of transmission
Directly through food and water contaminated with fecal material from carriers or persons with active infections

Signs and symptoms
• Painless, profuse, watery diarrhea (in adults, fluid loss may reach 1 liter/hour); may contain white flecks of mucus
• Effortless vomiting (without preceding nausea)
• Fluid and electrolyte losses
• Apathy
• Possible stupor or convulsions in small children
• Intense thirst, weakness, loss of skin turgor, wrinkled skin, sunken eyes, pinched facial expression, muscle cramps (especially in the extremities), cyanosis, oliguria, tachycardia, tachypnea, thready or absent peripheral pulses, falling blood pressure, fever, and inaudible, hypoactive bowel sounds

Diagnostic tests
• Culture of *V. cholerae* from feces or vomitus indicates cholera.
• Definitive diagnosis requires agglutination and other clear reactions to group- and type-specific antisera.
• Dark-field microscopic examination of fresh feces showing rapidly moving bacilli (like shooting stars) allows for quick, tentative diagnosis.
• Immunofluorescence also allows for rapid diagnosis.

Treatment
Improved sanitation and the administration of cholera vaccine to travelers in endemic areas can control this disease. Unfortunately, the vaccine now available confers only 60% to 80% immunity and is effective for only 3 to 6 months. Consequently, vaccination is impractical for residents of endemic areas.

Treatment requires rehydration by rapid I.V. infusion of large amounts (50 to 100 ml/minute) of isotonic saline solution, alternating with isotonic sodium bicarbonate or sodium lactate. Potassium may be added to the I.V. solution.

When I.V. infusions have corrected hypovolemia, fluid infusion decreases to a rate sufficient to maintain normal pulse and skin turgor or to replace fluid lost through diarrhea. An oral glucose-electrolyte solution can substitute for I.V. infusions. In mild cholera, oral fluid replacement is adequate. If symptoms persist despite fluid and electrolyte replacement, treatment includes tetracycline.

Clinical implications
• Wear a gown and gloves when giving physical care, and wash your hands before entering and after leaving the patient's room.
• Monitor output (including stool volume) and I.V. infusion accurately. To detect overhydration, carefully observe neck veins and auscultate the lungs (fluid loss in cholera is massive, and improper replacement may cause potentially fatal renal insufficiency).
• Protect the patient's family by administering oral tetracycline, if ordered.
• Advise anyone traveling to an endemic area to boil all drinking water and avoid uncooked vegetables. If the physician orders a cholera vaccine, tell

the patient that he will need a booster 3 to 6 months later for continuing protection.

Complications

If treatment is delayed or inadequate, cholera may lead to metabolic acidosis, uremia, and possibly coma and death.

Chronic granulomatous disease

Description

In chronic granulomatous disease (CGD), abnormal neutrophil metabolism impairs phagocytosis—one of the body's chief defense mechanisms—resulting in increased susceptibility to low-virulent or nonpathogenic organisms, such as *Nocardia, Staphylococcus epidermidis, Escherichia coli*, and *Aspergillus*. Phagocytes attracted to sites of infection can engulf these invading organisms but are unable to destroy them. Patients with CGD may develop granulomatous inflammation, which leads to ischemic tissue damage. Usually, the patient with CGD displays signs and symptoms by age 2, associated with infections of the skin, lymph nodes, lungs, liver, and bone.

Causes

CGD is usually inherited as an X-linked trait. A variant form—probably autosomal recessive—also exists. The genetic defect may be linked to deficiency of the enzyme NADH, NADPH oxidase, or NADH reductase.

Signs and symptoms

• Skin infection is characterized by small, well-localized areas of tenderness. Seborrheic dermatitis of the scalp and axilla is also common.
• Lymph node infection typically causes marked lymphadenopathy, with draining lymph nodes and hepatosplenomegaly.
• Liver abscess may be recurrent and multiple with abdominal tenderness, fever, anorexia, and nausea.
• Osteomyelitis causes localized pain and fever.
• Symptoms of pneumonia and periodontal disease may also be present.

Diagnostic tests

• The nitroblue tetrazolium (NBT) test, which assesses killing ability of neutrophils, confirms the diagnosis. Patients with CGD show impaired NBT reduction.
• Other laboratory values may support the diagnosis or help monitor disease activity.

Treatment and clinical implications

Early, aggressive treatment of infection is the chief goal in caring for a patient with CGD. Areas of suspected infection should be biopsied or cultured. Broad-spectrum antibiotics usually are started immediately, without waiting for results of cultures. Confirmed abscesses may be drained or surgically removed. Provide meticulous wound care after such treatment, including irrigation or packing.

Many patients with CGD receive a combination of I.V. antibiotics, frequently extended beyond the usual 10- to 14-day course. However, for fungal infections with *Aspergillus* or *Nocardia*, treatment involves amphotericin B in gradually increasing doses to achieve a maximum cumulative dose. During I.V. drug therapy, monitor the patient's vital signs frequently. Rotate the I.V. site every 48 to 72 hours.

To help treat life-threatening or antibiotic-resistant infection, or to help localize infection, the patient may receive granulocyte transfusions—usually once daily until the crisis has passed. During such transfusions, watch for fever and chills (these effects can sometimes be prevented by premedication with acetaminophen). Transfusions should not be given within 6 hours before or after amphotericin B to avoid severe pulmonary edema and possible respiratory arrest.

If prophylactic antibiotics are ordered, teach the patient and his family how to administer them properly and how to recognize adverse effects. Advise them to promptly report any signs or symptoms of infection. Stress the importance of good nutrition and hygiene, especially meticulous skin and mouth care.

During hospitalizations, encourage the patient to continue activities of daily living as much as possible. Try to arrange for a tutor to help the child keep up with his schoolwork.

Chronic mucocutaneous candidiasis

Description
Chronic mucocutaneous candidiasis is a form of candidiasis (moniliasis) that usually develops during the first year of life but occasionally may occur as late as the twenties. Affecting males and females, it is characterized by repeated infection with Candida albicans. In some patients, an autoimmune response affecting the endocrine system may induce various endocrinopathies.

Despite chronic candidiasis, patients rarely die of systemic infection. Instead, they usually die of hepatic or endocrine failure. Prognosis for chronic mucocutaneous candidiasis depends on the severity of the associated endocrinopathy. Patients with associated endocrinopathy rarely live beyond their thirties.

Causes
Although no characteristic immunologic defects have been identified, it is felt that this disorder may result from an inherited defect in cell-mediated (T-cell) immunity. (Humoral immunity, mediated by B cells, is intact.)

Signs and symptoms
• Large, circular lesions affecting the skin, mucous membranes, nails, and vagina
• Endocrine abnormalities, most commonly tetany related to hypoparathyroidism

Diagnostic tests
• Circulating T-cell count is usually normal, but it may be decreased.
• Delayed hypersensitivity tests to Candida are not found in most patients, even during the infectious stage.
• Laboratory test values may be abnormal because of an endocrinopathy and may include hypocalcemia, abnormal hepatic function studies, hyperglycemia, iron deficiency, and abnormal vitamin B_{12} absorption (pernicious anemia).

Treatment and clinical implications
Treatment aims to control infection but is not always successful. Topical antifungal agents are frequently ineffective against chronic mucocutaneous candidiasis. Miconazole and nystatin are sometimes useful, but ultimately fail to control this infection.

Systemic infections may not be fatal, but they are serious enough to warrant vigorous treatment. Oral ketoconazole and injected thymosin have had some positive effect. Oral or intramuscular iron replacement may be necessary.

Teach the patient about the progressive manifestations of the disease, and emphasize the importance of seeing an endocrinologist for regular checkups. Treatment may also include plastic surgery, when possible, and counseling to help the patient cope with disfigurement.

Complications

Most patients eventually develop endocrinopathies. Hypoparathyroidism, Addison's disease, hypothyroidism, diabetes, and pernicious anemia may occur. Psychiatric disorders are likely because of disfigurement and multiple endocrine aberrations.

Chronic obstructive pulmonary disease
(COPD, chronic obstructive lung disease [COLD])

Description

Chronic obstructive pulmonary disease (COPD) is chronic airway obstruction that usually results from emphysema, chronic bronchitis, asthma, or any combination of these disorders. Usually, more than one of these underlying conditions coexist. Most frequently, bronchitis and emphysema occur together. The most common chronic lung disease, COPD affects an estimated 17 million Americans, and its incidence is rising. It affects men more frequently than women, probably because until recently men were more likely to smoke heavily. It does not always produce symptoms and causes only minimal disability in many patients. However, COPD tends to worsen with time. It ranks fifth among the major causes of death in the United States.

Causes
• Emphysema
• Chronic bronchitis
• Asthma
• Bronchiectasis
• Cystic fibrosis

Risk factors
• Cigarette smoking (by far the most important)
• Recurrent or chronic respiratory infection
• Allergies
• Possible familial and hereditary factors (such as deficiency of alpha$_1$-antitrypsin)

Signs and symptoms
• The typical patient has no symptoms until middle age, when his ability to exercise or do strenuous work gradually starts to decline, and he begins to develop a productive cough.
• Eventually the patient develops dyspnea on minimal exertion.

Teaching Topics in Chronic Obstructive Pulmonary Disease

• An explanation of the disease process
• Preparation for pulmonary function tests, chest X-rays, and other diagnostic studies
• Exercise program
• Importance of diet and adequate hydration
• Drugs and their administration
• How to use an oral inhaler
• Chest physiotherapy at home
• Oxygen therapy at home
• Pursed-lip breathing exercises
• Importance of avoiding bronchial irritants, such as cigarette smoke
• How to modify activities of daily living
• Sexual counseling
• Warning signs and prevention of respiratory infection
• Availability of support groups, such as the American Lung Association

Types of COPD

DISEASE	CAUSES AND PATHO-PHYSIOLOGY	CLINICAL FEATURES
Emphysema • Abnormal irreversible enlargement of air spaces distal to terminal bronchioles caused by destruction of alveolar walls, resulting in decreased elastic recoil properties of lungs • Most common cause of death from respiratory disease in the United States	• Cigarette smoking, deficiency of alpha$_1$-antitrypsin • Recurrent inflammation associated with release of proteolytic enzymes from cells in lungs causes bronchiolar and alveolar wall damage and, ultimately, destruction. Loss of lung supporting structure results in decreased elastic recoil and airway collapse on expiration. Destruction of alveolar walls decreases surface area for gas exchange.	• Insidious onset, with dyspnea the predominant symptom • *Other signs and symptoms* of long-term disease: chronic cough, anorexia, weight loss, malaise, "barrel chest," use of accessory muscles of respiration, prolonged expiratory period with grunting, pursed-lip breathing and tachypnea, peripheral cyanosis, and digital clubbing • *Complications* include recurrent respiratory tract infections, cor pulmonale, and respiratory failure.
Chronic bronchitis • Excessive mucus production with productive cough for at least 3 months a year for 2 successive years • Only a minority of patients with the clinical syndrome of chronic bronchitis develop significant airway obstruction.	• Severity of disease related to amount and duration of smoking; respiratory infection exacerbates symptoms. • Hypertrophy and hyperplasia of bronchial mucous glands, increased goblet cells, damage to cilia, squamous metaplasia of columnar epithelium, and chronic leukocytic and lymphocytic infiltration of bronchial walls; widespread inflammation, distortion, narrowing of airways, and mucus within the airways produce resistance in small airways and cause severe ventilation-perfusion imbalance.	• Insidious onset, with productive cough and exertional dyspnea predominant symptoms • *Other signs and symptoms:* colds associated with increased sputum production and worsening dyspnea that take progressively longer to resolve; copious sputum (gray, white, or yellow); weight gain from edema; cyanosis; tachypnea; wheezing; prolonged expiratory time; use of accessory muscles of respiration

CONFIRMING DIAGNOSTIC MEASURES	MANAGEMENT
• *Physical examination:* hyperresonance on percussion, decreased breath sounds, expiratory prolongation, quiet heart sounds • *Chest X-ray:* in advanced disease, flattened diaphragm, reduced vascular markings at lung periphery, overaeration of lungs, vertical heart, enlarged antero-posterior chest diameter, large retrosternal air space • *Pulmonary function tests:* increased residual volume, total lung capacity, and compliance; decreased vital capacity, diffusing capacity, and expiratory volumes • *Arterial blood gases:* reduced PO_2 with normal PCO_2 until late in disease • *EKG:* tall, symmetrical P waves in leads II, III, and aVF; vertical QRS axis; signs of right ventricular hypertrophy late in disease • *RBC:* increased hemoglobin late in disease when persistent severe hypoxia is present	• Bronchodilators, such as aminophylline, to reverse bronchospasm and promote mucociliary clearance • Antibiotics to treat respiratory infection; influenza vaccine to prevent influenza; and Pneumovax to prevent pneumococcal pneumonia • Adequate fluid intake and, in selected patients, chest physiotherapy to mobilize secretions • O_2 at low-flow settings to treat hypoxia • Avoidance of smoking and air pollutants
• *Physical examination:* rhonchi and wheezes on auscultation, expiratory elongation; neck vein distention, pedal edema • *Chest X-ray:* may show hyperinflation and increased bronchovascular markings • *Pulmonary function tests:* increased residual volume, decreased vital capacity and forced expiratory volumes, normal static compliance and diffusing capacity • *Arterial blood gases:* decreased PO_2; normal or increased PCO_2 • *Sputum:* contains many organisms and neutrophils • *EKG:* may show atrial dysrhythmias; peaked P waves in leads II, III, and aVF; and, occasionally, right ventricular hypertrophy	• Antibiotics for infections • Avoidance of smoking and air pollutants • Bronchodilators to relieve bronchospasm and facilitate mucociliary clearance • Adequate fluid intake and chest physiotherapy to mobilize secretions • Ultrasonic or mechanical nebulizer treatments to loosen secretions and aid in mobilization • Occasionally, patients respond to corticosteroids. • Diuretics for edema • Oxygen for hypoxia

(continued)

Types of COPD (continued)

DISEASE	CAUSES AND PATHO-PHYSIOLOGY	CLINICAL FEATURES
Asthma • Increased bronchial reactivity to a variety of stimuli, which produces episodic bronchospasm and airway obstruction • Asthma with onset in adulthood: in most cases, without distinct allergies; asthma with onset in childhood: in most cases, associated with definite allergens. Status asthmaticus is an acute asthma attack with severe bronchospasm that fails to clear with bronchodilator therapy. • *Prognosis:* More than half of asthmatic children become asymptomatic as adults; more than half of asthmatics with onset after age 15 have persistent disease, with occasional severe attacks.	• Possible mechanisms include allergy (family tendency, seasonal occurrence); allergic reaction results in release of mast cell vasoactive and bronchospastic mediators. • Upper airway infection, exercise, anxiety, and rarely, coughing or laughing can precipitate an asthma attack. • Paroxysmal airway obstruction associated with nasal polyps may be seen in response to aspirin or indomethacin ingestion. • Airway obstruction from spasm of bronchial smooth muscle narrows airways; inflammatory edema of the bronchial wall and inspissation of tenacious mucoid secretions are also important, particularly in status asthmaticus.	• History of intermittent attacks of dyspnea and wheezing • Mild wheezing progresses to severe dyspnea, audible wheezing, chest tightness (a feeling of not being able to breathe), and cough productive of thick mucus. • *Other signs:* prolonged expiration, intercostal and supraclavicular retraction on inspiration, use of accessory muscles of respiration, flaring nostrils, tachypnea, tachycardia, perspiration, and flushing; patients often have symptoms of eczema and allergic rhinitis ("hay fever"). • Status asthmaticus, unless treated promptly, can progress to respiratory failure.

Diagnostic tests

(See *Types of COPD,* pp. 152 to 155, and "Bronchiectasis" and "Cystic Fibrosis.")

Treatment and clinical implications

Treatment is designed to relieve symptoms and prevent complications. Because most COPD patients receive outpatient treatment, they need comprehensive patient teaching to help them comply with therapy and understand the nature of this chronic, progressive disease. If programs in pulmonary rehabilitation are available, encourage the patient to enroll.

• Urge the patient to stop smoking and to avoid other respiratory irritants. Suggest that he install an air conditioner with an air filter in his home; it may prove helpful.

• Explain that bronchodilators alleviate bronchospasm and enhance mucociliary clearance of secretions.

CONFIRMING DIAGNOSTIC MEASURES	MANAGEMENT
• *Physical examination:* usually normal between attacks; auscultation shows rhonchi and wheezing throughout lung fields on expiration and, at times, inspiration; absent or diminished breath sounds during severe obstruction. Loud bilateral wheezes may be grossly audible; chest is hyperinflated. • *Chest X-ray:* hyperinflated lungs with air trapping during attack; normal during remission • *Sputum:* presence of Curschmann's spirals (casts of airways), Charcot-Leyden crystals, and eosinophils • *Pulmonary function tests:* during attacks, decreased forced expiratory volume, which improves significantly after inhaled bronchodilator; increased residual volume and, occasionally, total lung capacity; may be normal between attacks • *Arterial blood gases:* decreased Po_2; decreased, normal, or increased Pco_2 (in severe attack) • *EKG:* sinus tachycardia during an attack; severe attack may produce signs of cor pulmonale (right axis deviation, peaked P wave), which resolve after the attack. • *Skin tests:* may identify allergens	• Aerosol containing beta-adrenergic agents such as metaproterenol or albuterol; also, oral beta-adrenergic agents (terbutaline) and oral methylxanthines (aminophylline); occasionally, inhaled, oral, or I.V. corticosteroids • *Emergency treatment:* O_2 therapy, corticosteroids, and bronchodilators such as subcutaneous epinephrine, I.V. aminophylline, and inhaled agents such as metaproterenol. • Monitor for deteriorating respiratory status, and note sputum characteristics; provide adequate fluid intake and O_2, as ordered. • *Prevention:* Tell the patient to avoid possible allergens and to use antihistamines, decongestants, inhalation of cromolyn powder, and oral or aerosol bronchodilators, as ordered. Explain the influence of stress and anxiety on asthma and frequent association with exercise (particularly running) and cold air.

Familiarize the patient with prescribed bronchodilators.

• Administer antibiotics, as ordered, to treat respiratory infections. Stress the need to complete the prescribed course of antibiotic therapy. Teach the patient and his family how to recognize early signs of infection. Warn the patient to avoid contact with persons with respiratory infections. Encourage good oral hygiene to help prevent infection. Pneumococcal vaccination and annual influenza vaccinations are important preventive measures.

• To strengthen the muscles of respiration, teach the patient to take slow, deep breaths and exhale through pursed lips.

• To help mobilize secretions, teach the patient how to cough effectively. If the patient with copious secretions has difficulty mobilizing secretions, teach his family how to perform postural drainage and chest physiotherapy. If secretions are thick, urge the patient to drink 12 to 15 glasses of fluid a day. A home humidifier may be beneficial, particularly in the winter.

• Administer low concentrations of oxygen, as ordered. Perform blood gas analysis to determine O_2 need and to avoid CO_2 narcosis. If the patient is to continue oxygen therapy at home, teach him how to use the equipment correctly. Patients with COPD rarely require more than 2 to 3 liters/minute to maintain adequate oxygenation.

• Emphasize the importance of a balanced diet. Because the patient may tire easily when eating, suggest frequent, small meals, and consider using oxygen, administered by nasal cannula, during meals.

• Help the patient and his family adjust their life-styles to accommodate the limitations imposed by this debilitating chronic disease. Instruct the patient to allow for daily rest periods and to exercise daily as his physician directs.

• As COPD progresses, encourage the patient to discuss his fears.

• To help prevent COPD, advise all people, especially those with a family history of COPD or those in its early stages, not to smoke.

• Assist in the early detection of COPD by urging persons to have periodic physical examinations, including spirometry and medical evaluation of a chronic cough, and to seek treatment for recurring respiratory infections promptly. (See *Teaching Topics in Chronic Obstructive Pulmonary Disease*, p. 151.)

Cirrhosis

Description

Cirrhosis is a chronic hepatic disease characterized by diffuse destruction and fibrotic regeneration of hepatic cells. As necrotic tissue yields to fibrosis, this disease alters liver structure and normal vasculature, impairs blood and lymph flow, and ultimately causes hepatic insufficiency. It is twice as common in men as in women and is especially prevalent among malnourished chronic alcoholic patients over age 50. Mortality is high; many patients die within 5 years of onset. (See *Portal Hypertension and Esophageal Varices,* and *Circulation in Portal Hypertension,* p. 158.)

Causes

• Portal, nutritional, or alcoholic cirrhosis (Laennec's cirrhosis), the most common type, results from malnutrition, especially of dietary protein, and chronic alcohol ingestion.

• Biliary cirrhosis results from bile duct diseases.

• Postnecrotic (posthepatitic) cirrhosis stems from various types of hepatitis.

• Pigment cirrhosis may stem from disorders such as hemochromatosis.

• Cardiac cirrhosis (rare) is liver damage caused by right heart failure.

• Idiopathic cirrhosis (about 10% of patients) has no known cause.

Signs and symptoms

Gastrointestinal (usually early and vague)

Anorexia, indigestion, nausea and vomiting, constipation or diarrhea, or dull abdominal ache

Respiratory

Pleural effusion, limited thoracic expansion

Central nervous system

Progressive symptoms of hepatic encephalopathy: lethargy, mental changes, slurred speech, asterixis (flapping tremor), peripheral neuritis, paranoia, hallucinations, extreme obtundation, and coma

Hematologic

Bleeding tendencies (nosebleeds, easy bruising, bleeding gums), anemia

Endocrine

Testicular atrophy, menstrual irregularities, gynecomastia, or loss of chest and axillary hair

Portal Hypertension and Esophageal Varices

Portal hypertension—elevated pressure in the portal vein—occurs when blood flow meets increased resistance. The disorder is a common result of cirrhosis but may also stem from mechanical obstruction and occlusion of the hepatic veins (Budd-Chiari syndrome). As portal pressure rises, blood backs up into the spleen and flows through collateral channels to the venous system, bypassing the liver. Consequently, portal hypertension produces splenomegaly with thrombocytopenia, dilated collateral veins (esophageal varices, hemorrhoids, or prominent abdominal veins), and ascites. Nevertheless, in many patients the first sign of portal hypertension is bleeding from esophageal varices—dilated tortuous veins in the submucosa of the lower esophagus. Such varices often cause massive hematemesis, requiring emergency treatment to control hemorrhage and prevent hypovolemic shock.

• *Endoscopy* identifies the ruptured varix as the bleeding site and excludes other potential sources in the upper GI tract.

• *Angiography* may aid diagnosis but is less precise than endoscopy.

• *Vasopressin* infused into the superior mesenteric artery may temporarily stop bleeding; when angiography is unavailable, vasopressin may be infused by I.V. drip, diluted with 5% dextrose in water (except in patients with coronary vascular disease), but this route is usually less effective.

• *A Minnesota or Sengstaken-Blakemore tube* may also help control hemorrhage by applying pressure on the bleeding site. Iced saline lavage through the tube may help control bleeding.

The use of vasopressin or a Minnesota or Sengstaken-Blakemore tube is a temporary measure, especially in the patient with a severely deteriorated liver. Fresh blood and fresh frozen plasma, if available, are preferred for blood transfusions, to replace clotting factors. Treatment with lactulose promotes elimination of old blood from the GI tract and combats excessive production and accumulation of ammonia.

Appropriate surgical bypass procedures include portosystemic anastomosis, splenorenal shunt, and mesocaval shunt. Emergency shunts carry a mortality of 25% to 50%. Clinical evidence suggests that the portosystemic bypass does not prolong the patient's survival time; however, he will eventually die of hepatic coma rather than of hemorrhage.

Care for the patient who has portal hypertension with esophageal varices focuses on careful monitoring for signs and symptoms of hemorrhage and subsequent hypotension, compromised oxygen supply, and altered level of consciousness.

• Monitor vital signs, urine output, and central venous pressure to determine fluid volume status.

• Assess level of consciousness frequently.

• Provide emotional support and reassurance in the wake of massive GI bleeding, which is always a frightening experience.

• Keep the patient as quiet and comfortable as possible, but remember that tolerance for sedatives and tranquilizers may be decreased because of liver damage.

• Clean the patient's mouth, which may be dry and flecked with dried blood.

• Carefully monitor the patient with a Minnesota or Sengstaken-Blakemore tube in place for persistent bleeding in gastric drainage, signs of asphyxiation from tube displacement, proper inflation of balloons, and correct traction to maintain tube placement.

Circulation in Portal Hypertension

As portal pressure rises, blood will back up into the spleen and flow through collateral channels to the venous system, bypassing the liver and causing esophageal varices.

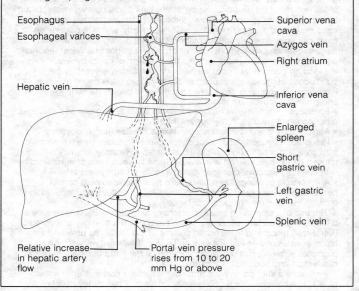

- Esophagus
- Esophageal varices
- Hepatic vein
- Superior vena cava
- Azygos vein
- Right atrium
- Inferior vena cava
- Enlarged spleen
- Short gastric vein
- Left gastric vein
- Splenic vein
- Relative increase in hepatic artery flow
- Portal vein pressure rises from 10 to 20 mm Hg or above

Skin
Severe pruritus, extreme dryness, poor tissue turgor, abnormal pigmentation, spider angiomas, palmar erythema, possibly jaundice

Hepatic
Jaundice, hepatomegaly, ascites, edema of the legs

Miscellaneous
Musty breath, enlarged superficial abdominal veins, muscle atrophy, pain in the right upper abdominal quadrant that worsens when the patient sits up or leans forward, palpable liver or spleen, temperature of 101° to 103° F. (38.3° to 39.4° C.), bleeding from esophageal varices

Diagnostic tests
- Liver biopsy, the definitive test for cirrhosis, detects destruction and fibrosis of hepatic tissue.
- Liver scan shows abnormal thickening and a liver mass.
- Cholecystography and cholangiography visualize the gallbladder and the biliary duct system, respectively.
- Splenoportal venography visualizes the portal venous system.
- Percutaneous transhepatic cholangiography differentiates extrahepatic from intrahepatic obstructive jaundice and discloses hepatic pathology and presence of gallstones.
- White blood cell count, hemoglobin and hematocrit, albumin, serum electrolytes, and cholinesterase levels are decreased.
- Globulin, serum ammonia, total bilirubin, alkaline phosphatase, serum

Managing Ascites: The LeVeen Shunt

A welcome alternative to traditional medical and surgical treatments, the LeVeen shunt drains ascitic fluid into the superior vena cava. Inserted under sedation and local anesthesia, the shunt consists of a peritoneal tube, a venous tube, and a one-way valve controlling fluid flow. The valve opens when intraperitoneal pressure exceeds superior vena caval pressure by at least 3 cm H_2O—which occurs on inspiration. Use of an abdominal binder and inspiration against resistance via a blow bottle enhance fluid drainage. The one-way valve prevents backflow of blood into the tubing, thus eliminating the risk of clotting and shunt occlusion.

Nursing care
Postoperative care includes the following:
- Teach the patient to take deep breaths against resistance for 15 minutes, four times daily.
- Check incision wounds (one on the right side of the abdomen and one in the right subclavian area) for bleeding, redness, swelling, drainage, and hematoma formation.
- Apply dry, sterile dressings.
- Monitor vital signs frequently, and watch for signs of hypovolemia or hypervolemia.
- Measure abdominal girth, and weigh the patient daily.
- Apply a firm abdominal binder 24 hours after surgery to enhance drainage.
- Record intake and output.
- Monitor complete blood count and serum electrolyte, blood urea nitrogen, creatinine, and albumin levels daily.
- Administer antibiotics, diuretics, and potassium replacements, as ordered.
- Watch for complications, such as leakage of ascitic fluid from incisions, subcutaneous bleeding, disseminated intravascular coagulation, wound infection, septicemia, shunt occlusion, and cardiac overload.

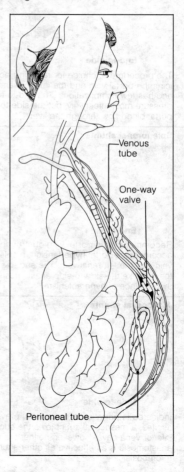

Venous tube

One-way valve

Peritoneal tube

Surgical Shunts for Portal Hypertension

Shunting procedures aim to reduce portal pressure and control bleeding esophageal varices by diverting blood from the portal venous system collateral vessels. However, these procedures carry significant risks, including hepatic encephalopathy, hemorrhage, and liver failure.

Portacaval shunts

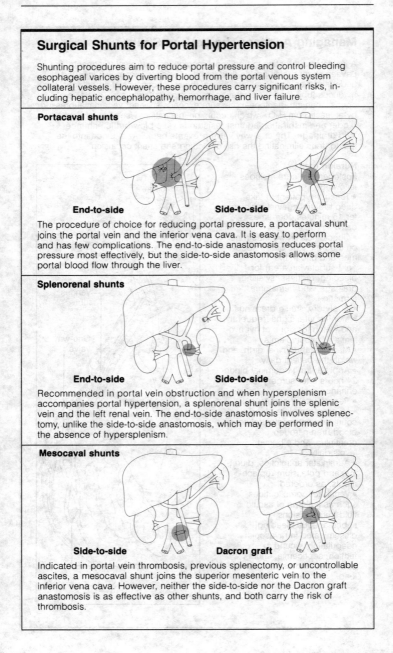

End-to-side   **Side-to-side**

The procedure of choice for reducing portal pressure, a portacaval shunt joins the portal vein and the inferior vena cava. It is easy to perform and has few complications. The end-to-side anastomosis reduces portal pressure most effectively, but the side-to-side anastomosis allows some portal blood flow through the liver.

Splenorenal shunts

End-to-side   **Side-to-side**

Recommended in portal vein obstruction and when hypersplenism accompanies portal hypertension, a splenorenal shunt joins the splenic vein and the left renal vein. The end-to-side anastomosis involves splenectomy, unlike the side-to-side anastomosis, which may be performed in the absence of hypersplenism.

Mesocaval shunts

Side-to-side   **Dacron graft**

Indicated in portal vein thrombosis, previous splenectomy, or uncontrollable ascites, a mesocaval shunt joins the superior mesenteric vein to the inferior vena cava. However, neither the side-to-side nor the Dacron graft anastomosis is as effective as other shunts, and both carry the risk of thrombosis.

glutamic-oxaloacetic transaminase (SGOT) and serum glutamic-pyruvic transaminase (SGPT), and lactate dehydrogenase levels are increased.

• Anemia, neutropenia, and thrombocytopenia are present. Prothrombin and partial thromboplastin times are prolonged.

• Vitamins A, B_{12}, C, and K; folic acid; and iron are decreased.

• Bromsulphalein excretion and glucose tolerance tests may yield abnormal results.

• Galactose tolerance and urine bilirubin tests are positive.

• Fecal urobilinogen is greater than 40 to 280 mg/24 hours; urine urobilinogen is greater than 0 to 1.16 mg/24 hours.

Treatment

Treatment is designed to remove or alleviate the underlying cause of cirrhosis, prevent further liver damage, and prevent or treat complications. The patient may benefit from a high-protein diet, but developing hepatic encephalopathy mandates restricted protein intake. In addition, sodium is usually restricted to 200 to 500 mg/day and fluids to 1,000 to 1,500 ml/day.

If the patient's condition continues to deteriorate, he may need tube feedings or hyperalimentation. Other supportive measures include supplemental vitamins—A, B complex, D, and K—to compensate for the liver's inability to store them, and vitamin B_{12}, folic acid, and thiamine for deficiency anemia. Rest, moderate exercise, and avoidance of exposure to infections and toxic agents are essential. When absolutely necessary, antiemetics, such as trimethobenzamide or benzquinamide, may be given for nausea; vasopressin, for esophageal varices; and diuretics, such as furosemide or spironolactone, for edema. However, diuretics require careful monitoring, because fluid and electrolyte imbalance may precipitate hepatic encephalopathy.

Paracentesis and infusions of salt-poor albumin may alleviate ascites. A LeVeen shunt may be used. (See *Managing Ascites: The LeVeen Shunt*, p. 159.) Surgical procedures include ligation of varices, splenectomy, esophagogastric resection, and surgical shunts to relieve portal hypertension. (See *Surgical Shunts for Portal Hypertension*.) Programs for preventing cirrhosis usually emphasize avoidance of alcohol.

Clinical implications

• Check skin, gums, stools, and vomitus regularly for bleeding. Apply pressure to injection sites to prevent bleeding. Warn the patient against taking aspirin, straining at stool, and blowing his nose or sneezing too vigorously. Suggest using an electric razor and soft toothbrush.

• Observe closely for signs of behavioral or personality changes. Report

---

Teaching Topics in Cirrhosis

• An explanation of how cirrhosis causes irreversible damage to liver cells
• Complications of cirrhosis and their warning signs
• Preparation for diagnostic tests, including liver scan and biopsy, and serum, urine, and stool studies, to confirm or evaluate cirrhosis
• Dietary measures and elimination of alcohol
• Importance of taking medication as prescribed, because of the liver's impaired ability to detoxify substances
• Preparation for portosystemic shunt, if necessary
• Measures to reduce the risk of bleeding and infection
• Availability of support groups

increasing stupor, lethargy, hallucinations, or neuromuscular dysfunction. Watch for asterixis, a sign of developing hepatic encephalopathy.

• To assess fluid retention, weigh the patient and measure abdominal girth daily, inspect ankles and sacrum for dependent edema, and accurately record intake and output.

• To prevent skin breakdown associated with edema and pruritus, avoid using soap when you bathe the patient. Instead, use lubricating lotion or moisturizing agents. Handle the patient gently, and turn and reposition him frequently to keep skin intact.

• Tell the patient that rest and good nutrition will conserve energy and decrease metabolic demands on the liver. Urge him to eat frequent small meals. Stress the need to avoid infections and abstain from alcohol. Refer the patient to Alcoholics Anonymous, if necessary. (See *Teaching Topics in Cirrhosis,* p. 161.)

Complications
• Ascites
• Bleeding varices
• Hepatic encephalopathy
• Hepatorenal syndrome

Cleft lip and palate

Description
Cleft lip and cleft palate deformities occur in 1 in every 800 births. They originate in the second month of pregnancy, when the front and sides of the face and the palatine shelves fuse imperfectly. Cleft deformities fall into four categories: clefts of the lip (unilateral or bilateral); clefts of the palate (along the midline); unilateral clefts of the lip, alveolus (gum pad), and palate, which are twice as common on the left side as on the right; and bilateral clefts of the lip, alveolus, and palate. Cleft lip with or without cleft palate is more common in boys. Cleft palate alone is more common in girls.

Causes
Genetic disorder resulting from multifactorial (polygenic) errors

Signs and symptoms
• A cleft lip can range from a simple notch to a complete cleft, extending from the lip through the floor of the nostril, on either side of the midline.

• A cleft palate may be partial or complete. A complete cleft includes the soft palate, the bones of the maxilla, and the alveolus on one or both sides of the premaxilla.

• A double cleft—the severest of all cleft deformities—runs from the soft palate forward to either side of the nose, separating the maxilla and premaxilla into free-moving segments. The tongue and other muscles can displace these bony segments, enlarging the cleft.

• In Pierre Robin syndrome, micrognathia and glossoptosis coexist with cleft palate.

Treatment
Treatment consists of surgical correction, but the timing of surgery varies.

When a wide horseshoe defect makes surgery impossible, a contoured speech bulb is attached to the posterior of a denture to occlude the nasopharynx and help the child develop intelligible speech. Surgery must be coupled with speech therapy. Because the palate is essential to speech, structural changes, even in a repaired cleft, can permanently affect speech patterns. To compound the problem, children with cleft palates often have hearing difficulties because of middle ear damage or infections.

Clinical implications
• Never place a child with Pierre Robin syndrome on his back, because his tongue can fall back and obstruct his airway. Train such an infant to sleep on his side. All other infants with cleft palate can sleep on their backs without difficulty.

• Maintain adequate nutrition for normal growth and development. Experiment with feeding devices. An infant with a cleft palate has an excellent appetite but often has trouble feeding because of air leaks around the cleft and nasal regurgitation. In most cases, he feeds better from a nipple with a flange that occludes the cleft, a lamb's nipple (a big soft nipple with large holes), or a regular nipple with enlarged holes.

Teach the mother to hold the infant in a near-sitting position, with the flow directed to the side or back of the infant's tongue. Tell her to burp the infant frequently, because he tends to swallow a lot of air.

• Encourage the mother of an infant with cleft lip to breast-feed if the cleft does not prevent effective sucking. Breast-feeding an infant with a cleft palate or one who has just had corrective surgery is impossible. (Postoperatively, the infant cannot suck for up to 6 weeks.) However, if the mother desires, suggest that she use a breast pump to express breast milk and then feed it to her baby from a bottle.

• Following surgery, record intake and output, and maintain good nutrition. To prevent atelectasis and pneumonia, the physician may gently suction the nasopharynx (this may be necessary before surgery, too). Restrain the infant to stop him from hurting himself. Elbow restraints allow the infant to move his hands while keeping them away from his mouth. When necessary, use an infant seat to keep the infant in a comfortable sitting position. Hang toys within reach of restrained hands.

• Surgeons sometimes place a curved metal Logan bow over a repaired cleft lip to minimize tension on the suture line. Remove the gauze before feedings, and replace it frequently. Moisten it with normal saline solution until the sutures are removed. Check institutional policy to confirm this procedure.

• Help parents deal with their feelings about the child's deformity. Start by telling them about it immediately and showing them their child as soon as possible. Because society places undue importance on physical appearance, parents often feel shock, disappointment, and guilt when they see the child. Help them by being calm and providing positive information. Direct parents' attention to their child's assets; show them what is "right" about their baby. Stress the fact that surgical repairs can be made. Include the parents in the care and feeding of the child right from the start to encourage normal bonding. Provide instructions, emotional support, and reassurance that parents will need to take proper care of the child at home. Refer them to a social worker who can guide them to community resources.

Clubfoot
(Talipes)

Description

Clubfoot is the most common congenital disorder of the lower extremities. In talipes equinovarus, the foot points downward (equinus) and turns inward (varus), and the front of the foot curls toward the heel (forefoot adduction). The deformity varies greatly in severity.

Clubfoot has an incidence of approximately 1 per 1,000 live births and is twice as common in boys as in girls. Usually it is bilateral. It may be associated with other birth defects. Clubfoot is correctable with prompt treatment.

Causes

• A combination of genetic and environmental factors in utero appears to cause clubfoot.

• It may be secondary to paralysis, poliomyelitis, or cerebral palsy in older children.

Signs and symptoms
- Deformed talus
- Shortened Achilles tendon
- Shortened and flattened calcaneus
- Possible underdeveloped calf muscles with soft-tissue contractures at the site of the deformity
- Resistance to manual efforts to push the foot into normal position

Diagnostic tests
X-rays show superimposition of the talus and the calcaneus and ladderlike appearance of the metatarsals in true clubfoot.

Treatment
Treatment for clubfoot is administered in three stages: correcting the deformity, maintaining the correction until the foot regains normal muscle balance, and observing the foot closely for several years to prevent recurrence. The ideal time to begin treatment is during the first few days and weeks of life—when the foot is most malleable. An infant's foot contains large amounts of cartilage; the muscles, ligaments, and tendons are supple.

Clubfoot deformities are usually corrected in sequential order: forefoot adduction first, then varus (or inversion), then equinus (or plantar flexion). Trying to correct all three deformities at once only results in a misshapen, rocker-bottomed foot. Forefoot adduction is corrected by uncurling the front of the foot away from the heel (forefoot abduction); the varus deformity is corrected by turning the foot so that the sole faces outward (eversion); and finally, the equinus deformity is corrected by casting the foot with the toes pointing up (dorsiflexion). This last correction may have to be supplemented with a subcutaneous tenotomy of the Achilles tendon and posterior capsulotomy of the ankle joint.

Several therapeutic methods have been tested and found effective in correcting clubfoot. The first is simple manipulation and casting, whereby the foot is gently manipulated into a partially corrected position, then held there in a cast for several days or weeks. After the cast is removed, the foot is manipulated into an even better position and casted again. This procedure is repeated as many times as necessary. In some cases, the shape of the cast can be transformed through a series of wedging maneuvers (Kite method), instead of changing the cast each time.

After correction of clubfoot, proper foot alignment should be maintained through exercise, night splints, and orthopedic shoes. With manipulating and casting, correction usually takes about 3 months.

Resistant clubfoot may require surgery. Older children with recurrent or neglected clubfoot will need surgery. Whenever clubfoot is severe enough to require surgery, it is rarely totally correctable; however, surgery can usually ameliorate the deformity.

Clinical implications
The primary concern is early recognition of clubfoot, preferably in newborn infants. Follow these guidelines:
- Look for any exaggerated attitudes in an infant's feet. Make sure you can recognize the difference between true clubfoot and apparent clubfoot. (The foot with apparent clubfoot moves easily.) Do not use excessive force in trying to manipulate a clubfoot.
- Stress the importance of prompt treatment to parents. Make sure they understand that clubfoot demands immediate therapy and orthopedic supervision until growth is completed.
- After casting, elevate the child's feet with pillows. Check the toes every 1 to 2 hours for temperature, color, sensation, motion, and capillary refill time. Watch for edema. Before a child in a clubfoot cast is discharged, teach parents to recognize circulatory impairment.

• Insert plastic petals over the top edges of a new cast while it is still wet, to keep urine from soaking and softening the cast. When the cast is dry, "petal" the edges with adhesive tape to keep out plaster crumbs and prevent skin irritation. Perform good skin care under the cast edges every 4 hours. After washing and drying the skin, rub it with alcohol. (Do not use oils or powders; they tend to macerate the skin.)

• Warn parents of an older child not to let the foot part of the cast get soft and thin from wear. If it does, much of the correction may be lost.

• When the Kite method is being used, check circulatory status frequently. Circulation may be impaired because of increased pressure on tissues and blood vessels. The equinus correction especially places considerable strain on ligaments, blood vessels, and tendons.

• After surgery, elevate the child's feet with pillows to decrease swelling and pain. Report any signs of discomfort or pain immediately. Try to locate the source of pain—it may result from cast pressure, not the incision. If bleeding occurs under the cast, circle the location and mark the time on the cast. If bleeding spreads, report it.

• Explain to the older child and his parents that in older children, surgery can improve clubfoot but cannot totally correct it.

• Emphasize the need for long-term orthopedic care to maintain correction. Teach parents prescribed exercises that the child can do at home. Urge them to make the child wear corrective shoes and splints during naps and at night, as ordered. Make sure they understand that treatment for clubfoot continues during the entire growth period. Permanent correction takes time and patience.

Coal workers' pneumoconiosis
(Black lung disease, coal miner's pneumoconiosis, miners' asthma, anthracosis, anthracosilicosis)

Description
A progressive nodular pulmonary disease, coal workers' pneumoconiosis (CWP) occurs in two forms. Simple CWP is characterized by small lung opacities; in complicated CWP, also known as progressive massive fibrosis (PMF), masses of fibrous tissue occasionally develop in the lungs of patients with simple CWP. The risk of developing CWP depends upon duration of exposure to coal dust (usually 15 years or longer), intensity of exposure (dust count, particle size), location of the mine, silica content of the coal (anthracite coal has the highest silica content), and the worker's susceptibility. Incidence of CWP is highest among anthracite coal miners in the eastern United States. Prognosis varies.

Causes
Inhalation and prolonged retention of respirable coal dust particles (less than 5 microns in diameter)

Signs and symptoms
Simple CWP is asymptomatic. Signs and symptoms of PMF include the following:
• Exertional dyspnea that progresses
• Cough, productive of milky, gray, clear, or coal-flecked sputum
• Barrel chest
• Hyperresonant lungs with areas of dullness, diminished breath sounds, rales, rhonchi, and wheezes

Diagnostic tests
• In simple CWP, chest X-rays show small opacities (less than 10 mm in diameter), which may be present in all

lung zones but are more prominent in the upper lung zones.

• In PMF, chest X-rays show one or more large opacities (1 to 5 cm in diameter), possibly exhibiting cavitation.

• Pulmonary function studies yield the following results:

—Vital capacity (VC): normal in simple CWP; decreased in PMF

—Forced expiratory volume in one second (FEV_1): decreased in complicated disease

—Residual volume and total lung capacity (RV and TLC): normal in simple CWP; decreased in PMF

—Diffusing capacity for carbon monoxide (DLCO): significantly decreased in complicated CWP as alveolar septae are destroyed and pulmonary capillaries obliterated

• Arterial blood gas studies yield the following results:

—PO_2: normal in simple CWP; decreased in complicated disease

—PCO_2: normal in simple CWP, but may decrease from hyperventilation; may also increase if the patient is hypoxic and has severe impairment of alveolar ventilation

Treatment and clinical implications

Respiratory symptoms may be relieved through bronchodilator therapy with theophylline or aminophylline (if bronchospasm is reversible), oral or inhaled sympathomimetic amines (metaproterenol), corticosteroids (oral prednisone or an aerosol form of beclomethasone), or cromolyn sodium aerosol. Chest physiotherapy techniques, such as controlled coughing and segmental bronchial drainage, with chest percussion and vibration, help remove secretions.

Other measures include increased fluid intake (at least 3 liters/day) and respiratory therapy, such as aerosol therapy, inhaled mucolytics, and intermittent positive-pressure breathing (IPPB). Diuretics, digitalis preparations, and salt restriction may be in-

dicated in cor pulmonale. In severe cases, it may be necessary to administer oxygen by cannula or mask (1 to 2 liters/minute) if the patient has chronic hypoxia or by mechanical ventilation if PO_2 cannot be maintained above 40 mm Hg. Respiratory infections require prompt administration of antibiotics.

• Teach the patient to prevent infections by avoiding crowds and persons with respiratory infections, and by receiving influenza and pneumococcal vaccines.

• Encourage the patient to stay active to avoid deterioration in his physical condition, but to pace his activities and practice relaxation techniques.

Complications
• Pulmonary hypertension
• Right ventricular hypertrophy
• Cor pulmonale
• Pulmonary tuberculosis
• Possible chronic bronchitis and emphysema in cigarette smokers

Coarctation of the aorta

Description
Coarctation is a narrowing of the aorta, usually just below the left subclavian artery, near the site where the ligamentum arteriosum (the remnant of the ductus arteriosus, a fetal blood vessel) joins the pulmonary artery to the aorta. The obstructive process causes hypertension in the aortic branches above the constriction (arteries that supply the arms, neck, and head) and diminished pressure in the vessels below the constriction. Usually, prognosis depends on the severity of associated cardiac anomalies. Prognosis for isolated coarctation is good if corrective surgery is performed before this condition induces severe systemic hypertension or degenerative changes in the aorta.

Causes

May develop as a result of spasm and constriction of the smooth muscle in the ductus arteriosus as it closes

Signs and symptoms

Cardinal signs

—Resting systolic hypertension
—Absent or diminished femoral pulses
—Wide pulse pressure

Other possible symptoms in infancy

—Tachypnea
—Dyspnea
—Pallor
—Tachycardia
—Failure to thrive
—Cardiomegaly and hepatomegaly

Other possible symptoms in adolescence

—Dyspnea
—Claudication
—Headache
—Epistaxis
—Visible aortic pulsation in the suprasternal notch
—Continuous systolic murmur (accentuated S_2 and S_3)

Diagnostic tests

• Chest X-ray may demonstrate left ventricular hypertrophy, congestive heart failure (CHF), a wide ascending and descending aorta, and notching of the undersurfaces of the ribs from extensive collateral circulation.

• EKG may eventually reveal left ventricular hypertrophy.

• Echocardiography may show increased left ventricular muscle thickness, coexisting aortic valve abnormalities, and the coarctation site.

• Cardiac catheterization and aortography are indicated. Cardiac catheterization evaluates collateral circulation and measures pressure in the right and left ventricles and in the ascending and descending aorta (on both sides of the obstruction). Aortography locates the site and extent of coarctation.

Treatment

For an infant with CHF caused by coarctation of the aorta, treatment consists of medical management with digoxin and diuretics. If medical management fails, surgery may be needed. Usually, the child's condition determines the timing of the surgery. Signs of CHF or hypertension may call for early surgery. If these signs do not appear, surgery usually occurs during the preschool years.

Before the operation, the child may require endocarditis prophylaxis, or if the child is older and has previously undetected coarctation, he may need antihypertensive therapy. During surgery, a flap of the left subclavian artery is used to reconstruct an unobstructed aorta.

Clinical implications

• When coarctation in an infant requires rapid digitalization, monitor vital signs closely and watch for digitalis toxicity (poor feeding, vomiting).

• Balance intake and output carefully, especially if the infant is receiving diuretics with fluid restriction.

• Since the infant may not be able to maintain proper body temperature, regulate environmental temperature with an overbed warmer, if needed.

• Monitor blood glucose levels to detect possible hypoglycemia, which may occur as glycogen stores become depleted.

• Offer the parents emotional support and an explanation of the disorder. Also explain diagnostic procedures, surgery, and drug therapy. Tell parents what to expect postoperatively.

• For an older child, assess the blood pressure in his extremities regularly, explain any exercise restrictions, stress the need to take medications properly and to watch for adverse effects, and teach him about tests and other procedures.

After corrective surgery, follow these guidelines:

• Monitor blood pressure closely, using an intraarterial line. Take blood pressure in all extremities. Monitor intake and output.

• If the patient develops hypertension and requires nitroprusside or trimethaphan, administer it, as ordered, by continuous I.V. infusion, using an infusion pump. Watch for severe hypotension, and regulate the dosage carefully.

• Provide pain relief, and encourage a gradual increase in activity.

• Promote adequate respiratory functioning through turning, coughing, and deep breathing.

• Watch for abdominal pain or rigidity and signs of GI or urinary bleeding.

• If an older child needs to continue antihypertensive therapy after surgery, teach him and his parents about it.

• Stress the importance of continued endocarditis prophylaxis.

Complications

Restricted blood flow through the narrowed aorta increases the pressure load on the left ventricle and causes dilation of the proximal aorta and ventricular hypertrophy. Untreated, this condition may lead to left heart failure and, rarely, to cerebral hemorrhage and aortic rupture. If ventricular septal defect accompanies coarctation, blood shunts left to right, straining the right heart. That leads to pulmonary hypertension and, eventually, right heart hypertrophy and failure.

Coccidioidomycosis
(Valley fever, San Joaquin Valley fever)

Description

Coccidioidomycosis, a fungal infection, occurs primarily as a respiratory infection, although generalized dissemination may occur. In the United States, coccidioidomycosis is endemic in the Southwest. It is most prevalent during warm, dry months. The pri-

mary pulmonary form is usually self-limiting and rarely fatal. The rare secondary (progressive, disseminated) form produces abscesses throughout the body and carries a mortality of up to 60%, even with treatment. Such dissemination is more common in dark-skinned men, pregnant women, and patients who are receiving immunosuppressive therapy.

Cause

The fungus *Coccidioides immitis*

Mode of transmission

• Inhalation of *C. immitis* spores found in the soil in endemic areas

• Inhalation of *C. immitis* spores from dressings or plaster casts of infected persons

Signs and symptoms
Primary form
—Dry cough
—Pleuritic chest pain
—Pleural effusion
—Fever
—Sore throat
—Chills
—Malaise
—Headache
—Itchy macular rash
—Possible tender red nodules (erythema nodosum) on the legs, especially the shins, with joint pain in the knees and ankles (particularly in white women)
Disseminated form
—Fever
—Abscesses throughout the body
—Possible bone pain
—Possible decreased level of consciousness
Either form
—Possible hemoptysis, with or without chest pain

Diagnostic tests

Typical clinical features and skin and serologic studies confirm the diagnosis.

• A positive coccidioidin skin test occurs in the primary form and sometimes in the disseminated form.

• In the first week of illness, complement fixation for IgG antibodies, or in the first month, positive serum precipitins (immunoglobulins), also establish the diagnosis.

• Examination or, more recently, immunodiffusion testing of sputum, pus from lesions, and a tissue biopsy may show *C. immitis* spores.

• The presence of antibodies in pleural and joint fluid, and a rising serum or body fluid antibody titer indicate dissemination.

• Other abnormal laboratory results include increased white blood cell (WBC) count, eosinophilia, and increased erythrocyte sedimentation rate.

• Chest X-ray shows bilateral diffuse infiltrates.

• In coccidioidal meningitis, examination of cerebrospinal fluid shows WBC count increased to more than 500/cu mm (due primarily to mononuclear leukocytes), increased protein, and decreased glucose. Ventricular fluid obtained from the brain may contain complement fixation antibodies.

After diagnosis, the results of serial skin tests, blood cultures, and serologic testing may document the effectiveness of therapy.

Treatment

Usually, mild primary coccidioidomycosis requires only bed rest and relief of symptoms. Severe primary disease and dissemination, however, also require long-term I.V. infusion or, in central nervous system (CNS) dissemination, intrathecal administration of amphotericin B and possibly excision or drainage of lesions. Severe pulmonary lesions may require lobectomy. Miconazole and ketoconazole show promise.

Clinical implications

• Do not wash off the circle marked on the skin for serial skin tests, since this aids in reading test results.

• In mild primary disease, encourage bed rest and adequate fluid intake. Record the amount and color of sputum. Watch for shortness of breath, which may point to pleural effusion. In patients with arthralgia, provide analgesics, as ordered.

• Coccidioidomycosis requires strict secretion precautions if the patient has draining lesions. "No-touch" dressing technique and careful handwashing are essential.

• In CNS dissemination, monitor carefully for decreased level of consciousness or change in mood or affect.

• Before intrathecal administration of amphotericin B, explain the procedure to the patient, and reassure him that he will receive analgesics before a lumbar puncture. If the patient is to receive amphotericin B intravenously, infuse it slowly, as ordered; rapid infusion may cause circulatory collapse. During infusion, monitor vital signs (temperature may rise but should return to normal within 1 to 2 hours). Watch for decreased urine output, and monitor laboratory results for elevated blood urea nitrogen and serum creatinine levels, elevated creatinine, and hypokalemia. Tell the patient to immediately report hearing loss, tinnitus, dizziness, and all signs of toxicity. To ease adverse effects of amphotericin B, give antiemetics and antipyretics, as ordered.

Complications

Meningitis

Cold injuries

Description

Cold injuries result from overexposure to cold air or water and occur in two major forms: localized injuries (such as frostbite) and systemic injuries (such as hypothermia). In hypothermia, the core body temperature drops below 95° F. (35° C.). Untreated or improperly treated frostbite can lead to gangrene and may necessitate amputation. Severe hypothermia can be fatal.

Causes
Frostbite
—Prolonged exposure to dry temperatures far below freezing
Hypothermia
—Near-drowning in cold water
—Prolonged exposure to cold temperatures

Risk factors
The risk of serious cold injuries, especially hypothermia, is increased by the following:
• Youth
• Old age
• Lack of insulating body fat
• Wet or inadequate clothing
• Drug abuse
• Cardiac disease
• Smoking
• Fatigue
• Hunger and depletion of caloric reserves
• Excessive alcohol intake, which draws blood into capillaries and away from body organs

Signs and symptoms
Superficial frostbite (affects skin and subcutaneous tissue)
—Upon returning to a warm place, burning, tingling, numbness, swelling, and a mottled, blue-gray skin color
Deep frostbite (extends beyond subcutaneous tissue)
—Skin white until thawed; then purplish blue
—Pain, skin blisters, tissue necrosis, and gangrene
Mild hypothermia
—Body temperature 89.6° to 95° F. (32° to 35° C.)
—Severe shivering
—Slurred speech
—Amnesia

Moderate hypothermia
—Body temperature 82.4° to 89.6° F. (28° to 32° C.)
—Unresponsiveness
—Muscle rigidity
—Peripheral cyanosis
—With improper rewarming, signs of shock
Severe hypothermia
—Body temperature 77° to 82.4° F. (25° to 28° C.)
—Loss of deep tendon reflexes
—Ventricular fibrillation
—Lack of palpable pulse or audible heart sounds
—Possible dilated pupils
—Cardiopulmonary arrest and death with body temperature below 77° F. (25° C.)

Treatment and clinical implications
To treat localized cold injuries, follow these guidelines:
• Remove constrictive clothing and jewelry. Slowly rewarm the affected part in tepid water (about 100° to 108° F. [37.8° to 42.2° C.]). Give the patient warm fluids to drink. *Never* rub the injured area; this aggravates tissue damage.
• When the affected part begins to rewarm, the patient will feel pain, so give analgesics, as ordered. Check for a pulse. Be careful not to rupture any blebs. If the injury is on the foot, place cotton or gauze sponges between the toes to prevent maceration. Instruct the patient not to walk.
• If the injury has caused an open skin wound, give antibiotics and tetanus prophylaxis, as ordered.
• If pulse fails to return, the patient may develop compartment syndrome and need fasciotomy to restore circulation. If pain and edema persist, expect to give tolazoline intraarterially to create temporary sympathectomy. If gangrene occurs, prepare for amputation.
• Before discharge, tell the patient about possible long-term effects: increased sensitivity to cold, burning and

Preventing Cold Injuries

• In cold weather, wear mittens (not gloves); windproof, water-resistant, many-layered clothing; two pairs of socks (cotton next to skin, then wool); and a scarf and a hat that cover the ears (to avoid substantial heat loss through the head).
• Before anticipated prolonged exposure to cold, do not drink alcohol or smoke, and get adequate food and rest.
• If caught in a severe snowstorm, find shelter early or increase physical activity to maintain body warmth.

tingling, and increased sweating. Warn against smoking, because it causes vasoconstriction and slows healing.

To treat systemic hypothermia, follow these guidelines:
• If there is no pulse or respiration, begin cardiopulmonary resuscitation (CPR) immediately and, if necessary, continue it for 2 to 3 hours. (Remember: Hypothermia helps protect the brain from anoxia, which normally accompanies prolonged cardiopulmonary arrest. Therefore, even after the patient has been unresponsive for a long time, resuscitation may be possible, especially after cold-water near-drownings.) Perform CPR until the patient is adequately rewarmed.
• Move the patient to a warm area, remove wet clothing, and keep him dry. If he is conscious, give warm fluids with high sugar content, such as tea with sugar. If the patient's core temperature is above 89.6° F. (32° C.), use external warming techniques. Bathe him in water that is 104° F. (40° C.), cover him with a heating blanket set at 97.9° to 99.9° F. (36.6° to 37.7° C.), and cautiously apply hot water bottles at 104° F. to groin and axillae, guarding against burns.
• If the patient's core temperature is below 89.6° F. (32° C.), use internal and external warming methods. Rewarm his body core and surface 1° to 2° F. per hour concurrently. (If you rewarm the surface first, rewarming shock can cause potentially fatal ven-

tricular fibrillation.) To warm inhalations, provide oxygen heated to 107.6° to 114.8° F. (42° to 46° C.). Infuse I.V. solutions that have passed through a warming coil at 98.6° F. (37° C.), and give nasogastric lavage with normal saline solution that has been warmed to the same temperature. Assist with peritoneal lavage, using a normal saline solution (full or half strength) warmed to 98.6° F.; in severe hypothermia, assist with heart/lung bypass at controlled temperatures and thoracotomy with direct cardiac warm-saline bath.
• Throughout treatment, monitor arterial blood gases, intake and output, central venous pressure, temperature, and cardiac and neurologic status every half hour. Monitor laboratory results such as complete blood count, blood urea nitrogren, electrolyte levels, prothrombin time, and partial thromboplastin time.
• Patients who have developed cold injuries because of inadequate clothing or housing may need referral to a community social service agency. (See *Preventing Cold Injuries*.)

Colorado tick fever

Description
Colorado tick fever, a benign infection, occurs in the Rocky Mountain region of the United States, mostly in April and May at lower altitudes and in June and July at higher altitudes.

Because of occupational or recreational exposure, it is more common in men than in women. Colorado tick fever apparently confers long-lasting immunity against infection. The incubation period is 3 to 6 days. After abrupt onset, symptoms subside after several days, then return within 2 to 3 days and continue for 3 more days before slowly disappearing. Complete recovery usually follows.

Cause
Colorado tick fever virus, an arbovirus

Mode of transmission
A hard-shelled wood tick called *Dermacentor andersoni* transmits the disease to humans. The adult tick acquires the virus when it bites infected rodents, and remains permanently infective.

Signs and symptoms
• Abrupt onset of chills and fever, with temperature of 104° F. (40° C.)
• Severe aching of back, arms, and legs
• Lethargy
• Headache with eye movement
• Possible photophobia, abdominal pain, nausea, and vomiting
• Rarely, petechial or maculopapular rashes and central nervous system involvement

Treatment and clinical implications
After correct removal of the tick, supportive treatment relieves symptoms, combats secondary infection, and maintains fluid balance.
• Carefully remove the tick by grasping it with forceps or gloved fingers and pulling gently. Be careful not to crush the tick's body. Keep it for identification. Thoroughly wash the wound with soap and water. If the tick's head remains embedded, surgical removal is necessary. Give a tetanus-diphtheria booster, as ordered.
• Be alert for secondary infection.

• Monitor fluid and electrolyte balance, and provide replacement accordingly.
• Reduce fever with antipyretics and tepid sponge baths.
• To prevent tickborne infection, tell the patient to avoid tick bites by wearing protective clothing (long pants tucked into boots) and carefully checking his body and scalp for ticks several times a day when in infested areas.

Colorectal cancer

Description
Colorectal cancer is the second most common visceral neoplasm in the United States and Europe. It tends to progress slowly and remains localized for a long time. Consequently, it is potentially curable in 75% of patients if early diagnosis allows resection before nodal involvement. With improved diagnosis, overall 5-year survival rate is nearing 50%.

Causes
Unknown

Risk factors
• Other diseases of the digestive tract
• Age (over 40)
• History of ulcerative colitis (average 11- to 17-year interval before onset of cancer)
• Familial polyposis (cancer almost always develops by age 50)
• Possibly, diet high in animal fat, especially beef, and low in fiber

Signs and symptoms
Right colon involvement
—Black, tarry stools
—Anemia
—Abdominal aching, pressure, or dull cramps
—With disease progression, weakness and fatigue
—Exertional dyspnea, vertigo
—Eventually, diarrhea or obstipation
—Anorexia, weight loss

—Vomiting and other signs of intestinal obstruction
—Possible palpable tumor
Left colon involvement
—Rectal bleeding
—Intermittent abdominal fullness or cramping
—Rectal pressure
—With disease progression, obstipation, diarrhea, or ribbon- or pencil-shaped stools
—Typically, pain relief with passage of stool or flatus
—Eventually, dark or bright-red blood in feces and mucus in or on stools
Rectal involvement
—Change in bowel habits (first symptom). Frequently begins with an urgent need to defecate on arising ("morning diarrhea") or obstipation alternating with diarrhea
—Blood or mucus in stool
—Sense of incomplete evacuation
—Pain. Late in the disease, pain begins as a feeling of rectal fullness that later becomes a dull, and sometimes constant, ache confined to the rectum or sacral region.
Late involvement
—Pallor
—Cachexia
—Ascites
—Hepatomegaly
—Lymphangiectasis

Diagnostic tests
• Tumor biopsy confirms the diagnosis.
• Digital examination can detect almost 15% of colorectal cancers.
• Hemoccult (guaiac) test can detect blood in stools.
• Proctoscopy or sigmoidoscopy can detect up to 66% of colorectal cancers.
• Colonoscopy permits visual inspection (and photographs) of the colon up to the ileocecal valve, and gives access for polypectomies and biopsies of suspected lesions.
• Intravenous pyelography verifies bilateral renal function and checks for any displacement of the kidneys, ureters, or bladder.

• Barium X-ray, utilizing dual contrast with air, can locate lesions that are undetectable manually or visually.
• Carcinoembryonic antigen (CEA) measurement, though not specific or sensitive enough for early diagnosis, is helpful in monitoring patients before and after treatment to detect metastasis or recurrence.

Treatment
The most effective treatment for colorectal cancer is surgery to remove the malignant tumor, adjacent tissues, and any lymph nodes that may contain cancer cells. The type of surgery depends on the location of the tumor.
• Right hemicolectomy (in advanced disease), for a tumor in the cecum and ascending colon, may include resection of the terminal segment of the ileum, cecum, ascending colon, and right half of the transverse colon with corresponding mesentery.
• For a tumor in the proximal and middle transverse colon, the procedure may be right colectomy (includes the transverse colon and mesentery corresponding to midcolic vessels) or segmental resection of the transverse colon and associated midcolic vessels.
• For a tumor in the sigmoid colon, surgery is usually limited to the sigmoid colon and mesentery.
• For a tumor in the upper rectum, the procedure is anterior or low anterior resection (newer method, using a stapler, allows for resections much lower than were previously possible).
• For a tumor in the lower rectum, abdominoperineal resection and permanent sigmoid colostomy are done.
  Chemotherapy is indicated for patients with metastasis, residual disease, or a recurrent inoperable tumor. Radiation therapy induces tumor regression and may be used before or after surgery. Immunotherapy using BCG (bacille Calmette-Guérin) vaccine is still experimental.

Clinical implications

Before colorectal surgery, monitor the patient's diet modifications, laxatives, enemas, and antibiotics—all used to cleanse the bowel and to decrease abdominal and perineal cavity contamination during surgery. If the patient is to have a colostomy, teach him and his family what he needs to know about the procedure:

• Emphasize that the stoma will be red, moist, and swollen, and that postoperative swelling will eventually subside.

• Show a diagram of the intestine before and after surgery, stressing how much of the bowel remains intact. Supplement your teaching with instruction booklets (available for a fee from the United Ostomy Association and free from various companies that manufacture ostomy supplies). Arrange a postoperative visit from a recovered ostomate.

• Prepare the patient for postoperative I.V. lines, nasogastric tube, and indwelling (Foley) catheter.

• Discuss the importance of cooperation during coughing and deep-breathing exercises.

After surgery, explain to the patient's family the importance of their positive reactions to the patient's adjustment. Consult with an enterostomal therapist, if available, for questions on setting up a regimen for the patient.

Encourage the patient to look at the stoma and participate in its care as soon as possible. Teach good hygiene and skin care. Allow him to shower or bathe as soon as the incision heals. If appropriate, instruct the patient with a sigmoid colostomy to do his own irrigation as soon as he can after surgery. Advise him to schedule irrigation for the time of the day when he normally evacuated before surgery. Many patients find that irrigating every 1 to 3 days is necessary for regulation. If flatus, diarrhea, or constipation occurs, eliminate suspected causative foods from the patient's diet. He may reintroduce them later.

After several months, many ostomates establish control with irrigation and no longer need to wear a pouch. A stoma cap or gauze sponge placed over the stoma protects it and absorbs mucoid secretions.

Before achieving such control, the patient can resume physical activities, including sports, providing there is no threat of injury to the stoma or surrounding abdominal muscles. He can place a pouch or stoma cap (if regulated) over the stoma when swimming. However, he should avoid heavy lifting, as herniation or prolapse may occur because of weakened muscles in the abdominal wall. A structured, gradually progressive exercise program to strengthen abdominal muscles may be instituted under the physician's supervision.

Schedule a visiting nurse to call on the patient at home to check on his physical care. Suggest sexual counseling for male patients; most are impotent after an abdominoperineal resection and suffer fear of rejection.

Anyone who has had colorectal cancer runs an increased risk of developing another primary cancer and should have yearly screening and follow-up testing, as well as a diet high in fiber (bulk).

Common variable immunodeficiency
(Acquired hypogammaglobulinemia, agammaglobulinemia with Ig-bearing B cells)

Description

Common variable immunodeficiency is characterized by progressive deterioration of B-cell (humoral) immunity, resulting in increased susceptibility to infection. Unlike X-linked hypogammaglobulinemia, this disorder usually causes symptoms after infancy and childhood, between ages 25 and 40. It affects men and women equally and usually does not interfere with normal life span or with normal pregnancy and offspring. Common variable immunodeficiency may be associated with autoimmune diseases, such as systemic lupus erythematosus, rheumatoid arthritis, hemolytic anemia, and pernicious anemia, and with malignancies, such as leukemia and lymphoma.

Causes

Unknown

Signs and symptoms

• Chronic pyogenic bacterial infections, such as sinopulmonary infections
• Conjunctivitis
• Intestinal infestation by *Giardia lamblia* with malabsorption

Diagnostic tests

• Serum IgM, IgA, and IgG levels, detected by immunoelectrophoresis, are decreased.
• B-cell counts are normal.
• Antigenic stimulation confirms an inability to produce specific antibodies.
• Cell-mediated immunity may be intact or delayed.
• X-rays usually show signs of chronic lung disease or sinusitis.

Treatment and clinical implications

Injection of immune globulin (usually weekly to monthly) helps maintain immune response. Because these injections are very painful, give them deep into a large muscle mass, such as the gluteal or thigh muscles, and massage well. If the dose is more than 1.5 ml, divide it and inject it into more than one site. For frequent injections, rotate the injection sites. Because immune globulin is composed primarily of IgG, the patient may also need fresh frozen plasma infusions to provide IgA and IgM.

Antibiotics are the mainstay for combating infection. Regular X-rays and pulmonary function studies help monitor infection in the lungs; chest physiotherapy may be ordered to forestall or help clear such infection.

To help prevent severe infection, teach the patient and his family how to recognize its early signs. Warn them to avoid crowds and persons who have active infections. Also stress the importance of good nutrition and regular follow-up care.

Complement deficiencies

Description

Complement is a series of circulating enzymatic serum proteins with nine functional components, labeled C1 through C9. When the immunoglobulins IgG or IgM react with antigens as part of an immune response, they activate C1, which then combines with C4, initiating the classic complement pathway, or cascade, or an alternative complement pathway. Complement then combines with the antigen-antibody complex and undergoes a sequence of complicated reactions that amplifies the immune response against the antigen. This complex process is called complement fixation.

Complement deficiency or dysfunction may increase susceptibility to infection and also seems related to certain autoimmune disorders. Prognosis varies with the abnormality and the severity of associated diseases.

Causes

• Primary complement deficiencies (rare) are inherited as autosomal recessive traits, except for deficiency of

C1 esterase inhibitor, which is autosomal dominant.
• Secondary complement deficiencies may follow complement-fixing (complement-consuming) immunologic reactions, such as drug-induced serum sickness, acute streptococcal glomerulonephritis, and acute active systemic lupus erythematosus.

Signs and symptoms
Clinical effects vary with the specific deficiency.
• C2 and C3 deficiencies and C5 familial dysfunction increase susceptibility to bacterial infection (which may involve several body systems simultaneously).
• C5 dysfunction, a familial defect in infants, causes failure to thrive, diarrhea, and seborrheic dermatitis.
• C1 esterase inhibitor deficiency (hereditary angioedema) may cause periodic swelling in the face, hands, abdomen, or throat, with potentially fatal laryngeal edema.

Diagnostic tests
• Total serum complement level (CH50) is low in various complement deficiencies.
• Specific assays may be done to confirm deficiency of specific complement components.

Treatment
Primary complement deficiencies have no known cure. Associated infection, collagen vascular disease, or renal disease requires prompt, appropriate treatment. Transfusion of fresh frozen plasma to provide replacement of complement components is controversial, because replacement therapy does not cure complement deficiencies and any beneficial effects are transient. Bone marrow transplant may be helpful but can cause a potentially fatal graft-versus-host (GVH) reaction. Anabolic steroids and antifibrinolytic agents are frequently used to reduce acute swelling in patients with C1 esterase inhibitor deficiency.

Clinical implications
• Teach the patient (or his family, if he is a child) the importance of avoiding infection, how to recognize its early signs and symptoms, and the need for prompt treatment if it occurs.
• After bone marrow transplant, monitor the patient closely for signs of transfusion reaction and GVH reaction.
• Meticulous patient care can speed recovery and prevent complications. For example, a patient with renal infection needs careful monitoring of intake and output, tests for serum electrolyte levels and acid-base balance, and observation for signs of renal failure.
• When caring for a patient with hereditary angioedema, be prepared for emergency management of laryngeal edema. Keep airway equipment on hand.

Concussion

Description
By far the most common head injury, concussion causes temporary neural dysfunction. Most concussion victims recover completely within 24 to 48 hours. Repeated concussions, however, exact a cumulative toll on the brain.

Causes
A sudden and forceful blow to the head that is not hard enough to cause a cerebral contusion, such as from a punch in the head, a motor vehicle accident, a fall to the ground, or a child abuse injury

Signs and symptoms
• Short-term loss of consciousness
• Vomiting
• Anterograde and retrograde amnesia
• Irritability
• Lethargy

What to Do after Concussion

Dear Patient:
You have suffered a concussion, which does not appear to have caused any serious brain injury. For safety's sake, however, follow these instructions:
• Return to the hospital immediately if you experience a persistent or worsening headache, forceful or constant vomiting, blurred vision, any change in personality, abnormal eye movements, staggering gait, or twitching.
• Don't take anything stronger than aspirin or acetaminophen for a headache.
• If vomiting occurs, eat lightly until it stops. (*Occasional* vomiting is normal after concussion.)
• Relax for 24 hours. Then, if you feel well, resume normal activities.
• Give this note to your parents, guardian, spouse, or roommate: *Wake the patient every 2 hours during the night, and ask him his name, where he is, and whether he can identify you. If you can't awaken him, or he can't answer these questions, or if he has convulsions, bring him back to the hospital immediately.*

• Dizziness
• Unusual behavior
• Severe headache
• In children, lethargy and somnolence in a few hours
• Postconcussion syndrome (headache, dizziness, vertigo, anxiety, fatigue that may persist for several weeks after the injury)

Diagnostic tests
Skull X-rays and computed tomography may rule out fractures and more serious injuries.

Treatment and clinical implications
• Obtain a thorough history of the trauma from the patient (if he is not suffering from amnesia), his family, eyewitnesses, or ambulance personnel. Ask whether the patient lost consciousness and, if so, for how long.
• Monitor vital signs, and check for additional injuries. Palpate the skull for tenderness or hematomas.
• If the patient has altered consciousness or if a neurologic examination reveals abnormalities, the injury may be more severe than a concussion. He should be admitted for neurologic consultation.
• If a neurologic examination reveals no abnormalities, observe the patient in the emergency department. Check vital signs, level of consciousness, and pupil size every 15 minutes.
• If his condition worsens or fluctuates, he should be admitted for neurosurgical consultation.
• The patient who is stable after 4 or more hours of observation can be discharged (with a head injury instruction sheet) in the care of a responsible adult. (See *What to Do after Concussion.*)

Congenital anomalies of the ureter, bladder, and urethra

Description
Congenital anomalies of the ureter, bladder, and urethra are among the

Types of Genitourinary Anomalies

DUPLICATED URETER

PATHOPHYSIOLOGY
- Most common ureteral anomaly
- *Complete,* a double collecting system with two separate pelvises, each with its own ureter and orifice
- *Incomplete* (y type), two separate ureters join before entering bladder

CLINICAL FEATURES
- Persistent or recurrent infection
- Frequency, urgency, or burning on urination
- Diminished urine output
- Flank pain, fever, and chills

DIAGNOSIS AND TREATMENT
- Intravenous pyelography
- Voiding cystoscopy
- Cystoureterography
- Retrograde pyelography
- Surgery for obstruction, reflux, or severe renal damage

RETROCAVAL URETER (PREURETERAL VENA CAVA)

PATHOPHYSIOLOGY
- Right ureter passes behind the inferior vena cava before entering the bladder. Compression of the ureter between the vena cava and the spine causes dilation and elongation of the pelvis; hydroureter, hydronephrosis; fibrosis and stenosis of ureter in the compressed area.
- Relatively uncommon; higher incidence in males

CLINICAL FEATURES
- Right flank pain
- Recurrent urinary tract infection
- Renal calculi
- Hematuria

DIAGNOSIS AND TREATMENT
- Intravenous or retrograde pyelography demonstrates superior ureteral enlargement with spiral appearance.
- Surgical resection and anastomosis of ureter with renal pelvis, or reimplantation into bladder

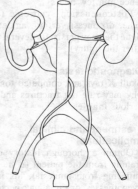

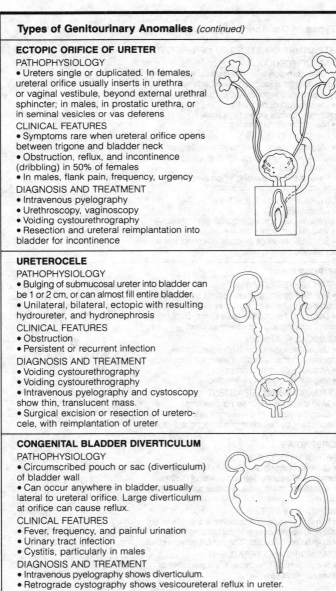

Types of Genitourinary Anomalies (continued)

ECTOPIC ORIFICE OF URETER

PATHOPHYSIOLOGY
• Ureters single or duplicated. In females, ureteral orifice usually inserts in urethra or vaginal vestibule, beyond external urethral sphincter; in males, in prostatic urethra, or in seminal vesicles or vas deferens

CLINICAL FEATURES
• Symptoms rare when ureteral orifice opens between trigone and bladder neck
• Obstruction, reflux, and incontinence (dribbling) in 50% of females
• In males, flank pain, frequency, urgency

DIAGNOSIS AND TREATMENT
• Intravenous pyelography
• Urethroscopy, vaginoscopy
• Voiding cystourethrography
• Resection and ureteral reimplantation into bladder for incontinence

URETEROCELE

PATHOPHYSIOLOGY
• Bulging of submucosal ureter into bladder can be 1 or 2 cm, or can almost fill entire bladder.
• Unilateral, bilateral, ectopic with resulting hydroureter, and hydronephrosis

CLINICAL FEATURES
• Obstruction
• Persistent or recurrent infection

DIAGNOSIS AND TREATMENT
• Voiding cystourethrography
• Voiding cystourethrography
• Intravenous pyelography and cystoscopy show thin, translucent mass.
• Surgical excision or resection of uretero-cele, with reimplantation of ureter

CONGENITAL BLADDER DIVERTICULUM

PATHOPHYSIOLOGY
• Circumscribed pouch or sac (diverticulum) of bladder wall
• Can occur anywhere in bladder, usually lateral to ureteral orifice. Large diverticulum at orifice can cause reflux.

CLINICAL FEATURES
• Fever, frequency, and painful urination
• Urinary tract infection
• Cystitis, particularly in males

DIAGNOSIS AND TREATMENT
• Intravenous pyelography shows diverticulum.
• Retrograde cystography shows vesicoureteral reflux in ureter.
• Surgical correction for reflux

(continued)

Types of Genitourinary Anomalies *(continued)*

STRICTURE OR STENOSIS OF URETER

PATHOPHYSIOLOGY
• Most common site, the distal ureter above ureterovesical junction; less common, ureteropelvic junction; rare, the midureter
• Discovered during infancy in 25% of patients; before puberty in most
• More common in males

CLINICAL FEATURES
• Megaloureter or hydroureter (enlarged ureter), with hydronephrosis when stenosis occurs in distal ureter
• Hydronephrosis alone when stenosis occurs at ureteropelvic junction

DIAGNOSIS AND TREATMENT
• Ultrasound
• Intravenous and retrograde pyelography
• Voiding cystography
• Surgical repair of stricture. Nephrectomy for severe renal damage

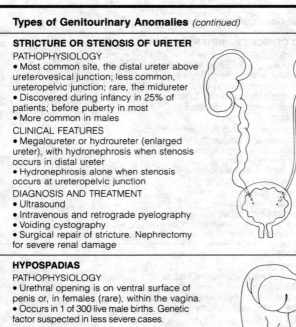

HYPOSPADIAS

PATHOPHYSIOLOGY
• Urethral opening is on ventral surface of penis or, in females (rare), within the vagina.
• Occurs in 1 of 300 live male births. Genetic factor suspected in less severe cases.

CLINICAL FEATURES
• Usually associated with chordee, making normal urination with penis elevated impossible
• Absence of ventral prepuce
• Vaginal discharge in females

DIAGNOSIS AND TREATMENT
• Mild disorder requires no treatment.
• Surgical repair of severe anomaly usually necessary before child reaches school age

EPISPADIAS

PATHOPHYSIOLOGY
• Urethral opening on dorsal surface of penis; in females, a fissure of the upper wall of urethra
• A rare anomaly; usually develops in males; often accompanies bladder exstrophy

CLINICAL FEATURES
• In mild cases, orifice appears along dorsum of glans; in severe cases, along dorsum of penis.
• In females, bifid clitoris and short, wide urethra

DIAGNOSIS AND TREATMENT
• Surgical repair, in several stages, almost always necessary

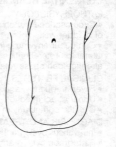

Types of Genitourinary Anomalies *(continued)*

EXSTROPHY OF BLADDER

PATHOPHYSIOLOGY
- Absence of anterior abdominal and bladder wall allows the bladder to protrude onto abdomen.
- In males, associated epispadias and undescended testes; in females, cleft clitoris, separated labia, or absent vagina
- Skeletal or intestinal anomalies possible

CLINICAL FEATURES
- Obvious at birth, with urine seeping onto abdominal wall from abnormal ureteral orifices
- Surrounding skin is excoriated; exposed bladder mucosa ulcerated; infection; associated abnormalities

DIAGNOSIS AND TREATMENT
- Intravenous pyelography
- Surgical closure of defect, and bladder and urethra reconstruction during infancy to allow pubic bone fusion; alternative treatment includes protective dressing and diapering; urinary diversion eventually necessary for most patients

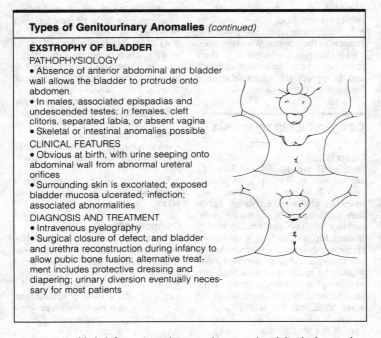

most common birth defects, occurring in about 5% of all births. Some of these abnormalities are obvious at birth; others are not apparent and are recognized only after they produce symptoms.

Causes

Unknown (For signs and symptoms, diagnostic tests, and treatment, see *Types of Genitourinary Anomalies*, pp. 178 to 181.)

Clinical implications

- Since these anomalies are not always obvious at birth, carefully evaluate the newborn's urogenital function. Document the amount and color of urine, voiding pattern, strength of stream, and any indications of infection, such as fever and urine odor. Tell parents to watch for these signs at home.
- In all children, watch for signs of obstruction, such as dribbling, oli-

guria or anuria, abdominal mass, hypertension, fever, bacteriuria, or pyuria.
- Monitor renal function daily; record intake and output accurately.
- Follow strict aseptic technique in handling cystostomy tubes or indwelling (Foley) catheters.
- Make sure that ureteral, suprapubic, or urethral catheters remain in place and do not become contaminated. Document type, color, and amount of drainage.
- Apply sterile saline pads to protect the exposed mucosa of the newborn with bladder exstrophy. Do not use heavy clamps on the umbilical cord, and avoid dressing or diapering the infant. Place the infant in an incubator, and direct a stream of saline mist onto the bladder to keep it moist. Use warm water and mild soap to keep the surrounding skin clean. Rinse well, and

keep the area as dry as possible to prevent excoriation.
• Provide reassurance and emotional support to the parents. When possible, allow them to participate in their child's care to promote normal bonding. As appropriate, suggest or arrange for genetic counseling.

Congenital hip dysplasia

Description
Congenital hip dysplasia (CHD), an abnormality of the hip joint present from birth, is the most common disorder that affects the hip joints of children under age 3. It can be unilateral or bilateral. This abnormality occurs in three forms of varying severity: unstable hip dysplasia, in which the hip is positioned normally but can be dislocated by manipulation; subluxation or incomplete dislocation, in which the femoral head rides on the edge of the acetabulum; and complete dislocation, in which the femoral head is totally outside the acetabulum.

Congenital hip subluxation or dislocation can cause abnormal acetabular development and permanent disability. About 85% of affected infants are girls.

Causes
Unproven theories exist concerning the causes of CHD.
• Hormones that relax maternal ligaments in preparation for labor may also cause laxity of infant ligaments around the capsule of the hip joint.
• Dislocation is 10 times more common after breech delivery (malpositioning in utero) than after cephalic delivery.

Signs and symptoms
• In newborns, no gross deformity or pain. However, in complete dysplasia, the hip rides above the acetabulum,

causing the leg on the affected side to appear shorter or the affected hip more prominent.
• As the child grows older and begins to walk, uncorrected bilateral dysplasia may cause him to sway from side to side ("duck waddle"); unilateral dysplasia may produce a limp.
• If corrective treatment is not begun before age 2, degenerative hip changes, lordosis, joint malformation, and soft-tissue damage may occur.
• An extra thigh fold on the affected side suggests subluxation or dislocation.
• The buttock fold on the affected side is typically higher in a child with dysplasia.

Diagnostic tests
• A positive Ortolani's or Trendelenburg's sign confirms the diagnosis. (See *Ortolani's and Trendelenburg's Signs*.)
• X-rays show the location of the femur head and a shallow acetabulum; X-rays can also monitor the progress of the disease or treatment.

Treatment
The earlier the infant receives treatment, the better his chances are for normal development. Treatment varies with the patient's age. In infants younger than 3 months, treatment includes gentle manipulation to reduce the dislocation, followed by holding the hips in a flexed and abducted position with a splint-brace or harness, to maintain the reduction. The infant must wear this apparatus continuously for 2 to 3 months and then wear a night splint for another month, so the joint capsule can tighten and stabilize in correct alignment.

If treatment does not begin until after age 3 months, it may include bilateral skin traction (in infants) or skeletal traction (in children who have started walking) in an attempt to reduce the dislocation by gradually abducting the hips. If traction fails, gentle closed reduction under general

Ortolani's and Trendelenburg's Signs

• To test for Ortolani's sign, place the infant on his back, with his hip flexed and in abduction. Adduct the hip while pressing the femur downward. This will dislocate the hip. Then, abduct the hip while moving the femur upward. If you hear a click or feel a jerk (produced by the femoral head moving over the acetabular rim), this indicates subluxation in an infant younger than 1 month; this sign indicates subluxation or complete dislocation in an older infant.

• To elicit Trendelenburg's sign, have the child rest his weight on the side of the dislocation and lift his other knee. His pelvis drops on the normal side because of weak abductor muscles in the affected hip. However, when the child stands with his weight on the normal side and lifts the other knee, the pelvis remains horizontal; these phenomena make up a positive Trendelenburg's sign.

anesthesia can further abduct the hips. The child is then placed in a hip-spica cast for 4 to 6 months. If closed treatment fails, open reduction, followed by immobilization in a hip-spica cast for an average of 6 months, or osteotomy may be considered.

In children age 2 to 5, treatment is difficult and includes skeletal traction and subcutaneous adductor tenotomy. Treatment begun after age 5 rarely restores satisfactory hip function.

Clinical implications

• Teach parents how to splint or brace the hips correctly, as ordered. Stress the need for frequent checkups.

• Listen sympathetically to the parents' expressions of anxiety and fear. Explain possible causes of CHD, and give reassurance that early, prompt treatment will probably result in complete correction.

• During the child's first few days in a cast or splint-brace, encourage his parents to stay with him as much as possible to calm and reassure him, because his restricted movement will make him irritable.

• Instruct parents to remove braces and splints while bathing the infant but to replace them immediately afterward. Stress good hygiene; parents should bathe and change the infant frequently and wash his perineum with

warm water and soap at each diaper change.

If treatment requires a hip-spica cast, follow these guidelines:

• When transferring the child immediately after casting, use your palms to avoid making dents in the cast. Such dents predispose the patient to pressure sores. Remember that the cast needs 24 to 48 hours to dry naturally. Do not use heat to make it dry faster, because heat also makes it more fragile.

• Immediately after the cast is applied, use a plastic sheet to protect it from moisture around the perineum and buttocks. Cut the sheet in strips long enough to cover the outside of the cast, and tuck them about a finger length beneath the cast edges. Using overlapping strips of tape, tack the corner of each petal to the outside of the cast. Remove the plastic under the cast every 4 hours; then wash, dry, and retuck it. Disposable diapers folded lengthwise over the perineum may also be used.

• Position the child either on a Bradford frame elevated on blocks, with a bedpan under the frame, or on pillows to support the child's legs. Keep the cast dry, and change diapers often.

• Wash and dry the skin under the cast edges every 2 to 4 hours, and rub it with alcohol. Do not use oils or pow-

Teaching Topics in CHD

- An explanation of the type of dysplasia: instability, subluxation, or dislocation
- Clinical tests to screen for CHD
- Importance of treatment to ensure a normal gait and to avoid degenerative joint disease later in life
- An explanation of selected treatment: external splinting, application of traction, surgery (open or closed reduction)
- Hip-spica cast care, if needed

ders; they can macerate skin.
- Turn the child every 2 hours during the day and every 4 hours at night. Check color, sensation, and motion of the infant's legs and feet. Be sure to examine all his toes. Notify the physician of dusky, cool, or numb toes.
- Shine a flashlight under the cast every 4 hours to check for objects and crumbs. Check the cast daily for odors, which may herald infection. Record temperature daily.
- If the child complains of itching, he may benefit from diphenhydramine. Or you may aim a blow-dryer set on cool at the cast edges to relieve itching. Do not scratch or probe under the cast. Investigate any persistent itching.
- Provide adequate nutrition, and maintain adequate fluid intake to avoid renal calculi and constipation, both complications of inactivity.
- If the child is very restless, apply a jacket restraint to keep him from falling out of bed or off the frame.
- Provide adequate stimuli to promote growth and development. If the child's hips are abducted in a froglike position, tell parents that he may be able to fit on a kiddy car. Encourage parents to let the child sit at a table by seating him on pillows on a chair, to put him on the floor for short periods of play, and to let him play with other children his age.

- Tell parents to watch for signs that the child is outgrowing the cast, such as cyanosis, cool extremities, or pain. (See *Teaching Topics in CHD*.)

Congestive heart failure

Description

Congestive heart failure (CHF) is a syndrome characterized by myocardial dysfunction that leads to impaired pump performance (diminished cardiac output) or to frank heart failure and abnormal circulatory congestion. Congestion of systemic venous circulation may result in peripheral edema or hepatomegaly. Congestion of pulmonary circulation may cause pulmonary edema, an acute life-threatening emergency. (See *Managing Pulmonary Edema*, p. 186.) Pump failure usually occurs in a damaged left ventricle (left heart failure) but may happen in the right ventricle, either as primary failure or secondary to left heart failure. Sometimes, left and right heart failure develop simultaneously.

CHF may be acute (as a direct result of myocardial infarction), but it is usually a chronic disorder associated with retention of salt and water by the kidneys. Advances in diagnostic and therapeutic techniques have greatly improved the outlook for patients with CHF, but prognosis still depends on the underlying cause and its response to treatment.

Causes
Cardiovascular
—Arteriosclerotic heart disease
—Myocardial infarction
—Hypertension
—Rheumatic heart disease
—Congenital heart disease
—Ischemic heart disease
—Cardiomyopathy
—Valvular diseases
—Dysrhythmias

—Noncompliance with treatment for heart disease

Noncardiovascular
—Pregnancy and childbirth
—Increased environmental temperature or humidity
—Severe physical or mental stress
—Thyrotoxicosis
—Acute blood loss
—Pulmonary embolism
—Severe infection
—Chronic obstructive pulmonary disease

Signs and symptoms
Left heart failure
—Dyspnea (exertional at first; possible paroxysmal nocturnal dyspnea, Cheyne-Stokes respirations, and orthopnea)
—Tachycardia
—Fatigue
—Muscle weakness
—Edema and weight gain
—Irritability
—Restlessness
—Shortened attention span
—Ventricular gallop heard over the apex
—Bibasilar rales
Right heart failure
—Edema (initially dependent, but may progress)
—Distended and rigid neck veins
—Hepatomegaly (may eventually lead to anorexia, nausea, and vague abdominal pain)
—Occasional ascites
—Ventricular heave

Diagnostic tests
• EKG reflects heart strain or enlargement, or ischemia. It may also reveal atrial enlargement, tachycardia, and extrasystoles, suggesting CHF.
• Chest X-ray shows increased pulmonary vascular markings, interstitial edema, or pleural effusion and cardiomegaly.
• Pulmonary artery monitoring demonstrates elevated pulmonary artery pressure and pulmonary capillary wedge pressure, which reflect left ventricular end-diastolic pressure, in left heart failure, and elevated right atrial pressure or central venous pressure in right heart failure.
• Cardiac blood pool imaging shows a decreased ejection fraction in left heart failure.
• Cardiac catheterization may show ventricular dilatation, coronary artery occlusion, and valvular disorders (such as aortic stenosis) in both left and right heart failure.
• Echocardiography may show ventricular hypertrophy, decreased contractility, and valvular disorders in both left and right heart failure. Serial echocardiograms may help assess the patient's response to therapy.

Treatment
• Diuresis to reduce total blood volume and circulatory congestion
• Prolonged bed rest
• Digitalis to strengthen myocardial contractility or, in acute failure, a positive inotropic agent such as I.V. dopamine or dobutamine
• Vasodilators to increase cardiac output by reducing impedance to ventricular outflow (afterload)
• Antiembolism stockings to prevent venostasis and possible thromboembolism formation
• Sodium-restricted diet and smaller, more frequent meals
• Oxygen therapy

After recovery, the patient usually must continue taking digitalis and diuretics and must remain under medical supervision. If the patient with valve dysfunction has recurrent acute CHF, surgical replacement may be necessary.

Clinical implications
During the acute phase of CHF, follow these guidelines:
• Place the patient in the Fowler position and give him supplemental oxygen to help him breathe more easily.

Managing Pulmonary Edema

INITIAL STAGE SYMPTOMS
• Persistent cough
• Slight dyspnea or orthopnea
• Exercise intolerance
• Restlessness and anxiety
• Crackles at lung bases
• Diastolic gallop

SPECIAL CONSIDERATIONS
• Check color and amount of expectoration.
• Position patient for comfort, and elevate head of bed.
• Auscultate chest for rales and S_3.
• Medicate, as ordered.
• Monitor apical and radial pulses.
• Assist patient to conserve strength.
• Provide emotional support (through all stages) for patient and family.

ACUTE STAGE SYMPTOMS
• Acute shortness of breath
• Respirations—rapid, noisy (audible wheeze, crackles)
• Cough—more intense and productive of frothy, blood-tinged sputum
• Cyanosis—cold, clammy skin
• Tachycardia—dysrhythmias
• Hypotension

SPECIAL CONSIDERATIONS
• Administer supplemental oxygen, as necessary (preferably by high concentration mask or intermittent positive-pressure breathing [IPPB]).
• Insert I.V. line, if not already done.
• Aspirate nasopharynx, as needed.
• Apply rotating tourniquets.
• Give nitrates, morphine, and potent diuretics (e.g., furosemide), as ordered.
• Insert indwelling (Foley) catheter.
• Calculate intake and output accurately.
• Draw blood to measure arterial blood gases.
• Attach cardiac monitor leads, and observe EKG.
• Reassure the patient.
• Keep resuscitation equipment available at all times.

ADVANCED STAGE SYMPTOMS
• Decreased level of consciousness
• Ventricular dysrhythmias; shock
• Diminished breath sounds

SPECIAL CONSIDERATIONS
• Be prepared for cardioversion.
• Assist with intubation and mechanical ventilation, and resuscitate, if necessary.

• Weigh the patient daily (this is the best index of fluid retention), and check for peripheral edema. Also, carefully monitor I.V. intake and urine output (especially in the patient receiving diuretics), vital signs (for increased respiratory rate, heart rate, and narrowing pulse pressure), and mental status. Auscultate the heart for abnormal sounds (S_3 gallop) and the lungs for crackles and rhonchi. Report changes immediately.
• Frequently monitor blood urea nitrogen and serum creatinine, potassium, sodium, chloride, and magnesium levels.
• When using rotating tourniquets, check the patient's radial and pedal pulses frequently to ensure that the tourniquets are not applied too tightly. At the completion of tourniquet therapy, remove one tourniquet at a time to prevent a sudden upsurge in circulating volume.
• To prevent deep vein thrombosis from vascular congestion, assist the patient with range-of-motion exercises. Enforce bed rest, and apply antiembolism stockings. Watch for calf pain and tenderness.

To prepare the patient for discharge, follow these guidelines:
• Advise the patient to avoid foods high in sodium, such as canned or commercially prepared foods and dairy products, to curb fluid overload.
• Instruct the patient that the potas-

Teaching Topics in CHF

- An explanation of the disorder
- Preparation for chest X-ray, EKG, cardiac blood pool imaging, and other diagnostic tests
- Activity restrictions and energy conservation methods
- Dietary sodium and fluid restrictions
- Medications and their use
- Preparation for pulmonary artery catheterization, rotating tourniquets, or other necessary acute care procedures
- Measures to relieve symptoms and minimize complications
- Similarity of risk factors for CHF and other cardiovascular disorders
- Sources of information and support

sium he loses through diuretic therapy must be replaced by taking a prescribed potassium supplement and eating high-potassium foods, such as bananas, apricots, and orange juice.
- Stress the need for regular checkups.
- Stress the importance of taking digitalis exactly as prescribed. Tell the patient to watch for and immediately report signs of toxicity, such as anorexia, vomiting, and yellow vision.
- Tell the patient to notify the physician if his pulse is unusually irregular or less than 60 beats per minute; if he experiences dizziness, blurred vision, shortness of breath, a persistent dry cough, palpitations, increased fatigue, paroxysmal nocturnal dyspnea, swollen ankles, or decreased urine output; or if he gains 3 to 5 lb (1.35 to 2.25 kg) in a week.

Complications
- Thromboembolism
- Cerebral insufficiency
- Renal insufficiency, with severe electrolyte imbalance (See *Teaching Topics in CHF.*)

Conjunctivitis

Description
Conjunctivitis, an inflammation of the conjunctiva, usually occurs as benign, self-limiting pinkeye. It may also be chronic, possibly indicating degenerative changes or damage from repeated acute attacks. In the Western hemisphere, conjunctivitis is probably the most common eye disorder.

Causes
- Bacterial infection
- Viral infection
- Chlamydial infection
- Less commonly, parasitic disease
- Rarely, fungal infection
- Allergy
- Occupational irritants
- Idiopathic but associated with certain systemic diseases, such as erythema multiforme and thyroid disease

Signs and symptoms
- Hyperemia of the conjunctiva
- Discharge possible (mucopurulent with bacteria infection, minimal with viral infection)
- Tearing
- Pain
- Photophobia with corneal involvement
- Itching and burning
- Sensation of a foreign body in the eye with acute bacterial infection
- Accompanying sore throat or fever possible in children

Diagnostic tests
- Stained smears of conjunctival scrapings reveal predominant mono-

cytes if the cause is a virus. Polymorphonuclear cells (neutrophils) predominate if the cause is bacteria; eosinophils, if the cause is allergy.
• Culture and sensitivity tests identify the causative bacterial organism and indicate appropriate antibiotic therapy.

Treatment

Treatment of conjunctivitis varies with the cause. Bacterial conjunctivitis requires topical application of the appropriate antibiotic or sulfonamide. Viral conjunctivitis resists treatment, but sulfonamide or broad-spectrum antibiotic eye drops may prevent secondary infection. Herpes simplex infection usually responds to treatment with idoxuridine or vidarabine ointment, but the infection may persist for 2 to 3 weeks. Treatment of vernal (allergic) conjunctivitis includes administration of vasoconstrictor eye drops, such as epinephrine; cold compresses to relieve itching; and, occasionally, oral antihistamines.

Instillation of 1% silver nitrate into the eyes of newborns prevents gonococcal conjunctivitis.

Clinical implications

• Teach proper hand-washing technique, because some forms of conjunctivitis are highly contagious. Stress the risk of spreading infection to family members by sharing washcloths, towels, and pillows. Warn against rubbing the infected eye, which can spread the infection to the other eye and to other persons.
• Apply warm compresses and therapeutic ointment or drops, as ordered. Do not irrigate the eye; this will spread infection. Have the patient wash his hands before he uses the medication, and use clean washcloths or towels so he does not infect his other eye.
• Teach the patient to instill eye drops and ointments correctly—without touching the bottle tip to his eye or lashes.
• Stress the importance of safety

glasses for the patient who works near chemical irritants.
• Notify public health authorities if cultures show *Neisseria gonorrhoeae*.

Conversion disorder
(Hysterical neurosis, conversion type)

Description

In a conversion disorder, emotional conflicts are repressed and converted into sensory, motor, or visceral symptoms such as blindness, paresthesias, tics, or paralysis. The patient's loss of physical function is involuntary. Usually, only one symptom develops.

The symptom serves one of two purposes. It can prevent expression or perception of an internal conflict. (For example, the spouse who does not wish to acknowledge her murderous rage develops vocal cord paralysis.) Or, it can help the patient gain support or avoid unpleasant activity. (A soldier may develop blindness when ordered into combat.)

The symptom itself is usually not life-threatening, but its complications, such as contractures, muscle wasting, decubitus ulcers, and dramatically altered life-style, can be severely disruptive and debilitating.

Causes

Recent severe psychological stress—a traumatic event the patient feels unable to handle

Signs and symptoms

• The most striking characteristic of a conversion disorder is the sudden onset of a debilitating symptom that prevents normal function of the affected body part.
• The patient does not consciously control the symptom. For example, he cannot move a leg even though he is trying.

Factitious Disorders

Factitious disorders are severely psychopathologic conditions marked by the intentional, repetitious simulation of a physical or mental illness for the purpose of obtaining medical treatment. Factitious illness may or may not be associated with overt mental symptoms.

Chronic factitious illness with physical symptoms (Münchausen's syndrome) has the following essential clinical features:
• Convincing presentation of feigned physical illness
• Voluntary production of symptoms
  Associated features include the following:
• Wandering from hospital to hospital (frequently covering great distances)
• Extensive knowledge of medical terminology
• Pathologic lying
• Evidence of prior treatment, including surgery
• Shifting complaints and symptoms
• Demanding and disruptive behavior
• Drug abuse
• Eagerness to undergo hazardous and painful procedures
• Discharge against medical advice to avoid detection
• Poor interpersonal relationships
• Usual refusal of psychiatric examination

Many patients have a history of deprivation and rejection, and poor identity formation. The patient may be seeking warmth and acceptance but can inspire anger.

Factitious illness with mental symptoms is extremely rare. Its essential features are the following:
• Voluntary production of symptoms suggesting a mental disorder, in the absence of malingering
• Actively seeking admission to a mental hospital
• Symptoms suggesting simultaneous organic, affective, and schizophrenic disorders

• Oddly, the patient does not show the affect and concern that such a severe symptom usually elicits.

Diagnostic tests
• Laboratory tests and diagnostic procedures do not show an organic cause.
• Thorough physical examination rules out any physical cause.

Treatment
Effective treatment relieves the symptom and returns the patient to normal function. The patient needs to know that his symptom has no organic cause, though its effect is no less real. He should be helped to understand the time relationship between the stress and the symptom. Psychiatric treatment is strongly indicated to help the patient understand his underlying psychological conflict and to resolve the stress in a more suitable way. When conflict is resolved, the symptom soon disappears.

Clinical implications
• Help the patient maintain integrity of the affected system. Regularly exercise paralyzed limbs to prevent muscle wasting and contractures.
• Change the bedridden patient's position frequently to prevent decubitus ulcers.
• Ensure adequate nutrition, even if the patient complains of GI distress.

• Provide a supportive environment, and encourage the patient to discuss the stress that provoked the conversion disorder. Do not force the patient to talk, but convey a caring and concerned attitude to help him share his feelings.

• Do not insist that the patient use the affected system. That will only anger him and prevent a therapeutic relationship.

• Add your support to the recommendation for psychiatric care.

• Include the patient's family in all aspects of care. They may be part of the patient's stress, and they are essential to support the patient and help him regain normal function. (See also *Factitious Disorders*, p. 189.)

Corneal abrasion

Description
A corneal abrasion is a scratch on the surface epithelium of the cornea. It is the most common eye injury. With treatment, prognosis is usually good. However, a corneal scratch produced by a fingernail, a piece of paper, or other organic substance may cause a persistent lesion. The epithelium does not always heal properly, and a recurrent corneal erosion may develop, with delayed effects more severe than the original injury.

Causes
Foreign body

Risk factors
• Failure to wear protective glasses in hazardous occupations
• Falling asleep while wearing hard contact lenses

Signs and symptoms
• Redness
• Increased tearing
• Sensation of "something in the eye"

• Pain disproportionate to the size of the injury
• Possible diminished visual acuity

Diagnostic tests
• Staining the cornea with fluorescein stain confirms the diagnosis. The injured area appears green when examined with a flashlight.
• Slit-lamp examination discloses the depth of the abrasion.
• Examining the eye with a flashlight may reveal a foreign body on the cornea. The eyelid must be everted to check for a foreign body embedded under the lid.
• A test to determine visual acuity provides a medical baseline and legal safeguard before beginning treatment.

Treatment and clinical implications
Removal of a deeply embedded foreign body is done with a foreign body spud, using a topical anesthetic. A rust ring on the cornea can be removed with an ophthalmic burr after applying a topical anesthetic. When only partial removal is possible, re-epithelialization lifts the ring again to the surface and allows complete removal the following day.

Treatment also includes instillation of broad-spectrum antibiotic eye drops in the affected eye every 3 to 4 hours. Initial application of a pressure patch prevents further corneal irritation when the patient blinks.

• Assist with examination of the eye. Check visual acuity before beginning treatment.
• If a foreign body is visible, irrigate the eye with normal saline solution.
• Tell the patient with an eye patch to leave the patch in place for 24 to 48 hours. Warn that wearing a patch alters depth perception, so advise caution in everyday activities, such as climbing stairs or stepping off a curb.
• Reassure the patient that the corneal epithelium usually heals in 24 to 48 hours.

• Stress the importance of instilling antibiotic eye drops, as ordered, because an untreated corneal infection can lead to ulceration and permanent loss of vision. Teach the patient the proper way to instill eye medications.

• Emphasize the importance of wearing safety glasses as necessary to protect eyes from flying fragments. Also review instructions for wearing and caring for contact lenses, if appropriate, to prevent further trauma.

Corneal ulcers

Description

A major cause of blindness worldwide, ulcers produce corneal scarring or perforation. They occur in the central or marginal areas of the cornea, vary in shape and size, and may be single or multiple. Marginal ulcers are the most common. Prompt treatment (within hours of onset) can prevent visual impairment.

Causes

• Bacterial, viral, or fungal infections are the most common causes.

• Other causes include trauma, exposure, reactions to bacterial infections, toxins, and allergens.

Signs and symptoms

• Typically, corneal ulceration begins with pain (aggravated by blinking), followed by increased tearing.

• Eventually, central corneal ulceration produces pronounced visual blurring.

• The eye may appear injected.

• Purulent discharge is possible with a bacterial ulcer.

• A hypopyon (accumulation of white cells or pus in the anterior chamber) may produce cloudiness or color change.

Diagnostic tests

• Patient history that possibly indicates trauma and flashlight examination that reveals an irregular corneal surface suggest corneal ulcer.

• Fluorescein dye, instilled in the conjunctival sac, stains the outline of the ulcer and confirms the diagnosis.

• Culture and sensitivity testing of corneal scraping may identify the causative bacteria or fungus and indicate appropriate antibiotic or antifungal therapy.

Treatment and clinical implications

Prompt treatment is essential for all forms of corneal ulcer, to prevent complications and permanent visual impairment. Usually, treatment consists of systemic and topical broad-spectrum antibiotics until culture results identify the causative organism. The goals of treatment are to eliminate the underlying cause of the ulcer and to relieve pain.

• In infection by *Pseudomonas aeruginosa,* polymyxin B and gentamicin are administered topically and by subconjunctival injection, or carbenicillin and tobramycin are administered I.V. Because this type of corneal ulcer spreads so rapidly, it can cause corneal perforation and loss of the eye within 48 hours. Immediate treatment and isolation of hospitalized patients are required. *Note:* Treatment of a corneal ulcer caused by bacterial infection should *never* include an eye patch, since patching creates a dark, warm, moist environment ideal for bacterial growth.

• In infections by herpes simplex type 1 virus, idoxuridine or vidarabine is applied topically every hour. Corneal ulcers resulting from a viral infection often recur; in this case, trifluridine becomes the treatment of choice.

• In infection by varicella-zoster virus, topical sulfonamide ointment is applied three or four times daily to prevent secondary infection. These lesions are unilateral, following the

pathway of the fifth cranial nerve, and are quite painful. Give analgesics, as ordered. Associated anterior uveitis requires cycloplegic eye drops. Watch for signs of secondary glaucoma (increased intraocular pressure, transient vision loss, and halos around lights).
• In infection by fungi, treatment is topical instillation of natamycin for *Fusarium, Cephalosporium*, and *Candida*.
• In hypersensitivity reactions, topical corticosteroids, such as dexamethasone and hydrocortisone, are administered.
• In hypovitaminosis A, treatment aims to correct dietary deficiency or GI malabsorption of vitamin A.
• In neurotropic ulcers or exposure keratitis, treatment is frequent instillation of artificial tears or lubricating ointments and use of a plastic bubble eye shield.

Corns and calluses

Description
A corn is a horny mass of condensed epithelial cells overlying a bony prominence. A callus is a thickening of the epidermis. Corns and calluses are usually located on areas of repeated trauma, in most cases the feet. Prognosis is good with proper foot care.

Causes
Corns
—External pressure, as from ill-fitting shoes
—Internal pressure, as from a protruding underlying bone
Calluses
—External pressure or friction experienced by manual laborers or guitarists, for example

Signs and symptoms
• Both corns and calluses cause pain.
• "Soft" corns appear as whitish thickenings and are commonly found between the toes—most often in the fourth interdigital web.
• "Hard" corns are sharply delineated and conical, and appear most frequently over the dorsolateral aspect of the fifth toe.
• Calluses have indefinite borders and may be quite large.

Treatment
Surgical debridement may be performed to remove the nucleus of a corn, usually under a local anesthetic. In intermittent debridement, keratolytics—usually 40% salicylic acid plasters—are applied to affected areas. Injections of corticosteroids beneath the corn may be necessary to relieve pain. However, the simplest and best treatment is essentially preventive—avoidance of trauma. Corns and calluses disappear after the source of trauma has been removed. Metatarsal pads may redistribute weight-bearing to different areas of the foot; corn pads may prevent painful pressure.

Patients with persistent corns or calluses require referral to a podiatrist or dermatologist. Those with corns or calluses caused by a bony malformation, as in arthritis, require orthopedic consultation.

Clinical implications
• Teach the patient how to apply salicylic acid plasters. Make sure the plaster is large enough to cover the affected area. Place the sticky side down on the foot, then cover the plaster with adhesive tape. Plasters are usually taken off after an overnight application but may be left in place for as long as 7 days. After removing the plaster, the patient should soak the area in water and abrade the soft, macerated skin with a towel or pumice stone. He should then reapply the plaster and repeat the entire procedure until he has removed all the hyperkeratotic skin. Warn the patient against removing

corns or calluses with a sharp instrument, such as a razor blade.
• Advise the patient to wear properly fitted shoes. Suggest the use of metatarsal or corn pads to relieve pressure. Refer to a podiatrist, dermatologist, or orthopedist, if necessary.
• Assure the patient that good foot care can correct this condition.

Coronary artery disease

Description

Coronary artery disease (CAD) is an umbrella term for various diseases that reduce or halt blood flow in the coronary arteries, causing a decrease in oxygen and nutrients that reach the myocardium. CAD claims more lives yearly than any other disease.

Typically, CAD strikes more whites than blacks, and more men than women. It is more prevalent in industrial than in underdeveloped countries and affects more affluent than poor people.

Causes
• Atherosclerosis (by far the most common)
• Arteritis
• Coronary artery spasm. (See *Cor-*

Coronary Artery Spasm

In coronary artery spasm, a spontaneous, sustained contraction of one or more coronary arteries causes ischemia and dysfunction of the heart muscle. This disorder also causes Prinzmetal's angina and even myocardial infarction in patients with unoccluded coronary arteries.

The direct cause of coronary artery spasm is unknown, but possible contributing factors include the following:
• Intimal hemorrhage into the medial layer of the blood vessel
• Hyperventilation
• Elevated catecholamine levels
• Fatty buildup in lumen

The major symptom of coronary artery spasm is angina. But unlike classic angina, this pain commonly occurs spontaneously and may not be related to physical exertion or emotional stress; it is also more severe, usually lasts longer, and may be cyclic, frequently recurring every day at the same time. Such ischemic episodes may cause dysrhythmia, altered heart rate, lower blood pressure, and, occasionally, fainting caused by diminished cardiac output. Spasm in the left coronary artery may result in mitral valve prolapse, producing a loud systolic murmur and, possibly, pulmonary edema, with dyspnea, crackles, and hemoptysis.

After diagnosis by coronary angiography and EKGs, the patient may receive calcium channel blockers (verapamil, nifedipine, or diltiazem) to reduce coronary artery spasm and to decrease vascular resistance, and nitrates (nitroglycerin or isosorbide dinitrate) to relieve chest pain.

When caring for a patient with coronary artery spasm, explain all necessary procedures and teach him how to take his medications safely. For calcium antagonist therapy, monitor blood pressure, pulse rate, and EKG patterns to detect dysrhythmias. For nifedipine and verapamil therapy, monitor digoxin levels and check for signs of digitalis toxicity. Because nifedipine may cause peripheral and periorbital edema, watch for fluid retention.

Because coronary artery spasm is sometimes associated with atherosclerotic disease, advise the patient to stop smoking, avoid overeating, use alcohol sparingly, and maintain a balance between exercise and rest.

onary Artery Spasm, p. 193.)
• Certain infectious diseases
• Congenital defects in the coronary vascular system

Risk factors
• Family history of heart disease
• Obesity
• Smoking
• High-fat, high-carbohydrate diet
• Sedentary life-style
• Type A personality
• Diabetes
• Hypertension
• Hyperlipoproteinemia

Signs and symptoms
• Chest discomfort (angina) is the classic symptom. Burning, squeezing, or crushing tightness in the substernal or precordial chest may radiate to the left arm, neck, jaw, or shoulder blade. Angina most frequently follows physical exertion but may also follow emotional excitement, exposure to cold, or a large meal. The angina is not as severe or as long as with acute myocardial infarction and is often relieved by nitroglycerin.
• Other possible symptoms include nausea, vomiting, weakness, diaphoresis, and cool extremities.

Diagnostic tests
• EKG during angina shows ischemia and possibly dysrhythmias, such as premature ventricular contraction. EKG is apt to be normal when the patient is pain-free. Dysrhythmias may occur without infarction, secondary to ischemia.
• Treadmill or bicycle exercise test may provoke chest pain and EKG signs of myocardial ischemia in response to physical exertion.
• Coronary angiography reveals coronary artery stenosis or obstruction, collateral circulation, and shows the condition of the arteries beyond the narrowing.
• Myocardial perfusion imaging with thallium-201 during treadmill exercise detects ischemic areas of the myocardium, visualized as "cold spots."
• Serum lipid studies detect and classify hyperlipemia.

Treatment
The goal of treatment in patients with angina is either to reduce myocardial oxygen demand or increase oxygen supply. Therapy consists primarily of nitrates, such as nitroglycerin (given sublingually, P.O., transdermally, or topically in ointment form), isosorbide dinitrate (sublingually or P.O.), beta-adrenergic blockers (P.O.), or calcium channel blockers (P.O.). Obstructive lesions may necessitate coronary artery bypass surgery using vein grafts. Angioplasty may be performed during cardiac catheterization to compress fatty deposits and relieve occlusion in patients with no calcification and partial occlusion. (See *Relieving Occlusions with Angioplasty*.) This procedure carries a certain risk, but morbidity is lower than it is for surgery. Laser angioplasty, a newer procedure, corrects occlusion by melting fatty deposits.

Because CAD is so widespread, prevention is of incalculable importance. Dietary restrictions aimed at reducing intake of calories (in obesity) and of salt, fats, and cholesterol serve to minimize the risk, especially when supplemented with regular exercise. Abstention from smoking and reduction of stress are also beneficial. Other preventive actions include control of hypertension (with sympathetic blocking agents, such as methyldopa and propranolol, or diuretics, such as hydrochlorothiazide); control of elevated serum cholesterol or triglyceride levels (with antilipemics such as clofibrate); and measures to minimize platelet aggregation and the danger of blood clots (with aspirin or sulfinpyrazone).

Relieving Occlusions with Angioplasty

For a patient with an occluded coronary artery, percutaneous transluminal coronary angioplasty (PTCA) can open it without opening the chest—an important advantage over bypass surgery. First, coronary angiography must confirm the presence and location of the arterial occlusion. Then, the physician threads a guide catheter through the patient's femoral artery into the coronary artery under fluoroscopic guidance, as shown below.

When angiography shows the guide catheter positioned at the occlusion site, the physician carefully inserts a smaller double-lumen balloon catheter through the guide catheter and directs the balloon through the occlusion (lower left). A marked pressure gradient will be obvious.

The physician alternately inflates and deflates the balloon until an angiogram verifies successful arterial dilation (lower right) and the pressure gradient has decreased.

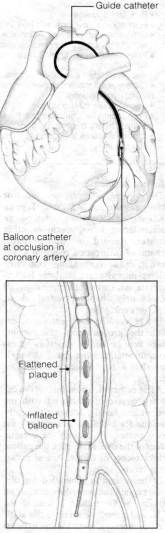

Guide catheter

Balloon catheter at occlusion in coronary artery

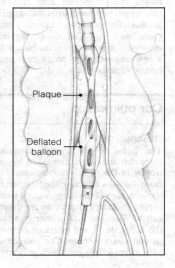

Plaque

Deflated balloon

Flattened plaque

Inflated balloon

Teaching Topics in CAD

• An explanation of disease mechanisms: atherosclerosis and coronary artery spasm
• Risk factor analysis
• How angina develops and how to treat and prevent it
• Importance of treating CAD to prevent complications, such as myocardial infarction, dysrhythmias, and congestive heart failure
• Preparation for diagnostic tests, such as EKG, angiography, and serum lipid studies
• Recommended exercise program
• Dietary restrictions to lower serum low-density lipoprotein levels and control hypertension
• Use of prescribed drugs
• Preparation for percutaneous transluminal coronary angioplasty or coronary artery bypass grafting, if ordered
• Other measures to reduce risk factors: reducing stress, controlling weight, quitting smoking

Clinical implications

• During anginal episodes, monitor blood pressure and heart rate. Take an EKG during anginal episodes before administering nitroglycerin or other nitrates. Record duration of pain, amount of medication required to relieve it, and accompanying symptoms.
• Keep nitroglycerin available for immediate use. Instruct the patient to call immediately whenever he feels chest, arm, or neck pain.
• Before cardiac catheterization, explain the procedure to the patient. Make sure he knows why it is necessary, understands the risks, and realizes that it may indicate a need for surgery.
• After catheterization, review the expected course of treatment with the patient and family. Monitor the catheter site for bleeding. Also, check for distal pulses. To counter the diuretic effect of the dye, make sure the patient drinks plenty of fluids. Assess potassium levels.
• If the patient is scheduled for surgery, explain the procedure to him and his family. Give them a tour of the ICU, and introduce them to the staff.
• After surgery, provide meticulous I.V., pulmonary artery catheter, and endotracheal tube care. Monitor blood pressure, intake and output, breath sounds, chest tube drainage, and EKG, watching for signs of ischemia and dysrhythmias. Also, observe for and treat chest pain. Give vigorous chest physiotherapy and guide the patient in pulmonary toilet.
• Before discharge, stress the need to follow the prescribed drug regimen (antihypertensives, nitrates, antilipemics, for example), exercise program, and diet. Encourage regular, moderate exercise. Refer the patient to a smoking cessation program if necessary. (See *Teaching Topics in CAD*.)

Cor pulmonale

Description

The World Health Organization defines chronic cor pulmonale as hypertrophy of the right ventricle resulting from diseases affecting the function or the structure of the lungs, except when these pulmonary alterations are the result of diseases that primarily affect the left side of the heart or of congenital heart disease. Cor pulmonale affects middle-aged to elderly men more often than women, but its incidence in women is increasing. Prognosis is usually poor.

Causes

Cor pulmonale is caused by pulmonary hypertension, which can result from the following:

• Chronic obstructive pulmonary disease (COPD—most common)

• Restrictive lung diseases such as pneumoconiosis, cystic fibrosis, interstitial pneumonitis, bronchiectasis, scleroderma, and sarcoidosis

• Loss of lung tissue after extensive lung surgery

• Pulmonary vascular diseases such as recurrent thromboembolism, primary pulmonary hypertension, schistosomiasis, and pulmonary vasculitis

• Respiratory insufficiency without pulmonary disease, as seen in chest wall disorders such as kyphoscoliosis, neuromuscular incompetence from muscular dystrophy and amyotrophic lateral sclerosis, polymyositis, and spinal cord lesions above C6

• Obesity hypoventilation syndrome (Pickwickian syndrome) and upper airway obstruction

• Living at high altitudes (chronic mountain sickness)

• In children, cystic fibrosis, hemosiderosis, upper airway obstruction, scleroderma, extensive bronchiectasis, neurologic diseases affecting respiratory muscles, or abnormalities of the respiratory control center

Signs and symptoms

Early

These signs and symptoms are associated with an underlying disorder:

—Chronic productive cough

—Exertional dyspnea

—Fatigue

—Wheezing

—Weakness

Progressive

—Dyspnea at rest

—Tachypnea

—Orthopnea

—Edema

—Right upper quadrant discomfort

Right ventricular failure

—Dependent edema

—Distended neck veins

—Hepatomegaly

—Parasternal or epigastric cardiac impulse

—Hepatojugular reflux

—Tachycardia

—Possible weak pulse and hypotension

Diagnostic tests

• Pulmonary artery pressure measurements (by pulmonary artery catheter) show increased right ventricular and pulmonary artery pressures as a result of increased pulmonary vascular resistance. Both right ventricular systolic and pulmonary artery systolic pressures are greater than 30 mm Hg. Pulmonary artery diastolic pressure is greater than 15 mm Hg.

• Echocardiography or angiography indicates right ventricular enlargement.

• Chest X-ray shows large central pulmonary arteries and suggests right ventricular enlargement.

• Arterial blood gases show decreased Po_2 (frequently less than 70 mm Hg and never more than 90 mm Hg).

• EKG frequently shows dysrhythmias such as premature atrial and ventricular contractions and atrial fibrillation during severe hypoxia; it may also show right bundle branch block, right axis deviation, prominent P waves and inverted T wave in right precordial leads, and right ventricular hypertrophy.

• Pulmonary function tests show results consistent with the underlying pulmonary disease.

• Hematocrit is frequently greater than 50%.

Treatment

Treatment of cor pulmonale is designed to reduce hypoxemia, increase

the patient's exercise tolerance, and, when possible, correct the underlying condition. In addition to bed rest, treatment may include the following:
• Digitalis glycoside (digoxin)
• Antibiotics when respiratory infection is present
• Potent pulmonary artery vasodilators such as diazoxide, nitroprusside, or hydralazine in primary pulmonary hypertension
• Oxygen by mask or cannula in concentrations ranging from 24% to 40%, depending on arterial P_{O_2}, as necessary. (Patients with underlying COPD usually should not receive high concentrations of oxygen because of possible subsequent respiratory depression.)
• In acute cases, possible mechanical ventilation
• Low-salt diet, restricted fluid intake, and diuretics such as furosemide to reduce edema. (Occasionally, cor pulmonale may require phlebotomy to reduce red cell mass.)
• Anticoagulation with small doses of heparin, since there may be increased risk of thromboembolism

Depending on the underlying cause, some variations in treatment may be indicated. For example, a tracheotomy may be necessary if the patient has an upper airway obstruction, and steroids may be used in patients with vasculitis or an autoimmune phenomenon.

Clinical implications
• Provide small, frequent feedings rather than three heavy meals.
• Prevent fluid retention by limiting the patient's fluid intake to 1 to 2 liters/day and providing a low-sodium diet.
• Monitor serum potassium levels closely if the patient is receiving diuretics. Low serum potassium levels can potentiate the risk of dysrhythmias associated with digitalis.

• Watch the patient for signs of digitalis toxicity; monitor for cardiac dysrhythmias.
• Reposition bedridden patients frequently to prevent atelectasis.
• Provide meticulous respiratory care, including oxygen therapy and, for COPD patients, pursed-lip breathing exercises. Periodically measure arterial blood gases and watch for signs of respiratory failure.
• Before discharge, make sure the patient understands the importance of maintaining a low-salt diet, weighing himself daily, and watching for and immediately reporting edema.
• Instruct the patient to allow himself frequent rest periods and to do his breathing exercises regularly.
• If the patient needs suctioning or supplemental oxygen therapy at home, refer him to a social service agency that can help him obtain the necessary equipment. As necessary, arrange for follow-up examinations.
• Since pulmonary infection frequently exacerbates COPD and cor pulmonale, tell the patient to watch for and immediately report early signs of infection. Tell the patient to avoid crowds and persons known to have pulmonary infections, especially during the flu season.
• Warn the patient to avoid nonprescribed medications, such as sedatives, that may depress the ventilatory drive.

Corrosive esophagitis and stricture

Description
Corrosive esophagitis is inflammation and damage to the esophagus after ingestion of a caustic chemical. The chemical may damage only the mucosa or submucosa or may damage all layers of the esophagus. Similar to a burn, this injury may be temporary or may lead to a permanent stricture (narrowing or stenosis) of the esophagus that

is correctable only through surgery. Severe injury can quickly lead to esophageal perforation, mediastinitis, and death from infection, shock, and massive hemorrhage (due to aortic perforation). In children, household chemical ingestion is accidental. In adults, it is usually a suicide attempt or gesture.

Causes
• Ingestion of lye or other strong alkalies (most common)
• Ingestion of strong acids

Signs and symptoms
• May be asymptomatic
• Intense pain in the mouth and anterior chest
• Salivation
• Inability to swallow
• Tachypnea
• With severe damage, bloody vomitus containing pieces of esophageal tissue
• With esophageal perforation and mediastinitis, crepitation
• With laryngeal damage, inability to speak
• Fever (suggests secondary infection)

Diagnostic tests
Physical examination, revealing oropharyngeal burns (including white membranes and edema of the soft palate and uvula), and a history of chemical ingestion usually confirm the diagnosis. Two procedures are helpful in evaluating the severity of the injury:
• Endoscopy (in the first 24 hours after ingestion) delineates the extent and location of the esophageal injury and assesses the depth of the burn. This procedure may also be performed a week after ingestion to assess stricture development.
• Barium swallow (1 week after ingestion and every 3 weeks thereafter) may identify segmental spasm or fistula but does not always show mucosal injury.

Treatment
The type and amount of the chemical ingested must be identified; this may sometimes be done by examining empty containers of the ingested material or by calling the poison control center.

Conservative treatment for corrosive esophagitis and stricture includes monitoring the victim's condition; administering corticosteroids, such as prednisone and hydrocortisone, to control inflammation and inhibit fibrosis; and administering a broad-spectrum antibiotic, such as ampicillin, to protect the corticosteroid-immunosuppressed patient against infection by his own mouth flora.

Current treatment includes administering corticosteroids and antibiotics and performing endoscopy early. It may also include bouginage. This procedure involves passing a slender, flexible, cylindrical instrument called a bougie into the esophagus to dilate it and minimize stricture. Some physicians begin bouginage immediately and continue it regularly to maintain a patent lumen and prevent stricture. Others delay it for a week to avoid the risk of esophageal perforation.

Surgery is necessary immediately for esophageal perforation, or later to correct stricture untreatable with bouginage. Corrective surgery may involve transplanting a piece of the colon to the damaged esophagus. Even after surgery, however, stricture may recur at the site of the anastomosis.

Supportive treatment includes I.V. therapy to replace fluids or total parenteral nutrition while the patient cannot swallow, gradually progressing to clear liquids and a soft diet.

Clinical implications
If you are the first health care professional to see the person who has ingested a corrosive chemical, the quality of your emergency care will be critical. To meet this challenge, follow these important guidelines:

• Do not induce vomiting or lavage, because they will expose the esophagus and oropharynx to injury a second time.

• Do not perform gastric lavage. The corrosive chemical may cause further damage to the mucous membrane of the GI lining.

• Provide vigorous support of vital functions, as needed, such as oxygen, mechanical ventilation, I.V. fluids, and treatment for shock, depending on severity of injury.

• Carefully observe and record intake and output.

• Before X-rays and endoscopy, explain the procedures to the patient to lessen anxiety and to obtain cooperation during the tests.

• Since the adult who has ingested a corrosive agent has usually done so with suicidal intent, encourage and assist him and his family to seek psychological counseling.

• Provide emotional support for parents whose child has ingested a chemical. They will be distraught and may feel guilty about the accident. After the emergency and without emphasizing blame, teach appropriate preventive measures, such as locking accessible cabinets and keeping all corrosive agents out of a child's reach.

Cri du chat syndrome
(Cat's cry syndrome, 5p-syndrome)

Description
Cri du chat syndrome is a rare congenital disorder characterized by a catlike cry in infancy, and severe mental and physical retardation. Many cri du chat infants do not live past their first year. Of those who do survive, some may live to adulthood. An infant with this disorder usually has a normal prenatal history and birth.

Causes
Abnormal deletion of the short arm of chromosome 5 ($5p-$)

Signs and symptoms
Clinical features, such as the following, strongly suggest the diagnosis:

• Abnormally small size at birth

• Microencephaly

• Wide-set eyes, receding chin, high-arched palate, round face, and decreased muscle tone, which makes feeding difficult

• High-pitched catlike cry that appears soon after birth and later disappears

• Other symptoms: low-set ears, simian crease, epicanthal folds, severe mental retardation (IQ less than 50), and associated defects, such as congenital heart disease, joint and bone deformities, and inguinal hernia

Diagnostic tests
A karyotype showing deleted short arm of chromosome 5 confirms the diagnosis.

Treatment
No specific treatment exists. Individualized treatment includes evaluation and treatment of congenital heart and eye defects. When these infants survive past their first year, management is primarily nonmedical and emphasizes education, training in self-care and socialization, recreational and social services, vocational training, and custodial arrangements.

Clinical implications
• Because an affected infant is usually a poor eater, closely monitor fluid intake and output, caloric intake, and weight. To help him meet caloric requirements, offer small feedings frequently. Large meals are apt to tire him because of his decreased muscle tone.

• Amniocentesis can detect cri du chat syndrome prenatally. Encourage parents of such a child to seek genetic counseling. If the father is the translocation carrier, artificial insemination may be a viable alternative.

• Explain the child's potential so that his family can understand and accept long-term plans (including whether or not to institutionalize the child). Refer the parents to an infant stimulation program, which will help their child reach his potential. To avoid rejection or overprotection of such a child, help the parents set realistic goals.

• If parents have trouble coping, refer them for psychological counseling.

Crohn's disease
(Regional enteritis, granulomatous colitis)

Description
Crohn's disease is an inflammation of any part of the GI tract (usually the terminal ileum) that extends through all layers of the intestinal wall. It may also involve regional lymph nodes and the mesentery. Crohn's disease is most prevalent in adults aged 20 to 40.

Causes
The exact cause is unknown. Possible causes include allergies, immune disorders, lymphatic obstruction, infection, and genetic factors.

Signs and symptoms
Clinical effects vary according to the location and extent of inflammation, and at first may be mild and nonspecific.
Acute
—Right lower abdominal quadrant pain
—Cramping
—Tenderness
—Flatulence
—Nausea
—Fever
—Diarrhea
—Bleeding (usually mild; may be massive)

Chronic
—Diarrhea
—Four to six stools a day
—Right lower quadrant pain
—Steatorrhea
—Marked weight loss
—Rarely, clubbing of fingers
—Possible weakness, lack of ambition, and inability to cope with everyday stress

Diagnostic tests
• Laboratory findings in most cases indicate increased white blood cell count and erythrocyte sedimentation rate, hypokalemia, hypocalcemia, hypomagnesemia, and decreased hemoglobin.

• Barium enema showing the string sign (segments of stricture separated by normal bowel) supports this diagnosis.

• Sigmoidoscopy and colonoscopy may show patchy areas or inflammation, thus helping to rule out ulcerative colitis.

• Biopsy results confirm the diagnosis.

Treatment
Treatment is symptomatic. In debilitated patients, therapy includes I.V. hyperalimentation to maintain nutrition while resting the bowel. Drug therapy may include anti-inflammatory corticosteroids, immunosuppressive agents such as azathioprine, and antibacterial agents such as sulfasalazine. Metronidazole has proved to be effective in some patients. Opium tincture and diphenoxylate may help combat diarrhea but are contraindicated in patients with significant intestinal obstruction. Effective treatment requires important changes in life-style: physical rest, restricted fiber diet (no fruit or vegetables), and elimination of dairy products for lactose intolerance.

Surgery may be necessary to correct bowel perforation, massive hemorrhage, fistulas, or acute intestinal obstruction. Colectomy with ileostomy is frequently necessary in patients with extensive disease of the large intestine and rectum.

Clinical implications
• Record fluid intake and output (including the amount of stool), and weigh the patient daily. Watch for dehydration and maintain fluid and electrolyte balance. Be alert for signs of intestinal bleeding (bloody stools). Check stools daily for occult blood.
• If the patient is receiving steroids, watch for adverse effects such as GI bleeding. Remember that steroids can mask signs of infection.
• Check hemoglobin and hematocrit regularly. Give iron supplements and blood transfusions, as ordered.
• Give analgesics, as ordered.
• Provide good patient hygiene and meticulous mouth care.
• Watch for fever and pain on urination, which may signal bladder fistula. Abdominal pain, fever, and hard, distended abdomen may indicate intestinal obstruction.
• Before ileostomy, arrange for a visit by an enterostomal therapist.
• After surgery, frequently check the patient's I.V. line and nasogastric tube for proper functioning. Monitor vital signs and fluid intake and output. Watch for wound infection. Provide meticulous stoma care, and teach it to the patient and family. Realize that ileostomy changes the patient's body image; offer reassurance and emotional support.
• Stress the need for a severely restricted diet and bed rest, which may be trying, particularly for the young patient. Encourage him to try to reduce tension. If stress is clearly an aggravating factor, refer him for counseling.

Complications
• Intestinal obstruction
• Fistula formation between the small bowel and the bladder

• Perianal and perirectal abscesses and fistulas
• Intra-abdominal abscesses
• Perforation
• Possible skin disorders, joint problems, and liver disease
• Increased risk of carcinoma

Croup

Description
Croup is a severe inflammation and obstruction of the upper airway after an upper respiratory infection. Onset of the acute stage is rapid, usually occurs at night, and may be precipitated by exposure to cold air. Croup must always be distinguished from epiglottitis. Croup is a childhood disease affecting boys more often than girls (typically between ages 3 months and 3 years). It usually occurs during the winter. Recovery is usually complete.

Causes
• Viral infection, especially parainfluenza (most common)
• Bacterial infection

Mode of transmission
• Inhalation of infected airborne particles
• Contact with infected secretions

Signs and symptoms
• Hoarse or muffled vocal sounds
• Fever
• Inspiratory stridor
• Distinctive harsh, barking cough
• Varying degrees of respiratory distress

Diagnostic tests
If necessary, tests may include the following:
• Throat cultures to identify or rule out bacterial infection
• Neck X-ray to show areas of upper airway narrowing and edema in subglottic folds

• Laryngoscopy to reveal inflammation and obstruction in epiglottal and laryngeal areas

Treatment
For most children with croup, home care with rest, cool humidification during sleep, and antipyretics such as acetaminophen relieve symptoms. However, respiratory distress that interferes with oral hydration requires hospitalization and parenteral fluid replacement to prevent dehydration. If bacterial infection is the cause, antibiotic therapy is necessary. Oxygen therapy may also be required.

Clinical implications
Monitor and support respiration, and control fever. Because croup is so frightening to the child and his family, provide support and reassurance.
• Carefully monitor cough and breath sounds, hoarseness, severity of retractions, inspiratory stridor, cyanosis, respiratory rate and character (especially prolonged and labored respirations), restlessness, fever, and cardiac rate.
• Keep the child as quiet as possible, but avoid sedation, because it may depress respiration. If the patient is an infant, position him in an infant seat or prop him up with a pillow. Place an older child in the Fowler position. If an older child requires a cool mist tent to help him breathe, explain why it is needed.
• Isolate patients suspected of having respiratory syncytial virus and parainfluenza infections, if possible. Wash your hands carefully before leaving the room, to avoid transmission to other children, particularly infants. Instruct parents and others involved in the care of these children to take similar precautions.
• Control fever with sponge baths and antipyretics. Keep a hypothermia blanket on hand for temperatures above 102° F. (38.9° C.). Watch for seizures

in infants and young children with high fevers. Give I.V. antibiotics, as ordered.
• Relieve sore throat with soothing, water-based ices such as fruit sherbet and ice pops. Avoid thicker, milk-based fluids if the child is producing heavy mucus or has great difficulty in swallowing. Apply petrolatum or another ointment around the nose and lips to soothe irritation from nasal discharge and mouth breathing.
• Maintain a calm, quiet environment and offer reassurance. Explain all procedures and answer any questions.

When croup does not require hospitalization, follow these guidelines:
• Provide thorough patient and family teaching for effective home care. Suggest the use of a cool humidifier (vaporizer). To relieve croupy spells, tell parents to carry the child into the bathroom, shut the door, and turn on the hot water. Breathing warm, moist air quickly eases an acute spell of croup.
• Warn parents that ear infections and pneumonia are complications of croup that may appear about 5 days after recovery. Stress the importance of reporting earache, productive cough, high fever, or increased shortness of breath immediately.

Cryptococcosis
(Torulosis, European blastomycosis)

Description
Cryptococcosis is an infectious disease caused by a fungus. It usually begins as an asymptomatic pulmonary infection but disseminates to extrapulmonary sites, usually to the central nervous system (CNS), but also to the skin, bones, prostate gland, liver, or kidneys. With treatment, prognosis in pulmonary cryptococcosis is good. However, untreated pulmonary disease may lead to CNS infection, which

is invariably fatal within 3 years of diagnosis. Treatment dramatically reduces mortality but does not always reverse neurologic deficit, such as paralysis and hydrocephalus.

Cause
The fungus *Cryptococcus neoformans*

Mode of transmission
Inhalation of *C. neoformans* in particles of dust contaminated by pigeon feces that harbor this organism

Risk factors
Immunologic compromise

Signs and symptoms
• Typically, pulmonary cryptococcosis is asymptomatic.
• Onset of CNS involvement (cryptococcal meningitis) is gradual and causes progressively severe frontal and temporal headache, diplopia, blurred vision, dizziness, ataxia, aphasia, vomiting, tinnitus, memory changes, inappropriate behavior, irritability, psychotic symptoms, convulsions, and fever.
• If untreated, symptoms progress to coma and death (usually a result of cerebral edema or hydrocephalus).
• Skin involvement produces red facial papules and other skin abscesses, with or without ulcerations.
• Bone involvement produces painful osseous lesions of the long bones, skull, spine, and joints.

Diagnostic tests
• Routine chest X-ray showing a pulmonary lesion may point to cryptococcosis; however, this infection usually escapes diagnosis until it disseminates.
• The diagnosis is confirmed by identification of *C. neoformans* by culture of sputum, urine, prostatic secretions, bone marrow aspirate or biopsy, or pleural biopsy; and in CNS infection, by an India ink preparation of cerebrospinal fluid (CSF) and culture.
• Blood cultures are positive only in

severe infection.
• Antigen titers are increased in serum and CSF.
• Other CSF findings may include increased pressure, protein, and white blood cell count in CNS infection and moderately decreased glucose level in about half of patients.

Treatment
Pulmonary cryptococcosis requires close medical observation for a year after diagnosis. Treatment is unnecessary unless extrapulmonary lesions develop or pulmonary lesions progress.

Treatment of disseminated infection calls for I.V. (or, in CNS infection, intrathecal) amphotericin B for 3 to 6 months, or for a 6-week course of oral flucytosine with amphotericin B. Supportive measures and acetazolamide can decrease CSF pressure.

Clinical implications
• Cryptococcosis does not necessitate isolation. However, amphotericin B administered intrathecally requires strict aseptic technique.
• Check vital functions, and note changes in mental status, orientation, pupillary response, and motor function. Watch for headache, vomiting, and nuchal rigidity.
• Before giving I.V. amphotericin B, check for phlebitis. Infuse slowly, and dilute as ordered. Rapid infusion may cause circulatory collapse. Before therapy, draw serum electrolytes to determine baseline renal status. During drug therapy, watch for decreased urine output, elevated blood urea nitrogen and creatinine levels, and hypokalemia. Monitor complete blood count, urinalysis, magnesium, potassium, and hepatic function. Ask the patient to report hearing loss, tinnitus, or dizziness.
• Give analgesics and antiemetics, as ordered.
• Provide psychological support to help the patient cope with long-term hospitalization.

- Advise patients to avoid pigeons. Support programs for pigeon control.

Complications
- Optic atrophy
- Ataxia
- Hydrocephalus
- Deafness
- Paralysis
- Personality changes
- Chronic brain syndrome

Cushing's syndrome

Description
Cushing's syndrome is a cluster of clinical abnormalities caused by excessive levels of adrenocortical hormones (particularly cortisol) or related corticosteroids and, to a lesser extent, androgens and aldosterone. Its unmistakable signs include rapidly developing adiposity of the face (moon face), neck, and trunk, and purple striae on the skin. Cushing's syndrome is most common in females. Prognosis depends on the underlying cause; it is poor in untreated persons and in those with untreatable ectopic adrenocorticotropic hormone- (ACTH-) producing carcinoma or metastatic adrenal carcinoma.

Causes
- Pituitary hypersecretion (Cushing's disease)
- ACTH-producing tumor in another organ (particularly bronchogenic or pancreatic carcinoma)
- Administration of synthetic glucocorticoids or ACTH
- Adrenal tumor, which is usually benign in adults (less common cause)
- Adrenal carcinoma (most common cause in infants)

Signs and symptoms
Like other endocrine disorders, Cushing's syndrome induces changes in multiple body systems, depending on the adrenocortical hormone involved.

Clinical effects may include the following signs and symptoms:
- Musculoskeletal system: muscle weakness, skeletal growth retardation in children
- Skin: purplish striae; fat pads above the clavicles, over the upper back (buffalo hump), on the face (moon face), and throughout the trunk, with slender arms and legs; little or no scar formation; poor wound healing; acne and hirsutism in women
- Central nervous system (CNS): irritability and emotional lability, ranging from euphoric behavior to depression or psychosis; insomnia
- Cardiovascular system: hypertension; bleeding, petechiae, and ecchymosis related to capillary weakness
- Immune system: increased susceptibility to infection, decreased resistance
- Renal and urinary systems: sodium and secondary fluid retention, ureteral colic
- Reproductive system: increased androgen production, causing gynecomastia in males and clitoral hypertrophy, mild virilism, and amenorrhea or oligomenorrhea in females

Diagnostic tests
- A low-dose dexamethasone suppression test confirms the diagnosis.
- A high-dose dexamethasone suppression test can determine if Cushing's syndrome results from pituitary dysfunction (Cushing's disease).
- Plasma steroid levels are consistently elevated, not reflecting a normal diurnal variation.
- 24-hour urine steroid levels show elevated free cortisol levels.
- A stimulation test with administration of metyrapone shows an excess secretion of plasma ACTH in Cushing's disease as measured by levels of urinary compound S or 17-hydroxycorticosteroids. With an adrenal or nonendocrine ACTH-secreting tumor, steroid levels remain stable or fall.
- Ultrasound, computed tomography (CT) scan, or angiography localize ad-

renal tumors.
• CT scan of the head identifies pituitary tumors.

Treatment

Management to restore hormone balance and reverse Cushing's syndrome may necessitate radiation or drug therapy or surgery. For example, pituitary-dependent Cushing's syndrome with adrenal hyperplasia and severe cushingoid symptoms—such as psychosis, poorly controlled steroid diabetes, osteoporosis, and severe pathologic fractures—may require bilateral adrenalectomy, hypophysectomy, or pituitary irradiation. Nonendocrine ACTH-producing tumors require excision of the tumor, followed by drug therapy (mitotane, metyrapone, or aminoglutethimide) to decrease cortisol levels if symptoms persist.

Aminoglutethimide and cyproheptadine decrease cortisol levels and have been beneficial for many cushingoid patients. Aminoglutethimide alone, or in combination with metyrapone, may also be useful in metastatic adrenal carcinoma.

Before surgery, the patient with cushingoid symptoms needs special management to control hypertension, edema, diabetes, and cardiovascular manifestations and to prevent infection. Glucocorticoid administration on the morning of surgery can help prevent acute adrenal insufficiency during surgery.

Cortisol therapy is essential during and after surgery, to help the patient tolerate the physiologic stress imposed by removal of the pituitary or adrenals. If normal cortisol production resumes, steroid therapy may be gradually tapered and eventually discontinued. However, bilateral adrenalectomy or total hypophysectomy mandates lifelong steroid replacement therapy to correct hormonal deficiencies. Patients with pituitary-dependent Cushing's disease may develop Nelson's syndrome (pituitary chromophobe adenoma) after bilateral adrenalectomy.

Clinical implications

Patients with Cushing's syndrome require painstaking assessment and vigorous supportive care.
• Frequently monitor vital signs, especially blood pressure. Carefully observe the hypertensive patient who also has cardiac disease.
• Check laboratory reports for hypernatremia, hypokalemia, hyperglycemia, and glycosuria.
• Because the cushingoid patient is likely to retain sodium and water, check for edema, and monitor daily weight and intake and output carefully. To minimize weight gain, edema, and hypertension, ask the dietitian to provide a diet that is high in protein and potassium but low in calories, carbohydrates, and sodium.
• Watch for infection—a particular problem in Cushing's syndrome.
• If the patient has osteoporosis and is bedridden, carefully perform passive range-of-motion exercises.
• Remember, Cushing's syndrome produces emotional lability. Record incidents that upset the patient, and try to prevent such situations, if possible. Help him get the physical and mental rest he needs—by sedation, if necessary. Offer support to the emotionally labile patient throughout the difficult testing period.
• After bilateral adrenalectomy and pituitary surgery, give meticulous postoperative care.
• Report wound drainage or temperature elevation immediately. Use strict aseptic technique in changing the patient's dressings.
• Administer analgesics and replacement steroids, as ordered.
• Monitor urine output, and check vital signs carefully, watching for signs of shock (decreased blood pressure, increased pulse rate, pallor, and cold, clammy skin). To counteract shock, give vasopressors and increase the rate of I.V. fluids, as ordered. Because mitotane, aminoglutethimide, and me-

tyrapone decrease mental alertness and produce physical weakness, assess neurologic and behavioral status, and warn the patient of CNS adverse effects. Also watch for severe nausea, vomiting, and diarrhea.

• Check laboratory reports for hypoglycemia from removal of the source of cortisol, a hormone that maintains blood glucose levels.

• Check for abdominal distention and return of bowel sounds following adrenalectomy.

• Check regularly for signs of adrenal hypofunction—orthostatic hypotension, apathy, weakness, fatigue—that indicate inadequate steroid replacement.

• In the patient undergoing pituitary surgery, check for and immediately report signs of increased intracranial pressure (confusion, agitation, changes in level of consciousness, nausea, and vomiting). Watch for hypopituitarism.

• Provide comprehensive teaching to help the patient cope with lifelong treatment.

• Advise the patient to take replacement steroids with antacids or meals, to minimize gastric irritation. (Usually, it is helpful to take two thirds of the dosage in the morning and the remaining third in the early afternoon to mimic diurnal adrenal secretion.)

• Tell the patient to carry a medical identification card and to report immediately any physiologically stressful situations, such as infections, which necessitate increased dosage.

• Instruct the patient to watch closely for signs of inadequate steroid dosage (fatigue, weakness, dizziness) and overdosage (severe edema, weight gain). Emphatically warn against discontinuing steroid dosage, because that may produce a fatal adrenal crisis.

Complications
• Steroid diabetes
• Pathologic fractures
• Osteoporosis
• Peptic ulcer

Cystic fibrosis
(Mycoviscidosis)

Description
Cystic fibrosis, a chronic disease, is a generalized dysfunction of the exocrine glands, affecting multiple organ systems with varying severity. The underlying biochemical defect probably reflects an alteration in a protein or enzyme. In fact, cystic fibrosis accounts for almost all cases of pancreatic enzyme deficiency in children. It is the most common fatal genetic disease of white children.

The immediate causes of symptoms in cystic fibrosis are increased viscosity of bronchial, pancreatic, and other mucous gland secretions and consequent obstruction of glandular ducts. About 50% of affected children die by age 16. Of the rest, some survive to age 30.

Cause
Genetic (transmitted as an autosomal recessive trait)

Signs and symptoms
The clinical effects of cystic fibrosis may become apparent soon after birth or may take years to develop.
Sweat gland dysfunction
—This is the most consistent abnormality. Muscular weakness, twitching, and other symptoms are associated with hyponatremia and hypochloremia.
Respiratory dysfunction
—Wheezing
—Dry, nonproductive paroxysmal cough
—Dyspnea
—Tachypnea
—Barrel chest
—Cyanosis
—Clubbing of the fingers and toes
GI dysfunction
—Abdominal distention
—Vomiting
—Malabsorption of fat and protein.

Stools are characteristically frequent, bulky, foul-smelling, and pale. Other abnormalities include poor weight gain, poor growth, ravenous appetite, distended abdomen, thin extremities, and sallow skin with poor turgor.

Diagnostic tests
- Sweat test shows elevated levels of sodium and chloride and can confirm the diagnosis.
- Examination of duodenal contents for pancreatic enzymes and stools for trypsin can confirm pancreatic insufficiency. Trypsin is absent in more than 80% of children with cystic fibrosis.
- Chest X-rays, pulmonary function tests, and arterial blood gas determinations assess the patient's pulmonary status.
- Sputum culture can detect concurrent infectious diseases.

Treatment and clinical implications
Since cystic fibrosis has no cure, the aim of treatment is to help the child lead a life as normal as possible. The child's family needs instruction about the disease and its complications; referral for genetic counseling will also be helpful. The emphasis of treatment depends on the organ systems involved.
- To combat sweat electrolyte losses, treatment includes generous salting of foods and, during hot weather, administration of salt supplements.
- To offset pancreatic enzyme deficiencies, treatment includes oral pancreatic enzymes with meals and snacks. The child's diet should be low in fat but high in protein and calories, and should include supplements of water-miscible, fat-soluble vitamins (A, D, E, and K).
- Pulmonary dysfunction management includes physical therapy, postural drainage, and breathing exercises several times daily, to aid removal of secretions from lungs. Patients with cystic fibrosis should not receive antihistamines, because these drugs have a drying effect on mucous membranes, making expectoration of mucus difficult or impossible. Aerosol therapy includes intermittent nebulizer treatments before postural drainage, to loosen secretions.

Treatment of pulmonary infection requires the following measures:
- Loosening and removal of mucopurulent secretions, using an intermittent nebulizer and postural drainage to relieve obstruction
- Aggressive use of broad-spectrum antimicrobials (usually with acute pulmonary infections, because prophylactic use produces resistant bacterial strains)
- Oxygen therapy as needed

Hot, dry air increases vulnerability to respiratory infections, so cystic fibrosis patients benefit from air conditioners and humidifiers.

Throughout this illness, follow these guidelines:
- Thoroughly explain all treatment measures and teach the patient and his family about his disease.
- Provide much-needed emotional support. Be flexible with care and visiting hours during hospitalization to allow continuation of schooling and friendships.
- For further information and support, refer the patient and his family to the Cystic Fibrosis Foundation.

Complications
- Electrolyte depletion can eventually induce fatal shock dysrhythmias, especially in hot weather, when sweating is profuse.
- Deficiencies of fat-soluble vitamins (A, D, E, and K) lead to clotting problems, retarded bone growth, and delayed sexual development. Males may experience azoospermia; females may experience secondary amenorrhea.
- Respiratory involvement causes recurring bronchitis and pneumonia. (Pneumonia, emphysema, or atelectasis usually causes death.)
- Rectal prolapse occurs secondary to malnutrition and wasting of perirectal

supporting tissues.
- Pancreatic insufficiency results in insufficient insulin production, abnormal glucose tolerance, and glycosuria.
- Biliary obstruction and fibrosis may prolong neonatal jaundice.
- In some patients, cirrhosis and portal hypertension may lead to esophageal varices, episodes of hematemesis, and occasionally hepatomegaly.

Cystinuria

Description
Cystinuria is an inborn error of amino acid transport in the kidneys and intestine that allows excessive urinary excretion of cystine and other dibasic amino acids and results in recurrent cystine renal calculi. It is the most common defect of amino acid transport. With proper treatment, prognosis is good.

Cause
Inherited as an autosomal recessive defect

Signs and symptoms
The clinical effects of cystinuria result from cystine or mixed cystine calculi.
- Flank pain
- Nausea
- Vomiting
- Abdominal distention
- Hematuria
- Costovertebral angle tenderness or tenderness over the kidneys

Diagnostic tests
The following tests confirm the diagnosis:
- Chemical analysis of calculi shows cystine crystals with a variable amount of calcium. Pure cystine calculi are radiolucent on X-ray, but most contain some calcium. These calculi are light yellow or brownish-yellow and granular; they may be large.
- Blood studies may show elevated white blood cell count, especially with

a urinary tract infection, and elevated clearance of cystine, lysine, arginine, and ornithine.
- Urinalysis with amino acid chromatography indicates aminoaciduria, consisting of cystine, lysine, arginine, and ornithine. Urine pH is usually less than 5.0.
- Microscopic examination of urine shows hexagonal, flat cystine crystals. When glacial acetic acid is added to chilled urine, cystine crystals resemble benzene rings.
- Cyanide-nitroprusside test yields positive results. In cystinuria, a urine specimen made alkaline by adding ammonia turns magenta when nitroprusside is added to it.
- Excretory urography determines renal function.
- Kidney-ureter-bladder X-rays determine size and location of calculi.

Treatment
No effective treatment exists to decrease cystine excretion. Increasing fluid intake to maintain a minimum 24-hour urine volume of 3,000 ml and to reduce urine cystine concentration is the primary means of dissolving excess cystine and preventing cystine calculi. Sodium bicarbonate and an alkaline-ash diet (high in vegetables and fruit, low in protein) alkalinize urine, increasing cystine solubility. However, this therapy may provide a favorable environment for formation of calcium phosphate calculi. Penicillamine can also increase cystine solubility but should be used with caution because of its toxic adverse effects and the high incidence of allergic reaction. Treatment may also include surgical removal of renal calculi, when necessary, and appropriate measures to prevent and treat urinary tract infections.

Clinical implications
- Emphasize the need to maintain increased, evenly spaced fluid intake, even through the night.
- Teach the patient how to recognize signs of renal calculi and urinary tract

infection, and tell him to report any symptoms immediately.

• Teach the patient to check urine pH and record the results.

• Carefully monitor sodium bicarbonate administration, because metabolic alkalosis may develop. Arterial bicarbonate level can be estimated by subtracting 2 from the serum CO_2 level.

Complications
• Urinary tract infection
• Ureteral obstruction with hydronephrosis

Cytomegalovirus infection
(Generalized salivary gland disease, cytomegalic inclusion disease [CID])

Description
Cytomegalovirus (CMV) infection occurs worldwide. About four out of five people over age 35 have been infected with cytomegalovirus, usually during childhood or early adulthood. In most of these people, the disease is so mild that it is overlooked. However, CMV infection during pregnancy can be hazardous to the fetus, possibly leading to stillbirth, brain damage, and other birth defects, or to severe neonatal illness.

Cause
Cytomegalovirus, a virus belonging to the herpes family

Mode of transmission
Transmission occurs through human contact with infected secretions, including sexual contact and travel across the placenta of an infected pregnant woman. (CMV has been found in the saliva, urine, semen, breast milk, feces, blood, and vaginal and cervical secretions of infected persons.)

Risk factors
• Immunodeficient patients, especially those who have received trans-

planted organs, run a 90% chance of contracting CMV infection.

• Recipients of blood transfusions from donors with positive CMV antibodies are at some risk.

Signs and symptoms
• Most adults exhibit mild, nonspecific clinical signs and symptoms, or none at all.

• Some adults develop mononucleosis with 3 or more weeks of irregular high fever.

• Immunodeficient patients and those receiving immunosuppressive therapy may develop symptoms of pneumonia (such as fever, cough, and dyspnea) or symptoms of other secondary infections.

Treatment
Treatment aims to relieve symptoms and prevent complications. Most important, parents of children with severe congenital CMV infection need emotional support and counseling to help them accept and cope with the possibility of brain damage or death.

Clinical implications
To help prevent CMV infection, follow these guidelines:

• Warn immunodeficient patients and pregnant women to avoid any individuals with confirmed or suspected CMV infection. (Maternal CMV infection can cause fetal abnormalities such as hydrocephaly, microphthalmia, seizures, encephalitis, hepatosplenomegaly, hematologic changes, microcephaly, and blindness.)

• Urge patients with CMV infection to wash their hands thoroughly to prevent spreading it. It is especially important to stress this with young children, who are usually unconcerned with personal hygiene.

• Be careful when handling urine and saliva or articles contaminated with these or other body secretions. Dispose of such articles properly. Mark contaminated linens for special handling.

Dacryocystitis

Description

Dacryocystitis is a common infection of the lacrimal sac. In adults, it results from an obstruction (dacryostenosis) of the nasolacrimal duct (most often in women over age 40) or from trauma; in infants, it results from congenital atresia of the nasolacrimal duct. Dacryocystitis can be acute or chronic and is usually unilateral.

Causes

• The most common infecting organism in acute dacryocystitis is *Staphylococcus aureus* or, occasionally, beta-hemolytic streptococcus.

• In chronic dacryocystitis, *Streptococcus pneumoniae* and, sometimes, a fungus—such as *Candida albicans*—are the causative organisms.

Signs and symptoms

The hallmark symptom, which occurs in both forms, is constant tearing.

Acute form
—Inflammation and tenderness over the nasolacrimal sac
—Possible purulent discharge with pressure over the nasolacrimal sac

Chronic form
—Possible mucoid discharge with pressure over the tear sac

Diagnostic tests

• Culture of the discharged material demonstrates the causative organism.

• White blood cell count may be elevated in the acute form.

• X-ray after injection of radiopaque medium (dacryocystography) locates the atresia.

Treatment

Treatment of acute dacryocystitis consists of application of warm compresses, and topical and systemic antibiotic therapy. Chronic dacryocystitis may eventually require dacryocystorhinostomy.

Therapy for nasolacrimal duct obstruction in an infant consists of careful massage of the area over the lacrimal sac four times a day for 2 to 3 months. If this fails to open the duct, dilatation of the punctum and probing of the duct are necessary. Postoperative management requires a pressure patch over the area of the eye.

Clinical implications

• Stress the need for precise compliance with prescribed antibiotic therapy.

• Tell the adult patient what to expect after surgery. He must lie on the operative side, with his arm behind him and his head tilted forward on a pillow, to facilitate drainage of blood. This position keeps the sinuses on the opposite side free of secretions and aids breathing.

• Monitor blood loss by counting dressings used to collect the blood.

• Apply ice compresses postoperatively. After the patch is removed (24 to 48 hours after surgery), place a small adhesive bandage over the suture line to protect it from damage.

Decompression sickness
("The bends," caisson disease)

Description

Decompression sickness is a painful and sometimes fatal condition that results from abrupt change in air or water pressure that causes nitrogen to spill out of tissues faster than it can be diffused through respiration. It causes gas bubbles to form in blood and body tissues, which produce characteristic symptoms. Usually, victims are scuba divers who ascend too quickly from water deeper than 33' and pilots and passengers of unpressurized aircraft who ascend too quickly to high altitudes.

Causes

An abrupt change from an environment of higher pressure to one of lower pressure

Signs and symptoms

Usually, symptoms appear during or within 30 minutes of rapid decompression, although they may be delayed up to 24 hours.

• "The bends." This is deep and usually constant joint and muscle pain so severe that it may be incapacitating.

• Transitory neurologic disturbances. These include difficult urination (from bladder paralysis), hemiplegia, deafness, visual disturbances, dizziness, aphasia, paresthesia and hyperesthesia of the legs, unsteady gait, and possibly coma.

• Respiratory distress. Known as "the chokes," this includes chest pain, retrosternal burning, and a cough that may become paroxysmal and uncontrollable.

Such symptoms may persist for days and result in dyspnea, cyanosis, fainting, and occasionally shock. Other symptoms include decreased temperature, pallor, itching, burning, mottled skin, fatigue, and possible tachypnea.

Treatment and clinical implications

Treatment consists of supportive measures, with recompression and oxygen administration, followed by gradual decompression. Recompression takes place in a hyperbaric chamber (not available in all hospitals), in which air pressure is increased to 2.8 absolute atmospheric pressure over 1 to 2 minutes. This rapid rise in pressure reduces the size of the circulating nitrogen bubbles, and relieves pain and other symptoms. During recompression, intermittent oxygen administration, with periodic maximal exhalations, promotes gas bubble diffusion. Once symptoms subside and diffusion is complete, a slow air pressure decrease in the chamber allows for gradual, safe decompression.

Supportive measures include fluid replacement in hypovolemic shock and sometimes corticosteroids to reduce the risk of spinal edema. Narcotics are contraindicated, because they further depress impaired respiration.

• To avoid oxygen toxicity during recompression, tell the patient to alternate breathing oxygen for 5 minutes with breathing air for 5 minutes.

• If the patient with bladder paralysis needs catheterization, monitor intake and output accurately.

• To prevent decompression sickness, advise divers and fliers to follow the U.S. Navy's ascent guidelines.

Decubitus ulcers
(Pressure sores, bedsores)

Description

Decubitus ulcers are localized areas of cellular necrosis that occur most frequently in the skin and subcutaneous tissue over bony prominences. These ulcers may be superficial (caused by local skin irritation with subsequent surface maceration) or

Special Aids for Preventing and Treating Decubitus Ulcers

Pressure relief aids

• *Gel flotation pads* disperse pressure over a greater skin surface area; convenient and adaptable for home and wheelchair use.

• *Water mattress* distributes body weight equally but is heavy and awkward; "mini" water beds (partially filled rubber gloves or plastic bags) help in small areas, such as heels.

• *Alternating pressure mattress* contains tubelike sections, running lengthwise, that deflate and reinflate, changing areas of pressure. Use mattress with a single untucked sheet, because layers of linen decrease its effectiveness.

• *Eggcrate mattress* minimizes area of skin pressure with its alternating areas of depression and elevation: soft, elevated foam areas cushion skin; depressed areas relieve pressure. This mattress should be used with a single, loosely tucked sheet and is adaptable for home and wheelchair use. If the patient is incontinent, cover mattress with the provided plastic sleeve.

• *Spanco mattress* has polyester fibers with silicon tubes to decrease pressure without limiting the patient's position. It has no weight limitation.

• *Sheepskin* is soft, dry, absorbent, and easy to clean. It should be in direct contact with the patient's skin. It is available in sizes to fit elbows and heels and is adaptable to home use.

• *Clinitron bed* supports the patient at a subcapillary pressure point and provides a warm, relaxing therapeutic airflow. The bed is filled with beads that move when the air flows. It eliminates friction and maceration.

• *Turning bed* (such as Stryker or Foster frame, CircOlectric bed, and Roto-Rest) is ineffective without adjuvant therapy. It also limits free movement and is expensive.

Topical agents

• Gentle soap
• Dakin's solution
• Zinc oxide cream
• Absorbable gelatin sponge
• Granulated sugar (mechanical irritant to enhance granulation)
• Dextranomer (inert, absorbing beads)
• Karaya gum patches
• Topical antibiotics (*only* when infection is confirmed by culture and sensitivity tests)
• Silver sulfadiazine cream (antimicrobial agent)
• Povidone-iodine packs (remain in place until dry)
• Water vapor–permeable dressings

Avoid these skin-damaging agents

• Harsh alkali soaps
• Alcohol-based products (can cause vasoconstriction)
• Tincture of benzoin (may cause painful erosions)
• Hexachlorophene (may irritate the central nervous system)
• Petrolatum gauze

deep (originating in underlying tissue). Deep lesions frequently go undetected until they penetrate the skin. By then, they have usually caused subcutaneous damage.

Causes

Pressure, particularly over bony prominences, interrupts normal circulatory function and causes most decubitus ulcers.

Risk factors

- Altered mobility
- Inadequate nutrition
- Breakdown in skin or subcutaneous tissue as a result of edema, incontinence, fever, pathologic conditions, or obesity

Signs and symptoms

Stage I
—Redness of the skin
Stage II (superficial damage)
—Blistered, peeling, or cracked skin
Stage III (a full thickness of the skin is lost)
—Broken skin
—Possible subcutaneous tissue damage
—Possible serous or bloody drainage
Stage IV (full thickness of the skin and subcutaneous tissues are destroyed)
—Deep craterlike ulcer
—Fascia tissue exposure
—Connective tissue, bone, or muscle are exposed and may be damaged.

Diagnostic tests

Wound culture and sensitivity testing of the exudate may identify infecting organisms and antibiotics that may be needed.

Treatment and clinical implications

Successful treatment must relieve pressure on the affected area, keep the area clean and dry, and promote healing.

- During each shift, check the skin of bedridden patients for possible changes in color, turgor, temperature, and sensation. Examine an existing ulcer for any change in size or degree of damage. When using pressure relief aids or topical agents, explain their function to the patient.
- Prevent pressure sores by repositioning the bedridden patient at least every 2 hours around the clock. Minimize the effects of a shearing force by using a footboard and by not raising the head of the bed to an angle that exceeds 60 degrees. Keep the patient's knees slightly flexed for short periods. Perform passive range-of-motion exercises, or encourage the patient to do active exercises, if possible.
- To prevent pressure sores in immobilized patients, use pressure relief aids on their beds.
- Give meticulous skin care. Keep the skin clean and dry without the use of harsh soaps. Gently massaging the skin around—not on—the affected area promotes healing. Rub moisturizing lotions into the skin thoroughly to prevent maceration of the skin surface. Frequently change the bed linens of patients who are diaphoretic or incontinent.
- Clean open lesions with a 3% solution of hydrogen peroxide or normal saline solution. Dressings, if needed, should be porous and lightly taped to healthy skin. Debridement of necrotic tissue may be necessary to allow healing. One method is to apply open wet dressings and allow them to dry on the ulcer. Removal of the dressings mechanically debrides exudate and necrotic tissue. Other methods include surgical debridement with a fine scalpel blade and chemical debridement using proteolytic enzyme agents.
- Encourage adequate intake of food and fluids to maintain body weight and promote healing. Consult with the dietary department to provide a diet that promotes tissue granulation. Encourage the debilitated patient to eat frequent, small meals that include protein- and calorie-rich supplements. Assist weakened patients with their meals.

Complications

Infection. (See *Special Aids for Preventing and Treating Decubitus Ulcers*, p. 213.)

Depression

Description

Major depression, a recurring syndrome of persistent sad, dysphoric mood with accompanying symptoms, may be a primary disorder, a response to systemic disease, or a drug reaction. Diagnosis is made primarily on observation and patient history. Depression is difficult to treat, especially in children, adolescents, elderly persons, or those with a history of chronic disease, but the effectiveness of treatment has been improved.

Causes

The multiple causes of depression are controversial and not completely understood. Current research suggests

---

Other Affective Disorders

DYSTHMYIC DISORDER (DEPRESSIVE NEUROSIS)

This common affliction is marked by feelings of depression that have persisted at least 2 years in adults (and at least 1 year in children and adolescents). It causes persistent depressive symptoms that are not sufficiently severe or prolonged to meet the criteria for major depression. No psychotic features are present.

Symptoms may be relatively continuous or separated by intervening periods of normal mood that last a few days to a few weeks but not longer than a few months. At least three of the following symptoms are present:

- Insomnia or hypersomnia
- Low energy level or chronic tiredness
- Feelings of inadequacy, loss of self-esteem, or self-deprecation
- Decreased effectiveness or productivity at home, work, or school
- Decreased attention, concentration, or ability to think clearly
- Social withdrawal
- Loss of interest in or enjoyment of pleasurable activities
- Irritability or excessive anger (in children, hostility to parents)
- Inability to respond with apparent pleasure to praise or rewards
- Less active or talkative than usual, or feelings of sluggishness or restlessness
- Pessimistic attitude toward the future, brooding about past events
- Tearfulness or crying, self-pity
- Recurrent thoughts of death or suicide

CYCLOTHYMIC DISORDER

This disorder describes patients who have moderate or transient symptoms of bipolar disorder, major depression, or mania. These patients have normal moods for months at a time. The essential feature of cyclothymic disorder is a chronic mood disturbance of at least 2 years' duration involving numerous periods of depression and hypomania that are not sufficiently severe or prolonged to meet the criteria for a major depressive or manic episode.

A cyclothymic disorder commonly precedes a bipolar disorder. Psychotic features, such as delusions and hallucinations, are absent.

ATYPICAL AFFECTIVE DISORDER

This disorder produces manic symptoms that are less severe and less prolonged than those required for a diagnosis of bipolar or cyclothymic disorders.

possible genetic, familial, biochemical, physical, psychological, and social causes. In many patients, the history identifies a specific personal loss or severe stress that probably interacts with an individual's predisposition to major depression.

Signs and symptoms
• According to the *DSM-III* classification, the primary feature of major depression is a relatively persistent and prominent dysphoric mood, with loss of interest in usual activities and pastimes, which may shift periodically to anger or anxiety.
• The second diagnostic requirement, according to the *DSM-III* classification, is the daily presence of at least four of the following symptoms for at least 2 weeks:
—Appetite disturbance (weight loss of at least 1 lb/week without dieting, or significant appetite or weight increase)
—Sleep disturbance (insomnia or hypersomnia)
—Energy loss, fatigue
—Psychomotor agitation or retardation (hyperactive or slowed behavior)
—Loss of interest or pleasure in activities, decreased sex drive
—Feelings of worthlessness, self-reproach, excessive guilt
—Difficulty in concentration, decision making, or thinking
—Recurrent suicidal thoughts, suicide attempts, or death wishes
Note: Acute depression involves recent onset of four or five of these behaviors and dysphoric mood. Chronic depression involves the same symptoms in milder form, present for 2 or more months. (See also *Other Affective Disorders,* p. 215.)

Diagnostic tests
The following tests support the diagnosis:
• Beck Depression Scale and other psychological tests
• Dexamethasone suppression test

• EEG, which shows evidence of sleep disturbance

Treatment
The primary treatment methods—psychotherapy, drug and somatic therapy (including electroconvulsive therapy [ECT])—along with possible adjuvant therapies aim to relieve depressive symptoms. Research confirms the effectiveness of antidepressant drug therapy, which, when combined with psychotherapy, is more effective than either method alone. Drug therapy usually includes tricyclic antidepressants (TCAs) and monoamine oxidase (MAO) inhibitors. TCAs produce fewer adverse effects and so are usually the preferred treatment. Drug treatment may include sedatives if the patient suffers insomnia. Careful monitoring is required to prevent hoarding of doses.

In severely depressed or suicidal patients who do not respond to other treatments, ECT may improve mood dramatically. However, ECT should be prescribed only after a complete evaluation, including history, physical examination, chest X-ray, and EKG. ECT may cause adverse effects—dysrhythmias, fractures, confusion, drowsiness, temporary memory loss, sluggish respirations, and occasionally permanent memory loss or learning difficulties. Consequently, before such treatment, safety, long-term risk, and the patient's rights associated with ECT should be discussed thoroughly with the patient and his family.

Clinical implications
The depressed patient needs a therapeutic relationship, with encouragement to talk and boost self-esteem.
• Encourage the patient to talk about and write down his feelings. Show him he is important by setting aside uninterrupted time each day to listen attentively and respectfully, allowing time for sluggish responses.

Suicide Prevention Guidelines

• **Assess for clues to suicide:** suicidal thoughts, threats, and messages; hoarding medication; talking about death and feelings of futility; giving away prized possessions; changing behavior, especially as depression begins to lift.

• **Provide a safe environment:** Check patient areas and correct dangerous conditions, such as exposed pipes, windows without safety glass, and access to the roof or open balconies.

• **Remove dangerous objects:** belts, razors, suspenders, light cords, glass, knives, nail files, clippers.

• **Consult with staff:** Recognize and document both verbal and nonverbal suicidal behaviors; keep the physician informed; share data with all staff; clarify the patient's specific restrictions; assess risk and plan for observation; clarify day and night staff responsibilities and frequency of consultation.

• **Observe suicidal patients:** Be alert when patients are using sharp objects (shaving), taking medication, or using the bathroom (to prevent hanging or other injury). Assign the patient to a room near nurses' station and with another patient. Observe acutely suicidal patients continuously.

• **Maintain personal contact:** Suicidal patients feel alone and without resources or hope. Encourage continuity of care and consistency of primary nurses. Building emotional ties to others is the ultimate technique for preventing suicide.

• Provide a structured routine, including noncompetitive activities, to build the patient's self-confidence and encourage interaction with others. Help him avoid isolation by urging him to join group activities and socialize.

• Reassure him that he can help ease his depression by expressing his feelings, participating in pleasurable activities, and improving grooming and hygiene.

• Ask the patient if he thinks of death or suicide. Such thoughts signal an immediate need for consultation and assessment. Failure to detect suicidal thoughts early may encourage a patient to attempt suicide.

• Record all observations of and conversations with the patient, because they are valuable for evaluating his response to treatment.

• While caring for the patient's psychological needs, do not forget his physical needs. If he is too depressed to take care of himself, help him with

personal hygiene. Encourage him to eat, or feed him if necessary. If he is constipated, add high-fiber foods to his diet, offer small, frequent feedings, and encourage physical activity and fluid intake. Offer warm milk or back rubs at bedtime to improve sleep.

• To prevent possible suicide, watch carefully for signs of suicidal ideation or intent. (See *Suicide Prevention Guidelines*.)

• If drug treatment fails, the physician may order ECT. A course of ECT usually includes two or three treatments per week for 3 to 4 weeks. Before each ECT, give the patient a sedative, and insert a nasal or oral airway. Monitor vital signs. Offer support by talking calmly or by gently touching the patient's arm. Afterward, he may be drowsy and have transient amnesia, but he should be alert, with a good memory, within 30 minutes (or at the latest, 6 to 8 hours).

Dermatitis

Description

Dermatitis, or inflammation of the skin, occurs in several forms: atopic (discussed here), contact, chronic, seborrheic, nummular, exfoliative, and stasis dermatitides. Atopic dermatitis (atopic or infantile eczema, neurodermatitis constitutionalis, Besnier's prurigo) is a chronic inflammatory response frequently associated with other atopic diseases, such as bronchial asthma, allergic rhinitis, and chronic urticaria. It usually develops in infants and toddlers between ages 1 month and 1 year, commonly in those with strong family histories of atopic

Dermatitis and Eczema

TYPE	CAUSES	SIGNS AND SYMPTOMS
Contact dermatitis	• Mild irritants: chronic exposure to detergents or solvents • Strong irritants: damage on contact with acids or alkalies • Allergens: sensitization after repeated exposure	• Mild irritants and allergens: erythema, and small vesicles that ooze, scale, and itch • Strong irritants: blisters and ulcerations • Classic allergic response: clearly defined lesions, with straight lines following points of contact • Severe allergic reaction: marked edema of affected areas
Chronic dermatitis	• Usually unknown but may result from progressive contact dermatitis • Secondary factors: trauma, infections, redistribution of normal flora, photosensitivity, and food sensitivity, which may perpetuate this condition	• Thick, lichenified, single or multiple lesions on any part of the body (in most cases, on the hands) • Inflammation and scaling • Recurrence follows long remissions.
Seborrheic dermatitis	• Unknown; stress and neurologic conditions may be predisposing factors.	• Eruptions in areas with many sebaceous glands (usually scalp, face, and trunk) and in skin folds • Itching, redness, and inflammation of affected areas; lesions may appear greasy; fissures may occur. • Indistinct, occasionally yellowish, scaly patches from excess stratum corneum (Dandruff may be a mild seborrheic dermatitis.)

disease. These children often acquire other atopic disorders as they grow older. Typically, this form of dermatitis subsides spontaneously by age 3 and stays in remission until prepuberty (ages 10 to 12), when it frequently flares up again.

Causes

The cause of atopic dermatitis is still unknown. However, several theories attempt to explain its pathogenesis. One theory suggests an underlying metabolically or biochemically induced skin disorder genetically linked to elevated serum IgE levels. Another suggests defective T-cell function.

• Exacerbating factors of atopic dermatitis include irritants, infections (commonly by *Staphylococcus au-*

DIAGNOSIS	TREATMENT AND INTERVENTION
• Patient history • Patch testing to identify allergens • Shape and distribution of lesions suggest contact dermatitis.	• Elimination of known allergens and decreased exposure to irritants; wearing protective clothing, such as gloves; and washing immediately after contact with irritants or allergens • Topical anti-inflammatory agents (including steroids), systemic steroids for edema and bullae, antihistamines, and local applications of Burow's solution (for blisters) • Sensitization to topical medications may occur. • Other nursing intervention similar to atopic dermatitis
• No characteristic pattern or course; diagnosis relies on detailed patient history and physical findings.	• Same as for contact dermatitis • Antibiotics for secondary infection • Avoidance of excessive washing and drying of hands, and of accumulation of soaps and detergents under rings • Use of emollients with topical steroids
• Patient history and physical findings, especially distribution of lesions in sebaceous gland areas, confirm seborrheic dermatitis. • Diagnosis must rule out psoriasis.	• Removal of scales with frequent washing and shampooing with selenium sulfide suspension (most effective), zinc pyrithione, or tar and salicylic acid shampoo • Application of fluorinated steroids to nonhairy areas

(continued)

Dermatitis and Eczema *(continued)*

TYPE	CAUSES	SIGNS AND SYMPTOMS
Nummular dermatitis	• Possibly precipitated by stress or by dryness, irritants, or scratching	• Round, nummular (coin-shaped) lesions, usually on arms and legs, with distinct borders of crusts and scales • Possible oozing and severe itching • Summertime remissions common, with wintertime recurrence
Localized neurodermatitis (lichen simplex chronicus, essential pruritus)	• Chronic scratching or rubbing of a primary lesion or insect bite, or other skin irritation	• Intense, sometimes continual scratching • Thick, sharp-bordered, possibly dry, scaly lesions, with raised papules • Usually affects easily reached areas, such as ankles, lower legs, anogenital area, back of neck, and ears
Exfoliative dermatitis	• Usually, preexisting skin lesions progress to exfoliative stage, such as in contact dermatitis, drug reaction, lymphoma, or leukemia.	• Generalized dermatitis, with acute loss of stratum corneum, and erythema and scaling • Sensation of tight skin • Hair loss • Possible fever, sensitivity to cold, shivering, gynecomastia, and lymphadenopathy
Stasis dermatitis	• Secondary to peripheral vascular diseases affecting legs, such as recurrent thrombophlebitis and resultant chronic venous insufficiency	• Varicosities and edema common, but obvious vascular insufficiency not always present • Usually affects the lower leg, just above internal malleolus, or sites of trauma or irritation • Early signs: dusky red deposits of hemosiderin in skin, with itching and dimpling of subcutaneous tissue. Later signs: edema, redness, and scaling of large area of legs • Fissures, crusts, and ulcers may develop.

DIAGNOSIS	TREATMENT AND INTERVENTION
• Physical findings and patient history confirm nummular dermatitis; a middle-aged or older patient may have a history of atopic dermatitis. • Diagnosis must rule out fungal infections, atopic or contact dermatitis, and psoriasis.	• Elimination of known irritants • Measures to relieve dry skin: increased humidification; limited frequency of baths and use of bland soap and bath oils; and application of emollients • Application of wet dressings in acute phase • Topical steroids (occlusive dressing or intralesional injections) for persistent lesions • Tar preparations and antihistamines to control itching • Antibiotics for secondary infection • Other nursing intervention similar to atopic dermatitis
• Physical findings confirm diagnosis.	• Lesions disappear about 2 weeks after scratching stops. • Fixed dressing or Unna's boot, to cover affected area • Steroids under occlusion or by intralesional injection • Antihistamines and open wet dressings • Emollients • Inform patient about underlying cause.
• Diagnosis requires identification of the underlying cause.	• Hospitalization, with protective isolation and hygienic measures to prevent secondary bacterial infection • Open wet dressings, with colloidal baths • Bland lotions over topical steroids • Maintenance of constant environmental temperature to prevent chilling or overheating • Careful monitoring of renal and cardiac status • Systemic antibiotics and steroids • Other intervention similar to atopic dermatitis
• Diagnosis requires positive history of venous insufficiency and physical findings, such as varicosities.	• Measures to prevent venous stasis: avoidance of prolonged sitting or standing, use of support stockings, and weight reduction in obesity • Corrective surgery for underlying cause • After ulcer develops, encourage rest periods, with legs elevated; open wet dressings; Unna's boot (zinc gelatin dressing provides continuous pressure to affected areas); antibiotics for secondary infection after wound culture.

reus), and some allergens (pollen, wool, silk, fur, ointments, detergent, and certain foods, particularly wheat, milk, and eggs).
• Flare-ups may occur in response to extremes in temperature and humidity, sweating, and stress.

Signs and symptoms
An intensely pruritic, often excoriated, maculopapular rash commonly found on the face and antecubital and popliteal areas

Diagnostic tests
Laboratory tests reveal eosinophilia and elevated serum IgE levels.

Treatment and clinical implications
Effective treatment of atopic lesions consists of eliminating allergens and avoiding irritants, extreme temperature changes, and other precipitating factors. Local and systemic measures relieve itching and inflammation. Topical application of a corticosteroid cream, especially after bathing, frequently alleviates inflammation. Between steroid doses, application of petrolatum can help retain moisture. Systemic corticosteroid therapy should be used only during extreme exacerbations. Weak tar preparations and ultraviolet B light therapy are used to increase the thickness of the stratum corneum. Antibiotics are appropriate if a bacterial agent has been cultured.
• Warn that drowsiness is possible with the use of antihistamines to relieve daytime itching. If nocturnal itching interferes with sleep, suggest methods for inducing natural sleep, such as drinking a glass of warm milk, to prevent overuse of sedatives.
• Complement medical treatment by helping the patient set up an individual schedule and plan for daily skin care. Instruct the patient to limit bathing, according to the severity of the lesions. Tell him to bathe with a special nonfatty soap and tepid water but to avoid using any soap when lesions are acutely inflamed. Advise the patient to shampoo frequently and apply corticosteroid cream afterward, to keep his fingernails short to limit excoriation and secondary infections caused by scratching, and to lubricate his skin after a tub bath.
• To help clear lichenified skin, apply occlusive dressings (such as plastic film) intermittently, and secure them with nonallergenic tape.
• Inform the patient that irritants, such as detergents and wool, and emotional stress exacerbate atopic dermatitis.
• Be careful not to show any anxiety or revulsion when touching the lesions during treatment. Help the patient accept his altered body image, and encourage him to verbalize his feelings. Remember, coping with disfigurement is extremely difficult, especially for children and adolescents.
• Arrange for counseling, if necessary, to help the patient deal with the disease more effectively.

Dermatophytosis
(Ringworm)

Description
Dermatophytosis may affect the scalp (tinea capitis), body (tinea corporis), nails (tinea unguium), feet (tinea pedis), groin (tinea cruris), and bearded skin (tinea barbae). With effective treatment, the cure rate is very high, but about 20% of infected persons develop chronic conditions.

Causes
Tinea infections (except for tinea versicolor) result from dematophytes (fungi) of the genera *Trichophyton, Microsporum,* and *Epidermophyton.*

Mode of transmission
• Directly, through contact with infected lesions
• Indirectly, through contact with contaminated articles such as shoes, towels, or shower stalls

Signs and symptoms
Lesions vary in appearance and duration.
• Tinea capitis is characterized by small, spreading papules on the scalp, causing patchy hair loss with scaling. Papules may progress to inflamed, pus-filled lesions (kerions).
• Tinea corporis produces flat lesions on the skin at any site except the scalp, bearded skin, or feet. Lesions may be dry and scaly or moist and crusty. As they enlarge, their centers heal, causing the classic ring-shaped appearance.
• Tinea unguium (onychomycosis) typically starts at the tip of one or more toenails (fingernail infection is less common) and produces gradual thickening, discoloration, and crumbling of the nail, with accumulation of subungual debris. Eventually, the nail may be destroyed completely.
• Tinea pedis (athlete's foot) causes scaling and blisters between the toes. Severe infection may result in inflammation, with severe itching and pain on walking. A dry, squamous inflammation may affect the entire sole.
• Tinea cruris (jock itch) produces red, raised, sharply defined, itchy lesions in the groin that may extend to buttocks, inner thighs, and external genitalia.

Diagnostic tests
• Microscopic examination of lesion scrapings prepared in potassium hydroxide solution usually confirms tinea infection.
• Wood's light examination confirms diagnosis of some types of tinea capitis.
• Culture identifies the infecting organism.

Treatment
Tinea infections usually respond to treatment with griseofulvin P.O., which is especially effective in tinea infections of the skin, hair, and nails; tinea pedis requires concomitant use of a topical agent. (Griseofulvin is contraindicated in the patient with porphyria; it may also necessitate an increase in dosage during anticoagulant [warfarin] therapy.) Also effective is topical application of antifungals such as clotrimazole, miconazole, haloprogin, or tolnaftate for localized infections. Supportive measures include open wet dressings, removal of scabs and scales, and application of keratolytics such as salicylic acid to soften and remove hyperkeratotic lesions of the heels or soles.

Clinical implications
Management of tinea infections requires application of topical agents, observation for sensitivity reactions, observation for secondary bacterial infections, and patient teaching.

Diabetes insipidus
(Pituitary diabetes insipidus)

Description
Diabetes insipidus results from a deficiency of circulating vasopressin (also called antidiuretic hormone [ADH]). This uncommon condition occurs equally among both sexes, usually between ages 10 and 20. In uncomplicated diabetes insipidus, prognosis is good. With adequate water replacement, patients usually lead normal lives. In cases complicated by an underlying disorder, such as breast cancer, prognosis varies.

Causes
Primary form
—Familial or idiopathic
Secondary form
—Intracranial neoplastic or metastatic lesions

—Hypophysectomy or other neuro-surgery

—Head trauma, which damages the neurohypophyseal structures

—Infection

—Granulomatous disease

—Vascular lesions

Signs and symptoms

• Extreme polyuria (usually 4 to 16 liters/day of dilute urine, but sometimes as much as 30 liters/day)

• Extreme thirst

• Slight to moderate nocturia

• Fatigue (in severe cases)

• Dehydration (characterized by poor tissue turgor, dry mucous membranes, constipation, muscle weakness, dizziness, and hypotension)

Diagnostic tests

• Urinalysis reveals almost colorless urine of low osmolality (50 to 200 mOsm/kg, less than that of plasma) and low specific gravity (less than 1.005).

• A water restriction test confirms the diagnosis by demonstrating renal inability to concentrate urine (evidence of vasopressin deficiency).

• Subcutaneous injection of 5 units of aqueous vasopressin produces decreased urine output with increased specific gravity.

Treatment

Until the cause of diabetes insipidus can be identified and eliminated, administration of various forms of vasopressin or of a vasopressin stimulant can control fluid balance and prevent dehydration.

Clinical implications

• Record fluid intake and output carefully. Maintain fluid intake to prevent severe dehydration. Watch for signs of hypovolemic shock, and monitor blood pressure and heart and respiratory rates regularly, especially during the water deprivation test. Check weight daily. If the patient is dizzy or has muscle weakness, keep the side rails up and assist with walking.

• Monitor urine specific gravity between doses. Watch for a decrease in specific gravity, with increasing urine output, indicating the return of polyuria and necessitating administration of the next dose or a dosage increase.

• Observe the patient receiving chlorpropamide for signs of hypoglycemia. Tell the patient about possible drug adverse effects. Make sure caloric intake is adequate; keep orange juice or another carbohydrate handy to treat hypoglycemic attacks. Watch for decreasing urine output and increasing specific gravity between doses. Check laboratory values for hyponatremia and hypoglycemia.

• If constipation develops, add more bulk foods and fruit juices to the diet. If necessary, obtain an order for a mild laxative such as milk of magnesia. Provide meticulous skin and mouth care; apply petrolatum, as needed, to cracked or sore lips.

• Before discharge, teach the patient how to monitor intake and output. Instruct him to administer vasopressin I.M. or by nasal insufflation only after onset of polyuria—not before—to prevent excessive fluid retention and water intoxication. Tell him to report weight gain; it may mean dosage is too high. Recurrence of polyuria, as reflected on the intake and output sheet, indicates dosage is too low.

• Because of its viscosity, warn the patient never to administer vasopressin tannate while the suspension is cold. Show him how to warm the vial in his hands and to rotate it gently to disperse the active particles throughout the oil.

• Identify all patients with coronary artery disease; they need special periodic evaluations, because vasopressin constricts the arteries.

• Advise the patient to wear a medical identification bracelet and to carry his medication with him at all times.

Diabetes mellitus

Description
A chronic disease of insulin deficiency or resistance, diabetes mellitus is characterized by disturbances in carbohydrate, protein, and fat metabolism. A leading cause of death by disease in the United States, this syndrome contributes to about 50% of myocardial infarctions and about 75% of strokes, as well as to renal failure and peripheral vascular disease. It is also the leading cause of new blindness.

This condition occurs in two forms: insulin-dependent diabetes mellitus (IDDM, ketosis-prone, Type I, or juvenile diabetes) and the more prevalent noninsulin-dependent diabetes mellitus (NIDDM, ketosis-resistant, Type II, or maturity-onset diabetes). IDDM usually occurs before age 30 (although it may occur at any age); the patient is usually thin and requires exogenous insulin and dietary management to achieve control. Conversely, NIDDM usually occurs in obese adults after age 40 and is most frequently treated with diet and exercise (possibly in combination with hypoglycemic drugs), although treatment may include insulin therapy.

Causes
Recent studies show that certain cases of IDDM are viral in origin, but heredity strongly influences most diabetes. Precipitating factors include the following:

• Obesity, which causes resistance to endogenous insulin

• Physiologic or emotional stress, which causes prolonged elevation of stress hormone levels (cortisol, epinephrine, glucagon, and growth hormone), resulting in elevated blood glucose levels and in turn placing increased demands on the pancreas

• Pregnancy and oral contraceptives, which increase levels of estrogen and placental hormones (insulin antagonists)

• Other medications that are known insulin antagonists, including thiazide diuretics, adrenal corticosteroids, and phenytoin

Signs and symptoms
• Fatigue
• Polyuria related to hyperglycemia
• Polydipsia
• Dry mucous membranes and poor skin turgor
• Weight loss in IDDM
• Polyphagia in IDDM

Diagnostic tests
• Fasting plasma glucose above 140 mg/dl, or with normal fasting glucose, a blood glucose level above 200 mg/dl during the first 2 hours of a glucose tolerance test (GTT) confirms the diagnosis.

• Ophthalmologic examination may show diabetic retinopathy.

• Cortisone GTT may be done to elicit stress-induced diabetes.

• Other tests include blood insulin level determination, urine testing for glucose and acetone, and glycosylated hemoglobin (hemoglobin A_{1c}) determination.

Treatment
Effective treatment normalizes blood glucose level and prevents complications. In IDDM, these goals are achieved with insulin replacement that mimics normal pancreatic function. Current means of insulin replacement include mixed, split doses of regular and NPH insulin injected twice a day; premeal injections of short-acting regular insulin with intermediate NPH injections at bedtime; and continuous subcutaneous insulin infusion (insulin pump). An additional treatment, pancreas transplantation, is still experimental.

Diabetic therapy also requires a strict diet carefully planned to meet

Teaching Topics in Diabetes Mellitus

• An explanation of the pathology underlying Type I or Type II diabetes (depending on which type the patient has)
• The relationship between good diabetes management and health
• Preparation for the oral glucose tolerance test and any other scheduled diagnostic tests
• Dietary restrictions, such as exchange lists and the timing of meals and insulin injections
• Exercise program and precautions
• Medications and how to administer them properly
• Techniques for obtaining blood and urine samples
• Self-testing of glucose and ketone levels
• Sick-day precautions
• Foot and skin care
• Signs and symptoms of hyperglycemia and hypoglycemia
• Preventive measures for reducing long-term complications, such as visiting a podiatrist and ophthalmologist regularly
• Sources of additional information and support

---

nutritional needs, to control blood glucose levels, and to reach and maintain appropriate body weight. For the obese diabetic, weight reduction is a dietary goal. In IDDM, the calorie allotment may be high, depending on growth stage and activity level. To be successful, however, the diet must be followed consistently, and meals must be eaten at regular times.

Patients with NIDDM may require oral hypoglycemics. These medications stimulate endogenous insulin production and may also increase insulin sensitivity at the cellular level.

Clinical implications

• Emphasize from the start that compliance with the prescribed program is essential. Tailor your teaching to the patient's needs, abilities, and developmental stage. (See *Teaching Topics in Diabetes Mellitus*.)
• Watch for acute complications of diabetes and diabetic therapy, especially hypoglycemia (vagueness, slow cerebration, dizziness, weakness, pallor, tachycardia, diaphoresis, seizures, and coma); immediately give carbo-

hydrates in the form of fruit juice, hard candy, honey, or, if the patient is unconscious, glucagon or dextrose I.V. Also be alert for signs of ketoacidosis (acetone breath, dehydration, weak and rapid pulse, Kussmaul's respirations) and hyperosmolar coma (polyuria, thirst, neurologic abnormalities, stupor). These hyperglycemic crises require I.V. fluids, insulin, and, possibly, potassium replacement.
• Monitor diabetic control by testing urine for glucose and acetone and obtaining blood glucose levels. (Urine glucose tests should be reported in mg/dl glucose instead of plus values.) A patient with NIDDM may test once daily using the glucose oxidase method (such as Tes-Tape). A patient with IDDM may test four times a day using the 2-drop copper sulfate reduction method (such as Clinitest) and an acetone test. A patient with renal disease (in whom urine testing is unreliable) should monitor control of blood glucose using a glucose-monitoring device.
• Watch for diabetic effects on the cardiovascular system, such as cerebral vascular, coronary artery, and peripheral vascular disease. Treat all inju-

ries, cuts, and blisters (particularly on the lower extremities) meticulously. Stay alert for signs of urinary tract infection, renal failure, and Kimmelstiel-Wilson syndrome (protein and red blood cells in urine, edema). The latter results from vascular deterioration in the kidneys and is a leading cause of death in young adults with diabetes. Urge regular ophthalmologic examinations for early detection of diabetic retinopathy.

• Assess the patient for signs of diabetic neuropathy (numbness or pain in arms and legs, footdrop, neurogenic bladder). Emphasize the need for personal safety, because decreased sensation can mask injuries. Minimize complications by maintaining strict blood glucose control.

• To prevent diabetes, teach persons at high risk to avoid precipitating factors; for example, females with family histories of diabetes should have thorough medical counseling about the use of contraceptives and the risks of pregnancy. Advise genetic counseling for young adults with diabetes who are planning families.

• Further information about diabetes and patient-teaching aids may be obtained from the Juvenile Diabetes Foundation, the American Diabetes Association, the American Association of Diabetes Educators, and the manufacturers of products used by diabetic patients.

Complications

• In ketoacidosis or hyperglycemic hyperosmolar nonketotic coma, dehydration may cause hypovolemia and shock.

• Long-term effects of diabetes may include retinopathy, nephropathy, atherosclerosis, and peripheral and autonomic neuropathy. Peripheral neuropathy usually affects the feet and may cause numbness.

DiGeorge's syndrome
(Congenital thymic hypoplasia or aplasia)

Description

DiGeorge's syndrome is a congenital disorder known typically by the partial or total absence of cell-mediated immunity that results from a deficiency of T lymphocytes. The thymus may be absent or underdeveloped and abnormally located, and the parathyroids may be absent. The disorder characteristically produces life-threatening hypocalcemia that may be associated with cardiovascular and facial anomalies. Patients rarely live beyond age 2 without fetal thymic transplant; however, prognosis improves when fetal thymic transplant, correction of hypocalcemia, and repair of cardiac anomalies are possible.

Causes

DiGeorge's syndrome is probably caused by abnormal fetal development of the third and fourth pharyngeal pouches (12th week of gestation) that interferes with the formation of the thymus. This syndrome has been associated with maternal alcoholism and resultant fetal alcohol syndrome.

Signs and symptoms

• Facial anomalies such as low-set ears, notched ear pinnae, fish-shaped mouth, undersized jaw, and abnormally wide-set eyes with antimongoloid eyelid formation

• Cardiovascular abnormalities such as cyanosis

• Hypocalcemia with tetany

• Indications of infection such as fever and coughing

Diagnostic tests

• Sheep cell test shows decreased or absent T lymphocytes.

• Chest X-ray reveals an absent thymus.

- Serum calcium level is decreased.
- Serum phosphorus level is elevated.
- Parathyroid studies show absence of parathyroid hormone.

Treatment and clinical implications

Life-threatening hypocalcemia must be treated immediately. It is unusually resistant and requires aggressive treatment—for example, with a rapid I.V. infusion of 10% solution of calcium gluconate. During infusion, monitor heart rate and watch carefully to avoid infiltration. Remember that calcium supplements must be given with vitamin D (sometimes also with parathyroid hormone) to ensure effective calcium utilization. After hypocalcemia is under control, fetal thymic transplant may restore normal cell-mediated immunity. Cardiac anomalies require surgical repair when possible.

A patient with DiGeorge's syndrome also needs a low-phosphorus diet and careful preventive measures for infection. Teach the parents of such an infant to watch for signs of infection and have it treated immediately, to keep the infant away from crowds or any other potential sources of infection, and to provide good hygiene and adequate nutrition and hydration.

Diphtheria

Description

Diphtheria is an acute, highly contagious toxin-mediated infection that usually infects the respiratory tract, primarily involving the tonsils, nasopharynx, and larynx. Currently, both cutaneous and wound diphtheria are seen more frequently in the United States and are often caused by nontoxigenic strains. The GI and urinary tracts, conjunctivae, and ears are rarely involved. Due to effective immunization, diphtheria is rare in many parts of the world, including the United States.

Cause

Corynebacterium diphtheriae, a gram-positive rod

Mode of transmission

Infection is transmitted by intimate contact or by airborne respiratory droplets from apparently healthy carriers or convalescing patients. Many more people carry this disease than contract active infection.

Signs and symptoms

The following are characteristic indications:
- Thick, patchy, grayish green membrane over the mucous membranes of the pharynx, larynx, tonsils, soft palate, and nose. Attempts to remove the membrane usually cause bleeding, which is highly characteristic of diphtheria.
- Fever
- Sore throat
- Rasping cough
- Hoarseness
- In the cutaneous form, skin lesions that resemble impetigo

Diagnostic tests

Throat culture or culture of other suspect lesions shows *C. diphtheriae*. This and examination showing the characteristic membrane confirm the diagnosis.

Treatment

Treatment must begin based on clinical findings without waiting for confirmation by culture. Standard treatment includes diphtheria antitoxin administered I.M. or I.V.; antibiotics such as penicillin or erythromycin, to eliminate the organisms from the upper respiratory tract and other sites, and to terminate the carrier state; and measures to prevent complications.

Clinical implications

Diphtheria requires comprehensive supportive care with psychological support.

• To prevent the spread of this disease, stress the need for strict isolation. Teach proper disposal of nasopharyngeal secretions. Maintain infection precautions until after two consecutive negative nasopharyngeal cultures—at least 1 week after drug therapy stops.

• Treatment of exposed individuals with antitoxin remains controversial, but suggest that family members later receive diphtheria toxoid (usually given as combined diphtheria and tetanus toxoids [DT] or a combination including pertussis vaccine [DPT] for children under age 6) if they have not been immunized.

• Administer drugs, as ordered. Although it is time-consuming and hazardous, desensitization should be attempted if tests are positive, because diphtheria antitoxin is the only specific treatment available. Because mortality increases directly with delay in antitoxin administration, the antitoxin is given before laboratory confirmation of diagnosis if sensitivity tests are negative.

• Before giving diphtheria antitoxin, which is made from horse serum, obtain eye and skin tests to determine sensitivity.

• After giving antitoxin or penicillin, be alert for anaphylaxis, and keep epinephrine 1:1,000 and resuscitative equipment handy. In patients who receive erythromycin, watch for thrombophlebitis.

• Monitor respirations carefully, especially in laryngeal diphtheria (usually, such patients are in a high-humidity or croup tent). Watch for signs of airway obstruction, and be ready to give immediate life support, including intubation and tracheotomy.

• Watch for signs of shock, which can develop suddenly.

• Obtain cultures, as ordered.

• If neuritis develops, tell the patient it is usually transient. Be aware that peripheral neuritis may not develop until 2 to 3 months after onset of illness.

• Be alert for signs of myocarditis, such as development of heart murmurs or EKG changes. Ventricular fibrillation is a common cause of sudden death in diphtheria patients.

• Assign a primary nurse to increase the effectiveness of isolation. Give reassurance that isolation is temporary.

• Stress the need for childhood immunizations to all parents. Report all cases to local public health authorities.

Complications

Laryngeal diphtheria may cause airway obstruction, which can progress to suffocation if untreated. Other complications include myocarditis, neurologic involvement (primarily affecting motor fibers but possibly also sensory neurons), renal involvement, and pulmonary involvement (bronchopneumonia) caused by *C. diphtheriae* or other superinfecting organisms.

Dislocated or fractured jaw

Description

Dislocation of the jaw is a displacement of the temporomandibular joint. Fracture of the jaw is a break in one or both of the two maxillae (upper jawbones) or the mandible (lower jawbone). Treatment can usually restore jaw alignment and function.

Causes

• Simple fractures or dislocations are usually caused by a manual blow along the jawline.

• More serious compound fractures often result from motor vehicle accidents.

Signs and symptoms

• Malocclusion (most obvious sign)
• Mandibular pain

- Swelling
- Ecchymosis
- Loss of function
- Asymmetry
- Possible anesthesia or paresthesia of the chin and lower lip with mandibular fracture
- Infraorbital paresthesia with maxillary fractures

Diagnostic tests
X-rays confirm the diagnosis.

Treatment
As in all trauma, check first for a patient airway, adequate ventilation, and pulses. Then control hemorrhage, and check for other injuries. As necessary, maintain airway patency with an oropharyngeal airway, nasotracheal intubation, or a tracheotomy. Relieve pain with analgesics, as needed. After the patient is stabilized, surgical reduction and fixation by wiring restores mandibular and maxillary alignment. Maxillary fractures may also require reconstruction and repair of soft-tissue injuries. Teeth or bone are never removed during surgery unless removal is unavoidable. If the patient has lost teeth from trauma, the surgeon will decide whether they can be reimplanted. If they can, he will reimplant them within 6 hours, while they are still viable. Dislocations are usually manually reduced under anesthesia.

Clinical implications
After reconstructive surgery, follow these guidelines:
- Position the patient on his side, with his head slightly elevated. A nasogastric tube is usually in place, with low suction to remove gastric contents and prevent nausea, vomiting, and aspiration of vomitus. As necessary, suction the nasopharynx through the nose, or by pulling the cheek away from the teeth and inserting a small suction catheter through any natural gap between teeth.
- If the patient is not intubated, provide nourishment through a straw. If

a natural gap occurs between teeth, insert the straw there; if not, one or two teeth may have to be extracted. However, such extraction is avoided when possible. Start with clear liquids; after the patient can tolerate fluids, offer milk shakes, eggnog, broth, juices, blenderized foods, and commercial nutritional supplements.
- If the patient is unable to tolerate oral fluids, I.V. therapy can maintain hydration.
- Administer antiemetics, as ordered, to minimize nausea and prevent aspiration of vomitus (a very real danger in a patient whose jaw is wired). Keep a pair of wire cutters at the bedside to snip the wires if the patient vomits.
- A dental water-pulsator may be used for mouth care while the wires are intact.
- Because the patient will have difficulty talking while his jaw is wired, provide a Magic Slate or pencil and paper, and suggest appropriate diversions.

Dislocations and subluxations

Description
Dislocations displace joint bones so their articulating surfaces totally lose contact. Subluxations partially displace the articulating surfaces. Dislocations and subluxations occur at the joints of the shoulders, elbows, wrists, digits, hips, knees, ankles, and feet. They may accompany fractures of the joints and may result in deposition of fracture fragments between joint surfaces. Prompt reduction can limit the resulting damage to soft tissue, nerves, and blood vessels.

Causes
- Congenital anomaly
- Trauma
- Disease of surrounding joint tissues

Signs and symptoms
• Deformity around the joint
• Altered length of the involved extremity
• Impaired joint mobility
• Point tenderness
• Extreme pain, in trauma

Diagnostic tests
X-rays, along with patient history and clinical examination, confirm or rule out fracture.

Treatment
Immediate reduction (before tissue edema and muscle spasm make reduction difficult) can prevent additional tissue damage and vascular impairment. Closed reduction consists of manual traction, under general anesthesia, or local anesthesia and sedatives. During such reduction, meperidine I.V. controls pain; diazepam I.V. controls muscle spasm and facilitates muscle-stretching during traction. Occasionally, such injuries require open reduction under regional block or general anesthesia. Such surgery may include wire fixation of the joint, skeletal traction, and ligament repair.

After reduction, a splint, cast, or traction immobilizes the joint. Usually, immobilizing the digits for 2 weeks, hips for 6 to 8 weeks, and other dislocated joints for 3 to 6 weeks allows surrounding ligaments to heal.

Clinical implications
• Until reduction immobilizes the dislocated joint, do not attempt manipulation. Apply ice to ease pain and edema. Splint the extremity "as it lies," even if the angle is awkward. If severe vascular compromise is present or is indicated by pallor, pain, loss of pulses, paralysis, and paresthesia, an immediate orthopedic examination is necessary.

• When a patient receives meperidine I.V. or diazepam I.V., he may develop respiratory depression or even respiratory arrest. So during reduction, keep an airway and Ambu bag in the room, and monitor respirations closely.
• To avoid injury from a dressing that is too tight, instruct the patient to report numbness, pain, cyanosis, or coldness of the extremity below the cast or splint.
• To avoid skin damage, watch for signs of pressure injury (pressure, pain, or soreness) both inside and outside the dressing.
• After removal of the cast or splint, inform the patient that he may gradually return to normal use of the joint.
• A dislocated hip needs immediate reduction. At discharge, stress the need for follow-up visits to detect aseptic femoral head necrosis from vascular damage.

Complications
Even in the absence of concomitant fracture, the displaced bone may damage surrounding muscles, ligaments, nerves, and blood vessels, and may cause bone necrosis, especially if reduction is delayed.

Disseminated intravascular coagulation
(Consumption coagulopathy, defibrination syndrome)

Description
Disseminated intravascular coagulation (DIC) is a grave coagulopathy that occurs as a complication of diseases and conditions that accelerate clotting, causing small blood vessel occlusion, organ necrosis, depletion of circulating clotting factors and platelets, and activation of the fibrinolytic system. (See also *Mechanisms of DIC,* p. 232.) That, in turn, can provoke severe hemorrhage. Clotting in the microcirculation usually affects the kidneys and

Mechanisms of DIC

Regardless of how DIC begins, the typical accelerated clotting results in generalized activation of prothrombin and a consequent excess of thrombin. Excess thrombin converts fibrinogen to fibrin, producing fibrin clots in the microcirculation. This process consumes exorbitant amounts of coagulation factors (especially fibrinogen, prothrombin, platelets, and Factor V and Factor VIII), causing hypofibrinogenemia, hypoprothrombinemia, thrombocytopenia, and deficiencies in Factor V and Factor VIII. Circulating thrombin activates the fibrinolytic system, which lyses fibrin clots into fibrin degradation products. The hemorrhage that occurs may be due largely to the anticoagulant activity of fibrin degradation products, as well as depletion of plasma coagulation factors.

extremities but may occur in the brain, lungs, pituitary and adrenal glands, and GI mucosa. DIC is usually an acute condition but may be chronic in cancer patients. Prognosis depends on early detection and treatment, the severity of the hemorrhage, and treatment of the underlying disease or condition.

Causes

In many patients, the triggering mechanisms may be the entrance of foreign protein into the circulation, and vascular endothelial injury. It is not clear why the following disorders may lead to DIC, nor is it certain that they share a common mechanism:

Infection
—Gram-negative or gram-positive septicemia
—Viral, fungal, or rickettsial infection
—Protozoal infection (falciparum malaria)

Obstetric complications
—Abruptio placentae
—Amniotic fluid embolism
—Retained dead fetus

Neoplastic disease
—Acute leukemia
—Metastatic carcinoma

Tissue necrosis
—Extensive burns and trauma
—Brain tissue destruction
—Transplant rejection
—Hepatic necrosis

Others
—Heatstroke
—Shock
—Poisonous snakebite
—Cirrhosis
—Fat embolism
—Incompatible blood transfusion
—Cardiac arrest
—Intraoperative cardiopulmonary bypass
—Giant hemangioma
—Severe venous thrombosis
—Purpura fulminans

Signs and symptoms

- Abnormal bleeding, without an accompanying history of a serious hemorrhagic disorder. Principal signs of such bleeding include cutaneous oozing, petechiae, ecchymoses, hematomas, bleeding from sites of surgical or invasive procedures (such as incisions or I.V. sites) and from the GI tract.
- Acrocyanosis
- Signs of acute tubular necrosis
- Related or possible: nausea, vomiting, dyspnea, oliguria, convulsions, coma, shock, failure of major organ systems, and severe muscle, back, and abdominal pain

Diagnostic tests

Abnormal bleeding in the absence of a known hematologic disorder suggests DIC. Initial laboratory findings supporting a tentative diagnosis of DIC include the following:

- Prolonged prothrombin time: >15 seconds
- Prolonged partial thromboplastin time: > 60 to 80 seconds

• Decreased fibrinogen levels: < 150 mg/dl
• Decreased platelet count: < 100,000/cu mm
• Increased fibrin degradation products: frequently > 100 mcg/ml

Other supportive data include positive fibrin monomers, diminished levels of Factors V and VIII, fragmentation of red blood cells (RBCs), and decreased hemoglobin (< 10 grams/dl). Assessment of renal status demonstrates reduction in urine output (< 30 ml/hour), and elevated blood urea nitrogen (> 25 mg/100 dl) and serum creatinine (> 1.3 mg/100 dl) levels.

Final confirmation of the diagnosis may be difficult, because many of these test results also occur in other disorders (primary fibrinolysis, for example). Additional diagnostic measures determine the underlying disorder.

Treatment

Successful management of DIC necessitates prompt recognition and adequate treatment of the underlying disorder. Treatment may be supportive (when the underlying disorder is self-limiting, for example) or highly specific. If the patient is not actively bleeding, supportive care alone may reverse DIC. However, active bleeding may require heparin I.V. and administration of blood, fresh-frozen plasma, platelets, or packed RBCs to support hemostasis.

Clinical implications

Patient care must focus on early recognition of principal signs of abnormal bleeding, prompt treatment of the underlying disorders, and prevention of further bleeding.
• To prevent clots from dislodging and causing fresh bleeding, do not scrub bleeding areas. Use pressure, cold compresses, and topical hemostatic agents to control bleeding.
• Protect the patient from injury. Enforce complete bed rest during bleed-

ing episodes. If the patient is very agitated, pad the side rails.
• Check all I.V. and venipuncture sites frequently for bleeding. Apply pressure to injection sites for at least 10 minutes. Alert other personnel to the patient's tendency to hemorrhage.
• Monitor intake and output hourly in acute DIC, especially when administering blood products. Watch for transfusion reactions and signs of fluid overload. To measure the amount of blood lost, weigh dressings and linen, and record drainage. Weigh the patient daily, particularly if there is renal involvement.
• Watch for bleeding from the GI and genitourinary tracts. If you suspect intra-abdominal bleeding, measure the patient's abdominal girth at least every 4 hours, and monitor closely for signs of shock.
• Monitor the results of serial blood studies (particularly hematocrit, hemoglobin, and coagulation times).
• Explain all diagnostic tests and procedures to the patient. Allow time for questions.
• Inform the family of the patient's progress. Prepare them for his appearance (I.V. lines, nasogastric tubes, bruises, dried blood). Provide emotional support for the patient and family. As needed, enlist the aid of a social worker, chaplain, and other members of the health care team in providing such support.

Diverticular disease

Description

In diverticular disease, bulging pouchlike herniations (diverticula) in the GI wall push the mucosal lining through the surrounding muscle. The most common site for diverticula is the sigmoid colon, but they may develop anywhere, from the proximal end of the pharynx to the anus. Other typical sites

Meckel's Diverticulum

In Meckel's diverticulum, a congenital abnormality, a blind tube, like the appendix, opens into the distal ileum near the ileocecal valve. This disorder results from failure of the intra-abdominal portion of the yolk sac to close completely during fetal development. It occurs in 2% of the population, mostly in males.

Uncomplicated Meckel's diverticulum produces no symptoms, but complications cause abdominal pain, especially around the umbilicus, and dark red melena. The lining of the diverticulum may be either gastric mucosa or pancreatic tissue. This disorder may lead to peptic ulceration, perforation, and peritonitis, and may resemble acute appendicitis.

Meckel's diverticulum may also cause bowel obstruction when a fibrous band that connects the diverticulum to the abdominal wall, the mesentery, or other structures snares a loop of the intestine. This may cause intussusception into the diverticulum, or volvulus near the diverticular attachment to the back of the umbilicus or another intra-abdominal structure. Meckel's diverticulum should be considered in cases of GI obstruction or hemorrhage, especially when routine GI X-rays are negative.

Treatment is surgical resection of the inflamed bowel, and antibiotic therapy if infection is present.

---

are the duodenum, near the pancreatic border or the ampulla of Vater, and the jejunum. Diverticular disease of the stomach is rare and is frequently a precursor of peptic or neoplastic disease. Diverticular disease of the ileum (Meckel's diverticulum) is the most common congenital anomaly of the GI tract. (Also see *Meckel's Diverticulum.*)

Diverticular disease has two clinical forms. In diverticulosis, diverticula are present but do not cause symptoms. In diverticulitis, diverticula are inflamed and may cause potentially fatal obstruction, infection, or hemorrhage. In diverticulitis, retained undigested food mixed with bacteria accumulates in the diverticular sac, forming a hard mass (fecalith). This substance cuts off the blood supply to the thin walls of the sac, making them more susceptible to attack by colonic bacteria.

Causes

Diverticula probably result from high intraluminal pressure on areas of weakness in the GI wall, where blood vessels enter. Diet, especially highly refined foods, may be a contributing factor. Lack of roughage reduces fecal residue, narrows the bowel lumen, and leads to higher intra-abdominal pressure during defecation.

Signs and symptoms
Diverticulosis
This disorder is usually asymptomatic but may cause the following symptoms:
—Recurrent left lower abdominal quadrant pain relieved by defecation or passage of flatus
—Alternating constipation and diarrhea
—Difficult defecation
Diverticulitis
—Moderate left lower abdominal quadrant pain
—Mild nausea
—Gas
—Irregular bowel habits
—Low-grade fever
—Leukocytosis
—Rupture of the diverticuli (can occur in severe diverticulitis)
—Fibrosis and adhesions (may occur in chronic diverticulitis)

Diagnostic tests

• Upper GI series confirms or rules out diverticulosis of the esophagus and upper bowel.

• Barium enema confirms or rules out diverticulosis of the lower bowel.

• Biopsy rules out cancer; however, a colonoscopic biopsy is not recommended during acute diverticular disease because of the strenuous bowel preparation it requires.

• Blood studies may show elevated erythrocyte sedimentation rate in diverticulitis, especially if the diverticula are infected.

Treatment

Asymptomatic diverticulosis usually does not necessitate treatment. Intestinal diverticulosis with pain, mild GI distress, constipation, or difficult defecation may respond to a liquid or bland diet, stool softeners, and occasional doses of mineral oil. These measures relieve symptoms, minimize irritation, and lessen the risk of progression to diverticulitis. After pain subsides, patients also benefit from a high-residue diet and bulk-forming laxatives, such as psyllium.

Treatment of mild diverticulitis without signs of perforation must prevent constipation and combat infection. It may include bed rest, a liquid diet, stool softeners, a broad-spectrum antibiotic, meperidine to control pain and relax smooth muscle, and an antispasmodic, such as propantheline, to control muscle spasms.

Diverticulitis that is refractory to medical treatment requires a colon resection to remove the involved segment. Complications that accompany diverticulitis may require a temporary colostomy to drain abscesses and rest the colon, followed by later anastomosis.

Patients who hemorrhage need blood replacement and careful monitoring of fluid and electrolyte balance. Such bleeding usually stops spontaneously. If it continues, angiography for catheter placement and infusion of vasopressin into the bleeding vessel is effective. Rarely, surgery may be required.

Clinical implications

Management of uncomplicated diverticulosis chiefly involves thorough patient teaching about bowel and dietary habits.

• Explain what diverticula are and how they form.

• Make sure the patient understands the importance of dietary roughage and the harmful effects of constipation and straining at stool. Encourage increased intake of foods high in undigestible fiber. Advise the patient to relieve constipation with stool softeners or bulk-forming laxatives. But caution against taking bulk-forming laxatives without plenty of water; if swallowed dry, they may absorb enough moisture in the mouth and throat to swell and obstruct the esophagus or trachea.

• If the patient with diverticulosis is hospitalized, observe his stools carefully for frequency, color, and consistency; keep accurate pulse and temperature charts, because they may signal developing inflammation or complications.

Management of diverticulitis depends on severity of symptoms, as follows:

• In mild disease, administer medications, as ordered; explain diagnostic tests and preparations for such tests; observe stools carefully; and maintain accurate records of temperature, pulse, respirations, and intake and output.

• Monitor carefully if the patient requires angiography and catheter placement for vasopressin infusion. Inspect the insertion site frequently for bleeding, check pedal pulses frequently, and keep the patient from flexing his legs at the groin.

• Watch for vasopressin-induced fluid

Teaching Topics in Diverticular Disease

• An explanation of diverticula: a bulging of the intestinal mucosa through the surrounding muscle
• Possible complications
• Preparation for tests to confirm diverticular disease, such as an upper GI and small bowel series, barium enema, and proctosigmoidoscopy
• Importance of high-fiber foods, constipation prevention, and weight control
• Medications to relieve symptoms, including bulk-forming laxatives and anticholinergics, and avoidance of nonprescription medications
• Preparation for colon resection, if necessary
• Measures to prevent or control symptoms—avoiding activities that increase intra-abdominal pressure and using bowel regulation techniques

---

retention (apprehension, abdominal cramps, convulsions, oliguria, or anuria) and severe hyponatremia (hypotension; rapid, thready pulse; cold, clammy skin; and cyanosis).

After surgery to resect the colon, follow these guidelines:
• Watch for signs of infection. Provide meticulous wound care, because the area may be infected already from perforation. Check drain sites frequently for signs of infection (pus on dressing, foul odor) or fecal drainage. Change dressings as necessary.
• Keep the nasogastric tube patent. If it becomes dislodged, notify the surgeon immediately. Do not attempt to reposition it yourself.
• As needed, teach colostomy care, and arrange for a visit by an enterostomal therapist. (Also see *Teaching Topics in Diverticular Disease*.)

Complications
• Perforation
• Infection
• Abscess
• Peritonitis
• Bowel obstruction
• Fistula
• Hemorrhage (may be a result of diverticulitis or, in elderly patients, a rare complication of diverticulosis)

Down's syndrome
(Mongolism, trisomy 21)

Description
Down's syndrome is a congenital condition characterized by varying degrees of mental retardation and multiple defects. It is associated with other congenital disorders, especially congenital heart defects. Overall, Down's syndrome occurs in 1 in 650 live births, but the incidence increases with maternal age, especially after age 35.

Life expectancy for patients with Down's syndrome has increased significantly because of improved treatment for related complications. Nevertheless, up to one third die before they are 10 years old. Mortality is highest in patients with congenital heart disease.

Causes
• Trisomy 21 is the usual cause. This is an aberration in which chromosome 21 has three copies instead of the normal two because of faulty meiosis (nondisjunction), resulting in a karyotype of 47 chromosomes instead of the normal 46.
• An unbalanced translocation in which the long arm of chromosome 21

breaks and attaches to another chromosome is the cause in about 4% of cases.

Signs and symptoms
• Hypotonia (readily apparent at birth)
• Mental retardation (IQ between 30 and 50; intellectual development slowing with age)
• Craniofacial anomalies (slanting, almond-shaped eyes [epicanthic folds]; protruding tongue and small, open mouth; a single transverse palmar crease [simian crease]; small white spots [Brushfield's spots] on the iris; strabismus; small skull; flat nasal bridge; slow dental development, with abnormal or absent teeth; flattened face; small external ears; short neck; and occasionally cataracts)
• Dry, sensitive skin with decreased elasticity
• Umbilical hernia
• Short stature
• Short extremities with broad, flat, and squarish hands and feet
• Small, inward-curving little finger
• Wide space between the first and second toe
• Abnormal fingerprints and footprints
• Impaired reflex development, posture, coordination, and balance
• Poorly developed genitalia
• Delayed puberty (Females may menstruate and be fertile. Males are infertile, with low serum testosterone levels; in many, the testicles fail to descend.)
• High susceptibility to acute and chronic infections

Diagnostic tests
• A karyotype showing the chromosome abnormality can confirm the diagnosis.
• Amniocentesis allows prenatal diagnosis; 80% of all amniocenteses are done for this purpose and are recommended for pregnant women past age 35. Amniocentesis is indicated for a pregnant woman of any age when either she or the father carries a translocated chromosome.

Treatment
Down's syndrome has no known cure. Life expectancy has increased considerably as a result of surgery to correct heart defects and other related congenital abnormalities, and antibiotic therapy for recurrent infections. Plastic surgery may be done to correct the characteristic facial traits, especially the protruding tongue. Benefits beyond improved appearance include improved speech, reduced susceptibility to dental caries, and fewer orthodontic problems. Down's syndrome patients may be cared for at home and attend special education classes or, if profoundly retarded, may be institutionalized. As adults, some may work in sheltered workshops. Other adults are capable of independent living.

Clinical implications
Support for the parents of a child with Down's syndrome is vital. By following the guidelines listed below, you can help them meet their child's physical and emotional needs.
• Establish a trusting relationship with parents, and encourage communication during the difficult period soon after diagnosis and when parents face the difficult decision of whether or not to care for their child at home.
• Teach parents the importance of a balanced diet. Stress the need for patience when feeding their child, because he may have difficulty sucking and may be less demanding and seem less eager to eat than normal babies.
• Encourage parents to hold and nurture their child, even though their first reaction may be to reject him because he is not normal.
• Emphasize the importance of adequate exercise and maximal environmental stimulation, and refer them for infant stimulation classes, which may begin at age 3 months.

• Assist parents in setting realistic goals for their child. His mental development may seem normal at first, but warn parents not to view this early development as a sign of future progress. By the time he is 1 year old, his development will clearly lag behind that of normal children. Help them view their child's successful achievements positively, even though he is slow. The Denver Developmental Screening Test for noninstitutionalized Down's children can help chart progress.

• Refer parents and older siblings for genetic counseling, and, if necessary, for psychological counseling, to help them evaluate future risks and adopt a positive outlook.

• Warn parents not to overlook the emotional needs of other children in the family.

Complications

Problems associated with Down's syndrome include the following:

• Congenital heart disease (septal defects or pulmonary or aortic stenosis)
• Duodenal atresia, megacolon
• Pelvic bone abnormalities
• Acute leukemia
• Alzheimer's syndrome

Drug abuse and dependence

Description

The National Institute of Drug Abuse defines this condition as the use of a legal or illegal drug that causes physical, mental, emotional, or social harm. Dependence is marked by physiologic changes—primarily tolerance and withdrawal symptoms. (See also *Drug Abuse or Dependence?*) Persons predisposed to drug abuse tend to have few mental or emotional resources against stress and a low tolerance for frustration. They demand immediate relief of tension or distress, which they receive from taking the abused drug.

Taking the drug gives them pleasure by relieving tension, abolishing loneliness, achieving a temporarily peaceful or euphoric state, or simply by relieving boredom. Drug abuse commonly involves the use of cocaine; however, many drugs are being abused. Abusers range from young students who experiment with hallucinogens and marijuana to adults who overuse tranquilizers and other prescription drugs. The most dangerous form of drug abuse is that in which several drugs are mixed—sometimes with alcohol and various other chemicals. Prognosis varies with the drug and the extent of abuse.

Causes

The exact causes of drug abuse are difficult to identify, but it sometimes follows the use of drugs for relief of physical pain. In young people it frequently follows experimentation with drugs as a result of peer pressure. Health care professionals are at special risk of drug abuse and dependence because of their easy access to drugs.

Signs and symptoms

Clinical effects vary according to the substance used, duration, and dosage. (See *Signs and Symptoms of Drug Abuse*, pp. 240 and 241.)

Diagnostic tests

Diagnosis depends largely on a history that shows a pattern of pathologic use of a substance, related impairment in social or occupational function, and duration of abnormal use and impairment for at least 1 month. A urine or blood screen can determine the amount of the substance present.

Treatment

Treatment of acute drug intoxication is symptomatic and depends on the drug ingested. (See *Treatment of Drug*

Drug Abuse or Dependence?

For most classes of substances, pathologic use is divided into abuse and dependence, as defined below according to *DSM-III.*

ABUSE	DEPENDENCE
A pattern of pathologic use, as manifested by inability to reduce or control intake despite: • a physical disorder that the user knows is made worse by using the substance • need for daily use of the substance for adequate function • episodes of a complication of intoxication (alcoholic blackouts, opiate overdose) • impairment in social or occupational function caused by substance use • minimal duration of disturbance at least 1 month.	A severe form of substance use with physiologic dependence shown by tolerance and withdrawal symptoms: • Tolerance means markedly increased amounts of the addicting substance are needed to achieve the desired effect, or regular use of the same dose produces a markedly diminished effect. • Withdrawal is a substance-specific syndrome provoked by stopping or reducing substance intake.

Intoxication, pp. 242 and 243.) It includes fluid replacement therapy and nutritional and vitamin supplements, if indicated; detoxification with the same drug or a pharmacologically similar drug (exceptions: cocaine, hallucinogens, and marijuana are not used for detoxification); sedatives to induce sleep; anticholinergics and antidiarrheal agents to relieve GI distress; antianxiety drugs for severe agitation, especially in cocaine abusers; and treatment of medical complications.

Treatment of drug dependence commonly involves a triad of care: detoxification, long-term rehabilitation (up to 2 years), and aftercare. The latter means a lifetime of abstinence, usually aided by participation in Narcotics Anonymous or a similar self-help group.

Detoxification, the controlled and gradual withdrawal of an abused drug, is achieved through substitution of a drug with similar action. Such gradual replacement of the abused drug controls the effects of withdrawal, reducing the patient's discomfort and

associated risks. Depending on the abused drug, detoxification is managed on an inpatient or an outpatient basis. For example, withdrawal from general depressants can produce hazardous effects, such as grand mal seizures, status epilepticus, and hypotension; the severity of these effects determines whether the patient can be safely treated as an outpatient or requires hospitalization. Withdrawal from depressants usually does not require detoxification. Opiate withdrawal causes severe physical discomfort and can even be life-threatening. To minimize these effects, chronic opiate abusers are frequently detoxified with methadone substitution.

To ease withdrawal from opiates, general depressants, and other drugs, useful nonchemical measures may include psychotherapy, exercise, relaxation techniques, and nutritional support. Sedatives and tranquilizers may be administered temporarily to

Signs and Symptoms of Drug Abuse

DRUG
Opiates
Codeine, heroin, meperidine, morphine, opium
(Butorphanol and pentazocine, though not narcotics, have similar effects and addictive potential.)
CLINICAL FEATURES
• *Acute:* coma, hypotension, tachycardia, pinpoint pupils
• *Chronic* (after injection): needle marks, scars from skin abscesses, thrombophlebitis
• *Withdrawal:* sweating, nausea, vomiting, diarrhea, anxiety, insomnia, dilated pupils, runny nose, tearing eyes, yawning, goose bumps, persistent back and abdominal pain, anorexia, cold flashes, spontaneous orgasm, fever, tachycardia, rising blood pressure and respiratory rate
COMPLICATIONS
• Viral hepatitis (resulting in hepatic dysfunction), osteomyelitis, pulmonary edema, bacterial endocarditis, coma (resulting in organic brain damage or seizures), secondary infection
• Physical and psychological dependence

DRUG
Amphetamines
Amphetamine, dextroamphetamine, methamphetamine
CLINICAL FEATURES
• *After high doses:* anxiety, hyperactivity, irritability, muscle tension, aggressive or violent behavior, paranoia, psychotic symptoms resembling schizophrenia, fever, hypertension, dilated pupils, tachycardia, convulsions, cardiovascular collapse, hallucinations
• *After injection:* needle marks, thrombophlebitis
• *Withdrawal:* depression, overwhelming fatigue. Long-term use yields a rapidly developing delusional syndrome resembling paranoid schizophrenia.
COMPLICATIONS
• Little or no physical dependence, but tolerance and psychological dependence possible

DRUG
Cocaine
CLINICAL FEATURES
• *Acute intoxication* (after I.V. injection): tremors, seizures, convulsions, delirium, potentially fatal cardiovascular or respiratory failure
• *Chronic intoxication:* hallucinations, dilated pupils, tachycardia, tachypnea, muscle twitching, violent behavior, nasal septum damage
• *Withdrawal:* depression, irritability, disorientation, tremors, muscle weakness
COMPLICATIONS
• Psychological dependence

DRUG
Barbiturates
Amobarbital, pentobarbital, secobarbital.
(Methaqualone is not a barbiturate, but symptoms and treatment are similar.)
CLINICAL FEATURES
• *Acute intoxication:* progressive central nervous system and respiratory depression
• *Chronic intoxication:* slurred speech, impaired coordination, decreased mental alertness and attention span, impaired judgment, memory disturbances, depressed pulse rate and tendon reflexes, mood swings, nystagmus or strabismus, diplopia, dizziness, hypotension, dehydration, aggressive or suicidal behavior
• *Withdrawal:* anxiety, irritability,

grand mal seizures, status epilepticus, orthostatic hypotension, tachycardia, auditory and visual disturbances
COMPLICATIONS
• Apnea, shock, coma, death
• Physical dependence and psychological dependence

DRUG
Phencyclidine (PCP)
CLINICAL FEATURES
• *Acute intoxication:* apnea, status epilepticus, paralysis, numbness, hallucinations, anxiety, dissociative reaction, paranoid or violent behavior, coma, death
• *Chronic intoxication:* confusion, fatigue, irritability, depression, hallucinations
COMPLICATIONS
• Psychological dependence, but no physical dependence

DRUG
Cannabis
Hashish, marijuana, tetrahydrocannabinol (THC)
CLINICAL FEATURES
• *Acute transient reaction* (rare): panic and paranoid reactions (with first-time use); pseudopsychotic reaction (with THC)
COMPLICATIONS
• Psychological dependence, but no physical dependence

DRUG
Hallucinogens
LSD, mescaline, psilocybin
CLINICAL FEATURES
• *Acute intoxication ("bad trip"):* anxiety, frightening hallucinations, and depression (possible suicidal tendencies)
COMPLICATIONS
• Psychological dependence, but no physical dependence

help the patient cope with insomnia, anxiety, and depression.

After withdrawal, rehabilitation is needed to prevent recurrence of drug abuse. Rehabilitation programs are available for both inpatients and outpatients; they usually last a month or longer and may include individual, group, and family psychotherapy. During and after rehabilitation, participation in a drug-oriented self-help group may be helpful. The largest such group is Narcotics Anonymous. Three new groups have been formed recently: Potsmokers Anonymous, Pills Anonymous, and Cocaine Anonymous.

Naltrexone (Trexan), a newly released drug, is used to help outpatient opiate abusers maintain abstinence. By blocking the opiate euphoria, it helps prevent readdiction. It is most useful in a comprehensive rehabilitation program.

Clinical implications

Patient care for drug abusers must focus not only on restoring physical health, but also on educating the patient and his family about drug abuse and dependence, providing support, and encouraging participation in drug treatment programs and self-help groups. Specific interventions may vary, depending on the drug abused, but commonly include the following measures:
• Observe the patient for signs and symptoms of withdrawal.
• During the patient's withdrawal from any drug, maintain a quiet, safe environment. Remove harmful objects from the room, and use restraints judiciously. Use side rails for the comatose patient. Reassure the anxious patient that medication will control most symptoms of withdrawal.
• Closely monitor visitors who might

Treatment of Drug Intoxication

DRUG
Opiates
TREATMENT
• Immediate goal is to prevent shock and maintain respirations by endotracheal intubation and mechanical ventilation and administration of oxygen, I.V. fluids, and plasma expanders.
• Naloxone (Narcan) is administered until central nervous system (CNS) depressant effects are reversed.
SPECIAL CONSIDERATIONS
• Observe the patient continuously, and closely monitor for hypoxemia because narcotics may impair respiratory drive. Auscultate the lungs frequently for rales, which could indicate pulmonary edema in the patient receiving I.V. fluids and plasma expanders.
• Before giving naloxone, apply secure restraints. Patient may be disoriented and agitated as he emerges from coma.
• Monitor cardiac rate and rhythm, being alert for atrial fibrillation.
• Be alert for signs of withdrawal.

DRUG
Amphetamines
TREATMENT
• If the drug was taken orally, vomiting is induced or gastric lavage performed; activated charcoal and a sodium or magnesium sulfate cathartic are also given.
• Ammonium chloride or ascorbic acid may be given I.V. to acidify the patient's urine and lower his urine pH to 5.0.
• Therapeutic drugs may include mannitol to force diuresis; a short-acting barbiturate, such as pentobarbital, to control stimulant-induced seizure activity; haloperidol or chlorpromazine to treat agitation or assaultive behavior; and an alpha-adrenergic blocking agent, such as phentolamine (Regitine), for hypertension.

SPECIAL CONSIDERATIONS
• Restrain the patient to keep him from injuring himself and others—especially if he is paranoid or hallucinating.
• Watch for cardiac dysrhythmias. Notify the physician if these develop, and expect to give propranolol (Inderal) or lidocaine to treat tachydysrhythmias or ventricular dysrhythmias, respectively.
• Treat hyperthermia with tepid sponge baths or a hypothermia blanket, as ordered.
• Provide a quiet environment to avoid overstimulation.
• Be alert for signs and symptoms of withdrawal.
• Take suicide precautions, especially if the patient shows signs of withdrawal.
• Closely monitor neurologic status, because haloperidol and chlorpromazine lower the seizure threshold.

DRUG
Cocaine
TREATMENT
• If cocaine was ingested, treatment includes induction of vomiting, gastric lavage, and activated charcoal followed by a saline cathartic.
• An antipyretic may be given to reduce fever; an anticonvulsant, such as diazepam (Valium), to prevent seizures; and propranolol to treat tachycardia.
SPECIAL CONSIDERATIONS
• Monitor respirations and blood pressure closely.
• Monitor cardiac rate and rhythm—ventricular fibrillation and cardiac standstill can occur as a direct cardiotoxic result of cocaine. Defibrillate and initiate cardiopulmonary resuscitation, if indicated.
• Calm the patient by talking to him in a quiet room.
• Observe for seizures, take seizure precautions, and administer ordered medication.

DRUG
Barbiturates
TREATMENT

• Immediate goal is to restore CNS and respiratory function and prevent shock.
• Treatment usually includes induction of vomiting or gastric lavage, if the patient ingested the drug within 4 hours; endotracheal intubation; I.V. fluids to correct hypotension and dehydration; vasopressors for phenobarbital overdose; and I.V. sodium bicarbonate to promote diuresis and counteract intoxication.
• Gastric lavage or administration of activated charcoal followed by a cathartic is usually recommended to eliminate the toxic drug.
• During detoxification, a pentobarbital challenge test determines the patient's tolerance level. An appropriate pentobarbital dose lessens withdrawal symptoms until dosage can gradually be reduced and finally totally withdrawn.
• Extreme intoxication may require dialysis.

SPECIAL CONSIDERATIONS
• Perform frequent neurologic assessments. Check pulse rate, temperature, skin color, and reflexes frequently.
• Notify the physician if you see signs of respiratory distress or pulmonary edema.
• Watch for and report signs of withdrawal.
• Protect the patient from injuring himself, and provide symptomatic relief of withdrawal symptoms, as ordered.

DRUG
Phencyclidine (PCP)
TREATMENT

• If the drug was taken orally, vomiting is induced or gastric lavage performed; activated charcoal is repeatedly instilled and removed.

• Acidic diuresis is performed by acidifying the patient's urine with ascorbic acid to increase excretion of the drug. This is continued for 2 weeks, because signs and symptoms may recur when fat cells release their stores of PCP.
• Therapeutic drugs may include diazepam and haloperidol to control agitation or psychotic behavior; diazepam to control seizures; propranolol for hypertension and tachycardia; and nitroprusside for severe hypertension.
• If the patient develops renal failure, hemodialysis is performed.

SPECIAL CONSIDERATIONS
• Provide a quiet, safe environment with dimmed lights.
• Be aware that overt attempts to reassure an aggressive patient often provoke more aggressive behavior.
• Closely monitor the patient's intake and output; maintain adequate hydration to promote PCP excretion; report diminished urinary output or abnormal renal function tests.
• Take suicide precautions as needed.

DRUG
Hallucinogens
TREATMENT

• Diazepam may be given to control seizures.
• If the drug was taken orally, vomiting is induced or gastric lavage performed; activated charcoal and a cathartic are given.

SPECIAL CONSIDERATIONS
• Reorient the patient repeatedly to time, place, and person.
• Restrain the patient, as ordered, to protect him from injuring himself and others.
• Calm the patient by sequestering him in a quiet room and talking to him in a soothing tone.

bring the patient drugs from the outside.

• Develop self-awareness and an understanding and positive attitude toward the patient. Control your reactions to the patient's undesirable behaviors—commonly, dependency, manipulation, anger, frustration, and alienation.

• Set limits for dealing with demanding, manipulative behavior.

• Carefully monitor and promote adequate nutritional intake.

• Administer medications carefully to prevent hoarding by the patient.

• Refer the patient for detoxification and rehabilitation, as appropriate.

• Encourage family members to seek help whether or not the abuser seeks it. You can suggest private therapy or community mental health clinics.

Complications

Chronic abuse of drugs, especially by I.V. use, can lead to life-threatening complications that include the following:

• Bacterial endocarditis
• Hepatitis
• Thrombophlebitis
• Pulmonary emboli
• Gangrene
• Malnutrition
• GI disturbances
• Respiratory infections
• Musculoskeletal dysfunction
• Trauma
• Psychosis

Dysfunctional uterine bleeding

Description

Dysfunctional uterine bleeding (DUB) refers to abnormal endometrial bleeding without recognizable organic lesions. Prognosis varies with the cause. DUB is the indication for almost 25% of gynecologic surgery.

Causes

DUB usually results from an imbalance in the hormonal-endometrial relationship, where persistent and unopposed stimulation of the endometrium by estrogen occurs. Disorders that cause sustained high estrogen levels include the following:

• Polycystic ovary syndrome
• Obesity
• Immaturity of the hypothalamic-pituitary-ovarian mechanism (in postpubertal teenagers)
• Anovulation (in women in their late thirties or early forties)
• Hormone-producing ovarian tumors

Signs and symptoms

Any of the following symptoms may occur:

• Metrorrhagia (episodes of vaginal bleeding between menses)
• Hypermenorrhea (heavy or prolonged menses, longer than 8 days)
• Chronic polymenorrhea (menstrual cycle of less than 18 days)
• Anemia

Diagnostic tests

• Dilatation and curettage (D&C) and biopsy results confirm the diagnosis by revealing endometrial hyperplasia.
• Hematocrit and hemoglobin levels determine the need for blood or iron replacement.

Treatment

High-dose estrogen-progestogen combination therapy (oral contraceptives), the primary treatment, is designed to control endometrial growth and reestablish a normal cyclic pattern of menstruation. These drugs are usually administered four times daily for 5 to 7 days, even though bleeding usually stops in 12 to 24 hours. (The patient's age and the cause of bleeding help determine the drug choice and dosage.) In patients over age 35, endometrial biopsy is necessary before the start of estrogen therapy to rule out endometrial adenocarcinoma. Progestogen therapy is a necessary alternative in some women, such as those susceptible to the adverse effects of estrogen (thrombophlebitis, for example).

If drug therapy is ineffective, a D&C serves as a supplementary treatment, through removal of a large portion of the bleeding endometrium. Also, a D&C can help determine the original cause of hormonal imbalance and can aid in planning further therapy. Regardless of the primary treatment, the patient may need iron replacement or transfusions of packed cells or whole blood, as indicated, because of anemia caused by recurrent bleeding.

Clinical implications
• Explain the importance of adhering to the prescribed hormonal therapy. If a D&C is ordered, explain this procedure and its purpose.
• Stress the need for regular checkups to assess treatment.

Dysrhythmias
(Arrhythmias)

Description
In cardiac dysrhythmias, abnormal electrical conduction or automaticity changes heart rate and rhythm. Dysrhythmias vary in severity, from those that are mild, asymptomatic, and require no treatment (such as sinus arrhythmia, in which heart rate increases and decreases with respiration) to catastrophic ventricular fibrillation, which necessitates immediate resus-

---

Cardiac Dysrhythmias

Normal sinus rhythm (NSR) in adults

• Ventricular and atrial rates of 60 to 100 beats per minute (BPM)
• QRS complexes and P waves regular and uniform
• P-R interval 0.12 to 0.2 seconds
• QRS duration < 0.12 seconds
• Identical atrial and ventricular rates, with constant P-R interval

Sinus arrhythmia

CAUSES
• Usually a normal variation of NSR; associated with sinus bradycardia
DESCRIPTION
• Slight irregularity of heartbeat, usually corresponding to respiratory cycle
• Rate increases with inspiration and decreases with expiration.
TREATMENT
• None

Sinus tachycardia

CAUSES
• Normal physiologic response to fever, exercise, anxiety, pain, dehydration; may also accompany shock, left ventricular failure, cardiac tamponade, anemia, hyperthyroidism, hypovolemia, pulmonary embolus
• May result from treatment with vagolytic and sympathetic stimulating drugs
DESCRIPTION
• Rate > 100 BPM; rarely, > 160 BPM
• Every QRS wave follows a P wave.
TREATMENT
• Correct underlying cause.

(continued)

Cardiac Dysrhythmias *(continued)*

Sinus bradycardia

CAUSES
- Increased intracranial pressure; increased vagal tone from bowel straining, vomiting, intubation, mechanical ventilation; sick sinus syndrome or hypothyroidism
- Treatment with beta-blockers and sympatholytic drugs
- May be normal in athletes

DESCRIPTION
- Rate < 60 BPM
- A QRS complex follows each P wave.

TREATMENT
- For low cardiac output, dizziness, weakness, altered level of consciousness, or low blood pressure, 0.5 mg atropine every 5 minutes to total of 2 mg
- Temporary pacemaker or isoproterenol, if atropine fails

Sinoatrial (SA) arrest or block (sinus arrest)

CAUSES
- Vagal stimulation; digitalis or quinidine toxicity
- In many cases, a sign of sick sinus syndrome

DESCRIPTION
- NSR interrupted by unexpectedly prolonged P-P interval, frequently terminated by an escape beat or return to NSR
- QRS complexes uniform but irregular

TREATMENT
- A pacemaker for repeated episodes

Wandering atrial pacemaker

CAUSES
- Seen in rheumatic pericarditis as a result of inflammation involving the SA node, digitalis toxicity, and sick sinus syndrome

DESCRIPTION
- Rate varies
- QRS complexes uniform in shape but irregular in rhythm
- P waves irregular with changing configuration, indicating they are not all from sinus node or single atrial focus
- P-R interval varies from short to normal.

TREATMENT
- Patient should use digitalis cautiously.
- No other treatment

Premature atrial contraction (PAC)

CAUSES
- Congestive heart failure, ischemic heart disease, acute respiratory failure, or chronic obstrutive pulmonary disease (COPD)
- May result from treatment with digitalis, aminophylline, or adrenergic drugs; or from anxiety or caffeine ingestion
- Occasional PAC may be normal.

DESCRIPTION
- Premature, abnormal-looking P waves
- QRS complexes follow, except in very early or blocked PACs.
- P wave frequently buried in the preceding T wave or can be identified in the preceding T wave

TREATMENT
- If more than six times per minute or frequency is increasing, give digitalis. quinidine, or propranolol;

after revascularization surgery, propranolol.
• Eliminate known causes, such as caffeine or drugs.

Paroxysmal atrial tachycardia (PAT) or paroxysmal supraventricular tachycardia (PSVT)

CAUSES
• Intrinsic abnormality of atrioventricular (AV) conduction system
• Congenital accessory atrial conduction pathway
• Physical or psychological stress; hypoxia; hypokalemia; caffeine, marijuana, stimulants; digitalis toxicity

DESCRIPTION
• Heart rate > 140 BPM; rarely exceeds 250 BPM
• P waves regular but aberrant; difficult to differentiate from preceding T wave
• Onset and termination of dysrhythmia occur suddenly.
• May cause palpitations and light-headedness

TREATMENT
• Vagal maneuvers, sympathetic blockers (propranolol, quinidine), or calcium blockers (verapamil) to alter AV node conduction
• Elective cardioversion, if patient is symptomatic and unresponsive to drugs

Atrial flutter

CAUSES
• Heart failure, valvular heart disease, pulmonary embolism, digitalis toxicity, postoperative revascularization

DESCRIPTION
• Ventricular rate depends on

degree of AV block (usually 60 to 100 BPM).
• Atrial rate 250 to 400 BPM and regular
• QRS complexes uniform in shape, but often irregular in rate
• P waves may have sawtooth configuration.

TREATMENT
• Digitalis (unless dysrhythmia is caused by digitalis toxicity), propranolol, or quinidine
• May require synchronized cardioversion, atrial pacemaker, or vagal stimulation

Atrial fibrillation

CAUSES
• Congestive heart failure, COPD, hyperthyroidism, sepsis, pulmonary embolus, mitral stenosis, digitalis toxicity (rarely), atrial irritation, postcoronary bypass or valve replacement surgery

DESCRIPTION
• Atrial rate > 400 BPM
• Ventricular rate varies.
• QRS complexes uniform in shape but at irregular intervals
• P-R interval indiscernible
• No P waves, or P waves appear as erratic, irregular baseline F waves.
• Irregular QRS rate

TREATMENT
• Digitalis and quinidine to slow ventricular rate, and quinidine to convert rhythm to NSR; diuretics, such as furosemide, for congestive heart failure
• May require elective cardioversion for rapid rate

(continued)

Cardiac Dysrhythmias *(continued)*

AV junctional rhythm (nodal rhythm)

CAUSES
- Digitalis toxicity, inferior wall myocardial infarction or ischemia, hypoxia, vagal stimulation
- Acute rheumatic fever
- Valve surgery

DESCRIPTION
- Ventricular rate usually 40 to 60 BPM (60 to 100 BPM is accelerated junctional rhythm)
- P waves may precede, be hidden within (absent), or follow QRS; if visible, they are altered.
- QRS duration is normal, except in aberrant conduction.
- Patient may be asymptomatic unless ventricular rate is very slow.

TREATMENT
- Symptomatic
- Atropine, with slow rate
- If patient is taking digitalis, it is discontinued.

Premature junctional contractions (PJC), premature nodal contractions

CAUSES
- Myocardial infarction or ischemia, digitalis toxicity, caffeine or amphetamine ingestion

DESCRIPTION
- QRS complexes of uniform shape but premature
- P waves irregular, with premature beat; may precede, be hidden within, or follow QRS

TREATMENT
- Correct underlying cause.
- Quinidine or disopyramide, as ordered
- If patient is taking digitalis, it may be discontinued.

First-degree AV block

CAUSES
- Inferior myocardial ischemia or infarction, hypothyroidism, digitalis toxicity, potassium imbalance

DESCRIPTION
- P-R interval prolonged > 0.20 seconds
- QRS complex normal

TREATMENT
- Patient should use digitalis cautiously.
- Correct underlying cause. Otherwise, be alert for increasing block.

Second-degree AV block *Mobitz Type I* (Wenckebach)

CAUSES
- Inferior wall myocardial infarction, digitalis toxicity, vagal stimulation

DESCRIPTION
- P-R interval becomes progressively longer with each cycle until QRS disappears (dropped beat). After a dropped beat, P-R interval is shorter. Ventricular rate is irregular; atrial rhythm, regular.

TREATMENT
- Atropine, if patient is symptomatic
- Discontinue digitalis.

Second-degree AV block *Mobitz Type II*

CAUSES
- Degenerative disease of conduction system, ischemia of AV node in anterior myocardial infarction, digitalis toxicity, anteroseptal infarction

DESCRIPTION
• P-R interval is constant, with QRS complexes dropped
• Ventricular rhythm may be irregular, with varying degree of block.
• Atrial rate regular
TREATMENT
• Temporary pacemaker, sometimes followed by permanent pacemaker
• Atropine, for slow rate
• If patient is taking digitalis, it is discontinued.

Third-degree AV block (complete heart block)

CAUSES
• Ischemic heart disease or infarction, postsurgical complications of mitral valve replacement, digitalis toxicity, hypoxia sometimes causing syncope from decreased cerebral blood flow (as in Stokes-Adams syndrome)
DESCRIPTION
• Atrial rate regular; ventricular rate, slow and regular
• No relationship between P waves and QRS complexes
• No constant P-R interval
• QRS interval normal (nodal pacemaker); wide and bizarre (ventricular pacemaker)
TREATMENT
• Usually requires temporary pacemaker, followed by permanent pacemaker
• Epinephrine or isoproterenol

Junctional tachycardia (nodal tachycardia)

CAUSES
• Digitalis toxicity, myocarditis, cardiomyopathy, myocardial ischemia or infarct

DESCRIPTION
• Onset of rhythm frequently sudden, occurring in bursts
• Ventricular rate > 100 BPM
• Other characteristics same as junctional rhythm
TREATMENT
• Vagal stimulation
• Propranolol, quinidine, digitalis (if cause is not digitalis toxicity)
• Elective cardioversion

Premature ventricular contraction (PVC)

CAUSES
• Heart failure; old or acute myocardial infarction or contusion with trauma; myocardial irritation by ventricular catheter, such as a pacemaker; hypoxia, as in anemia and acute respiratory failure; drug toxicity (digitalis, aminophylline, tricyclic antidepressants, beta-adrenergics [isoproterenol or dopamine]); electrolyte imbalances (especially hypokalemia); psychological stress
DESCRIPTION
• Beat occurs prematurely, usually followed by a complete compensatory pause after PVC; irregular pulse.
• QRS complex wide and distorted
• Can occur singly, in pairs, or in threes; can alternate with normal beats; focus can be from one or more sites.
• PVCs are most ominous when clustered, multifocal, with R wave on T pattern.
TREATMENT
• Lidocaine I.V. bolus and drip infusion; procainamide I.V. If induced by digitalis toxicity, stop this drug; if induced by hypokalemia, give potassium chloride I.V. Many other drugs may be used.

(continued)

Cardiac Dysrhythmias (continued)

Ventricular tachycardia (VT)

CAUSES
• Myocardial ischemia, infarction, or aneurysm; ventricular catheters; digitalis or quinidine toxicity; hypokalemia; hypercalcemia; anxiety

DESCRIPTION
• Ventricular rate 140 to 220 BPM; may be regular
• QRS complexes are wide, bizarre, and independent of P waves.
• Usually no visible P waves
• Can produce chest pain, anxiety, palpitations, dyspnea, shock, coma, and death

TREATMENT
• CPR (if pulses are absent) followed by lidocaine I.V. (bolus and drip infusion) and countershock. Use synchronized cardioversion if pulse is present.
• Bretylium tosylate and procainamide

Ventricular fibrillation

CAUSES
• Myocardial ischemia or infarction, untreated ventricular tachycardia, electrolyte imbalances (hypokalemia and alkalosis, hyperkalemia and hypercalcemia), digitalis or quinidine toxicity, electric shock, hypothermia

DESCRIPTION
• Ventricular rhythm rapid and chaotic

• QRS complexes wide and irregular; no visible P waves
• Loss of consciousness, with no peripheral pulses, blood pressure, or respirations; possible seizures; sudden death

TREATMENT
• CPR
• Asynchronized countershock (200 to 300 watts/second) twice; if rhythm does not return, reshock (300 to 400 watts/second).
• Lidocaine or bretylium tosylate I.V. or procainamide

Ventricular standstill (asystole)

CAUSES
• Acute respiratory failure, myocardial ischemia or infarction, ruptured ventricular aneurysm, aortic valve disease, or hyperkalemia

DESCRIPTION
• Primary ventricular standstill—regular P waves, no QRS complexes
• Secondary ventricular standstill—QRS complexes wide and slurred, occurring at irregular intervals; agonal heart rhythm
• Loss of consciousness, with no peripheral pulses, blood pressure, or respirations

TREATMENT
• CPR
• Endotracheal intubation; pacemaker should be available.
• Epinephrine, calcium gluconate, sodium bicarbonate, isoproterenol, and atropine
• Cardiac monitoring

citation. Dysrhythmias are usually classified according to their origin (ventricular or supraventricular). Their clinical significance depends on their effect on cardiac output and blood pressure, partially influenced by the site of origin.

Causes
Dysrhythmias may be congenital or

may result from the following:
- Myocardial anoxia
- Myocardial infarction
- Hypertrophy of heart muscle fiber because of hypertension or valvular heart disease
- Toxic doses of cardioactive drugs such as digoxin and other cardiotonic glycosides
- Degeneration of conductive tissue necessary to maintain normal heart rhythm (sick sinus syndrome)

(See also *Cardiac Dysrhythmias*, pp. 245 to 250.)

Clinical implications

- Assess an unmonitored patient for rhythm disturbances. If the patient's pulse is abnormally rapid, slow, or irregular, watch for signs of hypoperfusion, such as hypotension and diminished urine output.
- Document any dysrhythmias in a monitored patient, and assess for possible causes and effects.
- When life-threatening dysrhythmias develop, rapidly assess the level of consciousness, respirations, and pulse, and initiate cardiopulmonary resuscitation (CPR), if indicated.
- Evaluate for altered cardiac output resulting from dysrhythmias. Consider potentially progressive or ominous dysrhythmias in determining your course of action. Administer medications, as ordered, and prepare to assist with medical procedures (for example, cardioversion), if indicated.
- Monitor for predisposing factors—such as fluid and electrolyte imbalance—and signs of drug toxicity, especially with digoxin. If you suspect drug toxicity, report such signs to the physician immediately and withhold the next dose.
- To prevent dysrhythmias in a postoperative cardiac patient, provide adequate oxygen and reduce heart work

---

Holter Monitoring

Tape-recorded ambulatory electrocardiography (Holter monitoring) permits monitoring of all cardiac cycles over a prescribed period (usually 24 hours). This type of monitoring has proven useful for patients recuperating from myocardial infarctions, receiving antiarrhythmic drugs, or using pacemakers. It can record rate, rhythm, and conduction abnormalities as well as cardiac responses to typical environmental stimuli and is especially useful in diagnosing dysrhythmias. Holter monitoring has many advantages:
- With minimal equipment, the patient can be hooked up to one or more EKG leads. (Equipment includes the monitor, its carrying case, a belt, skin electrodes, alcohol swabs, a blank cassette tape, a patient diary, and a test analysis report.)
- Leads are recorded on a tape in a portable cassette recorder that the patient can wear easily. After the recorder is connected to a cardiac monitor for test readings, the electrodes are attached to the patient, and he goes through a typical day with the Holter monitor in place. He is encouraged to engage in activities that usually precipitate symptoms and is instructed to keep a diary of the exact times of symptoms and activities and of any medication he takes, so the impact of these factors can be correlated with EKG patterns.
- With a high-speed computer scanner, the physician can review 24 hours of tape in minutes to detect important rhythm changes. He can also correlate the patient's symptoms, such as light-headedness, with the documented dysrhythmias.
- The Holter monitor can capture a sporadic dysrhythmia that an office or stress-test EKG might miss.

Teaching Topics in Dysrhythmias

- An explanation of normal cardiac conduction
- An explanation of the patient's specific dysrhythmia
- Preparation for diagnostic tests, such as EKG, serum electrolyte studies, and electrophysiologic studies
- Activity instructions: regular exercise, appropriate warnings
- General dietary restrictions: moderate use of alcohol, caffeine, and tobacco; increased or decreased potassium intake, as ordered
- Antiarrhythmic drug use
- Applicable treatment methods: carotid sinus massage, Valsalva's maneuver, temporary pacemaker implantation, electrocardioversion
- Preparation for permanent pacemaker implantation, if necessary
- Guidelines for pacemaker use and maintenance, if necessary
- How to take pulse rate
- Sources of additional information and support

load, while carefully maintaining metabolic, neurologic, respiratory, and hemodynamic status.

• To avoid temporary pacemaker malfunction, install a fresh battery before each insertion. Carefully secure the external catheter wires and the pacemaker box. Assess the threshold daily. Watch closely for premature contractions, a sign of myocardial irritation.

• To avert permanent pacemaker malfunction, restrict the patient's activity after insertion, as ordered. Monitor the pulse rate regularly, and watch for signs of decreased cardiac output.

• Warn the patient about environmental hazards, as indicated by the pacemaker manufacturer. Although hazards may not present a problem, 24-hour Holter monitoring may be helpful in doubtful situations. (See also *Holter Monitoring*, p. 251.) Tell the patient to report light-headedness or syncope, and stress the importance of regular checkups. (See also *Teaching Topics in Dysrhythmias*.)

Eardrum perforation

Description
Perforation of the eardrum is a rupture of the tympanic membrane.

Causes
• Trauma (the usual cause, including deliberate or accidental insertion of objects [cotton swabs, bobby pins] or sudden excessive changes in pressure resulting from explosion, a blow to the head, flying, or diving)
• Untreated otitis media
• Acute otitis media in children

Signs and symptoms
• Sudden onset of severe earache
• Sudden onset of bleeding from the ear
• Hearing loss
• Tinnitus
• Vertigo
• Purulent otorrhea. Occurrence within 24 to 48 hours of injury signals infection.

Diagnostic tests
• Direct visualization of the perforated tympanic membrane with an otoscope confirms eardrum perforation.
• Audiometric testing is usually done.
• Voluntary facial movements are tested to rule out facial nerve damage.
• Culture of ear drainage may be ordered.

Treatment and clinical implications
If there is bleeding from the ear, use a sterile, cotton-tipped applicator to absorb the blood, and check for purulent drainage or evidence of cerebrospinal fluid leakage. *Irrigation of the ear is absolutely contraindicated*.

Apply a sterile dressing over the outer ear, and refer the patient to an ear specialist. A large perforation with uncontrolled bleeding may require immediate surgery to approximate the ruptured edges. Treatment may include a mild analgesic, a sedative to decrease anxiety, and an oral antibiotic.

Find out the cause of the injury, and report suspected child abuse. Before discharge, tell the patient not to blow his nose or allow water to enter his ear canal until the perforation heals.

Complications
• Infection
• Hearing loss

Ectopic pregnancy

Description
Ectopic pregnancy is the implantation of the fertilized ovum outside the uterine cavity. The most common site is the fallopian tube (more than 90% of ectopic implantations occur in the fimbria, ampulla, or isthmus), but other possible sites may include the interstitium, tubo-ovarian ligament, ovary,

---

Preventing Ectopic Pregnancy

To prevent ectopic pregnancy, follow these guidelines:
• Advise prompt treatment of pelvic infections to prevent diseases of the fallopian tubes.
• Inform patients who have undergone surgery involving the fallopian tubes or those with confirmed pelvic inflammatory disease that they are at an increased risk for ectopic pregnancy.
• Tell the patient who is vulnerable to ectopic pregnancy to delay using an intrauterine device until after she has completed her family.

---

abdominal viscera, and internal cervical os. In whites, ectopic pregnancy occurs in 1 in 200 pregnancies; in nonwhites, 1 in 120. Maternal prognosis is good with prompt diagnosis, appropriate surgical intervention, and control of bleeding. Rarely, in cases of abdominal implantation, the fetus may survive to term. Usually, subsequent intrauterine pregnancy is achieved.

Causes
Conditions that prevent or retard the passage of the fertilized ovum through the fallopian tube and into the uterine cavity include the following:
• Endosalpingitis
• Tubal diverticula
• Tumors pressing against the tube
• Previous surgery such as tubal ligation or resection
• Adhesions from previous abdominal or pelvic surgery
• Transmigration of the ovum (from one ovary to the opposite tube), resulting in delayed implantation
• Rarely, congenital defects in the reproductive tract or ectopic endometrial implants in the tubal mucosa
• Use of an intrauterine device (IUD) may increase the risk of an ectopic pregnancy.

Signs and symptoms
• Symptoms may be those of normal pregnancy, or there may be no symptoms other than mild abdominal pain (the latter is especially likely in abdominal pregnancy).

• Amenorrhea or abnormal menses, followed by slight vaginal bleeding, and unilateral pelvic pain over the mass may occur after fallopian tube implantation.

Diagnostic tests
The following tests confirm the diagnosis:
• Serum pregnancy test shows presence of human chorionic gonadotropin.
• Real-time ultrasonography determines intrauterine pregnancy or ovarian cyst (performed if serum pregnancy test is positive).
• Culdocentesis is performed if ultrasonography detects the absence of a gestational sac in the uterus. Fluid is aspirated from the vaginal cul-de-sac to detect free blood in the peritoneum.
• Laparoscopy reveals pregnancy outside the uterus (performed if culdocentesis is positive).
• Exploratory laparotomy confirms and treats the ectopic pregnancy by removing the affected fallopian tube (salpingectomy) and controlling bleeding.
• Decreased hemoglobin and hematocrit caused by blood loss support the diagnosis.

Treatment
If culdocentesis is positive for blood in the peritoneum, laparotomy and salpingectomy are indicated, possibly preceded by laparoscopy. Patients who wish to have children can undergo microsurgical repair of the fallopian tube.

The ovary is saved, if possible; however, ovarian pregnancy necessitates oophorectomy. Interstitial pregnancy may require hysterectomy; abdominal pregnancy requires a laparotomy to remove the fetus, except in rare cases, when the fetus survives to term or calcifies undetected in the abdominal cavity.

Supportive treatment includes transfusion with whole blood or packed cells to replace excessive blood loss, administration of broad-spectrum antibiotics I.V. for septic infection, administration of supplemental iron P.O. or I.M., and institution of a high-protein diet.

Clinical implications

Patient care measures include careful monitoring and assessment of vital signs and vaginal bleeding, preparing the patient with excessive blood loss for emergency surgery, and providing blood replacement and emotional support and reassurance.

• Record the location and character of the pain, and administer analgesics, as ordered. (Remember, however, that analgesics may mask the symptoms of intraperitoneal rupture of the ectopic pregnancy.)

• Check the amount, color, and odor of vaginal bleeding. Ask the patient the date of her last menstrual period and to describe the character of this period.

• Observe for signs of pregnancy (enlarged breasts, soft cervix).

• Provide a quiet, relaxing environment, and encourage the patient to freely express her feelings of fear, loss, and grief. (See also *Preventing Ectopic Pregnancy*.)

Complications

Rupture of the tube causes life-threatening complications, which include hemorrhage, shock, and peritonitis.

Signs and symptoms of these complications include the following:

• Sharp lower abdominal pain, possibly radiating to the shoulders and neck, frequently precipitated by activities that increase abdominal pressure, such as a bowel movement

• Extreme pain upon motion of the cervix and palpation of the adnexa during pelvic examination

• Tender, boggy uterus

Electric shock

Description

When an electric current passes through the body, the damage it does depends on the intensity of the current (amperes, milliamperes, or microamperes); the resistance of the tissues it passes through; the kind of current (AC, DC, or mixed); and the frequency and duration of current flow. Electric current can cause injury in three ways: true electrical injury as the current passes through the body, arc or flash burns from current that does not pass through the body, and thermal surface burns caused by associated heat and flames. Usually, the cause of electrical injuries is either obvious or suspected. However, an accurate history can define the voltage and the length of contact. Prognosis depends on the site and extent of damage, the patient's state of health, and the speed and adequacy of treatment.

Causes

• Usually, accidental contact with exposed parts of electrical appliances or wiring

• Lightning

• Electric arcs from high-voltage power lines or machines

Signs and symptoms

Severe electric shock usually causes muscle contraction, loss of consciousness, and loss of reflex control, sometimes with respiratory paralysis.

• Hyperventilation may follow initial muscle contraction after momentary shock.

• Ventricular fibrillation or other dysrhythmias that progress to fibrillation or myocardial infarction may occur if even the smallest electric current passes through the heart.

• Burns, local tissue coagulation and necrosis may occur if electric shock is from a high-frequency current (which generates more heat in tissues than a low-frequency current).

• Serious burns can occur with low-frequency current if contact with the current is concentrated in a small area (for example, when a toddler bites into an electrical cord).

Preventing Electric Shock

The increased use in the hospital of electrical medical devices, many of which are connected directly to the patient, has raised serious concern for electrical safety and has led to the development of electrical safety standards. But even well-designed equipment with reliable safety features can cause electric shock if mishandled.

Prevent electric shock by being alert for electrical hazards:

• Check for cuts, cracks, or frayed insulation on electrical cords, call buttons (also check for warm call buttons), and electrical devices attached to the patient's bed; keep these away from hot or wet surfaces and sharp corners.

• Do not set glasses of water, damp towels, or other wet items on electrical equipment. Wipe up accidental spills before they leak into electrical equipment.

• Avoid using extension cords, because they may circumvent the ground; if they are absolutely necessary, do not place them under carpeting or in areas where they will be walked on.

• Make sure ground connections on electrical equipment are intact. Line cord plugs should have three prongs; the prongs should be straight and firmly fixed. Check that prongs fit wall outlets properly and that outlets are not loose or broken. Do not use adapters on plugs.

• Report faulty equipment promptly to maintenance personnel. If a machine sparks, smokes, seems unusually hot, or gives you or your patient a slight shock, unplug it immediately if doing so will not endanger the patient's life. Check inspection labels and report equipment overdue for inspection.

• Be especially careful when using electrical equipment near patients with pacemakers or direct cardiac lines, because a cardiac catheter or pacemaker can create a direct, low-resistance path to the heart; even a small shock may cause ventricular fibrillation.

• Remember: Dry, calloused, unbroken skin offers more resistance to electric current than mucous membranes, an open wound, or thin, moist skin.

• Make sure defibrillator paddles are free of dry, caked gel before applying fresh gel, because poor electrical contact can cause burns. Also, do not apply too much gel. If the gel runs over the edge of the paddle and touches your hands, you will receive some of the defibrillator shock, and the patient will lose some of the energy in the discharge.

• Tell patients how to avoid electrical hazards at home and at work. Advise parents of small children to put safety guards on all electrical outlets and to keep children away from electrical devices. Warn all patients not to use electrical appliances while showering or wet. Also warn them *never* to touch electrical appliances while touching faucets, or cold-water pipes in the kitchen, because in many cases these pipes provide the ground for all circuits in the house.

Treatment and clinical implications

Immediate emergency treatment includes separating the victim from the current source, quick assessment of vital functions, and emergency measures, such as cardiopulmonary resuscitation (CPR) and defibrillation.

• To separate the victim from the current source, immediately turn it off or unplug it. If that is not possible, pull the victim free with a nonconductive device, such as a loop of dry cloth or rubber, a dry rope, or a leather belt.

• Quickly assess vital functions. If you do not detect a pulse or breathing, start CPR at once. Monitor the patient's cardiac rhythm continuously, and obtain a 12-lead EKG.

• Because internal tissue destruction may be much greater than skin damage indicates, give I.V. lactated Ringer's solution, as ordered, to maintain a urine output of 50 to 100 ml/hour. Insert an indwelling urinary catheter, and send the first specimen to the laboratory.

• Measure intake and output hourly and watch for tea- or port wine-colored urine, which occurs when coagulation necrosis and tissue ischemia liberate myoglobin and hemoglobin. These proteins can precipitate in the renal tubules, causing tubular necrosis and renal shutdown. To prevent that, give mannitol, as ordered.

• Administer sodium bicarbonate, as directed, to counteract acidosis caused by widespread tissue destruction and anaerobic metabolism.

• Assess the patient's neurologic status frequently, because central nervous system damage may result from ischemia or demyelination. Because a spinal cord injury may follow cord ischemia or a compression fracture, watch for sensorimotor deficits.

• Check for neurovascular damage in the extremities by assessing peripheral pulses and capillary refill and by asking about numbness, tingling, or pain. Elevate any injured extremities.

• Apply a temporary sterile dressing, and admit the patient for surgical debridement and observation, as needed. Frequent debridement and use of topical and systemic antibiotics can help reduce the risk of infection. As ordered, prepare the patient for grafting or, if his injuries are extreme, for amputation. (Also see *Preventing Electric Shock*.)

Complications

• Contusions, fractures, and other injuries can result from violent muscle contractions or falls during shock.

• Other complications include renal shutdown, residual hearing impairment, cataracts, and vision loss (may persist after severe electric shock).

Encephalitis

Description

Encephalitis is an inflammatory condition of the brain. Depending on the cause, the severity of encephalitis may range from subclinical to fatal. In this disorder, intense lymphocytic infiltration of brain tissues and the leptomeninges causes cerebral edema, degeneration of the brain's ganglion cells, and diffuse nerve cell destruction. During an encephalitis epidemic, diagnosis is readily made on clinical findings and patient history. However, sporadic cases are difficult to distinguish from other febrile illnesses, such as gastroenteritis or meningitis. Prognosis depends on the cause, the age and condition of the patient, and the extent of the inflammation.

Causes

• Arboviruses specific to rural areas are the usual cause.

• Enteroviruses such as Coxsackievirus, poliovirus, and echovirus are the most frequent cause in urban areas.

• Other causes include herpesvirus, mumps virus, adenoviruses, and demyelinating diseases after measles, varicella, rubella, or vaccination.

Mode of transmission
• The bite of an infected mosquito or tick is the usual mode of transmission.
• Other modes of transmission include ingestion of infected goat's milk or accidental injection or inhalation of the virus.

Signs and symptoms
Characteristic signs and symptoms
—Headache
—Nausea and vomiting
—Stiff neck and back
—Signs of meningeal irritation
Other neurologic disturbances
—Drowsiness
—Seizures
—Personality change
—Paralysis
—Weakness
—Ataxia
—Coma (may persist for days or weeks after the acute phase)

Diagnostic tests
• Identification of the virus in cerebrospinal fluid (CSF) or blood confirms this diagnosis.
• Serologic studies may show rising titers of complement-fixing antibodies in herpes encephalitis.
• CSF pressure is elevated, and despite inflammation, the fluid is frequently clear.
• White blood cell and protein levels in CSF are slightly elevated, but the glucose level remains normal.
• EEG reveals abnormalities.
• Computed tomography scan occasionally may be ordered to rule out cerebral hematoma.

Treatment
The antiviral agent vidarabine is effective only against herpes simplex encephalitis. Treatment of all other forms of encephalitis is entirely supportive. Drug therapy includes phenytoin or another anticonvulsant, usually given I.V.; glucocorticoids to reduce cerebral inflammation and resulting edema; sedatives for restlessness; and aspirin or acetaminophen to relieve headache

and reduce fever. Other supportive measures include adequate fluid and electrolyte intake to prevent dehydration, and appropriate antibiotics for associated infections, such as pneumonia or sinusitis. Isolation is unnecessary.

Clinical implications
During the acute phase of the illness, follow these guidelines:
• Assess neurologic function frequently. Observe level of consciousness and signs of increased intracranial pressure (ICP). Also watch for cranial nerve involvement (ptosis, strabismus, diplopia), abnormal sleep patterns, and behavior changes.
• Maintain adequate fluid intake to prevent dehydration, but avoid fluid overload, which may increase cerebral edema. Measure and record intake and output accurately.
• Give vidarabine by slow I.V. infusion only. Watch for adverse effects, such as tremors, dizziness, hallucinations, anorexia, nausea, vomiting, diarrhea, pruritus, rash, and anemia; also watch for adverse effects of other drugs. Check the infusion site frequently to avoid infiltration and phlebitis.
• Carefully position the patient to prevent joint stiffness and neck pain, and turn him frequently. Assist with range-of-motion exercises.
• Maintain adequate nutrition. It may be necessary to give the patient small, frequent meals or to supplement these meals with nasogastric tube or parenteral feedings.
• To prevent constipation and minimize the risk of increased ICP resulting from straining at stool, give a mild laxative or stool softener.
• Provide good mouth care.
• Maintain a quiet environment. Darkening the room may decrease photophobia and headache. If the patient naps during the day and is restless at night, plan daytime activities to minimize napping and promote sleep at night.

• Provide emotional support and reassurance, because the patient is apt to be frightened by the illness and frequent diagnostic tests.
• If the patient is delirious or confused, attempt to reorient him frequently. (Providing a calendar or a clock in the patient's room may be helpful.)
• Reassure the patient and his family that behavior changes caused by encephalitis usually disappear. If a neurologic deficit is severe and appears permanent, refer the patient to a rehabilitation program as soon as the acute phase has passed.

Complications
Severe inflammation with destruction of nerve tissue may result in a seizure disorder, loss of a specific sense, or other permanent neurologic problem.

Endocarditis
(Infective endocarditis, bacterial endocarditis)

Description
Endocarditis is an infection of the endocardium, heart valves, or cardiac prosthesis, resulting from bacterial (or, in I.V. drug abusers, fungal) invasion. This invasion produces vegetative growths on the heart valves, endocardial lining of a heart chamber, or the endothelium of a blood vessel that may embolize to the spleen, kidneys, central nervous system, and lungs.

Acute infective endocarditis usually results from bacteremia that follows septic thrombophlebitis, open-heart surgery involving prosthetic valves, or skin, bone, and pulmonary infections. This form of endocarditis also occurs in I.V. drug abusers. Subacute infective endocarditis typically occurs in persons with acquired valvular or congenital cardiac lesions. It can also

---

Prosthetic Valve Endocarditis

Increasing use of prosthetic heart valve implants has given rise to prosthetic valve endocarditis, an infection of the artificial valve along the suture line. This disorder can be either acute or subacute. Signs and symptoms usually are similar to those of other forms of endocarditis, although sometimes the only symptoms are fever and murmur from valve dysfunction. Treatment consists of antibiotic therapy and, in many cases, surgery to replace the infected prosthetic valve.

---

follow dental, genitourinary, gynecologic, and GI procedures.

Preexisting rheumatic endocardial lesions are a common predisposing factor in bacterial endocarditis. Rheumatic endocarditis commonly affects the mitral valve; less frequently, the aortic or tricuspid valve; and rarely, the pulmonic valve.

Untreated endocarditis is usually fatal, but with proper treatment, 70% of patients recover. Prognosis is worst when endocarditis causes severe valvular damage, leading to insufficiency and congestive heart failure, or when it involves a prosthetic valve. (Also see *Prosthetic Valve Endocarditis.*)

Causes
• Group A nonhemolytic streptococcus (rheumatic endocarditis), pneumococcus, staphylococcus, and rarely gonococcus are the most common causative organisms of acute infective endocarditis.
• *Staphylococcus aureus, Pseudomonas, Candida,* or usually harmless skin saprophytes are the usual causes of acute endocarditis in I.V. drug users.
• *Streptococcus viridans,* which normally inhabits the upper respiratory tract, and *Streptococcus faecalis* (en-

terococcus), which is usually found in GI and perineal flora, are the most common infecting organisms in subacute infective endocarditis.

Signs and symptoms
Early clinical features
These are usually nonspecific and include the following:
—Weakness
—Fatigue
—Weight loss
—Anorexia
—Arthralgia
—Night sweats
—Intermittent fever (may recur for weeks)
—Loud, regurgitant murmur. This murmur is typical of the underlying rheumatic or congenital heart disease. A suddenly changing murmur or the discovery of a new murmur in the presence of fever is a classic physical sign of endocarditis.
Other signs and symptoms
—Petechiae. These appear on the skin (especially common on the upper anterior trunk); the buccal, pharyngeal, or conjunctival mucosa; and the nails (splinter hemorrhages).
—Tender, raised, subcutaneous lesions on the fingers or toes (Osler's nodes; rare)
—Hemorrhagic areas with white centers on the retina (Roth's spots; rare)
—Purplish macules on the palms or soles (Janeway lesions; rare)
Subacute endocarditis
In about 30% of patients with subacute endocarditis, embolization from vegetating lesions or diseased valve tissue may produce typical features of splenic, renal, cerebral, or pulmonary infarction, or of peripheral vascular occlusion.
—Splenic infarction (pain in the upper left quadrant, radiating to the left shoulder; abdominal rigidity)
—Renal infarction (hematuria, pyuria, flank pain, decreased urine output)
—Cerebral infarction (hemiparesis, aphasia, or other neurologic deficits)

—Pulmonary infarction (most common in right-sided endocarditis, which often occurs among I.V. drug abusers and after cardiac surgery; cough, pleuritic pain, pleural friction rub, dyspnea, and hemoptysis)
—Peripheral vascular occlusion (numbness and tingling in an arm, leg, finger, or toe, or signs of impending peripheral gangrene)

Diagnostic tests
• Three or more blood cultures during a 24- to 48-hour period identify the causative organism in up to 90% of patients. The remaining 10% may have negative blood cultures, possibly suggesting fungal infection.
• White blood cell count is elevated.
• Histocytes (macrophages) are abnormal.
• Erythrocyte sedimentation rate is elevated.
• Normocytic, normochromic anemia may be found in subacute bacterial endocarditis.
• Rheumatoid factor occurs in about half of all patients with endocarditis.
• Echocardiography may identify valvular damage.
• EKG may show atrial fibrillation and other dysrhythmias that accompany valvular disease.

Treatment
The goal of treatment is to eradicate the infecting organism. Therapy should start promptly and continue over several weeks. Antibiotic selection is based on sensitivity studies of the infecting organism—or the probable organism, if blood cultures are negative. I.V. antibiotic therapy usually lasts about 4 weeks.

Supportive treatment includes bed rest, aspirin for fever and aches, and sufficient fluid intake. Severe valvular damage, especially aortic regurgitation, or infection of a cardiac prosthesis may require corrective surgery if refractory heart failure develops.

Clinical implications

• Before giving antibiotics, obtain a patient history of allergies. Administer antibiotics on time to maintain consistent antibiotic blood levels. Check dilutions for compatibility with other medications the patient is receiving, and use a solution that is compatible with drug stability. (For example, add methicillin to a buffered solution.)

• To reduce the risk of I.V. site complications, rotate venous access sites.

• Watch for signs of embolization (hematuria, pleuritic chest pain, left upper quadrant pain, or paresis), a common occurrence during the first 3 months of treatment. Tell the patient to watch for and report these signs, which may indicate impending peripheral vascular occlusion or splenic, renal, cerebral, or pulmonary infarction.

• Monitor the patient's renal status (including blood urea nitrogen and serum, creatinine level, and urine output) to check for signs of renal emboli or drug toxicity.

• Observe for signs of congestive heart failure.

• Provide reassurance by teaching the patient and family about his disease and the need for prolonged treatment. Tell them to watch closely for fever, anorexia, and other signs of relapse about 2 weeks after treatment stops. Suggest quiet diversionary activities to prevent excessive physical exertion.

• Make sure susceptible patients understand the need for prophylactic antibiotics before, during, and after dental work, childbirth, and genitourinary, GI, or gynecologic procedures.

• Teach patients how to recognize symptoms of endocarditis, and tell them to notify the doctor immediately if such symptoms occur.

Endometriosis

Description

Endometriosis is the presence of endometrial tissue outside the lining of the uterine cavity. Such ectopic tissue is usually confined to the pelvic area, most commonly around the ovaries, uterovesical peritoneum, uterosacral ligaments, and the cul-de-sac, but it can appear anywhere in the body. Active endometriosis usually occurs between ages 30 and 40, especially in women who postpone childbearing. It is uncommon before age 20. Severe symptoms of endometriosis may have abrupt onset or may develop over many years. Usually, this disorder becomes progressively severe during the menstrual years; after menopause, it tends to subside.

Causes

The direct cause is unknown, but familial susceptibility or recent surgery that necessitated opening the uterus (such as a cesarean section) may predispose a woman to endometriosis. Although neither of these possible predisposing factors explains all the lesions in endometriosis or their location, research focuses on the following possible causes:

• Transportation: During menstruation, the fallopian tubes expel endometrial fragments that implant on the ovaries or pelvic peritoneum.

• Formation in situ: Inflammation or a hormonal change triggers metaplasia (differentiation of coelomic epithelium to endometrial epithelium).

• Induction: This is a combination of transportation and formation in situ and is the most likely cause. The endometrium chemically induces undifferentiated mesenchyma to form endometrial epithelium.

Signs and symptoms

• Acquired dysmenorrhea. This is the classic symptom of this disorder. It may produce constant pain in the lower abdomen and in the vagina, posterior pelvis, and back. Pain usually begins from 5 to 7 days before menses reaches

Staging Endometriosis

A point system created by the American Fertility Society (AFS) grades endometrial implants or adhesions according to size, character, and location. To determine the stage of endometrial involvement, compare the total number of assigned points to the staging scale below. A score of 1 to 5 indicates minimal involvement (Stage I endometriosis), whereas a score of more than 40 indicates severe involvement (Stage IV endometriosis).

AFS Point System				
Peritoneum	**Endometriosis**	<1 cm	1 to 3 cm	>3 cm
	Superficial	1	2	4
	Deep	2	4	6
Ovary	R Superficial	1	2	4
	R Deep	4	16	20
	L Superficial	1	2	4
	L Deep	4	16	20

Posterior cul-de-sac obliteration	Partial	Complete
	4	40

	Adhesions	<1.3 Enclosure	1.3 to 2.3 Enclosure	>2.3 Enclosure
Ovary	R Filmy	1	2	4
	R Dense	4	8	16
	L Filmy	1	2	4
	L Dense	4	8	16
Tube	R Filmy	1	2	4
	R Dense	4*	8*	16
	L Filmy	1	2	4
	L Dense	4*	8*	16

*If the fimbriated end of the fallopian tube is completely enclosed, change the point assignment to 16.

Staging Scale: Stage I (minimal)—1 to 5, Stage II (mild)—6 to 15 Stage III (moderate)—16 to 40, Stage IV (severe)—> 40

Reprinted with permission from the American Fertility Society, Birmingham, Alabama. © 1985

Teaching Topics in Endometriosis

- An explanation of benign endometrial tissue growth outside the uterus
- Importance of treatment to prevent or postpone complications, such as infertility
- How to recognize endometrioma rupture
- Preparation for laparoscopy and other scheduled tests
- Drugs to relieve pain
- Hormonal therapy, if indicated
- An explanation of surgery options, including their impact on childbearing
- How to relieve dyspareunia
- Effect of pregnancy on endometriosis
- Symptoms and prevention of anemia
- Availability of support groups, such as the Endometriosis Association

its peak and lasts for 2 to 3 days. It differs from primary dysmenorrheal pain, which is more cramping and is concentrated in the abdominal midline. However, the severity of pain does not necessarily indicate the extent of the disease.

- Multiple tender nodules. These occur on uterosacral ligaments or in the rectovaginal system. They enlarge and become more tender during menses.
- Ovarian enlargement

Other clinical features depend on the location of the ectopic tissue:

- Ovaries and oviducts: infertility and profuse menses
- Ovaries or cul-de-sac: deep-thrust dyspareunia
- Bladder: suprapubic pain, dysuria, hematuria
- Rectovaginal septum and colon: painful defecation, rectal bleeding with menses, pain in the coccyx or sacrum
- Small bowel and appendix: nausea and vomiting, which worsen before menses, and abdominal cramps
- Cervix, vagina, and perineum: bleeding from endometrial deposits in these areas during menses

Diagnostic tests

- Laparoscopy may confirm diagnosis and determine the stage of the disease.
- Barium enema rules out malignant or inflammatory bowel disease.

Treatment

Treatment varies according to the stage of the disease (see *Staging Endometriosis*) and the patient's age and desire to have children. Conservative therapy for young women who want to have children includes androgens, such as danazol, which produce a temporary remission in Stages I and II. Progestins and oral contraceptives also relieve symptoms.

When ovarian masses are present (Stages III and IV), surgery is necessary to rule out malignancy. Conservative surgery is possible, but the treatment of choice for women who do not want to bear children or for extensive disease (Stages III and IV) is a total abdominal hysterectomy with bilateral salpingo-oophorectomy.

Clinical implications

- Minor gynecologic procedures are contraindicated immediately before and during menstruation.
- Advise adolescents to use sanitary napkins instead of tampons; that can help prevent retrograde flow in girls with a narrow vagina or small introitus.
- Because infertility is a possible complication, advise the patient who wants children not to postpone childbearing.
- Recommend an annual pelvic examination and Pap smear to all patients. (See also *Teaching Topics in Endometriosis*.)

Complications
• Infertility is the primary complication.
• Spontaneous abortion may also occur.

Enterobiasis
(Pinworm, seatworm, or threadworm infection; oxyuriasis)

Description
Enterobiasis is a benign helminthic infection in which adult pinworms live in the intestine. Female worms migrate to the perianal region to deposit their ova. Enterobiasis infection and reinfection occurs most frequently in children between ages 5 and 14 and in certain institutionalized groups because of poor hygiene and frequent hand-to-mouth activity. Crowded living conditions frequently enhance its spread to several members of a family. Found worldwide, it is common even in temperate regions with good sanitation. It is the most prevalent helminthic infection in the United States.

Cause
The nematode *Enterobius vermicularis*

Mode of transmission
• Direct transmission occurs when the patient's hands transfer infective eggs from the anus to the mouth.
• Indirect transmission occurs when he comes in contact with contaminated articles, such as linens and clothing. The eggs remain viable for 2 or 3 days in contaminated bedclothes.

Signs and symptoms
There may be no symptoms, or intense perianal pruritus may occur, especially at night, disturbing sleep and causing irritability, scratching, skin irritation, and sometimes vaginitis.

Diagnostic tests
Identification of *Enterobius* ova recovered from the perianal area with a cellophane tape swab confirms enterobiasis.

Treatment
Drug therapy with pyrantel, piperazine, or mebendazole destroys these parasites. Effective eradication requires simultaneous treatment of family members and, in institutions, other patients.

Clinical implications
• If the patient receives pyrantel, tell him and his family that this drug colors the stool bright red and may cause vomiting (vomitus will also be red). The tablet form of this drug is coated with aspirin and should not be given to aspirin-sensitive patients.
• Before givine piperazine, obtain a history of convulsive disorders. Piperazine may aggravate these disorders and is contraindicated in a patient with such a history.
• To help prevent this disease, tell parents to bathe children daily (showers are preferable to tub baths) and to change underwear and bed linens daily. Educate children in proper personal hygiene, and stress the need for handwashing after defecation and before handling food. Discourage nail biting. If the child cannot stop, suggest that he wear gloves until the infection clears.
• Report *all* outbreaks of enterobiasis to school authorities.

Epicondylitis
(Tennis elbow, epitrochlear bursitis)

Description
Epicondylitis is inflammation of the forearm extensor supinator tendon fibers at their common attachment to the

lateral humeral epicondyle. Epicondylitis is common among tennis players or persons whose activities require a forceful grasp, wrist extension against resistance, or frequent rotation of the forearm. Because X-rays are almost always negative, diagnosis typically depends on clinical signs and symptoms and a patient history of playing tennis or engaging in similar activities.

Causes

It probably begins as a partial tear owing to repeated strain on the forearm near the lateral epicondyle of the humerus.

Signs and symptoms

• Elbow pain. This initial sign gradually worsens and frequently radiates to the forearm and back of the hand when grasping an object or twisting the elbow.
• Tenderness over the involved lateral or medial epicondyle or over the head of radius
• Weak grasp
• Rarely, local heat, swelling or restricted range of motion

Diagnostic tests

Reproduction of pain by wrist extension and supination with lateral involvement, or by flexion and pronation with medial epicondyle involvement can aid diagnosis.

Treatment

Treatment aims to relieve pain, usually by local injection of corticosteroid and a local anesthetic and by systemic anti-inflammatory therapy with aspirin or indomethacin. Supportive treatment includes an immobilizing splint from the distal forearm to the elbow, which generally relieves pain in 2 to 3 weeks; heat therapy, such as warm compresses, short-wave diathermy, and ultrasound (alone or in combination with diathermy); and physical therapy, such

as manipulation and massage to detach the tendon from the chronically inflamed periosteum. A "tennis elbow strap" has helped many patients. This strap, which is wrapped snugly around the forearm approximately 1" (2.5) cm below the epicondyle, helps relieve the strain on affected forearm muscles and tendons. If these measures prove ineffective, surgical release of the tendon at the epicondyle may be necessary. Untreated epicondylitis can become disabling.

Clinical implications

• Assess level of pain, range of motion, and sensory function. Monitor heat therapy to prevent burns.
• Advise the patient to take anti-inflammatory drugs with food to avoid GI irritation.
• Instruct the patient to rest the elbow until inflammation subsides.
• Remove the support daily, and gently move the arm to prevent stiffness and contracture.
• Instruct the patient to follow the prescribed exercise program. For example, he may stretch his arm and flex his wrist to the maximum, then press the back of his hand against a wall until he can feel a pull in his forearm, and hold this position for 1 minute.
• Advise the patient to warm up for 15 to 20 minutes before beginning any sports activity.
• Urge the patient to wear an elastic support or splint during any activity that stresses the forearm or elbow.

Epidermolysis bullosa

Description

Epidermolysis bullosa (EB) is a heterogenous group of disorders that affect the skin and mucous membranes, producing vesicles and bullae in response to normally harmless heat and frictional trauma. As many as 16 scarring and nonscarring forms may exist, including an acquired form (epidermoylsis acquisita bullosa) that develops after childhood and is not genetically inherited. All nonscarring forms produce a split above the basement membrane, the layer between the epidermis and dermis. Scarring forms produce a split below the basement membrane in the upper part of the dermis. Children with dystrophic EB have been found to have fewer—and abnormal—anchoring fibrils securing the epidermis to the dermis. These children also have more—and abnormal—collagenase, an enzyme that may destroy the anchoring fibrils. Some patients with EB simplex also have deficiencies of other enzymes involved in collagen synthesis.

Prognosis depends on the severity

Caring for Patients with EB

For neonates:
- Use DeLiss catheter or bulb syringe. Avoid wall suction.
- Use sheepskin or soft blanket, not harsh linen.
- Keep skin scrupulously clean, but avoid alcohol or iodine preparations and harsh antibacterial soaps.
- Use Isolette, not overhead warmer, to maintain normal temperature. Check temperature with axillary thermometer.
- Cover large areas of denuded skin with petrolatum gauze, and place strips of it between fingers and toes to delay fusion. Avoid tape; elastic bandages; or adherent, dry dressings.
- Release fluid in blisters by puncturing both sides with a sterile needle or small scissors. Press gently with a gauze pad. Apply wet soaks or antibiotic cream. *Do not* remove blister roof.
- Secure dressings with soft fleece or gauze bandages; remove them by soaking in warm water. Never use adhesive tape or pull clothing from skin.
- Encourage breast-feeding. For formula feeding, use unheated formula and a preemie nipple or rubber-tipped syringe.
- Bathe infant in foam-cushioned plastic tub. Avoid stainless steel basins and washcloths.
- Encourage parents to use infant stimulation techniques, such as music, talking, and mobiles. Encourage them to hold their newborn.

For infants and children:
- Keep child's environment safe by using skin lubricants, padded walkers and swings, and air conditioning. Dress child in soft clothing.
- Lift child from under the buttocks—never from under the arms.
- Provide sheepskin, air, or water mattress for sleeping, and do not place wool, sharp objects, or toys near child.
- Observe for signs of infection, but do not treat without a physician's order.
- Feed the child small portions of a high-protein, complex-carbohydrate diet at frequent intervals, giving him cool fluids, sherbet, or ice pops to soothe his throat before and after each feeding. Use medium-chain triglyceride oil or Polycose, an enteral nutritional supplement. Provide lactose-free products for children who cannot tolerate lactose. Avoid simple sugars, megadoses of vitamins or minerals, or hot, spicy, acidic, or hard-crusted foods.
- Promote good bowel habits with fresh fruits and vegetables, bran, and plenty of fluids. Avoid laxatives.
- Clean teeth with a soft toothbrush, gauze, or sponge.
- Encourage an exercise program of stretching or swimming. Avoid jogging or contact sports.

of the disease. In the nonscarring forms of EB, blisters eventually become less severe and less frequent as the patient matures. But the severe scarring forms commonly cause disability or disfigurement and may be fatal during infancy or childhood.

Causes
• Autosomal dominant inheritance causes the nonscarring forms of EB—except for junctional EB (EB Herlitz or EB letalis), which is recessively inherited.
• Autosomal recessive inheritance is responsible for the scarring forms of EB, except dominant dystrophic EB.
• Sometimes, EB occurs as a mutation in families with no history of blistering disorders.

Signs and symptoms
• Blisters may be generalized or may develop only on hands, feet, knees, or elbows. In some forms of EB, they develop in areas that have not been exposed to trauma or heat.
• Parturition causes widespread blistering and occasional sloughing of large areas of newborn skin.
• Newborns with the severe scarring forms that affect mucous membranes can develop sucking blisters as well as blistering in the GI, respiratory, or genitourinary tracts.
• Other findings may be fusion of fingers and toes, delayed tooth eruption, malformed or carious teeth, alopecia, abnormal nails, retarded growth, anemia, constipation, and malnutrition.

Diagnostic tests
• Skin biopsy of a freshly induced blister using immunofluorescence and electron microscopy confirms which type of EB is present.
• Fetoscopy and biopsy can confirm prenatal diagnosis of the severe scarring forms at 20 weeks' gestation.

Treatment
Phenytoin (Dilantin) may help in recessive dystrophic forms of EB, and corticosteroids and retinoids may help in other forms.

Supportive treatment consists of preventing infection and guarding the skin from trauma and friction through application of protective dressings and skin lubricants. A high-calorie diet containing vitamin and mineral supplements helps combat chronic malnutrition. Iron supplements or transfusions help counteract anemia. Occupational and physical therapy help prevent contractures and deformities.

Clinical implications
Because EB is a visible skin disorder, it tends to disrupt the patient's body image as well as his family's dynamics. In many such families, parents and siblings become overprotective, fostering overdependence in the patient. Parents must also deal with the burden of providing time-consuming personal care, as well as continual advocacy in their child's behalf. Sadly, these parents are sometimes unjustly accused of child abuse by strangers who assume the child's distressing appearance is a result of being burned or beaten.

To help the patient and his family deal with this disease, encourage parents to seek family counseling and join a support group. (Also see *Caring for Patients with EB*.)

Complications
• Infections
• Strictures and adhesions
• Basal cell and squamous cell carcinoma
• Pyloric atresia
• Ocular complications, including eyelid blisters, conjunctivitis, blepharitis, adhesions, and corneal opacities

Epididymitis

Description
This infection of the epididymis, the cordlike excretory duct of the testis, is one of the most common infections of the male reproductive tract. Usually, the causative organisms result from established urinary tract infection or prostatitis and reach the epididymis through the lumen of the vas deferens. Rarely, epididymitis is secondary to a distant infection, such as pharyngitis or tuberculosis, that spreads through the lymphatic system or, less commonly, the bloodstream. It usually affects adults and is rare before puberty. Epididymitis may spread to the testis itself.

Causes
• Pyogenic organisms such as staphylococci, *Escherichia coli*, and streptococci are the usual cause.
• Gonorrhea
• Syphilis
• Chlamydial infection
• Trauma (may reactivate a dormant infection or initiate a new one)
• Prostatectomy
• Chemical irritation (results from extravasation of urine through the vas deferens)

Signs and symptoms
Key signs and symptoms
—Pain
—Extreme tenderness
—Swelling in the groin and scrotum
Other clinical effects
—High fever
—Malaise
—Characteristic waddle (an attempt to protect the groin and scrotum when walking)

Diagnostic tests
Diagnosis requires the following laboratory tests:
• Urinalysis: Increased white blood cell (WBC) count indicates infection.
• Urine culture and sensitivity: Findings may identify the causative organism.
• Serum WBC count: Greater than 10,000/cu mm indicates infection.

Treatment
The goal of treatment is to reduce pain and swelling and combat infection.

Orchitis

Orchitis, infection of the testes, is a serious complication of epididymitis. This infection may also result from mumps, which may lead to sterility, or, less frequently, from another systemic infection, testicular torsion, or severe trauma. Its typical effects include unilateral or bilateral tenderness, gradual onset of pain, and swelling of the scrotum and testes. The affected testis may be red and hot. Nausea and vomiting also occur. Sudden cessation of pain indicates testicular ischemia, which may result in permanent damage to one or both testes.

Treatment consists of immediate antibiotic therapy or, in mumps orchitis, diethylstilbestrol (DES), which may relieve pain, swelling, and fever. Corticosteroids are still experimental. Severe orchitis may require surgery to incise and drain the hydrocele and to improve testicular circulation. Other treatment is similar to that for epididymitis. To prevent mumps orchitis, stress the need for prepubertal males to receive mumps vaccine (or gamma globulin injection after contracting mumps).

In epididymitis accompanied by orchitis, diagnosis must be made cautiously, because symptoms mimic those of testicular torsion, a condition requiring urgent surgical intervention.

Therapy must begin immediately, particularly in the patient with bilateral epididymitis, because sterility is always a threat. During the acute phase, treatment consists of bed rest, scrotal elevation with towel rolls or adhesive strapping, broad-spectrum antibiotics, and analgesics. An ice bag applied to the area may reduce swelling and relieve pain (heat is contraindicated, because it may damage germinal cells, which are viable only at or below normal body temperature). When pain and swelling subside and allow walking, an athletic supporter may prevent pain. Occasionally, corticosteroids may be prescribed to help counteract inflammation, but their use is controversial.

In the older patient undergoing open prostatectomy, bilateral vasectomy may be necessary to prevent epididymitis as a postoperative complication; however, antibiotic therapy alone may prevent it. When epididymitis is refractory to antibiotic therapy, epididymectomy under local anesthetic is necessary.

Clinical implications
• Watch closely for abscess formation (localized, hot, red, tender area) or extension of infection into the testes. Closely monitor temperature, and ensure adequate fluid intake.
• Since the patient is usually very uncomfortable, administer analgesics, as necessary. During bed rest, check frequently for proper scrotum elevation.
• Before discharge, emphasize the importance of completing the prescribed antibiotic therapy, even after symptoms subside.
• If the patient faces the possibility of sterility, suggest supportive counseling, as necessary.

Complications
• Orchitis (Also see *Orchitis*.)
• Sterility (a serious threat in bilateral epididymitis)
• Acute hydrocele (a possible reaction to the inflammatory process)

Epiglottitis

Description
Epiglottitis is an acute inflammation of the epiglottis that tends to cause airway obstruction. It typically strikes children between ages 2 and 8. A critical emergency, epiglottitis can prove fatal in 8% to 12% of victims unless it is recognized and treated promptly.

Causes
• Usually, *Hemophilus influenzae* type B
• Pneumococci
• Group A streptococci

Signs and symptoms
Sometimes preceded by an upper respiratory infection, epiglottitis may rapidly progress to complete upper airway obstruction within 2 to 5 hours.
• Laryngeal obstruction (principal symptom)
• High fever
• Stridor
• Sore throat
• Dysphagia
• Irritability
• Restlessness
• Drooling
• Typical posture. The child attempting to relieve severe respiratory distress may hyperextend his neck, sit up, and lean forward with mouth open, tongue protruding, and nostrils flaring as he tries to breathe. Inspiratory retractions and rhonchi may develop.
• Edematous bright-red epiglottis. Throat examination should not be done if obstruction is severe because complete airway obstruction can occur.

Diagnostic tests
Low lateral neck X-rays reveal the obstruction.

Treatment

A child with acute epiglottitis and airway obstruction requires emergency hospitalization; he may need emergency endotracheal intubation or a tracheotomy and should be carefully monitored in an intensive care unit. Respiratory distress that interferes with swallowing necessitates parenteral fluid administration to prevent dehydration. A patient with acute epiglottitis should always receive a 10-day course of parenteral antibiotics—usually ampicillin. If the child is allergic to penicillin or if there is a significant incidence of ampicillin-resistant endemic *H. influenzae*, chloramphenicol or another antibiotic may be substituted.

Clinical implications

Keep the following equipment available in case of sudden complete airway obstruction: a tracheotomy tray, endotracheal tubes, Ambu bag, oxygen equipment, and a laryngoscope, with blades of various sizes. Monitor arterial blood gases for hypoxia and hypercapnia. Watch for increasing restlessness, increasing cardiac rate, fever, dyspnea, and retractions, which may indicate a need for emergency tracheotomy.

After tracheotomy, anticipate the patient's needs, because he will not be able to cry or call out, and provide emotional support. Reassure the patient and his family that tracheotomy is a short-term intervention (usually from 4 to 7 days). Monitor the patient for rising temperature and pulse rate and hypotension—signs of secondary infection.

Epistaxis
(Nosebleed)

Description

Epistaxis may be a primary or secondary disorder. Such bleeding in children usually originates in the anterior nasal septum and tends to be mild. In adults, such bleeding is most likely to originate in the posterior septum and can be severe. Epistaxis is twice as common in children as in adults. Simple observation confirms epistaxis; inspection with a bright light and nasal speculum is necessary to locate the site of bleeding.

Causes

• Trauma from external or internal causes, such as a blow to the nose, nose picking, or insertion of a foreign body, is the usual cause.
• Polyps
• Acute or chronic infections (sinusitis or rhinitis, for example, which cause congestion and eventual bleeding of the capillary blood vessels)
• Inhalation of chemicals that irritate the nasal mucosa

Risk factors

• Anticoagulant therapy
• Hypertension
• Chronic use of aspirin
• High altitudes and dry climates
• Sclerotic vessel disease
• Hodgkin's disease
• Scurvy
• Vitamin K deficiency
• Rheumatic fever
• Blood dyscrasias, such as hemophilia, purpura, leukemia, and some anemias

Signs and symptoms

Clinical effects depend on the severity of the bleeding. Bleeding is considered severe if it persists longer than 10 minutes after pressure is applied and may cause blood loss as great as 1 liter/hour in adults.
• Usually, unilateral bleeding, except when caused by dyscrasias or severe trauma. Blood oozing from the nostrils usually originates in the anterior nose and is bright red. Blood from the back of the throat originates in the posterior

area and may be dark or bright red (often mistaken for hemoptysis because of expectoration)

• In severe epistaxis, blood seepage behind the nasal septum

• Possible blood in the middle ear and in the corners of the eyes in severe epistaxis

• Light-headedness, dizziness

• Slight respiratory distress

• Shock. Severe hemorrhage causes a drop in blood pressure, rapid and bounding pulse, dyspnea, pallor, and other indications of progressive shock.

Diagnostic tests

Relevant laboratory values include the following:

• Tests show a gradual reduction in hemoglobin and hematocrit; results are frequently inaccurate immediately after epistaxis because of hemoconcentration.

• Platelet count is decreased in a patient with blood dyscrasia.

• Prothrombin time and partial thromboplastin time show a coagulation time twice the control due to a bleeding disorder or anticoagulant therapy.

Treatment

For anterior bleeding, treatment consists of application of a cotton ball saturated with epinephrine to the bleeding site, external pressure, and cauterization by electrocautery or silver nitrate stick. If these measures do not control the bleeding, petrolatum gauze nasal packing may be needed.

For posterior bleeding, therapy includes gauze packing inserted through the nose, or postnasal packing inserted through the mouth, depending on the bleeding site. (Gauze packing usually remains in place for 24 to 48 hours; postnasal packing, 3 to 5 days.) An alternate method, the nasal balloon catheter, also controls bleeding effectively. Antibiotics may be appropriate if packing must remain in place for longer than 24 hours. If local measures fail to control bleeding, additional treatment may include supplemental vitamin K and, for severe bleeding, blood transfusions and surgical ligation of a bleeding artery.

Clinical implications

To control epistaxis, follow these guidelines:

• Elevate the patient's head 45 degrees.

• Compress the soft portion of the nostrils against the septum continuously for 5 to 10 minutes. Apply an ice collar or cold, wet compresses to the nose. If bleeding continues after 10 minutes of pressure, notify the physician.

• Administer oxygen, as needed.

• Monitor vital signs and skin color; record blood loss.

• Instruct the patient to breathe through his mouth. Tell him not to swallow blood, talk, or blow his nose.

• Keep vasoconstrictors, such as phenylephrine, handy.

• Reassure the patient and family that epistaxis usually looks worse than it is.

To prevent recurrence of epistaxis, follow these guidelines:

• Instruct the patient not to pick his nose or insert foreign objects in it. Emphasize the need for follow-up examinations and periodic blood studies after an episode of epistaxis. Advise prompt treatment of nasal infection or irritation, to prevent recurring nose trauma.

• Suggest humidifiers for persons who live in dry climates or at high elevations or whose homes are heated with circulating hot air.

Erectile dysfunction
(Impotence)

Description

Erectile dysfunction refers to a man's inability to attain or maintain penile erection sufficient to complete intercourse. The patient with primary im-

---

Teaching Topics in Impotence

- An explanation of the cause of impotence: psychological or physical
- The importance of treatment to prevent severe depression and psychosocial isolation
- Preparation for nocturnal penile tumescence monitoring, Doppler readings of penile blood pressure, and other diagnostic studies
- Discussion of treatment options, such as hormonal therapy, vasodilators, and penile implants
- Referral for psychiatric counseling, if appropriate

---

potence has never achieved a sufficient erection. Secondary impotence, which is more common and less serious than the primary form, implies that the patient has succeeded in completing intercourse in the past. Secondary erectile dysfunction is classified as follows.

- Partial: The patient is unable to achieve a full erection.
- Intermittent: The patient is sometimes potent with the same partner.
- Selective: The patient is potent only with certain women.

Some patients lose erectile function suddenly; others lose it gradually. If the cause is not organic, erection may still be achieved through masturbation. Transient periods of impotence are not considered dysfunctional and probably occur in half of adult men. Erectile dysfunction affects all age-groups but increases in frequency with age. Personal sexual history provides the most useful clues in differentiating between organic and psychogenic factors and between primary and secondary impotence. Prognosis depends on the severity and duration of impotence and the underlying cause.

Causes
Psychogenic factors
—Intrapersonal factors. These reflect personal sexual anxieties and usually involve guilt, fear, depression, or feelings of inadequacy resulting from previous traumatic sexual experience, rejection by parents or peers, exaggerated religious orthodoxy, abnormal mother-son intimacy, or homosexual experiences.

—Interpersonal factors. These reflect a disturbed sexual relationship and may stem from differences in sexual preferences between partners, lack of communication, insufficient knowledge of sexual function, or nonsexual personal conflicts.

—Stress. This may result in situational impotence, a temporary condition.

Organic factors
—Chronic diseases (cardiopulmonary disease, diabetes, multiple sclerosis, or renal failure, for example)
—Spinal cord trauma
—Complications of surgery
—Drug- or alcohol-induced dysfunction
—Rarely, genital anomalies or central nervous system defects

Signs and symptoms
Problems with penile erection always occur in this disorder. Other symptoms, may or may not be present, such as the following:
- Inability to attain or maintain penile erection
- Anxiety
- Sweating
- Palpitations
- Total disinterest in sexual activity (possible)
- Depression (may result from impotence or cause it)

Treatment

Sex therapy, largely directed at reducing performance anxiety, may effectively cure psychogenic impotence. Such therapy should include both partners.

The course and content of sex therapy for impotence depend on the specific cause of the dysfunction and the nature of the male-female relationship. Usually, therapy includes the concept of sensate focus, which restricts the couple's sexual activity and encourages them to become more attuned to the physical sensations of touching. Sex therapy also includes improving verbal communication skills, eliminating unreasonable guilt, and reevaluating attitudes toward sex and sexual roles.

Treatment of organic impotence focuses on reversing the cause, if possible. If not, psychological counseling may help the couple deal realistically with their situation and explore alternatives for sexual expression. Certain patients suffering from organic impotence may benefit from surgically inserted inflatable or noninflatable penile implants.

Clinical implications

• When you identify a patient with impotence or with a condition that may cause impotence, help him feel comfortable about discussing his sexuality. Assess his sexual health during your initial nursing history. When appropriate, refer him for further evaluation or treatment.

• After penile implant surgery, instruct the patient to avoid intercourse until the incision heals, usually in 6 weeks.

To help prevent impotence, follow these guidelines:

• Promote establishment of responsible health and sex education programs at primary, secondary, and college levels.

• Provide information about resuming sexual activity as part of discharge instructions for any patient with a condition that requires modification of daily activities. Such patients include those with cardiac disease, diabetes, hypertension, and chronic obstructive pulmonary disease, and all postoperative patients. (Also see *Teaching Topics in Impotence*.)

Erythroblastosis fetalis

Description

Erythroblastosis fetalis, a hemolytic disease of the fetus and newborn, stems from an incompatibility of fetal and maternal blood, resulting in maternal antibody activity against fetal red cells. During her first pregnancy, an Rh-negative female becomes sensitized (during delivery or abortion) by exposure to Rh-positive fetal blood antigens inherited from the father. A female may also become sensitized from receiving blood transfusions with alien Rh antigens, causing agglutinins to develop; from inadequate doses of $Rh_o(D)$; or from failure to receive $Rh_o(D)$ after significant fetal-maternal leakage from abruptio placentae.

Subsequent pregnancy with an Rh-positive fetus provokes increasing amounts of maternal agglutinins to cross the placental barrier, attach to Rh-positive cells in the fetus, and cause hemolysis and anemia. To compensate for this, the fetus steps up the production of red blood cells (RBCs), and erythroblasts (immature RBCs) appear in the fetal circulation. Extensive hemolysis results in the release of large amounts of unconjugated bilirubin, which the liver is unable to conjugate and excrete, causing hyperbilirubinemia and hemolytic anemia. To prevent the development of antibodies, $Rh_o(D)$ immune human globulin is given. (Also see *Prevention of Rh Isoimmunization*, p. 274.)

Intrauterine transfusions can save 40% of fetuses; however, in severe,

---

Prevention of Rh Isoimmunization

Administration of $Rh_0(D)$ immune human globu in to an unsensitized Rh-negative mother as soon as possible after the birth of an Rh-positive infant, or after a spontaneous or elective abortion, prevents complications in subsequent pregnancies.

The following patients should be screened for Rh isoimmunization or irregular antibodies:

• all Rh-negative mothers during their first prenatal visit and at 24, 28, 32, and 36 weeks' gestation
• all Rh-positive mothers with histories of transfusion, a jaundiced baby, stillbirth, cesarean birth, induced abortion, placenta previa, or abruptio placentae.

---

untreated erythroblastosis fetalis, prognosis is poor, especially if kernicterus develops. About 70% of these infants die, usually within the first week of life. Severely affected fetuses that develop hydrops fetalis—the most severe form of this disorder—are commonly stillborn. Even if they are delivered live, they rarely survive longer than a few hours. (See also *Hydrops Fetalis.*)

Causes
Rh isoimmunization, a condition that develops in 7% of all pregnancies. (Also see *ABO Incompatibility*, p. 276.)

Signs and symptoms
Mildly affected infant
—Jaundice (usually absent at birth but appears as soon as 30 minutes later or within 24 hours)
—Mild to moderate hepatosplenomegaly
—Pallor
Severely affected infants
—Jaundice (appears as soon as 30 minutes after birth or within 24 hours)
—Pallor
—Edema
—Petechiae
—Hepatosplenomegaly
—Grunting respirations
—Pulmonary rales
—Poor muscle tone

—Neurologic unresponsiveness
—Possible heart murmurs
—Bile-stained umbilical cord
—Yellow or meconium-stained amniotic fluid

Diagnostic tests
Diagnostic evaluation takes into account both prenatal and neonatal findings.
• Prenatal blood typing and screening titers determine changes in the degree of maternal immunization.
• A paternal blood test determines Rh type, blood group, and Rh zygosity.
• Amniotic fluid analysis may show an increase in bilirubin (indicating possible hemolysis) and elevations in anti-Rh titers.
• Radiologic studies may show fetal edema.
• Direct Coombs' test of umbilical cord blood measures RBC (Rh-positive) antibodies in the newborn. Results are positive only when the mother is Rh-negative and the fetus is Rh-positive.
• Decreased cord hemoglobin count (less than 10 g) signals severe disease.
• Many nucleated peripheral RBCs indicate disease in the newborn.

Treatment
Treatment depends on the degree of maternal sensitization and the effects of hemolytic disease on the fetus or newborn.

• Intrauterine-intraperitoneal transfusion is performed when amniotic fluid analysis suggests the fetus is severely affected and delivery is inappropriate because of fetal immaturity. A transabdominal puncture under fluoroscopy into the fetal peritoneal cavity allows infusion of group O, Rh-negative blood. This may be repeated every 2 weeks until the fetus is mature enough for delivery.

• Planned delivery is usually done 2 to 4 weeks before term date, depending on maternal history, serologic tests, and amniocentesis; labor may be induced from the 34th to 38th week of gestation. During labor, the fetus should be monitored electronically; capillary blood scalp sampling determines acid-base balance. Any indication of fetal distress necessitates immediate cesarean delivery.

• Phenobarbital administered during the last 5 to 6 weeks of pregnancy may lower serum bilirubin levels in the newborn.

• Exchange transfusion removes antibody-coated RBCs and prevents hyperbilirubinemia through removal of the infant's blood and replacement with fresh group O, Rh-negative blood.

• Albumin infusion aids in the binding of bilirubin, reducing the chances of hyperbilirubinemia.

• Phototherapy by exposure to ultraviolet light reduces bilirubin levels.

• Gamma globulin that contains anti-Rh-positive antibody ($Rh_o[D]$) can provide passive immunization, which prevents maternal Rh isoimmunization in Rh-negative females. However, it is ineffective if sensitization has already resulted from a previous pregnancy, abortion, or transfusion.

Clinical implications

Structure the care plan around close maternal and fetal observation, explanations of diagnostic tests and therapeutic measures, and emotional support.

• Reassure the parents that they are not at fault in having a child with erythroblastosis fetalis. Encourage them to express their fears concerning possible complications of treatment.

• Before intrauterine transfusion, explain the procedure and its purpose. Before the transfusion, obtain a baseline fetal heart rate through electronic monitoring. Afterward, carefully observe the mother for uterine contractions and fluid leakage from the puncture site. Monitor fetal heart rate

Hydrops Fetalis

Hydrops fetalis, the most severe form of erythroblastosis fetalis, causes extreme hemolysis, fetal hypoxia, heart failure (with possible pericardial effusion and circulatory collapse), edema (ranging from mild peripheral edema to anasarca), peritoneal and pleural effusions (with dyspnea and pulmonary rales), and green- or brown-tinged amniotic fluid (usually indicating a stillbirth).

Other distinctive characteristics of the infant with hydrops fetalis include enlarged placenta, marked pallor, hepatosplenomegaly, cardiomegaly, and ascites. Petechiae and widespread ecchymoses are present in severe cases, indicating concurrent disseminated intravascular coagulation. Radiologic studies may show the halo sign (edematous, elevated, subcutaneous fat layers) and the Buddha position (fetal legs are crossed).

Neonatal therapy for hydrops fetalis consists of maintaining ventilation by intubation, oxygenation, and mechanical assistance, when necessary; and removal of excess fluid to relieve severe ascites and respiratory distress. Other appropriate measures include exchange transfusion and maintenance of the infant's body temperature.

ABO Incompatibility

ABO incompatibility—a form of fetomaternal incompatibility—occurs between mother and fetus in about 25% of all pregnancies, with highest incidence among blacks. In about 1% of this number, it leads to hemolytic disease of the newborn. ABO incompatibility is more common than Rh isoimmunization, but, fortunately, it is less severe. Low antigenicity of fetal or newborn ABO factors may account for the milder clinical effects.

Each blood group has specific antigens on red blood cells and specific antibodies in serum. Maternal antibodies form against fetal cells when blood groups differ. Infants with group A blood, born of group O mothers, account for approximately 50% of all ABO incompatibilities. Unlike Rh isoimmunization, which always follows sensitization during a previous pregnancy, ABO incompatibility is likely to develop in a firstborn infant.

Clinical effects of ABO incompatibility include jaundice, which usually appears in the newborn in 24 to 48 hours, mild anemia, and hepatosplenomegaly.

Diagnosis is based on clinical symptoms in the newborn, a weak to moderately positive Coombs' test, and elevated serum bilirubin levels. Cord hemoglobin and indirect bilirubin levels indicate the need for exchange transfusion. An exchange transfusion is done with blood of the same group and Rh type as that of the mother. Fortunately, because infants with ABO incompatibility respond so well to phototherapy, exchange transfusion is seldom necessary.

Blood group	Antigens on RBCs	Antibodies in serum	Most common incompatible groups
A	A	Anti-B	Mother A, infant B or AB
B	B	Anti-A	Mother B, infant A or AB
AB	A and B	No antibodies	Mother AB, infant (no incompatibility)
O	No antigens	Anti-A and anti-B	Mother O, infant A or B

for tachycardia or bradycardia.
• During exchange transfusion, maintain the infant's body temperature by placing him under a heat lamp or overhead radiant warmer. Keep resuscitative and monitoring equipment handy, and warm blood before transfusion.
• Watch for complications of exchange transfusion, such as lethargy, muscular twitching, convulsions, dark urine, edema, and change in vital signs. Watch for postexchange serum bilirubin levels that are usually 50% of preexchange levels (although these levels may rise to 70% to 89% of preexchange levels because of rebound

effect). Within 30 minutes of transfusion, bilirubin may rebound, requiring repeat exchange transfusions.
• Measure intake and output. Observe for cord bleeding and complications, such as hemorrhage, hypocalcemia, sepsis, and shock. Report serum bilirubin and hemoglobin levels.
• To promote normal parental bonding, encourage parents to visit and to help care for the infant as frequently as possible.

Complications
• Kernicterus. This develops in about 10% of untreated infants. Symptoms include anemia, lethargy, poor suck-

ing ability, retracted head, stiff extremities, squinting, a high-pitched cry, and convulsions.

• **Neurologic damage.** Sensory impairment, mental deficiencies, and cerebral palsy may develop in survivors.

Esophageal cancer

Description

Esophageal cancer develops most commonly in men over 60 years of age. More than 8,000 cases are reported annually in the United States alone. Esophageal tumors are usually fungating and infiltrating. Most arise in squamous cell epithelium. A few are adenocarcinomas; fewer still are melanomas and sarcomas.

About half of squamous cell cancers occur in the lower portion of the esophagus, about 40% in the midportion, and the remaining 10% in the upper or cervical esophagus. Regardless of cell type, prognosis for esophageal cancer is grim. Five-year survival rates do not exceed 10%.

In most cases, the tumor partially constricts the lumen of the esophagus. Regional metastasis occurs early, by way of submucosal lymphatics, and, in many cases, the tumor fatally invades adjacent vital intrathoracic organs. If the patient survives primary extension, the liver and lungs are the usual sites of distant metastasis. Rarer sites of metastasis include bone, kidneys, and adrenals.

Causes

Unknown

Risk factors

• Chronic irritation from heavy smoking and excessive use of alcohol
• Stasis-induced inflammation, as in achalasia or stricture
• Previous head and neck tumors
• Nutritional deficiency, as in untreated sprue and Plummer-Vinson syndrome

Signs and symptoms

Early signs
—Dysphagia (occurs only after ingestion of solid food [especially meat])
—Weight loss
Later signs
—Constant dysphagia
—Pain on swallowing
—Hoarseness
—Coughing
—Glossopharyngeal neuralgia
—Esophageal obstruction (in late stages, sialorrhea, nocturnal aspiration, regurgitation, and inability to swallow even liquids)
—Cachexia

Diagnostic tests

Tests that confirm esophageal tumors include the following:
• Punch and brush biopsies
• Exfoliative cytologic tests
• Endoscopic examination of the esophagus

Tests that reveal structural and filling defects and reduced peristalsis include the following:
• X-rays of the esophagus with barium swallow
• Motility studies

Treatment

Whenever possible, treatment includes resection to maintain a passageway for food. This often involves radical surgery, such as esophagogastrectomy with jejunal or colonic bypass grafts. Palliative surgery may include a feeding gastrostomy. Treatment also consists of radiation, chemotherapy (for example, with bleomycin), or installation of prosthetic tubes (such as the Mousseau Barbin or Celestin's tubes) to bridge the tumor and alleviate dysphagia. Unfortunately, none of these methods is completely successful. Surgery can cause its own complications (anastomotic leak, fistula formation, pneumonia, empyema, malnutrition). Radiation can cause esophageal perforation, pneumonitis and fibrosis of the lungs, or myelitis of the spinal cord. Prosthetic tubes can become blocked or dislodged, causing a perforation of the mediastinum, or can precipitate tumor erosion.

Clinical implications
• Before surgery, answer the patient's questions, and offer reassurance by letting him know what to expect. Explain the procedures he will experience after surgery—closed chest drainage, nasogastric suctioning, and gastrostomy tubes.
• After surgery, monitor vital signs. Report any unexpected changes to the physician immediately. If surgery has included an anastomosis to the esophagus, position the patient flat on his back to prevent tension on the suture line.
• Your primary goal is to promote adequate nutrition—a difficult task in such patients. Assess the patient's nutritional and hydration status for possible supplementary parenteral feedings.
• Prevent aspiration of food by placing the patient in the Fowler position for meals and allowing plenty of time to eat. Provide high-calorie, high-protein, "blenderized" food, as needed. Because the patient will probably regurgitate some food, clean his mouth carefully after each meal. Keep mouthwash handy.
• If the patient has a gastrostomy tube, give food slowly—by gravity—in prescribed amounts (usually 200 to 500 ml). Offer something to chew before each feeding. This promotes gastric secretions and provides some semblance of normal eating.
• Instruct the family in gastrostomy tube care (checking tube patency before each feeding, providing skin care around the tube, keeping the patient upright during and after feedings).

• Provide emotional support for the patient and family; refer them to appropriate organizations such as the American Cancer Society.

Complications
Direct invasion of adjoining structures may lead to the following dramatic complications:
• Mediastinitis
• Tracheoesophageal or bronchoesophageal fistulas (causing an overwhelming cough induced by swallowing liquids)
• Aortic perforation with sudden exsanguination

Esophageal diverticula

Description
Esophageal diverticula are hollow outpouchings of one or more layers of the esophageal wall. They occur in three main areas: just above the upper esophageal sphincter (Zenker's, or pulsion), near the midpoint of the esophagus (traction), and just above the lower esophageal sphincter (epiphrenic). Esophageal diverticula usually occur in middle to late adulthood—although they can affect infants and children—and are three times more common in men than in women. Zenker's diverticula, the most common type, usually occurs in men over age 60. Epiphrenic diverticula usually occur in middle-aged men.

Causes
• Primary muscular abnormalities that may be congenital
• Inflammatory processes adjacent to the esophagus

Signs and symptoms
Midesophageal and epiphrenic diverticulum with an associated motor disturbance, such as achalasia or spasm
—Seldom produces symptoms

—Dysphagia and heartburn may occur.

Zenker's diverticulum
—Throat irritation initially (progressing to dysphagia and near-complete obstruction)
—Regurgitation (occurs soon after eating in early stages; delayed in later stages and may even occur during sleep, leading to food aspiration and pulmonary infection)
—Noise when liquids are swallowed
—Chronic cough
—Hoarseness
—Bad taste in the mouth or foul breath
—Rarely, bleeding

Diagnostic tests
• X-rays taken after a barium swallow usually confirm diagnosis by showing characteristic outpouching.
• Esophagoscopy can rule out another lesion; however, the procedure risks rupturing the diverticulum by passing the scope into it rather than into the lumen of the esophagus, a special danger with Zenker's diverticulum.

Treatment
Treatment of Zenker's diverticulum is usually palliative and includes a bland diet, thorough chewing, and drinking water after eating to flush the sac. However, severe symptoms or a large sac necessitates surgery to remove it or facilitate drainage. An esophagomyotomy may be necessary to prevent recurrence.

A midesophageal diverticulum seldom requires therapy except when esophagitis aggravates the risk of rupture. Then, treatment includes antacids and an antireflux regimen: keeping the head elevated, maintaining an upright position for 2 hours after eating, eating small meals, controlling chronic coughing, and avoiding constrictive clothing.

Epiphrenic diverticulum requires treatment of accompanying motor disorders, such as achalasia, by repeated dilatations of the esophagus; of acute spasm by anticholinergic administration and diverticulum excision; and of dysphagia or severe pain by surgical excision or suspending the diverticulum to promote drainage. Depending on the patient's nutritional status, treatment may also include insertion of a nasogastric tube (passed carefully to prevent perforation) and tube feedings to prepare for the stress of surgery.

Clinical implications
• Carefully observe and document symptoms.
• Regularly assess nutritional status (weight, caloric intake, appearance).
• If the patient regurgitates food and mucus, protect against aspiration by careful positioning (head elevated or turned to one side). To prevent aspiration, tell the patient to empty any visible outpouching in the neck by massage or postural drainage before retiring.
• If the patient has dysphagia, record well-tolerated foods and what circumstances ease swallowing. Provide a "blenderized" diet, with vitamin or protein supplements, and encourage thorough chewing.
• Teach the patient about this disorder. Explain treatment instructions and diagnostic procedures.

Exophthalmos
(Proptosis)

Description
Exophthalmos is the unilateral or bilateral bulging or protrusion of the eyeballs or their apparent forward displacement (with lid retraction). It is obvious on physical examination. Prognosis depends on the underlying cause.

Causes
Usual causes
—Graves' disease
—Trauma. (For example, fracture of the ethmoid bone, which allows air from the sinus to enter the orbital tissue, displacing soft tissue and the eyeball, is a cause of unilateral exophthalmos.)
—Hemorrhage
—Varicosities
—Thrombosis
—Aneurysms
—Edema
Other systemic and ocular causes
—Infection (orbital cellulitis, panophthalmitis, and infection of the lacrimal gland or orbital tissues)
—Tumors and neoplastic diseases (especially in children: rhabdomyosarcomas, leukemia, gliomas of the optic nerve, dermoid cysts, teratomas, metastatic neuroblastomas, and Burkitt's lymphoma; in adults: lacrimal gland tumors, mucoceles, meningiomas, and metastatic carcinomas)
—Parasitic cysts in surrounding tissue
—Extraocular muscle paralysis (relaxation of eyeball retractors, congenital macrophthalmia, and high myopia)

Signs and symptoms
• Bulging eyeball (common with diplopia if extraocular muscle edema causes misalignment)
• Visible sclera
• Infrequent blinking
   Other symptoms depend on the cause:
• Pain may accompany traumatic exophthalmos.
• Conjunctival hyperemia or chemosis may be caused by a tumor.
• Paresis of the muscles supplied by cranial nerves III, IV, and VI, limited ocular movement, and a septic-type

(high) fever may occur if exophthalmos is associated with cavernous sinus thrombosis.

Diagnostic tests
• Exophthalmometer readings confirm diagnosis by showing the degree of anterior projection and asymmetry between the eyes (normal bar readings range from 12 to 20 mm). Other diagnostic measures identify the cause.
• X-rays show orbital fracture or bony erosion by an orbital tumor.
• Computed tomography scan detects pathology (lesions of the optic nerve, orbit, or ocular muscle) in the area of the orbit that is, relatively, radiologically blind.
• Culture of discharge from cellulitis or panophthalmitis determines the infecting organism; sensitivity testing indicates appropriate antibiotic therapy.
• Biopsy of orbital tissue may be necessary if initial treatment fails.

Treatment
The goal of treatment is to correct the underlying cause. For example, eye trauma may require cold compresses for the first 24 hours, followed by warm compresses, and prophylactic antibiotic therapy. After edema subsides, surgery may be necessary. Eye infection requires treatment with broad-spectrum antibiotics during the 24 hours preceding positive identification of the organism, followed by specific antibiotics. A patient with exophthalmos resulting from an orbital tumor may initially benefit from antibiotic or corticosteroid therapy. Eventually, however, surgical exploration of the orbit and, depending on the tumor, excision of the tumor, enucleation, or exenteration may be necessary. When primary orbital tumors, such as rhabdomyosarcoma, cannot be

fully excised as encapsulated lesions, radiation and chemotherapy may be used.

Treatment of Graves' disease may include antithyroid drug therapy or partial or total thyroidectomy to control hyperthyroidism; initial high doses of systemic corticosteroids, such as prednisone, for optic neuropathy; and, if lid retraction is severe, application of protective lubricants.

Surgery may include lateral tarsorrhaphy (suturing the lateral sections of the eyelids together) to correct lid retraction, or Krönlein's operation (removal of the superior and lateral orbital walls) to decompress the orbit. Such decompression is necessary if vision is threatened.

Clinical implications
• Administer medication (steroids, antibiotics), as ordered, and carefully record the patient's response to therapy.
• Apply cold and warm compresses, as ordered, for fractures or other trauma.
• Provide postoperative care.
• Explain tests and procedures thoroughly to the patient and family.
• Give emotional support, especially to those with sudden exophthalmos.

Fanconi's syndrome
(de Toni-Fanconi syndrome)

Description
Fanconi's syndrome is a renal disorder that produces malfunctions of the proximal renal tubules, such as shortening of the connection to glomeruli by an abnormally narrow segment (swan's neck)—a result of the atrophy of epithelial cells and loss of proximal tubular mass volume. Idiopathic congenital Fanconi's syndrome is most prevalent in children and affects both sexes equally. Onset of the hereditary form usually occurs during the first 6 months of life, although another hereditary form also occurs in adults. The more serious adult form of this disease is acquired Fanconi's syndrome. Because treatment of Fanconi's syndrome is usually unsuccessful, it commonly leads to end-stage renal failure, and the patient may survive only a few years after its onset.

Causes
• Congenital
• Acquired, secondary to Wilson's disease, cystinosis, galactosemia, or exposure to a toxic substance (heavy metal poisoning)

Signs and symptoms
Infants
Birth weight may be low, but most symptoms appear at about age 6 months.
—Failure to thrive
—Weakness
—Dehydration (associated with polyuria, vomiting, and anorexia)
—Constipation
—Acidosis
—Cystine crystals in the cornea and conjunctiva
—Peripheral retinal pigment degeneration
—Yellow skin with little pigmentation, even in summer
—Slow linear growth
—Osteomalacia
—Acidosis
—Potassium loss
—Rarely, renal calculi
Adults
—Osteomalacia
—Muscle weakness
—Paralysis
—Metabolic acidosis

Diagnostic tests
• Evidence of excessive 24-hour urinary excretion of glucose, phosphate, amino acids, bicarbonate, and potassium is required for diagnosis. Generally, serum values are correspondingly decreased.
• Hyperchloremic acidosis and hypokalemia support the diagnosis. (*Caution:* Glucose tolerance test is contraindicated for these patients, because it may cause a fatal shocklike reaction.)
• Other results include elevated phosphorus and nitrogen levels with increased renal dysfunction, and increased alkaline phosphatase with rickets.

• Serum sample from a child with refractory rickets shows increased alkaline phosphatase level and, with renal dysfunction, decreased calcium level.

Treatment
Treatment is symptomatic, with replacement therapy appropriate to the patient's specific deficiencies. For example, a patient with rickets receives large doses of vitamin D; with acidosis and hypokalemia, supplements containing a flavored mixture of sodium and potassium citrate; and with hypocalcemia, calcium supplements (close monitoring is necessary to prevent hypercalcemia). When diminishing renal function produces hyperphosphatemia, treatment includes aluminum hydroxide antacids to bind phosphate in the intestine and prevent its absorption. Acquired Fanconi's syndrome requires treatment of the underlying cause. End-stage Fanconi's syndrome occasionally requires dialysis. Other treatment is symptomatic.

Clinical implications
• Help the patient with acquired Fanconi's syndrome or the parents of an infant with inherited Fanconi's syndrome understand the seriousness of this disease (including the possibility of dialysis) and the need to comply with drug and dietary therapy. If the patient has rickets, help him accept the changes in his body image.
• Because the prognosis for acquired Fanconi's syndrome is poor, the patient with this disorder may be apathetic about taking medication. Encourage compliance with therapy.
• Monitor renal function closely. Make sure 24-hour urine specimens are collected accurately. Watch for fluid and electrolyte imbalances, particularly hypokalemia and hyponatremia; disturbed regulatory function characterized by anemia and hypertension; and uremic symptoms characteristic of renal failure (oliguria, anorexia, vomiting, muscle twitching, and pruritus).
• Instruct the patient with acquired Fanconi's syndrome to follow a diet for chronic renal failure, as ordered.

Femoral and popliteal aneurysms
(Peripheral arterial aneurysms)

Description
Femoral and popliteal aneurysms are the end result of progressive atherosclerotic changes occurring in the walls (medial layer) of these major peripheral arteries. These aneurysmal formations may be fusiform (spindle-shaped) or saccular (pouchlike). Fusiform aneurysms occur three times more frequently. They may be single or multiple segmental lesions, in many cases affecting both legs, and may accompany other arterial aneurysms located in the abdominal aorta or iliac arteries. This condition occurs most frequently in men over age 50. Elective surgery before complications arise greatly improves prognosis.

Causes
• Secondary to atherosclerosis
• Rarely, congenital weakness in the arterial wall
• Trauma (blunt or penetrating)
• Bacterial infection
• Peripheral vascular reconstructive surgery (which causes "suture line" aneurysms, whereby a blood clot forms a second lumen; also called false aneurysms)

Signs and symptoms
• Pain in the popliteal space may occur when popliteal aneurysms are large enough to compress the medial popliteal nerve.
• Edema and venous distention occurs in popliteal aneurysms if the aneurysm compresses the vein.
• Symptoms of severe ischemia may occur in the leg or foot.

• A pulsating mass above or below the inguinal ligament found on bilateral palpation identifies femoral aneurysm. A firm, nonpulsating mass identifies thrombosis.

Diagnostic tests
• Arteriography is helpful in identifying aneurysms if positive identification cannot be made on palpation. It may also detect associated aneurysms, especially those in the abdominal aorta and the iliac arteries.
• Ultrasound can also help identify aneurysms in doubtful situations. It also may be helpful in determining the size of the popliteal or femoral artery.

Treatment
Femoral and popliteal aneurysms require surgical bypass and reconstruction of the artery, usually with an autogenous saphenous vein graft replacement. Arterial occlusion that causes severe ischemia and gangrene may require leg amputation.

Clinical implications
Before corrective surgery, follow these guidelines:
• Assess and record circulatory status, noting location and quality of peripheral pulses in the affected arm or leg.
• Administer prophylactic antibiotics or anticoagulants, as ordered.

After arterial surgery, follow these guidelines:
• Monitor carefully for early signs of thrombosis or graft occlusion (loss of pulse, decreased skin temperature and sensation, severe pain) and infection (fever).
• Palpate distal pulses at least every hour for the first 24 hours, then as frequently as ordered. Correlate these findings with preoperative circulatory assessment. Mark the sites on the patient's skin where pulses are palpable, to facilitate repeated checks.
• Help the patient walk soon after surgery, to prevent venostasis and possible thrombus formation.

To prepare the patient for discharge, follow these guidelines:
• Tell the patient to report immediately any recurrence of symptoms, since the saphenous vein graft replacement can fail or another aneurysm may develop.
• Explain to the patient with popliteal artery resection that swelling may persist for some time. If antiembolism stockings are ordered, make sure they fit properly, and teach the patient how to apply them. Warn against wearing constrictive apparel.
• If the patient is receiving anticoagulants, suggest measures to prevent bleeding, such as using an electric razor. Tell the patient to report any signs of bleeding immediately (bleeding gums, tarry stools, easy bruising). Explain the importance of follow-up blood studies to monitor anticoagulant therapy. Warn him to avoid trauma, tobacco, and aspirin.

Complications
The clinical course of untreated femoral and popliteal aneurysms is usually progressive, eventually leading to the following problems:
• Acute thrombosis within the aneurysmal sac. Symptoms include severe pain, loss of pulse and color, coldness in the affected leg or foot, and gangrene.
• Embolization of mural thrombus fragments. Distal petechial hemorrhages may develop from aneurysmal emboli.
• Rarely, the aneurysm may rupture.

Folic acid deficiency anemia

Description
Folic acid deficiency anemia is a common, slowly progressive megaloblastic anemia. It occurs most frequently in infants, adolescents, pregnant and lactating women, alcoholic persons, elderly persons, and in persons with malignant or intestinal diseases.

Causes

Folic acid deficiency anemia may result from the following:

- Alcohol abuse (may suppress metabolic effects of folate)
- Poor diet (common in alcoholic persons, elderly persons living alone, and infants, especially those with infections or diarrhea)
- Impaired absorption (the result of intestinal dysfunction in disorders such as celiac disease, tropical sprue, regional jejunitis, or bowel resection)
- Bacteria (the result of competition for available folic acid)
- Excessive cooking (can destroy a high percentage of folic acid in foods)
- Limited storage capacity (in infants)
- Prolonged drug therapy (anticonvulsants, estrogens)
- Increased folic acid requirement (occurs during pregnancy, during rapid growth in infancy [common because of recent increase in survival of premature infants], during childhood and adolescence [because of general use of folate-poor cow's milk], and in patients with neoplastic diseases and some skin diseases [chronic exfoliative dermatitis])

Signs and symptoms

Folic acid deficiency anemia gradually produces clinical features characteristic of other megaloblastic anemias, without the neurologic manifestations, unless it is associated with vitamin B_{12} deficiency.

- Progressive fatigue
- Shortness of breath
- Palpitations
- Weakness
- Glossitis
- Nausea
- Anorexia
- Headache
- Fainting
- Irritability
- Forgetfulness
- Pallor
- Slight jaundice

Foods High in Folic Acid Content

Folic acid (pteroylglutamic acid, folacin) is found in most body tissues, where it acts as a coenzyme in metabolic processes involving one carbon transfer. It is essential for formation and maturation of red blood cells, and for synthesis of deoxyribonucleic acid (DNA). Although its body stores are comparatively small (about 70 mg), this vitamin is plentiful in most well-balanced diets.

However, because it is water-soluble and heat-labile, it is easily destroyed by cooking. Also, approximately 20% of folic acid intake is excreted unabsorbed. Insufficient daily folic acid intake (< 50 mcg/day) usually induces folic acid deficiency within 4 months. Below is a list of foods high in folic acid content.

FOOD	mcg/100 g
Asparagus spears	109
Beef liver	294
Broccoli spears	54
Collards (cooked)	102
Mushrooms	24
Oatmeal	33
Peanut butter	57
Red beans	180
Wheat germ	305

Diagnostic tests

- The Schilling test and a therapeutic trial of vitamin B_{12} injections distinguish between folic acid deficiency anemia and pernicious anemia.
- Significant blood findings include macrocytosis, decreased reticulocyte count, abnormal platelets, and serum folate less than 4 mg/ml.

Treatment

Treatment consists primarily of folic acid supplements and elimination of contributing causes. Folic acid supplements may be given orally (usually 1 to 5 mg/day) or parenterally (to patients who are severely ill, have malabsorption, or are unable to take oral medication). Many patients respond favorably to a well-balanced diet. (Also see *Foods High in Folic Acid Content,* p. 286.)

Clinical implications
• Teach the patient to meet daily folic acid requirements by including a food from each food group in every meal. If the patient has a severe deficiency, explain that diet only reinforces folic acid supplementation and is not therapeutic by itself. Urge compliance with the prescribed course of therapy. Advise the patient not to stop taking the supplements when he begins to feel better.
• If the patient has glossitis, emphasize the importance of good oral hygiene. Suggest regular use of mild or diluted mouthwash and a soft toothbrush.
• Watch fluid and electrolyte balance, particularly in the patient who has severe diarrhea and is receiving parenteral fluid replacement therapy.
• Remember that anemia causes severe fatigue. Schedule regular rest periods until the patient is able to resume normal activity.
• To prevent folic acid deficiency anemia, emphasize the importance of a well-balanced diet high in folic acid. Identify alcoholic persons with poor dietary habits, and try to arrange for appropriate counseling. Tell mothers who are not breast-feeding to use commercially prepared formulas.

Folliculitis, furunculosis, and carbunculosis

Description
Folliculitis is a bacterial infection of the hair follicle that causes the formation of a pustule. The infection can be superficial (follicular impetigo or Bockhart's impetigo) or deep (sycosis barbae). Folliculitis may also lead to the development of furuncles (furunculosis), commonly known as boils, or carbuncles (carbunculosis), especially if exacerbated by irritation, pressure, friction, or perspiration. Prognosis depends on the severity of the infection and on the patient's physical condition and ability to resist infection. (Also see *Forms of Bacterial Skin Infection.*)

Causes
Coagulase-positive *Staphylococcus aureus* is the most common cause.

Risk factors
Predisposing factors include:
• An infected wound elsewhere on the body
• Poor personal hygiene
• Debilitation
• Diabetes
• Exposure to chemicals (cutting oils)
• Management of skin lesions with tar or with occlusive therapy, using steroids

Signs and symptoms
Folliculitis
—Pustules (usually appear on the scalp, arms, and legs in children; on the face of bearded men [sycosis barbae]; and on the eyelids [styes])
—Pain (may occur with deep folliculitis)
Furunculosis
—Hard, painful nodules (commonly develop on the neck, face, axillae, and buttocks; enlarge for several days and then rupture, discharging pus and necrotic material)
—Pain (subsides after rupture)
—Erythema and edema (may persist for several weeks)
Carbunculosis
—Extremely painful, deep abscesses. These drain through multiple openings onto the skin surface, usually around several hair follicles.
—Fever
—Malaise

Forms of Bacterial Skin Infection

Degree of hair follicle involvement in bacterial skin infection ranges from superficial erythema and pustule of a single follicle to deep abscesses (carbuncles) involving several follicles.

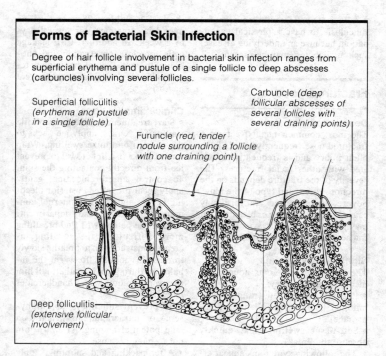

Superficial folliculitis *(erythema and pustule in a single follicle)*

Furuncle *(red, tender nodule surrounding a follicle with one draining point)*

Carbuncle *(deep follicular abscesses of several follicles with several draining points)*

Deep folliculitis *(extensive follicular involvement)*

Diagnostic tests
• Wound culture shows *S. aureus*.
• Complete blood count may show elevated white blood cell count (leukocytosis).

Treatment
Treatment of folliculitis consists of cleansing the infected area thoroughly with soap and water; applying hot, wet compresses to promote vasodilation and drainage of infected material from the lesions; and administering topical antibiotics, such as bacitracin and polymyxin B, and in recurrent infection, systemic antibiotics.

Furunculosis may also require incision and drainage of ripe lesions after application of hot, wet compresses, and topical antibiotics after drainage. Treatment of carbunculosis requires systemic antibiotics.

Clinical implications
Care for folliculitis, furunculosis, and carbunculosis is basically supportive, and emphasizes patient teaching of scrupulous personal and family hygiene, dietary modifications (reduced intake of sugars and fats), and precautions to prevent spreading infection.
• Caution the patient never to squeeze a boil, because that may cause it to rupture into the surrounding area.
• To avoid spreading bacteria to family members, urge the patient not to share his towel and washcloth. Tell him that these items should be boiled in hot water before being reused. The patient should change his clothes and bedsheets daily, and these also should be washed in hot water. Encourage the patient to change dressings frequently and to discard them promptly in paper bags.

• Advise the patient with recurrent furunculosis to have a physical examination, because an underlying disease, such as diabetes, may be present.

Fractured nose

Description
The most common facial fracture, a fractured nose frequently results from blunt injury and is frequently associated with other facial fractures. The severity of the fracture depends on the direction, force, and type of the blow. Severe, comminuted fracture may cause extreme swelling or bleeding that may jeopardize the airway and require tracheotomy during early treatment.

Signs and symptoms
The following symptoms appear immediately after injury:
• Possible nosebleed (ranges from minimal trickling to full nasal hemorrhage)
• Soft-tissue swelling (may quickly obscure the break)
  The following symptoms appear after several hours:
• Pain
• Periorbital ecchymosis
• Nasal displacement and deformity
• Possible clear fluid drainage (suggests a cerebrospinal fluid [CSF] leak)

Diagnostic tests
X-rays help confirm the diagnosis, which also requires palpation, clinical findings, and patient history.

Treatment
Treatment restores normal facial appearance and reestablishes bilateral nasal passage after swelling subsides. Reduction of the fracture corrects alignment; immobilization (intranasal packing and an external splint shaped to the nose and taped) maintains it. Such reduction is best accomplished in the operating room, with local anesthesia for adults and general anes-

thesia for children. Severe swelling may delay treatment for several days to a week. In addition, CSF leakage calls for close observation and antibiotic therapy. Septal hematoma requires incision and drainage to prevent necrosis.

Clinical implications
• Start treatment immediately. While waiting for X-rays, apply ice packs to the nose to minimize swelling. Wrap the ice packs in a light towel to prevent ice from directly contacting the skin. To control anterior bleeding, gently apply local pressure. Posterior bleeding is rare and requires internal tamponade in the emergency department.
• Since the patient will find breathing more difficult as the swelling increases, instruct him to breathe slowly through his mouth. To warm the inhaled air during cold weather, tell him to cover his mouth with a handkerchief or scarf.
• To prevent subcutaneous emphysema or intracranial air penetration (and potential meningitis), warn him not to blow his nose.
• After packing and splinting, apply ice in a plastic bag.
• Before discharge, tell the patient that ecchymosis should fade after about 2 weeks.

Complications
• Septal hematoma may lead to abscess formation, resulting in avascular and septal necrosis.
• Permanent nasal displacement, septal deviation, and obstruction may occur if treatment is inadequate or delayed.

Fractured skull

Description
A skull fracture is considered a neurosurgical condition, because possible damage to the brain is the first con-

cern, rather than the fracture itself. Skull fractures may be simple (closed) or compound (open) and may or may not displace bone fragments. Skull fractures are further described as linear, comminuted, or depressed. A linear fracture is a common hairline break, without displacement of structures; a comminuted fracture splinters or crushes the bone into several fragments; a depressed fracture pushes the bone toward the brain. Depressed fractures are of significance only if they compress underlying structures. In children, thinness and elasticity of the skull allow a depression without fracture. (Linear fracture across a suture line in an infant increases the possibility of epidural hematoma.)

Skull fractures are also classified according to location, such as a cranial vault fracture. A basilar fracture is at the base of the skull and involves the cribriform plate and the frontal sinuses. Because of the danger of grave complications, basilar fractures are usually far more serious than vault fractures.

Causes

Trauma is the usual cause:
• Traumatic blow to the head
• Motor vehicle accident
• Bad falls
• Severe beatings (especially in children)

Signs and symptoms

Symptoms reflect the severity and the extent of the head injury. Because some elderly patients may have brain atrophy, however, they have more space for brain swelling under the cranium and may not show signs of increased intracranial pressure (ICP).
• Dazed appearance (associated only with concussion in linear fractures)
• Persistent, localized headache
• Respiratory distress
• Alterations in level of consciousness
• Loss of consciousness (may last for hours, days, weeks, or indefinitely)

• Bleeding (may be profuse if scalp has been lacerated or torn away)
• Possible abrasions, contusions, lacerations, or avulsions
• Shock (may occur in severe head injury)
• Agitation and irritability
• Abnormal deep tendon reflexes
• Altered pupillary and motor response
• Hemiparesis
• Dizziness
• Convulsions
• Projectile vomiting
• Decreased pulse and respirations
• Possible blindness in sphenoidal fractures
• Possible unilateral deafness or facial paralysis in temporal fractures
• Commonly in basilar fractures, hemorrhage from the nose, pharynx, or ears; blood under the periorbital skin ("raccoon's eyes") and under the conjunctiva; and Battle's sign (supramastoid ecchymosis), sometimes with bleeding behind the eardrum
• Possible cerebrospinal fluid (CSF) or even brain tissue leakage from the nose or ears in basilar fractures. A halo sign—a blood-tinged spot surrounded by a lighter ring—from leakage of CSF may be found on the patient's bed linens.

Diagnostic tests

• Skull X-ray may locate the fracture (vault fractures are not visible or palpable).
• Using reagent strips, draining nasal or ear fluid is tested by dipstick for CSF. The tape turns blue if CSF is present; there is no change in the presence of blood alone. However, the tape will also turn blue if the patient is hyperglycemic.
• Cerebral angiography reveals vascular disruptions from internal pressure or injury.
• Computed tomography scan, echoencephalography, air encephalography, magnetic resonance imaging, and radioisotope scan disclose intracranial hemorrhage from ruptured blood ves-

sels (carotid arteries, venous sinuses) or cranial nerve injury, or indicate or localize subdural or intracerebral hematomas.

Treatment

Although occasionally even a simple linear skull fracture can tear an underlying blood vessel or cause a CSF leak, linear fractures usually require only supportive treatment, including mild analgesics (aspirin or acetaminophen), and cleansing and debridement of any wounds after local injection of procaine and shaving of the scalp around the wound. If the patient has not lost consciousness, he should be observed in the emergency room for at least 4 to 6 hours. After this observation period, if vital signs are stable, the patient can be discharged and should be given an instruction sheet for 24 to 48 hours of observation at home.

More severe vault fractures, especially depressed fractures, usually require a craniotomy to elevate or remove fragments that have been driven into the brain and to extract foreign bodies and necrotic tissue, thereby reducing the risk of infection and further brain damage. Cranioplasty follows the use of tantalum mesh or acrylic plates to replace the removed skull section. Antibiotic therapy and, in profound hemorrhage, blood transfusions are frequently required.

Basilar fractures call for immediate prophylactic antibiotics to prevent the onset of meningitis from CSF leaks, and close observation for secondary hematomas and hemorrhages. Surgery may be necessary. In addition, both basilar and vault fractures require dexamethasone I.V. or I.M. to reduce cerebral edema and minimize brain tissue damage.

Clinical implications

• Establish and maintain a patent airway; intubation may be necessary. Suction through the mouth, not the nose, to prevent introduction of bacteria in case a CSF leak is present.

• Obtain a complete history of the trauma from the patient, his family, eyewitnesses, and ambulance personnel. Ask whether the patient lost consciousness and, if so, for how long. Assist with diagnostic tests, including a complete neurologic examination, skull X-rays, and other studies. Check for abnormal reflexes, such as Babinski's sign.

• Look for CSF draining from the ears, nose, or mouth. Check bed linens for CSF leaks, and look for a halo sign. If the patient's nose is draining CSF, wipe it—*do not* let him blow it. If an ear is draining, cover it lightly with sterile gauze; *do not* pack it.

• Position a patient with a head injury so secretions can drain properly. With CSF leaks, elevate the head of the bed 30 degrees. Without CSF leaks, leave the head of the bed flat, but position the patient on his side or abdomen. Remember, however, that such a patient is at risk of increased ICP when not positioned on his back; be sure to keep his head properly aligned.

• Cover scalp wounds carefully with a sterile dressing; control any bleeding, as necessary.

• Take seizure precautions, but do not restrain the patient. Agitated behavior may be caused by hypoxia or increased ICP, so check for these. Speak in a calm, reassuring voice, and touch the patient gently. Do not make any sudden unexpected moves.

• Do not give narcotics or sedatives because they may depress respirations, increase CO_2, and lead to increased ICP, as well as mask changes in neurologic status. Give aspirin or another mild analgesic for pain, as ordered.

When a skull fracture requires surgery, follow these guidelines:

• Obtain consent, as needed, to shave the patient's head. Explain that you are doing this to provide a clean area for surgery. Type and cross match blood. Obtain orders for baseline laboratory studies, such as complete blood count, electrolytes, and urinalysis.

• After surgery, monitor vital signs and neurologic status frequently (usually every 5 minutes for 1 hour), and report any changes in level of consciousness. Because skull fractures and brain injuries heal slowly, do not expect dramatic postoperative improvement.

• Monitor intake and output frequently, and maintain indwelling (Foley) catheter patency. Take special care with fluid intake. Hypotonic fluids (even 5% dextrose in water) can increase cerebral edema. Their use should be restricted; give only as ordered.

• If the patient is unconscious, provide parenteral nutrition. (Remember, the patient may regurgitate and aspirate food if you use a nasogastric tube.)

If the fracture does not require surgery, follow these guidelines:

• Wear sterile gloves to examine the scalp laceration. With your finger, probe the wound for foreign bodies and palpable fracture. Gently cleanse lacerations and surrounding area. Cover with sterile gauze. Assist with suturing, if necessary.

• Provide emotional support for the patient and his family. Explain the need for procedures to reduce the risk of brain injury.

• Before discharge, instruct the patient's family to watch closely for changes in mental status, level of consciousness, or respirations, and to relieve the patient's headache with aspirin or acetaminophen. Tell the patient's family to return him to the hospital immediately if level of consciousness decreases, if headache persists after several doses of mild analgesics, if he vomits more than once, or if weakness develops in arms or legs.

• Teach the patient and his family how to care for his scalp wound. Emphasize the need for return for suture removal and follow-up evaluation.

Complications

• Meningitis and other infections can occur.

• Residual effects can occur depending on the extent of brain damage. These include convulsive disorders (epilepsy), hydrocephalus, and organic brain syndrome. Children may develop headaches, giddiness, easy fatigability, neuroses, and behavior disorders.

Fractures of the arm and leg

Description

Arm and leg fractures frequently cause substantial muscle, nerve, and other soft-tissue damage. Prognosis varies with extent of disablement or deformity, amount of tissue and vascular damage, adequacy of reduction and immobilization, and the patient's age, health, and nutrition. Children's bones usually heal rapidly and without deformity. Bones of adults in poor health and with impaired circulation may never heal properly. A history of trauma and suggestive findings on physical examination (including gentle palpation and failure of a cautious attempt by the patient to move parts distal to the injury) indicate a likely diagnosis of an arm or leg fracture. (Also see *Types of Fractures,* p. 292.)

Causes

• Major trauma—for example, a fall on an outstretched arm, a skiing accident, or child abuse (shown by multiple or repeated episodes of fractures)—is the most common cause.

• A cough or a sneeze can produce a fracture.

• Pathologic bone-weakening conditions such as osteoporosis, bone tumors, or metabolic disease can lead to fractures.

• Prolonged standing, walking, or running can cause stress fractures of the foot and ankle—usually in nurses, postal workers, soldiers, and joggers.

Types of Fractures

Incomplete: Break extends only partially through the bone; for example, in a greenstick fracture (more common in children), bone splinters fibers on one side of the bone, leaving the other side intact
Complete: Bone breaks into two or more pieces
Simple (closed): Overlying skin remains unbroken
Compound (open): Overlying skin is broken, creating the risk of infection
Nondisplaced: Fractured bones remain in alignment
Displaced: Break knocks bone ends out of alignment, creating the risk of muscle contractures and deformities
Transverse: Break runs transversely across the bone shaft
Oblique: Break runs across the bone on an angle
Spiral: Break winds around bone like a coil
Linear: Break runs the length of the bone
Comminuted: Bone shatters or is compressed into fragments
Impacted: Bone ends are driven into each other
Compression: Bone collapses (vertebrae) under excessive pressure
Avulsion: Overexertion tears a muscle or ligament away from a bone, pulling a small bone fragment with it
Depression: Trauma drives bone fragments inward

Signs and symptoms
Any of the following signs and symptoms may occur:
• Pain and point tenderness
• Pallor
• Pulse loss distal to fracture site
• Paresthesia distal to fracture site
• Paralysis distal to fracture site
• Deformity
• Swelling
• Discoloration
• Crepitus
• Loss of limb function
• Substantial blood loss and life-threatening hypovolemic shock (can occur in severe open fractures, especially of the femoral shaft)

Diagnostic tests
Anteroposterior and lateral X-rays of the suspected fracture, as well as X-rays of the joints above and below it, confirm the diagnosis.

Treatment
Emergency treatment consists of splinting the limb above and below the suspected fracture, applying a cold pack, and elevating the limb, to reduce edema and pain. In severe fractures that cause blood loss, direct pressure should be applied to control bleeding, and fluid replacement (including blood products) should be administered to prevent or treat hypovolemic shock.

After confirming diagnosis of a fracture, treatment begins with reduction (restoring displaced bone segments to their normal position), followed by immobilization by splint, cast, or traction. In closed reduction (manual manipulation), a local anesthetic (such as lidocaine) and an analgesic (such as meperidine I.M.) minimize pain. A muscle relaxant (such as diazepam I.V.) facilitates muscle stretching necessary to realign the bone. An X-ray confirms reduction and proper bone alignment. When closed reduction is impossible, open reduction during surgery reduces and immobilizes the fracture by means of rods, plates, or screws. After reduction, a plaster cast is usually applied.

When a splint or cast fails to maintain the reduction, immobilization requires skin or skeletal traction, using a series of weights and pulleys. In skin traction, elastic bandages and moleskin coverings are used to attach traction devices to the patient's skin. In skeletal traction, a pin or wire inserted through the bone distal to the fracture and attached to a weight allows more prolonged traction.

Treatment for open fractures also requires careful wound cleansing, tetanus prophylaxis, prophylactic antibiotics, and possibly surgery to repair soft-tissue damage.

Clinical implications
• Watch for signs of shock in the patient with a severe open fracture of a large bone, such as the femur.
• Offer reassurance. With any fracture the patient is apt to be frightened and in pain. Ease pain with analgesics, as needed. Help the patient set realistic goals for recovery.
• If the fracture requires long-term immobilization with traction, reposition the patient frequently to increase comfort and prevent decubitus ulcers. Assist with active range-of-motion exercises to prevent muscle atrophy. Encourage deep breathing and coughing to avoid hypostatic pneumonia.
• Urge adequate fluid intake to prevent urinary stasis and constipation. Watch for signs of renal calculi (flank pain, nausea, and vomiting).
• Give good cast care. While the cast is wet, support it with pillows. Observe for skin irritation near cast edges; check for foul odors or discharge. Tell the patient to report signs of impaired circulation (skin coldness, numbness, tingling, or discoloration) immediately. Warn against getting the cast wet, and instruct the patient not to insert foreign objects under the cast.
• Encourage the patient to start moving around as soon as he is able. Demonstrate how to use crutches properly.
• After cast removal, refer for physical therapy to restore limb mobility.

Complications
• Permanent deformity and dysfunction if bones fail to heal (nonunion) or heal improperly (malunion)
• Aseptic necrosis of bone segments from impaired circulation
• Hypovolemic shock as a result of blood vessel damage (especially likely to develop in patients with femoral fracture)
• Muscle contractures
• Renal calculi resulting from decalcification in prolonged immobility
• Fat embolism (See also *Fat Embolism.*)

Fat Embolism

A complication of long bone fracture, fat embolism may also follow severe soft-tissue bruising and fatty liver injury. Posttraumatic embolization may occur as bone marrow releases fat into the veins. The fat can lodge in the lungs, obstructing the pulmonary vascular bed, or pass into the arteries, eventually disturbing the central nervous system.

Fat embolism occurs 12 to 48 hours after injury, typically producing fever, tachycardia, tachypnea, blood-tinged sputum, cyanosis, anxiety, restlessness, altered level of consciousness, convulsions, coma, and a rash. Studies reveal decreased hemoglobin, increased serum lipase, leukocytosis, thrombocytopenia, hypoxemia, and fat globules in urine and sputum. A chest X-ray may show mottled lung fields and right ventricular dilation; an EKG, large S waves in lead I, large Q waves in lead III, and right axis deviation.

Although treatment is controversial, it may include steroids to reduce inflammation, heparin to clear lipemia, diazepam for sedation, and oxygen to correct hypoxemia. Expect to immobilize fractures early. As ordered, assist with endotracheal intubation and ventilation.

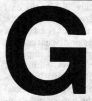

Galactosemia

Description

Galactosemia is any disorder of galactose metabolism. It occurs in two forms: classic galactosemia and galactokinase-deficiency galactosemia. In both forms of galactosemia, the inability to normally metabolize the sugar galactose (which is mainly formed by digestion of the disaccharide lactose that is present in milk) causes galactose accumulation. Although a galactose-free diet relieves most symptoms, galactosemia-induced mental impairment is irreversible. Some residual vision impairment may also persist. Galactosemia also can produce a short attention span, difficulty with spatial and mathematical relationships, and apathetic, withdrawn behavior.

Causes

Both forms are inherited as autosomal recessive defects.

• Classic galactosemia results from a defect in the enzyme galactose-1-phosphate uridyl transferase.

• Galactokinase-deficiency galactosemia, the rarer form of this disorder, stems from a deficiency of the enzyme galactokinase.

Signs and symptoms
Classic galactosemia

In children who are homozygous for the classic galactosemia gene, signs are evident at birth or within a few days after milk ingestion.

—Failure to thrive
—Vomiting
—Diarrhea
—Liver damage (evidenced by jaundice, hepatomegaly, cirrhosis, and ascites)
—Splenomegaly
—Galactosuria
—Proteinuria
—Aminoaciduria
—Cataracts (may be present at birth or develop later)
—Possible mental retardation, malnourishment, progressive hepatic failure, and death with continued ingestion of galactose or lactose-containing foods

Galactokinase-deficiency galactosemia

—Cataracts may be the only sign.

Diagnostic tests

• Deficiency of the enzyme galactose-1-phosphate uridyl transferase in red blood cells (RBCs) confirms classic galactosemia.

• Decreased RBC levels of galactokinase confirm galactokinase-deficiency galactosemia.

• Increased galactose levels in blood (normal value in children is less than 20 mg/dl) and urine (must use galactose oxidase to avoid confusion with other reducing sugars) support the diagnosis. Galactose measurements in blood and urine must be interpreted carefully, because some children who consume large amounts of milk have elevated plasma galactose concentrations and galactosuria but are not gal-

---

Diet for Galactosemia

Dear Parent:
If your child has galactosemia, make sure he follows a diet free of lactose.
He may eat:
• fish and animal products (except brains and mussels)
• fresh fruits and vegetables (except peas and lima beans)
• only bread and rolls made from cracked wheat.
He should avoid:
• dairy products
• puddings, cookies, cakes, pies
• food coloring
• instant potatoes
• canned and frozen foods (if lactose is listed as an ingredient).

This patient-teaching aid may be reproduced by office copier for distribution to patients.
© 1987, Springhouse Corporation.

---

actosemic. Also, newborns excrete galactose in their urine for about a week after birth; premature infants, even longer.
• Liver biopsy shows typical acinar formation.
• Liver enzymes (serum glutamic-oxaloacetic transaminase [SGOT], serum glutamic-pyruvic transaminase [SGPT]) are elevated.
• Urinalysis shows albumin in urine.
• Ophthalmoscopy reveals punctate lesions in the fetal lens nucleus.
• Amniocentesis permits prenatal diagnosis of galactosemia (recommended for heterozygous and homozygous parents).

Treatment and clinical implications

Elimination of galactose and lactose from the diet causes most effects to subside. The infant gains weight; liver anomalies, nausea, vomiting, galactosemia, proteinuria, and aminoaciduria disappear; and cataracts regress. To eliminate galactose and lactose from an infant's diet, replace cow's milk formula or breast milk with a meat-base or soybean formula. As the child grows, a balanced, galactose-free diet must be maintained. A pregnant woman who is heterozygous or homozygous for galactosemia should also follow a galactose-restricted diet. Such a diet supports normal growth and development and may delay symptoms in the newborn. (See also *Diet for Galactosemia*.)
• Teach the parents about dietary restrictions, and stress the importance of compliance. Warn them to read medication labels carefully and avoid giving any that contain lactose fillers.
• If the child has a learning disability, help parents secure educational assistance. Refer parents who want to have other children for genetic counseling. In some states, screening of all newborns for galactosemia is required by law.

Gallbladder and bile duct carcinoma

Description

Gallbladder carcinoma is rare, comprising less than 1% of all malignancies. It is normally found coincidentally in patients with cholecystitis; 1 in 400 cholecystectomies reveals malignancy. This disease is most prevalent in women over age 60. It is rapidly progressive and usually fatal. Patients seldom live a year after diagnosis. Poor prognosis is due to late diagnosis. Gallbladder cancer is usually not diagnosed until after cholecystectomy, when, in most cases, it is in an advanced, metastatic stage.

Lymph node metastasis is present in 25% to 70% of patients at diagnosis. Direct extension to the liver is common (in 46% to 89%). Direct extension to both the cystic and the common bile ducts, stomach, colon, duodenum, and jejunum also occurs, and produces obstructions. This tumor also spreads by portal or hepatic veins to the peritoneum, ovaries, and lower lung lobes.

Extrahepatic bile duct carcinoma is the cause of approximately 3% of all cancer deaths in the United States. It occurs in both men and women (incidence is slightly higher in men) between ages 60 and 70. The usual site is at the bifurcation in the common duct. Carcinoma at the distal end of the common duct is frequently confused with carcinoma of the pancreas. Characteristically, metastatic spread occurs to local lymph nodes, the liver, lungs, and the peritoneum.

Causes
Gallbladder carcinoma
Many consider gallbladder carcinoma a complication of gallstones. This inference, however, rests on circumstantial evidence from postmortem examinations. From 60% to 90% of gallbladder carcinoma patients also have gallstones, but postmortem data from patients with gallstones show gallbladder carcinoma in only 0.5%.
Bile duct carcinoma
The cause is unknown, but statistics do show an unexplained increased incidence of this carcinoma in patients with ulcerative colitis. This association may be due to a common cause—perhaps an immune mechanism, or chronic use of certain drugs by the colitis patient.

Signs and symptoms
Gallbladder carcinoma
—Signs of cholecystitis (pain in the epigastrium or right upper quadrant, weight loss, anorexia, nausea, vomiting, and jaundice)
—Chronic, progressively severe pain without fever
—Palpable gallbladder (right upper quadrant), with obstructive jaundice
—Possible hepatosplenomegaly
Bile duct carcinoma
—Profound jaundice (commonly the first sign)
—Chronic pain (in the epigastrium or right upper quadrant, radiating to the back)
—Other common symptoms, if associated with active cholecystitis: pruritus, skin excoriations, anorexia, weight loss, chills, and fever

Diagnostic tests
Gallbladder carcinoma
No test or procedure is, in itself, diagnostic of gallbladder carcinoma. However, the following laboratory tests support this diagnosis when they suggest hepatic dysfunction and extrahepatic biliary obstruction:
—Baseline studies include complete blood count, routine urinalysis, electrolyte studies, and enzymes.
—Liver function test results, including bilirubin, urine bile and bilirubin, and urobilinogen, are elevated in more than 50% of patients. Serum alkaline phosphatase levels are consistently elevated.
—Sulfur colloid liver-spleen scan
—Upper GI series shows abnormality of pylorus or duodenum.
—Occult blood in stools is linked to the associated anemia.
—Cholecystography may show stones or calcification—a "porcelain" gallbladder.
—Cholangiography may locate the site of common duct obstruction.
—Chest X-ray may show elevation

(displacement by the tumor) of right side of diaphragm.

Bile duct carcinoma
The following tests help confirm extrahepatic bile duct carcinoma:

—Liver function test results indicate biliary obstruction: elevated bilirubin (5 to 30 mg/dl), alkaline phosphatase, and blood cholesterol levels; prolonged prothrombin time; response to vitamin K.

—Barium studies, cholangiography, and endoscopic retrograde cannulation of the pancreas may help locate the obstruction but are not diagnostic.

Treatment
Surgical treatment of gallbladder cancer is essentially palliative. It includes cholecystectomy, common bile duct exploration, T-tube drainage, and wedge excision of hepatic tissue. If the cancer invades gallbladder musculature, the survival rate is less than 5%, even with massive resection. Although long-term survival (4 to 5 years) has been reported, few patients survive longer than 6 months after surgery.

Surgery is normally indicated to relieve obstruction and jaundice that result from extrahepatic bile duct carcinoma. The procedure depends on the site of the carcinoma and may include cholecystoduodenostomy or T-tube drainage of the common duct.

Other palliative measures for both kinds of carcinomas include radiation (mostly used for local and incisional recurrences) and chemotherapy (especially with 5-fluorouracil), both of which have limited effects.

Clinical implications
After biliary resection, follow these guidelines:
• Monitor vital signs.
• Use strict aseptic technique when caring for the incision and the surrounding area.
• Place the patient in the low Fowler position.
• Prevent respiratory problems by encouraging deep breathing and coughing. The high incision makes the patient want to take shallow breaths; using analgesics and splinting his abdomen with a pillow or an abdominal binder may aid in greater respiratory efforts.
• Monitor bowel sounds and bowel movements. Observe patient's tolerance to diet.
• Provide pain control.
• Check intake and output carefully. Watch for electrolyte imbalance. Monitor I.V. solutions to avoid overloading the cardiovascular system.
• Monitor the nasogastric tube, which will be in place for 24 to 72 hours postoperatively to relieve distention, and the T tube. Record amount and color of drainage each shift. Secure the T tube to minimize tension on it and prevent its being pulled out.
• Help the patient and his family cope with their initial fears and reactions to the diagnosis by offering information and support.
• Advise the patient of the adverse effects of both chemotherapy and radiation therapy. Monitor the patient on radiation therapy closely for adverse effects, and observe the patient receiving chemotherapy for adverse effects of cytotoxic drugs.

Gas gangrene

Description
Gas gangrene results from local infection. It is most frequently found in deep wounds, especially those in which tissue necrosis further reduces oxygen supply. When the causative bacteria invades soft tissues, it produces thrombosis of regional blood vessels, tissue necrosis, and localized edema. Such necrosis releases both carbon dioxide and hydrogen subcutaneously, producing interstitial gas bubbles. Gas gangrene most commonly occurs in the extremities and in abdominal wounds,

and less frequently in the uterus. True gas gangrene produces myositis and another form of this disease, involving only soft tissue, called anaerobic cellulitis. This rare infection is frequently fatal unless therapy begins immediately. However, with prompt treatment, 80% of patients with gas gangrene of the extremities survive. Prognosis is poorer for gas gangrene in other sites, such as the abdominal wall or the bowel. The usual incubation period is 1 to 4 days, but it can vary from 3 hours to 6 weeks or longer.

Causes
Anaerobic, spore-forming, gram-positive rod-shaped bacillus *Clostridium perfringens* (or another clostridial species), a normal inhabitant of the GI and the female genital tracts

Mode of transmission
Transmission occurs by entry of organisms during trauma or surgery.

Signs and symptoms
Most signs of infection develop within 72 hours of trauma or surgery.
Local
—Crepitation (the hallmark of gas gangrene)
—Severe, localized pain (swelling and discoloration, in many cases, dusky brown or reddish)
—Bullae and necrosis (occur within 36 hours from onset of symptoms)
—Finally, possible rupture of the skin over the wound reveals dark red or black necrotic muscle, a foul-smelling watery or frothy discharge, intravascular hemolysis, thrombosis of blood vessels, and evidence of infection spread.
Generalized
Signs of toxemia and hypovolemia include the following:
—Tachycardia
—Tachypnea
—Hypotension
—Moderate fever (usually not above 101° F. [38.3° C.])
—Pallor, prostration (patient motionless but still alert, oriented, and extremely apprehensive)
—Death (occurs suddenly, in many cases, during surgery for removal of necrotic tissue; may be preceded by delirium and coma; sometimes accompanied by profuse diarrhea and circulatory collapse)

Diagnostic tests
The following tests confirm the diagnosis:
• Anaerobic cultures of wound drainage showing *C. perfringens*
• Gram stain of wound drainage showing large, gram-positive, rod-shaped bacteria
• X-rays showing gas in tissues
• Blood studies showing leukocytosis

Treatment
Treatment includes careful observation for signs of myositis and cellulitis and immediate treatment if these signs appear; immediate wide surgical excision of all affected tissues and necrotic muscle in myositis (delayed or inadequate surgical excision is a fatal mistake); I.V. administration of high-dose penicillin; and, after adequate debridement, hyperbaric oxygenation,

---

Preventing Gas Gangrene

• Routinely take precautions to render all wound sites unsuitable for growth of clostridia by attempting to keep granulation tissue viable.
• Perform adequate debridement to reduce anaerobic growth conditions.
• Be alert for devitalized tissues, and notify the surgeon promptly.
• Position the patient to facilitate drainage, and eliminate all dead spaces in closed wounds.

if available. For 1 to 3 hours every 6 to 8 hours, the patient is placed in a hyperbaric chamber and is exposed to pressures designed to increase oxygen tension and prevent multiplication of the anaerobic *C. perfringens*. Surgery may be done within the hyperbaric chamber if the chamber is large enough.

Clinical implications

Careful observation may result in early diagnosis. Look for signs of ischemia (cool skin; pallor or cyanosis; sudden, severe pain; sudden edema; and loss of pulses in an involved limb).

After diagnosis, provide meticulous supportive care, following these guidelines:

• Throughout this illness, provide adequate fluid replacement, and assess pulmonary and cardiac function frequently. Maintain airway and ventilation.

• To prevent skin breakdown and further infection, give good skin care. After surgery, provide meticulous wound care.

• Psychological support is critical, because these patients can remain alert until death, knowing that death is imminent and unavoidable.

• Deodorize the room to control foul odor from the wound. Prepare the patient emotionally for a large wound after surgical excision, and refer him for physical rehabilitation, as necessary.

• Institute wound precautions. Dispose of drainage material properly (double-bag dressings in plastic bags for incineration), wear sterile gloves when changing dressings, and after the patient is discharged, have the room cleaned with a germicidal solution. (Also see *Preventing Gas Gangrene*.)

Gastric carcinoma

Description

Gastric carcinoma is common throughout the world and affects all races; however, unexplained geographic and cultural differences in incidence occur. The parts of the stomach affected by gastric carcinoma, listed in order of decreasing frequency, are the pylorus and antrum, the lesser curvature, the cardia, the body of the stomach, and the greater curvature. Gastric carcinoma infiltrates rapidly to regional lymph nodes, omentum, liver, and lungs by the following routes: walls of the stomach, duodenum, and esophagus; lymphatic system; adjacent organs; bloodstream; and peritoneal cavity.

In the United States during the past 25 years, incidence has decreased 50%, with the resulting death rate from gastric carcinoma one-third that of 30 years ago. This decrease has been attributed, without proof, to the improved and well-balanced diets most Americans enjoy. Incidence is higher in men over age 40. Prognosis depends on the stage of the disease at the time of diagnosis; however, overall, the 5-year survival rate is approximately 15%.

Causes

• Etiology is unknown.

• Genetic factors have been linked to this disease because it occurs more frequently among people with type A blood than among those with type O. Similarly, it occurs more frequently in people with a family history of such carcinoma.

• Dietary factors also seem related, including types of food preparation, physical properties of some foods, and certain methods of food preservation (especially smoking, pickling, or salting).

Risk factors

Predisposing factors include the following:

• Gastric atrophy
• Achlorhydria
• Hypochlorhydria
• Pernicious anemia

Dumping Syndrome

After gastric resection, rapid emptying of gastric contents into the small intestine produces the following:
• *Early dumping syndrome,* which may be mild or severe, occurs a few minutes after eating and lasts up to 45 minutes. Onset is sudden, with nausea, weakness, sweating, palpitations, dizziness, flushing, borborygmi, explosive diarrhea, and increased blood pressure and pulse rate.
• *Late dumping syndrome,* which is less serious, occurs 2 to 3 hours after eating. Similar symptoms include profuse sweating, anxiety, fine tremor of the hands and legs accompanied by vertigo, exhaustion, lassitude, palpitations, throbbing headache, faintness, sensation of hunger, glycosuria, and marked decrease in blood pressure and blood glucose level.
These symptoms may persist for 1 year after surgery or for the rest of the patient's life.

Signs and symptoms
The course of gastric cancer may be insidious or fulminating. Because chronic dyspepsia and epigastric discomfort are early signs, the patient typically treats himself with antacids until the symptoms of advanced stages appear.
• Weight loss
• Anorexia
• Feeling of fullness after eating
• Anemia
• Fatigue
• Possible blood in the stool
• Dysphagia and, later, vomiting (in many cases, coffee-ground vomitus); may be the first symptom if the carcinoma is in the cardia

Diagnostic tests
• Barium X-rays of the GI tract with fluoroscopy show changes (tumor or filling defect in the outline of the stomach; loss of flexibility and distensibility; and abnormal gastric mucosa with or without ulceration).
• Gastroscopy with fiberoptic endoscopy helps rule out other diffuse gastric mucosal abnormalities by allowing direct visualization and gastroscopic biopsy to evaluate gastric mucosal lesions.
• Photography with fiberoptic endoscopy provides a permanent record of gastric lesions that can later be used to determine disease progression and effect of treatment.
• Certain other studies may rule out specific organ metastases: computed tomography scans, chest X-rays, liver and bone scans, and liver biopsy.

Treatment
Surgery is frequently the treatment of choice. Excision of the lesion with appropriate margins is possible in over one third of patients. Even in patients whose disease is not considered surgically curable, resection offers palliation and improves potential benefits from chemotherapy and radiation.

The nature and extent of the lesion determine what kind of surgery is most appropriate. Common surgical procedures include subtotal gastric resection (subtotal gastrectomy) and total gastric resection (total gastrectomy). When carcinoma involves the pylorus and antrum, gastric resection removes the lower stomach and duodenum (gastrojejunostomy or Billroth II). If metastasis has occurred, the omentum and spleen may also have to be removed.

If gastric cancer has spread to the liver, peritoneum, or lymph glands, palliative surgery may include gastrostomy, jejunostomy, or gastric or partial gastric resection. Such surgery may temporarily relieve vomiting, nausea, pain, and dysphagia, while allowing enteral nutrition to continue.

Chemotherapy for GI malignancies may help to control symptoms and prolong survival. Adenocarcinoma of the stomach has responded to several agents, including 5-fluorouracil, carmustine (BCNU), and doxorubicin. Antiemetics can control nausea, which increases as the malignancy grows. In later stages, sedatives and tranquilizers may be necessary to control overwhelming anxiety. Narcotics are frequently necessary to relieve pain. However, morphine itself may produce nausea, so a synthetic derivative recently has been used more frequently.

Radiation has not been highly effective against carcinoma of the stomach but is still used occasionally. It should be given on an empty stomach, and should not be used preoperatively, because it may damage viscera and impede healing.

Patients for whom extensive spread of malignancy rules out surgery may benefit from a medical regimen. Antispasmodics and antacids may relieve distress.

Clinical implications

Before surgery, prepare the patient for its effects and explain postsurgical procedures such as nasogastric tube drainage and I.V. infusions.

- Reassure the patient who is having a partial gastric resection that he may eventually be able to eat normally. Prepare the patient who is having a total gastrectomy for slow recovery and only partial return to a normal diet.
- Include the family in all phases of the patient's care.
- Emphasize the importance of changing position every 2 hours and of deep breathing.
- After surgery, give meticulous supportive care to promote recovery and prevent complications.
- Regularly assist the patient with coughing, deep breathing, and turning. Hourly turning and judicious use of analgesic narcotics (these depress respiration) may prevent pulmonary problems, which may follow any type of gastrectomy. Oxygen may be needed, and intermittent positive-pressure breathing (IPPB) or incentive spirometry may be necessary for complete expansion of the lungs if the patient is not able to breathe effectively on his own.

- Proper positioning is important; the semi-Fowler position facilitates breathing and drainage.
- After gastrectomy, little (if any) drainage comes from the nasogastric tube, because no secretions form after the stomach is removed. Because the stomach's storage function has been eliminated, the patient frequently suffers from a dumping syndrome. (See also *Dumping Syndrome*.)
- Intrinsic factor is absent from gastric secretions, which leads to malabsorption of vitamin B_{12}. To prevent vitamin B_{12} deficiency, the patient needs to replace the vitamin the rest of his life, as well as take an iron supplement.
- During radiation treatment, encourage the patient to eat high-calorie, well-balanced meals. Offer fluids, such as orange juice, grapefruit juice, or ginger ale to minimize nausea and vomiting. Watch for radiation adverse effects (nausea, vomiting, hair loss, malaise, and diarrhea).
- Watch for complications of surgery.
- Patients who experience poor digestion and absorption after gastrectomy need a special diet: frequent feedings of small amounts of clear liquids, increasing to small, frequent feedings of bland food.
- After total gastrectomy, patients must eat small meals for the rest of their lives. (Some patients need pancreatin and sodium bicarbonate after meals to prevent or control steatorrhea and dyspepsia.)

• Wound dehiscence and delayed healing, stemming from decreased protein, anemia, and avitaminosis, occur frequently in cancer patients. Preoperative vitamin and protein replacement can prevent such complications. Parenteral administration of vitamin C may improve wound healing.

• Vitamin deficiency may result from obstruction, diarrhea, or an inadequate diet. Ascorbic acid, thiamine, riboflavin, nicotinic acid, and vitamin K supplements may be beneficial.

• Good nutrition promotes weight gain, strength, independence, and positive emotional outlook, and promotes tolerance for surgery, radiotherapy, or chemotherapy. Aside from meeting caloric needs, good nutrition also must provide adequate protein, fluid, and potassium intake to facilitate glycogen and protein synthesis.

• Anabolic agents, such as methandrostenolone, may induce nitrogen retention. Steroids, antidepressants, wine, or brandy may stimulate the appetite.

• When all treatment has failed, concentrate on keeping the patient comfortable and free of unnecessary pain, and provide as much psychological support as possible. Talk with family members, and answer any questions they may have. Tell them to let the patient talk about his future, but encourage them to maintain a realistic outlook. If the patient is going home, arrange for a visiting nurse or homemaker, if needed, as well as for his sickroom needs (for example, a bedside commode or a walker).

Gastritis

Description

Gastritis, an inflammation of the gastric mucosa, may be acute or chronic. Acute gastritis is the most common stomach disorder. In a person with epigastric discomfort or other GI symptoms (particularly bleeding), history

suggesting exposure to a GI irritant suggests gastritis. Gastritis is common in persons with pernicious anemia (as chronic atrophic gastritis). Although gastritis can occur at any age, it is more prevalent in elderly persons.

Causes

Acute gastritis
—Chronic ingestion of irritating foods or allergic reaction to them
—Alcoholic beverages
—Drugs such as aspirin
—Poisons, especially DDT, ammonia, mercury, and carbon tetrachloride
—Hepatic disorders such as portal hypertension
—GI disorders such as sprue
—Infectious diseases
—Curling's ulcer (after a burn)
—Cushing's ulcer
—GI injury (may be thermal [ingestion of hot fluid] or mechanical [swallowing a foreign object])
Corrosive gastritis
—Ingestion of strong acids or alkalies
Acute phlegmonous gastritis
—This results from a rare bacterial (usually streptococcal) infection of the stomach wall. (See also *Chronic Gastritis*.)

Signs and symptoms

• GI bleeding is the most common symptom.

• Mild epigastric discomfort (postprandial distress) may be the only symptom.

Diagnostic tests

Gastroscopy (frequently with biopsy) confirms the diagnosis when done before lesions heal (usually within 24 hours). However, gastroscopy is contraindicated after ingestion of a corrosive agent. X-rays rule out other diseases.

Treatment

Symptoms are usually relieved by eliminating the gastric irritant or other

Chronic Gastritis

Chronic gastritis results from recurring ingestion of an irritating substance or from pernicious anemia. The main types of chronic gastritis are fundal gland gastritis and chronic antral gastritis (pyloric gland gastritis). Fundal gland gastritis includes:

• Superficial gastritis—reddened edematous mucosa, with hemorrhages and small erosions
• Atrophic gastritis—inflammation in all stomach layers, with decreased number of parietal and chief cells
• Gastric atrophy—dull and nodular mucosa, with irregular, thickened, or nodular rugae.

Many patients with chronic gastritis, particularly those with chronic antral gastritis, have no symptoms. When symptoms develop, they are typically indistinct and may include loss of appetite, feeling of fullness, belching, vague epigastric pain, nausea, and vomiting. Diagnosis requires biopsy.

Usually no treatment is necessary, except for avoiding aspirin and spicy or irritating foods, and taking antacids if symptoms persist. If pernicious anemia is the underlying cause, vitamin B_{12} should be administered. Chronic gastritis frequently progresses to acute gastritis.

---

cause. For instance, the treatment for corrosive gastritis is neutralization with the appropriate antidote (emetics are contraindicated). Treatment for gastritis caused by other poisons includes emetics, anticholinergics such as methantheline bromide, histamine antagonists such as cimetidine, and antacids to relieve GI distress. When gastritis causes massive bleeding, treatment includes blood replacement; iced saline lavage, possibly with norepinephrine; angiography, with vasopressin infused in normal saline solution; and surgery. Treatment for bacterial gastritis includes antibiotics, bland diet, and an antiemetic. Treatment for acute phlegmonous gastritis is vigorous antibiotic therapy, followed by surgical repair.

Clinical implications
• Give antacids, anticholinergics, histamine antagonists, and antibiotics, as ordered.
• Explain all diagnostic procedures to the patient.

• If the patient is vomiting, give antiemetics and, as ordered, replace I.V. fluids. Monitor fluid intake and output, and watch electrolyte balance.
• Watch for signs of GI bleeding (hematemesis, melena, drop in hematocrit, bloody nasogastric drainage) or hemorrhagic shock (hypotension, tachycardia, or restlessness). In corrosive gastritis, watch for signs of obstruction, perforation, or peritonitis, such as nausea, vomiting, diarrhea, abdominal pain, or fever.
• Urge the patient to seek immediate attention for recurring symptoms (hematemesis, nausea, or vomiting).
• To prevent recurrence of gastritis, stress the importance of taking prescribed prophylactic medication exactly as ordered. Advise the patient to prevent gastric irritation by taking steroids with milk, food, or antacids; by taking antacids between meals and at bedtime; by avoiding aspirin-containing compounds; and by avoiding spicy foods, hot fluids, alcohol, caffeine, and tobacco.

Gastroenteritis
(Intestinal flu, traveler's diarrhea, viral enteritis, food poisoning)

Description
Gastroenteritis is an inflammation of the stomach and intestines accompanying numerous GI disorders. It occurs in persons of all ages and is a major cause of morbidity and mortality in underdeveloped nations. In the United States, gastroenteritis ranks second to the common cold as a cause of lost work time, and fifth as the cause of death among young children. It also can be life-threatening in elderly and debilitated persons.

Causes
Gastroenteritis has many possible causes, such as the following:
• Bacteria (responsible for acute food poisoning): *Staphylococcus aureus*, *Salmonella*, *Shigella*, *Clostridium botulinum*, *Escherichia coli*, *Clostridium perfringens*
• Amoebae, especially *Entamoeba histolytica*
• Parasites: *Ascaris*, *Enterobius*, and *Trichinella spiralis*
• Viruses (may be responsible for traveler's diarrhea): adenoviruses, echoviruses, or Coxsackieviruses
• Toxins: ingestion of plants or toadstools
• Drug reactions: antibiotics
• Enzyme deficiencies
• Food allergens

Signs and symptoms
Clinical manifestations vary depending on the pathologic organism and on the level of the GI tract involved. In children, elderly persons, and debilitated persons, intolerance to electrolyte and fluid losses leads to a higher mortality. However, gastroenteritis in adults is usually a self-limiting, nonfatal disease producing the following symptoms:

• Diarrhea
• Abdominal discomfort (ranging from cramping to pain)
• Nausea
• Vomiting
• Possible fever, malaise, and borborygmi

Diagnostic tests
Stool culture (by direct swab) or blood culture identifies causative bacteria or parasites.

Treatment
Treatment is usually supportive and consists of bed rest, nutritional support, and increased fluid intake. When gastroenteritis is severe or affects a young child or an elderly or debilitated person, treatment may necessitate hospitalization; specific antimicrobials; I.V. fluid and electrolyte replacement; bismuth-containing compounds, such as Pepto-Bismol; and antiemetics (P.O., I.M., or rectal suppository), such as prochlorperazine or trimethobenzamide.

Clinical implications
Administer medications, as ordered; correlate dosages, routes, and times appropriately with the patient's meals and activities (for example, give antiemetics 30 to 60 minutes before meals).
• If the patient can eat, replace lost fluids and electrolytes with broth, ginger ale, and lemonade, as tolerated. Vary the diet to make it more enjoyable, and allow some choice of foods. Warn the patient to avoid milk and milk products, which may provoke recurrence.
• Record intake and output carefully. Watch for signs of dehydration, such as dry skin and mucous membranes, fever, and sunken eyes.
• Wash hands thoroughly after giving care to avoid spreading infection.

• To ease anal irritation, provide warm sitz baths or apply witch hazel compresses.
• If food poisoning is probable, contact public health authorities.
• Teach good hygiene to prevent recurrence. Instruct patients to cook foods, especially pork, thoroughly; to refrigerate perishable foods, such as milk, mayonnaise, potato salad, and cream-filled pastry; always to wash hands with warm water and soap before handling food, especially after using the bathroom; to clean utensils thoroughly; to avoid drinking water or eating raw fruit or vegetables when visiting a foreign country; and to eliminate flies and roaches in the home.

Gaucher's disease

Description
Gaucher's disease, the most common lipidosis, causes an abnormal accumulation of glucocerebrosides in reticuloendothelial cells. It occurs in three forms: Type I (adult); Type II (infantile); and Type III (juvenile). Type II can prove fatal within 9 months of onset, usually from pulmonary involvement. Type I is 30 times more prevalent in Eastern Europeans of Jewish ancestry. Types II and III are less common. The adult form of Gaucher's disease is usually diagnosed while the patient is in his teens.

Cause
Gaucher's disease results from autosomal recessive inheritance and causes decreased activity of the enzyme glucocerebrosidase.

Signs and symptoms
All types
—Hepatosplenomegaly
—Bone lesions
Type I
—Thinning of cortices
—Pathologic fractures
—Collapsed hip joints
—Eventually, vertebral compression
—Severe episodic pain (possibly developing in the legs, arms, and back)
—Other clinical effects, including fever, abdominal distention, pneumonia, cor pulmonale (rarely), easy bruising and bleeding, anemia, and pancytopenia (rarely)
—Possible yellow pallor and brown-yellow pigmentation on the face and legs in older patients
Type II
—Motor dysfunction and spasticity at age 6 to 7 months
—Abdominal distention
—Strabismus
—Muscular hypertonicity
—Retroflexion of the head
—Neck rigidity
—Dysphagia
—Laryngeal stridor
—Hyperreflexia
—Seizures
—Respiratory distress
—Easy bruising and bleeding
Type III
—Convulsions
—Muscular hypertonicity
—Strabismus
—Poor coordination and mental ability
—Possible easy bruising and bleeding

Diagnostic tests
• Bone marrow aspiration showing Gaucher's cells and direct assay of glucocerebrosidase activity, which can be performed on venous blood, confirm this diagnosis.
• Serum acid phosphatase level is increased.
• Platelets are decreased.
• Serum iron level is decreased.
• EEG is abnormal in Type III after infancy.

Treatment and clinical implications
Treatment is mainly supportive and consists of vitamins, supplemental iron or liver extract to prevent anemia caused by iron deficiency and to al-

leviate other hematologic problems, blood transfusions for anemia, splenectomy for thrombocytopenia, and strong analgesics for bone pain. Enzyme replacement therapy is still experimental but looks promising.

• If the patient is confined to bed, prevent pathologic fractures by turning him carefully. If he is ambulatory, see that he is assisted when getting out of bed or walking.

• Observe closely for changes in pulmonary status.

• Explain all diagnostic tests and procedures to the patient or his parents. Help the patient accept the limitations imposed by this disorder.

• Recommend genetic counseling for parents who want to have another child.

Gender identity disorders

Description

Psychosexual disorders involving gender identity refer to an individual's persistent feelings of gender discomfort and inappropriateness of his or her anatomic sex. Gender identity may be defined as the intimate personal feelings one has about being male or female and includes three components: self-concept, perception of an ideal partner, and external presentation of masculinity and femininity through behavior, dress, and mannerisms.

Persons with gender identity disorder typically behave and present themselves as persons of the opposite sex, which they intensely desire to become. In both adults and children, this disorder is rare; it is often referred to as transsexualism in adults. Gender identity disorder should not be confused with the fairly common adult feeling of occasional sexual inadequacy or with the rejection of sexual stereotypes by behavior that is typically called "tomboy" or "sissy." Diagnosis rests on a careful history that confirms persistent and severe psychosexual dysphoria and a desire to be the opposite sex, persisting continuously for at least 2 years. (See also *Normal Differentiation of Gender Identity*.)

Causes

Current theories about the causes of gender identity disorders suggest a combination of predisposing factors.

• Chromosomal anomaly

• Hormonal imbalance (particularly in utero)

• Pathologic defects in early parent–child bonding and child-rearing practices (parents who consistently treat a child as one of the opposite biological sex significantly contribute to this disorder)

Signs and symptoms
Children

Gender identity disorders may be apparent at an early age.

—Expressed desire to be or insistence that he or she is of the opposite sex

—Expressed disgust with the genitals

—Expressed belief, frequently as an ardent hope, that the patient will become the opposite sex when grown

—School problems. These children, particularly boys, frequently suffer peer group rejection and have trouble in school because of social conflict. Girls may not experience social difficulties until early adolescence.

Adults

—Overwhelming desire to live as a person of the opposite sex

—Desire to be rid of genitals

—Psychological perception of being the opposite sex

—Commonly, dressing and engaging in activities typical of the opposite sex

—Heterosexual or homosexual preference in relationships

—Possible asexuality

—Often, coexisting depression, isolation, and anxiety

Normal Differentiation of Gender Identity

VARIABLE	SIGNIFICANCE
Chromosomal	Presence of XX or XY chromosome, the legal and medical definition of sex.
Gonadal	Structure of gonads in utero. With XY, testes differentiate; with XX, ovaries.
Hormonal	Male fetus produces androgen and testosterone; female normally produces none in utero. Drugs and stress may alter the amount and timing of hormone levels in the male and may stimulate hormone production in the female. This produces potential for infinite variety in genital and brain differentiation of the human fetus.
Internal organ formation	Hormones in the male fetus are responsible for disintegrating the Müllerian ducts and developing the Wolffian ducts into the prostate gland and seminal vesicles. Absence of hormones in the female causes Müllerian ducts to develop into the uterus, the inner two thirds of the vagina, and the fallopian tubes.
Formation of external organs	Every human fetus has a clitoris, labia, and vagina. Hormones in the male form the scrotum from the labia minora, and the penis from the labia majora and clitoris.
Sex assignment and rearing	Influence of genital appearance on labeling and psychosocial aspects of gender identity. Core gender identity is formed by age 3.
Self-concept, physiology of orgasm, puberty	Sexual fantasies and first activities associated with orgasm are believed to become "imprinted" on the nervous system, bonding imagery with self-concept. This accounts for individual preferences, normal or abnormal.

Treatment

Individual and family therapy are indicated for treatment of childhood gender identity disorders. Ideally, a therapist of the same sex may be useful for role-modeling purposes. The earlier this problem is diagnosed and treatment begins, the more hopeful the prognosis.

In adults, individual and couples therapy may help the patient to cope with the decision to live as the opposite sex or to cope with the knowledge that he or she will not be able to live as the opposite sex. Sex reassignment through hormonal and surgical treatment may be an option; however, surgical sex reassignment has not been as beneficial as first hoped. Severe psychological problems may persist after sex reassignment and sometimes lead to suicide. Further, these patients frequently have gender disorders as part of a larger pattern of depression and personality disorders, such as borderline personality disorder.

Female transsexuals have shown more stable patterns of adjustment with or without treatment.

Clinical implications

Nursing care of a person with gender identity disorder should include the following:

• A nonjudgmental approach in facial expression, tone of voice, and choice of words to convey acceptance of the individual's choices

• Respect for the patient's privacy and sense of modesty, particularly during procedures or examinations

• Observation for related or compounding problems such as suicidal thought or intent, depression, and anxiety

• The realization that treating such a patient with empathy does not threaten your own sexuality

• Referral of the patient for therapy, as appropriate

Genital herpes
(Venereal herpes)

Description

Genital herpes is an acute, inflammatory disease of the genitalia. This infection is one of the most common recurring disorders of the genitalia. Diagnosis is based on physical examination and patient history. Prognosis varies according to the patient's age, the strength of his immune defenses, and the infection site. Primary genital herpes is usually self-limiting but may cause painful local or systemic disease. In newborns, in patients with weak immune defenses, and in those with disseminated disease, genital herpes is frequently severe, with complications and a high mortality.

Cause

Herpes simplex II virus

Mode of transmission

• Sexual contact is the usual means of transmission.

• Contamination also occurs from infected toilet seats, towels, and bathtubs.

• Pregnant women may transmit the infection to newborns during vaginal delivery. Such transmitted infection may be localized (for instance, in the eyes) or disseminated, and may be associated with central nervous system involvement.

Signs and symptoms

• Fluid-filled, painless vesicles. These appear after a 3- to 7-day incubation period. In the female, they occur on the cervix (the primary infection site) and possibly on the labia, perianal skin, vulva, or vagina; in the male, on the glans penis, foreskin, or penile shaft. Extragenital lesions may occur in the mouth or anus.

• Extensive, shallow, painful ulcers. These create marked edema if vesicles rupture.

• Tender inguinal lymph nodes. These occur when ulcers develop.

• Other features of initial mucocutaneous infection: fever, malaise, dysuria, and, in the female, leukorrhea.

Diagnostic tests

• Demonstration of herpes simplex II virus in vesicular fluid, using tissue culture techniques, confirms genital herpes.

• Helpful but nondiagnostic measures include laboratory data showing increased antibody titers and atypical cells in smears of genital lesions.

Treatment

Acyclovir (Zovirax) has proven to be an effective treatment for genital herpes. Each of the three available dosage forms has a specific indication. A 5% acyclovir ointment is prescribed for first-time infections. I.V. administration may be required for patients who are hospitalized with severe genital herpes or who are immunocompromised and have potentially life-threatening herpes infections. Oral acyclovir may be prescribed for patients suffering from first-time infections or from recurrent outbreaks.

Clinical implications
• Encourage the patient to get adequate rest and nutrition and to keep the lesions dry, except for applying prescribed medications (using aseptic technique).
• Encourage the patient to avoid sexual intercourse during the active stage of this disease (while lesions are present). Urge the patient to seek medical examination for sexual partners.
• Advise the female patient to have a Pap smear taken every 6 months.
• Explain to the infected pregnant patient the risk to her newborn from vaginal delivery. Urge her to consider cesarean delivery.
• Refer patients to Herpes Resource Center, an American Social Health Association group, for support.

Complications
Rare complications—which usually arise from extragenital lesions—include the following:
• Hepatic keratitis, which may lead to blindness
• Potentially fatal herpes simplex encephalitis

Genital warts
(Venereal warts, condylomata acuminata)

Description
Genital warts consist of papillomas, with fibrous tissue overgrowth from the dermis and thickened epithelial coverings. Genital warts grow rapidly in the presence of heavy perspiration, poor hygiene, or pregnancy. They frequently accompany other genital infections. They are uncommon before puberty or after menopause.

Cause
Verruca vulgaris, the same papillomavirus that causes the common wart

Mode of transmission
Sexual contact is the usual mode of transmission.

Signs and symptoms
After a 1- to 6-month incubation period (usually 2 months), genital warts develop on moist surfaces: in males, on the subpreputial sac, within the urethral meatus, and less commonly on the penile shaft; in females, on the vulva and on vaginal and cervical walls. In both sexes, papillomas spread to the perineum and the perianal area. These painless warts start as tiny red or pink swellings that grow (sometimes to 4″ [10 cm]) and become pedunculated. Typically, multiple swellings give such warts a cauliflower appearance. If infected, these lesions become malodorous.

Diagnostic tests
Dark-field examination of scrapings from wart cells shows marked vascularization of epidermal cells, which helps to differentiate genital warts from condylomata lata.

Treatment
The initial goal of treatment is to eradicate associated genital infections. The warts may resolve spontaneously, but if treatment is necessary, topical drug therapy (20% podophyllum in tincture of benzoin or trichloroacetic acid) removes small warts. (Podophyllum is contraindicated in pregnancy.) Warts larger than 1″ (2.5 cm) are usually removed by surgery, cryosurgery, electrocautery, or 5-fluorouracil cream debridement. Rarely, the patient's warts are excised and used to prepare a vaccine, which is then injected into the patient's body to try to create antibodies. Carbon dioxide laser treatment has also been proven effective.

Clinical implications

• Tell the patient to wash off podophyllum with soap and water 4 to 6 hours after applying it. Recommend use of a condom during sexual intercourse until healing is complete. Advise the patient to protect the surrounding tissue with petrolatum before using trichloroacetic acid.

• Emphasize other preventive measures, such as avoiding sex with an infected partner and regularly washing genitalia with soap and water. To prevent vaginal infection, advise the female patient to avoid feminine hygiene sprays, frequent douching, tight pants, nylon underpants, or panty hose.

• Encourage examination of the patient's sexual partners. Also advise female patients to have a Pap smear taken every 6 months.

Giardiasis
(*Giardia* enteritis, lambliasis)

Description

Giardiasis is an infection of the small bowel. Mild infection may not produce intestinal symptoms. In untreated giardiasis, symptoms wax and wane. With treatment, recovery is complete. Giardiasis is most common in areas where sanitation and hygiene are poor. In the United States, it is most common in travelers who have recently returned from endemic areas and in campers who drink unpurified water from contaminated streams. Infection does not confer immunity, so reinfection may occur.

Cause

Giardia lamblia, a symmetrical flagellate protozoan that has two stages: a cystic stage and a trophozoite stage

Mode of transmission

• Ingestion of *G. lamblia* cysts in fecally contaminated water

• Fecal-oral transfer of *G. lamblia* cysts by an infected person. Probably because of frequent hand-to-mouth activity, children are more likely to become infected with *G. lamblia* than are adults.

Risk factor

Hypogammaglobulinemia

Signs and symptoms

• Chronic GI complaints, such as abdominal cramps

• Pale, loose, greasy, malodorous, frequent stools (from 2 to 10 daily) that contain mucus

• Possible fatigue and weight loss in chronic giardiasis

Diagnostic tests

• Laboratory examination of a fresh stool specimen for cysts or examination of duodenal aspirate for trophozoites confirms the diagnosis.

• Barium-enhanced X-ray of the small bowel may show mucosal edema and barium segmentation.

Treatment

Giardiasis responds readily to a 10-day course of metronidazole or a 7-day course of quinacrine and furazolidone P.O. Severe diarrhea may require parenteral fluid replacement to prevent dehydration if oral fluid intake is inadequate.

Clinical implications

• Inform the patient receiving metronidazole of expected adverse effects: commonly headache, anorexia, and nausea; and less commonly vomiting, diarrhea, and abdominal cramps. Warn against drinking alcoholic beverages, because these may provoke a disulfiram-like reaction. If the patient is a woman, ask if she is pregnant, because metronidazole is contraindicated during pregnancy.

• When talking to family members and other suspected contacts, emphasize the importance of stool examinations for *G. lamblia* cysts.

• Hospitalization may be required. If so, apply enteric precautions. A child or an incontinent adult patient will require a private room. When caring for such a patient, pay strict attention to handwashing, particularly after handling feces. Quickly dispose of fecal material. (Normal sewage systems can remove and process infected feces adequately.)

• Teach good personal hygiene, particularly proper hand-washing technique.

• To help prevent giardiasis, warn travelers to endemic areas not to drink water or eat uncooked and unpeeled fruits or vegetables (they may have been rinsed in contaminated water). Prophylactic drug therapy is not recommended. Advise campers to purify all stream water before drinking it.

• Report epidemic situations to public health authorities.

Glaucoma

Description

Glaucoma is a group of disorders characterized by abnormally high intraocular pressure (IOP), which can damage the optic nerve. Glaucoma occurs in three primary forms: chronic open-angle (primary), acute closed-angle, and congenital. It may also be secondary to other causes. In the United States, glaucoma affects 2% of the population over age 40 and accounts for 12% of all new cases of blindness. Its incidence is highest among blacks. Prognosis is good with early treatment. (See also *Blindness,* p. 312.)

Causes
Chronic open-angle glaucoma
This results from overproduction of aqueous humor or obstruction of its outflow through the trabecular meshwork or the canal of Schlemm. This form of glaucoma is frequently fa-

milial. It affects 90% of all patients with glaucoma.
Acute closed-angle glaucoma
Also called narrow-angle glaucoma, this form results from obstruction to the outflow of aqueous humor from anatomically narrow angles between the anterior iris and the posterior corneal surface, shallow anterior chambers, a thickened iris that causes angle closure on pupil dilation, or a bulging iris that presses on the trabeculae, closing the angle (peripheral anterior synechiae).
Congenital glaucoma
This form is inherited as an autosomal recessive trait.
Secondary glaucoma
This can result from uveitis, trauma, or drugs (such as steroids). Neovascularization in the angle can result from vein occlusion or diabetes.

Signs and symptoms
Patients within the IOP normal range of 8 to 21 mm Hg can develop signs and symptoms of glaucoma, and patients who have abnormally high pressure may have no clinical effects.
Chronic open-angle glaucoma
This is usually bilateral and slowly progressive. Onset is insidious. Symptoms appear late in the disease. They include the following:
—Mild aching in the eyes
—Gradual loss of peripheral vision
—Seeing halos around lights
—Reduced visual acuity, especially at night, that is uncorrectable with glasses
Acute closed-angle glaucoma
Typically, onset is rapid, constituting an ophthalmic emergency. Unless treated promptly, this form of glaucoma produces blindness in the affected eye in 3 to 5 days. Symptoms may include the following:
—Unilateral inflammation and pain
—Pressure over the eye

Blindness

Blindness affects 28 million people worldwide. In the United States, blindness is legally defined as optimal visual acuity of 20/200 or less in the better eye after best correction, or a visual field not exceeding 20 degrees in the better eye.

According to the World Health Organization, the most common causes of preventable blindness worldwide are trachoma, onchocerciasis (roundworm infection transmitted by a blackfly and other species of *Simulium*), and xerophthalmia (dryness of conjunctiva and cornea from vitamin A deficiency).

In the United States, the most common causes of acquired blindness are glaucoma, senile macular degeneration, and diabetic retinopathy. However, incidence of blindness from glaucoma is decreasing because of early detection and treatment. Rarer causes of acquired blindness include herpes simplex keratitis, cataracts, and retinal detachment.

—Moderate pupil dilation that is non-reactive to light
—Cloudy cornea
—Blurring and decreased visual acuity
—Photophobia
—Seeing halos around lights
—Nausea and vomiting

Diagnostic tests

• Tonometry (using an applanation, Schiotz, or pneumatic tonometer) measures the IOP and provides a baseline for reference.
• Fingertip tension also assesses IOP in acute closed-angle glaucoma. On gentle palpation of closed eyelids, one eye feels harder than the other.
• Slit-lamp examination is used to assess the anterior structures of the eye, including the cornea, iris, and lens.
• Gonioscopy determines the angle of the anterior chamber of the eye, enabling differentiation between chronic open-angle glaucoma and acute closed-angle glaucoma. The angle is normal in chronic open-angle glaucoma; however, in older patients partial closure of the angle may also occur, so that two forms of glaucoma coexist.
• Ophthalmoscopy provides visualization of the fundus, where cupping and atrophy of the optic disk are apparent in chronic open-angle glaucoma. These changes appear later in

uncontrolled chronic closed-angle glaucoma. A pale disk appears in acute closed-angle glaucoma.
• Perimetry permits determination of peripheral vision loss in chronic open-angle glaucoma.
• Fundus photography recordings are used to monitor the optic disk for any changes.

Treatment

For chronic open-angle glaucoma, treatment initially decreases IOP through administration of beta-blockers such as timolol (contraindicated for asthmatics or patients with bradycardia) or betaxolol (Betoptic), a beta$_1$-blocker; epinephrine; or diuretics such as acetazolamide. Drug treatment also includes miotic eye drops, such as pilocarpine, to facilitate outflow of aqueous humor.

Patients who are unresponsive to drug therapy may be candidates for argon laser trabeculoplasty (ALT) or a surgical filtering procedure called trabeculectomy, which creates an opening for aqueous outflow. In ALT, an argon laser beam is focused on the trabecular meshwork of an open angle. This produces a thermal burn that changes the surface of the meshwork and increases the outflow of aqueous humor. In trabeculectomy, a flap of sclera is dissected free to expose the trabecular meshwork. Then, this discrete tissue block is removed and a peripheral iridectomy is performed. This produces an opening for aqueous outflow under the conjunctiva, creating a filtering bleb.

Acute closed-angle glaucoma is an ocular emergency requiring immediate treatment to lower IOP. If pressure does not decrease with drug therapy, laser iridotomy or surgical peripheral iridectomy must be performed promptly to save the patient's vision. Iridectomy relieves pressure by excising part of the iris to reestablish aqueous humor outflow. A prophylactic iridectomy is performed a few days later on the normal eye. Preoperative drug therapy includes acetazolamide to lower IOP; pilocarpine to constrict the pupil, forcing the iris away from the trabeculae and allowing fluid to escape; and I.V. mannitol (20%) or oral glycerin (50%) to force fluid from the eye by making the blood hypertonic. Severe pain may necessitate narcotic analgesics.

Clinical implications

• Stress the importance of meticulous compliance with prescribed drug therapy to prevent disk changes, loss of vision, and an increase in IOP.
• For the patient with acute closed-angle glaucoma, give medications, as ordered, and prepare him physically and psychologically for laser iridotomy or surgery.
• Postoperative care after peripheral iridectomy includes cycloplegic eye drops to relax the ciliary muscle and to decrease inflammation, thus preventing adhesions. *Note:* Cycloplegics must be used only in the affected eye. The use of these drops in the normal eye may precipitate an attack of acute closed-angle glaucoma in that eye, threatening the patient's residual vision.
• Encourage ambulation immediately after surgery.
• Postoperative care after surgical filtering, includes dilation and topical steroids to rest the pupil.
• Stress the importance of glaucoma screening for early detection and prevention. All persons over age 35, especially those with family histories of glaucoma, should have an annual tonometric examination. (See also *Teaching Topics in Glaucoma.*)

Glomerulonephritis, acute poststreptococcal
(Acute glomerulonephritis)

Description

Acute poststreptococcal glomerulonephritis (APSGN) is a relatively com-

---

Teaching Topics in Glaucoma

• An explanation of the disorder: acute closed-angle or chronic open-angle glaucoma
• Intraocular pressure: what it is and why it needs to be lowered
• Preparation for gonioscopy, slit-lamp examination, or other nonroutine eye tests
• Importance of using prescribed eye drops in chronic open-angle glaucoma to prevent vision loss
• Administration of eye drops
• Argon laser trabeculoplasty and post-treatment instructions
• Surgical iridectomy for acute closed-angle glaucoma; trabeculectomy for chronic open-angle glaucoma

mon bilateral inflammation of the glomeruli. It follows a streptococcal infection of the respiratory tract or, less often, a skin infection, such as impetigo. APSGN is most common in boys ages 3 to 7 but can occur at any age. Up to 95% of children and up to 70% of adults with APSGN recover fully; the rest may progress to chronic renal failure within months.

Causes
APSGN results from the entrapment and collection of antigen–antibody complexes (produced in response to streptococcal infection) in the glomerular capillary membranes, inducing inflammatory damage and impeding glomerular function. Sometimes, the immune complexes further damage the glomerular membrane. The damaged and inflamed glomerulus loses the ability to be selectively permeable, and allows red blood cells (RBCs) and proteins to filter through as the glomerular filtration rate falls. Uremic poisoning may result.

Signs and symptoms
Usually, APSGN begins within 1 to 3 weeks after untreated pharyngitis. Symptoms include the following:
• Mild to moderate edema
• Proteinuria
• Azotemia
• Hematuria (urine is smoky or coffee-colored)
• Oliguria (less than 400 ml/24 hours)
• Fatigue
• Mild to severe hypertension
• Possible symptoms of pulmonary edema: shortness of breath, dyspnea, and orthopnea

Diagnostic tests
• Renal biopsy may be necessary to confirm diagnosis or assess renal tissue status.
• Blood values (elevated electrolytes, blood urea nitrogen [BUN], and serum creatinine levels) indicate renal failure if urinalysis results occur as described below.

• Urinalysis (RBCs, white blood cells, mixed cell casts, and protein) indicates renal failure when blood values occur as described.
• Elevated antistreptolysin-O titers (in 80% of patients), elevated streptozyme and anti-DNase B titers, and low serum complement levels verify recent streptococcal infection.
• Throat culture may also show group A beta-hemolytic streptococci.
• Kidney-ureter-bladder X-rays show bilateral kidney enlargement.

Treatment
The goals of treatment are relief of symptoms and prevention of complications. Vigorous supportive care includes bed rest, fluid and dietary sodium restrictions, and correction of electrolyte imbalances (possibly with dialysis, although this is rarely necessary). Therapy may include diuretics such as metolazone or furosemide, to reduce extracellular fluid overload, and an antihypertensive such as hydralazine. The use of antibiotics to prevent secondary infection or transmission to others is controversial.

Clinical implications
Because APSGN usually resolves within 2 weeks, patient care is primarily supportive.
• Check vital signs and electrolyte values. Monitor intake and output and daily weight. Assess renal function daily through serum creatinine and BUN levels, and urine creatinine clearance. Watch for and immediately report signs of acute renal failure (oliguria, azotemia, and acidosis).
• Consult the dietitian to provide a diet high in calories and low in protein, sodium, potassium, and fluids.
• Protect the debilitated patient against secondary infection by providing good nutrition, using good hygienic technique, and preventing contact with infected persons.
• Bed rest is necessary during the

acute phase. Allow the patient to resume normal activities gradually as symptoms subside.

• Provide emotional support for the patient and family. If the patient is on dialysis, explain the procedure fully.

• Advise the patient with a history of chronic upper respiratory tract infections to immediately report signs of infection (fever, sore throat).

• Tell the patient that follow-up examinations are necessary to detect chronic renal failure. Stress the need for regular blood pressure, urinary protein, and renal function assessments during the convalescent months to detect recurrence. After APSGN, gross hematuria may recur during nonspecific viral infections; abnormal urinary findings may persist for years.

• Encourage pregnant women with histories of APSGN to have frequent medical evaluations, because pregnancy further stresses the kidneys and increases the risk of chronic renal failure.

Glomerulonephritis, chronic

Description

Chronic glomerulonephritis is a slowly progressive, noninfectious disease characterized by inflammation of the renal glomeruli. This condition remains subclinical until the progressive phase begins. By the time it produces symptoms, chronic glomerulonephritis is usually irreversible. It results in eventual renal failure.

Causes

Primary renal disorders
—Membranoproliferative glomerulonephritis
—Membranous glomerulopathy
—Focal glomerulosclerosis
—Poststreptococcal glomerulonephritis

Systemic disorders
—Lupus erythematosus
—Goodpasture's syndrome
—Hemolytic-uremic syndrome

Signs and symptoms

This disease usually develops insidiously and asymptomatically, frequently over many years. At any time, however, it may suddenly become progressive.

Initial stage
—Nephrotic syndrome
—Hypertension
—Proteinuria
—Hematuria

Late stage
—Azotemia
—Nausea
—Vomiting
—Pruritus
—Dyspnea
—Malaise
—Fatigability
—Mild to severe anemia
—Severe hypertension (may cause cardiac hypertrophy, leading to congestive heart failure)

Diagnostic tests

• Urinalysis reveals proteinuria, hematuria, cylindruria, and red blood cell casts.

• Blood tests reveal rising blood urea nitrogen and serum creatinine levels, indicating advanced renal insufficiency.

• X-ray or ultrasound examination shows small kidneys.

• Kidney biopsy identifies underlying disease and provides data needed to guide therapy.

Treatment

Treatment is essentially nonspecific and symptomatic. The goals are to control hypertension with antihypertensives and a sodium-restricted diet, to correct fluid and electrolyte imbalances through restrictions and replacement, to reduce edema with diuretics such as furosemide, and to prevent congestive heart failure. Treatment may also include antibiotics (for symptomatic urinary tract infections), dialysis, or transplantation.

Clinical implications
Patient care is primarily supportive, focusing on continual observation and sound patient teaching.

• Accurately monitor vital signs, intake and output, and daily weight to evaluate fluid retention. Observe for signs of fluid, electrolyte, and acid-base imbalances.

• Ask the dietitian to plan low-sodium, high-calorie meals with adequate protein.

• Administer medications, as ordered, and provide good skin care (because of pruritus and edema) and oral hygiene. Instruct the patient to continue taking prescribed antihypertensives as scheduled, even if he is feeling better, and to report any adverse effects. Advise him to take diuretics in the morning, so that sleep will not be disrupted to void, and teach him how to assess ankle edema.

• Warn the patient to report signs of infection, particularly urinary tract infection, and to avoid contact with persons who have infections. Urge follow-up examinations to assess renal function.

• Help the patient adjust to this illness by encouraging him to express his feelings. Explain all necessary procedures beforehand, and answer the patient's questions about them.

Glycogen storage disease

Description
Glycogen storage diseases consist of at least eight distinct errors of metabolism that alter the synthesis or degradation of glycogen, the form in which glucose is stored in the body. Normally, muscle and liver cells store glycogen. Muscle glycogen is used in muscle contraction; liver glycogen can be converted into free glucose, which can then diffuse into the blood to increase blood glucose levels. The most common glycogen storage disease is Type I—von Gierke's, or hepatorenal glycogen storage disease.

Glycogen storage diseases manifest as dysfunctions of the liver, the heart, or the musculoskeletal system. Symptoms vary from mild and easily controlled hypoglycemia to severe organ involvement that may lead to cardiac and respiratory failure.

Causes
• Almost all glycogen storage diseases (Types I through V and Type VII) are inherited as autosomal recessive traits. The mode of transmission of Type VI is unknown; Type VIII may be an X-linked trait.

• Type I results from a deficiency of the liver enzyme glucose-6-phosphatase. This enzyme converts glucose-6-phosphate into free glucose and is necessary for the release of stored glycogen and glucose into the bloodstream, to relieve hypoglycemia.

Signs and symptoms
Clinical features of Type I glycogen storage disease may include the following:

Primary clinical features
—Hepatomegaly (also occurs in Types III, IV, VI, and VIII)
—Rapid onset of hypoglycemia and ketosis when food is withheld (also occurs in Types III, IV, VI, and VIII)

Other symptoms
—Infants: acidosis, hyperlipidemia, GI bleeding, coma. Infants may die of acidosis before age 2; if they survive past this age, with proper treatment, they may grow normally and live to adulthood, with only minimal hepatomegaly. However, there is a danger of adenomatous liver nodules, which may be premalignant.
—Children: low resistance to infection and, without proper treatment, short stature

Rare Forms of Glycogen Storage Disease

TYPE	CLINICAL FEATURES	DIAGNOSTIC TEST RESULTS
II (Pompe's) Absence of alpha-1,4-glucosidase (acid maltase)	• *Infants:* cardiomegaly, profound hypotonia, and, occasionally, endocardial fibroelastosis (usually fatal before age 1 because of cardiac or respiratory failure) • *Some infants and young children:* muscular weakness and wasting, variable organ involvement (slower progression, usually fatal by age 19) • *Adults:* muscle weakness without organomegaly (slowly progressive but not fatal)	• *Muscle biopsy:* increased concentration of glycogen with normal structure; alpha 1,4-glucosidase deficiency • *EKG* (in infants): large QRS complexes in all leads; inverted T waves; shortened P-R interval • *Electromyography* (in adults): muscle fiber irritability; myotonic discharges • *Amniocentesis:* alpha-1,4-glucosidase deficiency • *Placenta or umbilical cord examination:* alpha-1,4-glucosidase deficiency
III (Cori's) Absence of debranching enzyme (amylo-1,6-glucosidase) (*Note:* predominant cause of glycogen storage disease in Israel)	• *Young children:* massive hepatomegaly, which may disappear by puberty; growth retardation; moderate splenomegaly; hypoglycemia • *Adults:* progressive myopathy • Occasionally, moderate cardiomegaly, cirrhosis, muscle wasting, hypoglycemia	• *Liver biopsy:* deficient debranching activity; increased glycogen concentration • *Laboratory tests* (in children only): elevated serum glutamic-oxaloacetic transaminase (SGOT) or serum glutamic-pyruvic transaminase (SGPT); increased erythrocyte glycogen
IV (Andersen's) Deficiency of branching enzyme (amylo-1:4,1:6-transglucosidase) (*Note:* extremely rare)	• *Infants:* hepatosplenomegaly, ascites, muscle hypotonia; usually fatal before age 2 from progressive cirrhosis	• *Liver biopsy:* deficient branching enzyme activity; glycogen molecule has longer outer branches.
V (McArdle's) Deficiency of muscle phosphorylase	• *Children:* mild or no symptoms • *Adults:* muscle cramps and pain dur-	• *Serum lactate:* no increase in venous levels in sample drawn from extremity after ischemic

(continued)

Rare Forms of Glycogen Storage Disease *(continued)*

TYPE	CLINICAL FEATURES	DIAGNOSTIC TEST RESULTS
V (McArdle's) *(continued)*	ing strenuous exercise, possibly resulting in myoglobinuria and renal failure • *Older patients:* significant muscle weakness and wasting	exercise • *Muscle biopsy:* lack of phosphorylase activity; increased glycogen content
VI (Hers') Possible deficiency of hepatic phosphorylase	• Mild symptoms (similar to those of Type I), requiring no treatment	• *Liver biopsy:* decreased phosphorylase b activity; increased glycogen concentration
VII Deficiency of muscle phosphofructokinase	• Muscle cramps during strenuous exercise, resulting in myoglobinuria and possible renal failure • Reticulocytosis	• *Serum lactate:* no increase in venous levels in sample drawn from extremity after ischemic exercise • *Muscle biopsy:* deficient phosphofructokinase; marked rise in glycogen concentration • *Blood studies:* low erythrocyte phosphofructokinase activity; reduced half-life of red blood cells
VIII Deficiency of hepatic phosphorylase kinase	• Mild hepatomegaly • Mild hypoglycemia	• *Liver biopsy:* deficient phosphorylase b kinase activity; increased liver glycogen • *Blood study:* deficient phosphorylase b kinase in leukocytes

—Adolescents: gouty arthritis and nephropathy; chronic tophaceous gout; bleeding (especially epistaxis); small superficial vessels visible in skin; fat deposits in cheeks, buttocks, and subcutaneous tissues; poor muscle tone; enlarged kidneys; xanthomas over extensor surfaces of arms and legs; steatorrhea; multiple, bilateral, yellow lesions in fundi; and osteoporosis. (Also see *Rare Forms of Glycogen Storage Disease,* pp. 317 and 318, for a description of the various types of the disease.)

Diagnostic tests

• Liver biopsy confirms diagnosis by showing normal glycogen synthetase and phosphorylase activity but reduced or absent glucose-6-phosphatase activity. Glycogen structure is normal, but amounts are elevated.

• Muscle biopsy is one of the key tests

in diagnosing Type I glycogen storage disease.
• Laboratory studies of plasma demonstrate low glucose levels but high levels of free fatty acids, triglycerides, cholesterol, and uric acid. Serum analysis reveals high pyruvic and lactic acid levels.
• Injection of glucagon or epinephrine increases pyruvic and lactic acid levels but does not increase blood glucose levels. Glucose tolerance test curve typically shows depletional hypoglycemia and reduced insulin output.
• Prenatal diagnostic tests are available for Types II, III, and IV.

Treatment
For Type I, the aims of treatment are to maintain glucose homeostasis and prevent secondary consequences of hypoglycemia through frequent feedings and constant nocturnal nasogastric drip with Polycose, dextrose, or Vivonex. Treatment includes a low-fat diet, with normal amounts of protein and calories; carbohydrates should contain glucose or glucose polymers only.

Therapy for Type III includes frequent feedings and a high-protein diet. Type IV requires a high-protein, high-calorie diet; bed rest; diuretics; sodium restriction; and paracentesis, if necessary, to relieve ascites. Types V and VII require no treatment, but patients must avoid strenuous exercise. No treatment is necessary for Types VI and VIII, and no effective treatment exists for Type II.

Clinical implications
When managing Type I disease, follow these guidelines:
• Advise the patient or parents to include carbohydrate foods containing mainly starch in his diet and to sweeten foods with glucose only.
• Before discharge, teach the patient or family member how to pass a nasogastric tube, use a pump with alarm capacity, monitor blood glucose with Dextrostix, and recognize symptoms of hypoglycemia.
• Watch for and report signs of infection (fever, chills, myalgia) and of hepatic encephalopathy (mental confusion, stupor, asterixis, coma) caused by increased blood ammonia levels.

When managing other types of glycogen storage disease, follow these guidelines:
• Type II: Explain test procedures, such as electromyography and EEG, thoroughly.
• Type III: Instruct the patient to eat a high-protein diet (eggs, nuts, fish, meat, poultry, and cheese).
• Type IV: Watch for signs of hepatic failure (nausea, vomiting, irregular bowel function, clay-colored stools, right upper quadrant pain, jaundice, dehydration, electrolyte imbalance, edema, and changes in mental status, progressing to coma).
• When caring for patients with Types II, III, and IV, offer parents reassurance and emotional support. Recommend and arrange for genetic counseling, if appropriate.
• Types V through VIII: Care for these patients is minimal. Explain the disorder to the patient and his family, and help them accept the limitations imposed by the disease.

Goiter
(Nontoxic goiter)

Description
Simple goiter, or thyroid gland enlargement not caused by inflammation or a neoplasm, is commonly classified as endemic or sporadic. Endemic goiter usually results from geographically related nutritional factors. Areas in the United States where this nutritional deficiency is most common are called "goiter belts." They include the Mid-

west and the Pacific Northwest. Iodized salt prevents this deficiency. Sporadic goiter follows ingestion of certain drugs or foods and affects no particular segment of the population.

Goiter occurs when the thyroid gland cannot secrete enough thyroid hormone to meet metabolic requirements; as a result, the thyroid mass increases to compensate for inadequate hormone synthesis. Such compensation usually overcomes mild to moderate hormonal impairment.

Simple goiter is found most frequently in females, especially during adolescence, pregnancy, and menopause. With treatment, prognosis is good. Detailed patient history may reveal goitrogenic medications or foods, or endemic influence.

Causes

Inherited defects may cause insufficient thyroxine (T_4) synthesis or impaired iodine metabolism.

Endemic goiter
—Inadequate dietary intake of iodine

Sporadic goiter
—Ingestion of large amounts of goitrogenic foods. These are foods containing agents that decrease thyroxine production, such as rutabagas, cabbage, soybeans, peanuts, peaches, peas, strawberries, spinach, and radishes.

—Goitrogenic drugs. These include propylthiouracil iodides, phenylbutazone, para-aminosalicylic acid, cobalt, and lithium.

Signs and symptoms

• Thyroid enlargement. This may range from a single small nodule to massive multinodular goiter.
• Respiratory distress
• Dysphagia
• Swelling and distention of the neck
• Possible dizziness or syncope. Known as Pemberton's sign, this may occur when the patient raises his arms above his head, especially with a large goiter.

Diagnostic tests

• Thyroid-stimulating hormone (TSH) or triiodothyronine (T_3) serum concentration is high or normal.
• T_4 serum concentration is low-normal or normal.
• ^{131}I uptake is normal or increased (50% of the dose at 24 hours).
• Protein-bound iodine is low-normal or normal.
• Urinary excretion of iodine is low.

Treatment

The goal of treatment is to reduce thyroid hyperplasia. Exogenous thyroid hormone replacement (with levothyroxine, desiccated thyroid, or liothyronine) is the treatment of choice; it inhibits TSH secretion and allows the gland to rest. Small doses of iodide (Lugol's or potassium iodide solution) fequently relieve goiter that results from iodine deficiency. Sporadic goiter requires avoidance of known goitrogenic drugs or food. A large goiter unresponsive to treatment may require subtotal thyroidectomy.

Clinical implications

• Watch for progressive thyroid gland enlargement and for the development of hard nodules in the gland, which may indicate malignancy.
• To maintain constant hormone levels, instruct the patient to take prescribed thyroid hormone preparations at the same time each day. Also, tell him to watch for and immediately report signs of thyrotoxicosis: increased pulse rate, palpitations, nausea, vomiting, diarrhea, sweating, tremors, agitation, and shortness of breath.
• Instruct the patient with endemic goiter to use iodized salt to supply the daily 150 to 300 mcg iodine necessary to prevent goiter.
• Monitor the patient taking goitrogenic drugs for signs of sporadic goiter.

Gonorrhea

Description

A common venereal disease, gonorrhea is an infection of the genitourinary tract (especially the urethra and cervix) and occasionally of the rectum, pharynx, and eyes. After adequate treatment, prognosis in both males and females is excellent, although reinfection is common. Incidence of gonorrhea is especially prevalent among unmarried persons and young people, particularly between ages 19 and 25. Severe disseminated infection is more common in women than in men.

Causes

Neisseria gonorrhoeae

Mode of transmission

• Almost exclusively, transmission occurs through sexual contact with an infected person.
• Children born of infected mothers can contract gonococcal ophthalmia neonatorum during passage through the birth canal.
• Children and adults with gonorrhea can contract gonococcal conjunctivitis by touching their eyes with contaminated hands.

Signs and symptoms

Most common

Most females remain asymptomatic, but inflammation and a greenish-yellow discharge from the cervix are the most common symptoms. Males may be asymptomatic, but the following symptoms usually develop after a 3- to 6-day incubation period.
—Symptoms of urethritis, including dysuria and purulent urethral discharge
—Redness and swelling at the site of infection

Other symptoms

These vary according to the site involved.

—Urethra: dysuria, urinary frequency and incontinence, purulent discharge, itching, red and edematous meatus
—Vulva: occasional itching, burning, and pain caused by exudate from an adjacent infected area. Vulval symptoms tend to be more severe before puberty or after menopause.
—Vagina (most common site in children over age 1): engorgement, redness, swelling, and profuse purulent discharge
—Pelvis: severe pelvic and lower abdominal pain, muscular rigidity, tenderness, and abdominal distention. As infection spreads, nausea, vomiting, fever, and tachycardia may develop in patients with salpingitis or pelvic inflammatory disease (PID)
—Liver: right upper quadrant pain in patients with perihepatitis
—Eyes: adult conjunctivitis (most common in men), with unilateral conjunctival redness and swelling; and gonococcal ophthalmia neonatorum, with lid edema, bilateral conjunctival infection, and abundant purulent discharge 2 to 3 days after birth
—Other possible symptoms: pharyngitis; tonsillitis; rectal burning, itching, and bloody mucopurulent discharge

Diagnostic tests

• Culture from the site of infection (urethra, cervix, rectum, or pharynx), grown on Thayer-Martin or Transgrow medium, usually establishes diagnosis by isolating the organism.
• Gram stain showing gram-negative diplococci supports the diagnosis and may be sufficient to confirm gonorrhea in males.
• Confirmation of gonococcal arthritis requires identification of gram-negative diplococci in smears of joint fluid and skin lesions. Complement fixation and immunofluorescent assays of serum reveal antibody titers four times normal.
• Culture of conjunctival scrapings confirms gonococcal conjunctivitis.

Treatment

Treatment of choice for uncomplicated gonorrhea (including gonorrhea during pregnancy) is 1 gram of probenecid P.O. to block penicillin excretion from the body, followed in 30 minutes by I.M. administration of 4.8 million units of aqueous procaine penicillin injected at two separate sites in a large muscle mass. If the patient is allergic to penicillin, tetracycline P.O. (contraindicated in pregnant women) or spectinomycin I.M. may be substituted.

Gonorrhea complicated by severe PID or septicemia requires I.V. antibiotic therapy with doxycycline and cefoxitin for 4 to 6 days, followed by doxycycline P.O. for an additional 4 to 6 days. Outpatient therapy may consist of cefoxitin I.M., amoxicillin P.O., or ampicillin P.O. (each with probenecid), followed by doxycycline P.O. for 10 to 14 days. Treatment of gonococcal conjunctivitis requires I.V. administration of penicillin G, accompanied by irrigation of the eye with penicillin G and saline solution.

To confirm cure of gonococcal infection, follow-up cultures are necessary 4 to 7 days after treatment and again in 6 months, or before delivery in pregnant women.

Routine instillation of 1% silver nitrate or erythromycin drops into the eyes of newborns has greatly reduced the incidence of gonococcal ophthalmia neonatorum.

Clinical implications

• Warn the patient that until cultures prove negative, he is still infectious and can transmit gonococcal infection. Double-bag all soiled dressings and contaminated instruments; wear gloves when handling contaminated material and giving patient care. If the patient is being treated as an outpatient, advise the family to take precautions against infection. Isolate the patient with eye infection.
• In the patient with gonococcal arthritis, apply moist heat to ease pain in affected joints.
• Urge the patient to inform sexual contacts of his infection so they can seek treatment also. Report all cases to public health authorities for follow-up on sexual contacts.
• Routinely instill 2 drops of 1% silver nitrate or erythromycin in the eyes of all newborns immediately after birth. Check newborns of infected mothers for signs of infection. Take specimens for culture from the infant's eyes, pharynx, and rectum.
• To prevent gonorrhea, tell patients to avoid anyone *suspected* of being infected, to use condoms during intercourse, and to avoid sharing washcloths or douche equipment.

Complications

Untreated gonorrhea can spread through the blood to the joints, tendons, meninges, and endocardium. Other complications of untreated disease include the following:
• Gonococcal septicemia (more common in females than in males)
• Sterility
• Corneal ulceration and blindness
• Arthritis

Goodpasture's syndrome

Description

Goodpasture's syndrome is a chronic relapsing pulmonary hemosiderosis, usually associated with glomerulonephritis. Abnormal production and deposition of antibody to glomerular basement membrane (GBM) activates the complement and inflammatory responses, resulting in glomerular and alveolar tissue damage. This syndrome may occur at any age but is most common in men between ages 20 and 30. Prognosis improves with aggressive immunosuppressive and antibiotic therapy and with dialysis or renal transplantation.

Causes

The cause is unknown but the following are possibilities:

• Exposure to hydrocarbons or type 2 influenza

• Genetic predisposition because of the high incidence of HLA-DRw2 in these patients

Signs and symptoms

The following signs and symptoms may occur:

• Malaise
• Fatigue
• Pallor
• Slight dyspnea
• Cough (may produce blood-tinged sputum to hemoptysis to frank pulmonary hemorrhage)
• Hematuria
• Peripheral edema
• Progressive renal failure

Diagnostic tests

• Measurement of circulating anti-GBM antibody by radioimmunoassay and linear staining of GBM and alveolar basement membrane by immunofluorescence confirm Goodpasture's syndrome.

• Immunofluorescence of alveolar basement membrane shows linear deposition of immunoglobulin, C3, and fibrinogen.

• Immunofluorescence of GBM also shows linear deposition of immunoglobulin and detects circulating anti-GBM antibody. This finding distinguishes Goodpasture's from other pulmonary renal syndromes such as Wegener's granulomatosis, polyarteritis, and systemic lupus erythematosus.

• Lung biopsy shows interstitial and intraalveolar hemorrhage with hemosiderin-laden macrophages.

• Chest X-ray reveals pulmonary infiltrates in a diffuse, nodular pattern, and renal biopsy frequently shows focal necrotic lesions and cellular crescents.

• Creatinine and blood urea nitrogen

(BUN) levels typically are elevated two to three times normal.

• Urinalysis may reveal red blood cells and cellular casts, which typify glomerular inflammation. Granular casts and proteinuria may also be observed.

Treatment

Treatment aims to remove antibody by plasmapheresis and to suppress antibody production with immunosuppressive drugs. Patients with renal failure may benefit from dialysis or transplantation. Aggressive ultrafiltration helps relieve pulmonary edema that may aggravate pulmonary hemorrhage. High-dose I.V. steroids also help control pulmonary hemorrhage.

Clinical implications

• Promote adequate oxygenation by elevating the head of the bed and administering humidified oxygen. Encourage the patient to conserve his energy. Assess respirations and breath sounds regularly. Note sputum quantity and quality.

• Monitor vital signs, arterial blood gases, hematocrit, and coagulation studies.

• Transfuse blood and administer steroids, as ordered. Observe closely for drug adverse effects.

• Assess renal function by monitoring symptoms, intake and output, daily weight, creatinine clearance, and BUN and creatinine levels.

• Teach the patient and his family what signs and symptoms to expect and how to relieve them. Carefully describe other treatment measures, such as dialysis.

Gout
(Gouty arthritis)

Description

Gout is a metabolic disease marked by increased amounts of uric acid, leading to urate deposits, called tophi, that cause painfully arthritic joints. It can strike any joint but favors those in the feet and legs. Gout develops in four stages: asymptomatic, acute, intercritical, and chronic. Primary gout usually occurs in men older than age 30 and in postmenopausal women. Secondary gout occurs in elderly persons.

Gout follows an intermittent course and often leaves patients totally free of symptoms for years between attacks. It can lead to chronic disability or incapacitation and, rarely, severe hypertension and progressive renal disease. Prognosis is good with treatment.

Causes

Primary gout

The exact cause is unknown, but it appears to be linked to a genetic defect in purine metabolism, which causes overproduction of uric acid (hyperuricemia), retention of uric acid, or both.

Secondary gout

This develops in association with other conditions (such as obesity, diabetes mellitus, hypertension, sickle-cell anemia, and renal disease). Hyperuricemia results from the breakdown of nucleic acids. It can also follow drug therapy (especially with hydrochlorothiazide or pyrazinamide) that interferes with urate excretion.

Signs and symptoms

Asymptomatic stage

No symptoms are apparent, but serum uric acid levels rise.

Acute stage

The first acute attack strikes suddenly and peaks quickly. It usually involves only one or a few joints. Mild acute attacks frequently subside quickly but tend to recur at irregular intervals. Severe attacks may persist for days or weeks. Patients may have a second attack within 6 months to 2 years, but in some the second attack is delayed for 5 to 10 years. Delayed acute attacks are sometimes accompanied by fever. A migratory acute attack sequentially

strikes various joints and the Achilles tendon, and is associated with either subdeltoid or olecranon bursitis.

Common symptoms of this stage include the following:

—Inflammation of the metatarsophalangeal joint of the great toe (usually becomes inflamed first [podagra]) followed by inflammation of the instep, ankle, heel, knee, or wrist joints

—Extreme pain in affected joints (especially common during first attack)

—Hot tender joints. Affected joints appear inflamed, dusky red, or cyanotic.

—Possible low-grade fever

Intercritical stage

Symptom-free

Chronic stage

Eventually, chronic polyarticular gout—the final, unremitting stage of this disease—sets in, with the following symptoms:

—Persistent, painful polyarthritis. Large, subcutaneous tophi form in cartilage, synovial membranes, tendons, and soft tissue. Fingers, hands, knees, feet, ulnar sides of the forearms, the helix of the ear, Achilles tendons, and, rarely, internal organs such as the kidneys and myocardium may be affected.

—Possible ulceration of the skin over tophi. A white, chalky exudate or pus may be released.

Diagnostic tests

• Aspiration of synovial fluid (arthrocentesis) or of tophaceous material reveals needlelike intracellular crystals of sodium urate. The presence of monosodium urate monohydrate crystals in synovial fluid taken from an inflamed joint or tophus establishes the diagnosis.

• Serum uric acid level is above normal, but this is not specifically diagnostic of gout.

• Urinary uric acid level is usually higher in secondary gout than in primary gout.

• Initially, X-ray examinations are normal. However, in chronic gout, X-

Pseudogout

Pseudogout, or calcium pyrophosphate disease, results when calcium pyrophosphate crystals collect in periarticular joint structures. Without treatment, it leads to permanent joint damage in about half of the patients it affects, most of whom are elderly.

Like gout, pseudogout causes abrupt joint pain and swelling—most commonly affecting the knee, wrist, ankle, and other peripheral joints. These recurrent, self-limiting attacks may be triggered by stress, trauma, surgery, severe dieting, thiazide therapy, and alcohol abuse. Associated symptoms are similar to those of rheumatoid arthritis.

Diagnosis of pseudogout depends on joint aspirations and synovial biopsy to detect calcium pyrophosphate crystals. X-rays reveal calcific densities in the fibrocartilage and linear markings along bone ends. Blood tests may detect an underlying endocrine or metabolic disorder.

Effective treatment of pseudogout may include joint aspiration to relieve fluid pressure; instillation of steroids; administration of analgesics, phenylbutazone, salicylates, or other nonsteroidal anti-inflammatory agents; and, if appropriate, treatment of the underlying endocrine or metabolic disorder.

---

rays show damage of the articular cartilage and subchondral bone. Outward displacement of the overhanging margin from the bone contour characterizes gout.

Treatment

Correct management seeks to terminate an acute attack, reduce hyperuricemia, and prevent recurrence, complications, and the formation of renal calculi. Treatment for the patient with acute gout consists of bed rest; immobilization and protection of the inflamed, painful joints; and local application of heat or cold. Analgesics, such as acetaminophen, relieve the pain associated with mild attacks, but acute inflammation requires concomitant treatment with colchicine (P.O. or I.V.) every hour for 8 hours, until the pain subsides or nausea, vomiting, cramping, or diarrhea develops. Phenylbutazone or indomethacin in therapeutic doses may be used instead, but this therapy is less specific. Resistant inflammation may require corticosteroids or corticotropin (I.V. or I.M.), or joint aspiration and intraarticular corticosteroid injection.

Treatment for chronic gout aims to decrease serum uric acid levels. Maintenance therapy with allopurinol is frequently used to suppress uric acid formation or control uric acid levels, preventing further attacks. However, this powerful drug should be used cautiously in patients with renal failure. Colchicine prevents recurrent acute attacks until uric acid returns to a normal level, but it does not reduce the acid level. Uricosuric agents—probenecid and sulfinpyrazone—promote uric acid excretion and inhibit its accumulation, but their value is limited in patients with renal impairment. These medications should not be given to patients with renal calculi.

Adjunctive therapy emphasizes a few dietary restrictions, primarily the avoidance of alcohol and purine-rich foods. Obese patients should try to lose weight, because obesity places additional stress on painful joints.

In some cases, surgery may be necessary to improve joint function or correct deformities. Tophi must be excised and drained if they become infected or ulcerated. They can also be excised to prevent ulceration, improve the patient's appearance, or make it easier for him to wear shoes or gloves.

Clinical implications

• Encourage bed rest, but use a bed cradle to keep bedclothes off extremely sensitive, inflamed joints.

• Give pain medication, as needed, especially during acute attacks. Apply hot or cold packs to inflamed joints. Administer anti-inflammatory medication and other drugs, as ordered. Watch for adverse effects. Be alert for GI disturbances with colchicine.

• Urge the patient to drink plenty of fluids (up to 2 liters a day) to prevent formation of renal calculi. When forcing fluids, record intake and output accurately. Be sure to monitor serum uric acid levels regularly. Alkalinize urine with sodium bicarbonate or another agent, if ordered.

• Watch for acute gout attacks 24 to 96 hours after surgery. Even minor surgery can precipitate an attack. Before and after surgery, administer colchicine to help prevent gout attacks, as ordered.

• Make sure the patient understands the importance of checking serum uric acid levels periodically. Tell him to avoid purine-rich foods, such as anchovies, liver, sardines, kidneys, sweetbreads, lentils, and alcoholic beverages—especially beer and wine—which raise the urate level. Explain the principles of a gradual weight-reduction diet to obese patients. Such a diet features foods containing moderate amounts of protein and very little fat.

• Advise the patient receiving allopurinol, probenecid, and other drugs to report any adverse effects immediately. (Adverse effects may include drowsiness, dizziness, nausea, vomiting, urinary frequency, and dermatitis.) Warn the patient taking probenecid or sulfinpyrazone to avoid aspirin or any other salicylate. Their combined effect causes urate retention. (Also see *Pseudogout,* p. 325.)

• Inform the patient that long-term colchicine therapy is essential during the first 3 to 6 months of treatment with uricosuric drugs or allopurinol.

Complications

• Secondary joint degeneration with eventual erosions, deformity, and disability

• Urolithiasis

• Kidney involvement, with associated tubular damage, leading to chronic renal dysfunction

• Hypertension

Granulocytopenia and lymphocytopenia
(Agranulocytosis and lymphopenia)

Description

Granulocytopenia is characterized by a marked reduction in the number of circulating granulocytes. Although this implies that all granulocytes (neutrophils, basophils, eosinophils) are reduced, granulocytopenia usually refers to decreased neutrophils. This disorder, which can occur at any age, is associated with infections and ulcerative lesions of the throat, GI tract, other mucous membranes, and skin. Its severest form is known as agranulocytosis.

Lymphocytopenia, a rare disorder, is a deficiency of circulating lymphocytes (leukocytes produced mainly in lymph nodes).

In both granulocytopenia and lymphocytopenia, the total white blood cell (WBC) count may reach dangerously low levels, leaving the body unprotected against infection. Prognosis in both disorders depends on the underlying cause and whether it can be treated. Untreated, severe granulocytopenia can be fatal in 3 to 6 days.

Causes
Granulocytopenia
—Radiation
—Drug therapy. This is a common adverse effect of antimetabolites and al-

kylating agents and may occur in the patient who is hypersensitive to phenothiazines, sulfonamides (and some sulfonamide derivatives, such as chlorothiazide), antibiotics, and antiarrhythmic drugs. Drug-induced granulocytopenia usually develops slowly and typically correlates with dosage and duration of therapy.
—Aplastic anemia
—Bone marrow malignancies
—Heredity (infantile genetic agranulocytosis)
—Splenic sequestration
—Infections that destroy peripheral blood cells and other infections, such as infectious mononucleosis
—Drugs that act as haptens (that is, carry antigens that attack blood cells and cause acute idiosyncratic or non-dose-related drug reactions)

Lymphocytopenia
—Thymic dysplasia or ataxia-telangiectasia
—Radiation
—Chemotherapy
—Postsurgical thoracic duct drainage
—Intestinal lymphangiectasia
—Impaired intestinal lymphatic drainage (as in Whipple's disease)
—Elevated plasma corticoid levels
—Other associated disorders: Hodgkin's disease, leukemia, aplastic anemia, sarcoidosis, myasthenia gravis, lupus erythematosus, protein-calorie malnutrition, renal failure, terminal cancer, tuberculosis, and severe combined immunodeficiency disease (SCID) in infants

Signs and symptoms

Granulocytopenia
—Slowly progressive fatigue and weakness
—Sudden onset of signs of overwhelming infection. Onset of fever, chills, tachycardia, anxiety, headache, and extreme prostration follows fatigue and weakness.
—Ulcers in the mouth or colon
—Pharyngeal ulceration, possibly with associated necrosis
—Pneumonia

—Septicemia, possibly leading to mild shock
—Idiosyncratic drug reaction: abrupt onset of signs of infection without slowly progressive fatigue and weakness

Lymphocytopenia
—Patients may exhibit enlarged lymph nodes, spleen, and tonsils and signs of an associated disease.

Diagnostic tests

Granulocytopenia
—Marked reduction in neutrophils (less than 500/cu mm) and WBC count lower than 2,000/cu mm, with few observable granulocytes on complete blood count (CBC), confirm granulocytopenia.
—Examination of bone marrow usually shows a scarcity of granulocytic precursor cells beyond the most immature forms, but this finding may vary, depending on the cause.

Lymphocytopenia
—A lymphocyte count less than 1,500/cu mm in adults or less than 3,000/cu mm in children indicates lymphocytopenia.
—Bone marrow and lymph node biopsies help establish the diagnosis.

Treatment

Effective management of granulocytopenia must include identification and elimination of the cause, if possible. Treatment must also control infection until the bone marrow can generate more leukocytes. That frequently means drug or radiation therapy must be discontinued and antibiotic treatment begun immediately, even while awaiting results of culture and sensitivity tests. Treatment may also include antifungal preparations and transfusion of WBC concentrate. Spontaneous restoration of leukocyte production in bone marrow usually occurs within 1 to 3 weeks.

Treatment of lymphocytopenia includes eliminating the cause (such as alkylating drugs or thoracic drainage) and managing any underlying disorders (such as Hodgkin's disease). For infants with SCID, therapy may include bone marrow transplantation.

Clinical implications
• Monitor vital signs frequently. Obtain cultures from blood, throat, urine, and sputum, as ordered. Give antibiotics, as scheduled.
• Explain the necessity of protective isolation (preferably with laminar airflow) to the patient and family. Teach proper hand-washing technique and correct use of gowns and masks. Prevent patient contact with staff members or visitors with respiratory tract infections.
• Maintain adequate nutrition and hydration, because malnutrition aggravates immunosuppression. Make sure the patient with mouth ulcerations receives a high-calorie liquid diet (for example, high-protein milk shakes). Offer a straw to make drinking less painful.
• Provide warm saline solution gargles and rinses, analgesics, and anesthetic lozenges, because good oral hygiene promotes patient comfort and facilitates the healing process.
• Ensure adequate rest, which is essential to the mobilization of the body's defenses against infection. Provide good skin and perineal care.
• Monitor CBC and differential, blood culture results, serum electrolyte levels, intake and output, and daily weight.
• To help detect granulocytopenia and lymphocytopenia in the early, most treatable stages, monitor the WBC count of any patient receiving radiation or chemotherapy. After the patient has developed bone marrow depression, he must zealously avoid exposure to infection.
• Advise the patient with known or suspected sensitivity to a drug that may lead to granulocytopenia or lymphocytopenia to alert medical personnel to this sensitivity in the future.

Guillain-Barré syndrome
(Infectious polyneuritis, Landry-Guillain-Barré syndrome, acute idiopathic polyneuritis)

Description
Guillain-Barré syndrome is an acute, rapidly progressive, and potentially fatal form of polyneuritis. The major pathologic effect is segmental demyelination of the peripheral nerves. Because this syndrome causes inflammation and degenerative changes in both the posterior (sensory) and anterior (motor) nerve roots, signs of sensory and motor losses occur simultaneously. Recovery is spontaneous and complete in about 95% of patients, but mild motor or reflex deficits in the feet and legs may persist. Prognosis is best when symptoms clear between 15 and 20 days after onset.

Causes
Precisely what causes Guillain-Barré syndrome is unknown, but it may be a cell-mediated immunologic attack on peripheral nerves in response to a virus. Precipitating factors may include the following:
• Mild febrile illness
• Surgery
• Rabies or swine influenza vaccination
• Viral illness
• Hodgkin's disease or some other malignancy
• Systemic lupus erythematosus

Signs and symptoms
• Muscle weakness (the major neurologic sign). This usually appears in the legs first (ascending type), then extends to the arms and facial nerves in 24 to 72 hours. It sometimes develops in the arms first (descending

type), or in the arms and legs simultaneously. In milder forms of this disease, muscle weakness may be absent.
• Paresthesia (common)
• Other possible features: facial diplegia (possibly with ophthalmoplegia [ocular paralysis]), dysphagia or dysarthria, and, less often, weakness of the muscles supplied by the 11th cranial (spinal accessory) nerve
• Hypotonia and areflexia

Diagnostic tests
• Cerebrospinal fluid (CSF) protein level begins to rise several days after onset of signs and symptoms, peaking in 4 to 6 weeks.
• White blood cell count in CSF remains normal, but in severe disease CSF pressure may rise above normal.
• Complete blood cell shows leukocytosis and immature forms early in the illness, but blood studies soon return to normal.
• Electromyography may show repeated firing of the same motor unit, instead of widespread sectional stimulation.
• Nerve conduction velocities are slowed soon after paralysis develops.

Treatment
Treatment is primarily supportive, consisting of endotracheal intubation or tracheotomy if the patient has difficulty clearing secretions. A trial dose of prednisone may be tried if the course of the disease is relentlessly progressive. If prednisone produces no noticeable improvement after 7 days, the drug is discontinued. Plasma exchange for patients with Guillain-Barré syndrome is currently under investigation.

Clinical implications
• Watch for ascending sensory loss, which precedes motor loss. Also, monitor vital signs and level of consciousness.
• Assess and treat respiratory dysfunction. If respiratory muscles are weak, take serial vital capacity recordings. Use a spirometer with a mouthpiece or a face mask for bedside testing.
• Obtain arterial blood gas measurements. Because neuromuscular disease results in primary hypoventilation with hypoxemia and hypercapnia, watch for PO_2 below 70 mm Hg, which signals respiratory failure. Be alert for signs of rising PCO_2 (confusion, tachypnea).
• Auscultate breath sounds, turn and position the patient, and encourage coughing and deep breathing. Begin respiratory support at the first sign of dyspnea (in adults, vital capacity less than 800 ml; in children, less than 12 ml/kg body weight) or decreasing PO_2.
• If respiratory failure becomes imminent, establish an emergency airway with an endotracheal tube, as ordered.
• Give meticulous skin care to prevent skin breakdown and contractures.
• Perform passive range-of-motion exercises within the patient's pain limits, perhaps using a Hubbard tank. When the patient's condition stabilizes, change to gentle stretching and active assistance exercises.
• To prevent aspiration, test the gag reflex, and elevate the head of the bed before the patient eats. If the gag reflex is absent, give nasogastric feedings until this reflex returns.
• As the patient regains strength and can tolerate a vertical position, be alert for postural hypotension. Monitor blood pressure and pulse and, if necessary, apply toe-to-groin elastic bandages or an abdominal binder to prevent postural hypotension.
• Inspect the patient's legs regularly for signs of thrombophlebitis, a common complication of Guillain-Barré syndrome. To prevent thrombophlebitis, apply antiembolism stockings and give prophylactic anticoagulants, as ordered.

• If the patient has facial paralysis, give eye and mouth care every 4 hours.
• Watch for urinary retention. Measure and record intake and output every 8 hours, and offer the bedpan every 3 to 4 hours. Encourage adequate fluid intake (2,000 ml/day), unless contraindicated. If urinary retention develops, begin intermittent catheterization, as ordered. Because the abdominal muscles are weak, the patient may need manual pressure on the bladder (Credé's method) before he can urinate.
• To prevent and relieve constipation, offer prune juice and a high-bulk diet. If necessary, give daily or alternateday suppositories (glycerin or bisacodyl), or Fleet enemas, as ordered.
• Before discharge, prepare a home care plan. Teach the patient how to transfer from bed to wheelchair, from wheelchair to toilet or to tub, and how to walk short distances with a walker or a cane. Teach the family how to help him eat, compensating for facial weakness, and how to help him avoid skin breakdown. Stress the need for a regular bowel and bladder routine.
• Refer the patient for physical therapy, as needed.

Complications
• Mechanical ventilatory failure
• Aspiration
• Pneumonia
• Sepsis
• Joint contractures
• Deep vein thrombosis
• In unexplained autonomic nervous system involvement, sinus tachycardia or bradycardia, hypertension, postural hypotension, or loss of bladder and bowel sphincter control

H

Hallux valgus

Description

Hallux valgus is a lateral deviation of the great toe at the metatarsophalangeal joint. It occurs with medial enlargement of the first metatarsal head and bunion formation (bursa and callus formation at the bony prominence).

Causes

- Congenital or familial
- Acquired, in degenerative arthritis
- Prolonged pressure, especially from narrow-toed, high-heeled shoes that compress the forefoot

Signs and symptoms

- Red, tender bunion
- Angulation of the great toe away from the midline of the body toward the other toes
- Possible in an advanced stage: a flat, splayed forefoot, severely curled toes (hammer toes), and a small bunion on the fifth metatarsal. (See *Hammer Toe*, p. 332.)

Diagnostic tests

X-rays confirm diagnosis by showing medial deviation of the first metatarsal and lateral deviation of the great toe.

Treatment

In the very early stages of acquired hallux valgus, good foot care and proper shoes may eliminate the need for further treatment. Other useful measures for early management include felt pads to protect the bunion, foam pads or other devices to separate the first and second toes at night, and a supportive pad and exercises to strengthen the metatarsal arch. Early treatment is vital in patients predisposed to foot problems, such as those with rheumatoid arthritis or diabetes mellitus. If the disease progresses to severe deformity with disabling pain, bunionectomy is necessary.

After surgery, the toe is immobilized in its corrected position in one of two ways: with a soft compression dressing (which may cover the entire foot or just the great toe and the second toe, and which serves as a splint) or with a short cast (such as a light slipper spica cast). The patient may need crutches or controlled weight-bearing. Depending on the extent of surgery, some patients walk on their heels a few days after surgery; others must wait 4 to 6 weeks to bear weight on the affected foot. Supportive treatment may include physical therapy, such as warm compresses, soaks, and exercises, and analgesics to relieve pain and stiffness.

Clinical implications

Before surgery, obtain a patient history and assess the neurovascular status of the foot (temperature, color, sensation, blanching sign). If necessary, teach the patient how to walk with crutches.

After bunionectomy, follow these guidelines:

- Apply ice to reduce swelling. In-

Hammer Toe

In hammer toe, the toe assumes a clawlike pose from hyperextension of the metatarsophalangeal joint, flexion of the proximal interphalangeal joint, and hyperextension of the distal interphalangeal joint, usually under pressure from hallux valgus displacement. This causes a painful corn on the back of the interphalangeal joint and on the bone end, and a callus on the sole of the foot, both of which make walking painful. Hammer toe may be mild or severe, and can affect one toe or all five, as in clawfoot (which also causes a very high arch).

Hammer toe can be congenital (and familial) or acquired from constantly wearing short, narrow shoes, which put pressure on the end of the long toe. Acquired hammer toe is commonly bilateral and often develops in children who rapidly outgrow shoes and socks.

In young children, or adults with early deformity, repeated foot manipulation and splinting of the affected toe relieve discomfort and may correct the deformity. Other treatment includes protection of protruding joints with felt pads, corrective footwear (open-toed shoes and sandals, or special shoes that conform to the shape of the foot), the use of a metatarsal arch support, and exercises, such as passive manual stretching of the proximal interphalangeal joint. Severe deformity requires surgical fusion of the proximal interphalangeal joint in a straight position.

---

crease negative venous pressure and reduce edema by supporting the foot with pillows, elevating the foot of the bed, or putting the bed in a Trendelenburg position.

• Record the neurovascular status of the toes, including the patient's ability to move them (dressing may inhibit movement), every hour for the first 24 hours, then every 4 hours. Report any change in neurovascular status to the surgeon immediately.

• Prepare the patient for walking by having him dangle his foot over the side of the bed for a short time before he gets up, allowing a gradual increase in venous pressure. If crutches are needed, supervise the patient in using them, and make sure he masters this skill before discharge. The patient also should have a proper cast shoe or boot to protect the cast or dressing.

• Before discharge, instruct the patient to limit activities, to rest frequently with his feet elevated, to elevate his feet whenever he feels pain or has edema, and to wear wide-toed shoes and sandals after the dressings are removed.

• Teach proper foot care, such as cleanliness, massages, and cutting toenails straight across to prevent ingrown nails and infection.

• Suggest exercises to do at home to strengthen foot muscles, such as standing at the edge of a step on the heel, then raising and inverting the top of the foot.

• Stress the importance of follow-up care and prompt medical attention for painful bunions, corns, and calluses.

Heat syndrome

Description

Heat syndrome may develop when heat loss mechanisms fail to offset heat production and the body retains heat. Normally, humans adjust to excessive temperatures by complex cardiovascular and neurologic changes, which are coordinated by the hypothalamus. Heat loss offsets heat production to regulate the body temperature. Heat loss occurs by evaporation (sweating) or vasodilation, which permits cooling of the body's surface by radiation, conduction, and convection. Heat syndrome falls into three categories: heat cramps, heat exhaustion, and heatstroke.

Causes

Environmental or internal conditions may increase heat production or impair heat dissipation.

Heat production increases with the following:

- Exercise
- Infection
- Drugs such as amphetamines

Heat loss decreases with the following:

- High temperatures or humidity
- Lack of acclimatization
- Excess clothing
- Obesity
- Dehydration
- Cardiovascular disease
- Sweat gland dysfunction
- Drugs such as phenothiazines and anticholinergics (For signs and symptoms and treatment, see *How to Manage Heat Syndrome,* pp. 334 and 335.)

Clinical implications

Heat illnesses are easily preventable, so it is important to educate patients about causes. This information is espceially vital for athletes, laborers, and soldiers in field training.

- Advise patients to avoid heat syndrome by taking the following precautions in hot weather: wear loose-fitting, lightweight clothing; rest frequently; avoid hot places; and drink adequate fluids.
- Advise patients who are obese, elderly, or taking drugs that impair heat regulation to avoid overheating.
- Tell patients who have had heat cramps or heat exhaustion to exercise gradually and to increase their salt and water intake.

- Tell patients with heatstroke that residual hypersensitivity to high temperatures may persist for several months.

Hemophilia

Description

Hemophilia is a hereditary bleeding disorder resulting from deficiency of specific clotting factors. After a person with hemophilia forms a platelet plug at a bleeding site, clotting factor deficiency impairs his capacity to form a stable fibrin clot. Hemophilia A (classic hemophilia), which affects more than 80% of all hemophiliacs, results from deficiency of Factor VIII. Hemophilia B (Christmas disease), which affects 15% of hemophiliacs, results from deficiency of Factor IX. (Recent evidence suggests that hemophilia may actually result from nonfunctioning Factors VIII and IX, rather than from their deficiency.)

Severity and prognosis of hemophilia vary with the degree of deficiency and the site of bleeding. The overall prognosis is best in mild hemophilia, which does not cause spontaneous bleeding and joint deformities. Advances in treatment have greatly improved prognosis, and many hemophiliacs live normal life spans. Surgical procedures can be done safely under the guidance of a hematologist at special treatment centers for hemophiliacs.

Cause

Hemophilia A and B are inherited as X-linked recessive traits. This means that female carriers have a 50% chance of transmitting the gene to each daughter and a 50% chance of transmitting the gene to each son. Daughters who received the gene would be carriers; sons who received it would be born with hemophilia.

How to Manage Heat Syndrome

TYPE AND PREDISPOSING FACTORS	SIGNS AND SYMPTOMS
Heat cramps	
• Commonly affect young adults • Strenuous activity without training or acclimatization • Normal to high temperature or high humidity	• Muscle twitching and spasms, weakness, severe muscle cramps • Nausea • Normal temperature or slight fever • Normal CNS findings • Diaphoresis
Heat exhaustion	
• Commonly affects young people • Physical activity without acclimatization • Decreased heat dissipation • High temperature and humidity	• Muscle cramps (infrequent) • Nausea and vomiting • Decreased blood pressure • Thready, rapid pulse • Cool, pallid skin • Headache, mental confusion, syncope, giddiness • Oliguria, thirst • No fever
Heatstroke	
• Exertional heatstroke commonly affects young, healthy people who are involved in strenuous activity. • Classic heatstroke commonly affects elderly, inactive people who have cardiovascular disease or who take drugs that influence temperature regulation. • High temperature and humidity without any wind	• Hypertension, followed by hypotension • Atrial or ventricular tachycardia • Hot, dry, red skin, which later turns gray; no diaphoresis • Confusion, progressing to seizures and loss of consciousness • Temperature higher than 104° F. (40° C.) • Dilated pupils • Slow, deep respiration; then Cheyne-Stokes respiration

MANAGEMENT

• Hospitalization is usually unnecessary.
• To replace fluid and electrolytes, give salt tablets and balanced electrolyte drink.
• Loosen patient's clothing, and have him lie down in a cool place. Massage his muscles. If muscle cramps are severe, start an I.V. infusion with normal saline solution, as ordered.

• Hospitalization is usually unnecessary.
• *Immediately* give salt tablets and balanced electrolyte drink.
• Loosen patient's clothing, and put him in a shock position in a cool place. Massage his muscles. If cramps are severe, start an I.V. infusion, as ordered.
• If needed, give oxygen.

• Initiate ABCs of life support.
• To lower body temperature, cool rapidly with ice packs on arterial pressure points and hypothermia blankets.
• To replace fluids and electrolytes, start an I.V. infusion, as ordered.
• Hospitalization is needed.
• Insert nasogastric tube to prevent aspiration.
• Give diazepam to control seizures; chlorpromazine I.V. to reduce shivering; or mannitol to maintain urine output, as ordered.
• Monitor temperature, intake, output, and cardiac status. Give dobutamine, as ordered, to correct cardiogenic shock. (Vasoconstrictors are contraindicated.)

Signs and symptoms
Mild hemophilia
—No spontaneous bleeding
—No bleeding after minor trauma
—Prolonged bleeding after major trauma or surgery
Moderate hemophilia
—Only occasional episodes of spontaneous bleeding
—Excessive bleeding after surgery or trauma
Severe hemophilia
—Spontaneous bleeding or severe bleeding after minor trauma. This may produce large subcutaneous and deep intramuscular hematomas.
—Bleeding into joints and muscles. This causes pain, swelling, extreme tenderness, and possibly permanent deformity.

Diagnostic tests
Characteristic findings in hemophilia A include the following:
• Factor VIII assay 0% to 30% of normal
• Prolonged activated partial thromboplastin time (PTT)
• Normal platelet count and function, bleeding time, and prothrombin time.
    Characteristic findings in hemophilia B include the following:
• Deficient Factor IX assay
• Baseline coagulation results similar to hemophilia A, with normal Factor VIII.
    In hemophilia A or B, the degree of factor deficiency determines severity:
• Mild hemophilia: factor levels 5% to 40% of normal
• Moderate hemophilia: factor levels 1% to 5% of normal
• Severe hemophilia: factor levels less than 1% of normal.

Treatment
Hemophilia is not curable, but treatment can prevent crippling deformities and prolong life expectancy. Correct treatment quickly stops bleeding by increasing plasma levels of deficient clotting factors to help prevent disabling deformities that result from re-

Factor Replacement Products

Cryoprecipitate
- Contains Factor VIII (70 to 100 units/bag). Does not contain Factor IX.
- Can be stored frozen up to 12 months but must be used within 6 hours after it thaws.
- Given through a blood filter. Compatible with normal saline solution only.

Lyophilized Factor VIII or IX
- Freeze-dried.
- Can be stored up to 2 years at about 36° to 46° F. (2° to 8° C.); up to 6 months at room temperature not exceeding 88° F. (31° C.).
- Labeled with exact units of Factor VIII or IX contained in vial.
- Vials range from 200 to 1,500 units of Factor VIII or IX each and contain 20 to 40 ml after reconstitution with diluent.
- Collected from large donor pools, so may cause hepatitis.
- No blood filter needed. Usually given via slow I.V. push through a butterfly infusion set.

Fresh frozen plasma
- Contains Factor VIII (approximately 0.75 unit/ml) and Factor IX (approximately 1 unit/ml). Not practical to use for most hemophiliacs because a large volume is needed to raise factors to hemostatic levels.
- Can be stored frozen up to 12 months but must be used within 2 hours after it thaws.
- Given through a blood filter. Compatible with normal saline solution only.

peated bleeding into muscles and joints.

In hemophilia A, cryoprecipitated antihemophilic factor (AHF), lyophilized AHF, or both given in doses large enough to raise clotting factor levels above 25% of normal can permit normal hemostasis. Before surgery, AHF is administered to raise clotting factors to hemostatic levels. Levels are then kept within a normal range until the wound has completely healed.

In hemophilia B, administration of Factor IX concentrate during bleeding episodes increases Factor IX levels.

A patient who undergoes surgery needs careful management by a hematologist with expertise in care of the hemophiliac. The patient will require deficient factor replacement before and after surgery, possibly even for minor surgery such as a dental extraction. (See *Factor Replacement Products.*) In addition, epsilon-aminocaproic acid is frequently used for oral bleeding to inhibit the active fibrinolytic system present in the oral mucosa.

Preventive treatment teaches the patient how to avoid trauma, manage minor bleeding, and recognize bleeding that requires immediate medical intervention. Genetic counseling helps those who are carriers understand how this disease is transmitted.

Clinical implications
During bleeding episodes, follow these guidelines:
- Give deficient clotting factor or plasma, as ordered. The body uses up AHF in 48 to 72 hours, so repeat infusions, as ordered, until bleeding stops.
- Apply cold compresses or ice bags and raise the injured part.
- To prevent recurrence of bleeding, restrict activity for 48 hours after bleeding is under control.
- Control pain with an analgesic, such as acetaminophen, propoxyphene, codeine, or meperidine, as ordered. Avoid I.M. injections because of pos-

sible hematoma formation at the injection site. Aspirin and aspirin-containing medications are contraindicated, since they decrease platelet adherence and may increase the bleeding.

• If there is bleeding into a joint, immediately elevate the joint.

After bleeding episodes and surgery, follow these guidelines:
• Watch closely for signs of further bleeding, such as increased pain and swelling, fever, or symptoms of shock.
• Closely monitor PTT.
• To restore mobility in an affected joint, begin range-of-motion exer-

---

Parent-Teaching Aid

Managing Hemophilia

Dear Parents:
Your child has hemophilia, a lifelong condition that requires special care.
• Notify your doctor immediately after even minor injury, but especially after injury to the head, neck, or abdomen. Such injuries may require special blood factor replacement. Also, check with your doctor before you allow dental extractions or any other surgery. Get the names of other doctors you can contact in case your regular doctor isn't available.
• Teach your child the importance of regular, careful toothbrushing to prevent any need for dental surgery. Have him use a soft toothbrush to avoid gum injury.
• Always watch for signs of severe internal bleeding, such as severe pain or swelling in a joint or muscle, stiffness, decreased joint movement, severe abdominal pain, blood in urine, black tarry stools, and severe headache.
• Because your child receives blood components, he risks hepatitis and AIDS. Make sure he receives the vaccine against hepatitis. Watch for early signs of this disease, which may appear 3 weeks to 6 months after treatment with blood components: headache, fever, decreased appetite, nausea, vomiting, abdominal tenderness, and pain over the liver.
• Make sure your child wears a medical identification bracelet at all times.
• *Never give him aspirin!* It can aggravate his tendency to bleed. Give acetaminophen instead.
• Protect your child from injury, but avoid unnecessary restrictions that impair his normal development. For example, for a toddler, sew padded patches into the knees and elbows of clothing to protect these joints during frequent falls. You must forbid an older child to participate in contact sports such as football, but you can encourage him to swim or to play golf.
• After injury, apply cold compresses or ice bags and elevate the injured part, or apply light pressure to the bleeding site. To prevent recurrence of bleeding after treatment, restrict activity for 48 hours after bleeding is under control.
• If you've been trained to administer blood factor components at home to avoid frequent hospitalization, know proper venipuncture and infusion techniques, and don't delay treatment during bleeding episodes. Keep blood factor concentrate and infusion equipment with you at all times, even when you're on vacation. Don't let your child miss routine follow-up examinations at your local hemophilia center. To answer your questions about the vulnerability of future offspring, get genetic counseling. Your daughters should have genetic screening to determine if they're hemophilia carriers.
  For more information, contact the National Hemophilia Foundation.

cises, if ordered, at least 48 hours after the bleeding is controlled. Tell the patient to avoid placing weight on the joint until bleeding stops and swelling subsides.
• Teach parents special precautions to prevent bleeding episodes. Reassure them that with proper management, their child can lead a productive life.
• Refer new or suspected patients to a hemophilia treatment center for evaluation. The center will devise a treatment and management plan for the patient's primary care physician and serve as a resource for medical personnel, dentists, school personnel, or anyone else involved in the patient's care. (See *Parent-Teaching Aid: Managing Hemophilia,* p. 337.)

Complications
• Bleeding near peripheral nerves may cause peripheral neuropathies, pain, paresthesias, and muscle atrophy.
• If bleeding impairs blood flow through a major vessel, it can cause ischemia and gangrene.
• Pharyngeal, lingual, intracardial, intracerebral, and intracranial bleeding all may lead to shock and death.

Hemophilus influenzae infection

Description
Hemophilus influenzae infection causes diseases in many organ systems but most frequently attacks the respiratory system. It is a common cause of epiglottitis, laryngotracheobronchitis, pneumonia, bronchiolitis, otitis media, and meningitis. Less often, it causes bacterial endocarditis, conjunctivitis, facial cellulitis, septic arthritis, and osteomyelitis. *H. influenzae* pneumonia is an increasingly common nosocomial infection, affecting about half of all children before age 1 and virtually all children by age 3. A promising new vaccine may reduce this number.

Cause
H. influenzae, a small, gram-negative, pleomorphic aerobic bacillus

Signs and symptoms
• High fever
• Generalized malaise
• Signs and symptoms of pharyngeal, laryngeal, tracheal, or bronchial infection or bronchopneumonia

Diagnostic tests
• Isolation of the organism, usually by blood culture, confirms *H. influenzae* infection.
• Other laboratory findings include polymorphonuclear leukocytosis (15,000 to 30,000/mm^3); leukopenia (2,000 to 3,000/mm^3) in young children with severe infection.

Treatment
H. influenzae infections usually respond to a 2-week course of ampicillin (resistant strains are becoming more common) or chloramphenicol.

Clinical implications
• Maintain adequate respiratory function through proper positioning, humidification (croup tent) in children, and suctioning, as needed. Monitor rate and type of respirations. Watch for signs of cyanosis and dyspnea; they necessitate intubation or a tracheotomy. For home treatment, suggest using a room humidifier or breathing moist air from a shower or bath, as necessary.
• Check the patient's history for drug allergies before administering antibiotics. Monitor CBC for signs of bone marrow depression when therapy includes chloramphenicol.
• Monitor intake (including I.V. infusions) and output. Watch for signs of dehydration, such as decreased skin turgor, parched lips, concentrated urine, decreased urine output, and increased pulse.
• Organize your physical care measures beforehand, and do them quickly to avoid disrupting the patient's rest.

• Take preventive measures, such as giving *H. influenzae* vaccine to children aged 2 (or younger) to 6, maintaining respiratory isolation, using proper hand-washing technique, properly disposing of respiratory secretions, placing soiled tissues in a plastic bag, and decontaminating all equipment.

Hemorrhoids

Description

Hemorrhoids are varicosities in the superior or inferior hemorrhoidal venous plexus. Dilation and enlargement of the superior plexus produce internal hemorrhoids; dilation and enlargement of the inferior plexus produce external hemorrhoids, which may protrude from the rectum. Physical examination confirms external hemorrhoids. Proctoscopy confirms internal hemorrhoids and rules out rectal polyps.

Cause

Hemorrhoids probably result from increased intravenous pressure in the hemorrhoidal plexus.

Risk factors

• Occupations that require prolonged standing or sitting
• Straining due to constipation, diarrhea, coughing, sneezing, or vomiting
• Heart failure
• Hepatic disease
• Alcoholism
• Anorectal infections
• Loss of muscle tone due to old age, rectal surgery, or episiotomy
• Anal intercourse
• Pregnancy

Signs and symptoms

Patients may be asymptomatic, but painless, intermittent bleeding which occurs on defecation is the characteristic symptom. Other symptoms include the following:
• Possible pruritus
• Possible discomfort and prolapse in response to any increase in intraabdominal pressure
• Sudden rectal pain and a large, firm, subcutaneous lump with thrombosed external hemorrhoids

Treatment

Treatment depends on the type and severity of the hemorrhoid and on the patient's overall condition. Generally, treatment includes measures to ease pain, combat swelling and congestion, and regulate bowel habits. Patients can relieve constipation by increasing the amount of raw vegetables, fruit, and whole grain cereal in the diet or by using stool softeners. Venous congestion can be prevented by avoiding prolonged sitting on the toilet. Local swelling and pain can be decreased with local anesthetic agents (lotions, creams, or suppositories), astringents, or cold compresses, followed by warm sitz baths or thermal packs. Rarely, the patient with chronic, profuse bleeding may require blood transfusion.

Other nonsurgical treatments include injection of a sclerosing solution to produce scar tissue that decreases prolapse, manual reduction, and hemorrhoid ligation or freezing.

Hemorrhoidectomy, the most effective treatment, is necessary for most patients with severe bleeding, intolerable pain and pruritus, and large prolapse.

Clinical implications

• To prepare the patient for hemorrhoidectomy, administer an enema, as ordered (usually 2 to 4 hours before surgery), and record the results. Shave the perianal area, and clean the anus and surrounding skin.
• Postoperatively, check for signs of prolonged rectal bleeding, administer adequate analgesics, and provide sitz baths, as ordered.
• As soon as the patient can resume

oral feedings, administer a bulk medication, such as psyllium, about 1 hour after the evening meal, to ensure a daily stool. Warn against using stool-softening medications soon after hemorrhoidectomy, since a firm stool acts as a natural dilator to prevent anal stricture resulting from the scar tissue. (Some patients may need repeated digital dilation to prevent such narrowing.)

• Keep the wound site clean to prevent infection and irritation.

• Before discharge, stress the importance of regular bowel habits and good anal hygiene. Warn against too vigorous wiping with washcloths and using harsh soaps. Encourage the use of medicated astringent pads and white toilet paper (the fixative in colored paper can irritate the skin).

Hepatic coma
(Hepatic encephalopathy)

Description
Hepatic coma is a neurologic syndrome that develops as a complication of chronic liver disease. Most common in patients with cirrhosis, this syndrome is due primarily to ammonia intoxication of the brain. It may be acute and self-limiting, or chronic and progressive. In advanced stages, prognosis is extremely poor despite vigorous treatment.

Causes
Rising blood ammonia levels may result from the following:

• Portal hypertension, which shunts portal blood past the liver

• Surgically created portal-systemic shunts

• Cirrhosis

• Excessive protein intake

• Sepsis

• Constipation or gastrointestinal hemorrhage

• Bacterial action on protein and urea.

Certain other factors heighten the brain's sensitivity to ammonia intoxication, including:

• Fluid and electrolyte imbalance (especially metabolic alkalosis)

• Hypoxia

• Azotemia

• Impaired glucose metabolism

• Infection

• Administration of sedatives, narcotics, and general anesthetics

Signs and symptoms
Clinical manifestations of hepatic encephalopathy vary (depending on the severity of neurologic involvement) and develop in four stages.

• Prodromal stage: Early symptoms are often overlooked because they are so subtle. They include slight personality changes (disorientation, forgetfulness, slurred speech) and a slight tremor.

• Impending stage: Tremor progresses into asterixis (liver flap or flapping tremor), the hallmark of hepatic coma. Asterixis is characterized by quick, irregular extensions and flexions of the wrists and fingers when the wrists are held out straight and the hands flexed upward. Lethargy, aberrant behavior, and apraxia also occur.

• Stuporous stage: Hyperventilation occurs, and the patient is stuporous but noisy and abusive when aroused.

• Comatose stage: Signs include hyperactive reflexes, a positive Babinski's sign, fetor hepaticus (musty, sweet breath odor), and coma.

Diagnostic tests
• Serum ammonia levels are increased in venous and arterial blood. This, along with clinical features and a positive history of liver disease, confirms the diagnosis.

• EEG shows slow waves as the disease progresses.

• Serum bilirubin is increased.

• Prothrombin time is prolonged.

Treatment

Effective treatment stops the progression of encephalopathy by reducing blood ammonia levels. Such treatment eliminates ammonia-producing substances from the gastrointestinal tract by administration of neomycin to suppress bacterial flora (preventing them from converting amino acids into ammonia), sorbitol-induced catharsis to produce osmotic diarrhea, continuous aspiration of blood from the stomach, reduction of dietary protein intake, and administration of lactulose to reduce blood ammonia levels.

Treatment may also include potassium supplements (80 to 120 mEq/day, P.O. or I.V.) to correct alkalosis (from increased ammonia levels), especially if the patient is taking diuretics. Sometimes, hemodialysis can temporarily clear toxic blood. Exchange transfusions may provide dramatic but temporary improvement; however, these require a particularly large amount of blood. Salt-poor albumin may be used to maintain fluid and electrolyte balance, replace depleted albumin levels, and restore plasma.

Clinical implications

• Frequently assess and record the patient's level of consciousness. Continually orient him to place and time. Remember to keep a daily record of the patient's handwriting to monitor progression of neurologic involvement.
• Monitor intake, output, and fluid and electrolyte balance. Check daily weight and measure abdominal girth. Watch for, and immediately report, signs of anemia (decreased hemoglobin), infection, alkalosis (increased serum bicarbonate), and gastrointestinal bleeding (melena, hematemesis).
• Give drugs, as ordered, and watch for side effects.
• Ask the dietary department to provide the specified low-protein diet,

with carbohydrates supplying most of the calories. Provide good mouth care.
• Promote rest, comfort, and a quiet atmosphere. Discourage stressful exercise.
• Use restraints, if necessary, but avoid sedatives. Protect the comatose patient's eyes from corneal injury by using artificial tears or eye patches.
• Provide emotional support for the patient's family in the terminal stage of encephalopathy.

Hepatitis, nonviral

Description

Nonviral inflammation of the liver (toxic or drug-induced hepatitis) is a form of hepatitis that usually results from exposure to certain chemicals or drugs. In toxic hepatitis, liver damage (diffuse fatty infiltration of liver cells and necrosis) usually occurs within 24 to 48 hours following exposure to toxic agents. Alcohol, anoxia, and preexisting liver disease exacerbate the toxic effects of some of these agents. Drug-induced (idiosyncratic) hepatitis may stem from a hypersensitivity reaction unique to the affected individual, but toxic hepatitis appears indiscriminately with exposure. Most patients recover from nonviral hepatitis, although a few develop fulminating hepatitis or cirrhosis.

Causes

• Various hepatotoxins—carbon tetrachloride, acetaminophen, trichloroethylene, poisonous mushrooms, vinyl chloride—can cause the toxic form of this disease.
• Drug-induced hepatitis may result from halothane, sulfonamides, isoniazid, methyldopa, and phenothiazines (cholestasis-induced hepatitis).

Signs and symptoms

• Anorexia
• Nausea and vomiting
• Jaundice

- Dark urine
- Hepatomegaly
- Possible abdominal pain
- Clay-colored stools or pruritus with the cholestatic form

Diagnostic tests
- Serum transaminases (SGOT, SGPT) are elevated.
- Total and direct serum bilirubin is elevated (with cholestasis).
- Alkaline phosphatase is elevated.
- WBC count is elevated.
- Eosinophils are increased in drug-induced nonviral hepatitis.
- Liver biopsy may help identify the underlying pathology, especially infiltration with WBCs and eosinophils.

Treatment and clinical implications
Effective treatment must remove the causative agent by lavage, catharsis, or hyperventilation, depending on the route of exposure. Dimercaprol may serve as an antidote for toxic hepatitis caused by gold or arsenic poisoning but does not prevent drug-induced hepatitis caused by other substances. Corticosteroids may be ordered for patients with the drug-induced type. Thioctic acid, an investigational drug, may be successful with mushroom poisoning. Preventive measures should include instructing the patient about the proper use of drugs and the proper handling of cleaning agents and solvents.

Hepatitis, viral

Description
Viral hepatitis is an acute inflammation of the liver. It is marked by liver cell destruction, necrosis, and autolysis. This disease has three forms: type A (infectious or short-incubation hepatitis), type B (serum or long-incubation hepatitis), and type non-A, non-B hepatitis. (See *Comparing Types of Hepatitis*.)

Cause
Hepatitis viruses

Signs and symptoms
Preicteric phase
—Fatigue and malaise
—Arthralgia, myalgia
—Headache
—Anorexia
—Photophobia
—Cough
—Nausea and vomiting
—Altered taste and smell
—Fever (may be associated with liver and lymph node enlargement)
Icteric phase
This phase lasts 1 to 2 weeks.
—Mild weight loss
—Dark urine
—Clay-colored stools
—Yellow sclera and skin
—Continued hepatomegaly with tenderness
Convalescent phase
This phase lasts 2 to 12 weeks or longer.
—Continued fatigue
—Flatulence
—Abdominal pain or tenderness
—Indigestion

Diagnostic tests
- The presence of hepatitis B surface antigens (HBsAg) and hepatitis B antibodies (anti-HBs) confirms a diagnosis of type B hepatitis.
- Detection of an antibody to type A hepatitis (anti-HAV) confirms diagnosis of type A hepatitis.
- Prothrombin time is prolonged (more than 3 seconds longer than normal indicates severe liver damage)
- Serum transaminases (SGOT, SGPT) are elevated.
- Serum alkaline phosphatase is slightly elevated.
- Serum and urine bilirubin is elevated (with jaundice).
- Serum albumin is low and serum globulin is high.
- Liver biopsy and scan shows patchy necrosis.

Comparing Types of Hepatitis

	TYPE A (infectious)	TYPE B (serum)	TYPE NON-A, NON-B
Age incidence	Children, young adults	Any age	Adults
Seasonal incidence	Fall, winter	Anytime	Anytime
Transmission	Food, water, semen, tears, stools, and possibly urine	Serum, blood and blood products, and semen	Serum, blood and blood products, and possibly food
Incubation	15 to 45 days	40 to 180 days	15 to 160 days
Onset	Sudden	Insidious	Insidious
Serum markers	Anti-HAV	HBsAg + anti-HBs	
Prognosis	Good	Worsens with age	Moderate
Carrier state	No	Yes	Unknown

Treatment

No specific treatment exists for hepatitis. The patient should rest in the early stages of the illness and combat anorexia by eating small meals high in calories and protein. (Protein intake should be reduced if signs of precoma—lethargy, confusion, mental changes—develop.) Large meals are usually better tolerated in the morning. Antiemetics (trimethobenzamide or benzquinamide) may be given ½ hour before meals to relieve nausea and prevent vomiting; phenothiazines have a cholestatic effect and should be avoided. If vomiting persists, the patient will require I.V. infusions.

In severe hepatitis, corticosteroids may give the patient a sense of well-being and may stimulate appetite, while decreasing itching and inflammation; however, their use in hepatitis is controversial.

Clinical implications

Base your care plan on supportive care, observation, and emotional support.

• Wear gloves when handling fluids and feces from a patient with type A hepatitis and when drawing blood from a patient with type B hepatitis.

• Inform visitors about isolation precautions.

• Encourage the patient to eat. Do not overload his meal tray; too much food on the tray will only diminish his appetite. And do not overmedicate; this too will diminish his appetite.

• Force fluids (at least 4,000 ml/day). Encourage the anorectic patient to drink fruit juices. Also offer chipped ice and effervescent soft drinks to promote adequate hydration without inducing vomiting.

• Record weight daily, and keep accurate intake and output records. Observe feces for color, consistency, frequency, and amount.

• Watch for signs of hepatic coma, de-

Preventing Viral Hepatitis

Immune globulin (IG)—or gamma globulin—is 80% to 90% effective in preventing type A hepatitis in contacts. In confirmed type A cases, IG should be given to high-risk contacts as soon as possible after exposure, but within 2 weeks after jaundice appears in the patients. Type A hepatitis is transmitted through the fecal-oral route; household, intimate, sexual, and institutional contacts are at high risk.

Most IG made in the United States contains low titers of antibody against type B hepatitis, which probably transmits some passive protection. However, a combination of hepatitis B vaccine (HB vaccine) and hepatitis B immune globulin (HBIG) currently offers the best protection after exposure to type B hepatitis. HB vaccine and HBIG should be given prophylactically to newborn infants whose mothers are HBsAg-positive. HBIG should be given I.M. after the infant has stabilized, preferably within 12 hours after birth; HB vaccine may be given I.M. at the same time in a different site, or within 7 days after birth. Infants of HBeAg-positive mothers need extra HBIG with the vaccine. HB vaccine and HBIG should be given prophylactically within 24 hours to persons who have had significant oral or percutaneous contact with an HBsAg-positive fluid. Sexual contact with an HBsAg-positive patient may require a single dose of HBIG if it can be given within 14 days of the last contact. If the patient remains HBsAg-positive 3 months after detection, the contact may need a second dose. If he becomes a chronic carrier, the contact may need HB vaccine. Homosexual men may need a dose of HBIG and the HB vaccine series.

hydration, pneumonia, vascular problems, and decubitus ulcers.

• With fulminant hepatitis, maintain electrolyte balance and a patent airway, and control bleeding. Be sure to correct hypoglycemia and any other complications while awaiting liver regeneration and repair.

• Report all cases of hepatitis to health officials. Ask the patient to name anyone he came in contact with recently.

• Before discharge, emphasize the importance of having regular medical checkups for at least 1 year. Be sure to warn the patient not to drink any alcohol during this time period, and teach him how to recognize signs of recurrence. Refer the patient for follow-up, as needed.
(See *Preventing Viral Hepatitis*.)

Complications

Complications include chronic hepatitis, which may be benign (chronic persistent hepatitis) or active (chronic aggressive hepatitis). About 25% of patients with chronic aggressive hepatitis die from hepatic failure. Life-threatening fulminant hepatitis develops in about 1% of patients, causing unremitting hepatic failure with encephalopathy. It progresses to coma and commonly leads to death within 2 weeks.

Hereditary fructose intolerance

Description

Hereditary fructose intolerance is an inability to metabolize fructose. After fructose is eliminated from the diet, symptoms subside within weeks. Older children and adults with hereditary fructose intolerance have normal intelligence and apparently normal liver and kidney function.

Cause
Transmitted as an autosomal recessive trait, hereditary fructose intolerance results from a deficiency in the enzyme fructose-1-phosphate aldolase.

Signs and symptoms
The following signs and symptoms appear shortly after dietary introduction of foods containing fructose or sugar, such as fruit:
• Nausea
• Vomiting
• Pallor
• Excessive sweating
• Cyanosis
• Tremor

Diagnostic tests
• A fructose tolerance test (using glucose oxidase or paper chromatography to measure glucose levels) usually confirms the diagnosis.
• Liver biopsy showing a deficiency in fructose-1-phosphate aldolase may be necessary for definitive diagnosis.
• Serum inorganic phosphorus levels are decreased.
• Urine studies may show fructosuria and albuminuria.

Treatment and clinical implications
Treatment of hereditary fructose intolerance consists of exclusion of fructose and sucrose (cane sugar or table sugar) from the diet. Tell the patient to avoid fruits containing fructose and vegetables containing sucrose (sugar beets, sweet potatoes, and peas), because sucrose is digested to glucose and fructose in the intestine.

Refer the patient and family for genetic and dietary counseling, as appropriate.

Complications
In newborns and young children, continuous ingestion of foods containing fructose may result in failure to thrive, hypoglycemia, jaundice, hyperbilirubinemia, ascites, hepatomegaly, dehydration, hypophosphatemia, albuminuria, aminoaciduria, seizures, convulsions, coma, febrile episodes, substernal pain, and anemia.

Hereditary hemorrhagic telangiectasia
(Rendu-Osler-Weber disease)

Description
Hereditary hemorrhagic telangiectasia is an inherited vascular disorder in which venules and capillaries dilate to form fragile masses of thin convoluted vessels (telangiectases), resulting in an abnormal tendency to hemorrhage. This disorder affects both sexes but may cause less severe bleeding in females. It rarely skips generations. In its homozygous state, it may be lethal.

Cause
Hereditary hemorrhagic telangiectasia is transmitted by autosomal dominant inheritance.

Signs and symptoms
• Localized aggregations of dilated capillaries. These appear on the skin of the face, ears, scalp, hands, arms, and feet; under the nails; and on the mucous membranes of the nose, mouth, and stomach.
• Frequent epistaxis, hemopytsis, and gastrointestinal bleeding
• Characteristic telangiectases. These are violet, bleed spontaneously, may be flat or raised, blanch on pressure, and are nonpulsatile.

Diagnostic tests
• Bone marrow aspiration showing depleted iron stores confirms secondary iron deficiency anemia; however, diagnosis rests on an established familial pattern of bleeding disorders and clinical evidence of telangiectasia and hemorrhage.

• Hypochromic, microcytic anemia is common; abnormal platelet function may also be found.

Treatment
Supportive therapy includes blood transfusions and the administration of supplemental iron. Ancillary treatment includes applying pressure and topical hemostatic agents to bleeding sites; excising bleeding sites (when accessible); and protecting the patient from trauma and unnecessary bleeding.

Parenteral administration of supplemental iron enhances absorption to maintain adequate iron stores and prevent gastric irritation. Administering antipyretics or antihistamines before blood transfusion and transfusing saline-washed cells, frozen blood, or other types of leukocyte-poor blood (instead of whole blood) may prevent febrile transfusion reactions.

Clinical implications
• If the patient is receiving a blood transfusion, stay with him during the first 15 minutes, for signs of febrile transfusion reaction (flushing, shaking chills, fever, headache, rash, tachycardia, hypertension), since he is quite susceptible to a reaction.
• Observe the patient for indications of gastrointestinal bleeding, such as hematemesis and melena. Instruct him to watch for and report such signs.
• If the patient requires an iron supplement, stress the importance of following dosage instructions and taking oral iron with meals to minimize gastric irritation. Warn that iron turns stools dark green or black.
• Teach the patient and family how to manage minor bleeding episodes, especially recurrent epistaxis, and to recognize major ones that necessitate emergency intervention.
• Refer the patient for genetic counseling, as appropriate.

Herniated disk
(Ruptured or slipped disk, herniated nucleus pulposus)

Description
Herniated disk occurs when all or part of the nucleus pulposus—the soft, gelatinous, central portion of an intervertebral disk—is forced through the weakened or torn outer ring (anulus fibrosus). When this happens, the extruded disk may impinge on spinal nerve roots as they exit from the spinal canal or on the spinal cord itself, resulting in back pain and other signs of nerve root irritation. Most herniation occurs in the lumbar and lumbosacral regions.

Causes
• Severe trauma or strain
• Intervertebral joint degeneration

Signs and symptoms
• The overriding symptom of lumbar herniated disk is severe low back pain that radiates to the buttocks, legs, and feet (usually unilaterally) and intensifies with Valsalva's maneuver, coughing, sneezing, or bending. Other symptoms include the following:
• Possible motor and sensory loss in the area innervated by the compressed spinal nerve root
• In later stages, weakness and atrophy of leg muscles

Diagnostic tests
• The straight-leg–raising test and its variants are perhaps the best tests for herniated disk. For the straight-leg–raising test, the patient lies supine while the examiner places one hand on the patient's ilium, to stabilize the pelvis, and the other hand under the ankle, then slowly raises the patient's leg. The test is positive only if the patient complains of posterior leg (sciatic) pain, not back pain. In LeSegue's test, the patient lies flat while the thigh and knee are flexed to a 90-degree angle.

Teaching Topics in Herniated Disk

- An explanation of the disorder, including how it causes back and leg pain
- Warning signs and symptoms of nerve root compression
- An explanation of procedures to confirm sciatica
- Preparation for X-rays, myelography, and possibly a CT scan
- Initial treatments, such as bed rest
- Back-strengthening exercises
- Importance of using proper body mechanics
- Medications and their administration
- Other pain-relief measures: heat or cold therapy, massage, TENS
- Chemonucleolysis, if performed
- Surgery (laminectomy or spinal fusion), if performed
- Postoperative exercises and wound care

Resistance and pain, as well as loss of ankle or knee-jerk reflex, indicate spinal root compression.

- X-rays of the spine are essential to rule out other abnormalities, but they may not diagnose herniated disk, since marked disk prolapse can be present despite a normal X-ray.
- Myelography or CT scan provides the most specific diagnostic information, showing spinal compression by the herniated disk.

Treatment

Unless neurologic impairment progresses rapidly, treatment is initially conservative and consists of several days of bed rest (possibly with pelvic traction), heat applications, and an exercise program. Aspirin reduces inflammation and edema at the site of injury; rarely, corticosteroids may be prescribed for the same purpose. Muscle relaxants, especially diazepam or methocarbamol, also may be beneficial.

A herniated disk that fails to respond to conservative treatment may necessitate surgery. The most common procedure, laminectomy, involves excision of a portion of the lamina and removal of the protruding disk. If lam-

inectomy does not alleviate pain and disability, a spinal fusion may be necessary to overcome segmental instability. Laminectomy and spinal fusion are sometimes performed concurrently to stabilize the spine.

Chemonucleolysis—injection of the enzyme chymopapain into the herniated disk to dissolve the nucleus pulposus—is a possible alternative to laminectomy. Microdiskectomy can also be used to remove fragments of nucleus pulposus.

Clinical implications

- If the patient requires myelography, provide necessary instructions and care.
- During conservative treatment, watch for any deterioration in neurologic status (especially during the first 24 hours after admission), which may indicate an urgent need for surgery.
- Use antiembolism stockings, as prescribed, and encourage the patient to move his legs, as allowed. Provide high-topped sneakers to prevent footdrop.
- Work closely with the physical therapy department to ensure a consistent regimen of leg- and back-strengthening exercises.
- Give plenty of fluids to prevent renal stasis, and remind the patient to cough, deep-breathe, and use blow bottles or

an incentive spirometer to preclude pulmonary complications.

• Provide good skin care, and assess bowel function regularly.

• After laminectomy, microdiskectomy, or spinal fusion, enforce bed rest, as ordered. Monitor vital signs, and check for bowel sounds and abdominal distention. Use logrolling technique to turn the patient.

• If a blood drainage system (such as Hemovac) is in use, check the tubing frequently for kinks and a secure vacuum. Empty the Hemovac at the end of each shift, as ordered, and record the amount and color of drainage.

• Report colorless moisture on dressings (possible cerebrospinal fluid leakage) or excessive drainage immediately. Observe neurovascular status of legs (color, motion, temperature, sensation).

• Administer analgesics, as ordered, especially 30 minutes before initial attempts at sitting or walking. Assist the patient during his first attempt to walk. Provide a straight-backed chair for limited sitting.

• Teach the patient who has undergone spinal fusion how to wear a brace. Assist with straight-leg–raising and toe-pointing exercises, as ordered. Before discharge, teach proper body mechanics—bending at the knees and hips (never at the waist), standing straight, carrying objects close to the body. Advise the patient to lie down when tired and to sleep on his side (never on his abdomen) on an extra-firm mattress or a bed board. Urge maintenance of proper weight to prevent lordosis caused by obesity.

• Before chemonucleolysis, make sure the patient is not allergic to meat tenderizers (chymopapain is a similar substance). Such an allergy contraindicates the use of this enzyme, which can produce severe anaphylaxis in a sensitive patient.

• After chemonucleolysis, enforce bed rest, as ordered. Administer analgesics and apply heat, as needed. Urge

the patient to cough and deep breathe. Assist with special exercises, and tell the patient to continue these exercises after discharge.

• Tell the patient who must receive a muscle relaxant of possible side effects, especially drowsiness. Warn him to avoid activities that require alertness until he has built up a tolerance to the drug's sedative effects.

• Provide emotional support. Try to cheer the patient during periods of frustration and depression. Assure him of his progress, and offer encouragement.

(See *Teaching Topics in Herniated Disk,* p. 347.)

Herpangina

Description

Herpangina is an acute infection that characteristically produces vesicular lesions on the mucous membranes of the soft palate, tonsillar pillars, and throat. Herpangina usually affects children under age 10 (except newborns).

Causes

Usually group A coxsackieviruses; less commonly, group B coxsackieviruses and echoviruses

Mode of transmission

Fecal-oral transfer

Signs and symptoms

• Sore throat
• Pain on swallowing
• Fever (temperature of 100° to 104° F. [37.8° to 40° C.] that persists for 1 to 4 days)
• Possible convulsions, headache, anorexia, vomiting, diarrhea, and pain in the stomach, back of the neck, legs, and arms
• Grayish white papulovesicles on the soft palate and, less commonly, on the tonsils, uvula, tongue, and larynx. These lesions grow from 1 to 2 mm in

diameter to large, punched out ulcers surrounded by small, inflamed margins.

Diagnostic tests
• Isolation of the virus from mouth washings or feces, and elevated specific antibody titer confirm the diagnosis.
• WBC count shows slight leukocytosis.

Treatment and clinical implications
Treatment for herpangina is entirely symptomatic, emphasizing measures to reduce fever and prevent convulsions and possible dehydration. Herpangina does not require isolation or hospitalization but does require careful hand washing and sanitary disposal of excretions.

Teach parents to give adequate fluids, enforce bed rest, and administer tepid sponge baths and antipyretics.

Herpes simplex

Description
Herpes simplex is a recurrent viral infection. Type I herpes affects the skin and mucous membranes and commonly produces cold sores and fever blisters. Type II herpes primarily affects the genital area. About 85% of all herpes infections are subclinical. The others produce localized lesions and systemic reactions. After the first infection, a patient is a carrier susceptible to recurrent infections, which may be provoked by fever, menses, stress, heat, and cold. However, in recurrent infections, the patient usually has no constitutional signs and symptoms.

In neonates, symptoms usually appear a week or two after birth. They range from localized skin lesions to disseminated infection of such organs as the liver, lungs, or brain. Up to 90% of infants with disseminated disease will die.

Cause
Herpesvirus hominis (HVH)

Mode of transmission
• Type I herpes is transmitted by oral and respiratory secretions.
• Type II herpes is transmitted by sexual contact. However, cross-infection may result from orogenital sex.
• Herpes may also rarely be transmitted to the fetus transplacentally. However, most neonatal infection is acquired from exposure to the mother's infected genital tract at the time of delivery.

Signs and symptoms
Type I herpes
—In primary infection, a brief period of prodromal tingling and itching, accompanied by fever and pharyngitis, is followed by eruption of vesicles on any part of the oral mucosa, especially the tongue, gums, and cheeks.
—Vesicles form on an erythematous base, then rupture and leave a painful ulcer, followed by a yellowish crust.
—Submaxillary lymphadenopathy, increased salivation, halitosis, anorexia, conjunctivitis, and fever may occur.
—Recurrence typically causes only the characteristic vesicular eruptions on the lips or buccal mucosa.
Type II herpes
—Typically painful, the initial attack produces fluid-filled vesicles in the genital area. These ulcerate and heal in 1 to 3 weeks.
—In primary infection, fever, regional lymphadenopathy, and dysuria may also occur.
—Recurrence causes characteristic vesicular eruptions.

Diagnostic tests
• Isolation of the virus from local lesions and histologic biopsy confirm the diagnosis; appearance of typical lesions suggests it.

• A rise in antibody levels and moderate leukocytosis may support the diagnosis.

Treatment

Symptomatic and supportive therapy is essential. Generalized primary infection usually requires an analgesic-antipyretic to reduce fever and relieve pain. Anesthetic mouthwashes, such as viscous lidocaine, may reduce the pain of gingivostomatitis, enabling the patient to eat and preventing dehydration. Drying agents, such as calamine lotion, make labial lesions less painful.

Refer patients with eye infections to an ophthalmologist. Topical corticosteroids are contraindicated in active infection, but idoxuridine, trifluridine, and vidarabine are effective.

A 5% acyclovir ointment may bring relief to patients with genital herpes or to immunosuppressed patients with HVH skin infections. Acyclovir I.V. helps treat more severe infections.

Clinical implications

• Because herpesviruses are extremely contagious, take appropriate precautions to avoid acquiring the infection and transmitting it to other patients.
• Teach the patient with genital herpes to use warm compresses or take sitz baths several times a day. Tell him to use a drying agent, such as povidone-iodine solution; to increase his fluid intake; and to avoid all sexual contact during the active stage.
• For pregnant women with type II herpes infection, recommend weekly viral cultures of the cervix and external genitalia starting at 32 weeks' gestation.
• Tell patients with cold sores not to kiss infants or people with eczema. (Those with genital herpes pose no risk to infants if their hygiene is meticulous.)
• Patients with central nervous system infection alone need no isolation.
• Encourage gynecologic follow-up

for females (especially adolescents) with genital herpes, since this condition is associated with an increased incidence of cervical cancer.

Complications

• In early pregnancy, type II herpes infection may cause spontaneous abortion or premature birth.
• Common complications in neonates include seizures, mental retardation, blindness, chorioretinitis, deafness, microcephaly, diabetes insipidus, and spasticity.
• Other complications may include encephalitis and keratoconjunctivitis.

Herpes zoster
(Shingles)

Description

Herpes zoster is an acute unilateral and segmental inflammation of the dorsal root ganglia caused by infection with the herpesvirus varicella-zoster (V-Z), which also causes chicken pox. This infection usually occurs in adults. It produces localized vesicular skin lesions confined to a dermatome, and severe neuralgic pain in peripheral areas innervated by the nerves arising in the inflamed ganglia.

Prognosis is good unless the infection spreads to the brain. Eventually, most patients recover completely except for possible scarring and, in corneal damage, visual impairment. Occasionally, neuralgia may persist for months or years.

Cause

Reactivation of the herpesvirus V-Z that has lain dormant in the cerebral ganglia (extramedullary ganglia of the cranial nerves) or the ganglia of posterior nerve roots since a previous episode of chicken pox.

Signs and symptoms

- Onset of herpes zoster is characterized by fever and malaise.
- Within 2 to 4 days, severe deep pain, pruritus, and paresthesia or hyperesthesia develop, usually on the trunk and occasionally on the arms and legs. Pain may be continuous or intermittent.
- Small, red, nodular skin lesions then usually erupt on the painful areas and commonly spread unilaterally around the thorax or vertically over the arms or legs. They quickly become vesicles filled with clear fluid or pus.
- About 10 days after they appear, the vesicles dry and form scabs.

Diagnostic tests

- Laboratory examination of vesicular fluid and infected tissue shows eosinophilic intranuclear inclusions and varicella virus.
- Lumbar puncture shows increased pressure; examination of CSF shows increased protein levels and, possibly, pleocytosis.

Treatment

The primary goal of treatment is to relieve itching and neuralgic pain with calamine lotion or another topical antipruritic; aspirin, possibly with codeine or another analgesic; and occasionally, application of collodion or tincture of benzoin to unbroken lesions. If bacteria have infected ruptured vesicles, treatment includes an appropriate systemic antibiotic.

Trigeminal zoster with corneal involvement calls for instillation of idoxuridine ointment or another antiviral agent. To help a patient cope with the intractable pain of postherpetic neuralgia, the doctor may order systemic corticosteroids—such as cortisone or possibly corticotropin—to reduce inflammation, or tranquilizers, sedatives, or tricyclic antidepressants with phenothiazines.

Researchers are studying two other drugs for treating herpes zoster. Acyclovir seems to stop progression of the skin rash and prevent visceral complications. Vidarabine reportedly speeds healing of lesions, decreases pain, and prevents the disease from spreading and developing complications.

As a last resort, transcutaneous peripheral nerve stimulation, cordotomy (used with limited succes in "suicidal pain"), or low-dose radiotherapy also may be considered.

Clinical implications

Your care plan should emphasize keeping the patient comfortable, maintaining meticulous hygiene, and preventing infection. During the acute phase, adequate rest and supportive care can promote proper healing of lesions.

- If calamine lotion has been ordered, apply it liberally to the lesions. If lesions are severe and widespread, apply a wet dressing.
- Instruct the patient to avoid scratching the lesions.
- If vesicles rupture, apply a cold compress, as ordered.
- To decrease the pain of oral lesions, tell the patient to use a soft toothbrush, eat a soft diet, and use saline solution mouthwash.
- To minimize neuralgic pain, never withhold or delay administration of analgesics. Give them exactly on schedule because the pain of herpes zoster can be severe. In postherpetic neuralgia, avoid narcotic analgesics because of the danger of addiction.
- Repeatedly reassure the patient that herpetic pain will eventually subside. Provide diversionary activity to take his mind off the pain and pruritus.

Complications

Geniculate herpes may cause vesicle formation in the external auditory canal, ipsilateral facial palsy, hearing loss, dizziness, and loss of taste. Trigeminal ganglion involvement causes eye pain and, possibly, corneal and scleral damage and impaired vision.

Rarely, oculomotor involvement causes conjunctivitis, extraocular weakness, ptosis, and paralytic mydriasis.

In rare cases, herpes zoster leads to generalized CNS infection, muscle atrophy, motor paralysis (usually transient), acute transverse myelitis, and ascending myelitis. More often, generalized infection causes acute urine retention and unilateral paralysis of the diaphragm. In postherpetic neuralgia, a complication most common in the elderly, intractable neurologic pain may persist for years. Scars may be permanent.

Hiatal hernia
(Hiatus hernia)

Description
Hiatal hernia is a defect in the diaphragm that permits a portion of the stomach to pass through the esophageal diaphragmatic opening, or hiatus, into the chest when intraabdominal pressure increases, as from ascites, pregnancy, obesity, constrictive clothing, bending, straining or coughing, Valsalva's maneuver, or extreme physical exertion.

Three types of hiatal hernia can occur: sliding hernia (the most common type), paraesophageal ("rolling") hernia, or mixed hernia, which includes features of the others. In a sliding hernia, both the stomach and the gastroesophageal junction slip up into the chest so that the gastroesophageal junction is above the diaphragmatic hiatus. In a paraesophageal hernia, a part of the greater curvature of the stomach rolls through the diaphragmatic defect. (See *Two Types of Hiatal Hernia.*) Treatment can prevent complications, such as strangulation of the herniated intrathoracic portion of the stomach.

Cause
Muscle weakening associated with the following:

- Aging
- Esophageal carcinoma
- Kyphoscoliosis
- Trauma
- Certain surgical procedures
- Congenital diaphragmatic malformations

Signs and symptoms
Sliding hiatal hernia
Symptoms occur in the presence of an incompetent gastroesophageal sphincter.
—Pyrosis (heartburn). This occurs from 1 to 4 hours after eating and is aggravated by increased intraabdominal pressure. It may be accompanied by regurgitation or vomiting.
—Retrosternal or substernal chest pain. This occurs most often after meals or at bedtime and is aggravated by reclining, belching, and increased intraabdominal pressure.
Paraesophageal hiatal hernia
—Typically asymptomatic
—Possible feeling of fullness in the chest or pain resembling angina pectoris

Diagnostic tests
- Chest X-ray occasionally shows an air shadow behind the heart with a large hernia; infiltrates are seen in lower lobes if the patient has aspirated gastric contents.
- In a barium study, the hernia may appear as an outpouching containing barium at the lower end of the esophagus. (Small hernias are difficult to recognize.) Diaphragmatic abnormalities are seen.
- Endoscopy and biopsy differentiate between hiatal hernia, varices, and other small gastroesophageal lesions; identify the mucosal junction and the edge of the diaphragm indenting the esophagus; and can rule out malignancy.
- Esophageal motility studies assess the presence of esophageal motor abnormalities before surgical repair of the hernia.

- Measurement of pH assesses for reflux of gastric contents.
- Acid perfusion (Bernstein) test indicates that heartburn results from esophageal reflux when perfusion of hydrochloric acid through the nasogastric tube provokes this symptom.
- CBC may show hypochromic microcytic anemia when bleeding from esophageal ulceration occurs.
- Stool guaiac test may be positive.
- Analysis of gastric contents may reveal blood.

Treatment

The primary goals of treatment are to relieve symptoms by minimizing or correcting the incompetent cardia and to manage and prevent complications. Medical therapy is used first, because symptoms usually respond to it and because hiatal hernia tends to recur after surgery. Such therapy attempts to modify or reduce reflux by changing the quantity or quality of gastric contents; by strengthening the gastroesophageal sphincter muscle pharmacologically; or by decreasing the amount of reflux through gravity. Treatment also includes restricting any activity that increases intraabdominal pressure (coughing, straining, bending), giving antiemetics and cough suppressants, avoiding constrictive clothing, modifying the diet, giving stool softeners or laxatives to prevent straining at stool, and discouraging smoking, which stimulates gastric acid production. Modifying the diet means eating small, frequent, bland meals at least 2 hours before lying down (no bedtime snack); eating slowly; and avoiding spicy foods, fruit juices, alcoholic beverages, and coffee.

Antacids modify the fluid refluxed into the esophagus and are probably the best treatment for intermittent reflux. Intensive antacid therapy may call for hourly administration; however, the choice of antacid should take

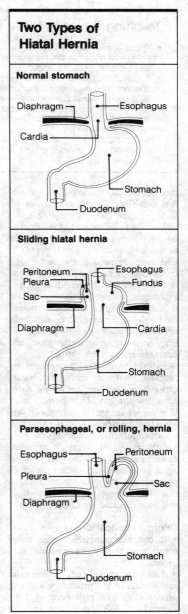

Two Types of Hiatal Hernia

Normal stomach

Diaphragm — Esophagus
Cardia
Stomach
Duodenum

Sliding hiatal hernia

Peritoneum — Esophagus
Pleura — Fundus
Sac
Diaphragm — Cardia
Stomach
Duodenum

Paraesophageal, or rolling, hernia

Esophagus — Peritoneum
Pleura — Sac
Diaphragm
Stomach
Duodenum

Teaching Topics in Hiatal Hernia

• An explanation of hiatal hernia as muscle weakness of the diaphragm opening that encircles the distal esophagus and stomach
• Possible complications: esophagitis, gastritis, and aspiration pneumonia
• Preparation for tests to confirm hiatal hernia, such as barium swallow, endoscopy, and esophageal manometry
• Preoperative instruction for hernia repair, if necessary
• Meal scheduling, size, and contents
• Use of antacids, cholinergics, and other drugs to relieve symptoms and prevent complications
• Positioning, cessation of smoking, and avoidance of activities that increase intraabdominal pressure

into consideration the patient's bowel function. Cimetidine also modifies the fluid refluxed into the esophagus.

To reduce the amount of reflux, the overweight patient should lose weight to decrease intraabdominal pressure. Elevating the head of the bed 6″ (15 cm) reduces gastric reflux by gravity.

Drug therapy to strengthen gastroesophageal sphincter tone may include a cholinergic agent, such as bethanechol. Metoclopramide has also been used to stimulate smooth muscle contraction, increase sphincter tone, and decrease reflux after eating.

Failure to control symptoms by medical means, or onset of complications, requires surgical repair. Also, a paraesophageal hiatal hernia, even if it causes no symptoms, needs surgical treatment because of the high risk of strangulation. Techniques vary greatly, but most create an artificial closing mechanism at the gastroesophageal junction to strengthen the lower esophageal sphincter's barrier function. The surgeon may use an abdominal or a thoracic approach.

Clinical implications
• To enhance compliance with treatment, teach the patient about this disorder.
• If surgery is scheduled, reinforce the explanation of the procedure and any preoperative and postoperative considerations. Tell the patient that he probably will not be allowed to eat or drink and will have a nasogastric tube in place, with low suction, for 2 to 3 days postoperatively.
• After surgery, carefully record intake and output, including nasogastric or wound drainage.
• While the nasogastric tube is in place, provide meticulous mouth and nose care. Give ice chips to moisten oral mucous membranes. (Remember to include this ice in your intake and output record.)
• If the surgeon used a thoracic approach, the patient will have chest tubes in place. Carefully observe chest tube drainage and respiratory status, and perform chest physiotherapy.
• Before discharge, tell the patient what foods he can eat (he may require a bland diet), and recommend small, frequent meals. Warn against activities that cause increased intraabdominal pressure, and advise a slow return to normal functions. Tell him he will probably be able to resume regular activity in 6 to 8 weeks.

Complications
• Esophagitis
• Stricture
• Bleeding
• Aspiration
• Strangulation
• Incarceration
(See *Teaching Topics in Hiatal Hernia*.)

Hirschsprung's disease
(Congenital megacolon, congenital aganglionic megacolon)

Description
Hirschsprung's disease is a congenital disorder of the large intestine, characterized by the absence or marked reduction of parasympathetic ganglion cells in the colorectal wall. This disorder impairs intestinal motility and causes severe, intractable constipation. Without prompt treatment, an infant with colonic obstruction may die within 24 hours from enterocolitis that leads to severe diarrhea and hypovolemic shock. With prompt treatment, the prognosis is good.

Causes
Hirschsprung's disease is believed to be a familial, congenital defect.

Signs and symptoms
Newborn
—Failure to pass meconium within 24 to 48 hours
—Bile-stained or fecal vomiting
—Abdominal distention
—Irritability
—Feeding difficulties
—Failure to thrive
—Dehydration (pallor, loss of skin turgor, dry mucous membranes, sunken eyes)
—Overflow diarrhea
—Rectal examination revealing a rectum empty of stool and, when the examining finger is withdrawn, an explosive gush of malodorous gas and liquid stool
Older child
—Intractable constipation
—Abdominal distention
—Easily palpated fecal masses
—Failure to grow in severe cases
Adult (rare)
—Abdominal distention
—Rectal bleeding
—Chronic intermittent constipation

Diagnostic tests
• Rectal biopsy provides definitive diagnosis by showing absence of ganglion cells.
• In older infants, barium enema showing a narrowed segment of distal colon with a sawtooth appearance and a funnel-shaped segment above it confirms the diagnosis and assesses the extent of intestinal involvement.
• Rectal manometry detects failure of the internal anal sphincter to relax and contract.
• Upright plain films of the abdomen show marked colonic distention.

Treatment
Surgical treatment involves pulling the normal ganglionic segment through to the anus. However, such corrective surgery is usually delayed until the infant is at least 10 months old and better able to withstand it. Management of an infant until the time of surgery consists of daily colonic lavage to empty the bowel. If total obstruction is present in the newborn, a temporary colostomy or ileostomy is necessary to decompress the colon. A preliminary bowel preparation with an antibiotic, such as neomycin or nystatin, is necessary before surgery.

Clinical implications
Before emergency decompresson surgery, follow these guidelines:
• Maintain fluid and electrolyte balance, and prevent shock. Provide adequate nutrition, and hydrate with I.V. fluids, as needed. Transfusions may be necessary to correct shock or dehydration.
• Relieve respiratory distress by keeping the patient in an upright position (place an infant in an infant seat).

After colostomy or ileostomy, follow these guidelines:
• Place the infant in a heated incubator, with the temperature set at 98° to 99° F. (36.6° to 37.2° C.), or in a radiant warmer. Monitor vital signs, watching for sepsis and enterocolitis (increased respiratory rate with ab-

dominal distention).
• Carefully monitor and record fluid intake and output (including drainage from ileostomy or colostomy) and electrolyte levels. Ileostomy is especially likely to cause excessive electrolyte losses. Also, measure and record nasogastric drainage, and replace fluids and electrolytes, as ordered. Check stools carefully for excess water—a sign of fluid loss.
• Check urine for specific gravity, glucose (hyperalimentation may lead to osmotic diuresis), and blood.
• To prevent aspiration pneumonia and skin breakdown, turn and reposition the patient often. Also, suction the nasopharynx frequently.
• Keep the area around the stoma clean and dry, and cover it with dressings or a colostomy or ileostomy appliance to absorb drainage. Use aseptic technique until the wound heals.
• Oral feeding can begin when bowel sounds return.
• Teach parents to recognize the signs of fluid loss and dehydration and of enterocolitis.
• Before discharge, if possible, make sure the parents consult with an enterostomal therapist for valuable tips on colostomy and ileostomy care.

Before corrective surgery, follow these guidelines:
• At least once a day, perform colonic lavage with normal saline solution to evacuate the colon, since ordinary enemas and laxatives will not clean it adequately. Keep accurate records of how much lavage solution is instilled. Repeat lavage until the return solution is completely free of fecal particles.
• Administer antibiotics for bowel preparation, as ordered.

After corrective surgery, follow these guidelines:
• Keep the wound clean and dry, and check for significant inflammation (some inflammation is normal). Do not use a rectal thermometer or suppository until the wound has healed. After 3 to 4 days, the infant will have a first bowel movement, a liquid stool, which

will probably create discomfort. Record the number of stools.
• Check urine for blood, especially in a boy. Extensive surgical manipulation may cause bladder trauma.
• Watch for signs of possible anastomotic leaks (sudden development of abdominal distention unrelieved by gastric aspiration, temperature spike, extreme irritability), which may lead to pelvic abscess.
• Begin oral feedings when active bowel sounds return and nasogastric drainage decreases. Start with clear fluids, increasing bulk as tolerated.
• Instruct parents to watch for foods that increase the number of stools and to avoid offering these foods. Reassure them that their child will probably gain sphincter control and be able to eat a normal diet. But warn that complete continence may take several years to develop and constipation may recur at times.
• Because an infant with Hirschsprung's disease needs surgery and hospitalization so early in life, parents have difficulty establishing an emotional bond with their child. To promote bonding, encourage them to participate in their child's care as much as possible.

Complications
In infants, the main cause of death is enterocolitis, caused by fecal stagnation that leads to bacterial overgrowth, production of bacterial toxins, intestinal irritation, profuse diarrhea, hypovolemic shock, and perforation.

Histoplasmosis
(Ohio Valley disease, Central Mississippi Valley disease, Appalachian Mountain disease, Darling's disease)

Description
Histoplasmosis is a fungal infection. In the United States, it occurs in three

forms: primary acute histoplasmosis, progressive disseminated histoplasmosis (acute disseminated or chronic disseminated disease), and chronic pulmonary (cavitary) histoplasmosis, which produces cavitations in the lung similar to those in pulmonary tuberculosis.

The incubation period is from 5 to 18 days, although chronic pulmonary histoplasmosis may progress slowly for many years.

Prognosis varies with each form. Primary acute disease is benign. Progressive disseminated disease is fatal in approximately 90% of patients. Without proper chemotherapy, chronic pulmonary histoplasmosis is fatal in 50% of patients within 5 years.

Cause

The fungus *Histoplasma capsulatum*

Mode of transmission

- Inhalation of *H. capsulatum* spores
- Invasion of *H. capsulatum* spores after minor skin trauma

Signs and symptoms

Primary acute histoplasmosis
—Possibly asymptomatic
—Fever
—Malaise
—Headache
—Myalgia
—Anorexia
—Cough
—Chest pain

Progressive disseminated histoplasmosis
—Hepatosplenomegaly
—General lymphadenopathy
—Anorexia
—Weight loss
—Fever
—Possible ulceration of the tongue, palate, epiglottis, and larynx, with resulting pain, hoarseness, and dysphagia

Chronic pulmonary histoplasmosis
—Productive cough
—Dyspnea
—Occasional hemoptysis
—Weight loss
—Extreme weakness
—Breathlessness
—Cyanosis

Diagnostic tests

- Histoplasmin skin test is positive. This, along with a history of exposure to contaminated soil in an endemic area, and miliary calcification in the lung or spleen, indicates exposure to histoplasmosis.
- Rising complement fixation and agglutination titers (more than 1:32) strongly suggest histoplasmosis.
- Morphologic examination of tissue biopsy and culture of *H. capsulatum* (from sputum in acute primary and chronic pulmonary histoplasmosis; from bone marrow, lymph node, blood, and infection sites in progressive disseminated histoplasmosis) is required for diagnosis. However, cultures take several weeks to grow these organisms. Faster diagnosis is possible with stained biopsies using Gomori's stains (methenamine silver) or periodic acid-Schiff reaction.

Treatment

Treatment consists of antifungal therapy, surgery, and supportive care.

- Antifungal therapy is most important. Except for asymptomatic primary acute histoplasmosis (which resolves spontaneously), histoplasmosis requires high-dose or long-term (10-week) therapy with amphotericin B or ketoconazole.
- Surgery includes lung resection to remove pulmonary nodules, a shunt for increased intracranial pressure, and cardiac repair for constrictive pericarditis.
- Supportive care includes oxygen for respiratory distress, glucocorticoids for adrenal insufficiency, and parenteral fluids for dysphagia from oral or laryngeal ulcerations. Histoplasmosis does not require isolation.

Clinical implications

Patient care is primarily supportive.

• Give drugs, as ordered, and teach patients about possible side effects. Since amphotericin B may cause chills, fever, nausea, and vomiting, give appropriate antipyretics and antiemetics, as ordered.

• Patients with chronic pulmonary or progressive disseminated histoplasmosis also need psychological support because of long-term hospitalization. As needed, refer them to a social worker or an occupational therapist. Help parents of children with this disease arrange for a visiting teacher.

• Teach persons in endemic areas to watch for early signs of this infection and to seek treatment promptly. To help prevent histoplasmosis, instruct persons who risk occupational exposure to contaminated soil to wear face masks.

Complications

Progressive disseminated histoplasmosis may cause endocarditis, meningitis, pericarditis, and adrenal insufficiency.

Hodgkin's disease

Description

Hodgkin's disease is a neoplastic disease characterized by painless, progressive enlargement of lymph nodes, the spleen, and other lymphoid tissue—resulting from proliferation of lymphocytes, histiocytes, eosinophils, and Reed-Sternberg cells. The latter cells are its special histologic feature. Untreated, Hodgkin's disease follows a variable but relentlessly progressive and ultimately fatal course. Recent advances in therapy make Hodgkin's disease potentially curable, even in advanced stages, and appropriate treatment yields a 5-year survival rate in approximately 90% of patients.

Cause

Unknown

Signs and symptoms

• Painless swelling in one of the cervical lymph nodes is usually the first sign. Occasionally, this early sign appears in another lymph node.

• Pruritus

• Persistent fever, night sweats, fatigue, weight loss, and malaise may occur first in older patients.

• Pel-Ebstein fever pattern (intermittent fever of several days' duration, alternating with afebrile periods) is a rare symptom.

• Late-stage symptoms include edema of the face and neck, possible jaundice, nerve pain, enlargement of retroperitoneal nodes, and nodular infiltration of the spleen, liver, and bones.

Diagnostic tests

The same tests are used for diagnosis and for staging.

• Lymph node biopsy checks for abnormal histiocyte proliferation and nodular fibrosis and necrosis.

• Other appropriate tests include bone marrow, liver, and spleen biopsies; and routine chest X-ray, abdominal CT scan, lung scan, bone scan, and lymphangiography, to detect lymph node or organ involvement.

• Hematologic tests show mild to severe normocytic anemia; normochromic anemia (in 50%); elevated, normal, or reduced WBC count; and differential showing any combination of neutrophilia, lymphocytopenia, monocytosis, and eosinophilia.

• A staging laparotomy is necessary for patients under age 55 or those without obvious Stage III or Stage IV disease, lymphocyte predominance subtype histology, or medical contraindications. (See *The Stages of Hodgkin's Disease*.)

Treatment

Appropriate therapy (chemotherapy and/or radiation, varying with the stage

The Stages of Hodgkin's Disease

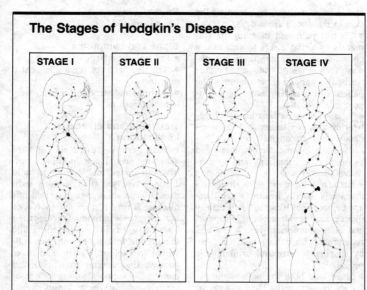

STAGE I STAGE II STAGE III STAGE IV

STAGE I
Disease limited to a single lymph node region or to a single extralymphatic organ

STAGE II
Disease in two or more nodes on the same side of the diaphragm; involvement of an extralymphatic organ and one or more node regions, or of the spleen

STAGE III
Disease present on both sides of the diaphragm; accompanied by involvement of the spleen, or of an extralymphatic organ, or both

STAGE IV
Diffuse or disseminated involvement of one or more extralymphatic organs or tissues, with or without associated lymph node involvement

of the disease) depends on careful physical examination, accurate histologic interpretation, and proper clinical staging. Correct treatment allows longer survival and even induces an apparent cure in many patients. Radiation therapy is used alone for Stage I and Stage II and in combination with chemotherapy for Stage III. Chemotherapy is used for Stage IV, sometimes inducing a complete remission. Use of these drugs may require concomitant antiemetics, sedatives, or antidiarrheals to combat gastrointestinal side effects.

Clinical implications
Because many patients with Hodgkin's disease receive radiation or chemotherapy as outpatients, tell the patient to observe the following precautions:
• Watch for and report radiation and chemotherapy side effects (particularly anorexia, nausea, vomiting, and diarrhea).
• Minimize radiation side effects by maintaining good nutrition (aided by eating small, frequent meals of favorite foods); drinking plenty of fluids; pacing activities to counteract ther-

apy-induced fatigue; and keeping the skin in irradiated areas dry.

• Control pain and bleeding of stomatitis by using a soft toothbrush, a cotton swab, or an anesthetic mouthwash such as viscous lidocaine (as prescribed); by applying petrolatum to the patient's lips; and by avoiding astringent mouthwashes.

• If a woman patient is of childbearing age, advise her to delay pregnancy until prolonged remission, because radiation and chemotherapy can cause genetic mutations and spontaneous abortions.

• Because the patient with Hodgkin's disease is usually healthy when therapy begins, he is likely to be especially distressed. Provide emotional support and offer appropriate counseling and reassurance. Ease the patient's anxiety by sharing your optimism about his prognosis.

• Make sure both the patient and his family know that the local chapter of the American Cancer Society is available for information, financial assistance, and supportive counseling.

Homosexuality, ego-dystonic

Description

Ego-dystonic homosexuality is the preference for a sexual partner of the same sex that causes psychological pain, negative emotions, and the desire for compliance with heterosexual social standards. Homosexuals affected by this have a persistent desire to change their sexual orientation rather than a brief difficulty with adjustment to homosexual impulses. Weak or absent heterosexual impulses are found in both adolescents and adults with this disorder. A history of the individual's sexual practices and feelings about them is essential for establishing this diagnosis.

Cause
Unknown

Signs and symptoms
• Psychological pain
• Negative feelings regarding sexual practice
• Wishing and striving for heterosexual relationships

Treatment and clinical implications

Psychotherapy directed toward achieving acceptance, building a positive self-image, and learning to build a supportive social network is indicated. Some sources suggest that this disorder is time-limited and that, with maturity, these individuals accept their homosexuality. Good listening and therapeutic techniques help the individual to explore, clarify, and make choices. Encouraging participation in community support groups for homosexuals and working on family acceptance are also useful.

Hookworm disease
(Uncinariasis)

Description

Hookworm disease is an infection of the upper intestine. Sandy soil, high humidity, a warm climate, and failure to wear shoes all favor its transmission. In the United States, hookworm disease is most common in the Southeast. Although this disease can cause cardiopulmonary complications, it is rarely fatal, except in debilitated persons or infants under age 1.

Causes
• *Ancylostoma duodenale*, found in the eastern hemisphere
• *Necator americanus*, found in the western hemisphere

Mode of transmission
Direct skin penetration (usually in the foot) by hookworm larvae in soil con-

taminated with feces that contain hookworm ova

Signs and symptoms
Usually, there are few symptoms.
• Irritation, pruritus, and edema at the site of entry
• Possible fever, sore throat, crackles,and cough when the larvae reach the lungs
• Possible fatigue, nausea, weight loss, dizziness, melena, and uncontrollable diarrhea with intestinal infection
• Passage of worms in stool

Diagnostic tests
• Identification of hookworm ova in the stool confirms the diagnosis.
• Hemoglobin level 5 to 9 g in severe disease
• Leukocyte count as high as 47,000/mm^3
• Eosinophil count 500 to 700/mm^3

Treatment
Treatment for hookworm infection includes administering mebendazole or pyrantel and providing an iron-rich diet or iron supplements to prevent or correct anemia.

Clinical implications
• Obtain a complete history, with special attention to travel or residency in endemic areas. Note the sequence and onset of symptoms. Interview the family and other close contacts to see if they too have any symptoms.
• Carefully assess the patient, noting signs of entry, lymphedema, and respiratory status.
   If the patient has confirmed hookworm infestation, follow these guidelines:
• Segregate the incontinent patient.
• Wash your hands thoroughly after every patient contact.
• Closely monitor intake and output. Note quantity and frequency of diarrheal stools. Dispose of feces promptly, and wear gloves when doing so.

• To help assess nutritional status, weigh the patient daily. To combat malnutrition, emphasize the importance of good nutrition, with particular attention to foods high in iron and protein. If the patient receives iron supplements, explain that they will darken stools. Administer anthelmintics on an empty stomach, but without a purgative.
• To help prevent reinfection, educate the patient in proper hand-washing technique and sanitary disposal of feces. Tell him to wear shoes in endemic areas.

Complications
In severe and chronic infection, anemia from blood loss may led to cardiomegaly (a result of increased oxygen demands), heart failure, and generalized massive edema.

Huntington's disease
(Huntington's chorea, hereditary chorea, chronic progressive chorea, adult chorea)

Description
Huntington's disease is a hereditary disease in which degeneration in the cerebral cortex and basal ganglia causes chronic progressive chorea and mental deterioration, ending in dementia. Either sex can transmit and inherit the disease. Each child of a parent with this disease has a 50% chance of inheriting it; however, the child who does not inherit it cannot pass it on to his own children. The average age of onset is 35.

Cause
The specific cause is unknown. The disease is inherited as an autosomal dominant trait.

Signs and symptoms
• Gradual development of severe choreic movements, which are rapid,

often violent, and purposeless. Initially, they are unilateral and more prominent in the face and arms than in the legs.

• Dementia, which may be mild at first, eventually severely disrupts the personality.

• Ultimately, musculoskeletal control is lost.

Diagnostic tests

No reliable confirming test exists for Huntington's disease.

• Pneumoencephalography shows characteristic butterfly dilation of the brain's lateral ventricles.

• CT scan shows brain atrophy.

Treatment and clinical implications

Since Huntington's disease has no known cure, treatment is supportive, protective, and symptomatic. Tranquilizers, as well as chlorpromazine, haloperidol, or imipramine, help control choreic movements but cannot stop mental deterioration. They also alleviate discomfort and depression, making the patient easier to manage. However, tranquilizers increase rigidity. To control choreic movements without rigidity, choline may be prescribed. Institutionalization is often necessary because of mental deterioration.

• Provide physical support by attending to the patient's basic needs, such as hygiene, skin care, bowel and bladder care, and nutrition. Increase this support as mental and physical deterioration makes him increasingly immobile.

• Offer emotional support to the patient and family. Teach them about the disease, and listen to their concerns and special problems. Keep in mind the patient's dysarthria, and allow him extra time to express himself, thereby decreasing frustration. Teach the family to participate in the patient's care.

• Stay alert for possible suicide attempts. Control the patient's environment to protect him from suicide or

self-inflicted injury. Pad the side rails of the bed, but avoid restraints, which may cause the patient to injure himself during violent, uncontrolled movement.

• Make sure families receive genetic counseling. All affected family members should realize that each of their offspring has a 50% chance of inheriting this disease.

• Refer the patient and family to appropriate community organizations: visiting nurse services, social services, psychiatric counseling, or a long-term care facility.

• For more information about this degenerative disease, refer the patient and family to the Committee to Combat Huntington's Disease or the National Huntington's Disease Association.

Hyaline membrane disease (Respiratory distress syndrome)

Description

Hyaline membrane disease is an acute lung disease of the newborn, characterized by airless alveoli and inelastic lungs. Also called respiratory distress syndrome (RDS), it is the most common cause of neonatal mortality. RDS occurs in premature infants and, if untreated, is fatal within 72 hours of birth in up to 14% of infants weighing less than 5½ lb (2,500 g). It occurs more often in infants of diabetic mothers, those delivered by cesarean section, and those delivered suddenly after antepartum hemorrhage. Aggressive management using mechanical ventilation can improve the prognosis, but a few infants who survive have bronchopulmonary dysplasia. Mild RDS slowly subsides after 3 days.

Cause

Deficiency of pulmonary surfactant with resulting widespread alveolar collapse

Signs and symptoms

- Rapid, shallow breathing within minutes or hours of birth
- Intercostal, subcostal, or sternal retractions
- Nasal flaring
- Audible expiratory grunting
- Possible hypotension, peripheral edema, and oliguria
- Apnea, bradycardia, and cyanosis in severe disease
- Pallor
- Frothy sputum
- Low body temperature

Diagnostic tests

- Chest X-ray may be normal for the first 6 to 12 hours (in 50% of newborns with RDS) but later shows a fine reticulonodular pattern.
- Arterial blood gas (ABG) measurements show decreased PO_2 with normal, decreased, or increased PCO_2 and decreased pH (a combination of respiratory and metabolic acidosis).
- Amniocentesis allows determination of the lecithin/sphingomyelin (L/S) ratio, which helps to assess prenatal lung development and the risk of RDS when a cesarean section is necessary before the 36th week of gestation.

Treatment

Treatment of an infant with RDS requires vigorous respiratory support. Warm, humidified, oxygen-enriched gases are administered by oxygen hood or, if such treatment fails, by mechanical ventilation. Severe cases may require mechanical ventilation with positive end-expiratory pressue (PEEP) or continuous positive airway pressure (CPAP), administered by tightly fitted face mask or, when absolutely necessary, endotracheal intubation. Treatment also includes the following:

- A radiant infant warmer or isolette for thermoregulation
- I.V. fluids and sodium bicarbonate to control acidosis and maintain fluid and electrolyte balance
- Tube feedings or hyperalimentation to maintain adequate nutrition if the infant is too weak to eat.

Clinical implications

Infants with RDS require continual assessment and monitoring in an intensive care nursery.

- Closely monitor ABG levels as well as fluid intake and output. If the infant has an umbilical catheter (arterial or venous), check for arterial hypotension or abnormal central venous pressure. Watch for complications, such as infection, thrombosis, or decreased circulation to the legs. If the infant has a transcutaneous PO_2 monitor (an accurate method for determining PO_2), change the site of the lead placement every 2 to 4 hours to avoid burning the skin.
- Weigh the infant once or twice daily. To evaluate his progress, assess skin color, rate and depth of respirations, severity of retractions, nostril flaring, frequency of expiratory grunting, frothing at the lips, and restlessness.
- Regularly assess the effectiveness of oxygen or ventilator therapy. Evaluate every change in fraction of inspired oxygen, PEEP, or CPAP by measuring ABG levels 20 minutes after each change. Be sure to adjust PEEP or CPAP, as indicated by ABG readings.
- When the infant is on mechanical ventilation, watch carefully for signs of barotrauma (increase in respiratory distress, subcutaneous emphysema) and accidental disconnection from the ventilator. Check ventilator settings frequently. Be alert for signs of complications of PEEP or CPAP therapy, such as decreased cardiac output, pneumothorax, and pneumomediastinum. Mechanical ventilation increases the risk of infection in premature infants, so preventive measures are essential.

• As needed, arrange for follow-up care with a neonatal ophthalmologist to check for retinal damage.

• Teach the parents about their infant's condition and, if possible, let them participate in his care (using aseptic technique), to encourage normal parent-infant bonding. Advise parents that full recovery may take up to 12 months. When the prognosis is poor, prepare the parents for the infant's impending death, and offer emotional support.

• Help reduce mortality in RDS by early detection of respiratory distress. Recognize intercostal retractions and grunting, especially in a premature infant, as signs of RDS, and make sure the infant receives immediate treatment.

Hydatidiform mole

Description

Hydatidiform mole is an uncommon chorionic tumor of the placenta. Its early signs—amenorrhea and uterine enlargement—mimic normal pregnancy; however, it eventually causes vaginal bleeding. Hydatidiform mole occurs most commonly in women over age 45. With prompt diagnosis and appropriate treatment, the prognosis is excellent; however, approximately 10% of patients with hydatidiform mole develop chorionic malignancy. Recurrence is possible in about 2% of cases.

Cause

Unknown

Signs and symptoms

• Uterine growth more rapid than usual in early pregnancy
• Absence of fetal heart sounds
• Vaginal bleeding (blood may contain hydatid vesicles)
• Lower abdominal cramps
• Hyperemesis likely

Diagnostic tests

• Histologic examination of passed hydatid vesicles establishes the diagnosis.

• Confirmation requires dilatation and curettage (D&C)

• Ultrasound assesses uterine contents. Use of a Doppler ultrasonic flowmeter demonstrates the absence of fetal heart tones.

• Pregnancy test shows elevated human chorionic gonadotropin (HCG) serum levels 100 or more days after the last menstrual period.

• Arteriography shows typical early venous shadows.

Treatment

Hydatidiform mole necessitates uterine evacuation via D&C or, if this is ineffective, abdominal hysterectomy or suction curettage. Before evacuation, oxytocin I.V. promotes uterine contractions.

Postoperative treatment varies, depending on the amount of blood lost and complications. If no complications develop, hospitalization is usually brief, and normal activities can be resumed quickly, as tolerated.

Because of the possibility of choriocarcinoma after hydatidiform mole, scrupulous follow-up care is essential. Such care includes monitoring HCG levels until they return to normal and taking chest X-rays to check for lung metastasis. Most doctors advise postponing another pregnancy until at least 1 year after HCG levels return to normal.

Clinical implications

• Preoperatively, observe for signs of complications, such as hemorrhage and uterine infection, and vaginal passage of hydatid vesicles. Save any expelled tissue for laboratory analysis.

• Postoperatively, monitor vital signs, especially blood pressure, and check blood loss.

• Provide patient and family teaching, and give emotional support. Encourage the patient to express her feelings, and help her through the grieving for her lost infant.

• Instruct the patient to promptly report any new symptoms (for example, hemoptysis, cough, suspected pregnancy, nausea, vomiting, and vaginal bleeding).

• Stress the need for regular follow-up by HCG and chest X-ray monitoring, for early detection of possible malignant changes.

• Explain to the patient that she must use contraceptives to prevent pregnancy for at least 1 year after HCG levels return to normal and regular ovulation and menstrual cycles are reestablished.

Complications
• Preeclampsia
• Anemia
• Infection
• Spontaneous abortion
• Uterine rupture
• Choriocarcinoma

Hydrocephalus

Description
Hydrocephalus is an excessive accumulation of cerebrospinal fluid (CSF) within the ventricular spaces of the brain. It occurs most often in newborns, but it can also occur in adults. In infants, hydrocephalus enlarges the head. In both infants and adults, resulting compression can damage brain tissue. Without surgery, the prognosis is poor. Mortality may result from increased intracranial pressure in persons of all ages. Infants may also die prematurely of infection and malnutrition. With early detection and surgical intervention, the prognosis improves but remains guarded. Even after surgery, such complications as mental retardation, impaired motor function, and vision loss can persist. (See *Normal Circulation of CSF*, p. 366.)

Causes
Obstruction of CSF flow (noncommunicating hydrocephalus)
—Faulty fetal development
—Infection (syphilis, granulomatous diseases, meningitis)
—Tumor
—Cerebral aneurysm
—Blood clot
Faulty reabsorption of CSF (communicating hydrocephalus)
—Surgery to repair a myelomeningocele
—Adhesions between meninges at the base of the brain
—Meningeal hemorrhage
Overproduction of CSF
This rare cause results from a tumor in the choroid plexus.

Signs and symptoms
Infants
—Enlargement of the head
—Distended scalp veins
—Thin, shiny, fragile-looking scalp skin
—Underdeveloped neck muscles
—In severe hydrocephalus, depressed orbital roof, downward displacement of the eyes, and prominent sclera
—Possible high-pitched, shrill cry; abnormal muscle tone in the legs; irritability; anorexia; vomiting
Older children and adults
—Decreased level of consciousness
—Ataxia
—Incontinence
—Impaired intellect

Diagnostic tests
• Skull X-rays show thinning of the skull, separation of sutures, and widening of fontanelles.
• Ventriculography shows enlargement of the brain's ventricles.
• Angiography, pneumoencephalography, CT scan, and magnetic resonance imaging can differentiate between hydrocephalus and intracranial lesions and can also demonstrate the Arnold-Chiari deformity, which

Normal Circulation of CSF

Cerebrospinal fluid (CSF) is produced from blood in a capillary network (choroid plexus) in the brain's lateral ventricles. From the lateral ventricles, CSF flows through the interventricular foramen (foramen of Monro) to the third ventricle. From there, it flows through the aqueduct of Sylvius to the fourth ventricle and through the foramina of Luschka and Magendie to the cisterna of the subarachnoid space.

Then, the fluid passes under the base of the brain, upward over the brain's upper surfaces, and down around the spinal cord. Eventually, CSF reaches the arachnoid villi, where it is reabsorbed into venous blood at the venous sinuses.

Normally, the amount of fluid produced (about 500 ml/day) equals the amount absorbed. The average amount circulated at one time is 150 to 175 ml.

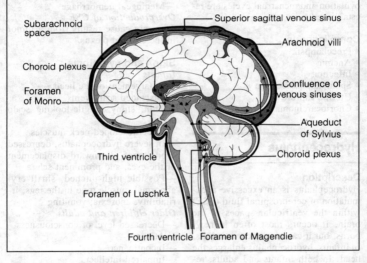

Subarachnoid space
Choroid plexus
Foramen of Monro
Third ventricle
Foramen of Luschka
Fourth ventricle Foramen of Magendie

Superior sagittal venous sinus
Arachnoid villi
Confluence of venous sinuses
Aqueduct of Sylvius
Choroid plexus

occurs with hydrocephalus (See *Arnold-Chiari Syndrome*.)

Treatment

Surgical correction is the only treatment for hydrocephalus. Usually, such surgery consists of insertion of a ventriculoperitoneal shunt, which transports excess fluid from the lateral ventricle into the peritoneal cavity. A less common procedure is insertion of a ventriculoatrial shunt, which drains fluid from the brain's lateral ventricle into the right atrium of the heart,

where the fluid makes its way into the venous circulation.

Complications of surgery include shunt infection, septicemia (after ventriculoatrial shunt), adhesions and paralytic ileus, shunt migration, peritonitis, and intestinal perforation (with peritoneal shunt).

Clinical implications

On initial assessment, obtain a complete history from the patient or the family. Note general behavior, especially irritability, apathy, or decreased level of consciousness. Perform a neurologic assessment. Ask the patient if he has headaches, and watch for projectile vomiting; both are signs of increased intracranial pressure. Also watch for convulsions. Note changes in vital signs.

Before surgery to insert a shunt, follow these guidelines:

• Encourage maternal-infant bonding when possible.

• Check fontanelles for tension or fullness, and measure and record head circumference. On the patient's chart, draw a picture showing where to measure the head so that other staff members measure it in the same place, or mark the forehead with ink.

• To prevent postfeeding aspiration and hypostatic pneumonia, place the infant on his side and reposition him every 2 hours, or prop him up in an infant seat.

• To prevent skin breakdown, make sure his earlobe is flat, and place a sheepskin or rubber foam under his head.

• When turning the infant, move his head, neck, and shoulders with his body, to reduce strain on his neck.

• Feed the infant slowly.

After surgery, follow these guidelines:

• Place the infant on the side opposite the operative site, with his head level with his body unless the physician's orders specify otherwise.

• Check temperature, pulse rate, blood pressure, and level of consciousness. Also check fontanelles for fullness daily. Watch for vomiting, which may be an early sign of increased intracranial pressure and shunt malfunction.

• Watch for signs of infection, especially meningitis. Check the dressing often for drainage.

• Listen for bowel sounds after ventriculoperitoneal shunt insertion.

• Teach parents to watch for signs of shunt malfunction, infection, and paralytic ileus. Tell them that shunt insertion requires periodic surgery to lengthen the shunt as the child grows older, to correct malfunctioning, or to treat infection.

• Check the infant's growth and development periodically, and help the parents set goals consistent with the child's ability and potential. Help parents focus on their child's strengths, not his weaknesses. Discuss special education programs, and emphasize the infant's need for sensory stimulation appropriate for his age.

Hydronephrosis

Description

Hydronephrosis is an abnormal dilation of the renal pelvis and the calyces of one or both kidneys. It is caused by an obstruction of urine flow in the genitourinary tract. If obstruction is in the

---

Arnold-Chiari Syndrome

Arnold-Chiari syndrome commonly accompanies hydrocephalus, especially when a myelomeningocele is also present. In this condition, an elongation or tonguelike downward projection of the cerebellum and medulla extends through the foramen magnum into the cervical portion of the spinal canal, impairing CSF drainage from the fourth ventricle.

In addition to signs and symptoms of hydrocephalus, infants with this syndrome have nuchal rigidity, noisy respirations, irritability, vomiting, weak sucking reflex, and a preference for hyperextending the neck.

Treatment requires surgery to insert a shunt like that used in hydrocephalus. Surgical decompression of the cerebellar tonsils at the foramen magnum is sometimes indicated.

urethra or bladder, hydronephrosis is usually bilateral; if obstruction is in a ureter, it is usually unilateral. Although partial obstruction and hydronephrosis may not produce symptoms initially, increased pressure behind the obstruction eventually results in symptomatic renal dysfunction.

Cause
Any type of obstructive uropathy—most commonly, benign prostatic hypertrophy, urethral strictures, and calculi

Signs and symptoms
Clinical features of hydronephrosis vary with the cause of the obstruction. Any of the following may occur:
• No symptoms
• Mild pain and slightly decreased urinary flow
• Severe, colicky renal pain
• Dull flank pain that may radiate to the groin. Unilateral obstruction may cause pain on only one side, usually in the flank area.
• Hematuria
• Pyuria
• Dysuria
• Alternating oliguria and polyuria
• Complete anuria
• Nausea and vomiting
• Abdominal fullness
• Pain on urination
• Dribbling
• Hesitancy

Diagnostic tests
Intravenous pyelography, retrograde pyelography, renal ultrasound, and renal function studies are necessary to confirm the diagnosis.

Treatment
The goals of treatment are to preserve renal function and prevent infection through surgical removal of the obstruction, such as dilation for stricture of the urethra or prostatectomy for benign prostatic hypertrophy. If renal function has already been affected, therapy may include a diet low in protein, sodium, and potassium. This diet is designed to stop the progression of renal failure before surgery. Inoperable obstructions may necessitate decompression and drainage of the kidney, using a nephrostomy tube placed temporarily or permanently in the renal pelvis. Concurrent infection requires appropriate antibiotic therapy.

Clinical implications
• Explain hydronephrosis, as well as the purpose of diagnostic procedures.
• Administer medication for pain, as needed and prescribed.
• Postoperatively, closely monitor intake and output, vital signs, and fluid and electrolyte status. Watch for a rising pulse rate and cold, clammy skin, which indicate possible impending hemorrhage and shock. Monitor renal function studies daily.
• If a nephrostomy tube has been inserted, check it frequently for bleeding and patency. Irrigate the tube only as ordered, and do not clamp it.
• If the patient is to be discharged with a nephrostomy tube in place, teach him how to care for it properly.
• To prevent progression of hydronephrosis to irreversible renal disease, urge older men (especially those with family histories of benign prostatic hypertrophy or prostatitis) to have routine medical checkups. Teach them to recognize and report symptoms of hydronephrosis (colicky pain, hematuria) or urinary tract infection.

Complications
• Infection (pyelonephritis)
• Paralytic ileus, with acute obstruction

Hyperaldosteronism

Description
Hyperaldosteronism is a condition characterized by hypersecretion of al-

dosterone by the adrenal cortex, occurring as a primary disease of the adrenal cortex or, more often, as a secondary disorder in response to various extraadrenal pathologic processes often associated with increased plasma renin activity.

Aldosterone hypersecretion causes excessive reabsorption of sodium and water and excessive renal excretion of potassium.

Causes
Primary hyperaldosteronism
—Benign adrenal adenoma
—Unknown cause
—Adrenocortical hyperplasia (in children) or carcinoma
Secondary hyperaldosteronism
—Renal artery stenosis
—Wilms' tumor
—Pregnancy
—Oral contraceptives
—Nephrotic syndrome
—Cirrhosis with ascites
—Idiopathic edema
—Congestive heart failure
—Bartter's syndrome
—Salt-losing nephritis

Signs and symptoms
Any of the following may occur:
• Hypertension
• Muscle weakness
• Tetany
• Paresthesias
• Dysrhythmias
• Fatigue
• Headache
• Polyuria
• Polydipsia
• Visual disturbances

Diagnostic tests
• Low plasma renin level after volume depletion by diuretic administration and upright posture, and a high plasma aldosterone level after volume expansion by salt loading confirm primary (Conn's) hyperaldosteronism in a hypertensive patient without edema.
• Serum bicarbonate level is often elevated, with ensuing alkalosis from hydrogen and potassium ion loss in the distal renal tubules.
• Other tests show markedly increased urinary aldosterone levels; increased plasma aldosterone levels; and, in secondary hyperaldosteronism, increased plasma renin levels.
• A suppression test is useful to differentiate between primary and secondary hyperaldosteronism. During this test, the patient receives desoxycorticosterone P.O. for 3 days, while plasma aldosterone levels and urinary metabolites are continually measured. These levels decrease in secondary hyperaldosteronism but remain the same in primary hyperaldosteronism. Simultaneously, renin levels are low in primary disease and high in secondary disease.
• Other helpful diagnostic evidence includes an increase in plasma volume of 30% to 50% above normal, EKG signs of hypokalemia (ST segment depression and U waves), chest X-ray showing left ventricular hypertrophy from chronic hypertension, and localization of tumor by adrenal angiography or CT scan.

Treatment
Although treatment for primary hyperaldosteronism may include unilateral adrenalectomy, administration of a potassium-sparing diuretic—spironolactone—and sodium restriction may control the disease without surgery. Bilateral adrenalectomy reduces blood pressure for most patients with idiopathic primary hyperaldosteronism. However, some degree of hypertension persists in most patients, even after surgery, necessitating treatment with spironolactone or another antihypertensive. Such patients also require lifelong adrenal hormone replacement.

Treatment of secondary hyperaldosteronism must include correction of the underlying cause.

Clinical implications

• Monitor and record urinary output, blood pressure, weight, and serum potassium levels.

• Watch for signs of tetany (muscle twitching, Chvostek's sign) and for hypokalemia-induced cardiac dysrhythmias, paresthesia, or weakness. Give potassium replacements, as ordered, and keep calcium gluconate I.V. available.

• Ask the dietitian to provide a low-sodium, high-potassium diet.

• After adrenalectomy, watch for weakness, hyponatremia, rising serum potassium levels, and signs of adrenal insufficiency, especially hypotension.

• If the patient is taking spironolactone, advise him to watch for signs of hyperkalemia. Tell him that impotence and gynecomastia may follow long-term use.

• Tell the patient who requires steroid hormone replacement therapy to wear a Medic Alert bracelet.

Hyperbilirubinemia
(Neonatal jaundice)

Description

Hyperbilirubinemia is marked by elevated serum bilirubin levels and mild jaundice. It can be physiologic (with jaundice the only symptom) or pathologic (resulting from an underlying disease). Physiologic jaundice is very common and is self-limiting. Prognosis for pathologic jaundice varies, depending on the cause. Untreated, severe hyperbilirubinemia may result in kernicterus, a neurologic syndrome caused by deposition of unconjugated bilirubin in the brain cells and characterized by severe neural symptoms. Survivors may develop cerebral palsy, epilepsy, or mental retardation; or they may have relatively minor sequelae, such as perceptual-motor handicaps and learning disorders.

Causes

• Factors that disrupt bilirubin conjugation and usurp albumin-binding sites, including such drugs as aspirin, tranquilizers, and sulfonamides and such conditions as hypothermia, anoxia, hypoglycemia, and hypoalbuminemia

• Decreased hepatic function, which results in reduced bilirubin conjugation

• Increased erythrocyte production or breakdown from hemolytic disorders, or Rh or ABO incompatibility

• Biliary obstruction or hepatitis that results in blockage of normal bile flow

• Enzyme deficiency (inhibited glucuronyltransferase conjugating activity)

(See also *Underlying Causes of Hyperbilirubinemia*.)

Signs and symptoms

Jaundice is the predominant sign.

Diagnostic tests

• Increased serum bilirubin levels, along with jaundice, confirm the diagnosis.

• Besides a detailed history, blood testing of the infant and mother (blood group incompatibilities, hemoglobin level, direct Coombs' test, hematocrit) may be needed to determine the underlying cause of hyperbilirubinemia.

Treatment

Depending on the underlying cause, treatment may include phototherapy, exchange transfusions, albumin infusion, and possibly drug therapy. Phototherapy is the treatment of choice for physiologic jaundice and for pathologic jaundice from erythroblastosis fetalis (after the initial exchange transfusion). Phototherapy uses fluorescent light to decompose bilirubin in the skin by oxidation. It is usually discontinued after bilirubin levels fall below 10 mg/dl and continue to decrease for 24 hours. However, phototherapy is rarely the only treatment for pathologic jaundice.

Underlying Causes of Hyperbilirubinemia

When jaundice occurs during the 1st day of life:
- Blood type incompatibility (Rh, ABO, other minor blood groups)
- Intrauterine infection (rubella, cytomegalic inclusion disease, toxoplasmosis, syphilis, and, occasionally, such bacteria as *Escherichia coli,* staphylococcus, *Pseudomonas, Klebsiella, Proteus,* and streptococcus)

When jaundice occurs during the 2nd or 3rd day of life:
- Infection (usually from gram-negative bacteria)
- Polycythemia
- Enclosed hemorrhage (skin bruises, subdural hematoma)
- Respiratory distress syndrome (hyaline membrane disease)
- Heinz-body anemia from drugs and toxins (vitamin K_3, sodium nitrate)
- Transient neonatal hyperbilirubinemia
- Abnormal RBC morphology
- Red cell enzyme deficiencies (glucose-6-phosphate dehydrogenase, hexokinase)
- Physiologic jaundice
- Blood group incompatibilities

When jaundice occurs during the 4th and 5th days of life:
- Breast-feeding, respiratory distress syndrome, maternal diabetes
- Crigler-Najjar syndrome (congenital nonhemolytic icterus)
- Gilbert's syndrome

When jaundice occurs after 1 week of life:
- Herpesvirus infection
- Pyloric stenosis
- Hypothyroidism
- Neonatal giant cell hepatitis
- Infection (usually acquired in neonatal period)
- Bile duct atresia
- Galactosemia
- Choledochal cyst

Text adapted and reproduced with permission from Rita G. Harper and Jing Ja Yoon, *Handbook of Neonatology,* 2nd ed. © 1987 by Year Book Medical Publishers, Inc., Chicago.

An exchange transfusion replaces the infant's blood with fresh blood (less than 48 hours old), removing some of the unconjugated bilirubin in serum. Possible indications for exchange transfusions include hydrops fetalis, polycythemia, erythroblastosis fetalis, marked reticulocytosis, drug toxicity, and jaundice that develops within the first 6 hours after birth.

Other therapy for excessive bilirubin levels may include albumin administration (1 g/kg of 25% salt-poor albumin), which provides additional albumin for binding unconjugated bilirubin. This may be done 1 to 2 hours before exchange or as a substitute for a portion of the plasma in the transfused blood.

Drug therapy, which is rare, usually consists of phenobarbital administered to the mother before delivery and to the newborn several days after delivery. This drug stimulates the hepatic glucuronide conjugating system.

Clinical implications

• Reassure parents that most infants experience some degree of jaundice. Explain hyperbilirubinemia, its causes, diagnostic tests, and treatment. Also explain that the infant's stool contains some bile and may be greenish.

• Assess and record the infant's jaundice, and note the time it began. Report the jaundice and serum bilirubin levels immediately.

For the infant receiving phototherapy, follow these guidelines:

• Keep a record of how long each bilirubin light bulb is in use, since these bulbs require frequent changing for optimum effectiveness.

• Undress the infant so that his entire body surface is exposed to the light rays. Keep him 18″ to 30″ (45 to 75 cm) from the light source. Protect his eyes with shields that filter the light.

• Monitor and maintain the infant's body temperature; high and low temperatures predispose him to kernicterus. Remove him from the light source every 3 to 4 hours, and take off the eye shields. Allow his parents to visit and feed him.

• When the infant's bilirubin level is less than 10 mg/dl and has been decreasing for 24 hours, discontinue phototherapy, as ordered. (The infant usually shows a decrease in serum bilirubin level 1 to 12 hours after the start of phototherapy.) Resume therapy, as ordered, if the serum bilirubin level increases several milligrams per deciliter, as it often does, from a rebound effect.

For the infant receiving exchange transfusions, follow these guidelines:

• Prepare an infant warmer and tray before the transfusion. Try to keep the infant quiet. Give him nothing by mouth for 3 to 4 hours before the procedure.

• Check the blood to be used for the exchange—type, Rh, age. Keep emergency equipment (resuscitation and intubation equipment and oxygen) available. During the procedure, monitor respiratory and heart rates every 15 minutes; check temperature every 30 minutes. Continue to monitor vital signs every 15 to 30 minutes for 2 hours.

• Measure intake and output. Observe for cord bleeding and such complications as hemorrhage, hypocalcemia, sepsis, and shock. Report serum bilirubin and hemoglobin levels. Bilirubin levels may rise, from a rebound effect, within 30 minutes after transfusion, necessitating repeat transfusions.

To prevent hyperbilirubinemia, follow these guidelines:

• Maintain oral intake. Do not skip any feedings, since fasting stimulates the conversion of heme to bilirubin.

• Administer $Rh_o(D)$ immune globulin (human), as ordered, to an Rh-negative mother after amniocentesis or— to prevent hemolytic disease in subsequent infants—to an Rh-negative mother after the birth of an Rh-positive infant or after spontaneous or elective abortion.

Hyperemesis gravidarum

Description

Unlike the transient nausea and vomiting normally experienced between the 6th and 12th weeks of pregnancy, hyperemesis gravidarum is severe and unremitting nausea and vomiting that persists after the first trimester. If untreated, it produces substantial weight loss; starvation; dehydration, with subsequent fluid and electrolyte imbalance (hypokalemia); and acid-base disturbances (acidosis and alkalosis). Prognosis is good with appropriate treatment.

Cause

Unknown

Signs and symptoms

Unremitting nausea and vomiting are the cardinal symptoms. Associated ef-

fects may include the following:
- Weight loss, emaciation
- Pale, dry, waxy, and possibly jaundiced skin
- Subnormal or elevated temperature
- Rapid pulse
- Fetid, fruity breath odor (acidosis)
- CNS symptoms, such as confusion, delirium, headache, lassitude, stupor, and possibly coma

Diagnostic tests
- Serum analysis shows decreased protein, chloride, sodium, and potassium levels and increased blood urea nitrogen levels.
- Other laboratory tests reveal ketonuria, slight proteinuria, and elevated hemoglobin and WBC levels.

Treatment
Hyperemesis gravidarum may necessitate hospitalization to correct electrolyte imbalance and prevent starvation. I.V. infusions maintain nutrition until the patient can tolerate oral feedings. She progresses slowly to a clear liquid diet, then a full liquid diet, and finally, to small, frequent meals of high-protein solid foods. A midnight snack helps stabilize blood glucose levels. Vitamin B supplements help correct vitamin deficiency.

When vomiting stops and electrolyte balance has been restored, the pregnancy usually continues without recurrence of hyperemesis gravidarum. Most patients feel better as they begin to regain normal weight, but some continue to vomit throughout the pregnancy, requiring extended treatment. If appropriate, some patients may benefit from consultations with clinical nurse specialists, psychologists, or psychiatrists.

Clinical implications
- Encourage the patient to eat. Suggest dry foods and decreased liquid intake during meals. Company and diversionary conversation at mealtime may be beneficial.
- Instruct the patient to remain upright for 45 minutes after eating to decrease reflux.
- Provide reassurance and a calm, restful atmosphere. Encourage the patient to discuss her feelings regarding her pregnancy.
- Before discharge, provide nutritional counseling.

Hyperparathyroidism

Description
Hyperparathyroidism is characterized by overactivity of one or more of the four parathyroid glands, resulting in excessive secretion of parathyroid hormone (PTH). Such hypersecretion of PTH promotes bone resorption and leads to hypercalcemia and hypophosphatemia. In turn, increased renal and gastrointestinal absorption of calcium occurs.

Hyperparathyroidism may be primary or secondary. In primary hyperparathyroidism, one or more of the parathyroid glands enlarge, increasing PTH secretion and elevating serum calcium levels.

In secondary hyperparathyroidism, excessive compensatory production of PTH stems from a hypocalcemia-producing abnormality outside the parathyroid gland, which causes a resistance to the metabolic action of PTH.

Causes
Primary hyperparathyroidism
—Single adenoma
—Genetic disorder
—Multiple endocrine neoplasia
Secondary hyperparathyroidism
—Rickets
—Vitamin D deficiency
—Chronic renal failure
—Phenytoin or laxative abuse

Signs and symptoms
Primary hyperparathyroidism
—Renal: symptoms of recurring nephrolithiasis, which may lead to renal

insufficiency

—Skeletal and articular: chronic low back pain and easy fracturing from bone degeneration; bone tenderness

—Gastrointestinal: pancreatitis, causing constant, severe epigastric pain radiating to the back; peptic ulcers, causing abdominal pain, hematemesis, nausea, and vomiting

—Neuromuscular: marked muscle weakness and atrophy, particularly in the legs

—CNS: psychomotor and personality disturbances, depression, overt psychosis, stupor, and possibly coma

—Other: skin necrosis, vision impairment from cataracts, polyuria, anemia, subcutaneous calcification

Secondary hyperparathyroidism

—May produce the same clinical features as above, with possible skeletal deformities of the long bones (rickets, for example) as well as other symptoms of the underlying disease

Diagnostic tests

Primary disease

—On radioimmunoassay, serum PTH level is high. Along with increased serum calcium level, this confirms the diagnosis.

—X-rays show diffuse demineralization of bones, bone cysts, outer cortical bone resorption, and subperiosteal erosion of the radial aspect of the middle fingers.

—Microscopic examination of the bone with such tests as X-ray spectrophotometry typically demonstrates increased bone turnover.

—Laboratory tests reveal elevated urine and serum calcium, chloride, and alkaline phosphatase levels, and decreased serum phosphorus level.

—Uric acid and creatinine levels may be increased along with basal acid secretion and serum immunoreactive gastrin.

—Serum amylase level is increased with acute pancreatitis.

Secondary disease

—Serum calcium level is normal or slightly decreased.

—Serum phosphorus levels are variable.

—Other laboratory values may identify the cause of secondary hyperparathyroidism.

Treatment

Treatment varies, depending on the cause of the disease. Treatment for primary hyperparathyroidism may include surgery to remove the adenoma or, depending on the extent of hyperplasia, all but half of one gland (the remaining part of the gland is necessary to maintain normal PTH levels). Such surgery may relieve bone pain within 3 days. However, renal damage may be irreversible.

Other treatments can decrease calcium levels preoperatively or if surgery is not feasible or necessary. Such treatments include forcing fluids; limiting dietary intake of calcium; promoting sodium and calcium excretion through forced diuresis, using normal saline solution (up to 6 liters in life-threatening circumstances), furosemide, or ethacrynic acid; and administering oral sodium or potassium phosphate, calcitonin, or mithramycin.

Therapy for potential postoperative magnesium and phosphate deficiencies includes I.V. administration of magnesium and phosphate, or sodium phosphate solution given P.O. or by retention enema. In addition, during the first 4 or 5 days after surgery, when serum calcium falls to low-normal levels, supplemental calcium may be necessary. Vitamin D or calcitriol may also be used to raise the serum calcium level.

Treatment of secondary hyperparathyroidism must correct the underlying cause of parathyroid hypertrophy and includes vitamin D therapy or, in the patient with renal disease, aluminum hydroxide for hyperphosphatemia. In the patient with renal failure, peritoneal dialysis is necessary to lower calcium levels and may have to continue for life. In the patient with chronic secondary hyperparathyroidism, the enlarged glands may not revert to normal size and function even after calcium levels have been controlled.

Clinical implications
Care emphasizes prevention of complications from the underlying disease and its treatment.
• During hydration to reduce serum calcium level, record intake and output accurately. Strain urine to check for stones. Monitor sodium, potassium, and magnesium levels frequently.
• Auscultate for lung sounds often. Listen for signs of pulmonary edema in the patient receiving large amounts of saline solution I.V., especially if he has pulmonary or cardiac disease.
• Since the patient is predisposed to pathologic fractures, take measures to avoid trauma.
• Watch for signs of peptic ulcer and administer antacids, as appropriate.
    After parathyroidectomy, follow these guidelines:
• Check frequently for respiratory distress, and keep a tracheotomy tray at bedside. Watch for postoperative complications, such as renal colic, acute psychosis, laryngeal nerve damage, or rarely, hemorrhage. Monitor intake and output carefully.
• Check for swelling at the operative site. Place the patient in semi-Fowler's position, and support his head and neck with sandbags to decrease edema, which may cause pressure on the trachea.
• Watch for signs of tetany. Keep calcium gluconate available for emergency I.V. administration. Encourage ambulation as soon as possible postoperatively, even though the patient may find this uncomfortable. Weight-bearing exercise speeds bone recalcification.
• Check laboratory results for low serum calcium and magnesium levels.
• Monitor mental status and watch for listlessness. In the patient with persistent hypercalcemia, check for muscle weakness and signs of psychosis.
• Before discharge, advise the patient of the possible side effects of drug therapy. Emphasize the need for periodic follow-up through laboratory blood tests. If hyperparathyroidism was not corrected surgically, warn the patient to avoid calcium-containing antacids and thiazide diuretics.

Complications
• Renal calculi, which may lead to renal failure
• Osteoporosis
• Pancreatitis
• Peptic ulcer

Hyperpituitarism
(Acromegaly and gigantism)

Description
A chronic, progressive disease marked by hormonal dysfunction and startling skeletal overgrowth, hyperpituitarism appears in two forms. Acromegaly occurs after epiphyseal closure, causing bone thickening and transverse growth and visceromegaly. Gigantism begins before epiphyseal closure and causes proportional overgrowth of all body tissues. Although the prognosis depends on the cause, this disease usually reduces life expectancy.

Cause
Oversecretion of human growth hormone (HGH), possibly from tumor of the anterior pituitary gland

Signs and symptoms
Acromegaly
—Gradual, marked enlargement of the bones of the face, jaw, and extremities
—Diaphoresis
—Oily skin
—Hirsutism
Gigantism
—Proportional overgrowth of all body tissues with remarkable height increases

Diagnostic tests

• Plasma HGH levels are increased on radioimmunoassay; however, a random sampling may be misleading.

• Glucose suppression test offers more reliable information.

• Skull X-rays, CT scan, arteriography, and pneumoencephalography determine the presence and extent of the pituitary lesion.

• Bone X-rays showing a thickening of the cranium (especially of frontal, occipital, and parietal bones) and of the long bones, as well as osteoarthritis in the spine, support this diagnosis.

Treatment

The aim of treatment is to curb overproduction of HGH through removal of the underlying tumor by cranial or transsphenoidal hypophysectomy or pituitary radiation therapy. In acromegaly, surgery is mandatory when a tumor causes blindness or other severe neurologic disturbances. Postoperative therapy often requires replacement of thyroid, cortisone, and gonadal hormones. Adjunctive treatment may include bromocriptine, which inhibits HGH synthesis.

Clinical implications

• Grotesque body changes characteristic of this disorder can cause severe psychological stress. Provide emotional support to help the patient cope with an altered body image.

• To promote maximum joint mobility, perform or assist with range-of-motion exercises.

• Evaluate muscle weakness, especially in the patient with late-stage acromegaly.

• Keep the skin dry. Avoid using an oily lotion, since the skin is already oily.

• Test urine for glucose. Check for signs of hyperglycemia.

• Be aware that a pituitary tumor may cause visual problems. If the patient has hemianopia, stand where he can see you.

• Remember that hyperpituitarism can cause inexplicable mood changes. Reassure the family that these mood changes result from the disease and can be modified with treatment.

• Before surgery, reinforce what the surgeon has told the patient, and try to allay the patient's fear with a clear and honest explanation of the scheduled operation. If the patient is a child, explain to parents that such surgery prevents permanent soft-tissue deformities but will not correct bone changes that have already taken place. Arrange for counseling, if necessary, to help the child and parents cope with these permanent defects.

• After surgery, diligently monitor vital signs and neurologic status.

• Check blood glucose levels often. Remember, HGH levels usually fall rapidly after surgery. Measure intake and output hourly, and report large increases. Transient diabetes insipidus, which sometimes occurs after surgery for hyperpituitarism, can cause such increases in urine output.

• Give good mouth care if the transsphenoidal approach was used. Nasal packing is kept in place for several days, and the patient must breathe through his mouth. (The surgical site is packed with a piece of tissue, generally taken from a midthigh donor site.)

• Watch for cerebrospinal fluid (CSF) leaks from the packed site. Look for increased external nasal drainage or drainage into the nasopharynx. CSF leaks may necessitate additional surgery for repair.

• Before discharge, emphasize the importance of continuing hormone replacement therapy, if ordered.

• Advise the patient to wear a medical identification bracelet at all times and to bring his hormone replacement schedule with him whenever he returns to the hospital.

• Instruct the patient to have follow-up examinations at least once a year for the rest of his life, since a slight chance exists that the tumor that caused his hyperpituitarism may recur.

Complications

Prolonged effects of excessive HGH secretion include bowlegs, barrel chest, arthritis, osteoporosis, kyphosis, hypertension, and arteriosclerosis. Both gigantism and acromegaly may also cause signs of glucose intolerance and clinically apparent diabetes mellitus, because of the insulin-antagonistic character of HGH.

Hypertension

Description

Hypertension, an intermittent or sustained elevation in diastolic or systolic blood pressure, occurs as two major types: essential (primary) hypertension, the most common; and secondary hypertension, which results from renal disease or another identifiable cause. Malignant hypertension is a severe, fulminant form of hypertension common to both types. Hypertension is a major cause of cerebrovascular accident, cardiac disease, and renal failure. Prognosis is good if this disorder is detected early and treatment begins before complications develop. Severely elevated blood pressure (hypertensive crisis) may be fatal (see *Hypertensive Crisis*).

Causes

Essential hypertension

No single cause is identifiable. This condition probably reflects an interaction of multiple homeostatic forces, including changes in renal regulation of sodium and extracellular fluids, in aldosterone secretion and metabolism, and in norepinephrine secretion and metabolism.

Hypertensive Crisis

Hypertensive crisis is an acute, life-threatening rise in blood pressure (diastolic usually over 120 mm Hg). It may develop in hypertensive patients after abrupt discontinuation of antihypertensive medication; increased salt consumption; increased production of renin, epinephrine, and norepinephrine; and added stress. This emergency requires immediate and vigorous treatment to lower blood pressure and thereby prevent cerebrovascular accident, left heart failure, and pulmonary edema.

Hypertensive crisis produces severe and widespread symptoms, including headache, drowsiness, mental clouding, vomiting, focal neurologic signs (such as paresthesias), and, if pulmonary edema is present, shortness of breath and hemoptysis. Treatment to rapidly lower blood pressure and thereby prevent hypertensive encephalopathy may include vasodilators, such as I.V. nitroprusside, hydralazine, or diazoxide; a potent diuretic, such as furosemide; and a sympathetic blocker, such as methyldopa, trimethaphan, or phentolamine.

In the early stages of antihypertensive I.V. therapy, monitor blood pressure and heart rate frequently (as often as every 1 to 3 minutes with some drugs) for a precipitous drop, indicating hypersensitivity to the prescribed medications. Maintain blood pressure level, as ordered.

Keep the patient calm; administer a sedative, as ordered. Record intake and output accurately, and, if necessary, explain the reasons for fluid restriction. Watch closely for hypotension, and, until blood pressure is stable at a desirable level, check for signs of heart failure, such as tachycardia, tachypnea, dyspnea, pulmonary crackles, S_3 or S_4 gallops, neck vein distention, cyanosis, edema, and oliguria.

Teaching Topics in Hypertension

• An explanation of the patient's type of hypertension: primary or secondary
• An explanation of how high blood pressure develops, including significant risk factors
• Normal blood pressure readings
• The importance of adhering to treatment measures to prevent potentially fatal complications, such as myocardial infarction
• Exercise program and precautions
• Dietary restrictions
• Use of antihypertensives, diuretics, and other prescribed medications
• Home blood pressure monitoring, including an explanation of systolic and diastolic pressures
• Other measures to reduce long-term complications, such as controlling weight, quitting smoking, and reducing stress
• Sources of information and support, such as the American Heart Association

Secondary hypertension
—Renal vascular disease
—Pheochromocytoma
—Primary hyperaldosteronism
—Cushing's syndrome
—Dysfunction of the thyroid, pituitary, or parathyroid glands
—Coarctation of the aorta
—Pregnancy
—Neurologic disorders

Risk factors
• Family history
• Race (more common in blacks)
• Stress
• Obesity
• High dietary intake of saturated fats or sodium
• Tobacco use
• Oral contraceptive use
• Sedentary life-style
• Aging

Signs and symptoms
Serial blood pressure measurements of more than 140/90 mm Hg in persons under age 50 or 150/95 mm Hg in persons over age 50 confirm hypertension. Other clinical effects are absent until complications develop from vascular changes.

Diagnostic tests
Patient history and the following ad-

ditional tests may show predisposing factors and help identify an underlying cause, such as renal disease:
• Urinalysis: Protein, RBCs, and WBCs may indicate glomerulonephritis.
• Intravenous pyelography: Renal atrophy indicates chronic renal disease; one kidney more than 5/8″ (1.5 cm) shorter than the other suggests unilateral renal disease.
• Serum potassium: Levels less than 3.5 mEq/liter may indicate adrenal dysfunction (primary hyperaldosteronism).
• BUN and creatinine: BUN normal or elevated to more than 20 mg/dl and creatinine normal or elevated to more than 1.5 mg/dl suggest renal disease.
Other tests help detect cardiovascular damage and other complications:
• EKG may show left ventricular hypertrophy or ischemia.
• Chest X-ray may show cardiomegaly.

Treatment
Although essential hypertension has no cure, drugs and modifications in diet and life-style can control it. Drug therapy usually begins with a diuretic alone. Beta-adrenergic blockers, other sympathetic blockers, or vasodilators may be added, as needed. Therapy may

also include angiotensin-converting enzyme and calcium channel blockers. Life-style and dietary changes may include weight loss, relaxation techniques, regular exercise, and restriction of sodium and saturated fat intake.

Treatment of secondary hypertension includes correcting the underlying cause and controlling hypertensive effects.

Clinical implications

• To encourage compliance with antihypertensive therapy, suggest that the patient establish a daily routine for taking medication. Warn that uncontrolled hypertension may cause stroke and heart attack. Tell him to report drug side effects. Also, advise him to avoid high-sodium antacids and over-the-counter cold and sinus medications, which contain harmful vasoconstrictors.

• Encourage a change in dietary habits. Help the obese patient plan a reducing diet; tell him to avoid high-sodium foods (pickles, potato chips, canned soups, cold cuts) and table salt.

• Help the patient examine and modify his life-style (for example, by reducing stress and exercising regularly).

• If a patient is hospitalized with hypertension, find out if he was taking prescribed medication. If not, ask why. If the patient cannot afford the medication, refer him to an appropriate social service agency. Tell the patient and family to keep a record of drugs used in the past, noting especially which ones were or were not effective. Suggest recording this information on a card so that the patient can show it to his physician.

• To help identify hypertension and prevent untreated hypertension, participate in public education programs dealing with hypertension and ways to reduce risk factors. Encourage public participation in blood pressure screening programs. Routinely screen all patients, especially those at risk (blacks and persons with family histories of hypertension, stroke, or heart attack).

(See *Teaching Topics in Hypertension*.)

Complications

• Brain: cerebrovascular accident
• Retina: blindness
• Heart: myocardial infarction and congestive heart failure
• Kidneys: proteinuria, edema, and eventually, renal failure

Hyperthyroidism
(Graves' disease, Basedow's disease, Parry's disease, thyrotoxicosis)

Description

Hyperthyroidism is a metabolic imbalance that results from thyroid hormone overproduction. The most common form of hyperthyroidism is Graves' disease, which increases thyroxine production, enlarges the thyroid gland (goiter), and causes multisystem changes. With treatment, most patients can lead normal lives. However, thyroid storm—an acute exacerbation of hyperthyroidism—is a medical emergency that may lead to cardiac, hepatic, or renal failure. (See *Other Forms of Hyperthyroidism*, p. 380.)

Cause

The cause of Graves' disease is unknown, but the disease is familial. It may be autoimmune. Antibodies to thyroglobulin or to thyroid microsomes are found in most patients with this disorder.

Signs and symptoms

Classic symptoms of Graves' disease include enlarged thyroid (goiter), nervousness, heat intolerance, weight loss despite increased appetite, sweating, diarrhea, tremor, palpitations, and possibly exophthalmos. (In thyroid storm, these symptoms can be accompanied by extreme irritability, hypertension, tachycardia, vomiting, temperature up to 106° F. [41.1° C.],

Other Forms of Hyperthyroidism

• *Toxic adenoma*—a small, benign nodule in the thyroid gland that secretes thyroid hormone—is the second most common cause of hyperthyroidism. The cause of toxic adenoma is unknown; incidence is highest in the elderly. Clinical effects are essentially similar to those of Graves' disease, except that toxic adenoma does not induce ophthalmopathy, pretibial myxedema, or acropachy. Presence of adenoma is confirmed by radioactive iodine (^{131}I) uptake and thyroid scan, which show a single hyperfunctioning nodule suppressing the rest of the gland. Treatment includes ^{131}I therapy or surgery to remove adenoma after antithyroid drugs achieve a euthyroid state.

• *Thyrotoxicosis factitia* results from chronic ingestion of thyroid hormone for thyrotropin suppression in patients with thyroid carcinoma, or from thyroid hormone abuse by persons who are trying to lose weight.

• *Functioning metastatic thyroid carcinoma* is a rare disease that causes excess production of thyroid hormone.

• *TSH-secreting pituitary tumor* causes overproduction of thyroid hormone.

• *Subacute thyroiditis* is a virus-induced granulomatous inflammation of the thyroid, producing transient hyperthyroidism associated with fever, pain, pharyngitis, and tenderness in the thyroid gland.

• *Silent thyroiditis* is a self-limiting, transient form of hyperthyroidism, with histologic thyroiditis but no inflammatory symptoms.

delirium, and coma.) Other symptoms include the following:

Central nervous system

Difficulty in concentrating, excitability or nervousness, fine tremor, shaky handwriting, clumsiness, and mood swings, ranging from occasional outbursts to overt psychosis

Skin, hair, and nails

Smooth, warm, flushed skin; fine, soft hair; premature graying and increased hair loss in both sexes; friable nails and onycholysis (distal nail separated from the bed); pretibial myxedema (dermopathy), producing thickened skin, accentuated hair follicles, raised red patches of skin that are itchy and sometimes painful, with occasional nodule formation

Cardiovascular system

Tachycardia; full, bounding pulse; wide pulse pressure; cardiomegaly; increased cardiac output and blood volume; visible point of maximal impulse; paroxysmal supraventricular tachycardia and atrial fibrillation (especially in the elderly); occasionally, systolic murmur at the left sternal border

Respiratory system

Dyspnea on exertion and at rest

Gastrointestinal system

Possible anorexia; nausea and vomiting; increased defecation; soft stools or, with severe disease, diarrhea; liver enlargement

Musculoskeletal system

Weakness, fatigue, and muscle atrophy; generalized or localized paralysis associated with hypokalemia; occasional acropachy—soft-tissue swelling, accompanied by underlying bone changes where new bone formation occurs

Reproductive system

In females, oligomenorrhea or amenorrhea, decreased fertility, higher incidence of spontaneous abortions; in males, gynecomastia; in both sexes, diminished libido

Eyes

Exophthalmos; occasional inflammation of conjunctivae, corneas, or eye muscles; diplopia; increased tearing

Diagnostic tests

• Radioimmunoassay showing increased serum triiodothyronine (T_3) and thyroxine (T_4) concentrations confirms the diagnosis. (This test is contraindicated if the patient is pregnant.)
• Thyroid scan reveals increased uptake of [131]I.
• Thyroid-releasing hormone (TRH) stimulation test indicates hyperthyroidism if thyroid-stimulating hormone (TSH) level fails to rise within 30 minutes after administration of TRH.
• Basal metabolic rate is elevated in hyperthyroidism, but this test has largely been superseded by the more reliable and efficient measurements of T_3 and T_4.
• Serum protein-bound iodine level is increased.
• Serum cholesterol and total lipid levels are decreased.
• Ultrasonography confirms subclinical ophthalmopathy.

Treatment

The primary forms of treatment for hyperthyroidism are antithyroid drugs, ^{131}I, and surgery. Appropriate treatment depends on the size of the goiter, the causes, the patient's age and parity, and how long surgery will be delayed (if it is planned).

Antithyroid drug therapy is used for children, young adults, pregnant women, and patients who refuse surgery or ^{131}I treatment. Thyroid hormone antagonists include propylthiouracil (PTU) and methimazole, which block thyroid hormone synthesis.

During pregnancy, antithyroid medication should be kept at the minimum dosage required to keep maternal thyroid function normal until delivery and to minimize the risk of fetal hypothyroidism—even though most infants of hyperthyroid mothers are born with mild and transient hyperthyroidism.

Another major form of therapy for hyperthyroidism is a single P.O. dose of [131]I—the treatment of choice for patients not planning to have children.

(Patients of reproductive age must give informed consent for this treatment, since small amounts of ^{131}I concentrate in the gonads.)

Subtotal (partial) thyroidectomy is indicated for the patient younger than age 40 who has a very large goiter and whose hyperthyroidism has repeatedly relapsed after drug therapy. Thyroidectomy removes part of the thyroid gland, thus decreasing its size and capacity for hormone production. Preoperatively, the patient may receive iodides (Lugol's solution or saturated solution of potassium iodide), antithyroid drugs, or high doses of propranolol, to help prevent thyroid storm. If euthyroidism is not achieved, surgery should be delayed and propranolol administered to decrease the systemic effects (cardiac dysrhythmias) caused by hyperthyroidism.

After ablative treatment with ^{131}I or surgery, patients require regular, frequent medical supervision for the rest of their lives, because they usually develop hypothyroidism, sometimes several years after treatment.

Therapy for hyperthyroid ophthalmopathy includes local applications of topical medications but may require high doses of corticosteroids, given systemically or, in severe cases, injected into the retrobulbar area. A patient with severe exophthalmos that causes pressure on the optic nerve may require surgical decompression to lessen pressure on the orbital contents.

Treatment of thyroid storm includes administration of an antithyroid drug such as PTU, propranolol I.V. to block sympathetic effects, a corticosteroid to inhibit the conversion of T_4 to T_3 and to replace depleted cortisol levels, and an iodide to block release of thyroid hormone. Supportive measures include nutrients, vitamins, fluid administration, and sedation, as necessary.

Clinical implications

Patients with hyperthyroidism require vigilant care to prevent acute exacer-

bations and complications.
• Record vital signs and weight. Monitor serum electrolytes, and check periodically for hyperglycemia and glycosuria. Carefully monitor cardiac function. Check level of consciousness and urinary output. If the patient is pregnant, tell her to watch closely during the first trimester for signs of spontaneous abortion (spotting, occasional mild cramps) and to report such signs to the physician immediately.
• Remember, extreme nervousness may produce bizarre behavior. Reassure the patient and family that such behavior subsides with treatment. Provide sedatives, as necessary.
• To promote weight gain, provide a balanced diet, with six meals a day. If the patient has edema, suggest a low-sodium diet.
• If iodine is part of the treatment, mix it with milk to prevent gastrointestinal distress, and administer it through a straw to prevent tooth discoloration.
• Watch for signs of thyroid storm. Check intake and output carefully to ensure adequate hydration and fluid balance. Closely monitor blood pressure, cardiac rate and rhythm, and temperature. If the patient has a high fever, reduce it with appropriate hypothermic measures (sponging, hypothermia blankets, and acetaminophen); avoid aspirin because it raises

thyroxine levels. Maintain an I.V. line and give drugs, as ordered.
• If the patient has exophthalmos or another ophthalmopathy, suggest sunglasses or eyepatches to protect his eyes from light. Moisten the conjunctivae often with isotonic eyedrops. Warn the patient with severe lid retraction to avoid sudden physical movements that might cause the lid to slip behind the eyeball.
  Thyroidectomy necessitates meticulous postoperative care to prevent complications:
• Check often for respiratory distress, and keep a tracheotomy tray at bedside.
• Watch for evidence of hemorrhage into the neck, such as a tight dressing with no blood on it. Change dressings and perform wound care, as ordered; check the *back* of the dressing for drainage. Keep the patient in semi-Fowler's position, and support his head and neck with sandbags to ease tension on the incision.
• Check for dysphagia or hoarseness from possible laryngeal nerve injury.
• Watch for signs of hypoparathyroidism (tetany, numbness), a complication that results from accidental removal of the parathyroid glands during surgery.
• Stress the importance of regular medical follow-up after discharge, since hypothyroidism may develop

---

Teaching Topics in Graves' Disease

• Pathophysiology of Graves' disease, including how excessive levels of thyroid hormone occur
• Complications, such as thyroid storm
• Blood tests and X-rays necessary to evaluate thyroid function
• Dietary measures to ensure sufficient caloric intake
• Activity restrictions to help counteract increased metabolism
• Relationship of stress to hormonal balance
• Medications and their administration
• Radioactive iodine therapy, if indicated
• Subtotal thyroidectomy, if indicated, and possible need for lifelong hormonal replacement therapy
• Eye care, if exophthalmos or visual changes occur

from 2 to 4 weeks postoperatively.

Drug therapy and ^{131}I therapy require careful monitoring and comprehensive patient teaching. (See *Teaching Topics in Graves' Disease*.)

Hypervitaminoses A and D

Description
Hypervitaminosis A is excessive accumulation of vitamin A; hypervitaminosis D, of vitamin D. Vitamins A and D are fat-soluble vitamins that accumulate in the body because they are not dissolved and excreted in the urine. A single dose of more than 1 million units of vitamin A can cause acute toxicity. Daily doses of 15,000 to 25,000 units taken over weeks or months have proven toxic in infants and children. For the same dose to produce toxicity in adults, ingestion over years is necessary. Ingestion of only 1,600 to 2,000 units of vitamin D is sufficient to cause toxicity.

These conditions usually respond well to treatment. They are most prevalent in infants and children, usually as a result of accidental or misguided overdosage by parents. A related, benign condition called hypercarotenemia results from excessive consumption of carotene, a chemical precursor of vitamin A.

Cause
Ingestion of excessive amounts of supplemental vitamin preparations

Signs and symptoms
Hypervitaminosis A
—Anorexia
—Irritability
—Headache
—Hair loss
—Malaise
—Itching
—Vertigo
—Bone pain
—Bone fragility
—Dry, peeling skin
—Possible hepatosplenomegaly and emotional lability
—Vomiting and transient hydrocephalus in acute toxicity
—Yellow or orange skin coloration with hypercarotenemia
Hypervitaminosis D
—Anorexia
—Headache
—Nausea
—Vomiting
—Weight loss
—Polyuria
—Polydipsia
—Hypercalcemia, with calcifications of soft tissues, and lethargy, confusion, and coma, if severe

Diagnostic tests
• Elevated serum vitamin A level (over 90 mcg/dl) confirms diagnosis of hypervitaminosis A.
• Increased serum carotene level (over 250 mcg/dl) confirms hypercarotenemia.
• Increased serum vitamin D level confirms hypervitaminosis D.
• Increased serum calcium level may suggest hypervitaminosis D.
• X-rays showing calcifications of tendons, ligaments, and subperiosteal tissues (in children) support a diagnosis of hypervitaminosis D.

Treatment
Withholding vitamin supplements usually corrects hypervitaminosis A quickly and hypervitaminosis D gradually. Hypercalcemia may persist for weeks or months after the patient stops taking vitamin D. Treatment for severe hypervitaminosis D may include glucocorticoids to control hypercalcemia and prevent renal damage. In the acute stage, diuretics or other emergency measures for severe hypercalcemia may be necessary. Hypercarotenemia responds well to dietary exclusion of foods high in carotene.

Clinical implications
• Keep the patient comfortable, and reassure him that symptoms will sub-

side after he stops taking the vitamin.
• Make sure the patient or the parents of a child with these conditions understand that vitamins are not innocuous. Explain the hazards associated with excessive vitamin intake. Point out that vitamin A and D requirements can easily be met with a diet containing dark green leafy vegetables, fruits, and fortified milk or milk products.
• To prevent hypervitaminosis A or D, monitor serum vitamin A levels in patients receiving doses above the recommended daily dietary allowance and serum calcium levels in patients receiving pharmacologic doses of vitamin D.

Hypochondriasis
(Hypochondriacal neurosis)

Description
The dominant feature of hypochondriasis is an unrealistic misinterpretation of the severity and significance of physical signs or sensations as abnormal. This leads to preoccupation with fear of having a serious disease, which persists despite medical reassurance to the contrary. Hypochondriasis allows the patient to assume a dependent sick role to ensure his needs are met. Such a patient is unaware of these unmet needs and is not consciously causing his symptoms. Hypochondriasis causes severe social and occupational impairment. It is not caused by other mental disorders, such as schizophrenia, affective disorder, or somatization disorder.

Hypochondriasis involves the danger of overlooking a serious organic disease, given the patient's previously unfounded complaints. It also has potential for significant complications or disabilities resulting from multiple evaluations, tests, and invasive procedures.

Cause
Hypochondriasis is not linked to any specific cause; however, it commonly develops in persons or relatives of those who have experienced an organic disease.

Signs and symptoms
The dominant feature of hypochondriasis is the misinterpretation of symptoms—usually multiple complaints that involve a single organ system—as signs of serious illness; however, as medical evaluation proceeds, complaints may shift and change. Symptoms can range from very specific to general, vague complaints and often reflect a preoccupation with normal body functions.

Diagnostic tests
• Projective psychological testing may show a preoccupation with somatic concerns; however, a complete history, including emphasis on current psychological stresses, is the most useful diagnostic tool.
• Various diagnostic tests may be performed to rule out underlying organic disease, but invasive procedures should be kept to a minimum.

Treatment
The goal of treatment is to help the patient continue to lead a productive life despite distressing symptoms and fears. After medical evaluation is complete, the patient should be told clearly that he does not have a serious disease, but that continued medical follow-up will help control his symptoms. Providing a diagnosis will not make hypochondriasis disappear, but it may ease some anxiety.

Regular outpatient follow-up can help the patient deal with his symptoms and is necessary to detect organic illness. As many as 30% of these patients later develop an organic disease. Unfortunately, because the patient can be quite demanding and irritating, consistent follow-up is often difficult. Typically, these patients do not acknowledge any psychological influence on their symptoms and resist psychiatric treatment.

Clinical implications
Provide a supportive relationship that lets the patient feel cared for and understood. The patient with hypochondriasis feels real pain and distress; do not deny his symptoms or challenge his behavior.
• Help the patient and family find new ways to deal with stress other than development of physical symptoms.
• If the patient is receiving a tranquilizer, both he and his family should know dosages, expected effects, and possible side effects (for example, drowsiness, fatigue, blurred vision, and hypotension).
• Warn the patient who is taking tranquilizers to avoid alcohol or other central nervous system depressants, since they may potentiate tranquilizer action. Warn him to take the drug only as prescribed, since larger or more frequent doses may lead to dependence; to avoid hazardous tasks until he has developed a tolerance to the tranquilizer's sedative effects; and to continue the tranquilizer as his doctor directs, since abrupt withdrawal may be hazardous.
• Recognize that the patient will never be symptom-free, and do not become angry when he will not give up his disease. Such anger can drive the patient away to yet another unnecessary medical evaluation.

Hypoglycemia

Description
Hypoglycemia is an abnormally low glucose level in the bloodstream. It occurs when glucose is used too rapidly, when the glucose release rate falls behind tissue demands, or when excessive insulin enters the bloodstream. Hypoglycemia is classified as reactive or fasting. Reactive hypoglycemia results from the reaction to the disposition of meals or the administration of excessive insulin. Fasting hypoglycemia causes discomfort during long periods of abstinence from food—for example, in the early morning hours before breakfast. Although hypoglycemia is a specific endocrine imbalance, its symptoms are often vague and depend on how quickly the patient's glucose levels drop. If not corrected, severe hypoglycemia may result in coma and irreversible brain damage.

Causes
Reactive hypoglycemia
—Too much insulin or oral hypoglycemic medication in diabetic patients
—Idiopathic
—Rapid small-intestine glucose absorption caused by gastrectomy or other GI procedures
—Impaired glucose tolerance, with early hyperglycemia followed by a delayed rise in insulin levels
Fasting hypoglycemia
—Exogenous factors, such as alcohol or drug ingestion
—Endogenous factors caused by organ damage, such as pancreatic tumor, hepatic disease, or renal disease

Signs and symptoms
• Hunger
• Weakness
• Cold sweats
• Shakiness
• Trembling
• Headache
• Irritability
• Tachycardia
• Pallor
• Possible blurred vision, confusion, motor weakness, hemiplegia, convulsions, or coma

Diagnostic tests
• A 5-hour glucose tolerance test may be administered to provoke reactive hypoglycemia. Laboratory testing to detect plasma insulin and plasma glu-

---

Teaching Topics in Hypoglycemia

- An explanation of the patient's type of hypoglycemia: fasting or reactive
- Emergency treatment of a hypoglycemic episode
- Symptoms of hypoglycemia and hyperglycemia
- Preparation for diagnostic tests to help distinguish between fasting and reactive hypoglycemia, such as a fasting plasma glucose test
- Dietary modifications to prevent alterations in blood glucose levels
- Weight reduction, if necessary
- Medications and their administration
- Surgery, if necessary
- Prevention of hypoglycemic episodes

---

cose levels may identify fasting hypoglycemia after a 12-hour fast.

- Dextrostix or Chemstrips provide quick screening methods for determining blood glucose level. A color change that corresponds to < 45 mg/dl indicates the need for a venous blood sample.
- Laboratory testing confirms diagnosis by showing decreased blood glucose values. The following values indicate hypoglycemia:

Full-term infants:
< 30 mg/dl before feeding
< 40 mg/dl after feeding
Pre-term infants:
< 20 mg/dl before feeding
< 30 mg/dl after feeding
Children and adults:
< 40 mg/dl before meal
< 50 mg/dl after meal

Treatment

For acute hypoglycemia, the first priority is to bring the patient's glucose level back to normal. If the patient is unconscious, an I.V. bolus of 50 ml of 50% dextrose is usually administered first. If the patient is conscious, a fast-acting carbohydrate, such as sweetened orange juice, non-diet soda, or candy, is administered.

When the patient's condition improves, in about 15 to 20 minutes, a snack should be given to prevent another hypoglycemic episode. Typically, the snack is a combination of a complex carbohydrate and protein,

such as peanut butter crackers. Effective long-term treatment of reactive hypoglycemia requires dietary modification to help delay glucose absorption and gastric emptying. Usually, this includes small, frequent meals; ingestion of complex carbohydrates, fiber, and fat; and avoidance of simple sugars, alcohol, and fruit drinks. The patient may also receive anticholinergic drugs to slow gastric emptying and intestinal motility and to inhibit vagal stimulation of insulin release.

For fasting hypoglycemia, surgery and drug therapy are usually required. In patients with insulinoma, removal of the tumor is the treatment of choice. Drug therapy may include nondiuretic thiazides, such as diazoxide, to inhibit insulin secretion; streptozocin; and hormones, such as glucocorticoids and long-acting glycogen.

Therapy for newborn infants who have hypoglycemia or risk developing it includes preventive measures. A hypertonic solution of 10% to 25% dextrose, calculated at 2 to 4 ml/kg of body weight and administered I.V., should correct a severe hypoglycemic state in newborns. To reduce the chance of hypoglycemia developing in high-risk infants, such infants should receive feedings—either breast milk or a solution of 5% to 10% glucose and water—as soon after birth as possible.

Clinical implications
• Watch for and report signs of hypoglycemia (such as poor feeding) in high-risk infants.
• Monitor infusion of hypertonic glucose in the newborn to avoid hyperglycemia, circulatory overload, and cellular dehydration. Terminate glucose solutions gradually to prevent hypoglycemia caused by hyperinsulinemia.
• Explain the purpose and procedure for any diagnostic tests. Collect blood samples at the appropriate times, as ordered.
• Monitor the effects of drug therapy, and watch for the development of any side effects.
• Teach the patient which foods to include in his diet (complex carbohydrates, fiber, fat) and which foods to avoid (simple sugars, alcohol). Refer the patient and family for dietary counseling, as appropriate. (See *Teaching Topics in Hypoglycemia*.)

Hypoparathyroidism

Description
Hypoparathyroidism is a deficiency of parathyroid hormone (PTH). Since the parathyroid glands primarily regulate calcium balance, hypoparathyroidism causes hypocalcemia, producing neuromuscular symptoms ranging from paresthesia to tetany. The clinical effects of hypoparathyroidism are usually correctable with replacement therapy. However, some complications of this disorder, such as cataracts and basal ganglion calcifications, are irreversible.

Causes
• Congenital absence or malfunction of the parathyroid glands
• Removal of or injury to one or more parathyroid glands during neck surgery or, rarely, from massive thyroid irradiation
• Ischemic infarction of the parathyroids during surgery or from disease, such as amyloidosis or neoplasms
• Suppression of normal gland function caused by hypercalcemia (reversible)
• Hypomagnesemia-induced impairment of hormone synthesis (reversible)

Signs and symptoms
• May be asymptomatic in mild cases
• Neuromuscular irritability
• Increased deep tendon reflexes
• Hyperirritability of the facial nerve (characteristic spasm when it is tapped [Chvostek's sign])
• Dysphagia
• Psychosis
• Mental deficiency in children
• Tetany
• Seizures
• Abdominal pain
• Dry, lusterless hair
• Spontaneous hair loss
• Brittle fingernails that develop ridges or fall out
• Dry, scaly skin
• Weakened tooth enamel, which causes teeth to stain, crack, and decay easily
• Dysrhythmias

Diagnostic tests
The following test results confirm the presence of hypoparathyroidism:
• Radioimmunoassay for parathyroid hormone: decreased PTH concentration
• Serum calcium: decreased level
• Serum phosphorus: increased level (more than 5.4 ml/dl)
• X-rays: increased bone density
• EKG: increased QT and ST intervals caused by hypocalcemia.

In addition, inflating a blood pressure cuff on the upper arm in excess of systolic blood pressure elicits Trousseau's sign (carpal spasm), providing clinical evidence of hypoparathyroidism.

Treatment

Treatment initially includes vitamin D, with or without supplemental calcium. Such therapy is usually lifelong, except in patients with the reversible form of the disease. If the patient cannot tolerate the pure form of vitamin D, alternatives include dihydrotachysterol, if renal function is adequate, and calcitriol, if renal function is severely compromised.

Acute life-threatening tetany calls for immediate I.V. administration of calcium gluconate to raise serum calcium levels. If the patient is awake and able to cooperate, he can help raise ionized serum calcium levels by breathing into a paper bag and then inhaling his own carbon dioxide; this produces hypoventilation and mild respiratory acidosis. Sedatives and anticonvulsants may control spasms until calcium levels rise. Chronic tetany calls for maintenance of serum calcium levels with oral calcium supplements.

Clinical implications

• While awaiting diagnosis of hypoparathyroidism in a patient with a history of tetany, maintain a patent I.V. line and keep calcium gluconate solution available. Because the patient is vulnerable to convulsions, observe seizure precautions. Also, keep a tracheotomy tray and an endotracheal tube at bedside, since laryngospasm may result from hypocalcemia.

• For the patient with tetany, administer 10% calcium gluconate by slow I.V. infusion (1 mg/minute), and maintain a patent airway. The patient may also require intubation and sedation with diazepam I.V. Monitor vital signs often after I.V. administration of diazepam to make certain blood pressure and heart rate return to normal.

• Advise the patient to follow a high-calcium, low-phosphorus diet, and tell him which foods are permitted.

• When caring for the patient with chronic disease, particularly a child, stay alert for minor muscle twitching (especially in the hands) and for signs of laryngospasm (respiratory stridor or dysphagia), since these effects may signal onset of tetany.

• For the patient on drug therapy, emphasize the importance of checking serum calcium levels at least three times a year. Instruct the patient to watch for signs of hypercalcemia and to keep medications away from light.

• Because the patient with chronic disease has prolonged QT intervals on EKG, watch for heart block and signs of decreasing cardiac output. Closely monitor the patient receiving both digitalis and calcium, since calcium potentiates the effect of digitalis. Stay alert for signs of digitalis toxicity (dysrhythmias, nausea, fatigue, visual changes).

• Instruct the patient with scaly skin to use creams to soften his skin. Also, tell him to keep his nails trimmed to prevent them from splitting.

Hypopituitarism
(Panhypopituitarism and dwarfism)

Description

Hypopituitarism is a complex syndrome marked by metabolic dysfunction, sexual immaturity, and growth retardation (when it occurs in childhood), resulting from a deficiency of the hormones secreted by the anterior pituitary gland. However, clinical manifestations do not become apparent until 75% of the gland is destroyed. Panhypopituitarism refers to a generalized condition caused by partial or total failure of all six of this gland's vital hormones—adrenocorticotropic hormone (ACTH), thyroid-stimulating hormone (TSH), luteinizing hormone (LH), follicle-stimulating hormone (FSH), human growth hormone (HGH), and prolactin. Prognosis may be good with adequate replacement therapy and correction of the underlying causes.

Causes
Primary hypopituitarism
—Tumor (most common)
—Congenital defects (hypoplasia or aplasia of the pituitary gland)
—Pituitary infarction (most often from postpartum hemorrhage)
—Partial or total hypophysectomy by surgery, irradiation, or chemical agents
—Rarely, granulomatous disease (tuberculosis, for example)
—Occasionally, no identifiable cause
Secondary hypopituitarism
—Deficiency of releasing hormones produced by the hypothalamus (either idiopathic or a possible result of infection, trauma, or tumor)

Signs and symptoms
Clinical features of hypopituitarism usually develop slowly and vary greatly with the severity of the disorder.
Adults
—Amenorrhea
—Impotence
—Infertility
—Decreased libido
—Tiredness
—Lethargy
—Sensitivity to cold
—Menstrual disturbances
—Hypoglycemia
—Anorexia
—Nausea
—Abdominal pain
—Hypotension
—Failure of lactation, menstruation, and growth of pubic and axillary hair with postpartum necrosis
Children
—Growth retardation
—Absence of secondary sexual characteristics during puberty

Diagnostic tests
• Radioimmunoassay showing decreased plasma levels of some or all pituitary hormones (except ACTH, which requires more sophisticated testing), accompanied by end-organ hypofunction, suggests pituitary failure and eliminates target gland disease.
• Failure of thyrotropin-releasing hormone administration to increase TSH or prolactin concentrations rules out hypothalamic dysfunction as the cause of hormonal deficiency.
• Provocative tests: To pinpoint the source of low hydroxycorticosteroid levels, P.O. administration of metyrapone blocks cortisol synthesis, which should stimulate pituitary secretion of ACTH. Insulin-induced hypoglycemia also stimulates ACTH secretion. Persistently low levels of ACTH indicate pituitary or hypothalamic failure. (These tests require careful medical supervision, because they may precipitate an adrenal crisis.)
• Persistently low HGH levels, despite provocative testing, confirm HGH deficiency. Testing includes administration of regular insulin (inducing hypoglycemia) or levodopa (causing hypotension). These drugs should provoke increased secretion of growth hormone.
• CT scan, pneumoencephalography, or cerebral angiography confirms the presence of intrasellar or extrasellar tumors.

Treatment
Replacement of hormones secreted by the target glands is the most effective treatment for hypopituitarism and panhypopituitarism. Hormonal replacement includes cortisol, thyroxine, and androgen or cyclic estrogen. Prolactin need not be replaced. The patient of reproductive age may benefit from administration of FSH and human chorionic gonadotropin to boost fertility.

HGH, obtained from cadaver pituitaries, is effective for treating dwarfism and stimulates growth increases as great as 4″ to 6″ (10 to 15 cm) in the first year of treatment. Growth rate tapers off in later years. After pubertal changes have occurred, the effects of HGH therapy are limited. (The National Pituitary Agency, which supplies HGH, currently withdraws treatment after the patient attains a height of 5' [152 cm].) Occasionally, a child becomes unresponsive to HGH therapy, even with larger doses, perhaps because of antibody formation against the hormone. In such patients, small doses of an androgen may again stimulate growth, but extreme caution is necessary to prevent premature closure of the epiphyses. Children with hypopituitarism may also need replacement of adrenal and thyroid hormones and, as they approach puberty, sex hormones.

Clinical implications
• Keep track of the results of all laboratory tests for hormonal deficiencies, and know what they mean. Until replacement therapy is complete, check for signs of thyroid deficiency (increasing lethargy), adrenal deficiency (weakness, orthostatic hypotension, hypoglycemia, fatigue, and weight loss), and gonadotropin deficiency (decreased libido, lethargy, and apathy).
• Record temperature, blood pressure, and heart rate every 4 to 8 hours. Check eyelids, nailbeds, and skin for pallor, which indicates anemia, a problem of panhypopituitarism.
• Prevent infection by giving meticulous skin care. Since the patient's skin is probably dry, use oil or lotion instead of soap. If body temperature is low, provide additional clothing and covers, as needed, to keep the patient warm.
• Darken the room if the patient has a tumor that is causing headaches and visual disturbances. Help with any activity that requires good vision, such as reading the menu.
• During insulin testing, monitor closely for signs of hypoglycemia (initially, slow cerebration, tachycardia, and nervousness, progressing to convulsions). Keep dextrose 50% in water available for I.V. administration to correct hypoglycemia rapidly.
• To prevent postural hypotension, be sure to keep the patient supine during levodopa testing.

• Instruct the patient to wear a medical identification bracelet. Teach him to administer steroids parenterally in case of an emergency.
• Refer the family of a child with dwarfism to appropriate community resources for psychological counseling, since the emotional stress caused by this disorder increases as the child becomes more aware of his condition.

Hypothyroidism in adults

Description
Hypothyroidism, a state of low serum thyroid hormone, results from hypothalamic, pituitary, or thyroid insufficiency. The disorder can progress to life-threatening myxedema coma—usually precipitated by infection, exposure to cold, or sedatives. Hypothyroidism is most prevalent in women.

Causes
• Thyroidectomy
• Irradiation therapy
• Inflammation
• Chronic, autoimmune thyroiditis (Hashimoto's disease)
• Inflammatory conditions, such as amyloidosis and sarcoidosis
• Pituitary failure to produce thyroid-stimulating hormone (TSH)
• Hypothalamic failure to produce thyrotropin-releasing hormone (TRH)
• Inborn errors of thyroid hormone synthesis
• Inability to synthesize thyroid hormone because of iodine deficiency (usually dietary)
• Use of antithyroid medications, such as propylthiouracil

Signs and symptoms
• Fatigue
• Forgetfulness
• Sensitivity to cold
• Unexplained weight gain
• Constipation

- Decreasing mental stability
- Dry, flaky, inelastic skin
- Puffy face, hands, and feet
- Periorbital edema
- Dry, sparse hair
- Thick, brittle nails
- Slow pulse rate
- Anorexia
- Abdominal distention
- Menorrhagia
- Decreased libido
- Infertility
- Ataxia
- Intention tremor
- Nystagmus
- Delayed reflex relaxation time (especially in the Achilles tendon)

Note: Clinical effects of myxedema coma include progressive stupor, hypoventilation, hypoglycemia, hyponatremia, hypotension, and hypothermia.

Diagnostic tests

- Radioimmunoassay showing low triiodothyronine (T_3) and thyroxine (T_4) levels confirms hypothyroidism.
- TSH level is increased in hypothyroidism because of thyroid insufficiency. TRH level is decreased because of hypothalamic or pituitary insufficiency.
- Serum cholesterol, carotene, alkaline phosphatase, and triglyceride levels are increased.

Note: In myxedema coma, laboratory tests may also show low serum sodium, and decreased pH and increased PCO_2 in arterial blood gases, indicating respiratory acidosis.

Treatment

Therapy for hypothyroidism consists of gradual thyroid replacement with levothyroxine (T_4), liothyronine (T_3), liotrix, or thyroid USP (desiccated). During myxedema coma, effective treatment supports vital functions while restoring euthyroidism. To support blood pressure and pulse rate, treatment includes I.V. administration of levothyroxine and hydrocortisone to correct possible pituitary or adrenal insufficiency. Hypoventilation necessitates oxygenation and vigorous respiratory support. Other supportive measures include careful fluid replacement and antibiotics for infection.

Clinical implications

To manage the hypothyroid patient, follow these guidelines:

- Provide a high-bulk, low-calorie diet and encourage activity. Administer cathartics and stool softeners, as needed.
- After thyroid replacement therapy begins, watch for symptoms of hyperthyroidism, such as restlessness, sweating, and excessive weight loss.
- Tell the patient to report any signs of aggravated cardiovascular disease, such as chest pain and tachycardia.
- To prevent myxedema coma, tell the patient to continue his course of antithyroid medication even if his symptoms subside. Warn the patient to report infection immediately and to make sure any doctor who prescribes drugs for him knows about the underlying hypothyroidism.

To manage the patient in myxedema coma, follow these guidelines for supportive care:

- Check frequently for signs of decreasing cardiac output, such as decreasing urinary output.
- Monitor temperature until stable. Provide extra blankets and clothing and a warm room to compensate for hypothermia. Rapid rewarming may cause vasodilation and vascular collapse.
- Record intake and output and daily weight. As treatment begins, urinary output should increase and body weight decrease; if not, report this immediately.
- Turn the edematous patient every 2 hours, and provide skin care, particularly around bony prominences, at least once a shift.
- Maintain a patent I.V. line. Monitor serum electrolyte levels carefully when administering I.V. fluids.

• Monitor vital signs carefully when administering T_4, since rapid correction of hypothyroidism can cause adverse cardiac effects. Report tachycardia immediately. Watch for hypertension and congestive heart failure in the elderly patient.

• Check arterial blood gas measurements for indications of hypoxia and respiratory acidosis to determine whether the patient needs ventilatory assistance.

• Since myxedema coma may have been precipitated by an infection, check possible sources of infection, such as blood or urine, and obtain sputum cultures.

Hypothyroidism in children
(Cretinism)

Description

Deficiency of thyroid hormone secretion during fetal development or early infancy results in infantile cretinism (congenital hypothyroidism). Early diagnosis and treatment allow the best prognosis. Infants treated before age 3 months usually grow and develop normally. Athyroid children who remain untreated beyond age 3 months and children with acquired hypothyroidism who remain untreated beyond age 2 suffer irreversible mental retardation. Their skeletal abnormalities are reversible with treatment.

Causes
Infants
—Congenital absence or underdevelopment of the thyroid gland
—Inherited enzymatic defect in the synthesis of thyroxine (T_4)
—Antithyroid drugs taken during pregnancy
Children older than age 2
—Chronic autoimmune thyroiditis

Signs and symptoms
Infants
—Excessive sleeping
—Hoarse crying
—General inactivity
—Abnormal deep tendon reflexes
—Hypotonic abdominal muscles
—Slow, awkward movements
—Constipation
—Jaundice
—Loud, noisy breathing
—Possible dyspnea and abnormal facial features
—Cold skin
—Slow pulse
Children older than age 2
—Short stature
—Obesity
—Abnormally large head
—Mental retardation, if untreated
—Delayed or accelerated sexual development in older children

Diagnostic tests

• Elevated level of serum thyroid-stimulating hormone (TSH), associated with low triiodothyronine (T_3) and T_4 levels, points to cretinism.

• Thyroid scan (^{131}I uptake test) shows decreased uptake levels and confirms the absence of thyroid tissue in athyroid children.

• Increased gonadotropin levels are compatible with sexual precocity in older children and may coexist with hypothyroidism.

• EKG shows bradycardia and flat or inverted T waves in untreated infants.

• Hip, knee, and thigh X-rays reveal absence of the femoral or tibial epiphyseal line and delayed skeletal development that is markedly inappropriate for the child's chronologic age. A low T_4 level that is associated with a normal TSH level suggests hypothyroidism secondary to hypothalamic or pituitary disease, a rare condition.

Treatment

Early detection is mandatory to prevent irreversible mental retardation and permit normal physical development. Treatment in infants younger than age 1 consists of replacement therapy with T_4 P.O., beginning with moderate doses. Dosage gradually increases to levels sufficient for lifelong maintenance. (A rapid increase in dosage may precipitate thyrotoxicity.) Doses are proportionately higher in children than in adults, because children metabolize thyroid hormone more quickly. Therapy in older children also includes T_4.

Clinical implications
Prevention, early detection, comprehensive parent teaching, and psychological support are essential. Know the early signs. Be especially wary if parents emphasize how good and how quiet their new baby is. After cretinism is diagnosed, provide supportive care during hormonal replacement.
• During early management of infantile cretinism, monitor blood pressure and pulse rate; report hypertension and tachycardia immediately. (Remember that infant heart rate is approximately 120 beats/minute.)
• If the infant's tongue is unusually large, position him on his side and observe him frequently to prevent airway obstruction.
• Check rectal temperature every 2 to 4 hours. Keep the infant warm and his skin moist.
• Inform parents that the child will require lifelong treatment with thyroid supplements. Teach them to recognize signs of overdose: rapid pulse rate, irritability, insomnia, fever, sweating, and weight loss.
• Provide support to help parents deal with a child who may be mentally retarded. Help them adopt a positive but realistic attitude and focus on their child's strengths rather than his weaknesses. Encourage them to provide stimulating activities to help the child reach maximum potential. Refer them to supportive community resources.
• To prevent infantile cretinism, emphasize the importance of adequate nutrition during pregnancy, including iodine-rich foods and the use of iodized salt or, in case of sodium restriction, an iodine supplement.

Hypovolemic shock
(Hypovolemic shock syndrome)

Description
In hypovolemic shock, reduced intravascular blood volume causes circulatory dysfunction and inadequate tissue perfusion. Without sufficient blood or fluid replacement, hypovolemic shock syndrome may led to irreversible cerebral and renal damage, cardiac arrest, and, ultimately, death. Hypovolemic shock syndrome necessitates early recognition of signs and symptoms and prompt, aggressive treatment to improve the prognosis. (See *Pathophysiology of Hypovolemic Shock*, p. 394.)

Causes
Acute blood loss—about one fifth of total volume—is the most common cause. Other causes include the following:
• Severe burns
• Intestinal obstruction
• Peritonitis
• Acute pancreatitis
• Ascites and dehydration from excessive perspiration
• Severe diarrhea or protracted vomiting
• Diabetes insipidus
• Diuresis or inadequate fluid intake

Signs and symptoms
• Hypotension, with narrowing pulse pressure
• Decreased sensorium
• Tachycardia
• Rapid, shallow respirations
• Reduced urinary output (less than 25 ml/hour)
• Cold, pale, clammy skin

Pathophysiology of Hypovolemic Shock

Normally, the body compensates for a loss of blood or fluid by constricting arteriolar beds, increasing heart rate and contractile force, and redistributing fluids. These compensatory mechanisms are effective enough to maintain stable vital signs, even after a 10% blood loss. But by the time blood or fluid loss reaches 15% to 25%, these mechanisms fail to maintain cardiac output, and blood pressure drops.

Baroreceptors (pressure-sensitive stretch receptors) in the aorta and carotid bodies trigger sympathetic nerve fibers. As a result, the adrenals release norepinephrine and epinephrine, causing vasoconstriction, which sharply reduces the blood flow to peripheral muscle and some of the vital organs (kidneys, liver, and lungs). Some cells, therefore, no longer receive oxygen, and cellular metabolism shifts from aerobic to anaerobic pathways, producing an accumulation of lactic acid, which is not metabolized to yield needed energy. Impaired renal or hepatic function causes this acid to accumulate and results in metabolic acidosis.

To compensate for metabolic acidosis, the patient hyperventilates to exhale more carbon dioxide and, in doing so, induces respiratory alkalosis. Since he may be unable to maintain the physical exertion required for hyperventilation, he may eventually need respiratory support, either oxygen by mask or mechanical ventilation.

Eventually, the compensatory mechanisms that serve to maintain acid-base balance fail, and cellular function is severely impaired, leading to cell death and subsequent organ failure.

Diagnostic tests

No single symptom or diagnostic test establishes the diagnosis or severity of hypovolemic shock.

• Serum potassium, serum lactate, and blood urea nitrogen levels are increased.

• Urine specific gravity is increased (more than 1.020). Urine osmolality also is increased.

• Blood pH and PO_2 levels are decreased; PCO_2 level is increased.

• In addition, gastroscopy, aspiration of gastric contents through a nasogastric tube, and X-rays identify internal bleeding sites.

• Coagulation studies may detect coagulopathy from disseminated intravascular coagulation (DIC).

Treatment

Emergency treatment measures consist of prompt, adequate blood and fluid replacement to restore intravascular volume and raise blood pressure. Saline solution, then possibly plasma proteins (albumin), other plasma expanders, or lactated Ringer's solution may produce volume expansion until whole blood can be matched. Application of medical antishock trousers may be helpful. Treatment may also include oxygen administration, identification of the bleeding site, control of bleeding by direct measures (such as pressure and elevation of an extremity), and possibly surgery.

Clinical implications

• Check for a patent airway and adequate circulation. Administer oxygen, as ordered. If blood pressure and heart rate are absent, start cardiopulmonary resuscitation.

• Place the patient flat in bed, with his legs elevated about 30 degrees to increase blood flow by promoting venous return to the heart.

• Record blood pressure, pulse rate, peripheral pulses, respirations, and other vital signs every 15 minutes. Monitor continuous EKG recording. When systolic blood pressure drops below 80 mm Hg, increase the oxygen flow rate, and notify the physician immediately. A progressive drop in blood pressure, accompanied by a thready pulse, generally signals inadequate cardiac output from reduced intravascular volume. Notify the physician, and increase the infusion rate.

• Start an I.V. infusion with normal saline or lactated Ringer's solution, using a large-bore catheter (14G), which allows easier administration of later blood transfusions. (*Caution:* Do not start an I.V. infusion in the legs of a patient in shock who has suffered abdominal trauma, since infused fluid may escape through the ruptured vessel into the abdomen.)

• An indwelling (Foley) catheter may be inserted to measure hourly urinary output. If output is less than 30 ml/hour in adults, increase the fluid infusion rate, but watch for signs of fluid overload. Notify the physician if urinary output does not improve. An osmotic diuretic may be ordered to increase renal blood flow and urinary output. Determine how much fluid to give by checking blood pressure, urinary output, central venous pressure, or pulmonary capillary wedge pressure.

• Draw an arterial blood sample to measure blood gas levels. Administer oxygen by face mask or airway to ensure adequate oxygenation of tissues. Adjust the oxygen flow rate to a higher or lower level, as blood gas measurements indicate.

• Watch for signs of impending coagulopathy (petechiae, bruising, and bleeding or oozing from gums or venipuncture sites).

• Explain all procedures and their purposes. Throughout these emergency measures, provide emotional support to the patient and family.

Complications
• DIC
• Decreased blood pressure (systolic below 80 mm Hg), usually resulting in inadequate coronary artery blood flow, cardiac ischemia, dysrhythmias, and other complications of low cardiac output

Idiopathic hypertrophic subaortic stenosis

Description

This primary disease of cardiac muscle is characterized by disproportionate, asymmetrical thickening of the interventricular septum, particularly in the anterior-superior part. In idiopathic hypertrophic subaortic stenosis (IHSS), cardiac output may be low, normal, or high, depending on whether stenosis is obstructive or nonobstructive. If cardiac output is normal or high, IHSS may go undetected for years. Low cardiac output may lead to potentially fatal congestive heart failure. The course of IHSS varies. Some patients demonstrate progressive deterioration. Others remain stable for several years.

Cause

Despite the designation idiopathic, IHSS is inherited in almost all cases as a non–sex-linked autosomal dominant trait.

Signs and symptoms

- Pain of angina pectoris
- Dysrhythmias
- Dyspnea
- Syncope
- Congestive heart failure
- Systolic ejection murmur (of medium pitch; heard along the left sternal border and at the apex)
- Double-impulse peripheral pulse (characteristic pulsus biferiens)
- With atrial fibrillation, irregular pulse

Diagnostic tests

- Echocardiography (most useful) shows increased thickness of the interventricular septum and abnormal motion of the anterior mitral leaflet during systole. Left ventricular outflow is occluded in obstructive IHSS.
- Cardiac catheterization reveals elevated left ventricular end-diastolic pressure and possibly mitral insufficiency.
- EKG usually demonstrates left ventricular hypertrophy, ST segment and T wave abnormalities, deep waves (due to hypertrophy, not infarction), left anterior hemiblock, ventricular dysrythmias, and possibly atrial fibrillation.
- Phonocardiography confirms an early systolic murmur.

Treatment

The goals of treatment of IHSS are to relax the ventricle and to relieve outflow tract obstruction. Propranolol, a beta-adrenergic blocking agent, slows heart rate and increases ventricular filling by relaxing the obstructing muscle, thereby reducing angina, syncope, dyspnea, and dysrhythmias. However, propranolol may aggravate symptoms of cardiac decompensation. Atrial fibrillation necessitates cardioversion to treat the dysrhythmia and, because of the high risk of systemic embolism, anticoagulant therapy until fibrillation subsides. Since vasodilators such as nitroglycerin reduce venous return by permitting pooling of blood in the periphery, decreasing ventricular volume and chamber size, and may cause further obstruction, they are contraindicated in patients with IHSS. Also contraindicated are sympathetic stimulators, such as isoproterenol, which enhance cardiac contractility and myocardial demands for oxygen, intensifying the obstruction.

If drug therapy fails, surgery is indicated. Ventricular myotomy (resection of the hypertrophied septum) alone or combined with mitral valve replacement may ease outflow tract obstruction and relieve symptoms. Ventricular myotomy is experimental, however. It may cause complications, such as complete heart block and ventricular septal defect.

Clinical implications
• Because syncope or sudden death may follow well-tolerated exercise, warn such patients against strenuous physical activity, such as running.
• Administer medication, as ordered. Warn the patient not to stop taking propranolol abruptly, since doing so may cause rebound effects, resulting in myocardial infarction or sudden death.
• Before dental work or surgery, administer prophylaxis for subacute bacterial endocarditis.
• Provide psychological support. If the patient is hospitalized for a long time, be flexible with visiting hours, and encourage occasional weekends away from the hospital, if possible. Refer the patient for psychosocial counseling to help him and his family accept his restricted life-style and poor prognosis.
• If the patient is a child of school age, urge his parents to arrange for him to continue his studies in the hospital.
• Since sudden cardiac arrest is possible, urge the patient's family to learn cardiopulmonary resuscitation.

Idiopathic thrombocytopenic purpura

Description
Thrombocytopenia that results from immunologic platelet destruction is known as idiopathic thrombocytopenic purpura (ITP). This form of thrombocytopenia may be acute (postviral thrombocytopenia) or chronic (Werlhof's disease, purpura hemorrhagica, essential thrombocytopenia, autoimmune thrombocytopenia). Acute ITP usually affects children between ages 2 and 6 and has a sudden onset. Chronic ITP mainly affects adults under age 50 and has an insidious onset. Prognosis for acute ITP is excellent. Prognosis for chronic ITP is good; transient remissions lasting weeks or even years are common, especially among women.

Causes
There is a possible autoimmune basis. Acute ITP usually follows a viral infection, such as rubella or chicken pox. ITP may also be drug-induced or associated with lupus erythematosus or pregnancy.

Signs and symptoms
• Petechiae
• Ecchymoses
• Mucosal bleeding from the mouth, nose, or gastrointestinal tract

Diagnostic tests
• Platelet count less than 20,000/mm³ and prolonged bleeding time suggest ITP.
• Platelet size and morphologic appearance may be abnormal.
• RBC count is decreased if bleeding has occurred.
• Bone marrow studies show an abundance of megakaryocytes (platelet precursors) and a shortened circulating platelet survival time (several hours or days rather than the usual 7 to 10 days).
• Occasionally, platelet antibodies

may be found in vitro, but this diagnosis is usually inferred from platelet survival data and the absence of an underlying disease.

Treatment

Corticosteroids, the initial treatment of choice, promote capillary integrity but are only temporarily effective in chronic ITP. Alternative treatments include immunosuppression (with vincristine sulfate, for example), plasmapheresis, and splenectomy in adults (85% successful). Before splenectomy, the patient may require blood, blood components, and vitamin K to correct anemia and coagulation defects. After splenectomy, he may need blood and component replacement, and platelet concentrate. Normally, however, platelets multiply spontaneously after splenectomy.

Clinical implications

Patient care for ITP focuses on teaching the patient to observe for petechiae, ecchymoses, and other signs of recurrence, especially following acute ITP. Closely monitor patients receiving immunosuppressives (often given before splenectomy) for signs of bone marrow depression, infection, mucositis, gastrointestinal tract ulceration, and severe diarrhea or vomiting.

Impetigo
(Impetigo contagiosa)

Description

A contagious, superficial skin infection, impetigo occurs in nonbullous and bullous forms. This vesiculopustular eruptive disorder spreads most easily among infants, young children, and the elderly. Impetigo can complicate chicken pox, eczema, or other skin conditions marked by open lesions.

Causes

• Beta-hemolytic streptococcus usually produces nonbullous impetigo.

• Coagulase-positive *Staphylococcus aureus* usually causes bullous impetigo.

Risk factors
• Poor hygiene
• Anemia
• Malnutrition

Signs and symptoms
Streptococcal impetigo
—This typically begins with a small red macule that turns into a vesicle, becoming pustular in a matter of hours. When the vesicle breaks, a characteristic thick, yellow crust forms from the exudate. Autoinoculation may cause satellite lesions to appear. Other symptoms include pruritus, burning, and regional lymphadenopathy.

Staphylococcal impetigo
—A thin-walled vesicle opens, and a thin, clear crust forms from the exudate. The lesion consists of a central clearing, circumscribed by an outer rim—much like a ringworm lesion—and commonly appears on the face or other exposed areas. It causes painless pruritus.

Diagnostic tests
• Microscopic visualization of the causative organism in a Gram's stain of vesicle fluid usually confirms infection, although characteristic lesions suggest impetigo.

• Culture and sensitivity testing of fluid or denuded skin may indicate the most appropriate antibiotic, but therapy should not be delayed for laboratory results, which can take 3 days.

• WBC count may be elevated in the presence of infection.

Treatment
Generally, treatment consists of systemic antibiotics (usually penicillin, or erythromycin for patients who are allergic to penicillin), which also help prevent glomerulonephritis. Therapy also includes removal of the exudate

Ecthyma

Ecthyma is a superficial skin infection that usually causes scarring. It generally results from infection by beta-hemolytic streptococcus. Ecthyma differs from impetigo in that its characteristic ulcer results from deeper penetration of the skin by the infecting organism (involving the lower epidermis and dermis), and the overlying crust tends to be piled high (1 to 3 cm). These lesions often occur on the posterior aspects of the thighs and buttocks. Autoinoculation can transmit ecthyma to other parts of the body, especially to sites that have been scratched open. (Ecthyma often results from the scratching of chigger bites.) Therapy is basically the same as for impetigo, beginning with removal of the crust, but response may be slower. Widespread ulcers may require parenteral antibiotics.

by washing the lesions two to three times a day with soap and water, or for stubborn crusts, warm soaks or compresses of normal saline or a diluted soap solution before application of topical antibiotics. Topical antibiotics are less effective than systemic antibiotics.

Clinical implications
• Urge the patient not to scratch, since this exacerbates impetigo. Advise parents to cut the child's fingernails. Give medications, as ordered; remember to check for penicillin allergy. Stress the need to continue prescribed medications even after lesions have healed.
• Teach the patient or family how to care for impetiginous lesions. To prevent further spread of this highly contagious infection, encourage frequent bathing using a bactericidal soap. Tell the patient not to share towels, washcloths, or bed linens with family members. Emphasize the importance of following proper hand-washing technique.
• Check family members for impetigo. If this infection is present in a school-age child, notify his school. (See *Ecthyma*.)

Complications
A rare but serious complication of streptococcal impetigo is glomerulonephritis.

Inclusion conjunctivitis
(Inclusion blennorrhea)

Description
A fairly common disease, inclusion conjunctivitis is an acute ocular inflammation. Although the disorder occasionally becomes chronic, prognosis is generally good.

Cause
Chlamydia trachomatis, which infects the urethra in males and cervix in females and is transmitted through sexual activity

Mode of transmission
• Contaminated cervical secretions infect the eyes of the neonate during birth.
• Rarely, an infected person transfers the virus from his genitourinary tract to his own eyes.

Signs and symptoms
Newborns
—Reddened lower eyelids
—Thick, purulent discharge
—Possible formation of pseudomembranes (can lead to conjunctival scarring)

Children and adults
—Follicles inside the lower eyelids
—Preauricular lymphadenopathy

Diagnostic tests
Examination of Giemsa-stained conjunctival scraping reveals cytoplasmic inclusion bodies in conjunctival epithelial cells, many polymorphonuclear leukocytes, and a negative culture for bacteria.

Treatment
Treatment consists of eye drops of 1% tetracycline in oil, erythromycin ophthalmic ointment, or sulfonamide eye drops five or six times daily for 2 weeks for infants, and oral tetracycline or erythromycin for 3 weeks for adults. In severe disease, adults may require concomitant systemic sulfonamide therapy.

Clinical implications
• Keep patient's eyes as clean as possible, using strict aseptic technique. Clean the eyes from the inner to the outer canthus. Apply warm soaks, as needed. Record amount and color of drainage.
• Remind the patient not to rub his eyes; rubbing can irritate them.
• If the patient's eyes are sensitive to light, keep the room dark or suggest that he wear dark glasses. Provide appropriate diversionary activities.

To prevent further spread of inclusion conjunctivitis, follow these guidelines:
• Wash hands thoroughly before and after administering eye medications.
• Suggest genital examination of the mother of an infected newborn or of any adult with inclusion conjunctivitis.
• Obtain a history of recent sexual contacts, so they can be examined for inclusion conjunctivitis.

Complications
Otitis media

Infantile autism

Description
Infantile autism is a severe developmental disorder marked by unresponsiveness to human contact, gross deficits in language development, and bizarre responses to various aspects of the environment. It becomes apparent before the child reaches age 30 months. Infantile autism is rare. It affects three to four times more males than females, most commonly the firstborn male. Prognosis is poor. (See also *Symbiotic Psychosis*, p. 401, and *Stress Disorders with Physical Manifestations*, pp. 402 and 403.)

Cause
The cause of infantile autism remain unclear but is thought to include psychological, physiologic, and sociologic factors.

Signs and symptoms
For diagnosis of infantile autism, symptoms must develop before age 30 months. They include the following:
• Unresponsiveness to people (primary characteristic)
• Becoming rigid or flaccid when held
• Crying when touched
• Smiling response delayed or absent
• No sign of recognition or affection for parents or caretakers
• Lack of stranger anxiety in later infancy
• Severe language impairment (possible muteness or use of immature speech patterns; commonly, echolalia, meaningless repetition of words or phrases, and pronoun reversal)
• Bizarre behavior patterns (may include screaming fits, rituals, rhythmic rocking, arm flapping, disturbed eating and sleeping patterns, and self-destructive behavior such as head banging)

Diagnostic tests
• The Denver Developmental Screen-

Symbiotic Psychosis

This pervasive developmental disorder, almost opposite in ego structure to infantile autism, becomes manifest at ages 2 to 5 years.

Signs and symptoms
This condition is marked by abnormal development of ego. The child with this psychosis does not see himself as a separate person. His ego is fused with that of a significant other, usually his mother. He can express himself verbally but does not need language to convey his ideas to her. (They seem to know each other's thoughts.) He functions at an immature level unless his mother is present; then, the two function as one (for example, when one is cold, both mother and child put on sweaters).

Special considerations
• Treatment is characteristically difficult and prolonged. It must involve both members of the symbiotic relationship. Plan your interventions to support the child and mother in developing separate interests, ideas, and goals.
• Help each to develop a separate identity. Encourage separate activities. Point out individual successes.
• Practice reality therapy with both. Point out separate body parts. ("This is your hand. This is your mother's hand." Or, "I'm going to bandage your foot. This is your foot. Your mother's foot has no cut.")

ing Test shows the autistic child to have delayed development, especially of social and language skills.
• IQ testing shows retardation in 70%, but low IQ scores may simply reflect inability to cooperate during the test. In autistic children who do cooperate, IQ tests often show average or superior intelligence.

Treatment
Treatment of autism is difficult and prolonged. It must begin early, continue for years (through adolescence), and involve the child, parents, teachers, and therapists in coordinated efforts to encourage social adjustment and speech development and to reduce self-destructive behavior. Positive reinforcement using food and other rewards can promote language and social skills. Providing pleasurable sensory and motor stimulation (jogging, playing with a ball) encourages appropriate behavior and helps eliminate inappropriate behavior. In children with a biochemical disorder (excessive dopamine blood levels), haloperidol often mitigates withdrawn and stereotypical behavior patterns, making the child more amenable to behavior modification therapies.

Treatment may take place in a psychiatric institution, in a specialized school, or in a day-care program, but the current trend is toward home treatment. Helping family members to develop strong one-to-one relationships with the autistic child often initiates responsive, imitative behavior. Because family members often feel inadequate and guilty, they may need counseling. Until the causes of infantile autism are known, prevention is not possible.

Clinical implications
• Encourage development of self-esteem. Show the child that he is accepted as a person. If he sits on the floor, sit on the floor with him.
• Reduce self-destructive behaviors. Physically stop the child from harming himself, while firmly saying "no."

Stress Disorders with Physical Manifestations

These disorders are usually outgrown by adolescence. Treatment involves determining the underlying cause, which is usually related to extreme stress in the parent-child relationship stemming from unrealistic demands on the child in terms of his developmental level.

DISORDER AND DEFINITION	CAUSES AND INCIDENCE	ASSOCIATED PROBLEMS	TREATMENT
Stuttering: abnormalities of the rhythm of speech, with repetitions and hesitations at the beginning of words; may involve associated movements of the respiratory muscles, shoulders, and face	• Possibly associated with mental dullness, poor social background, and history of birth trauma • Often occurs in children of average or superior intelligence who fear they cannot meet expectations of socially striving success-oriented families	• Low self-esteem • Tension, anxiety • Withdrawal from social situations because of fear of stuttering • Humiliation	• Usually outgrown • Evaluation and treatment by speech pathologist teaches the patient to place equal weight on each syllable in sentence, proper breathing technique and timing, and anxiety control.
Functional enuresis: involuntary voiding of urine, usually during the night (nocturnal enuresis)	• Normal in children until age 3 or 4; occurs in about 40% of children at this age • Persists in 22% at age 5; in 10% at age 10; and in 1% to 2% at age 20 • Persists longer in boys • Possibly related to stress in child's life: birth of sibling, move to new home, divorce, separation, hospitalization; faulty toilet training (inconsistent, demanding, punitive); or unrealistic, not age-appropriate responsibilities	• Low self-esteem • Social withdrawal from peers	• Parents should avoid punitive reactions that burden the child with additional stress and guilt. A matter-of-fact attitude helps the child learn to control his bladder function without undue stress. • If enuresis persists into late childhood, treatment may help. Tofranil can control or reduce enuresis. *Caution:* Tofranil can cause schizophrenia-like symptoms in young children. Dry-bed therapy may include use of a urine alarm apparatus (wet bell pad), social motivation, self-correction of accidents, and positive reinforcement.

Stress Disorders with Physical Manifestations *(continued)*

DISORDER AND DEFINITION	CAUSES AND INCIDENCE	ASSOCIATED PROBLEMS	TREATMENT
Functional encopresis: repeated evacuation of feces into clothes or inappropriate receptacles	• Associated with low intelligence, cerebral dysfunction, or other developmental symptoms, such as language lag • Common in anxious children from socially disadvantaged families with hostile, dependent mother-son relationship and distant, uninvolved father	• Repressed anger • Withdrawal from peers in social relationships • Loss of self-esteem	• Encourage child to come to parents when he has an "accident." Encourage parents to help the child by giving him clean clothes without criticism or punishment. • Medical examination should rule out physical disorder. • Child, adult, and family therapy can reduce anger over disappointment in child's development and parenting techniques.
Sleepwalking and sleep terror: In sleepwalking, the child calmly rises from bed in state of altered consciousness and walks about with no subsequent recollection of any dream content. In sleep terror, he wakes terrified, in a state of clouded consciousness, often unable to recognize parents and familiar surroundings. Visual hallucinations are common.	• Sleep terrors are a normal developmental event in 2- to 3-year-olds. • Usually occurring between 30 and 200 minutes of onset of sleep • Tachycardia, tachypnea, diaphoresis, dilated pupils, or piloerection associated with terror	• Fear of being alone	• Usually are self-limiting and subside within a few weeks • Make sure the child has access to his parents at night.

When he responds to your voice, give a primary reward (food). Later, substitute a secondary reward (verbal: "good;" or physical: a hug or pat on the back).

• Encourage appropriate use of language. Give positive reinforcement when the child indicates his needs correctly. Give verbal reinforcement at first ("good, okay, great"). Later, give physical reinforcement (hug him; pat his hand or his shoulder).

• Encourage self-care. For example, place a brush in his hand and guide his hand to brush his hair. Similarly, teach him to wash his hands and face.

• Encourage acceptance of minor environmental changes. Prepare the child for the change by telling him about it. Make the minor change: change the color of his bedspread or the placement of food on his plate. When he has accepted minor changes, move on to bigger ones.

• Support and assist parents. Refer the family to the National Society for Autistic Children for further assistance.

Infectious mononucleosis

Description
Infectious mononucleosis is an acute infectious disease that primarily affects young adults and children, although in children it is usually so mild that it is often overlooked. Characteristically, infectious mononucleosis produces fever, sore throat, and cervical lymphadenopathy (the hallmarks of the disease) as well as hepatic dysfunction, increased lymphocytes and monocytes, and development and persistence of heterophil antibodies. Infectious mononucleosis is probably contagious before symptoms develop and until fever subsides and oropharyngeal lesions disappear. Prognosis is excellent, and major complications are uncommon.

Cause
Epstein-Barr virus (EBV), a herpesvirus

Mode of transmission
• Oral-pharyngeal route
• Blood transfusion

Signs and symptoms
Prodromal
—Headache
—Malaise
—Fatigue
Characteristic
—Sore throat
—Cervical lymphadenopathy
—Fever
Possible
—Splenomegaly
—Hepatomegaly
—Stomatitis
—Exudative tonsillitis or pharyngitis
—Maculopapular rash in early phase

Diagnostic tests
The following abnormal laboratory results confirm the diagnosis.
• Leukocyte count increases 10,000 to 20,000/mm³ during the second and third weeks of illness. Lymphocytes and monocytes account for 50% to 70% of the total WBC count; 10% of the lymphocytes are atypical.
• Heterophil antibodies (agglutinins for sheep RBCs) in serum drawn during acute illness and at 3- to 4-week intervals rise to four times normal.
• Indirect immunofluorescence shows antibodies to EBV and cellular antigens. Such testing is usually more definitive than heterophil antibodies.
• Liver function studies are abnormal.

Treatment
Infectious mononucleosis resists prevention and antimicrobial treatment. Thus, therapy is essentially supportive: relief of symptoms, bed rest during the acute febrile period, and aspirin or another salicylate for headache and sore throat. If severe throat inflammation causes airway obstruction, steroids can be used to relieve swelling

and avoid tracheotomy. Splenic rupture, marked by sudden abdominal pain, requires splenectomy. About 20% of patients with infectious mononucleosis will also have streptococcal pharyngotonsillitis; these patients should receive antibiotic therapy for at least 10 days.

Clinical implications
Since uncomplicated infectious mononucleosis does not require hospitalization, patient teaching is essential. Convalescence may take several weeks, usually until the patient's WBC count returns to normal.
• During acute illness, stress the need for bed rest. If the patient is a student, tell him he may continue less demanding school assignments and see his friends but should avoid long, difficult projects until after recovery.
• To minimize throat discomfort, encourage the patient to drink milk shakes, fruit juices, and broths and also to eat cool, bland foods. Advise the use of saline gargles and acetaminophen as needed.

Complications
Major complications rarely occur, but they include the following:
• Splenic rupture
• Aseptic meningitis
• Encephalitis
• Hemolytic anemia
• Guillain-Barré syndrome

Infertility in females

Description
Infertility, the inability to conceive after regular intercourse for at least 1 year without contraception, affects approximately 10% to 15% of all couples in the United States. About 40% to 50% of all infertility is attributed to the female. (See also "Infertility in males," pp. 406 to 408.) Diagnosis requires a complete physical examination and health history, including specific questions on the patient's reproductive and sexual function, past diseases, mental state, previous surgery, types of contraception used in the past, and family history. Following extensive investigation and treatment, approximately 50% of infertile couples achieve pregnancy. Of the 50% who do not, 10% have no pathologic basis for infertility; the prognosis in this group becomes extremely poor if pregnancy is not achieved after 3 years.

Causes
• Any defect or malfunction of the hypothalamic-pituitary-ovarian axis, such as infections, tumors, or neurologic disease of the hypothalamus or pituitary gland
• Ovarian factors related to anovulation or oligo-ovulation
• Uterine abnormalities, which may include congenitally absent, bicornuate, or double uterus; leiomyomas; or Asherman's syndrome, in which the anterior and posterior uterine walls adhere because of scar tissue formation
• Tubal and peritoneal factors such as tubal loss or impairment secondary to ectopic pregnancy, or tubal occlusion due to salpingitis or peritubal adhesions
• Cervical factors such as infection and possibly cervical antibodies that immobilize sperm
• Psychological problems

Signs and symptoms
Inability to achieve pregnancy after having regular intercourse without contraception for at least 1 year

Diagnostic tests
The following tests assess ovulation:
• Basal body temperature graph shows a sustained elevation in body temperature postovulation until just before onset of menses, indicating the approximate time of ovulation.

• Endometrial biopsy, done on or about day 5 after the basal body temperature elevates, provides histologic evidence that ovulation has occurred.

• Progesterone blood levels, measured when they should be highest, can show a luteal phase deficiency.

The following procedures assess structural integrity of the fallopian tubes, the ovaries, and the uterus:

• Hysterosalpingography provides radiologic evidence of tubal obstruction and abnormalities of the uterine cavity after injection of radiopaque contrast medium through the cervix.

• Endoscopy confirms the results of hysterosalpingography and visualizes the endometrial cavity by hysteroscopy or explores the posterior surface of the uterus, fallopian tubes, and ovaries by culdoscopy. Laparoscopy allows visualization of the abdominal and pelvic areas.

Male-female interaction studies include the following:

• Postcoital test (Sims-Huhner test) examines the cervical mucus for motile sperm cells following intercourse that takes place at midcycle (as close to ovulation as possible).

• Immunologic or antibody testing detects spermicidal antibodies in the sera of the female. (Further research is being conducted in this area.)

Treatment

Treatment depends on identifying the underlying abnormality or dysfunction within the hypothalamic-pituitary-ovarian complex. In hyperactivity of hypoactivity of the adrenal or thyroid gland, hormone therapy is necessary. Progesterone deficiency requires progesterone replacement. Anovulation necessitates treatment with clomiphene, human menopausal gonadotropins, or human chorionic gonadotropin. Ovulation usually occurs several days after such administration. If mucous production decreases (a side effect of clomiphene), small doses of estrogen to improve the quality of cervical mucus may be given concomitantly.

Surgical restoration may correct certain anatomic causes of infertility, such as fallopian tube obstruction. Surgery may also be necessary to remove tumors located within or near the hypothalamus or pituitary gland. Endometriosis requires drug therapy (danazol or medroxyprogesterone, or noncyclic administration of oral contraceptives), surgical removal of areas of endometriosis, or a combination of both.

Artificial insemination has proven to be an effective alternative strategy for dealing with infertility problems. In vitro (test tube) fertilization has also been successful.

Clinical implications

Management includes providing the infertile couple with emotional support and information about diagnostic and treatment techniques.

An infertile couple may suffer loss of self-esteem. They may feel angry, guilty, or inadequate, and the diagnostic procedures for this disorder may intensify their fear and anxiety. You can help by explaining these procedures thoroughly. Above all, encourage the patient and her partner to talk about their feelings, and listen to what they have to say with a nonjudgmental attitude.

If the patient requires surgery, tell her what to expect postoperatively; this, of course, depends on which procedure is to be performed.

Infertility in males

Description

Male infertility may be suspected whenever a couple fails to achieve pregnancy after about 1 year of regular intercourse without contraceptive use. Approximately 40% to 50% of infertility problems in the United States are totally or partially attributed to the male. Detailed patient history may reveal abnormal sexual development, delayed puberty, infertility in previous relationships, and a medical history of prolonged fever, mumps, impaired nutritional status, previous surgery, or trauma to genitalia. (See also "Infertility in females," pp. 405 to 406.)

Causes
• Varicocele, a mass of dilated and tortuous varicose veins in the spermatic cord
• Semen disorders, such as volume or motility disturbances or inadequate sperm density
• Proliferation of abnormal or immature sperm, with variations in the size and shape of the sperm head
• Systemic disease, such as diabetes mellitus, neoplasms, hepatic and renal diseases, and viral disturbances, especially mumps orchitis
• Genital infection, such as gonorrhea, tuberculosis, and herpes
• Disorders of the testes, such as cryptorchidism, Sertoli-cell-only syndrome, varicocele, and ductal obstruction (caused by absence or ligation of vas deferens or infection)
• Genetic defects, such as Klinefelter's syndrome (chromosomal pattern XXY, eunuchoidal habitus, gynecomastia, small testes) or Reifenstein's syndrome (chromosomal pattern 46XY, reduced testosterone, azoospermia, eunuchoidism, gynecomastia, hypospadias).
• Immunologic disorders, such as autoimmune infertility or allergic orchitis
• Endocrine imbalance (rare) that disrupts pituitary gonadotropins, inhibiting spermatogenesis, testosterone production, or both (occurs in Kallmann's syndrome, panhypopituitarism, hypothyroidism, and congenital adrenal hyperplasia)

• Chemicals and drugs that can inhibit gonadotropins or interfere with spermatogenesis, such as arsenic, methotrexate, medroxyprogesterone acetate, nitrofurantoin, monoamine oxidase inhibitors, and some antihypertensives
• Sexual problems, such as erectile dysfunction, ejaculatory incompetence, or low libido
• Other factors, including age, occupation, and trauma to testes

Signs and symptoms
• Failure to impregnate a fertile woman is the most obvious indication.
• Clinical features may include atrophied testes; empty scrotum; scrotal edema; varicocele or anteversion of the epididymis; inflamed seminal vesicles; beading or abnormal nodes on the spermatic cord and vas; penile nodes, warts, plaques, or hypospadias; and prostatic enlargement, nodules, swelling, or tenderness.
• Possible psychological indications include troublesome negative emotions in a couple—anger, hurt, disgust, guilt, and loss of self-esteem.

Diagnostic tests
• Semen analysis is the most conclusive test.
• Gonadotropin assay determines integrity of the pituitary gonadal axis.
• Serum testosterone levels determine end organ response to LH.
• Urine 17-ketosteroid levels measure testicular function.
• Testicular biopsy helps clarify unexplained oligospermia and azoospermia.
• Vasography and seminal vesiculography may be necessary.

Treatment
When anatomic dysfunctions or infections cause infertility, treatment consists of correcting the underlying problem. A varicocele requires surgical repair or removal. For patients with sexual dysfunctions, treatment includes education, therapy or counseling (on sexual techniques, coital

frequency, and reproductive physiology), and proper nutrition, with vitamin supplements. Decreased FSH levels may respond to vitamin B therapy; decreased LH levels, to chorionic gonadotropin therapy. Normal or elevated LH requires low-dosage testosterone. Decreased testosterone levels, decreased semen motility, and volume disturbances may respond to chorionic gonadotropin.

Patients with oligospermia who have a normal history and physical examination, normal hormonal assays, and no signs of systemic disease require emotional support and counseling, adequate nutrition, multivitamins, and selective therapeutic agents, such as clomiphene, chorionic gonadotropin, and low-dosage testosterone. Obvious alternatives to such treatment are adoption and artificial insemination.

Clinical implications

• Educate the couple, as necessary, regarding reproductive and sexual functions and factors that may interfere with fertility, such as the use of lubricants and douches.

• Urge men with oligospermia to avoid habits that may interfere with normal spermatogenesis by elevating scrotal temperature, such as wearing tight underwear and athletic supporters, taking hot tub baths, or habitually riding a bicycle. Explain that cool scrotal temperatures are essential for adequate spermatogenesis.

• When possible, advise infertile couples to join group programs to share their feelings and concerns with other couples who have the same problem.

• Help prevent male infertility by encouraging patients to have regular physical examinations, to protect gonads during athletic activity, and to receive early treatment for venereal diseases and surgical correction for anatomic defects.

Influenza
(Grippe, flu)

Description

Influenza is an acute, highly contagious viral infection of the respiratory tract. It occurs in isolated cases, epidemics, and pandemics. Its severity is greatest in the very young, the elderly, and those with chronic diseases. New strains of the influenza virus emerge at regular intervals and are named according to their geographic origin.

Cause

One of three different types of *Myxovirus influenzae:* Type A, Type B, or Type C

Mode of transmission

Airborne droplet infection

Signs and symptoms

• Sudden onset of chills
• Temperature of 101° to 104° F. (38.3° to 40° C.)
• Headache
• Malaise
• Myalgia
• Nonproductive cough
• Occasionally, hoarseness, rhinitis, rhinorrhea
• Cervical adenopathy (likely in children)

Diagnostic tests

• Since signs and symptoms are not pathognomonic, isolation of *M. influenzae* through inoculation of chicken embryos (with nasal secretions from infected patients) is essential at the first sign of an epidemic.
• Nose and throat cultures and increased serum antibody titers help confirm these findings.
• After these measures confirm an influenza epidemic, diagnosis requires only observation of clinical signs and symptoms. Uncomplicated cases show decreased WBCs with an increase in lymphocytes.

Treatment

Treatment of uncomplicated influenza includes bed rest, adequate fluid intake, acetaminophen to relieve fever and muscle pain, and guaifenesin or another expectorant to relieve nonproductive coughing. Prophylactic antibiotics are not recommended, because they have no effect on the influenza virus.

Amantadine (an antiviral agent) has proven to be effective in reducing the duration of signs and symptoms in influenza A infection. In influenza complicated by pneumonia, supportive care (fluid and electrolyte supplements, oxygen, assisted ventilation) and treatment of bacterial superinfection with appropriate antibiotics are necessary.

Clinical implications

Unless complications occur, influenza does not require hospitalization. Like treatment, patient care focuses on relief of symptoms.

• Advise the patient to use mouthwashes and increase his fluid intake. Warm baths or heating pads may relieve myalgia. Give him nonnarcotic analgesics-antipyretics, as ordered.

• Screen visitors to protect the patient from bacterial infection and the visitor from influenza. Use respiratory precautions.

• Teach the patient proper disposal of tissues and proper hand-washing technique to prevent the virus from spreading.

• Watch for signs and symptoms of developing pneumonia, such as rales, another temperature rise, or coughing accompanied by purulent or bloody sputum. Assist the patient in a gradual return to his normal activities.

• Educate patients about influenza immunizations. For high-risk patients and health care personnel, suggest annual inoculations at the start of the flu season (late autumn). Remember, however, that such vaccines are made from chicken embryos and must not be given to persons who are hypersensitive to eggs, feathers, or chickens. The vaccine administered is based on the previous year's virus and is usually about 75% effective.

• All persons receiving the vaccine should be made aware of possible side effects (discomfort at the vaccination site, fever, malaise, and rarely Guillain-Barré syndrome).

• Although the vaccine has not been proven harmful to the fetus, it is not recommended for pregnant women, except those who are highly susceptible to influenza, such as those with chronic diseases.

Complications

Fever that persists longer than 3 to 5 days signals the onset of complications. The most common complication is pneumonia, which can be primary (influenza viral pneumonia) or secondary to bacterial infection. Influenza may also cause myositis, exacerbation of chronic obstructive pulmonary disease (COPD), Reye's syndrome, and, rarely, myocarditis, pericarditis, transverse myelitis, and encephalitis.

Inguinal hernia
(Rupture)

Description

In an inguinal hernia, the most common type of hernia, the large or small intestine, omentum, or bladder protrudes into the inguinal canal. Hernias can be reducible (if the hernia can be manipulated back into place with relative ease), incarcerated (if the hernia cannot be reduced because adhesions have formed in the hernial sac), or strangulated (part of the herniated intestine becomes twisted or edematous, seriously interfering with normal blood flow and peristalsis, and possibly leading to intestinal obstruction

Assessing for Inguinal Hernia

To detect a hernia in a male patient, the patient is asked to stand with his ipsilateral leg slightly flexed and his weight resting on the other leg. The examiner inserts an index finger into the lower part of the scrotum and invaginates the scrotal skin so that the finger advances through the external inguinal ring to the internal ring (about 1½" to 2" [4 to 4 cm] through the inguinal canal). The patient is then told to cough. If the examiner feels pressure against the fingertip, an indirect hernia exists; if he feels pressure against the side of the finger, a direct hernia exists.

and necrosis). Inguinal hernia can also be direct or indirect. Indirect inguinal hernia causes the abdominal viscera to protrude through the inguinal ring and follow the spermatic cord (in males), or round ligament (in females). Direct inguinal hernia results from a weakness in the fascial floor of the inguinal canal.

Causes
• Weak abdominal muscles, due to congenital malformation, trauma, or aging
• Increased intra-abdominal pressure (due to heavy lifting, pregnancy, obesity, or straining)

Signs and symptoms
• A lump appears over the herniated area when the patient stands or strains, and disappears when the patient is supine.
• Tension on the herniated area may cause a sharp, steady pain in the groin, which fades when the hernia is reduced.
• Strangulation produces severe pain.
• Palpation of the inguinal area while the patient is performing Valsalva's maneuver is needed to confirm the diagnosis. (See *Assessing for Inguinal Hernia*.)

Diagnostic tests
X-rays and a WBC count (may be elevated) are required for suspected bowel obstruction.

Treatment
If the hernia is reducible, the pain may be temporarily relieved by pushing the hernia back into place. A truss may keep the abdominal contents from protruding into the hernial sac, although it will not cure the hernia. This device is especially beneficial for an elderly or debilitated patient, since any surgery is potentially hazardous to him.

For infants, adults, and otherwise healthy elderly patients, herniorrhaphy is the treatment of choice. Herniorrhaphy replaces the contents of the hernial sac into the abdominal cavity and closes the opening. This procedure is often performed under local anesthesia in a short-term unit, or as a single-day admission. Another effective surgical procedure for repairing hernia is hernioplasty, which reinforces the weakened area with steel mesh, fascia, or wire.

A strangulated or necrotic hernia necessitates bowel resection. Rarely, an extensive resection may require temporary colostomy. In either case, bowel resection lengthens postoperative recovery and requires massive doses of antibiotics, parenteral fluids, and electrolyte replacement.

Clinical implications
• Apply a truss only after a hernia has been reduced. For best results, apply it in the morning, before the patient gets out of bed.
• To prevent skin irritation, tell the patient to bathe daily and apply liberal amounts of cornstarch or baby pow-

der. Warn against applying the truss over clothing, since this reduces its effectiveness and may make it slip.

• Watch for and immediately report signs of incarceration and strangulation. Do not try to reduce an incarcerated hernia, since this may perforate the bowel. If severe intestinal obstruction arises because of hernial strangulation, inform the physician immediately. A nasogastric tube may be inserted promptly to empty the stomach and relieve pressure on the hernial sac.

• Before surgery, closely monitor vital signs. Administer I.V. fluids, and analgesics for pain, as ordered. Control fever with acetaminophen or tepid sponge baths, as ordered. Place the patient in Trendelenburg's position to reduce pressure on the hernia site.

• Give special reassurance and support to a child scheduled for hernia repair. Encourage him to ask questions, and answer them as simply as possible. Offer appropriate diversions to distract him from the impending surgery.

• After surgery, make sure the patient voids within 8 to 12 hours. Check the incision and dressing at least three times a day for drainage, inflammation, or swelling. Check for normal bowel sounds and watch for fever.

• Observe carefully for postoperative scrotal swelling. To reduce such swelling, support the scrotum with a rolled towel and apply an ice bag.

• Encourage fluid intake to maintain hydration and prevent constipation. Teach deep-breathing exercises, and show the patient how to splint the incision before coughing.

• Before discharge, warn the patient against lifting or straining. In addition, tell him to watch for signs of infection (oozing, tenderness, warmth, redness) at the incision site, and to keep the incision clean and covered until the sutures are removed.

• Advise the patient not to resume normal activity or return to work without the surgeon's permission.

Complications
Partial or complete bowel obstruction

Insect bites and stings

Description
Among the most common traumatic complaints are insect bites and stings, the more serious of which include those of a tick, brown recluse spider, black widow spider, scorpion, bee, wasp, or yellow jacket. (See *Insect Bites and Stings,* pp. 412 to 415.)

Intestinal obstruction

Description
Intestinal obstruction is the partial or complete blockage of the lumen in the small or large bowel. Small bowel obstruction is far more common (90% of patients) and usually more serious. Complete obstruction in any part of the bowel, if untreated, can cause death within hours from shock and vascular collapse. Intestinal obstruction is most likely to occur after abdominal surgery or in persons with congenital bowel deformities. (See *Pathophysiology of Intestinal Obstruction,* p. 416.)

Causes
Mechanical
—Adhesions and strangulated hernias. These usually cause small bowel obstruction.
—Carcinomas. These usually cause large bowel obstruction.
—Foreign bodies (fruit pits, gallstones, worms)
—Compression
—Stenosis
—Intussusception
—Volvulus of the sigmoid or cecum

Insect Bites and Stings

GENERAL INFORMATION	CLINICAL FEATURES
Tick • Common in woods and fields throughout the United States • Attaches to host in any of its life stages (larva, nymph, adult). Fastens to host with its teeth, then secretes a cementlike material to reinforce attachment. • Flat, brown, speckled body about 0.25″ (6.25 mm) long; has eight legs • Also transmits diseases such as Rocky Mountain spotted fever	• Itching may be sole symptom; or after several days, host may develop tick paralysis (acute flaccid paralysis, starting as paresthesia and pain in legs and resulting in respiratory failure from bulbar paralysis).
Brown recluse (violin) spider • Common to south-central United States; usually found in dark areas (outdoor privy, barn, woodshed) • Dark brown violin on its back, three pairs of eyes; female more dangerous than male • Most bites occur between April and October.	Venom is coagulotoxic. Reaction begins within 2 to 8 hours after bite. • Localized vasoconstriction causes ischemic necrosis at bite site. Small, reddened puncture wound forms a bleb and becomes ischemic. In 3 to 4 days, center becomes dark and hard. Within 2 to 3 weeks, an ulcer forms. • Minimal initial pain increases over time. • Other symptoms: fever, chills, malaise, weakness, nausea, vomiting, edema, convulsions, joint pains, petechiae, cyanosis, phlebitis • Rarely, thrombocytopenia and hemolytic anemia develop and lead to death within first 24 to 48 hours (usually in a child or patient with previous history of cardiac disease). Prompt and appropriate treatment results in recovery.
Black widow spider • Common throughout the United States, particularly in warmer climates; usually found in dark areas (outdoor privy, barn, woodshed) • Female is coal black with a red or orange hourglass on her ventral side; she is larger than male (male does not bite). • Mortality less than 1% (increased risk among the	Venom is neurotoxic. Age, size, and sensitivity of patient determines severity and progression of symptoms • Pinprick sensation, followed by dull, numbing pain (may go unnoticed) • Edema and tiny, red bite marks • Rigidity of stomach muscles and severe abdominal pain (10 to 40 minutes after bite) • Muscle spasms in extremities • Ascending paralysis, causing difficulty in swallowing and labored, grunting respirations • Other symptoms: extreme restlessness, vertigo, sweating, chills, pallor, convulsions

TREATMENT	SPECIAL CONSIDERATIONS
• Removal of tick • Local antipruritics for itching papule • Mechanical ventilation for respiratory failure	• To remove tick, cover it with mineral, salad, or machine oil, or alcohol on a tissue or gauze pad. This blocks the tick's breathing pores and causes it to withdraw from the skin. If the tick does not disengage after the pad has been in place for ½ hour, carefully remove it with tweezers, taking care to remove all parts. • To reduce risk of being bitten, teach the patient to keep away from wooded areas, to wear protective clothes, and to carefully examine body for ticks after being outdoors. • Teach patients how to safely remove ticks.
• No known specific treatment • Combination therapy with corticosteroids, antibiotics, antihistamines, tranquilizers, I.V. fluids, and tetanus prophylaxis • Lesion excision in first 10 to 12 hours relieves pain. A split-thickness skin graft closes the wound. Without grafting, healing may take 6 to 8 weeks. • A large chronic ulcer may require skin grafting.	• Cleanse the lesion with a 1:20 Burow's aluminum acetate solution, and as ordered, apply antibiotic ointment. • Take complete patient history, including allergies and other preexisting medical problems. • Monitor vital signs, patient's general appearance, and any changes at bite site. • Reassure patient with disfiguring ulcer that skin grafting can improve appearance. • To prevent brown recluse bites, tell patients to spray areas of infestation with creosote at least every 2 months, to wear gloves and heavy clothes when working around woodpiles or sheds, to inspect outdoor working clothes for spiders before use, and to discourage children from playing near infested areas.
• Neutralization of venom using antivenin I.V., preceded by desensitization when skin or eye tests show sensitivity to horse serum • Calcium gluconate I.V. to control muscle spasms • Muscle relaxants like diazepam for severe muscle spasms • Adrenalin or antihistamines	• Take complete patient history, including allergies and other preexisting medical problems. • Have epinephrine and emergency resuscitation equipment on hand in case of anaphylactic reaction to antivenin. • Keep patient quiet and warm, and the affected part immobile. • Cleanse bite site with antiseptic, and apply ice to relieve pain and swelling, and to slow circulation. • Check vital signs frequently during first 12 hours after bite. Report any changes to

(continued)

Insect Bites and Stings *(continued)*

GENERAL INFORMATION	CLINICAL FEATURES
Black widow spider *(continued)* elderly, infants, and those with allergies)	(especially in children), hyperactive reflexes; hypertension, tachycardia, thready pulse, circulatory collapse, nausea, vomiting, headache, ptosis, eyelid edema, urticaria, pruritus, and fever
Scorpion • Common throughout the United States (30 different species); two deadly species in southwestern states • Curled tail with stinger on end; eight legs; 3″ (7.5 cm) long • Most stings occur during warmer months. • Mortality less than 1% (increased risk among the elderly and children)	*Local reaction:* • Local swelling and tenderness, sharp burning sensation, skin discoloration, paresthesia, lymphangitis with regional gland swelling *Systemic reaction* (neurotoxic): • Immediate sharp pain; hyperesthesia; drowsiness; itching of nose, throat, and mouth; impaired speech (due to sluggish tongue); generalized muscle spasms (including jaw muscle spasms, laryngospasms, incontinence, convulsions, nausea, vomiting, drooling) • Symptoms last from 24 to 78 hours. Bite site recovers last. • Anaphylaxis (rare) • Death may follow cardiovascular or respiratory failure. • Prognosis is poor if symptoms progress rapidly in first few hours.
Bee, wasp, and yellow jacket • When a honeybee (rounded abdomen) or a bumblebee (over 1″ [2.5 cm] long; furry, rounded abdomen) stings, its stinger remains in the victim; the bee flies away and dies. • A wasp or yellow jacket (slender body with elongated abdomen) retains its stinger and can sting repeatedly.	*Local reaction:* painful wound (protruding stinger from bees), edema, urticaria, pruritus *Systemic reaction* (anaphylaxis): symptoms of hypersensitivity usually appear within 20 minutes and may include weakness, chest tightness, dizziness, nausea, vomiting, abdominal cramps, and throat constriction. The shorter the interval between the sting and systemic symptoms, the worse the prognosis. Without prompt treatment, symptoms may progress to cyanosis, coma, and death.

TREATMENT	SPECIAL CONSIDERATIONS
• Oxygen by nasal cannula or mask • Tetanus immunization • Antibiotics to prevent infection	the physician. Symptoms usually subside in 3 to 4 hours. • When giving analgesics, monitor respiratory status. • To prevent black widow spider bites, tell patient to spray areas of infestation with creosote at least every 2 months, to wear gloves and heavy clothing when working around woodpiles or sheds, to inspect outdoor working clothes for spiders before putting them on, and to discourage children from playing near infested areas.
• Antivenin (made from cat serum), if available (contact Antivenin Lab, Arizona State University, Tempe, Arizona) • Calcium gluconate I.V. for muscle spasm • Phenobarbital I.M. for convulsions • Emetine subcutaneously to relieve pain (opiates such as morphine and codeine are contraindicated because they enhance the venom's effects)	• Take complete patient history, including allergies and other preexisting medical conditons. • Immobilize patient, and apply tourniquet proximal to sting. • Pack area extending beyond tourniquet in ice. After 5 minutes of ice pack, remove tourniquet. • Monitor vital signs. Watch closely for signs of respiratory distress. (Keep emergency resuscitation equipment available.)
• Antihistamines and corticosteroids (in urticaria) • Tetanus prophylaxis *In anaphylaxis:* • Oxygen by nasal cannula or mask • Epinephrine 1:1,000 subcutaneously or I.M. • In bronchospasm, aminophylline and hydrocortisone • In hypotension, epinephrine and isoproterenol	• If stinger is in place, scrape it off. Do not pull it; this action releases more toxin. • Cleanse the site and apply ice. • Watch the patient carefully for signs of anaphylaxis. Keep emergency resuscitation equipment available. • Tell patient who is allergic to bee stings to wear a medical identification bracelet or carry a card, and to carry an anaphylaxis kit. Teach him how to use the kit, and refer him to an allergist for hyposensitization. • To prevent bee stings, tell patient not to wear fragrant cosmetics during insect season, to avoid wearing bright colors and going barefoot, to avoid flowers and fruit that attract bees, and to use insect repellent.

—Tumors
—Atresia
Nonmechanical
—Paralytic ileus
—Electrolyte imbalances
—Toxicity
—Neurogenic abnormalities
—Thrombosis or embolism of mesenteric vessels (see *Paralytic [Adynamic] Ileus.*)

Signs and symptoms
Small bowel obstruction
—Colicky pain
—Nausea, vomiting
—Constipation
—Abdominal distention
—Vomiting fecal contents (in complete small bowel obstruction)
—On auscultation, bowel sounds, borborygmi, and rushes (occasionally loud enough to be heard without a stethoscope)
—On palpation, abdominal tenderness, with moderate distention
—Rebound tenderness when obstruction has caused strangulation with ischemia
Large bowel obstruction
Constipation may be the only clinical effect for days. Other symptoms include the following:
—Colicky abdominal pain
—Nausea (vomiting usually absent at first)
—Abdominal distention (degree may be dramatic)
—Eventually, continuous pain
—Possible fecal vomiting

Diagnostic tests
• X-rays confirm the diagnosis. Abdominal films show the presence and location of intestinal gas or fluid. In small bowel obstruction, a typical "stepladder" pattern emerges, with alternating fluid and gas levels apparent in 3 to 4 hours. In large bowel obstruction, barium enema reveals a distended, air-filled colon or a closed loop of sigmoid with extreme distention (in sigmoid volvulus).
• Laboratory results supporting this diagnosis include the following:
—Sodium, chloride, and potassium levels are decreased (due to vomiting).
—WBC count is slightly elevated (with necrosis, peritonitis, or strangulation).
—Serum amylase is increased (possibly from irritation of the pancreas).

Pathophysiology of Intestinal Obstruction

Intestinal obstruction develops in three forms:
• *simple:* blockage prevents intestinal contents from passing, with no other complications
• *strangulated:* blood supply to part or all of the obstructed section is cut off, in addition to blockage of the lumen
• *close-looped:* both ends of a bowel section are occluded, isolating it from the rest of the intestine.

In all three forms, the physiologic effects are similar: when intestinal obstruction occurs, fluid, air, and gas collect near the site. Peristalsis increases temporarily as the bowel tries to force its contents through the obstruction, injuring intestinal mucosa and causing distention at and above the obstruction site. This distention blocks the flow of venous blood and halts normal absorptive processes. As a result, the bowel begins to secrete water, sodium, and potassium into the fluid pooled in the lumen. Obstruction in the upper intestine results in metabolic alkalosis from dehydration and loss of gastric hydrochloric acid. Lower obstruction causes slower dehydration and loss of intestinal alkaline fluids, resulting in metabolic acidosis. Ultimately, intestinal obstruction may lead to ischemia, necrosis, and death.

Paralytic (Adynamic) Ileus

Paralytic ileus is a physiologic form of intestinal obstruction that usually develops in the small bowel after abdominal surgery. It causes decreased or absent intestinal motility that usually disappears spontaneously after 2 to 3 days. This condition can develop as a response to trauma, toxemia, or peritonitis, or as a result of electrolyte deficiencies (especially hypokalemia) and the use of certain drugs, such as ganglionic blocking agents and anticholinergics. It can also result from vascular causes, such as thrombosis or embolism. Excessive air swallowing may contribute to it, but paralytic ileus brought on by this factor alone seldom lasts more than 24 hours.

Clinical effects of paralytic ileus include severe abdominal distention, extreme distress, and possibly, vomiting. The patient may be severely constipated or may pass flatus and small, liquid stools. Paralytic ileus lasting longer than 48 hours necessitates intubation for decompression and nasogastric suctioning. Because of the absence of peristaltic activity, a weighted Cantor tube may be necessary in the patient with extraordinary abdominal distention. However, such procedures must be used with extreme caution, because any additional trauma to the bowel can aggravate ileus. When paralytic ileus results from surgical manipulation of the bowel, treatment may also include cholinergic agents, such as neostigmine or bethanechol.

When caring for patients with paralytic ileus, warn those receiving cholinergic agents to expect certain paradoxical side effects, such as intestinal cramps and diarrhea. Remember that neostigmine produces cardiovascular side effects, usually bradycardia and hypotension. Check frequently for returning bowel sounds.

Treatment

Preoperative therapy consists of correction of fluid and electrolyte imbalances, decompression of the bowel to relieve vomiting and distention, and treatment of shock and peritonitis. Strangulated obstruction usually necessitates blood replacement as well as I.V. fluid administration. Passage of a Levin tube, followed by use of the longer, weighted Miller-Abbott tube, usually accomplishes decompression, especially in small bowel obstruction. Close monitoring of the patient's condition determines duration of treatment. If the patient fails to improve or his condition deteriorates, surgery is necessary. In large bowel obstruction, surgical resection with anastomosis, colostomy, or ileostomy commonly follows decompression with a Levin tube.

Hyperalimentation may be appropriate if the patient suffers a protein deficit from chronic obstruction, postoperative or paralytic ileus, or infection. Drug therapy includes analgesics or sedatives, such as meperidine or phenobarbital (but not opiates, since they inhibit GI motility), and antibiotics for peritonitis caused by strangulation or infarction of the bowel.

Clinical implications

Effective management of intestinal obstruction, a life-threatening condition that often causes overwhelming pain and distress, requires skillful supportive care and keen observation.

• Monitor vital signs frequently. A drop in blood pressure may indicate reduced circulating blood volume due to blood loss from a strangulated hernia. Remember, as much as 10 liters of fluid can collect in the small bowel, drastically reducing plasma volume. Observe closely for signs of shock (pallor, rapid pulse, and hypotension).

• Stay alert for signs of metabolic alkalosis (changes in sensorium; slow, shallow respirations; hypertonic muscles; tetany) or acidosis (shortness of breath on exertion; disorientation; and, later, deep, rapid breathing, weakness, and malaise). Watch for signs and symptoms of secondary infection, such as fever and chills.

• Monitor urinary output carefully to assess renal function, circulating blood volume, and possible urinary retention due to bladder compresson by the distended intestine. If you suspect bladder compression, catheterize the patient for residual urine immediately after he has voided. Also measure abdominal girth frequently to detect progressive distention.

• Provide fastidious mouth and nose care if the patient has undergone decompression by intubation or if he has vomited. Look for signs of dehydration (thick, swollen tongue; dry, cracked lips; dry oral mucous membranes). Record amount and color of drainage from the decompression tube. Irrigate the tube, if necessary, with normal saline solution to maintain patency.

• If a weighted tube has been inserted, check periodically to make sure it is advancing. Help the patient turn from side to side (or walk around, if he can) to facilitate passage of the tube.

• Keep the patient in Fowler's position as much as possible to promote pulmonary ventilation and ease respiratory distress from abdominal distention. Listen for bowel sounds, and watch for signs of returning peristalsis (passage of flatus and mucus through the rectum).

• Explain all diagnostic and therapeutic procedures to the patient and answer any questions he may have. Make sure he understands that these procedures are necessary to relieve the obstruction and reduce pain. Tell the patient to lie on his left side for about a half hour before X-rays are taken. Prepare him and his family for the possibility of surgery, and provide emotional support and positive reinforcement afterward. Arrange for an enterostomal therapist to visit the patient who has had a colostomy.

Complications
• Metabolic alkalosis or metabolic acidosis
• Peritonitis
• Hypovolemic shock

Intussusception

Description
Intussusception is a telescoping (invagination) of a portion of the bowel into an adjacent distal portion. It occurs most often in infants. Intussusception may be fatal, especially if treatment is delayed more than 24 hours. Strangulation of the intestine usually occurs, with gangrene, shock, and perforation.

Causes
Infants
Unknown
Older children
—Polyps
—Alterations in intestinal motility
—Hemangioma
—Lymphosarcoma
—Lymphoid hyperplasia
—Meckel's diverticulum
Adults
—Benign or malignant tumors
—Polyps
—Meckel's diverticulum
—Gastroenterostomy with herniation
—Appendiceal stump

Signs and symptoms
Infants or children
—Intermittent attacks of colicky pain. These cause the child to scream, draw his legs up to his abdomen, turn pale and diaphoretic, and possibly display grunting respirations.
—Vomiting. Initially, stomach contents and, later, bile-stained or fecal material, are vomited.

—"Currant jelly" stools. Feces contain a mixture of blood and mucus.
—Tender, distended abdomen. There is a palpable, sausage-shaped abdominal mass. Often, the viscera are absent from the right lower quadrant.
Adults
—Intermittent colicky abdominal pain and tenderness
—Vomiting
—Diarrhea
—Occasionally constipation
—Bloody stools
—Weight loss
—With strangulation, excruciating pain, abdominal distention, and tachycardia

Diagnostic tests
• Barium enema confirms colonic intussusception when it shows the characteristic coiled spring sign; it also delineates the extent of intussusception.
• Upright abdominal X-rays may show a soft-tissue mass and signs of complete or partial obstruction, with dilated loops of bowel.
• WBC count up to 15,000/mm^3 indicates obstruction; greater than 15,000/mm^3, strangulation. If the count exceeds 20,000/mm^3, bowel infarction should be considered.

Treatment
In children, therapy may include hydrostatic reduction or surgery. Surgery is indicated for children with recurrent intussusception, for those who show signs of shock or peritonitis, and for those in whom symptoms have been present longer than 24 hours. In adults, surgery is always the treatment of choice.

During hydrostatic reduction, the radiologist drips a barium solution into the rectum from a height of not more than 3′ (0.9 m); fluoroscopy traces the progress of the barium. If the procedure is successful, the barium backwashes into the ileum, and the mass disappears. If not, the procedure is stopped, and the patient is prepared for surgery.

During surgery, manual reduction is attempted first. After compressing the bowel above the intussusception, the physician attempts to milk the intussusception back through the bowel. However, if manual reduction fails, or if the bowel is gangrenous or strangulated, the physician will perform a resection of the affected bowel segment. In addition, he will probably perform a prophylactic appendectomy.

Clinical implications
• Monitor vital signs before and after surgery. A change in temperature may indicate sepsis. Infants may become hypothermic at onset of infection. Rising pulse rate and falling blood pressure may be signs of peritonitis.
• Check intake and output. Watch for signs of dehydration and bleeding. If the patient is in shock, give blood or plasma, as ordered.
• A nasogastric tube is inserted to decompress the intestine and minimize vomiting. Monitor tube drainage, and replace volume lost, as ordered.
• After surgery, administer broad-spectrum antibiotics, as ordered, and give meticulous wound care. Most incisions heal without complications. However, closely check the incision for inflammation, drainage, or suture separation.
• Encourage the patient to cough productively by turning him from side to side. Take care to splint the incision when he coughs, or teach him to do so himself. In addition, make sure he takes 10 deep breaths an hour.
• Oral fluids may be resumed postoperatively when bowel sounds and peristalsis return, nasogastric tube drainage is minimal, the abdomen remains soft, and vomiting does not occur when the nasogastric tube is clamped briefly for a trial period. When the patient tolerates oral fluids well, the tube can be removed and the patient's diet gradually returned to normal, as tolerated.

• Check for abdominal distention after the patient resumes a normal diet, and monitor his general condition.

• Offer special reassurance and emotional support to the child and parents. This condition is considered a pediatric emergency, and parents are often unprepared for their child's hospitalization and possible surgery; they may feel guilty for not seeking medical aid when their child first began exhibiting symptoms. Similarly, the child is unprepared for an abrupt separation from his parents and familiar environment.

• To minimize the stress of hospitalization, encourage parents to participate in their child's care as much as possible. Be flexible about visiting hours.

Iron deficiency anemia

Description
Iron deficiency anemia is caused by an inadequate supply of iron for optimal formation of RBCs, resulting in smaller (microcytic) cells with less color on staining. Body stores of iron, including plasma iron, decrease, as does transferrin, which binds with and transports iron. Insufficient body stores of iron lead to a depleted RBC mass and, in turn, to a decreased hemoglobin concentration (hypochromia) and decreased oxygen-carrying capacity of the blood. Iron deficiency anemia occurs most commonly in premenopausal women, infants (particularly premature or low-birth-weight infants), children, and adolescents (especially girls).

Causes
• Inadequate dietary intake of iron (less than 1 to 2 mg/day), as in prolonged unsupplemented breast- or bottle-feeding of infants, or during periods of stress, such as rapid growth in children and adolescents
• Iron malabsorption, as in chronic diarrhea, partial or total gastrectomy, and malabsorption syndromes, such as celiac disease

---

Preventing Iron Deficiency Anemia

Public health professionals can play a vital role in the prevention of iron deficiency anemia by following these guidelines.
• Teach the basics of a nutritionally balanced diet—red meats, green vegetables, eggs, whole wheat, iron-fortified bread, and milk. (However, no food in itself contains enough iron to *treat* iron deficiency anemia; an average-sized person with anemia would have to eat at least 10 lb of steak daily to receive therapeutic amounts of iron.)
• Emphasize the need for high-risk individuals—such as premature infants, children under age 2, and pregnant women—to receive prophylactic oral iron, as ordered by a physician. (Children under age 2 should also receive supplemental cereals and formulas high in iron.)
• Assess a family's dietary habits for iron intake and note the influence of childhood eating patterns, cultural food preferences, and family income on adequate nutrition.
• Encourage families with deficient iron intake to eat meat, fish, or poultry; whole or enriched grain; and foods high in ascorbic acid.
• Carefully assess a patient's drug history, since certain drugs, such as pancreatic enzymes and vitamin E, may interfere with iron metabolism and absorption and since aspirin, steroids, and other drugs may cause gastrointestinal bleeding. (Teach patients who must take gastric irritants to take these medications with meals or milk.)

Supportive Management of Patients with Anemia

To meet the anemic patient's nutritional needs:
• If the patient is fatigued, urge him to eat small, frequent meals throughout the day.
• If he has oral lesions, suggest soft, cool, bland foods.
• If he has dyspepsia, eliminate spicy foods, and include milk and dairy products in his diet.
• If the patient is anorexic and irritable, encourage his family to bring his favorite foods from home (unless his diet is restricted) and to keep him company during meals if possible.

To set limitations on activities:
• Assess the effect of a specific activity by monitoring pulse rate during the activity. If the patient's pulse accelerates rapidly and he develops hypotension with hypernoia, diaphoresis, light-headedness, palpitations, shortness of breath, or weakness, the activity is too strenuous.
• Tell the patient to pace his activities, and to allow for frequent rest periods.

To decrease the patient's susceptibility to infection:
• Use strict aseptic technique.
• Isolate the patient from infectious persons.
• Instruct the patient to avoid crowds and other sources of infection. Encourage him to practice good hand-washing technique. Stress the importance of receiving necessary immunizations and prompt medical treatment for any sign of infection.

To prepare the patient for diagnostic testing:
• Explain erythropoiesis, the function of blood, and the purpose of diagnostic and therapeutic procedures.
• Tell the patient how he can participate in diagnostic testing. Give him an honest description of the pain or discomfort he will probably experience.
• If possible, schedule all tests to avoid disrupting the patient's meals, sleep, and visiting hours.

To prevent complications:
• Observe for signs of bleeding that may exacerbate anemia. Check stool for occult bleeding. Assess for ecchymoses, gingival bleeding, and hematuria. Monitor vital signs frequently.
• If the patient is confined to strict bed rest, assist with range-of-motion exercises and frequent turning, coughing, and deep breathing.
• If blood transfusions are needed for severe anemia (hemoglobin less than 5 g/100 ml), give washed RBCs, as ordered, in partial exchange if evidence of pump failure is present. Carefully monitor for signs of circulatory overload or transfusion reaction. Watch for a change in pulse rate, blood pressure, or respirations, or onset of fever, chills, pruritus, or edema. If any of these signs develop, stop the transfusion and notify the physician.
• Warn the patient to move about or change positions slowly to minimize dizziness induced by cerebral hypoxia.

• Blood loss secondary to drug-induced gastrointestinal bleeding (from anticoagulants, aspirin, steroids) or due to heavy menses, hemorrhage from trauma, gastrointestinal ulcers, malignancy, or varices

• Pregnancy, in which the mother's iron supply is diverted to the fetus for erythropoiesis

• Intravascular hemolysis-induced hemoglobinuria or paroxysmal nocturnal hemoglobinuria

• Mechanical erythrocyte trauma caused by a prosthetic heart valve

Signs and symptoms

There may be no symptoms initially.

• Dyspnea on exertion
• Fatigue
• Listlessness
• Pallor
• Inability to concentrate
• Irritability
• Headache
• Tachycardia
• Numbness and tingling of the extremities
• Neurologic pain
• Brittle, spoon-shaped nails and cracks at corners of mouth in chronic iron deficiency

Diagnostic tests

• Hemoglobin levels are decreased

Teaching Topics in Iron Deficiency Anemia

• Explanation of iron deficiency anemia (including roles played by iron and red blood cells, hemoglobin, and tissue oxygenation)
• Explanation of the cause of the patient's anemia
• Frequent blood tests to determine serum iron level
• Foods high in iron
• Daily iron supplements
• Importance of follow-up visits

(males, < 12 g/100 ml; females, < 10 g/100ml).

• Hematocrit levels are decreased (males, < 47%; females, < 42%)

• Serum iron levels are decreased, with high binding capacity.

• Serum ferritin levels are low.

• RBC count is low, with microcytic and hypochromic cells. (In early stages, RBC count may be normal, except in infants and children.)

• Mean corpuscular hemoglobin is decreased in severe anemia.

• Bone marrow studies reveal depleted or absent iron stores (on staining) and normoblastic hyperplasia.

Treatment

The first priority of treatment is to determine the underlying cause of anemia. Once this is determined, iron replacement therapy can begin. Treatment of choice is an oral preparation of iron or a combination of iron and ascorbic acid, which enhances iron absorption. In some cases, iron may have to be administered parenterally—for instance, if the patient is noncompliant with the oral preparation, if he needs more iron than he can take orally, if malabsorption prevents adequate iron absorption, or if a maximum rate of hemoglobin regeneration is desired.

Because total dose I.V. infusion of supplemental iron is painless and requires fewer injections, it is usually preferred to I.M. administration. Pregnant patients and geriatric patients with severe anemia, for example, should receive a total dose infusion of iron dextran in normal saline solution over 8 hours. To minimize the risk of an allergic reaction to iron, an I.V. test dose of 0.5 ml should be given first.

Clinical implications

• Monitor the patient's compliance with the prescribed iron supplement therapy. Advise the patient not to stop therapy even if he feels better, since

replacement of iron stores takes time.
• Advise the patient that milk or an antacid interferes with absorption but that vitamin C can increase absorption. Instruct the patient to drink liquid supplemental iron through a straw to prevent staining his teeth.
• Tell the patient to report any side effects of iron therapy, such as nausea, vomiting, diarrhea, or constipation, which may require a dosage adjustment.
• If the patient receives iron intravenously, monitor the infusion rate carefully, and observe for an allergic reaction. Stop the infusion and begin supportive treatment immediately if the patient shows signs of an adverse reaction. Also, watch for dizziness and headache and for thrombophlebitis around the I.V. site.
• Use the Z-track injection method when administering iron I.M. to prevent skin discoloration, scarring, and irritating iron deposits in the skin.
• Since an iron deficiency may recur, advise regular checkups. (See *Preventing Iron Deficiency Anemia*, p. 420; *Supportive Management of Patients with Anemia*, p. 421; and *Teaching Topics in Iron Deficiency Anemia*.)

Irritable bowel syndrome
(Spastic colon, spastic colitis)

Description

Irritable bowel syndrome is a common condition marked by chronic or periodic diarrhea, alternating with constipation, and accompanied by straining and abdominal cramps. Diagnosis of irritable bowel syndrome requires a careful history to determine contributing psychological factors, such as a recent stressful life change.

Diagnosis must also rule out other disorders, such as amebiasis, diverticulitis, colon cancer, and lactose intolerance. Prognosis is good. Supportive treatment or avoidance of a known irritant often relieves symptoms.

Causes
• Generally associated with psychological stress
• May result from physical factors, such as diverticular disease, ingestion of irritants (coffee, raw fruits or vegetables), lactose intolerance, abuse of laxatives, food poisoning, or colon cancer

Signs and symptoms
The following symptoms alternate with constipation or normal bowel function:
• Lower abdominal pain (usually relieved by defecation or passage of gas)
• Diarrhea (typically occurs during the day)
• Small stools that contain visible mucus
• Possible dyspepsia and abdominal distention

Diagnostic tests
These may include sigmoidoscopy, colonoscopy, barium enema, rectal biopsy, and stool examination for blood, parasites, and bacteria.

Treatment
Therapy aims to relieve symptoms and includes counseling to help the patient understand the relationship between stress and his illness. Strict dietary restrictions are not beneficial, but food irritants should be investigated. The patient should be instructed to avoid them. Rest and heat applied to the abdomen are helpful, as is judicious use of sedatives (phenobarbital) and antispasmodics (propantheline, diphenoxylate with atropine sulfate). With chronic use, however, the patient may become dependent on these drugs. If

Teaching Topics in Irritable Bowel Syndrome

• Explanation of the disorder and its causative factors
• Preparation for tests, such as barium enema and proctosigmoidoscopy, to rule out other disorders
• Dietary measures to prevent pain, constipation, and diarrhea
• Medication administration: anticholinergics and tranquilizers
• Other care measures: stress management, cessation of smoking, and development of a regular bowel routine

the cause of irritable bowel syndrome is chronic laxative abuse, bowel training may help correct the condition.

Clinical implications
Since the patient with irritable bowel syndrome is not hospitalized, focus your care on patient teaching.
• Tell the patient to avoid irritating foods, and encourage development of regular bowel habits.
• Help the patient deal with stress, and warn against dependence on sedatives or antispasmodics.
• Encourage regular checkups, since irritable bowel syndrome is associated with a higher-than-normal incidence of diverticulitis and colon cancer. For patients over age 40, emphasize the need for an annual sigmoidoscopy and rectal examination. (See *Teaching Topics in Irritable Bowel Syndrome*.)

J

Juvenile rheumatoid arthritis

Description
Affecting children under age 16, juvenile rheumatoid arthritis (JRA) is an inflammatory disorder of the connective tissues characterized by joint swelling and pain or tenderness. It may also involve organs such as the skin, heart, lungs, liver, spleen, and eyes, producing extraarticular signs and symptoms. There are three major types of JRA: systemic (Stills' disease or acute febrile type), polyarticular, and pauciarticular.

Cause
The cause of JRA remains puzzling. Research continues to test several theories, such as those linking JRA to genetic factors or to an abnormal immune response. Viral or bacterial (particularly streptococcal) infection, trauma, and emotional stress may be precipitating factors, but their relationship to JRA remains unclear.

Signs and symptoms
Persistent joint pain, typical rash, and fever point to JRA. A characteristic symptom is joint stiffness in the morning or after periods of inactivity. Growth disturbances may also occur, resulting in overgrowth or undergrowth adjacent to inflamed joints. Other specific signs and symptoms vary with the type of JRA.

Systemic JRA
—Joint pain
—Intermittent spiking fever (to 103° F. [39.4° C.] or higher)
—Possible rash (consists of small, pale or salmon pink macules, most commonly on the trunk and proximal extremities)
—Possible hepatosplenomegaly, lymphadenopathy, nonspecific abdominal pain, and manifestations of pleuritis, pericarditis, and myocarditis

Polyarticular JRA
—Swollen, tender, stiff joints (five or more joints involved in this type; clinical effects are usually symmetric and may be remittent or indolent)
—Possible low-grade fever with daily peaks
—Possible listlessness and weight loss
—Subcutaneous nodules on the elbows or heels
—Developmental retardation
—Possible lymphadenopathy and hepatosplenomegaly

Pauciarticular JRA
—Limited joint involvement (usually no more than four joints involved in this type)
—Chronic iridocyclitis in one subtype (may be asymptomatic or may produce pain, redness, blurred vision, and photophobia)
—Possible acute iritis

Diagnostic tests
Laboratory tests are useful for ruling out other inflammatory or even malignant diseases that can mimic JRA and for monitoring disease activity and response to therapy.
• CBC shows decreased hemoglobin,

neutrophilia, and thrombocytosis.
- Erythrocyte sedimentation rate, C-reactive protein, haptoglobin, immunoglobulins, and C3 complement may be elevated.
- ANA test may be positive in patients who have pauciarticular JRA with chronic iridocyclitis.
- RF is present in 15% of JRA cases, as compared with 85% of RA cases.
- Presence of HLA-B27 may forecast later development of ankylosing spondylitis.
- Early X-ray changes include soft-tissue swelling, effusion, and periostitis in affected joints. Later, osteoporosis and accelerated bone growth may appear, followed by subchondral erosions, joint space narrowing, bone destruction, and fusion.

Treatment and clinical implications

Successful management of JRA usually involves administration of anti-inflammatory drugs, physical therapy, carefully planned nutrition and exercise, and regular eye examinations. Both child and parents must be involved in therapy.

Aspirin is the initial drug of choice, with dosage based on the child's weight. However, other nonsteroidal anti-inflammatory drugs (NSAIDs) may also be used. If these prove ineffective, gold salts, hydroxychloroquine, and penicillamine may be tried. Because of adverse effects, steroids are generally reserved for treatment of systemic complications, such as pericarditis or iritis, that are resistant to NSAIDs. Corticosteroids and mydriatic drugs are commonly used for iridocyclitis. Low-dose cytotoxic drug therapy is currently being investigated.

Physical therapy promotes regular exercise to maintain joint mobility and muscle strength, thereby preventing contractures, deformity, and disability. Good posture, gait training, and joint protection are also beneficial. Splints help reduce pain, prevent contractures, and maintain correct joint alignment.

Parents and health care professionals should encourage the child to be as independent as possible and to develop a positive attitude toward school, social development, and vocational planning.

Regular slit-lamp examinations help ensure early diagnosis and treatment of iridocyclitis. Children with pauciarticular JRA with chronic iridocyclitis should be checked every 3 months during periods of active disease and every 6 months during remissions.

Generally, the prognosis for JRA is good, although disabilities can occur. Surgery is usually limited to soft-tissue releases to improve joint mobility. Joint replacement is delayed until the child has matured physically and can handle vigorous rehabilitation.

K

Keratitis

Description

Keratitis, or inflammation of the cornea, is usually unilateral. It may be acute or chronic, superficial or deep. Superficial keratitis is fairly common and may develop at any age. Prognosis is good, with treatment. Untreated, recurrent keratitis may lead to blindness.

Causes

Type I infection by *Herpesvirus hominis,* (dendritic keratitis) is the usual cause. Other causes include the following.
• Exposure of the cornea resulting from inability to close eyelids
• Congenital syphilis
• Bacterial or fungal infection (less common)

Signs and symptoms

• Opacities of the cornea
• Mild irritation
• Tearing
• Photophobia
• Possible blurred vision

Diagnostic tests

• Slit-lamp examination confirms keratitis.
• If keratitis is due to herpesvirus, staining the eye with a fluorescein strip reveals one or more small branchlike (dendritic) lesions, and touching the cornea with cotton reveals reduced corneal sensation.
• Vision testing may show slightly decreased acuity.

Treatment

Treatment of acute keratitis due to herpesvirus consists of idoxuridine eye drops and ointment or vidarabine ointment. Trifluridine is used to treat recurrent herpetic keratitis. A broad-spectrum antibiotic may prevent secondary bacterial infection. Chronic dendritic keratitis may respond more quickly to vidarabine. Long-term topical therapy may be necessary. (Corticosteroid therapy is contraindicated in dendritic keratitis or any other viral or fungal disease of the cornea.) Treatment for fungal keratitis consists of natamycin.

Keratitis due to exposure requires application of moisturizing ointment to the exposed cornea and of a plastic bubble eye shield or eye patch. Treatment for severe corneal scarring may include keratoplasty (cornea transplantation).

Clinical implications

• Look for keratitis in patients predisposed to cold sores. Explain that stress, trauma, fever, colds, and overexposure to the sun may trigger flare-ups.
• Protect the exposed corneas of unconscious patients by cleaning the eyes daily, applying moisturizing ointment, or covering the eyes with an eye shield.

Kidney cancer
(Nephrocarcinoma, renal cell carcinoma, hypernephroma, Grawitz's tumor)

Description
Kidney cancer usually occurs in older adults. Renal pelvic tumors and Wilms' tumor occur primarily in children. About 85% of kidney cancers are primary tumors; others are metastases.

Usually, kidney tumors are large, firm, nodular, encapsulated, unilateral, and solitary. Occasionally, they are bilateral or multifocal.

The incidence of this malignancy is rising, possibly as a result of exposure to environmental carcinogens as well as increased longevity. Overall, prognosis for kidney cancer has improved considerably, with the 5-year survival rate now at approximately 50% of patients and the 10-year survival rate at 18% to 23% of patients. (See *Staging Kidney Cancer*.)

Cause
Unknown

Signs and symptoms
Any of the following may occur:

Staging Kidney Cancer

Stage I: Tumor confined to kidney

Stage II: Perirenal spread confined to Gerota's space (fascia around the kidney)

Stage III: Spread to renal vein or inferior vena cava, with or without lymphatic involvement

Stage IV: Advanced disease, with spread to adjacent organs (except for adrenal glands) or metastases, usually to distant lymph nodes, lungs, liver, and bone

---

• Hematuria
• Constant abdominal or flank pain (may be dull or, if the cancer causes bleeding or clot formation, acute and colicky)
• Palpable mass (generally, smooth, firm, and nontender)
• Fever
• Hypertension
• Weight loss, edema in the legs, nausea, and vomiting. These symptoms point to advanced disease.

Diagnostic tests
• Studies to identify kidney cancer usually include CT scans, intravenous pyelography, retrograde pyelography, ultrasound studies, cystoscopy (to rule out associated bladder cancer), and nephrotomography or renal angiography to distinguish a kidney cyst from a tumor.
• Other relevant tests include liver function studies, showing increased alkaline phosphatase, bilirubin, transaminase, and prolonged prothrombin time. (Such results may point to liver metastasis, but if the tumor has not metastasized, these abnormalities reverse after tumor resection.)

Treatment
Radical nephrectomy, with or without regional lymph node dissection, offers the only chance of cure for a patient with kidney cancer. Since this disease is radiation resistant, radiation is used only when the tumor has spread into the perinephric region or the lymph nodes, or when the primary tumor or metastatic sites cannot be completely excised. Then, high radiation doses are usually necessary.

Clinical implications
Meticulous postoperative care, supportive treatment (including relief from associated symptoms and side effects) during radiation and chemotherapy, and psychological support can hasten recovery and minimize complications.

Before surgery, follow these guidelines:
• Encourage the patient to express his anxieties and fears. Assure him that his body will adapt to the loss of a kidney.
• Explain the possible side effects of radiation and chemotherapy.
• Teach the patient about the expected postoperative procedures, as well as diaphragmatic breathing, how to cough properly, and how to splint his incision while coughing.

After surgery, follow these guidelines:
• Encourage diaphragmatic breathing and coughing.
• Assist the patient with leg exercises to reduce the risk of phlebitis, and turn him every 2 hours.
• Check dressings often for excessive bleeding. Watch for signs of internal bleeding, such as restlessness, sweating, and increased pulse rate.
• Position the patient on the operative side to allow the pressure of adjacent organs to fill the dead space at the operative site and thus improve dependent drainage. If possible, assist the patient with walking within 24 hours after surgery.
• Maintain adequate fluid intake, and monitor intake and output. Monitor lab results for anemia, polycythemia, or abnormal blood chemistries that may point to bone or hepatic involvement or may result from radiation or chemotherapy.
• Symptomatically treat all drug side effects.
• When preparing a patient for discharge, stress the importance of compliance with any prescribed outpatient treatment. This includes an annual follow-up chest X-ray to rule out lung metastasis and intravenous pyelography every 6 to 12 months to check for contralateral tumors.

Complications
Hypercalcemia

Klinefelter's syndrome

Description
This relatively common genetic abnormality, probably the most common cause of hypogonadism, affects only males. It usually becomes apparent at puberty, when the secondary sex characteristics develop. Although the penis is normal, the testicles fail to mature, and degenerative testicular changes eventually result in irreversible infertility. Klinefelter's syndrome is also associated with a tendency toward mental deficiency. In addition, it is associated with increased incidence of pulmonary disease, varicose veins, and breast cancer. (See also *Turner's Syndrome,* p. 430.)

Cause
One or more extra X chromosomes

Signs and symptoms
Characteristic features apparent at puberty
—Small penis and prostate
—Small, firm testicles
—Sparse facial and abdominal hair
—Feminine distribution of pubic hair
—Sexual dysfunction (impotence, lack of libido)
—Gynecomastia, in less than 50% of patients
Other associated problems
—Mental retardation
—Osteoporosis
—Abnormal body build (long legs with short, obese trunk)
—Tall stature
—Tendency toward alcoholism, antisocial behavior, and other personality disorders

Diagnostic tests
• Chromosome analysis determined by culturing lymphocytes from peripheral blood confirms the diagnosis.
• Urinary 17-ketosteroids are decreased.
• Follicle-stimulating hormone (FSH)

Turner's Syndrome

In Turner's syndrome, the missing X chromosome (or missing part of the second X chromosome) may be lost from either ovum or sperm through nondisjunction or chromosome lag. Mixed aneuploidy may result from mitotic nondisjunction.

Incidence of Turner's syndrome is 1 per 2,500 to 1 per 7,000 births; 95% to 98% of fetuses with this syndrome are spontaneously aborted.

Turner's syndrome produces certain characteristic signs. At birth, 50% of infants with this syndrome measure below the third percentile in length. Commonly, they have swollen hands and feet, a wide chest with laterally displaced nipples, and a low hairline that becomes more obvious as they grow. They may have severe webbing of the neck; some have coarse, enlarged, prominent ears. Gonadal dysgenesis is seen at birth and typically causes sterility in adults.

Cardiovascular malformations occur in 10% to 40% of patients, but renal abnormalities are even more common. Short stature (usually under 59″ [150 cm]) is the most common adult sign.

Most patients have average or slightly below average intelligence; they commonly show space-form blindness, right-left disorientation for extrapersonal space, and defective figure drawing. They are typically immature, socially naive, and conforming.

Turner's syndrome can be diagnosed by chromosome analysis. Differential should rule out mixed gonadal dysgenesis, Noonan-Ehmke's syndrome, and other similar disorders.

Treatment should begin in early childhood and include hormonal therapy: androgens, human growth hormone, and, possibly, small doses of estrogen. Later, progesterone and estrogen can induce sexual maturation.

excretion is increased.
• Plasma testosterone levels after puberty are decreased.

Treatment and clinical implications

Depending on severity, treatment may include mastectomy in persistent gynecomastia, and supplemental testosterone in sexual dysfunction. However, not all patients need hormonal treatment. The testicular changes that lead to infertility cannot be prevented. But earlier treatment may be more effective.

Psychotherapy with sexual counseling is indicated when sexual dysfunction causes emotional maladjustment. If patients with the mosaic form (only some, not all, cells have the extra X chromosomes) of the syndrome are fertile, genetic counseling is essential,

since they may transmit this chromosomal abnormality.

Encourage such patients to discuss feelings of confusion and rejection that may arise, and reinforce their male identity. Improve compliance with hormone therapy by making sure they understand testosterone's benefits and side effects.

Kyphosis
(Roundback)

Description
Kyphosis is an anteroposterior curving of the spine that causes a bowing of the back, commonly at the thoracic level, but sometimes at the thoracolumbar or sacral level. Normally, the spine displays some convexity, but excessive thoracic kyphosis is patho-

logic. There are three types of kyphosis: congenital (rare), adolescent, and adult.

Causes

Adolescent kyphosis

—Growth retardation or a vascular disturbance in the vertebral epiphysis (usually at the thoracic level) during periods of rapid growth

—Congenital deficiency in the thickness of the vertebral plates

—Infection

—Inflammation

—Aseptic necrosis

—Disk degeneration

Adult kyphosis

—Aging and associated degeneration of intervertebral disks, atrophy, and osteoporotic vertebral collapse

—Endocrine disorders such as hyperparathyroidism, and Cushing's disease

—Prolonged steroid therapy

—Arthritis

—Paget's disease

—Polio

—Compression fracture of the thoracic vertebrae

—Metastatic tumor

—Plasma cell myeloma

—Tuberculosis

—Poor posture

Signs and symptoms

If kyphosis is caused by factors other than poor posture alone, the spine will not straighten out when the patient assumes a recumbent position.

Adolescent kyphosis

—May be asymptomatic

—Mild pain at the apex of the curve (about 50% of patients)

—Fatigue

—Tenderness or stiffness in the involved area or along the entire spine

—Prominent vertebral spinous processes at the lower dorsal and upper lumbar levels, with compensatory increased lumbar lordosis

—Hamstring tightness

Adult kyphosis

—Characteristic roundback appearance

—Possible pain, weakness of the back, and generalized fatigue

—Local tenderness (associated with recent compression fracture in senile osteoporosis; otherwise rare in adult kyphosis)

Diagnostic tests

• X-rays may show vertebral wedging, Schmorl's nodes, irregular end plates, and possibly mild scoliosis of 10° to 20°.

• Vertebral biopsy may be needed to evaluate other sites of bone disease, primary sites of malignancy, and infection.

Treatment

For kyphosis caused by poor posture alone, treatment may consist of therapeutic exercises, bed rest on a firm mattress (with or without traction), and a brace to straighten the kyphotic curve until spinal growth is complete.

Treatment for both adolescent and adult kyphosis also includes appropriate measures for the underlying cause and, possibly, spinal arthrodesis for relief of symptoms. Although rarely necessary, surgery may be recommended when kyphosis causes neurologic damage, a spinal curve greater than 60°, or intractable and disabling back pain in a patient with full skeletal maturity. Preoperative measures may include halo-femoral traction. Corrective surgery includes a posterior spinal fusion with spinal instrumentation, iliac bone grafting, and plaster immobilization. Anterior spinal fusion followed by immobilization in plaster may be necessary when kyphosis produces a spinal curve greater than 70°.

Clinical implications

Effective management of kyphosis necessitates first-rate supportive care for patients in traction or a brace, skillful patient teaching, and sensitive emotional support.

• Teach the patient with adolescent kyphosis caused by poor posture alone the prescribed therapeutic exercises and the fundamentals of good posture. Suggest bed rest when pain is severe. Encourage use of a firm mattress, preferably with a bed board. If the patient needs a brace, explain its purpose and teach him how and when to wear it. Teach good skin care. The patient should not use lotions, ointments, or powders where the brace contacts the skin. Warn that only the physician or orthotist should adjust the brace.

• If corrective surgery is needed, explain all preoperative tests thoroughly, as well as the need for postoperative traction or casting, if applicable. After surgery, check neurovascular status every 2 to 4 hours for the first 48 hours, and report any changes immediately. Turn the patient often by logrolling him.

• Offer pain medication every 3 or 4 hours for the first 48 hours. Institute blood product replacement, if ordered. Accurately measure fluid intake and output, including urine specific gravity. Insert a nasogastric tube and a Foley catheter.

• Give meticulous skin care. Change dressings as ordered.

• Provide emotional support. The adolescent patient is likely to exhibit mood changes and periods of depression. Maintain communication, and offer frequent encouragement and reassurance.

• Assist during removal of sutures and application of a new cast (usually about 10 days after surgery). Encourage gradual ambulation (often with the use of a tilt-table in the physical therapy department).

• At discharge, provide detailed, written cast care instructions. Tell the patient to report immediately pain, burning, skin breakdown, loss of feeling, tingling, numbness, or cast odor. Advise the patient to drink plenty of liquids to avoid constipation, and to report any illness (especially abdominal pain or vomiting) immediately.

Arrange for home visits by a social worker and a home care nurse.

Complications

• Rarely, kyphosis may induce neurologic damage: spastic paraparesis secondary to spinal cord compression or herniated nucleus pulposus.

• In adults, disk lesions called Schmorl's nodes may develop in the anteroposterior curvature of the spine. These are localized protrusions of nuclear material through the cartilage plates and into the spongy bone of the vertebral bodies. If the anterior portions of the cartilage are destroyed, bridges of new bone may form in the intervertebral space, causing ankylosis.

L

Labyrinthitis

Description

Labyrinthitis, an inflammation of the labyrinth of the inner ear, frequently incapacitates the patient by producing severe vertigo that lasts for 3 to 5 days. Symptoms gradually subside over a 3- to 6-week period. Viral labyrinthitis is often associated with upper respiratory tract infections.

Causes

• Organisms that cause acute febrile diseases, such as pneumonia, influenza, and especially chronic otitis media
• Toxic drugs

Signs and symptoms

• Severe vertigo with any movement of the head
• Sensorineural hearing loss
• Possible spontaneous nystagmus, with jerking movements of the eyes toward the unaffected ear; nausea, vomiting, and giddiness; and with severe bacterial infection, purulent drainage

Diagnostic tests

• Audiometric testing
• Culture and sensitivity testing, if purulent drainage is present
• Other possible tests: intracranial CT scan to rule out a brain lesion; caloric testing to rule out Ménière's disease

Treatment

Symptomatic treatment includes bed rest with the head immobilized between pillows, meclizine P.O. to control vertigo, and massive doses of antibiotics to combat diffuse purulent labyrinthitis. Oral fluids can prevent dehydration from vomiting. For severe nausea and vomiting, I.V. fluids may be necessary.

When conservative management fails, surgical excision of the cholesteatoma and drainage of the infected areas of the middle and inner ear are necessary. Prevention is possible by early and vigorous treatment of predisposing conditions, such as otitis media and local or systemic infection.

Clinical implications

• Keep the side rails up to prevent falls.
• If vomiting is severe, administer antiemetics, as ordered. Record intake and output, and give I.V. fluids, as ordered.
• Reassure the patient that recovery is certain but may take as long as 6 weeks. Tell the patient that during this time he should limit activities that vertigo may make hazardous, such as climbing a ladder or driving a car.

Laryngeal cancer

Description

The most common form of laryngeal cancer is squamous cell carcinoma (95%). Rare forms include adenocarcinoma, sarcoma, and others. Such cancer may be intrinsic or extrinsic. An intrinsic tumor is on the true vocal cords and does not have a tendency to spread, because underlying connective tissues lack lymph nodes. An extrinsic tumor is on another part of the larynx and tends to spread early.

Laryngeal cancer is classified according to its location: supraglottis (posterior surface of the epiglottis, aryepiglottic folds, false vocal cords), glottis (true vocal cords), and subglottis (downward extension from vocal cords [rare]).

Cause
Unknown

Risk factors
Major
—Smoking
—Alcoholism
Minor
—Chronic inhalation of noxious fumes
—Familial tendency
—History of frequent laryngitis and vocal straining

Signs and symptoms
Intrinsic tumor
—The earliest symptom is hoarseness that persists longer than 3 weeks.
Extrinsic tumor
—Lump in the throat
—Burning in the throat or pain when drinking citrus juice or hot liquid
Metastatic effects
—Dysphagia
—Dyspnea
—Cough
—Enlarged cervical lymph nodes
—Pain radiating to the ear

Diagnostic tests
• Indirect (mirror visualization) or direct laryngoscopy is required for hoarseness that lasts longer than 2 weeks.
• Firm diagnosis also requires xeroradiography, laryngoscopy, biopsy, laryngeal tomography, CT scan, or laryngography to define the borders of the lesion, and chest X-ray to detect metastases.

Treatment
In laryngeal cancer, the goal of treatment is to eliminate the cancer through surgery, radiation, or both, and to preserve speech. Surgical procedures vary with tumor size and can include cordectomy, partial or total laryngectomy, supraglottic laryngectomy, or total laryngectomy with laryngoplasty.

If speech preservation is not possible, speech rehabilitation may include esophageal speech or prosthetic devices. Surgical techniques to construct a new voice box are still experimental.

Clinical implications
Psychological support and good preoperative and postoperative care can minimize complications and speed recovery.

Before partial or total laryngectomy, follow these guidelines:
• Instruct the patient to maintain good oral hygiene. If appropriate, instruct the male patient to shave off his beard to facilitate postoperative care.
• Encourage the patient to verbalize his concerns before surgery temporarily cuts off effective verbal communication. Prepare him for this by helping him choose an alternative method of communication that he finds comfortable (such as pencil and paper, sign language, or alphabet board).
• If you are preparing the patient for total laryngectomy, arrange for a laryngectomee to visit him. Explain postoperative procedures (suctioning, nasogastric feeding, care of laryngectomy tube) and their results (breathing through neck, speech alteration). Also prepare him for other functional losses: he will not be able to smell, blow his nose, whistle, gargle, sip, or suck on a straw.

After partial laryngectomy, follow these guidelines:
• Give I.V. fluids and, usually, tube feedings for the first 2 days postop-

---

Neck Stoma Care

Dear Patient:
After you're discharged, you'll have to do your own neck stoma care.
• To prevent infection, wash your hands before touching your stoma.
• Then, wet a washcloth with warm water (don't use wet cotton or soap); wring it out, and place it over the stoma.
• To keep the stoma moist, apply petrolatum thinly around its edges. Wipe off any excess.
• Use a stoma bib (crocheted cover or cotton cloth) over the stoma to filter and warm air before it enters the stoma. Fasten the bib with a tie around your neck. You can wear an ascot, a turtleneck sweater, or a regular shirt (sew the second button from the top over the buttonhole as though it were fastened, to leave access for a handkerchief when coughing); you can also wear jewelry or scarves.
• If you're a man, be careful when shaving, as some of your sensory nerve endings may have been cut in surgery. These endings will regenerate in about 6 months.

---

eratively; then resume oral fluids. Keep the tracheostomy tube (inserted during surgery) in place until tissue edema subsides.
• Make sure the patient does not use his voice until the physician gives permission (usually 2 to 3 days postoperatively). Then caution the patient to whisper until healing is complete.

After total laryngectomy, follow these guidelines:
• As soon as he returns to his bed, position the patient on his side and elevate his head 30° to 45°. When you move him, remember to support the back of his neck to prevent tension on sutures and possible wound dehiscence.
• The patient will probably have a laryngectomy tube in place until his stoma heals (about 7 to 10 days). This tube is shorter and thicker than a tracheostomy tube but requires the same care.
• Watch for and report complications: fistula formation (redness, swelling, secretions on suture line), carotid ar-

tery rupture (bleeding), and tracheostomy stenosis (constant shortness of breath).
• Give frequent mouth care.
• Suction gently. Unless ordered otherwise, do not attempt deep suctioning, which could penetrate the suture line. Suction through both the tube and the patient's nose, since the patient can no longer blow air through his nose. Suction his mouth gently.
• After insertion of a drainage catheter (usually connected to a blood drainage system or a gastrointestinal drainage system), do not stop suction without the physician's consent. After catheter removal, check dressings for drainage.
• Give analgesics, as ordered. Keep in mind that narcotics depress respiration and inhibit coughing.
• If the physician orders nasogastric tube feeding, check tube placement, and elevate the patient's head to prevent aspiration. Be ready to suction after nasogastric tube removal or oral fluid intake, since the patient may have difficulty swallowing.
• Reassure the patient that speech re-

habilitation (laryngeal speech, esophageal speech [air bolus techniques], artificial larynx, various mechanical aids) can help him speak again. Encourage him to contact the American Speech and Hearing Association, the International Association of Laryngectomees, the American Cancer Society, or the local chapter of the Lost Chord Club or the New Voice Club.

• Support the patient through inevitable grieving. If he seems severely depressed, consider psychiatric referral. (See *Neck Stoma Care*, p. 435.)

Laryngitis

Description
A common disorder, laryngitis is acute or chronic inflammation of the vocal cords. Acute laryngitis may occur as an isolated infection or as part of a generalized bacterial or viral upper respiratory tract infection. Repeated attacks of acute laryngitis cause inflammatory changes associated with chronic laryngitis.

Causes
Acute laryngitis
—Infection
—Excessive use of the voice
—Inhalation of smoke or fumes
—Aspiration of caustic chemicals
Chronic laryngitis
—Upper respiratory tract disorders (sinusitis, bronchitis, nasal polyps, allergy)
—Mouth breathing
—Smoking
—Constant exposure to dust or other irritants
—Alcohol abuse

Signs and symptoms
Acute laryngitis
—Hoarseness
—Pain (especially when swallowing or speaking)
—Dry cough
—Fever
—Malaise
—Laryngeal edema
Chronic laryngitis
—Persistent hoarseness

Diagnostic tests
Indirect laryngoscopy confirms diagnosis by revealing exudate and red, inflamed, and occasionally hemorrhagic vocal cords, with rounded rather than sharp edges. Bilateral swelling may be present, which restricts movement but does not cause paralysis.

Treatment
Primary treatment consists of resting the voice. For viral infection, symptomatic care includes analgesics and throat lozenges for pain relief. Bacterial infection requires antibiotic therapy. Severe, acute laryngitis may necessitate hospitalization. Occasionally, when laryngeal edema results in airway obstruction, tracheotomy may be necessary. In chronic laryngitis, effective treatment must eliminate the underlying cause.

Clinical implications
• Explain to the patient why he should not talk, and place a sign over the bed to remind others of this restriction. Provide a Magic Slate or a pad and pencil for communication. Mark the intercom panel so other hospital personnel are aware the patient cannot answer. Minimize the need to talk by trying to anticipate the patient's needs.

• Suggest the patient maintain adequate humidification by using a vaporizer or humidifier during the winter, by avoiding air conditioning during the summer (because it dehumidifies), by using medicated throat lozenges, and by not smoking. Urge completion of prescribed antibiotics.

• Obtain a detailed patient history to help determine the cause of chronic laryngitis. Encourage modification of predisposing habits.

Lassa fever

Description
Lassa fever is an epidemic hemorrhagic fever caused by a virus. The disease is rare in the United States. Incidence is highest in western Africa. This highly fatal disorder kills 10% to 50% of its victims, but those who survive its early stages usually recover and acquire immunity to secondary attacks.

Cause
Lassa virus, an extremely virulent arenavirus

Mode of transmission
• The virus is transmitted to humans by contact with infected rodent urine, feces, and saliva.
• In the early stages, when the virus is in the throat, human transmission may occur through inhalation of infected droplets.

Signs and symptoms
• Fever that persists for 2 to 3 weeks
• Exudative pharyngitis
• Oral ulcers
• Lymphadenopathy with swelling of the face and neck
• Purpura
• Conjunctivitis
• Bradycardia
• Bleeding tendency
• Secondary bacterial infection

Diagnostic tests
• Isolation of the Lassa virus from throat washings, pleural fluid, or blood confirms the diagnosis.
• Specific antibody titer and recent travel to an endemic area support this diagnosis.

Treatment
Treatment of Lassa fever is primarily supportive. It includes administration of antibiotics (depending on the organism cultured) for secondary bacterial infection, I.V. colloids for shock, analgesics for pain, and antipyretics for fever. Infusion of immune plasma from patients who have recovered from Lassa fever may be useful in treatment, but studies of the benefits of this type of therapy are inconclusive.

Clinical implications
• Carefully monitor fluid and electrolytes, vital signs, and intake and output. Watch for and immediately report signs of infection or shock.
• Strict isolation is necessary for at least 3 weeks, until the patient's throat washings and urine are free of the virus.
• To prevent the spread of this contagious disease, carefully dispose of or disinfect all materials contaminated with the infected patient's urine, feces, respiratory secretions, or exudates. Watch known contacts closely for at least 3 weeks for signs of the disease.
• Provide good mouth care. Remember to clean the patient's mouth with a soft-bristled brush to avoid irritating mouth ulcers. Ask the dietary department to supply a soft, bland, nonirritating diet.
• Immediately report all cases of Lassa fever to public health authorities.
• Immediately contact the Viral Diseases Division of the Centers for Disease Control in Atlanta to get specific guidelines for managing suspected or confirmed cases of Lassa fever.

Complications
• Severe infection may cause hepatitis, myocarditis, pleural infection, encephalitis, and permanent unilateral or bilateral deafness.
• Capillary lesions may cause focal hemorrhage in the stomach, small intestine, kidneys, lungs, and brain and, possibly, hemorrhagic shock and peripheral vascular collapse.

Legg-Calvé-Perthes disease
(Coxa plana)

Description

Legg-Calvé-Perthes disease is ischemic necrosis leading to eventual flattening of the head of the femur due to vascular interruption. This usually unilateral condition occurs most frequently in boys aged 4 to 10 and tends to recur in families. The disease usually runs its course in 3 to 4 years when healing or regeneration is complete. It may lead to premature osteoarthritis later in life from misalignment of the acetabulum and the flattened femoral head.

Cause

Unknown

Signs and symptoms

- Persistent limp (the first indication; becomes progressively severe)
- Mild pain in the hip, thigh, or knee (aggravated by activity and relieved by rest)
- Muscle spasm
- Atrophy of upper thigh muscles
- Slight shortening of the leg
- Severely restricted abduction and rotation of the hip

Diagnostic tests

Hip X-rays taken every 3 to 4 months confirm the diagnosis, with findings that vary according to the stage of the disease.

Treatment

The aim of treatment is to protect the femoral head from further stress and damage by containing it within the acetabulum. After 3 months of bed rest, therapy may include reduced weight-bearing and bed rest in bilateral split counterpoised traction, then application of hip abduction splint or cast, or weight-bearing while a splint, cast, or brace holds the leg in abduction. Analgesics help relieve pain.

For a young child in the early stages of the disease, osteotomy and subtrochanteric derotation provide maximum confinement of the epiphysis within the acetabulum to allow return of the femoral head to normal shape and full range of motion. Proper placement of the epiphysis thus allows remolding with ambulation. Postoperatively, the patient requires a spica cast for about 2 months.

Clinical implications

- Monitor fluid intake and output. Maintain sufficient fluid balance. Provide a diet sufficient for growth but one that does not cause excessive weight gain, which might lead to cast change and ultimate loss of the corrective position.
- Provide good cast care.
- Watch for complications. Check toes for color, temperature, swelling, sensation, and motion. Report dusky, cool, numb toes immediately. Check the skin under the cast with a flashlight every 4 hours while the patient is awake. Check under the cast daily for odors, particularly after surgery, to detect skin breakdown or wound problems. Report persistent soreness.
- Administer analgesics, as ordered.
- Relieve itching by using a hair dryer (set on cool) at the cast edges; this also decreases dampness from perspiration. If itching becomes excessive, get an order for an antipruritic. *Never* insert an object under the cast to scratch.
- Provide emotional support. Explain all procedures and the need for bed rest, a cast, or braces to the child; encourage him to verbalize his fears and anxiety. Encourage parents to participate in their child's care. Teach them proper cast care and how to recognize signs of skin breakdown. Offer tips for making home management of the bedridden child easier. Tell them what special supplies are needed: pa-

jamas and trousers a size larger (open the side seam, and attach Velcro fasteners to close it), bedpan, adhesive tape, moleskin, and, possibly, a hospital bed.

• After removal of the cast, debride dry, scaly skin *gradually* by applying lotion after bathing.

• Stress the need for follow-up care to monitor rehabilitation. Also stress home tutoring and socialization to promote normal growth and development.

Legionnaires' disease

Description

Legionnaires' disease is an acute bronchopneumonia produced by a fastidious, gram-negative bacillus. This disease may occur epidemically or sporadically, usually in late summer or early fall. Its severity ranges from a mild illness, with or without pneumonitis, to multilobar pneumonia, with a mortality rate as high as 15%. A milder, self-limiting form (Pontiac syndrome) subsides within a few days but leaves the patient fatigued for several weeks; this form produces few or no respiratory symptoms, no pneumonia, and no fatalities.

Cause

Legionnaires' disease bacterium (LDB), recently named *Legionella pneumophilia*, an aerobic, gram-negative bacillus

Mode of transmission

The bacterium probably is transmitted by an airborne route. In past epidemics, it has spread through cooling towers or evaporation condensers in air-conditioning systems. However, LDB also flourishes in soil and excavation sites. It does not spread from person to person.

Risk factors

Legionnaires' disease is most likely to affect the following groups:

• Middle-aged to elderly persons
• Immunocompromised patients, (particularly those receiving corticosteroids) or those with lymphoma or other disorders associated with delayed hypersensitivity
• Patients with a chronic underlying disease, such as diabetes, chronic renal failure, or chronic obstructive pulmonary disease (COPD)
• Alcoholics
• Cigarette smokers (three to four times more likely to develop Legionnaires' disease than nonsmokers)

Signs and symptoms

• Prodromal signs and symptoms include diarrhea, anorexia, malaise, diffuse myalgias and generalized weakness, headache, recurrent chills, and an unremitting fever, which develops within 12 to 48 hours. Temperature may reach 105° F. (40.5° C.). Other symptoms include the following:
• Cough (initially nonproductive but eventually may produce grayish, nonpurulent, and occasionally blood-streaked sputum)
• Nausea and vomiting
• Disorientation, mild temporary amnesia
• Chest pain
• Dyspnea
• Tachypnea, and possibly bradycardia
• Fine rales, progressing to coarse rales

Diagnostic tests

• Chest X-ray shows patchy, localized infiltration, which progresses to multilobar consolidation (usually involving the lower lobes), pleural effusion, and in fulminant disease, opacification of the entire lung.
• WBC count is increased.
• Erythrocyte sedimentation rate is increased.
• SGOT, SGPT, and alkaline phos-

phatase show moderate increases.
- PO_2 and PCO_2 are decreased initially.
- Bronchial washings, blood and pleural fluid cultures, and transtracheal aspirates rule out other pulmonary infections.
- Definitive tests include direct immunofluorescence of respiratory tract secretions and tissue, culture of *L. pneumophilia*, and indirect fluorescent antibody testing of serum to compare samples taken during acute illness with convalescent samples drawn at least 3 weeks later. Convalescent serum showing a fourfold or greater rise in antibody titer for LDB confirms the diagnosis.

Treatment

Antibiotic treatment begins as soon as Legionnaires' disease is suspected and diagnostic material is collected. Treatment should not await laboratory confirmation. Erythromycin is the drug of choice, but if it is not effective alone, rifampin can be added to the regimen. If erythromycin is contraindicated, rifampin or rifampin with tetracycline may be used. Supportive therapy includes administration of antipyretics, fluid replacement, circulatory support with pressor drugs, if necessary, and oxygen administration by mask or cannula or by mechanical ventilation with positive end-expiratory pressure (PEEP).

Clinical implications

- Closely monitor respiratory status. Evaluate chest wall expansion, depth and pattern of respirations, cough, and chest pain. Watch for restlessness, which may indicate the patient is hypoxemic, requiring suctioning, repositioning, or more aggressive oxygen therapy.
- Continually monitor vital signs, arterial blood gases, level of consciousness, and dryness and color of lips and mucous membranes. Watch for signs of shock (decreased blood pressure, thready pulse, diaphoresis, clammy skin).

- Keep the patient comfortable; avoid chills and exposure to drafts. Provide frequent mouth care. If necessary, apply soothing cream to the nostrils.
- Replace fluid and electrolytes, as needed. The patient with renal failure may require dialysis.
- Provide mechanical ventilation and other respiratory therapy, as needed. Teach the patient how to cough effectively, and encourage deep breathing exercises. Stress the need to continue these until recovery is complete.
- Give antibiotic therapy, as ordered, and observe carefully for side effects.

Complications
- Hypoxia
- Hypotension
- Delirium
- Congestive heart failure
- Dysrhythmias
- Acute respiratory failure
- Renal failure
- Shock

Leprosy
(Hansen's disease)

Description

Leprosy is a chronic, systemic infection characterized by progressive cutaneous lesions. Leprosy occurs in three distinct forms. Lepromatous leprosy, the most serious type, causes damage to the upper respiratory tract, eyes, and testes, as well as the nerves and skin. Tuberculoid leprosy affects peripheral nerves and sometimes the surrounding skin, especially on the face, arms, legs, and buttocks. Borderline (dimorphous) leprosy has characteristics of both lepromatous and tuberculoid leprosy. Skin lesions are diffuse and poorly defined. The incubation period is unusually long—6 months to 8 years. With timely, correct treatment, prognosis is good. The disease is rarely fatal. Untreated, how-

Peripheral Nervous System Involvement in Leprosy

Mycobacterium leprae attacks the peripheral nervous system, especially the ulnar, radial, posterior-popliteal, anterior-tibial, and facial nerves. The central nervous system appears highly resistant. When the bacilli damage the skin's fine nerves, they cause anesthesia, anhidrosis, and dryness; if they attack a large nerve trunk, then motor nerve damage, weakness, and pain occur, followed by peripheral anesthesia, muscle paralysis, or atrophy. In later stages, clawhand, foot drop, and ocular complications—such as corneal insensitivity and ulceration, conjunctivitis, photophobia, and blindness—can occur. Injury, ulceration, infection, and disuse of the deformed parts cause scarring and contracture. Neurologic complications occur in both lepromatous and tuberculoid leprosies but are less extensive and develop more slowly in the lepromatous form.

ever, it can cause severe disability. The lepromatous type may lead to blindness and deformities. Borderline leprosy may deteriorate into lepromatous disease.

Cause
Mycobacterium leprae, an acid-fast bacillus that attacks cutaneous tissue and peripheral nerves

Mode of transmission
Presumably, transmission occurs through airborne respiratory droplets containing *M. leprae* or by inoculation through skin breaks (with a contaminated hypodermic or tattoo needle, for example). The disease is not highly contagious. Continuous, close contact is needed to transmit it.

Signs and symptoms
Lepromatous leprosy
—Early lesions appear as macules or papules. Later they form widespread plaques and nodules in the skin, conjunctiva, and sclera. Other symptoms include the following:
—Deterioration of fingers
—Destruction of nasal cartilage and bone
—Testicular atrophy
—Peripheral edema
—Hepatosplenomegaly
—Possible blindness

Tuberculoid leprosy
—Thickening of cutaneous nerves
—Anesthetic, saucer-shaped skin lesions with clearly defined borders
—Signs and symptoms of peripheral nervous system involvement. (See *Peripheral Nervous System Involvement in Leprosy*.)
Borderline leprosy
—Skin lesions are numerous, but smaller, less anesthetic, and less sharply defined than tuberculoid lesions.

Diagnostic tests
• Biopsies of skin lesions are diagnostic.
• Biopsies of peripheral nerves, or smears of the skin or of ulcerated mucous membranes, help confirm the diagnosis.
• Blood tests show increased erythrocyte sedimentation rate; decreased albumin, calcium, and cholesterol levels; and possibly anemia.

Treatment
Treatment consists of antimicrobial therapy using sulfones, primarily oral dapsone, which may cause hypersensitivity reactions. Hepatitis and exfoliative dermatitis, although uncommon, are especially dangerous reactions. If these reactions do occur,

sulfone therapy should be stopped immediately.

Failure to respond to sulfone, or the occurrence of respiratory involvement or other complications, requires use of alternative therapy, such as rifampin in combination with the investigational agent clofazimine or ethionamide. Clawhand, wristdrop, or footdrop may require surgical correction.

When a patient's disease becomes inactive, as determined by the morphologic and bacterial index, treatment continues according to the following schedule; tuberculoid—3 years; borderline—depends on the severity of the disease, but may be as long as 10 years; lepromatous—lifetime therapy.

Since erythema nodosum leprosum (ENL) is often considered a sign that the patient is responding to treatment, antimicrobial therapy should be continued. Thalidomide and clofazimine have been used successfully to treat ENL at the National Hansen's Disease Center (NHDC). However, this treatment requires a signed consent form and strict adherence to established NHDC protocols. Corticosteroids may also be given as part of ENL therapy.

Any patient suspected of having Hansen's disease may be referred to the NHDC at Carville, La. At this international research and educational center, patients undergo diagnostic studies and treatment and are educated about their disease. (Communicating accurate information about Hansen's disease to the general public, and especially to health care professionals, is a function of primary importance for the entire staff at the NHDC.) Patients are encouraged to return home as soon as their medical condition permits. The federal government pays the full cost of their medical and nursing care.

Clinical implications
Patient care is supportive and consists of measures to control acute infection, prevent complications, speed rehabilitation and recovery, and provide psychological support.

• Give antipyretics, analgesics, and sedatives, as needed. Watch for and report ENL or Lucio's phenomenon which produces generalized punched-out ulcers that may extend into muscle and fascia.

• Although leprosy is not highly contagious, take precautions against the possible spread of infection. Tell patients to cover coughs or sneezes with a paper tissue and to dispose of it properly. Take infection precautions when handling clothing or articles that have been in contact with open skin lesions.

• Patients with borderline or lepromatous leprosy may suffer associated eye complications, such as iridocyclitis and glaucoma. Decreased corneal sensation and lacrimation may also occur, requiring patients to use a tear substitute daily and protect their eyes to prevent corneal irritation and ulceration.

• Stress the importance of adequate nutrition and rest. Watch for fatigue, jaundice, and other signs of anemia and hepatitis.

• Tell the patient to be careful not to injure an anesthetized leg by putting too much weight on it. Advise testing bath water carefully to prevent scalding. To prevent ulcerations, suggest the use of sturdy footwear and soaking feet in warm water after any kind of exercise, even a short walk. Advise rubbing the feet with petrolatum, oil, or lanolin.

• For patients with deformities, an interdisciplinary rehabilitation program employing a physiotherapist and plastic surgeon may be necessary. Teach the patient and help him with prescribed therapies.

• Provide emotional support throughout threatment.

Complications
Occasionally, acute episodes intensify leprosy's slowly progressive course. It remains a matter of dispute whether

such exacerbations are part of the disease process or a reaction to therapy. ENL, seen in lepromatous leprosy, produces fever, malaise, lymphadenopathy, and painful red skin nodules, usually during antimicrobial treatment, although it may occur in untreated persons. In Mexico and other Central American countries, some patients with lepromatous disease develop Lucio's phenomenon. Leprosy may also lead to complications such as tuberculosis, malaria, secondary bacterial infection of skin ulcers, and amyloidosis.

Leukemia, acute

Description
Acute leukemia is a malignant proliferation of white blood cell precursors (blasts) in bone marrow or lymph tissue and their accumulation in peripheral blood, bone marrow, and body tissues. Its most common forms are acute lymphoblastic (lymphocytic) leukemia (ALL), involving abnormal growth of lymphocyte precursors (lymphoblasts); acute myeloblastic (myelogenous) leukemia (AML), involving rapid accumulation of myeloid precursors (myeloblasts); and acute monoblastic (monocytic) leukemia, or Schilling's type, involving marked increases in monocyte precursors (monoblasts). Other variants include acute myelomonocytic leukemia and acute erythroleukemia.

Untreated, acute leukemia is invariably fatal, usually because of complications that result from leukemic cell infiltration of bone marrow or vital organs. With treatment, prognosis varies. In ALL, treatment induces remissions in 90% of children (average survival time: 5 years) and in 65% of adults (average survival time: 1 to 2 years). Children between ages 2 and 8 have the best survival rate—about 50%—with intensive therapy. In AML, the average survival time is only

---

Predisposing Factors to Acute Leukemia

Although the exact causes of most leukemias remain unknown, increasing evidence suggests a combination of contributing factors.
Acute lymphoblastic leukemia
• familial tendency
• monozygotic twins
• congential disorders, such as Down's syndrome, Bloom's syndrome, Fanconi's anemia, ataxia-telangiectsia, and congenital agammaglobulinemia
• viruses.
Acute myeloblastic leukemia
• familial tendency
• monozygotic twins
• congenital disorders, such as Down's syndrome, Bloom's syndrome, Fanconi's anemia, ataxia-telangiectasia, and congenital agammaglobulinemia
• viruses.
Acute monoblastic leukemia
• unknown (irradiation, exposure to chemicals, heredity, and infections show little correlation to this disease).

---

1 year after diagnosis, even with aggressive treatment. In acute monoblastic leukemia, treatment induces remissions lasting 2 to 10 months in 40% of children. Adults survive only about 1 year after diagnosis, even with treatment.

Acute leukemia ranks 20th in causes of cancer-related deaths among people of all age groups. Among children, however, it is the most common form of cancer.

Cause
Unknown

Risk factors
Research on predisposing factors is not conclusive but points to some com-

bination of viruses (viral remnants have been found in leukemic cells), genetic and immunologic factors, and exposure to radiation and certain chemicals. (For more information, see *Predisposing Factors to Acute Leukemia*, p. 443.)

Signs and symptoms
Typical
—Sudden onset of high fever
—Abnormal bleeding (for example, nosebleeds, gingival bleeding, purpura, ecchymoses, petechiae)
—Easy bruising after minor trauma
—Prolonged menses
Nonspecific
—Low-grade fever
—Pallor
—Weakness and lassitude (may persist for days or months before appearance of other symptoms)
Possible with ALL, AML, and acute monoblastic leukemia
—Dyspnea
—Fatigue
—Malaise
—Tachycardia
—Palpitations
—Systolic ejection murmur
—Abdominal or bone pain
Characteristic of meningeal leukemia
—Confusion
—Lethargy
—Headache

Diagnostic tests
• Bone marrow aspiration typically shows a proliferation of immature WBCs and confirms the diagnosis.
• Bone marrow biopsy is performed in a patient with typical clinical findings but whose aspirate is dry or free of leukemic cells.
• CBC shows thrombocytopenia and neutropenia.
• Differential leukocyte count determines cell type.
• Lumbar puncture detects meningeal involvement.

Treatment
Systemic chemotherapy aims to eradicate leukemic cells and induce remission (restore normal bone marrow function). Chemotherapy varies.
• Meningeal leukemia—intrathecal instillation of methotrexate or cytarabine with cranial radiation
• ALL—vincristine and/or prednisone with intrathecal methotrexate or cytarabine; I.V. asparaginase, daunorubicin, and doxorubicin; maintenance with mercaptopurine and methotrexate
• AML—a combination of I.V. daunorubicin or doxorubicin, cytarabine, and oral thioguanine; or, if these fail to induce remission, a combination of cyclophosphamide, vincristine, prednisone, or methotrexate; high-dose cytarabine alone or with other drugs; amsacrine; 5-azacytidine and mitoxantrone (both investigational); maintenance with additional chemotherapy
• Acute monoblastic leukemia—cytarabine and thioguanine with daunorubicin or doxorubicin

Bone marrow transplant is now possible in some cases. Treatment also may include antibiotic, antifungal, and antiviral drugs and granulocyte injections to control infection, platelet transfusions to prevent bleeding, and red blood cell transfusions to prevent anemia.

Clinical implications
• Explain the disease course, treatment, and side effects.
• Teach the patient and his family how to recognize infection (fever, chills, cough, sore throat) and abnormal bleeding (bruising, petechiae), and how to stop bleeding (pressure, application of ice).
• Promote good nutrition. Explain that chemotherapy may cause weight loss and anorexia. Encourage the patient to eat and drink high-calorie, high-protein foods and beverages. However, chemotherapy and adjunctive prednisone may cause weight gain, so dietary

counseling and teaching are helpful.
• Help establish an appropriate rehabilitation program for the patient during remission.
• Watch for signs of meningeal leukemia. If these occur, know how to manage care after intrathecal chemotherapy. After such instillation, place the patient in the Trendelenburg position for 30 minutes. Force fluids, and keep the patient supine for 4 to 6 hours. Check the lumbar puncture site often for bleeding. If the patient receives cranial radiation, teach him about potential side effects, and do what you can to minimize them.
• Prevent hyperuricemia, a possible result of rapid chemotherapy-induced leukemic cell lysis. Force fluids to about 2 liters daily, and give acetazolamide, $NaHCO_3$ tablets, and allopurinol. Check urine pH often—it should be above 7.5. Watch for rash or other hypersensitivity reaction to allopurinol.
• Control infection by placing the patient in a private room and imposing reverse isolation, if necessary. (The benefits of reverse isolation are controversial.) Coordinate patient care so the leukemic patient does not come in contact with staff who also care for patients with infections or infectious diseases. Avoid using Foley catheters and giving I.M. injections, since they provide an avenue for infection. Screen staff and visitors for contagious diseases. Watch for and report any signs of infection.
• Monitor temperature every 4 hours; patients with fever over 101° F. (38° C.) and decreased WBC counts should receive prompt antibiotic therapy.
• Watch for bleeding; if it occurs, apply ice compresses and pressure, and elevate the extremity. Avoid giving I.M. injections, aspirin, and aspirin-containing drugs. Also avoid taking rectal temperatures, giving rectal suppositories, and doing digital examinations.
• Take measures to prevent constipation.

• Control mouth ulceration by checking often for obvious ulcers and gum swelling and by providing frequent mouth care and saline solution rinses. Tell the patient to use a soft toothbrush and to avoid hot, spicy foods and overuse of commercial mouthwashes. Also check the rectal area daily for induration, swelling, erythema, skin discoloration, or drainage.
• Provide psychological support by establishing a trusting relationship to promote communication. Allow the patient and his family to verbalize their anger and depression. Let the family participate in his care as much as possible.
• Minimize stress by providing a calm, quiet atmosphere that is conducive to rest and relaxation. For children particularly, be flexible with patient care and visiting hours to promote maximum interaction with family and friends and to allow time for schoolwork and play.
• For a patient whose disease is refractory to chemotherapy and who is in the terminal phase, provide supportive nursing care directed to comfort; management of pain, fever, and bleeding; and patient and family support. Provide the opportunity for religious counseling. Discuss the option of home or hospice care.

Leukemia, chronic granulocytic
(Chronic myelogenous [or myelocytic] leukemia [CML])

Description
Chronic granulocytic leukemia (CGL) is characterized by the abnormal overgrowth of granulocyte precursors (myeloblasts, promyelocytes, metamyelocytes, and myelocytes) in bone marrow, peripheral blood, and body tissues. CGL is most common in young and middle-aged adults.

CGL's clinical course proceeds in two distinct phases: the insidious chronic phase, with anemia and bleeding abnormalities and, eventually, the acute phase (blastic crisis), in which myeloblasts, the most primitive granulocyte precursors, proliferate rapidly. This disease is invariably fatal. Average survival time is 3 to 4 years after onset of the chronic phase and 3 to 6 months after onset of the acute phase.

Cause

Almost 90% of patients with CGL have the Philadelphia (Ph¹) chromosome, an abnormality discovered in 1960 in which the long arm of chromosome 22 is translocated, usually to chromosome 9. Radiation and carcinogenic chemicals may induce this chromosome abnormality. Myeloproliferative diseases also seem to increase the incidence of CGL, and some clinicians suspect that an unidentified virus causes this disease.

Signs and symptoms

Typically, CGL induces the following clinical effects:
• Anemia (fatigue, weakness, decreased exercise tolerance, pallor, dyspnea, tachycardia, and headache)
• Thrombocytopenia (resulting in bleeding and clotting disorders [retinal hemorrhage, ecchymoses, hematuria, melena, bleeding gums, nosebleeds, and easy bruising])
• Hepatosplenomegaly, with abdominal discomfort and pain
• Other symptoms include sternal and rib tenderness; low-grade fever; weight loss; anorexia; pain associated with renal calculi or gouty arthritis; occasionally, prolonged infection and ankle edema; and, rarely, priapism and symptoms of vascular insufficiency.

Diagnostic tests

• Chromosomal analysis of peripheral blood or bone marrow showing the Philadelphia chromosome and low leukocyte alkaline phosphatase levels confirm CGL in patients with typical clinical changes.
• WBC abnormalities include leukocytosis (leukocytes more than 50,000/mm³, ranging as high as 250,000/mm³), occasional leukopenia (leukocytes less than 5,000/mm³), neutropenia (neutrophils less than 1,500/mm³) despite high leukocyte count, and increased circulating myeloblasts.
• Hemoglobin is often below 20 g.
• Hematocrit is low (less than 30%).
• Thrombocytopenia is common (less than 50,000/mm³), but platelet levels may be normal or elevated.
• Serum uric acid may be more than 8 mg.
• Bone marrow aspirate or biopsy shows hypercellular bone marrow infiltration by increased numbers of myeloid elements (biopsy is done only if aspirate is dry). In the acute phase, myeloblasts predominate.

Treatment

Control of abnormal myeloid proliferation requires rigorous chemotherapy. During the chronic phase, outpatient chemotherapy induces remissions, and it is often continued at lower doses during remissions. Such chemotherapy usually includes busulfan and, occasionally, melphalan, other nitrogen mustards, thioguanine, and hydroxyurea.

Ancillary treatments may include the following:
• Local splenic radiation to reduce peripheral blood counts and splenic size, or splenectomy (controversial)
• Leukapheresis (selective leukocyte removal) to reduce leukocyte count
• Bone marrow transplant
• Allopurinol to prevent hyperuricemia, or colchicine to relieve gouty attacks caused by elevated serum uric acid
• Prompt treatment of infections that may result from chemotherapy-induced bone marrow suppression.

During the acute phase, treatment is the same as for acute myeloblastic leukemia (although it is less likely to induce remission) and emphasizes supportive measures and chemotherapy with doxorubicin or daunorubicin, thioguanine, cyclophosphamide, vincristine, methotrexate, cytarabine, or daunorubicin with prednisone. Despite vigorous treatment, CGL is rapidly fatal after onset of the acute phase.

Clinical implications

Throughout the chronic phase of CGL, follow these guidelines when the patient is hospitalized.

• If the patient has persistent anemia, plan your care to help avoid exhaustion. Schedule lab tests and physical care to allow frequent rest periods, and assist the patient with walking, if necessary. Regularly check the patient's skin and mucous membranes for pallor, petechiae, and bruising.

• To minimize bleeding, suggest a soft-bristle toothbrush, an electric razor, and other safety precautions.

• To minimize the abdominal discomfort of splenomegaly, provide small, frequent meals. For the same reason, prevent constipation by giving a stool softener or laxative, as needed. Ask the dietary department to provide a high-bulk diet, and maintain adequate fluid intake.

• To prevent atelectasis, stress the need for coughing and deep breathing exercises.

Because the patient with CGL often receives outpatient chemotherapy throughout the chronic phase, sound patient teaching is essential. Follow these guidelines:

• Explain expected side effects of chemotherapy; pay particular attention to dangerous side effects, such as bone marrow suppression.

• Tell the patient to watch for and immediately report signs and symptoms of infection: any fever over 100° F. (37.7° C.), chills, redness or swelling, sore throat, and cough.

• Instruct the patient to watch for signs of thrombocytopenia, to apply ice and pressure immediately to any external bleeding site, and to avoid aspirin and aspirin-containing compounds because of the risk of increased bleeding.

• Emphasize the importance of adequate rest to minimize the fatigue of anemia. To minimize the toxic effects of chemotherapy, stress the importance of a high-calorie, high-protein diet.

For information on treatment during the acute phase, see "Leukemia, acute," pp. 443 to 445.

Leukemia, chronic lymphocytic

Description

A generalized, progressive disease that is common in the elderly, chronic lymphocytic leukemia is marked by an uncontrollable spread of abnormal, small lymphocytes in lymphoid tissue, blood, and bone marrow. Nearly all patients with chronic lymphocytic leukemia are men over age 50. According to the American Cancer Society, chronic lymphocytic leukemia accounts for almost one third of new leukemia cases annually.

Cause

Although the cause of chronic lymphocytic leukemia is unknown, researchers suspect hereditary factors (higher incidence has been recorded within families), still-undefined chromosome abnormalities, and certain immunologic defects (such as ataxia-telangiectasia or acquired agammaglobulinemia). The disease does not seem to be associated with radiation exposure.

Signs and symptoms
Early stages
—Fatigue
—Malaise
—Fever

—Nodal involvement
—Susceptibility to infection
Advanced stages
—Severe fatigue
—Weight loss
—Hepatomegaly
—Splenomegaly
—Bone tenderness
—Edema
—Possible nodular eruptions on skin
—Pallor
—Dyspnea
—Tachycardia and palpitations
—Bleeding
—Weakness

Diagnostic tests
Typically, chronic lymphocytic leukemia is an incidental finding during a routine blood test that reveals numerous abnormal lymphocytes.
• WBC count is mildly but persistently elevated in early stages. Granulocytopenia is the rule, but the WBC count climbs as the disease progresses.
• Blood studies show hemoglobin count under 11 g, hypogammaglobulinemia, depressed serum globulins, neutropenia (under 1,500/mm³), lymphocytosis (over 10,000/mm³), and thrombocytopenia (under 150,000/mm³).
• Bone marrow aspiration and biopsy show lymphocytic invasion.

Treatment
Systemic chemotherapy includes alkylating agents, usually chlorambucil or cyclophosphamide, and sometimes steroids (prednisone) when autoimmune hemolytic anemia or thrombocytopenia occurs.

When chronic lymphocytic leukemia causes obstruction or organ impairment or enlargement, local radiation can be used to reduce organ size. Allopurinol can be given to prevent hyperuricemia, a relatively uncommon finding.

Prognosis is poor if anemia, thrombocytopenia, neutropenia, bulky lymphoadenopathy, and severe lympho-cytosis are present. Gross bone marrow replacement by abnormal lymphocytes is the most common cause of death, usually within 4 to 5 years after diagnosis.

Clinical implications
• Plan patient care to relieve symptoms and prevent infection. Clean the patient's skin daily with mild soap and water. Frequent soaks may be ordered. Watch for signs of infection: temperature over 100° F. (37.7° C.), chills, redness, or swelling of any body part.
• Watch for signs of thrombocytopenia (black tarry stools, easy bruising, nosebleeds, bleeding gums) and anemia (pale skin, weakness, fatigue, dizziness, palpitations). Advise the patient to avoid aspirin and products containing aspirin.
• Explain chemotherapy and its possible side effects. If the patient is to be discharged, tell him to avoid coming in contact with obviously ill persons, especially children with common contagious childhood diseases. Urge him to eat high-protein food and drink high-calorie beverages.
• Stress the importance of follow-up care, frequent blood tests, and taking all medications exactly as prescribed. Teach the patient the signs of recurrence (swollen lymph nodes in the neck, axilla, and groin; increased abdominal size or discomfort), and tell him to notify his physician immediately if he detects any of these signs.
• Provide emotional support and be a good listener. Most patients with chronic lymphocytic leukemia are elderly; some are frightened. Try to keep their spirits up by concentrating on little things like improving their personal appearance, providing a pleasant environment, asking questions about their families. If possible, provide opportunities for their favorite activities.

Complications
Opportunistic fungal, viral, and bacterial infections commonly occur in late stages.

Lichen planus

Description
Lichen planus is a nonmalignant, chronic, pruritic skin disease, typically affecting middle-aged persons. This relatively rare disorder usually resolves spontaneously in 6 to 18 months. In some patients, lichen planus may persist for several years.

Cause
Unknown

Signs and symptoms
• Skin lesions (common on arms or legs; evolve into the generalized eruption of flat, glistening, purple papules, marked with white lines or spots [Wickham's striae]; may be linear, due to scratching, or coalesce into plaques)
• Lesions of mucous membranes (especially the buccal mucosa), male genitalia, and sometimes the nails
• Mild to severe pruritus

Diagnostic tests
Although characteristic skin lesions frequently establish the diagnosis of lichen planus, confirmation may necessitate skin biopsy.

Treatment
Treatment is essentially symptomatic. The goal of therapy is to relieve itching with topical fluorinated steroids and occlusive dressings; intralesional injections of steroids; oatmeal baths; and antihistamines. Vitamin A in the form of retinoic acid may shrink lesions but is not generally recommended. Systemic corticosteroids, given in early acute stages, may shorten the duration of the disease. If a drug is suspected as the cause, it should be discontinued. Treatment of lichen planus associated with emotional stress may require counseling to identify stressors and teach more effective coping mechanisms.

Clinical implications
• Administer medications, as ordered, and inform the patient of possible side effects, especially drowsiness produced by antihistamines.
• Provide emotional suppport, and reassure the patient that lichen planus, although annoying, is usually a benign, self-limiting condition.

Listeriosis

Description
Listeriosis is an infection caused by a weakly hemolytic, gram-positive bacillus. It occurs most often in utero, in neonates (during the first 3 weeks of life), and in older or immunosuppressed adults. The infected fetus is usually stillborn or is born prematurely, almost always with lethal listeriosis. This infection produces milder illness in pregnant women and varying degrees of illness in older and immunosuppressed patients. Prognosis depends on the severity of underlying illness.

Cause
Listeria monocytogenes

Mode of transmission
• Primarily, in utero (through the placenta) or during passage through an infected birth canal
• Inhaling contaminated dust
• Drinking contaminated, unpasteurized milk
• Coming in contact with infected animals, contaminated sewage or mud, or soil contaminated with feces containing *L. monocytogenes*

Signs and symptoms
Contact with *L. monocytogenes* commonly causes a transient asymptomatic carrier state. Sometimes it produces bacteremia and a generalized febrile illness.

Pregnant women
—Malaise
—Chills
—Fever
—Back pain
—Abortion
—Premature delivery
—Stillbirth
Neonate
—Possible organ abscesses
—Meningitis (resulting in tense fontanelles, irritability, lethargy, convulsions, and coma)
Other adults
—Low-grade fever
—Personality changes
—Rarely, coma

Diagnostic tests
• A wet mount of the culture identifies the organism through its characteristic tumbling motility.
• Positive culture of blood, spinal fluid, drainage from cervical or vaginal lesions, or lochia from a mother with an infected infant. (Isolation of the organism from these specimens is often difficult.)
• WBC differential reveals monocytosis.

Treatment
The treatment of choice is ampicillin or penicillin I.V. for 3 to 6 weeks, possibly with gentamicin to increase its effectiveness. Alternative treatments include erythromycin, chloramphenicol, or tetracycline.

Ampicillin and penicillin G are best for treating meningitis due to *L. monocytogenes*, since they more easily cross the blood-brain barrier. Pregnant women require prompt, vigorous treatment to combat fetal infection.

Clinical implications
• Deliver specimens to the laboratory promptly. Because very few organisms may be present, take at least 10 cc of spinal fluid for culture.
• Use secretion precautions until a series of cultures of bodily discharges are negative. Be especially careful

when handling lochia from an infected mother and secretions from her infant's eyes, nose, mouth, and rectum, including meconium.
• Evaluate neurologic status at least every 2 hours. In an infant, check fontanelles for bulging.
• Maintain adequate I.V. fluid intake. Measure intake and output accurately.
• If the patient has CNS depression and becomes apneic, provide respiratory assistance, monitor respirations, and obtain frequent ABG measurements.
• Provide adequate nutrition by total parenteral nutrition, nasogastric tube feedings, or a soft diet, as ordered.
• Allow parents to see and, if possible, hold their infant in the ICU. Be flexible about visiting privileges. Keep parents informed of the infant's status and prognosis at all times.
• Reassure parents of an infected newborn who may feel guilty about the infant's illness.
• Educate pregnant women to avoid infective materials on farms where listeriosis is endemic among livestock.

Complications
• Circulatory collapse
• Shock
• Endocarditis
• Hepatosplenomegaly

Liver abscess

Description
A liver abscess occurs when bacteria or protozoa destroy hepatic tissue, producing a cavity, which fills with infectious organisms, liquefied liver cells, and leukocytes. Necrotic tissue then walls off the cavity from the rest of the liver.

Liver abscess is relatively uncommon. With a single abscess the mortality rate is 30% to 50%. This soars to more than 80% with multiple abscesses and to more than 90% with complications.

Causes
• In pyogenic liver abscesses, the common infecting organisms are *Escherichia coli, Klebsiella, Enterobacter* species, *Salmonella, Staphylococcus,* and enterococci.
• An amebic abscess results from infection with the protozoa *Entamoeba histolytica,* the organism that causes amebic dysentery.

Signs and symptoms
• Right abdominal and shoulder pain
• Weight loss
• Fever
• Chills
• Diaphoresis
• Nausea
• Vomiting
• Dyspnea and pleural pain (develop if the abscess extends through the diaphragm)
• Possible jaundice

Diagnostic tests
• A liver scan showing filling defects at the area of the abscess more than ¾" (1.9 cm), together with characteristic clinical features, confirms this diagnosis.
• Ultrasound scan of the liver may indicate defects caused by the abscess but is less definitive than a liver scan.
• In a chest X-ray, the diaphragm on the affected side appears raised and fixed.
• CT scan verifies diagnosis after liver scan or ultrasound.
• Relevant laboratory values include elevated serum transaminase (SGOT, SGPT), alkaline phosphatase, bilirubin, and WBC count (usually more elevated in pyogenic abscess than in amebic), and decreased serum albumin.
• Blood culture can identify the bacterial agent in pyogenic abscess. In amebic abscess, a stool culture and serologic and hemagglutination tests can isolate *E. histolytica.*

Treatment
If the organism causing the liver abscess is unknown, long-term antibiotic therapy begins immediately with aminoglycosides, cephalosporins, clindamycin, or chloramphenicol. If cultures demonstrate that the infectious organism is *E. coli,* treatment includes ampicillin. With *E. histolytica,* treatment includes emetine, chloroquine, or metronidazole. Therapy continues for 2 to 4 months. Surgery is usually avoided, but it may be done for a single pyogenic abscess or for an amebic abscess that fails to respond to antibiotics.

Clinical implications
• Provide supportive care, monitor vital signs (especially temperature), and maintain fluid and nutritional intake.
• Administer anti-infectives and antibiotics, as ordered, and watch for possible side effects. Stress the importance of compliance with therapy.
• Explain diagnostic and surgical procedures.
• Watch carefully for complications of abdominal surgery, such as hemorrhage or infection.

Complications
Rupture into the peritoneum, pleura, or pericardium

Liver cancer
(Primary hepatic carcinoma)

Description
Liver cancer is a rare form of cancer with a high mortality. Most primary liver tumors (90%) originate in the parenchymal cells and are hepatomas (hepatocellular carcinoma, primary lower-cell carcinoma). Some primary tumors originate in the intrahepatic bile ducts and are known as cholangiomas (cholangicarcinoma, cholangicellular carcinoma). Rarer tumors include a mixed-cell type, Kupffer cell sarcoma, and hepatoblastomas (which occur almost exclusively in children

and are usually resectable and curable). The liver is one of the most common sites of metastasis from other primary cancers, particularly colon, rectum, stomach, pancreas, esophagus, lung, and breast cancers and melanoma. In the United States, metastatic carcinoma occurs with more than 20 times the frequency of primary carcinoma.

Cause
The cause is unknown, but many consider it a congenital disease in children. Adult liver cancer may result from environmental exposure to carcinogens, such as the chemical compound aflatoxin (a mold that grows on rice and peanuts), thorium dioxide (a contrast dye medium used in liver radiography in the past), Senecio alkaloids, and possibly androgens and oral estrogens.

Risk factors
• Cirrhosis
• Exposure to hepatitis B virus

Signs and symptoms
• A mass in the right upper quadrant
• Tender, nodular liver on palpation
• Severe pain in the epigastrium or the right upper quadrant
• Bruit, hum, or rubbing sound if tumor involves a large part of the liver
• Weight loss, weakness, anorexia, fever
• Dependent edema
• Occasionally, jaundice or ascites
• Occasionally, metastasis (may move through venous system to lungs, from lymphatics to regional lymph nodes, or into portal veins)

Diagnostic tests
• Liver biopsy by needle or open biopsy is the confirming test.
• Serum transaminases (SGOT, SGPT), alkaline phosphatase, lactic dehydrogenase, and bilirubin all show abnormal liver function.
• Alpha-fetoprotein rises to a level above 500 mcg/ml.

• Chest X-ray may rule out metastasis.
• Liver scan may show filling defects.
• Arteriography may define large tumors.
• Blood studies may indicate increased retention of sodium (resulting in functional renal failure) and hypoglycemia, leukocytosis, hypercalcemia, or hypocholesterolemia.

Treatment
Because liver cancer is often in an advanced stage at diagnosis, few hepatic tumors are resectable. A resectable tumor must be a single tumor in one lobe, without cirrhosis, jaundice, or ascites. Resection is done by lobectomy or partial hepatectomy.

Radiation therapy for unresectable tumors is usually palliative. But because of the liver's low tolerance for radiation, this therapy has not increased survival.

Another method of treatment is chemotherapy with I.V. 5-fluorouracil, methotrexate, or doxorubicin or with regional infusion of 5-fluorouracil or floxuridine. Catheters are placed directly into the hepatic artery or left brachial artery for continuous infusion for 7 to 21 days, or permanent implantable pumps are used on an outpatient basis for long-term infusion.

Appropriate treatment for metastatic cancer of the liver may include resection by lobectomy or chemotherapy (with results similar to those in hepatoma). Liver transplantation is now a possible alternative for some patients.

Clinical implications
The patient care plan should emphasize comprehensive supportive care and emotional support.
• Control edema and ascites. Monitor the patient's diet throughout. Most patients need a special diet that restricts sodium, fluids (no alcohol allowed),

and protein. Weigh the patient daily, and note intake and output accurately.
• Watch for signs of ascites—peripheral edema, orthopnea, or dyspnea on exertion. If ascites is present, measure and record abdominal girth daily. To increase venous return and prevent edema, elevate the patient's legs whenever possible.
• Monitor respiratory function. Note any increase in respiratory rate or shortness of breath.
• Relieve fever. Administer sponge baths and aspirin suppositories if there are no signs of GI bleeding. Avoid acetaminophen, since the diseased liver cannot metabolize it. High fever indicates infection and requires antibiotics.
• Give meticulous skin care. Administer an antipruritic, such as diphenhydramine, for severe itching.
• Watch for encephalopathy. Many patients develop symptoms of ammonia intoxication, including confusion, restlessness, irritability, agitation, delirium, asterixis, lethargy, and, finally, coma. Monitor the patient's serum ammonia level, vital signs, and neurologic status. Be prepared to control ammonia accumulation with sorbitol (to induce osmotic diarrhea), neomycin (to reduce bacterial flora in the GI tract), lactulose (to control bacterial elaboration of ammonia), and sodium polystyrene sulfonate (to lower potassium level).
• If a transhepatic catheter is used to relieve obstructive jaundice, irrigate it frequently with prescribed solution (normal saline solution or sometimes 5,000 units of heparin in 500 ml of dextrose 5% in water). Monitor vital signs frequently for any indication of bleeding or infection.
• After surgery, give standard postoperative care. Watch for intraperitoneal bleeding and sepsis, which may precipitate coma. Monitor for renal failure by checking urine output, blood urea nitrogen, and creatinine levels hourly.

• Remember that throughout the course of this intractable illness, your primary concern is to keep the patient as comfortable as possible.

Lung abscess

Description
Lung abscess is a lung infection accompanied by pus accumulation and tissue destruction. It often has a well-defined border. The availability of effective antibiotics has made this condition much less common than it was in the past. Lung abscess is a manifestation of necrotizing pneumonia, often the result of aspiration of oropharyngeal contents. Poor oral hygiene with dental or gingival (gum) disease is strongly associated with putrid lung abscess.

Cause
Anaerobic or aerobic bacteria

Signs and symptoms
• Cough (may produce bloody, purulent, or foul-smelling sputum)
• Pleuritic chest pain
• Dyspnea
• Excessive sweating
• Chills
• Fever
• Headache
• Malaise
• Diaphoresis
• Weight loss
• Rales
• Diminished breath sounds

Diagnostic tests
• Chest X-ray shows a localized infiltrate with one or more clear spaces, usually containing air-fluid levels.
• Percutaneous aspiration of an abscess may be attempted or bronchoscopy may be used to obtain cultures

to identify the causative organism. Bronchoscopy is used only if abscess resolution is eventful and the patient's condition permits it.

• Blood cultures, Gram stain, and culture of sputum are also used to detect the causative organism. Leukocytosis (WBC count greater than 10,000/mm³) is commonly present.

Treatment

Treatment consists of prolonged antibiotic therapy, often lasting for months, until radiographic resolution or definite stability occurs. Symptoms usually disappear in a few weeks. Postural drainage may facilitate discharge of necrotic material into upper airways, where expectoration is possible. Oxygen therapy may relieve hypoxemia. Poor response to therapy requires resection of the lesion or removal of the diseased section of the lung. All patients need rigorous follow-up and serial chest X-rays.

Clinical implications

Care emphasizes aiding the patient with chest physiotherapy (including coughing and deep breathing), increasing fluid intake to loosen secretions, and providing a quiet, restful atmosphere.

• To prevent lung abscess in the unconscious patient and the patient with seizures, first prevent aspiration of secretions. Do this by suctioning the patient and by positioning him to promote drainage of secretions.

• Give good mouth care and encourage patients to practice good oral hygiene.

Complications

• Rupture into the pleural space, which results in empyema and, rarely, massive hemorrhage

• With chronic lung abscess, localized bronchiectasis

Lung cancer

Description

Lung cancer usually develops within the wall or epithelium of the bronchial tree. Its most common types are epidermoid (squamous cell) carcinoma, small-cell (oat cell) carcinoma, adenocarcinoma, and large-cell (anaplastic) carcinoma. Although prognosis is generally poor, it varies with cell type and the extent of spread at the time of diagnosis. Only 13% of patients with lung cancer survive 5 years after diagnosis. Lung cancer is the most common cause of cancer death in men and is fast becoming the most common cause in women, even though it is largely preventable.

Cause

Unknown

Risk factors

• Cigarette smoking

• Exposure to carcinogenic industrial and air pollutants (asbestos, uranium, arsenic, nickel, iron oxides, chromium, radioactive dust, and coal dust)

• Familial susceptibility

Signs and symptoms

Because early-stage lung cancer usually produces no symptoms, this disease is often in an advanced state at diagnosis.

Late-stage respiratory symptoms

—Epidermoid and small-cell carcinomas: smoker's cough, hoarseness, wheezing, dyspnea, hemoptysis, and chest pain

—Adenocarcinoma and large-cell carcinoma: fever, weakness, weight loss, anorexia, and shoulder pain

Symptoms due to hormonal changes

—Gynecomastia (possible with large-cell carcinoma)

—Bone and joint pain (possible with large-cell carcinoma and adenocarcinoma)

—Symptoms of Cushing's and carcinoid syndromes (possible with small-cell carcinoma)

—Symptoms of hypercalcemia, such as muscle pain and weakness (possible with epidermoid tumors)

Metastatic symptoms

—Bronchial obstruction: hemoptysis, atelectasis, pneumonitis, dyspnea

—Recurrent nerve invasion: hoarseness, vocal cord paralysis

—Chest wall invasion: piercing chest pain; increasing dyspnea; severe shoulder pain, radiating down arm

—Local lymphatic spread: cough, hemoptysis, stridor, pleural effusion

—Phrenic nerve involvement: dyspnea; shoulder pain; unilateral paralyzed diaphragm, with paradoxical motion

—Esophageal compression: dysphagia

—Vena caval obstruction: venous distention and edema of face, neck, chest, and back

—Pericardial involvement: pericardial effusion, tamponade, dysrhythmias

—Cervical thoracic sympathetic nerve involvement: miosis, ptosis, exophthalmos, reduced sweating

Diagnostic tests

• Chest X-ray usually shows an advanced lesion, but it can detect a lesion up to 2 years before symptoms appear. It also indicates tumor size and location.

• Sputum cytology, which is 75% reliable, requires specimen coughed up from lungs and tracheobronchial tree, not postnasal secretions or saliva.

• Bronchoscopy can locate the tumor site. Bronchoscopic washings provide material for cytologic and histologic examination. The flexible fiberoptic bronchoscope increases test effectiveness.

• Needle biopsy of the lungs employs biplane fluoroscopic visual control to detect peripherally located tumors.

This allows firm diagnosis in 80% of patients.

• Tissue biopsy of accessible metastatic sites includes supraclavicular and mediastinal node and pleural biopsy.

• Thoracentesis allows chemical and cytologic examination of pleural fluid.

• Additional studies include chest tomography, bronchography, esophagography, angiocardiography (contrast studies of bronchial tree, esophagus, and cardiovascular tissues).

• Tests to detect metastasis include bone scan (positive scan may lead to bone marrow biopsy; bone marrow biopsy is also recommended in small-cell carcinoma), CT scan of the brain, liver function studies, and gallium scan (noninvasive nuclear scan) of liver, spleen, and bone.

• After histologic confirmation, staging determines the extent of the disease and helps in planning treatment and understanding prognosis.

Treatment

Treatment—which consists of combinations of surgery, radiation, and chemotherapy—may improve prognosis and prolong survival. Nevertheless, because treatment usually begins at an advanced stage, it is largely palliative.

Surgery is the primary treatment for Stage I, Stage II, or selected Stage III squamous cell carcinoma, adenocarcinoma, and large-cell carcinoma, unless the tumor is nonresectable or other conditions (such as cardiac disease) rule out surgery. Surgery may include partial removal of a lung (wedge resection, lobectomy) or total removal (pneumonectomy, radical pneumonectomy).

Preoperative radiation therapy may reduce tumor bulk to allow for surgical resection, but this is of questionable value. Radiation therapy is ordinarily recommended for Stage I and Stage II lesions if surgery is contraindicated, and for Stage III lesions when the disease is confined to the involved hemithorax and the ipsilateral supraclavicular lymph nodes. Usually, radiation therapy is delayed until 1 month after surgery, to allow the wound to heal, and is then directed to the part of the chest most likely to develop metastatic lesions.

Several new chemotherapy combinations show promise. The combination of fluorouracil, vincristine, and mitomycin induces remission in 40% of patients with adenocarcinomas. Promising combinations for treating small-cell carcinomas include cyclophosphamide, doxorubicin, and vincristine (CAV); cyclophosphamide, doxorubicin, vincristine, and etoposide (CAVE); and etoposide and cisplatin (VP16).

Immunotherapy is still experimental. Nonspecific immunotherapy using bacille Calmette-Guérin (BCG) vaccine or possibly *Corynebacterium parvulum* appears the most promising.

In laser therapy, also largely experimental, a laser beam is directed through a bronchoscope to destroy local tumors.

Clinical implications

Comprehensive supportive care and patient teaching can minimize complications and speed recovery from surgery, radiation, and chemotherapy.

Before surgery, follow these guidelines:
• Supplement and reinforce what the physician has told the patient about the disease and the surgical procedure itself.
• Explain expected postoperative procedures, such as insertion of a Foley catheter, endotracheal tube, dressing changes, and I.V. therapy. Instruct the patient in coughing, deep diaphragmatic breathing, and range-of-motion exercises. Reassure him that analgesics and proper positioning will control postoperative pain.
• Explain preoperative measures.

After thoracic surgery, follow these guidelines:

• Maintain a patent airway, and monitor chest tubes to reestablish normal intrathoracic pressure and prevent postoperative and pulmonary complications.
• Check vital signs.
• Suction often, and encourage the patient to begin deep breathing and coughing as soon as possible. Check secretions often. Initially, sputum will be thick and dark with blood, but it should become thinner and grayish-yellow within a day.
• Monitor and record closed chest drainage. Keep chest tubes patent and draining effectively. Position the patient on the surgical side to promote drainage and lung reexpansion.
• Watch for and report foul-smelling discharge and excessive drainage on dressing. Usually, the dressing is removed after 24 hours, unless the wound appears infected.
• Monitor intake and output. Maintain adequate hydration.
• Watch for and treat infection, shock, hemorrhage, atelectasis, dyspnea, mediastinal shift, and pulmonary embolus.
• To prevent pulmonary embolus, apply antiembolism stockings and encourage range-of-motion exercises.

If the patient is receiving chemotherapy and radiation, follow these guidelines:
• Explain possible side effects of radiation and chemotherapy. Watch for and treat them. When possible, try to prevent them.
• Ask the dietary department to provide soft, nonirritating foods that are high in protein, and encourage the patient to eat high-calorie between-meal snacks.
• Give antiemetics and antidiarrheals, as needed.
• Schedule patient care to help the patient conserve his energy.
• Impose reverse isolation if the pa-

tient develops bone marrow suppression.

To prevent lung cancer, educate high-risk patients in ways to reduce their chances of developing lung cancer:

• Refer smokers who want to quit to local branches of the American Cancer Society, Smokenders, I Quit Smoking Clinics, or I'm Not Smoking Clubs. As an alternative, suggest group therapy, individual counseling, or hypnosis.

• Recommend that all heavy smokers over age 40 have a chest X-ray annually and sputum cytology every 6 months. Also encourage patients with recurring or chronic respiratory infections and those with chronic lung disease who detect any change in the character of a cough to see their physician promptly for evaluation.

Lyme disease

Description

A multisystemic disorder, Lyme disease is caused by a spirochete. It often begins in the summer with the classic skin lesion called erythema chronicum migrans (ECM). Weeks or months later, cardiac or neurologic abnormalities sometimes develop, possibly followed by arthritis.

Cause

The spirochete *Borrelia burgdorferi*

Mode of transmission

The minute tick *Ixodes dammini* or another tick in the Ixodidae family injects spirochete-laden saliva into the bloodstream or deposits fecal matter on the skin.

Signs and symptoms

Stage one

ECM is the characteristic sign. A red macule or papule develops; later more lesions may erupt, along with a malar rash, conjunctivitis, or diffuse urticaria. Then, lesions are replaced by small red blotches. Other symptoms include the following:

—Constant malaise and fatigue

—Intermittent headache, fever, chills, achiness, and regional lymphadenopathy

—Less commonly, symptoms of meningeal irritation, mild encephalopathy, hepatitis and migrating musculoskeletal pain

Stage two

This begins weeks or months later.

—Symptoms of fluctuating meningoencephalitis with peripheral and crainal neuropathy

—Facial palsy

—Cardiac abnormalities, such as fluctuating atrioventricular heart block

Stage three

This begins weeks or years later.

—Arthritis, with marked swelling, especially in the large joints

Diagnostic tests

• Because isolation of *B. burgdorferi* is unusual in humans and because indirect immunofluorescent antibody tests are marginally sensitive, diagnosis often rests on the characteristic ECM lesion and related clinical findings, especially in endemic areas.

• Blood tests showing mild anemia and elevated erythrocyte sedimentation rate, leukocyte count, serum IgM, and SGOT support the diagnosis.

Treatment

A 10- to 20-day course of oral tetracycline is the treatment of choice for adults. Penicillin and erythromycin are alternatives. Oral penicillin is usually prescribed for children. When given in the early stages, these drugs can minimize later complications. When given during the late stages, high-dose penicillin I.V. may be a successful treatment.

Clinical implications

• Take a detailed patient history, ask-

ing about travel to endemic areas and exposure to ticks.
• Check for drug allergies, and administer antibiotics carefully.
• For a patient with arthritis, help with range-of-motion and strengthening exercises, but avoid overexertion.
• Assess the patient's neurologic function and level of consciousness frequently. Watch for signs of increased intracranial pressure and cranial nerve involvement, such as ptosis, strabismus, and diplopia. Also check for cardiac abnormalities, such as dysrhythmias and heart block.

Lymphomas, malignant
(Non-Hodgkin's lymphomas, lymphosarcomas)

Description
Malignant lymphomas are a heterogeneous group of malignant diseases originating in lymph glands and other lymphoid tissue. Lymphomas are categorized by the Rappaport histologic classification according to the degree of cellular differentiation and the presence or absence of nodularity. Nodular lymphomas yield a better prognosis than the diffuse form of the disease, but prognosis is less hopeful in both than in Hodgkin's disease.

Cause
Unknown, although some theories suggest a viral source

Signs and symptoms
• Swelling of the lymph glands
• Enlarged tonsils and adenoids
• Painless rubbery nodes in the cervical supraclavicular area
• Possible dyspnea and coughing
• With disease progression, fatigue, malaise, weight loss, fever, and night sweats

Diagnostic tests
• Histologic evaluation of biopsied lymph nodes; of tonsils, bone marrow, liver, bowel, or skin; or, as needed, of tissue removed during exploratory laparotomy comfirms the diagnosis.
• Other relevant tests include bone and chest X-rays, lymphangiography, liver and spleen scan, CT scan of the abdomen, and intravenous pyelography.

Staging Malignant Lymphoma

Stage I: Involvement of a single lymph node region or of a single extralymphatic organ or site

Stage II: Involvement of two or more lymph node regions on the same side of the diaphragm, or localized involvement of an extralymphatic organ and one or more lymph node regions on the same side of the diaphragm

Stage III: Involvement of lymph node regions on both sides of the diaphragm, which may also be accompanied by localized involvement of an extralymphatic organ or site or by involvement of the spleen or both

Stage IV: Diffuse or disseminated involvement of one or more extralymphatic organs or tissues with or without associated lymph node enlargement.

Reprinted from *Manual for Staging of Cancer* (Chicago: American Joint Committee for Cancer Staging and End Results Reporting, 1983). Used with permission.

• Laboratory tests include CBC (may show anemia), uric acid (elevated or normal), serum calcium (elevated if bone lesions are present), serum protein (normal), and liver function studies. (See *Staging Malignant Lymphoma*.)

Treatment

Treatment for malignant lymphomas may include radiotherapy or chemotherapy. Radiotherapy is used mainly in the early localized stage of the disease. Total body irradiation is often effective for both nodular and diffuse lymphomas.

Chemotherapy is most effective with multiple combinations of antineoplastic agents. For example, cyclophosphamide, vincristine, and prednisone can induce complete remission in 70% to 80% of patients with nodular lymphoma and in 20% to 55% of patients with diffuse lymphoma. Other combinations—such as bleomycin, Adriamycin, Cytoxan, vincristine (Oncovin), and prednisone (BACOP)—induce prolonged remission and possible cure in patients with diffuse lymphoma.

• Observe the patient who is receiving radiation or chemotherapy for side effects (anorexia, nausea, vomiting, diarrhea). Consult with the dietitian, and plan small, frequent meals scheduled around the patient's treatment and including his favorite foods.

• If the patient cannot tolerate oral feedings, administer I.V. fluids and, if necessary, give antiemetics and sedatives, as ordered.

• Instruct the patient to keep irradiated skin dry.

• Provide emotional support by informing the patient and family about the prognosis and diagnosis and by listening to their concerns. If needed, refer them to the local chapter of the American Cancer Society for information and counseling. Stress the need for continued treatment and follow-up care.

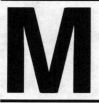

Malaria

Description
Malaria, an acute infectious disease, is endemic in tropical and subtropical regions. Falciparum malaria is the most severe form of the disease, and is the only fatal form. Untreated primary attacks last from a week to a month or longer. Relapses are common and can recur sporadically for several years. Susceptibility to the disease is universal.

Cause
Protozoa of the genus *Plasmodium*: *P. falciparum, P. vivax, P. malariae,* and *P. ovale*

Mode of transmission
• The bite of female *Anopheles* mosquitoes, which abound in humid, swampy areas. When an infected mosquito bites, it injects *Plasmodium* sporozoites into the wound.
• Blood transfusions from an infected person
• Infected street-drug paraphernalia

Signs and symptoms
• Chills
• Fever
• Diaphoresis
• Headache
• Myalgia alternating with periods of well-being
• Enlarged spleen

Diagnostic tests
• Laboratory identification of the parasites in RBCs of peripheral blood smears confirms the diagnosis.
• Indirect fluorescent serum antibody tests are used by the CDC to identify donors responsible for transfusion malaria. (These tests are unreliable in the acute phase, because antibodies can be undetectable for 2 weeks after onset.)
• Laboratory values show decreased hemoglobin level, normal to decreased leukocyte count (as low as 3,000/mm³), and protein and leukocytes in urine sediment.
• Serum values in falciparum malaria reflect disseminated intravascular coagulation (DIC): reduced number of platelets (20,000 to 50,000/mm³), prolonged prothrombin time (18 to 20 seconds), prolonged partial thromboplastin time (60 to 100 seconds), and decreased plasma fibrinogen.

Treatment
Malaria is best treated with chloroquine P.O. in all but disease caused by chloroquine-resistant *P. falciparum.* Within 24 hours after such therapy begins, symptoms and parasitosis decrease, and the patient usually recovers within 3 to 4 days. If the patient is comatose or vomiting frequently, chloroquine is given I.M. instead. Although rare, toxic reactions include gastrointestinal upset, pruritus, headache, and visual disturbances.

Malaria due to *P. falciparum,* which is resistant to chloroquine, requires treatment with quinine P.O. for 10 days, given concurrently with pyrimethamine and a sulfonamide, such as sulfadiazine. Relapses require the same treatment, or quinine alone, followed by tetracycline.

The only drug available in the United States that is effective against the hepatic stage of the disease is primaquine phosphate, given daily for 14 days. This drug can induce DIC from increased hemolysis of RBCs; consequently, it is contraindicated during an acute attack.

For travelers spending less than 3 weeks in areas where malaria exists, weekly prophylaxis includes chloroquine P.O. beginning 2 weeks before and ending 6 weeks after the trip. Chloroquine and sulfadoxine/pyrimethamine (Fansidar) may be ordered for those staying longer than 3 weeks, although combination treatment can have severe side effects. If the traveler is not sensitive to either component of Fansidar, he may be given a single dose to take if he has a febrile episode. Any traveler who develops acute febrile illness should seek prompt medical attention, even though he has received prophylaxis.

Clinical implications

• Obtain a detailed patient history, noting recent travel, foreign residence, blood transfusion, or drug addiction. Record symptom pattern, fever, type of malaria, and any systemic signs.

• Assess the patient on admission and daily thereafter for fatigue, fever, orthostatic hypotension, disorientation, myalgia, and arthralgia. Enforce bed rest during periods of acute illness.

• Protect the patient from secondary bacterial infection by following proper hand-washing and aseptic techniques. Protect yourself by wearing gloves when handling blood or body fluids containing blood. If DIC occurs, wear a gown and gloves while in contact with the patient. Discard needles and syringes in an impervious container designated for incineration. Double-bag all contaminated linen, and send

---

Preventing Malaria

• Drain, fill, and eliminate breeding areas of the *Anopheles* mosquito.
• Install screens in living and sleeping quarters in endemic areas.
• Use a residual insecticide on clothing and skin to prevent mosquito bites.
• Seek treatment for known cases.
• Question blood donors about a history of malaria or possible exposure to malaria. They *may* give blood if they have not taken any antimalarial drugs and are asymptomatic after 6 months outside an endemic area; they were asymptomatic after treatment for malaria over 3 years ago; or they were asymptomatic after receiving malaria prophylaxis over 3 years ago.
• Seek prophylactic drug therapy before traveling to an endemic area.

---

it to the laundry as an isolation item.

• To reduce fever, administer antipyretics, as ordered. Document onset of fever and its duration, and symptoms before and after episodes.

• Fluid balance is fragile, so keep a strict record of intake and output. Monitor I.V. fluids closely. Avoid fluid overload (especially with *P. falciparum*), since it can lead to pulmonary edema and the aggravation of cerebral symptoms. Observe blood chemistry levels for hyponatremia and increased BUN, creatinine, and bilirubin levels.

• Monitor urine output hourly, and maintain it at 40 to 60 ml/hour for an adult and at 15 to 30 ml/hour for a child. Immediately report any decrease in urine output or the onset of hematuria as a possible sign of renal failure. Be prepared to do peritoneal dialysis for uremia caused by renal failure. For oliguria, administer furosemide or mannitol I.V., as ordered.

• Slowly administer packed RBCs or whole blood, as ordered, while checking for rales, tachycardia, and shortness of breath.

• If humidified oxygen is ordered because of anemia, note the patient's response, particularly any changes in rate or character of respirations, or improvement in mucous membrane color.

• Watch for and immediately report signs of internal bleeding, such as tachycardia, hypotension, and pallor.

• Encourage frequent coughing and deep breathing, especially if the patient is on bed rest or has pulmonary complications. Record the amount and color of sputum.

• Watch for side effects of drug therapy, and take measures to relieve them.

• If the patient is comatose, make frequent, gentle changes in his position, and perform passive range-of-motion exercises every 3 to 4 hours. If the patient is unconscious or disoriented, use restraints, as needed, and keep an airway or padded tongue blade available.

• Provide emotional support and reassurance, especially in critical illness. Explain the procedures and treatment to the patient and his family. Listen sympathetically, and answer questions clearly. Suggest that other family members be tested for malaria. Emphasize the need for follow-up care to check the effectiveness of treatment and to manage residual problems.

• Report all cases of malaria to local public health authorities. (See *Preventing Malaria,* p. 461.)

Complications

• Hemolytic anemia is present in all but the mildest infections.

• Falciparum malaria produces persistent high fever, orthostatic hypotension, and massive erythrocytosis that leads to capillary obstruction at various sites.

—Cerebral: hemiplegia, convulsions, delirium, coma
—Pulmonary: coughing, hemoptysis

—Splanchnic: vomiting, abdominal pain, diarrhea, melena
—Renal: oliguria, anuria, uremia

• During blackwater fever (a complication of *P. falciparum* infection), massive intravascular hemolysis causes jaundice, hemoglobinuria, a tender and enlarged spleen, acute renal failure, and uremia. This dreaded complication is fatal in about 20% of patients.

Malignant melanoma

Description

A neoplasm that arises from melanocytes, malignant melanoma is relatively rare. It accounts for only 1% to 2% of all malignancies. The three types of melanoma are superficial spreading melanoma, nodular malignant melanoma, and lentigo malignant melanoma. Melanoma is slightly more common in women than in men, and is rare in children. Peak incidence occurs between ages 50 and 70, although the incidence in younger age-groups is increasing. Up to 70% of lesions arise from an existing nevus.

Melanoma spreads through the lymphatic and vascular systems and metastasizes to the regional lymph nodes, skin, liver, lungs, and central nervous system. Its course is unpredictable, however, and recurrence and metastases may not appear for more than 5 years after resection of the primary lesion. Prognosis varies with tumor thickness. Usually, superficial lesions are curable, while deeper lesions tend to metastasize. The Breslow level method measures tumor depth from the granular level of the epidermis to the deepest melanoma cell. Melanoma lesions less than 0.76 mm deep have an excellent prognosis, while deeper lesions (more than 0.76 mm) are at risk for metastasis. Prognosis is better for a tumor on an extremity (which is drained by one lymphatic network) than for one on the head, neck, or

Staging Malignant Melanoma

Primary tumor (T)

T_0 Tumor confined to epidermis (Clark level I)

T_1 Tumor invades papillary dermis (level II), or tumor of ≤ 0.75 mm thickness

T_2 Tumor extends to interface between papillary and reticular dermis (level III), or tumor of 0.76 to 1.5 mm thickness

T_3 Tumor extends into reticular dermis (level IV), or tumor of 1.51 to 4 mm thickness

T_4 Tumor invades subcutaneous tissue (level V), or tumor of ≥ 4.1 mm thickness, or satellite within 2 cm of a primary melanoma

Nodal involvement (N)

N_0 No evidence of regional lymph node involvement

N_1 Movable nodes (≤ 5 cm in diameter) involving one regional lymph node station, or no regional lymph node involvement with less than five in-transit (between primary tumor and primary lymph node drainage site) metastases beyond 2 cm from primary site

N_2 Involvement of more than one regional lymph node station, or regional nodes more than 5 cm in diameter or fixed, or five or more in-transit metastases, or any in-transit metastases beyond 2 cm from primary site with regional lymph node involvement

Distant metastasis (M)

M_0 No evidence of metastasis

M_1 Metastasis to skin or subcutaneous tissues beyond the site of primary lymph node drainage

M_2 Metastasis to any distant site other than skin or subcutaneous tissues

Reprinted from *Manual for Staging of Cancer* (Chicago: American Joint Committee for Cancer Staging and End Results Reporting, 1983). Used with permission.

trunk (drained by several networks). (See *Recognizing Potentially Malignant Nevi*, p. 464, and *Staging Malignant Melanoma*.)

Cause
Unknown

Risk factors
Several factors seem to influence the development of melanoma.

• Excessive exposure to sunlight. Melanoma is most common in sunny, warm areas and often develops on parts of the body that are exposed to the sun.

• Skin type. Most persons who develop melanoma have blond or red hair, fair skin, and blue eyes; are prone to sunburn; and are of Celtic or Scandinavian ancestry. Melanoma is rare among blacks; when it does develop, it usually arises in lightly pigmented areas (the palms, plantar surface of the feet, or mucous membranes).

• Hormonal factors. Pregnancy may increase risk and exacerbate growth.

• Family history. Melanoma occurs slightly more often within families.

• History of melanoma. A person who has had one melanoma is at greater risk of developing a second.

Signs and symptoms
Melanoma should be suspected when any skin lesion or nevus enlarges, changes color, becomes inflamed or sore, itches, ulcerates, bleeds, changes texture, or shows signs of surrounding pigment regression (halo nevus or vitiligo).

Superficial spreading melanoma
This is the most common type. It usually develops between ages 40 and 50,

Recognizing Potentially Malignant Nevi

Nevi (moles) are skin lesions that are commonly pigmented and may be hereditary. They begin to grow in childhood (occasionally they are congenital) and become more numerous in young adults. Up to 70% of patients with melanoma have a history of a preexisting nevus at the tumor site. Of these, approximately one third are reported to be congenital; the remainder develop later in life.

Changes in nevi (color, size, shape, texture, ulceration, bleeding, or itching) suggest possible malignant transformation. The presence or absence of hair within a nevus has no significance.

Types of nevi:
• *Junctional nevi* are flat or slightly raised and light to dark brown, with melanocytes confined to the epidermis. Usually, they appear before age 40. These nevi may change into compound nevi if junctional nevus cells proliferate and penetrate into the dermis.
• *Compound nevi* are usually tan to dark brown and slightly raised, although size and color vary. They contain melanocytes in both the dermis and epidermis, and they rarely undergo malignant transformation. Excision is necessary only to rule out malignant transformation or for cosmetic reasons.
• *Dermal nevi* are elevated lesions from 2 to 10 mm in diameter and vary in color from flesh to brown. They usually develop in older adults and generally arise on the upper part of the body. Excision is necessary only to rule out malignant transformation.
• *Blue nevi* are flat or slightly elevated lesions from 0.5 to 1 cm in diameter. They appear on the head, neck, arms, and dorsa of the hands and are twice as common in women as in men. Their blue color results from pigment and collagen, which reflect blue light but absorb other wavelengths, in the dermis. Excision is necessary to rule out pigmented basal cell epithelioma or melanoma, or for cosmetic reasons.
• *Dysplastic nevi* are generally greater than 5 mm in diameter, with irregularly notched or indistinct borders. Coloration is usually a variable mixture of tan and brown, sometimes with red, pink, and black pigmentation. No two lesions are exactly alike. They occur in great numbers (typically over 100 at a time), never singly, usually appearing on the back, scalp, chest, and buttocks. Dysplastic nevi are potentially malignant, especially in patients with a personal or familial history of melanoma. Skin biopsy confirms diagnosis; treatment is by surgical excision, followed by regular physical examinations (every 6 months) to detect any new lesions or changes in existing lesions.
• *Lentigo maligna* (melanotic freckles, Hutchinson freckles) is a precursor to malignant melanoma. (In fact, about one third of them eventually give rise to malignant melanoma.) Usually, they occur in persons over age 40, especially on exposed skin areas such as the face. At first, these lesions are flat tan spots, but they gradually enlarge and darken and develop black speckled areas against their tan or brown background. Each lesion may simultaneously enlarge in one area and regress in another. Histologic examination shows typical and atypical melanocytes along the epidermal basement membrane. Removal by simple excision (not electrodessication and curettage) is recommended.

and arises in areas where irritation is chronic. Characteristics include the following:

—Red, white, and blue color over a brown or black background

—Irregular, notched margin

—Irregular surface

—Small, elevated tumor nodules that may ulcerate and bleed

—Horizontal growth pattern.

Nodular malignant melanoma

This type usually develops between ages 40 and 50, grows vertically, invades the dermis, and metastasizes early.

—Usually polypoidal

—Uniformly dark discoloration, may be grayish; looks like a blackberry.

—Occasionally flesh colored. May have pigment flecks around the base, which may be inflamed.

Lentigo malignant melanoma

This relatively rare type develops over many years from a lentigo maligna on an exposed skin surface. The lesion, which is usually diagnosed between ages 60 and 70, looks like a large (1″ to 2½″ [3- to 6-cm]), flat freckle.

—Tan, brown, black, white, or slate color

—Scattered black nodules on the surface

—Possible ulceration, eventually

Treatment

A patient with malignant melanoma always requires surgical resection to remove the tumor. The extent of resection depends on the size and location of the primary lesion. Closure of a wide resection may necessitate a skin graft. If so, new plastic surgery techniques provide excellent cosmetic repair. Surgical treatment may also include regional lymphadenectomy.

Deep primary lesions may merit adjuvant chemotherapy and immunotherapy to eliminate or reduce the number of tumor cells. Although new drug therapies for primary and metastatic lesions are constantly being developed, their effectiveness awaits further clinical evaluation.

Radiation therapy is usually reserved for metastatic disease. It does not prolong survival but may reduce tumor size and relieve pain. Regardless of treatment, melanomas require close long-term follow-up to detect metastases and recurrences. Statistics show that 13% of recurrences develop more than 5 years after primary surgery.

Clinical implications

Management of the melanoma patient requires careful physical, psychological, and social assessment. Preoperative teaching, meticulous postoperative care, and psychological support can make the patient more comfortable, speed recovery, and prevent complications.

• After diagnosis, review the physician's explanation of treatment alternatives. Tell the patient what to expect before and after surgery, what the wound will look like, and what type of dressing will be used. Warn him that the donor site for a skin graft may be as painful as, if not more painful than, the tumor excision site itself. Honestly answer any questions he may have regarding surgery, chemotherapy, and radiation.

• After surgery, be careful to prevent infection. Check dressings often for excessive drainage, foul odor, redness, or swelling. If surgery included lymphadenectomy, minimize lymphedema by applying a compression stocking, and instruct the patient to keep the extremity elevated.

• During chemotherapy, know what side effects to expect and do what you can to minimize them. For instance, give an antiemetic, as ordered, to reduce nausea and vomiting.

• To prepare the patient for discharge, emphasize the need for close follow-up to detect recurrences early. Explain that recurrences and metastases, if they occur, are often delayed, so follow-up must continue for years. Tell him how to recognize signs of recurrence.

• Provide psychological support to

help the patient cope with anxiety. Encourage him to verbalize his fears. Answer his questions honestly without destroying hope.

• In advanced metastatic disease, control and prevent pain with consistent, regularly scheduled administration of analgesics. *Do not* wait to relieve pain until after it occurs.

• Make referrals for home care, social services, and spiritual and financial assistance, as needed.

• If the patient is dying, identify the needs of patient, family, and friends, and provide appropriate support and care.

• To help prevent malignant melanoma, stress the detrimental effects of overexposure to solar radiation, especially to fair-skinned, blue-eyed patients. Recommend that they use a sunblock or sunscreen. In all physical examinations, especially in fair-skinned persons, look for unusual nevi or other skin lesions.

Mallory-Weiss syndrome

Description

Mallory-Weiss syndrome involves mild to massive, usually painless bleeding from a tear in the mucosa or submucosa of the cardia or lower esophagus. It is most common in men over age 40, especially alcoholics.

Cause

Prolonged or forceful vomiting, probably when the upper esophageal sphincter fails to relax

Risk factors

• Excessive alcohol intake
• Coughing
• Straining during bowel movements
• Trauma
• Convulsions
• Childbirth
• Hiatal hernia
• Esophagitis
• Gastritis

• Atrophic gastric mucosa

Signs and symptoms

• Vomiting of blood or passing large amounts of blood rectally a few hours to several days after normal vomiting
• Possible epigastric or back pain

Diagnostic tests

• Fiber-optic endoscopy confirms the diagnosis.
• Angiography (selective celiac arteriography) can determine the bleeding site but not the cause. This is used when endoscopy is not available.
• Hematocrit helps quantify blood loss.

Treatment

Treatment varies with the severity of bleeding. Usually, gastrointestinal bleeding stops spontaneously, and requires supportive measures and careful observation but no definitive treatment. If bleeding continues, treatment may include the following:

• Angiography, with infusion of a vasoconstrictor (vasopressin) into the superior mesenteric artery or direct infusion into a vessel that leads to the bleeding artery
• Transcatheter embolization or thrombus formation with an autologous blood clot or other hemostatic material (insertion of artificial material, such as shredded absorbable gelatin sponge, or, less often, the patient's own clotted blood through a catheter into the bleeding vessel to aid thrombus formation)
• Surgery to suture each laceration (for massive recurrent or uncontrollable bleeding).

Clinical implications

• Evaluate respiratory status, monitor arterial blood gas measurements, and administer oxygen, as necessary.
• Assess the amount of blood loss, and record related symptoms, such as hematemesis and melena (including color, amount, consistency, and frequency). Monitor hematologic status

(hemoglobin, hematocrit, RBCs). Draw blood for coagulation studies (prothrombin time, partial thromboplastin time, and platelet count) and typing and cross matching. Try to keep 3 units of matched whole blood on hand at all times. Until blood is available, insert a large-bore (14G to 18G) I.V. line, and start a temporary infusion of normal saline solution.

• Monitor vital signs, central venous pressure, urinary output, and overall clinical status.

• Explain diagnostic procedures carefully to facilitate cooperation and promote psychological well-being.

• Keep the patient warm.

• Obtain a history of recent medications taken, dietary habits, and use of alcohol. Avoid giving medications that may cause nausea or vomiting. Administer antiemetics to prevent postoperative retching and vomiting.

• Reassure the patient that bleeding will subside.

• Advise the patient to avoid alcohol, aspirin, and other irritating substances.

Complications
In Mallory-Weiss syndrome, the blood vessels are only partially severed, preventing retraction and closure of the lumen. Massive bleeding—most likely when the tear is on the gastric side, near the cardia—may quickly lead to fatal shock.

Marfan's syndrome
(Arachnodactyly)

Description
Marfan's syndrome is a rare, inherited, degenerative, generalized disease of connective tissue that causes ocular, skeletal, and cardiovascular anomalies. Death is usually attributed to cardiovascular complications and may occur anytime from early infancy to adulthood, depending on the severity of the symptoms.

Causes
• Marfan's syndrome probably results from elastin and collagen abnormalities.

• It is inherited as an autosomal dominant trait.

Signs and symptoms
Diagnosis rests on typical clinical features and a history of the disease in close relatives. Signs and symptoms include the following:

• Excessively long tubular bones
• Arm span exceeding height
• Chest deformities
• Weakness of ligaments, tendons, and joint capsules
• Eye problems, especially crystalline lens displacement (ectopia lentis) and myopia
• Abnormal heart sounds
• Sparsity of subcutaneous fat
• Scoliosis

Diagnostic tests
X-rays identify skeletal abnormalities.

Treatment
Attempts to stop the degenerative process have met with little success. Therefore, treatment of Marfan's syndrome is basically symptomatic, such as surgical repair of aneurysms and of ocular deformities. In young patients with early dilation of the aorta, prompt treatment with propranolol can often decrease ventricular ejection and protect the aorta. Extreme dilation requires surgical replacement of the aorta and the aortic valve. Steroids and sex hormones have been successful (especially in girls) in inducing precocious puberty and early epiphyseal closure to prevent abnormal adult height. Genetic counseling is important, particularly since pregnancy and resultant increased cardiovascular work load can produce aortic rupture.

Clinical implications
• Provide supportive care, as appropriate for the patient's clinical status.
• Also provide information for the pa-

tient and his family about the course of this disease and its potential complications, such as lung disease and pneumothorax.

• Stress the need for frequent check-ups so that degenerative changes can be discovered and treated early.

• Emphasize the importance of taking prescribed medication as ordered.

• If recommended by the physician, encourage hormonal therapy to induce early epiphyseal closure, thus preventing abnormal adult height.

• Encourage normal adolescent development by telling the parents not to have unrealistic expectations for the child just because he is tall and looks older than his years.

Complications

• The most serious complications occur in the cardiovascular system and include weakness of the aortic media, leading to progressive dilation or dissecting aneurysm of the ascending aorta. Dilation appears first in the coronary sinuses and is often preceded by aortic regurgitation. Less common cardiovascular complications include mitral regurgitation and endocarditis.

• Other general problems include frequent hernia, cystic lung disease, and recurrent spontaneous pneumothorax.

Mastitis and breast engorgement

Description

Mastitis (parenchymatous inflammation of the mammary glands) and breast engorgement (congestion) are disorders that may affect lactating females. Mastitis occurs in about 1% of women postpartum, mainly in primiparas who are breast-feeding. It occurs occasionally in nonlactating females and rarely in males. All breast-feeding mothers develop some degree of engorgement, but it is especially likely to be severe in primiparas. Prognosis for both disorders is good.

Causes

Mastitis

—A pathogen, most commonly *Staphylococcus aureus*, from the infant's nose or pharynx invades breast tissue through a fissured or cracked nipple.

—Rarely, disseminated tuberculosis or the mumps virus is the cause.

Breast engorgement

—Venous and lymphatic stasis

—Alveolar milk accumulation

Risk factors

• A fissure or abrasion on the nipple

• Wearing a tight bra

• Prolonged intervals between breast-feedings

• Incomplete let-down reflex, usually due to emotional trauma

Signs and symptoms

Mastitis

—Fever (temperature of 101° F. [38.3° C.] or higher)

—Malaise

—Flulike symptoms

—Tender, hard, swollen, warm breasts

Breast engorgement

—Mild to severe pain

—Possible fever

—Swollen, rigid breast

Diagnostic tests

• Cultures of expressed milk in a lactating female confirm generalized mastitis.

• Cultures of breast skin surface confirm localized mastitis.

Treatment

Antibiotic therapy is the primary treatment for mastitis. Although symptoms usually subside 2 to 3 days after treatment begins, antibiotic therapy should continue for 10 days. Other appropriate measures include analgesics for pain. Rarely, when antibiotics fail to control the infection and mastitis progresses to breast abscess, incision and drainage of the abscess are necessary.

Treatment of breast engorgement is aimed at relieving discomfort and controlling swelling. It may include analgesics to alleviate pain, and ice packs and an uplift support to minimize edema. Rarely, oxytocin nasal spray may be necessary to release milk from the alveoli into the ducts. To facilitate breast-feeding, the mother may manually express excess milk before a feeding so the infant can grasp the nipple properly.

Clinical implications

If the patient has mastitis, follow these guidelines:

• Isolate the patient and her infant to prevent the spread of infection to other nursing mothers. Explain mastitis to the patient and why isolation is necessary.

• Assess and record the cause and amount of discomfort. Give analgesics, as needed.

• Reassure the mother that breast-feeding during mastitis will not harm her infant, since he is the source of the infection. Tell her to offer the infant the affected breast first to promote complete emptying of the breast and prevent clogged ducts.

• If an open abscess develops, tell her to stop breast-feeding with the affected breast and use a breast pump until the abscess heals. She should continue to breast-feed on the unaffected side. Suggest applying a warm, wet towel to the affected breast or taking a warm shower to relax and improve her ability to breast-feed.

• To prevent mastitis and relieve its symptoms, teach the patient good health care, breast care, and breast-feeding habits. Advise her to always wash her hands before touching her breasts.

If the patient has breast engorgement, follow these guidelines:

• Assess and record the level of discomfort. Give analgesics, and apply ice packs and a compression binder, as needed.

• Teach the patient how to express excess breast milk manually. She should do this just before nursing to enable the infant to get the swollen areola into his mouth. Caution against excessive expression of milk between feedings; this stimulates milk production and prolongs engorgement.

• Explain that because breast engorgement is due to the physiologic processes of lactation, breast-feeding is the best remedy for engorgement. Suggest breast-feeding every 2 to 3 hours and at least once during the night.

• Ensure that the mother wears a well-fitted nursing bra, usually a size larger than she normally wears.

Complications

Breast abscess

Mastoiditis

Description

Mastoiditis is a bacterial infection and inflammation of the air cells of the mastoid antrum. It is usually a complication of chronic otitis media and, less frequently, of acute otitis media. An accumulation of pus under pressure in the middle ear cavity results in necrosis of adjacent tissue and extension of the infection into the mastoid cells. Chronic systemic diseases or immunosuppression may also lead to mastoiditis. Prognosis is good with early treatment.

Cause

Bacteria that cause mastoiditis include pneumococcus (usually in children under age 6), *Hemophilus influenzae,* beta-hemolytic streptococci, staphylococci, and gram-negative organisms.

Signs and symptoms

• Dull ache and tenderness in the area of the mastoid process
• Low-grade fever
• Thick, purulent discharge that grad-

ually becomes more profuse
- Postauricular erythema and edema (may push the auricle out from the head)
- Possible conductive hearing loss
- Edema of the tympanic membrane

Diagnostic tests
X-rays of the mastoid area reveal hazy mastoid air cells. The bony walls between the cells appear decalcified.

Treatment
Treatment of mastoiditis consists of intense parenteral antibiotic therapy. If bone damage is minimal, myringotomy drains purulent fluid and provides a specimen of discharge for culture and sensitivity testing. Recurrent or persistent infection, or signs of intracranial complications necessitate simple mastoidectomy. This procedure involves removal of the diseased bone and cleansing of the affected area, after which a drain is inserted.

A chronically inflamed mastoid bone requires radical mastoidectomy (excision of the posterior wall of the ear canal, remnants of the tympanic membrane, and the malleus and incus [although these bones are usually destroyed by infection before surgery]). The stapes and facial nerve remain intact. Radical mastoidectomy, which is seldom necessary because of antibiotic therapy, does not drastically affect the patient's hearing because significant hearing loss precedes surgery. With either surgical procedure, the patient continues oral antibiotic therapy for several weeks after surgery and hospital discharge.

Clinical implications
- After simple mastoidectomy, give pain medication, as needed. Check wound drainage, and reinforce dressings (the surgeon usually changes the dressing daily and removes the drain in 72 hours). Check the patient's hearing, and watch for signs of complications, especially infection (either localized or extending to the brain); facial nerve paralysis, with unilateral facial drooping; bleeding; and vertigo, especially when the patient stands.
- After radical mastoidectomy, the wound is packed with petrolatum gauze or gauze treated with an antibiotic ointment. Give pain medication before the packing is removed, on the fourth or fifth postoperative day.
- Because of stimulation to the inner ear during surgery, the patient may feel dizzy and nauseated for several days afterward. Keep the side rails up, and assist the patient with ambulation. Also, give antiemetics, as ordered and as needed.
- Before discharge, teach the patient and family how to change the dressing and tell them to avoid getting it wet. Urge compliance with prescribed antibiotic treatment, and promote regular follow-up care.

Complications
- Meningitis
- Facial paralysis
- Brain abscess
- Suppurative labyrinthitis

Melasma
(Chloasma, mask of pregnancy)

Description
A patchy, hypermelanotic skin disorder, melasma poses a serious cosmetic problem. Although it tends to occur equally in all races, the light-brown color characteristic of melasma is most evident in dark-skinned whites. Melasma affects females more often than males. It may be chronic but is never life-threatening.

Cause
Unknown

Risk factors
Melasma may develop without any apparent predisposing factor. It may also

be related to the following:
• Increased hormonal levels associated with pregnancy, ovarian carcinoma, and the use of oral contraceptives
• Progestational agents, phenytoin, and mephenytoin
• Exposure to sunlight

Signs and symptoms

Typically, melasma produces large, brown, irregular patches, symmetrically distributed on the forehead, cheeks, and sides of the nose. Less commonly, these patches may occur on the neck, upper lip, and temples.

Treatment and clinical implications

Treatment consists primarily of application of bleaching agents containing 2% to 4% hydroquinone, to inhibit melanin synthesis. This preparation is applied twice daily for up to 8 weeks. Adjunctive measures include topical steroids, avoidance of sunlight, use of sunblockers, and discontinuation of oral contraceptives.
• Instruct the patient to avoid sunlight by using sunscreens and wearing protective clothing. Advise him that bleaching agents may achieve the desired effect but may require periodic treatments to maintain it. Cosmetics may help mask deep pigmentation.
• Reassure the patient that melasma is treatable. Serial photographs help show the patient that patches are improving.

Ménière's disease
(Endolymphatic hydrops)

Description

Ménière's disease is a labyrinthine dysfunction that usually affects adults between ages 30 and 60. Violent paroxysmal attacks occur, lasting from 10 minutes to several hours. After multiple attacks over several years, this disorder leads to residual tinnitus and hearing loss.

Cause

Unknown

Signs and symptoms

Characteristic effects
—Severe vertigo
—Tinnitus
—Sensorineural hearing loss
Other symptoms
These may occur during acute attacks:
—Severe nausea
—Vomiting
—Sweating
—Giddiness
—Nystagmus
—Loss of balance and falling to the affected side

Diagnostic tests

• Audiometric studies indicate a sensorineural hearing loss and loss of discrimination and recruitment.
• Electronystagmography and X-rays of the internal meatus may be necessary for differential diagnosis.

Treatment

Treatment with atropine may stop an attack in 20 to 30 minutes. Epinephrine or diphenhydramine may be necessary in a severe attack. Dimenhydrinate, meclizine, diphenhydramine, or diazepam may be effective in a milder attack.

Long-term management includes use of a diuretic or vasodilator, and restricted sodium intake. Prophylactic antihistamines or mild sedatives (phenobarbital, diazepam) may also be helpful. If Ménière's disease persists after more than 2 years of treatment or produces incapacitating vertigo, surgical destruction of the affected labyrinth may be necessary. This procedure permanently relieves symptoms but at the expense of irreversible hearing loss.

Clinical implications
- If the patient is in the hospital during an attack of Ménière's disease, advise him against reading and exposure to glaring lights.
- Keep the side rails of the bed up to prevent falls. Tell him not to get out of bed or walk without assistance.
- Instruct the patient to avoid sudden position changes and any tasks that vertigo makes hazardous, because an attack can begin quite rapidly.
- Before surgery, if the patient is vomiting, record fluid intake and output and characteristics of emesis. Administer antiemetics, as ordered, and give small amounts of fluid frequently.
- Explain diagnostic tests and offer reassurance and emotional support.
- After surgery, record intake and output carefully.
- Tell the patient to expect dizziness and nausea for 1 to 2 days after surgery.
- Give prophylactic antibiotics and antiemetics, as ordered.

Meningitis

Description
In meningitis, the brain and the spinal meninges become inflamed, usually as a result of bacterial infection. Such inflammation may involve all three meningeal membranes—the dura mater, the arachnoid, and the pia mater. Prognosis is good and complications are rare, especially if the disease is recognized early and the infecting organism responds to antibiotics. Prognosis is poorer for infants and the elderly. Mortality in untreated meningitis is 70% to 100%.

Causes
- Meningitis is almost always a complication of another bacterial infection—bacteremia (especially from pneumonia, empyema, osteomyelitis, and endocarditis), sinusitis, otitis media, encephalitis, myelitis, or brain abscess—usually caused by *Neisseria meningitidis, Hemophilus influenzae, Streptococcus (Diplococcus) pneumoniae,* and *Escherichia coli.*
- Meningitis may also follow skull fracture, a penetrating head wound, lumbar puncture, or ventricular shunting procedures.
- Aseptic meningitis may result from a virus or other organism. Sometimes, no causative organism can be found.

Signs and symptoms
- Fever
- Chills
- Malaise
- Headache
- Vomiting
- Nuchal rigidity
- Positive Brudzinski's and Kernig's signs
- Exaggerated and symmetrical deep tendon reflexes
- Opisthotonos
- Rarely, papilledema
- Other possible symptoms: sinus dysrhythmias; irritability; photophobia, diplopia, and other visual problems; delirium, deep stupor, and coma; twitching and seizures

Diagnostic tests
- Typical CSF findings (and positive Brudzinski's and Kernig's signs) usually establish the diagnosis. CSF pressure is elevated. CSF protein levels tend to be high and glucose levels may be low.
- CSF culture and sensitivity tests usually identify the infecting organism, unless it is a virus.
- Cultures of blood, urine, and nose and throat secretions; chest X-ray; or an EKG may uncover the primary sites of infection.
- CT scan can rule out cerebral hematoma, hemorrhage, or tumor.

Treatment
Treatment of meningitis includes appropriate antibiotic therapy and vig-

Aseptic Meningitis

Aseptic meningitis is a benign syndrome characterized by headache, fever, vomiting, and meningeal symptoms. It results from some form of virus infection, including enteroviruses (most common), arboviruses, herpes simplex virus, mumps virus, or lymphocytic choriomeningitis virus.

Aseptic meningitis begins suddenly with a fever up to 104° F. (40° C.), alterations in consciousness (drowsiness, confusion, stupor), and neck or spine stiffness, which is slight at first. (The patient experiences such stiffness when bending forward.) Other signs and symptoms include headaches, nausea, vomiting, abdominal pain, poorly defined chest pain, and sore throat.

Patient history of recent illness and knowledge of seasonal epidemics are essential in differentiating among the many forms of aseptic meningitis. Negative bacteriologic cultures and cerebrospinal fluid (CSF) analysis showing pleocytosis and increased protein levels suggest the diagnosis. Isolation of the virus from CSF confirms it.

Treatment is supportive, including bed rest, maintenance of fluid and electrolyte balance, analgesics for pain, and exercises to combat residual weakness. Isolation is not necessary. Careful handling of excretions and good hand-washing technique prevent spreading the disease.

orous supportive care. Usually, I.V. antibiotics are given for at least 2 weeks and are followed by oral antibiotics. Such antibiotics include penicillin G, ampicillin, or nafcillin. If the patient is allergic to penicillin, however, anti-infective therapy includes tetracycline, chloramphenicol, or kanamycin. Other drugs include a cardiac glycoside, such as digoxin, to control dysrhythmias, mannitol to decrease cerebral edema, an anticonvulsant (usually given I.V.) or a sedative to reduce restlessness, and aspirin or acetaminophen to relieve headache and fever.

Supportive measures include bed rest, hypothermia, and measures to prevent dehydration. Isolation is necessary if nasal cultures are positive. Of course, treatment includes appropriate therapy for any coexisting conditions, such as endocarditis or pneumonia.

To prevent meningitis, prophylactic antibiotics are sometimes used after ventricular shunting procedures, skull fracture, or penetrating head wounds. Their use is controversial.

Clinical implications

- Assess neurologic function often.
- Watch for deterioration. Be especially alert for a temperature increase up to 102° F. (38.9° C.), deteriorating level of consciousness, onset of seizures, and altered respirations, all of which may signal an impending crisis.
- Monitor fluid balance. Maintain adequate fluid intake to avoid dehydration, but avoid fluid overload because of the danger of cerebral edema. Measure central venous pressure, and record intake and output accurately.
- Position the patient carefully to prevent joint stiffness and neck pain. Turn him often, according to a planned positioning schedule. Assist with range-of-motion exercises.
- Maintain adequate nutrition and elimination.
- Ensure the patient's comfort. Maintain a quiet environment. Darkening the room may decrease photophobia. Relieve headache with a nonnarcotic analgesic, such as aspirin or acetaminophen, as ordered. (Narcotics interfere with accurate neurologic assessment.)
- Provide reassurance and support.

The patient may be frightened by his illness and frequent lumbar punctures. If he is delirious or confused, attempt to reorient him often. Reassure the family that the delirium and behavior changes caused by meningitis usually disappear. However, if a severe neurologic deficit appears permanent, refer the patient to a rehabilitation program as soon as the acute phase of this illness has passed.

• To help prevent development of meningitis, teach patients with chronic sinusitis or other chronic infections the importance of proper medical treatment. Follow strict aseptic technique when treating patients with head wounds or skull fractures. (See *Aseptic Meningitis*, p. 473.)

Mental retardation

Description
Mental retardation is defined by the American Association of Mental Retardation (AAMR) as "significantly subaverage general intellectual function coexisting with deficits in adaptive behavior and manifested during the developmental period (before age 18)." An estimated 1% to 3% of the population is mentally retarded. Individuals in this group have IQ scores below 70, associated with deficits in their ability to perform tasks required for personal independence.

Causes
The AAMR has grouped the causes of mental retardation into 10 categories (see *Causative Factors in Mental Retardation*). A specific cause is identifiable in only 25% of retarded persons.

Risk factors
• Deficient prenatal or perinatal care
• Inadequate nutrition
• Poor social environment
• Poor child-rearing practices

Signs and symptoms
Deviations from normal adaptive behaviors

Diagnostic tests
• A score below 70 on a standardized IQ test confirms mental retardation and predicts school performance. The recognized levels of mental retardation are as follows:
—Mild retardation, IQ 51 to 69
—Moderate retardation, IQ 36 to 51
—Severe retardation, IQ 20 to 36
—Profound retardation, IQ < 20.

• The Adaptive Behavior Scale evaluates self-help skills (toileting and eating), physical and social development, language, socialization, and time and number concepts. It also examines inappropriate behaviors (such as violent or destructive acts, withdrawal, or self-abusive or sexually aberrant behavior).

• Developmental screening tests, such as the Denver Developmental Screening Test, assess age-appropriate adaptive behaviors.

Treatment
Effective management of a mentally retarded patient requires an interdisciplinary team approach that provides complete, continuous, and coordinated services. A primary goal is to develop the patient's strengths as fully as possible, taking into account his interests, personal experiences, and resources. Another major goal is the development of adaptive social skills to help the patient function as normally as possible.

Mentally retarded children require special education and training, ideally beginning in infancy. Such education has been enormously beneficial and has been extended in recent years even to the profoundly retarded.

Prognosis for persons with mental retardation is related more to timing and aggressiveness of treatment, personal motivation, training opportunities, and associated conditions than to retardation itself. With good support

Causative Factors in Mental Retardation

- Infection and intoxication (congenital rubella, syphilis, lead poisoning, meningitis, encephalitis, insecticides, drugs, maternal viral infection)
- Trauma or physical agents (mechanical injury, asphyxia, hyperpyrexia)
- Disorders of metabolism or nutrition (phenylketonuria, hypothyroidism, Hurler's syndrome, galactosemia, Tay-Sachs disease)
- Gross brain disease, postnatal (neurofibromatosis, intracranial neoplasm)
- Diseases and conditions resulting from unknown prenatal influence (hydrocephalus, hydranencephaly, microcephaly)
- Gestational disorders (prematurity)
- Chromosomal abnormalities (Down's syndrome, Klinefelter's syndrome)
- Psychiatric disorders (autism)
- Environmental influences (cultural-familial retardation, poor nutrition, no medical care)
- Other conditions

Adapted from P. Chinn, et al., *Mental Retardation: A Life Cycle Approach*, 2nd ed. St. Louis: C.V. Mosby Co., 1979, p. 16. Reprinted by permission of Merrill Publishing Co., Columbus, Ohio

systems, many mentally retarded persons have become productive members of society. Successful management leads to independent functioning for some and a sheltered environment for others. Even those persons whose handicaps require total care benefit from appropriate stimulation and training.

Clinical implications
- Carefully assess the retarded person's health needs, plan activities to maximize abilities, and make referrals as needed. Remember that the mentally retarded child has all the ordinary needs of a normal child plus those created by his handicap. The child also needs affection, acceptance, stimulation, and prudent, consistent discipline; he is less able to cope if rejected, overprotected, or forced beyond his abilities.
- When caring for a hospitalized retarded patient, promote continuity of care by acting as liaison for parents and other health care professionals involved in his care. During hospitalization, continue training programs already in place, but remember that illness may bring on some regression in behavior and skills.

- Teach retarded adolescents how to deal with physical changes and sexual maturation. Encourage participation in appropriate sex education classes. Consider that the retarded person may find it difficult to express his sexual concerns because of limited verbal skills.
- Provide coordinated advice, support, and practical help for the family. Suggest that the family contact the AAMR and the National Association for Retarded Citizens for more information and referral to sources of community support.

Metabolic acidosis

Description
Metabolic acidosis, a physiologic state of excess acid accumulation and deficient base bicarbonate, is produced by an underlying pathologic disorder. Symptoms result from the body's attempts to correct the acidotic condition through compensatory mecha-

nisms in the lungs, kidneys, and cells. Metabolic acidosis is more prevalent among children, who are vulnerable to acid-base imbalance because their metabolic rates are faster and their ratios of water to body weight are lower. Severe or untreated metabolic acidosis can be fatal.

Causes
• Diabetic ketosis
• Starvation
• Chronic alcoholism
• Low-carbohydrate, high-fat diet
• Renal insufficiency and failure
• Lactic acidosis
• Diarrhea and intestinal malabsorption
• Addison's disease
• Biliary fistulas
• Salicylate intoxication
• Exogenous poisoning

Signs and symptoms
• Headache and lethargy
• Kussmaul's respirations
• Disorientation
• Drowsiness (may progress to stupor and coma)
• Possible nausea, vomiting, anorexia, or diarrhea

Diagnostic tests
• Arterial pH below 7.35 confirms metabolic acidosis.
• In severe acidotic states, pH may fall to 7.10, and PCO_2 in arterial blood gas levels may be normal or < 34 mm Hg as compensatory mechanisms take hold.
• HCO_3 may be < 22 mEq/liter.
• Urine pH is < 4.5 in the absence of renal disease.
• Serum potassium is > 5.5 mEq/liter from chemical buffering.
• Glucose is > 150 mg/dl in diabetes.
• Serum ketone bodies are elevated in diabetes mellitus.
• Plasma lactic acid is elevated in lactic acidosis.
• Anion gap > 14 mEq/liter indicates metabolic acidosis (diabetic ketoacidosis, aspirin overdose, alcohol poisoning).

Treatment
Treatment for metabolic acidosis includes sodium bicarbonate I.V. to neutralize blood acidity, careful evaluation and correction of electrolyte imbalances, and, ultimately, correction of the underlying cause. For example, in diabetic ketoacidosis, low-dose continuous I.V. insulin infusion is recommended.

Clinical implications
• Keep sodium bicarbonate ampules handy for emergency administration. Frequently monitor vital signs, laboratory results, and level of consciousness, since changes can occur rapidly.
• In diabetic acidosis, watch for secondary changes due to hypovolemia, such as decreasing blood pressure.
• Record intake and output accurately to monitor renal function. Watch for signs of excessive serum potassium—weakness, flaccid paralysis, and dysrhythmias, possibly leading to cardiac arrest. After treatment, check for overcorrection to hypokalemia.
• Because metabolic acidosis commonly causes vomiting, position the patient to prevent aspiration. Be prepared for possible convulsions (seizure precautions).
• Provide good oral hygiene. Use sodium bicarbonate washes to neutralize mouth acids, and lubricate the patient's lips with lemon and glycerine swabs.
• To prevent metabolic acidosis, carefully observe patients receiving I.V. therapy or those who have intestinal tubes in place, and those suffering from shock, hyperthyroidism, hepatic disease, circulatory failure, or dehydration. Teach the patient with diabetes how to routinely test urine for sugar and acetone, and encourage strict adherence to insulin or oral hypoglycemic therapy.

Metabolic alkalosis

Description

A clinical state marked by decreased amounts of acid or increased amounts of base bicarbonate, metabolic alkalosis causes metabolic, respiratory, and renal responses. It produces characteristic symptoms—most notably, hypoventilation. This condition is always secondary to an underlying cause. With early diagnosis and prompt treatment, prognosis is good. Untreated metabolic alkalosis may lead to coma and death.

Causes

Acid loss
—Vomiting
—Hyperadrenocorticism
—Hyperaldosteronism
—Cushing's disease
—Nasogastric tube drainage or lavage without adequate electrolyte replacement
—Use of steroids and certain diuretics
Base retention
—Excessive intake of bicarbonate of soda or other antacids
—Milk-alkali syndrome
—Excessive I.V. infusions with high concentrations of bicarbonate

Signs and symptoms

• Hypoventilation
• Irritability
• Twitching
• Confusion
• Possible tetany
• Nausea and vomiting
• Dysrhythmias
• Weakness
• Leg cramps
• Paresthesias
• Possible progression to convulsions and coma

Diagnostic tests

• Blood pH level > 7.45 and HCO_3 > 29 mEq/liter confirm the diagnosis.
• P_{CO_2} > 45 mm Hg indicates attempts at respiratory compensation.
• Serum electrolyte levels show decreased potassium and chloride levels.
• Urine pH is usually about 7.
• Urinalysis reveals alkalinity after the renal compensatory mechanism begins to excrete bicarbonate.
• EKG may show low T wave, merging with a P wave, and atrial tachycardia.

Treatment and clinical implications

The goal of treatment is to correct the underlying cause of metabolic alkalosis. Therapy for severe alkalosis may include cautious administration of ammonium chloride I.V. to release hydrogen chloride and restore concentration of extracellular fluid and chloride levels. Potassium chloride and normal saline solution (except in the presence of congestive heart failure) are usually sufficient to replace losses from gastric drainage. Electrolyte replacement with potassium chloride and discontinuation of diuretics correct metabolic alkalosis resulting from potent diuretic therapy.

Structure your care plan around cautious I.V. therapy, keen observation, and strict monitoring of the patient's status.

• Dilute potassium when giving I.V. solutions containing potassium salts. Monitor the infusion rate to prevent damage to blood vessels. Watch for signs of phlebitis.
• When administering ammonium chloride 0.9%, limit the infusion rate to 1 liter in 4 hours; faster administration may cause RBC hemolysis. Avoid overdosage, since it may cause overcorrection to metabolic acidosis. Do not give ammonium chloride with signs of hepatic or renal disease.
• Watch closely for signs of muscle weakness, tetany, or decreased activity. Monitor vital signs frequently, and record intake and output to evaluate respiratory, fluid, and electrolyte sta-

tus. Remember, respiratory rate usually decreases in an effort to compensate for alkalosis. Hypotension and tachycardia may indicate electrolyte imbalance, especially hypokalemia.

• Observe seizure precautions.

• To prevent metabolic alkalosis, warn patients against overusing alkaline agents. Irrigate nasogastric tubes with isotonic saline solution instead of plain water to prevent loss of gastric electrolytes. Monitor I.V. fluid concentrations of bicarbonate or lactate. Teach patients with ulcers to recognize signs of milk-alkali syndrome: a distaste for milk, anorexia, weakness, and lethargy.

Migraine headache

Description
Migraine headaches are recurring, throbbing, vascular headaches that usually begin to appear in childhood or adolescence and continue throughout adulthood. They are more common in females and have a strong familial incidence. They often occur during a period of relaxation following physical or psychological stress.

Cause
The cause is unknown, but allergic reactions, excess carbohydrates, iodine-rich foods, alcohol, bright lights, or loud noises may trigger attacks.

Signs and symptoms
See *Clinical Features of Migraine Headaches.*

Diagnostic tests
May include skull X-rays, EEG, CT scan, and brain scan to rule out other causes of headache

Treatment
Ergotamine alone or with caffeine is the most effective treatment. These drugs and other analgesics work best when taken early in the course of an attack. If nausea and vomiting make oral administration impossible, drugs may be given as rectal suppositories. Drugs that can help prevent migraine headache include propranolol and calcium channel blockers such as verapamil and diltiazem.

Clinical implications
• Obtain a complete patient history: duration and location of the headache; time of day it usually begins; nature of the pain; concurrence with other symptoms, such as blurred vision; precipitating factors, such as tension, menstruation, loud noises, menopause, or alcohol; medications being taken, such as oral contraceptives; or prolonged fasting.

• Using the history as a guide, help the patient avoid exacerbating factors. Advise him to lie down in a dark, quiet room during an attack and to place ice packs on his forehead or a cold cloth over his eyes.

• Instruct the patient to take the prescribed medication at the onset of migraine symptoms, to prevent dehydration by drinking plenty of fluids after nausea and vomiting subside, and to use other headache relief measures.

• The patient with migraine usually needs to be hospitalized only if nausea and vomiting are severe enough to induce dehydration and possible shock.

Multiple endocrine neoplasia
(Wermer's syndrome, Sipple's syndrome)

Description
Multiple endocrine neoplasia (MEN) is a hereditary disorder in which two or more endocrine glands develop hyperplasia, adenoma, or carcinoma concurrently or consecutively. Two of the types that occur are well documented; a third may exist. MEN I

Clinical Features of Migraine Headaches

TYPE	SIGNS AND SYMPTOMS
Common migraine *(most prevalent, 85%)* Usually occurs on weekends and holidays	• Prodromal symptoms (fatigue, nausea and vomiting, fluid imbalance) precede headache by about a day. • Sensitivity to light and noise (most prominent feature) • Headache pain (unilateral or bilateral, aching or throbbing) lasts longer than in classic migraine.
Classic migraine *(incidence 10%)* Usually occurs in compulsive personalities and within families	• Prodromal symptoms include visual disturbances, such as zig-zag lines and bright lights (most common), sensory disturbances (tingling of face, lips, and hands), or motor disturbances (staggering gait). • Recurrent and periodic headaches
Hemiplegic and ophthalmoplegic migraine *(rare)* Usually occurs in young adults	• Severe, unilateral pain • Extraocular muscle palsies (involving third cranial nerve) and ptosis • With repeated headaches, possible permanent third cranial nerve injury • In hemiplegic migraine, neurologic deficits (hemiparesis, hemiplegia) may persist after headache subsides.
Basilar artery migraine Occurs in young women before their menstrual periods	• Prodromal symptoms usually include partial vision loss followed by vertigo; ataxia; dysarthria; tinnitus; and, sometimes, tingling of fingers and toes, lasting from several minutes to almost an hour. • Headache pain, severe occipital throbbing, vomiting

(Wermer's syndrome) involves hyperplasia and adenomatosis of the parathyroids, islet cells of the pancreas, pituitary, and, rarely, adrenals and thyroid gland. MEN II (Sipple's syndrome) involves medullary carcinoma of the thyroid, with hyperplasia and adenomatosis of the adrenal medulla (pheochromocytoma) and parathyroids. MEN I is the most common form.

Cause
MEN usually results from autosomal dominant inheritance.

Signs and symptoms
Clinical effects of MEN may develop in various combinations and orders, depending on the glands involved. Any of the following may occur:

MEN I
—Symptoms of peptic ulcer or Zollinger-Ellison syndrome such as epigastric pain (most common)
—Symptoms of hypoglycemia
—Symptoms of hyperparathyroidism, including hypercalcemia
—Symptoms of pituitary hypofunc-

tion, such as amenorrhea, impotence, infertility, or less frequently, hyperfunction, such as acromegaly

MEN II

—With thyroid carcinoma, symptoms such as enlarged thyroid mass

—With ectopic ACTH, symptoms of Cushing's syndrome

—With tumors of the adrenal medulla, symptoms such as headache, tachydysrhythmias, and hypotension

—With adenomatosis or hyperplasia of the parathyroids, symptoms of renal calculi

Diagnostic tests

• Tests used to investigate symptoms of pituitary tumor, hypoglycemia, hypercalcemia, or gastrointestinal hemorrhage may lead to a diagnosis of MEN.

• Diagnostic tests must be used to evaluate carefully each affected endocrine gland. For example, radioimmunoassay showing increased levels of gastrin in patients with peptic ulcer and Zollinger-Ellison syndrome suggests the need for follow-up studies for MEN I, since 50% of patients with Zollinger-Ellison syndrome have MEN.

Treatment

Treatment must eradicate the tumors. Subsequent therapy controls residual symptoms. In MEN I, peptic ulceration is usually the most urgent clinical feature, so primary treatment emphasizes control of bleeding or resection of necrotic tissue. In hypoglycemia caused by insulinoma, P.O. administration of diazoxide or glucose can keep blood glucose within acceptable limits. However, subtotal (partial) pancreatectomy is frequently required. Because all parathyroid glands have the potential for neoplastic enlargement, subtotal parathyroidectomy may also be required, along with transphenoidal hypophysectomy. In MEN II, treatment for adrenal medullary tumor includes antihypertensives and resection of the tumor.

Clinical implications

Supportive care depends on the body system involved.

• If MEN involves the pancreas, monitor blood and urine glucose levels frequently. If it affects the adrenal glands, monitor blood pressure closely, especially during drug therapy.

• Manage peptic ulcers, hypoglycemia, and other complications, as needed.

• If pituitary tumor is suspected, watch for signs of pituitary trophic hormone dysfunction, which may affect any of the endocrine glands. Also, be aware that pituitary apoplexy (sudden severe headache, altered level of consciousness, visual disturbances) may occur.

Multiple myeloma
(Malignant plasmacytoma, plasma cell myeloma, myelomatosis)

Description

Multiple myeloma is a disseminated neoplasm of marrow plasma cells that infiltrates bone to produce osteolytic lesions throughout the skeleton (flat bones, vertebrae, skull, pelvis, ribs); in late stages, it infiltrates the internal organs (liver, spleen, lymph nodes, lungs, adrenal glands, kidneys, skin, and gastrointestinal tract). Prognosis is usually poor, because diagnosis is often made after the disease has already infiltrated the vertebrae, pelvis, skull, ribs, clavicles, and sternum. By then, skeletal destruction is widespread. Without treatment, it leads to vertebral collapse. Early diagnosis and treatment prolong the lives of many patients by 3 to 5 years, but 52% of patients die within 3 months of diagnosis, and 90%, within 2 years.

Cause

Unknown

Signs and symptoms

Severe, constant back pain that increases with exercise is the earliest symptom. Other symptoms include the following:
- Achiness
- Joint swelling and tenderness
- Fever
- Malaise
- Slight evidence of peripheral neuropathy, such as paresthesias
- Pathologic fractures
- With disease progression, anemia, weight loss, thoracic deformities, and loss of height

Diagnostic tests

- CBC shows moderate or severe anemia. The differential may show 40% to 50% lymphocytes but seldom more than 3% plasma cells. Rouleaux formation (often the first clue) seen on differential smear results from elevation of the erythrocyte sedimentation rate.
- Urine studies may show Bence Jones protein and hypercalciuria. Absence of Bence Joines protein does not rule out multiple myeloma; however, its presence almost invariably confirms the disease.
- Bone marrow aspiration detects myelomatous cells (abnormal number of immature plasma cells).
- Serum electrophoresis shows an elevated globulin spike that is electrophoretically and immunologically abnormal.
- X-rays during early stages may show only diffuse osteoporosis. Eventually, they show multiple, sharply circumscribed osteolytic (punched out) lesions, particularly on the skull, pelvis, and spine—the characteristic lesions of multiple myeloma.
- Intravenous pyelography (IVP) can assess renal involvement.

Treatment

Long-term treatment of multiple myeloma consists mainly of chemotherapy to suppress plasma cell growth and control pain. Combinations of mel-phalan and prednisone or of cyclophosphamide and prednisone are used. Adjuvant local radiation reduces acute lesions, such as collapsed vertebrae, and relieves localized pain. Other treatment usually includes a melphalan-prednisone combination in high intermittent doses or low continuous daily doses, and analgesics for pain. If the patient develops spinal cord compression, he may require a laminectomy; if he has renal complications, he may need dialysis.

Because the patient may have bone demineralization and may lose large amounts of calcium into blood and urine, he is a prime candidate for renal stones, nephrocalcinosis, and eventually renal failure due to hypercalcemia. Hypercalcemia is managed with hydration, diuretics, corticosteroids, oral phosphate, and mithramycin I.V. to decrease serum calcium levels.

Clinical implications

- Encourage the patient to drink 3,000 to 4,000 ml of fluids daily, particularly before IVP. Monitor fluid intake and output (daily output should not be less than 1,500 ml).
- Encourage the patient to walk (immobilization increases bone demineralization). Give analgesics, as ordered, to lessen pain. Never allow the patient to walk unaccompanied; be sure that he uses a walker or other supportive aid to prevent falls. Since he is particularly vulnerable to pathologic fractures, he may be fearful. Give reassurance, and allow him to move at his own pace.
- Prevent complications by watching for fever or malaise, which may signal the onset of infection, and for signs of other problems, such as severe anemia and fractures. If the patient is bedridden, change his position every 2 hours. Give passive range-of-motion and deep breathing exercises. When he can tol-

erate them, promote active exercises.
• If possible, get the patient out of bed within 24 hours after laminectomy. Check for hemorrhage, motor or sensory deficits, and loss of bowel or bladder function. Position the patient as ordered, maintain alignment, and log-roll when turning.
• Provide much-needed emotional support for the patient and his family, as they are likely to be very anxious. Help relieve their anxiety by truthfully informing them about diagnostic tests (including painful procedures, such as bone marrow aspiration and biopsy), treatment, and prognosis. If needed, refer them to an appropriate community resource for additional support.

Complications
• Infection
• Renal failure
• Hematologic imbalance
• Fractures
• Hypercalcemia
• Hyperuricemia
• Dehydration

Multiple sclerosis

Description
Multiple sclerosis (MS) is characterized by exacerbations and remissions caused by progressive demyelination of the white matter of the brain and the spinal cord. It is a major cause of chronic disability in young adults. Sporadic patches of demyelination in various parts of the central nervous system induce widely disseminated and varied neurologic dysfunction. Diagnosis requires evidence of multiple neurologic attacks and characteristic remissions and exacerbations.

Prognosis is variable. MS may progress rapidly, disabling the patient by early adulthood or causing death within months of onset. However, 70% of patients lead active, productive lives with prolonged remissions.

Cause
The exact cause of MS is unknown, but current theories suggest a slow-acting viral infection, an autoimmune response of the nervous system, or an allergic response to an infectious agent.

Signs and symptoms
Signs and symptoms are extremely variable and include the following:.
• Visual disturbances, such as optic neuritis, diplopia, ophthalmoplegia, and blurred vision
• Sensory impairment, such as paresthesias
• Muscle dysfunction, such as weakness, paralysis ranging from monoplegia to quadriplegia, spasticity, hyperreflexia, intention tremor, gait ataxia
• Urinary disturbances, such as incontinence, frequency, urgency, and frequent infections
• Emotional lability, such as mood swings, irritability, euphoria, or depression
• Associated signs and symptoms: poorly articulated or scanning speech, and dysphagia

Diagnostic tests
Since diagnosis is so difficult, periodic testing and close observation are necessary, perhaps for years, depending on the course of the disease.
• EEG showing abnormalities occurs in one third of patients.
• Lumbar puncture shows elevated gamma globulin fraction of IgG but normal total protein levels in cerebrospinal fluid (CSF). Elevated CSF gamma globulin is significant only when serum gamma globulin levels are normal; it reflects hyperactivity of the immune system because of chronic demyelination. Oligoclonal bands of immunoglobulin can be detected when CSF gamma globulin is examined by electrophoresis.
• Psychological testing may be needed.
• Various other neurological tests such

Teaching Topics in Multiple Sclerosis

- Explanation of the effects of demyelination on sensory and motor function
- Preparation for tests, such as a computed tomography scan, cerebrospinal fluid analysis, and evoked potential studies, to rule out other disorders
- Administration of drugs to relieve symptoms
- Preparation for stereotaxic thalamotomy, if ordered
- Balancing activity and rest
- Energy conservation
- Measures for minimizing neurologic deficits
- Dietary adjustments (such as semisolid foods) and proper elimination
- Bladder/bowel retraining to correct incontinence
- Self-catheterization technique or Credé's maneuver to correct urinary retention
- Precipitating factors for exacerbations
- Referral for financial and sexual counseling
- Sources of additional information and support

as CT scans and evoked potential studies may be performed to rule out other disorders.

Treatment

The aim of treatment is to shorten exacerbations and, if possible, relieve neurologic deficits, so the patient can resume a normal life-style. Because MS is thought to have allergic and inflammatory causes, ACTH, prednisone, or dexamethasone is used to reduce the associated edema of the myelin sheath during exacerbations. ACTH and corticosteroids seem to relieve symptoms and hasten remission but do not prevent future exacerbations.

Other drugs used with ACTH and corticosteroids include chlordiazepoxide to mitigate mood swings, baclofen or dantrolene to relieve spasticity, and bethanechol or oxybutynin to relieve urinary retention and minimize frequency and urgency. During acute exacerbation, supportive measures include bed rest, comfort measures such as massages, prevention of fatigue, prevention of decubitus ulcers, bowel and bladder training (if necessary), treatment of bladder infections with antibiotics, physical therapy, and counseling.

Clinical implications

Appropriate care depends on the severity of the disease and the symptoms.

- Assist with physical therapy. Increase patient comfort with massages and relaxing baths. Make sure bathwater is not too hot, since it may temporarily intensify otherwise subtle symptoms. Assist with active, resistive, and stretching exercises to maintain muscle tone and joint mobility, decrease spasticity, improve coordination, and boost morale.
- Educate the patient and family concerning the chronic course of MS. Emphasize the need to avoid stress, infections, and fatigue and to maintain independence by developing new ways of performing daily activities. Tell the patient to avoid exposure to infections.
- Stress the importance of eating a nutritious, well-balanced diet that contains sufficient roughage to prevent constipation.
- Evaluate the need for bowel and bladder training during hospitalization. Encourage adequate fluid intake and regular urination. Eventually, the patient may require urinary drainage by self-catheterization or, in men, condom drainage. Teach the correct use of suppositories to help establish a reg-

ular bowel schedule.

• Watch for drug side effects. For instance, dantrolene may cause muscle weakness and decreased muscle tone.

• Promote emotional stability. Help the patient establish a daily routine to maintain optimal functioning. Activity level is regulated by tolerance level. Encourage daily physical exercise and regular rest periods to prevent fatigue.

• Inform the patient that exacerbations are unpredictable, necessitating physical and emotional adjustments in life-style.

• For more information, refer him to the National Multiple Sclerosis Society. (See *Teaching Topics in Multiple Sclerosis,* p. 483.)

Mumps
(Infectious or epidemic parotitis)

Description
Mumps is an acute viral disease characterized by swelling of the parotid glands. It is most prevalent in children between ages 5 and 9. Prognosis for complete recovery is good, although mumps sometimes causes complications.

Cause
Paramyxovirus

Mode of transmission
• Airborne droplets
• Direct contact

Signs and symptoms
The clinical features of mumps vary widely. An estimated 30% of susceptible people have subclinical illness.
Prodromal
—Myalgia
—Anorexia
—Malaise
—Headache
—Low-grade fever

Subsequent
—Parotid gland swelling and tenderness
—Earache, aggravated by chewing
—Temperature of 101° to 104° F. (38.3° to 40° C.)
—Pain when chewing or when drinking sour or acidic liquids
—Possible swelling of one or more of the other salivary glands

Diagnostic tests
Serologic antibody testing can verify the diagnosis when parotid or other salivary gland enlargement is absent. If comparison between a blood specimen obtained during the acute phase of illness and another specimen obtained 3 weeks later shows a fourfold rise in antibody titer, the patient most likely had mumps.

Treatment
Treatment includes analgesics for pain, antipyretics for fever, and adequate fluid intake to prevent dehydration from fever and anorexia. If the patient cannot swallow, consider I.V. fluid replacement.

Clinical implications
• Stress the need for bed rest during the febrile period. Give analgesics, and apply warm or cool compresses to the neck to relieve pain. Give antipyretics and tepid sponge baths for fever. To prevent dehydration, encourage the patient to drink fluids; to minimize pain and anorexia, advise him to avoid spicy, irritating foods and those that require a lot of chewing. During the acute phase, observe the patient closely for signs of CNS involvement, such as altered level of consciousness and nuchal rigidity.

• Because the mumps virus is present in the saliva throughout the course of the disease, respiratory isolation is recommended until symptoms subside.

• Emphasize the importance of routine immunization with live attenuated mumps virus (paramyxovirus) at age

15 months and for susceptible patients (especially males) who are approaching or are past puberty. Remember, immunization within 24 hours of exposure may prevent or attenuate the actual disease. Immunity against mumps lasts at least 12 years. An actual attack of mumps almost always confers lifelong immunity.

• Report all cases of mumps to local public health authorities.

Complications
• Epididymo-orchitis
• Mumps meningitis
• Less commonly, pancreatitis, deafness, arthritis, myocarditis, encephalitis, pericarditis, oophoritis, and nephritis

---

Muscular dystrophy

Description
Muscular dystrophy is actually a group of congenital disorders characterized by progressive symmetrical wasting of skeletal muscles without neural or sensory defects. Paradoxically, these wasted muscles tend to enlarge because of connective tissue and fat deposits, giving an erroneous impression of muscle strength. Four main types of muscular dystrophy occur: pseudohypertrophic (Duchenne's) muscular dystrophy, which accounts for 50% of all cases; facioscapulohumeral (Landouzy-Dejerine) dystrophy; limb-girdle (Erb's) dystrophy; and a mixed type. Characteristic abnormalities of gait and other voluntary movements, with a typical medical and family history, suggest this diagnosis. Prognosis varies. Duchenne's muscular dystrophy generally strikes during early childhood and results in death within 10 to 15 years of onset. Facioscapulohumeral and limb-girdle dystrophies usually do not shorten life expectancy. The mixed type progresses rapidly and is usually fatal within 5 years after onset.

Causes
• Duchenne's muscular dystrophy is an X-linked recessive disorder.
• Facioscapulohumeral dystrophy is an autosomal dominant disorder.
• Limb-girdle muscular dystrophy may be inherited in several ways but is usually an autosomal recessive disorder.
• The mixed type does not appear to be inherited.

Signs and symptoms
Duchenne's muscular dystrophy
—Early signs include delay in learning to walk, frequent falls, or intermittent calf pain.
—Waddling gait appears at age 3 to 4 and becomes pronounced by age 6.
—Later findings include lordosis, with abdominal protrusion, Gowers' sign, and equinovarus foot position.
—With disease progression, symptoms include rapid muscle wasting, contractures, obesity, and possibly tachycardia from cardiac muscle weakening and pulmonary symptoms.
—The child is usually wheelchair-bound by age 12.
Facioscapulohumeral dystrophy
—Early signs include progressive weakness and atrophy of facial, shoulder, and arm muscles; slight lordosis; and pelvic instability.
—Waddling gait appears late.
Limb-girdle dystrophy
—Muscle weakness first appears in the upper arm and pelvic muscles.
—Other symptoms include winging of the scapulae, lordosis with abdominal protrusion, waddling gait, poor balance, and inability to raise the arms.
Mixed dystrophy
—This affects all voluntary muscles and causes rapidly progressive deterioration.

Diagnostic tests
• A muscle biopsy showing fat and connective tissue deposits confirms the diagnosis.

• Electromyography often shows short, weak bursts of electrical activity in affected muscles, but this is not conclusive. With a positive muscle biopsy, however, electromyography can help rule out neurogenic muscle atrophy by showing intact muscle innervation.

• Other relevant laboratory results in Duchenne's muscular dystrophy include increased urinary creatinine excretion and elevated serum levels of creatinine phosphokinase (CPK), lactate dehydrogenase, and transaminases. Usually, the rise in CPK level occurs before muscle weakness becomes severe and is a good early indicator of Duchenne's muscular dystrophy. These diagnostic tests are also useful for genetic screening, since unaffected carriers of Duchenne's muscular dystrophy also show elevated CPK and other enzyme levels.

Treatment

No treatment can stop the progressive muscle impairment of muscular dystrophy, but orthopedic appliances, exercise, physical therapy, and surgery to correct contractures can help preserve mobility and independence. Family members who are carriers of muscular dystrophy should receive genetic counseling regarding the risk of transmitting this disease.

Clinical implications

Comprehensive long-term care and follow-up, patient and family teaching, and psychological support can help the patient and family deal with this disorder.

• When respiratory involvement occurs in Duchenne's muscular dystrophy, encourage coughing, deep-breathing exercises, and diaphragmatic breathing. Teach parents how to recognize early signs of respiratory complications.

• Encourage and assist with active and passive range-of-motion exercises. Advise the patient to avoid long periods of bed rest and inactivity. If necessary, limit TV viewing and other sedentary activities. Refer the patient for physical therapy.

• Because inactivity may cause constipation, encourage adequate fluid intake, increase dietary bulk, and obtain an order for a stool softener. Since such a patient is prone to obesity because of reduced physical activity, help him and his family plan a low-calorie, high-protein, high-fiber diet.

• Always allow the patient plenty of time to perform even simple physical tasks, since he is apt to be slow and awkward.

• Encourage communication between family members to help them deal with the emotional strain this disorder produces. Provide emotional support to help the patient cope with continual changes in body image.

• Help the child with Duchenne's muscular dystrophy maintain peer relationships and realize his intellectual potential by encouraging his parents to keep him in a regular school as long as possible.

• If necessary, refer adult patients for sexual counseling. Refer those who must learn new job skills for vocational rehabilitation. (Contact your state's Department of Labor for more information.) For information on social services and financial assistance, refer these patients and their families to the Muscular Dystrophy Association, Inc.

Myasthenia gravis

Description

Myasthenia gravis produces sporadic but progressive weakness and abnormal fatigability of striated (skeletal) muscles, which are exacerbated by exercise and repeated movement but improved by anticholinesterase drugs. Usually, this disorder affects muscles innervated by the cranial nerves (face,

---

Teaching Topics in Myasthenia Gravis

- Explanation of the autoimmune process that impairs transmission of nerve impulses
- Warning symptoms of myasthenic crisis
- Preparation for tests that confirm myasthenia gravis, such as the Tensilon test, electromyography, and nerve conduction studies
- Antimyasthenic drugs and their administration
- Coordination of activities with drug administration schedule to take advantage of peak muscle strength
- Preparation for plasmapheresis or thymectomy, if necessary
- Dietary measures to compensate for muscle weakness
- Factors that increase symptoms and the risk of infection
- Sources of additional information and support

---

lips, tongue, neck, and throat), but it can affect any muscle group. Frequently, myasthenia gravis coexists with immunologic and thyroid disorders. In fact, 15% of myasthenic patients have thymomas.

Myasthenia gravis follows an unpredictable course of recurring exacerbations and periodic remissions. There is no known cure. Drug treatment has improved prognosis and allows patients to lead relatively normal lives, except during exacerbations. When the disease involves the respiratory system, it may be life-threatening.

Cause

Myasthenia gravis is thought to be an autoimmune disorder that impairs transmission of nerve impulses.

Signs and symptoms

- Gradually progressive skeletal muscle weakness and fatigue are the cardinal symptoms. Typically, weakness is mild upon awakening but worsens during the day.
- Early signs may include weak eye closure, ptosis, and diplopia; a blank, masklike facies; difficulty chewing and swallowing; hanging jaw; and bobbing head.
- Respiratory muscle involvement may lead to symptoms of respiratory failure.

Diagnostic tests

- Electromyography, with repeated neural stimulation, may help confirm this diagnosis.
- Tensilon test is the classic proof of myasthenia gravis, showing improved muscle function after an I.V. injection of edrophonium or neostigmine. In myasthenic patients, muscle function improves within 30 to 60 seconds and lasts up to 30 minutes. However, longstanding ocular muscle dysfunction often fails to respond to such testing.
- Tensilon test also can differentiate a myasthenic crisis from a cholinergic crisis (caused by acetylcholine overactivity at the neuromuscular junction, possibly due to anticholinesterase overdose).
- Other tests may include nerve conduction studies and a CT scan of the chest.

Treatment

Treatment is symptomatic. Anticholinesterase drugs, such as neostigmine and pyridostigmine, counteract fatigue and muscle weakness and allow about 80% of normal muscle function. These drugs become less effective as the disease worsens, however. Corticosteroids may be beneficial in relieving symptoms.

Plasmapheresis may be performed

in some patients. Patients with thymomas require thymectomy, which may lead to remission in adult-onset myasthenia.

Acute exacerbations that cause severe respiratory distress necessitate emergency treatment. Tracheotomy, positive-pressure ventilation, and vigorous suctioning to remove secretions usually bring improvement in a few days. Because anticholinesterase drugs are not effective in myasthenic crisis, they are discontinued until respiratory function begins to improve. Such crisis requires immediate hospitalization and vigorous respiratory support.

Clinical implications
• Establish an accurate neurologic and respiratory baseline. Thereafter, monitor tidal volume and vital capacity regularly. The patient may need a ventilator and frequent suctioning to remove accumulating secretions.
• Be alert for signs of an impending crisis (increased muscle weakness, respiratory distress, difficulty in talking or chewing).
• Evenly space administration of drugs, and give them on time, as ordered, to prevent relapses. Be prepared to give atropine for anticholinesterase overdose or toxicity.
• Plan exercise, meals, patient care, and activities to make the most of energy peaks. For example, give medication 20 to 30 minutes before meals to facilitate chewing or swallowing. Allow the patient to participate in his care.
• When swallowing is difficult, give soft, solid foods instead of liquids to lessen the risk of choking.
• Patient teaching is essential, since myasthenia gravis is usually a lifelong condition. Help the patient plan daily activities to coincide with energy peaks. Stress the need for frequent rest periods throughout the day. Emphasize that periodic remissions, exacerbations, and day-to-day fluctuations are common.

• Teach the patient how to recognize side effects and signs of toxicity of anticholinesterase drugs (headaches, weakness, sweating, abdominal cramps, nausea, vomiting, diarrhea, excessive salivation, and bronchospasm) and corticosteroids.
• Warn the patient to avoid strenuous exercise, stress, infection, and needless exposure to the sun or cold weather. All of these things may worsen signs and symptoms.
• Advise the patient with diplopia that an eye patch or glasses with one frosted lens may be helpful.
• For more information and an opportunity to meet myasthenics who lead full, productive lives, refer the patient to the Myasthenia Gravis Foundation. (See *Teaching Topics in Myasthenia Gravis*, p. 487.)

Mycosis fungoides
(Malignant cutaneous reticulosis, granuloma fungoides)

Description
Mycosis fungoides (MF) is a rare, chronic, malignant T cell lymphoma that originates in the reticuloendothelial system of the skin, eventually affecting lymph nodes and internal organs. In the United States, it strikes more than 1,000 patients of all races annually; most are between ages 40 and 60. Unlike other lymphomas, MF allows an average life expectancy of 7 to 10 years after diagnosis. If correctly treated, particularly before it has spread past the skin, MF may go into remission for many years. However, after MF has reached the tumor stage, progression to severe disability or death is rapid.

Cause
Unknown

Signs and symptoms
• The first sign of MF may be generalized erythroderma, possibly associated with itching.
• Eventually, MF evolves into varied combinations of infiltrated, thickened, or scaly patches, tumors, or ulcerations.

Diagnostic tests
• Biopsy permits histologic confirmation of lymphoma cell infiltration of the skin.
• A finger-stick smear shows Sézary cells (abnormal circulating lymphocytes), which may be present in the erythrodermic variants of MF (Sézary syndrome).
• Blood chemistries screen for visceral dysfunction.
• Chest X-ray, liver-spleen scanning, lymphangiography, and lymph node biopsy also help to stage the disease— a necessary prerequisite to treatment. (See *Staging Mycosis Fungoides*.)

Treatment
Treatment of MF may include topical, intralesional, or systemic corticosteroid therapy; phototherapy; methoxsalen photochemotherapy; radiation; topical, intralesional, or systemic mechlorethamine hydrochloride; and other systemic chemotherapy.

Application of topical mechlorethamine hydrochloride (nitrogen mustard) is the preferred treatment for inducing remission in pretumorous stages. Preliminary I.V. infusions of small amounts of mechlorethamine hydrochloride are given before beginning this treatment to reduce the risk of allergic sensitization. However, the value of this practice has not been definitely established.

Total body electron-beam radiation, which is less toxic to internal organs than standard photon-beam radiation, has induced remission in some patients with early-stage MF.

Chemotherapy is used primarily for patients with advanced-stage MF. Chemotherapeutic agents used include

---

Staging Mycosis Fungoides

Magnitude of skin involvement (T):
T_0 Clinically or histopathologically suspicious lesions
T_1 Premycotic lesions, papules, or plaques involving less than 10% of the skin surface
T_2 Premycotic lesions, papules, or plaques involving more than 10% of the skin surface
T_3 One or more tumors of the skin
T_4 Extensive, often generalized erythroderma

Status of peripheral lymph nodes (N):
N_0 Clinically normal; no pathologic involvement
N_1 Clinically abnormal; no pathologic involvement
N_2 Clinically normal; pathologic involvement
N_3 Clinically abnormal; pathologic involvement

Status of visceral organs (M):
M_0 No pathologic involvement
M_1 Pathologic involvement

---

cyclophosphamide, chlorambucil, methotrexate (with or without folinic acid rescue), doxorubicin, vincristine, and bleomycin.

Clinical implications
• If the patient applying nitrogen mustard has difficulty reaching all skin surfaces, give assistance. But wear gloves to prevent contact sensitization.
• If the patient is receiving drug treatment, report side effects, particularly infection, immediately.
• If the patient is receiving radiation, he will probably develop alopecia and erythema. Suggest that he wear a wig until hair regrowth begins, and suggest or give medicated oil baths to ease erythema.

• Because pruritus is often worse at night, the patient may need larger bedtime doses of antipruritics or sedatives, as ordered, to ensure a good night's sleep. When the patient has had a difficult night's sleep, postpone early morning care to allow him more sleep.

• The patient with pruritus has an overwhelming need to scratch—often to the point of removing epidermis and replacing pruritus with pain, which some patients find easier to endure. Realize that you cannot keep such a patient from scratching. The best you can do is help minimize the damage. Advise the patient to keep fingernails short and clean and to wear a pair of white gloves when itching is unbearable.

• The malignant skin lesions are likely to make the patient depressed, fearful, and self-conscious. Fully explain the disease and its stages to help the patient and family understand and accept the disease. Provide reassurance and support by demonstrating a positive but realistic attitude. Reinforce your verbal support by touching the patient without any hint of anxiety or distaste.

Myelitis and acute transverse myelitis

Description

Myelitis, or inflammation of the spinal cord, can result from several diseases. Poliomyelitis affects the cord's gray matter and produces motor dysfunction. Leukomyelitis affects only the white matter and produces sensory dysfunction. These types of myelitis can attack any level of the spinal cord, causing partial destruction or scattered lesions. Acute transverse myelitis, which affects the entire thickness of the spinal cord, produces both motor and sensory dysfunctions. This form of myelitis, which has a rapid onset, is the most devastating. The prognosis depends on the severity of cord damage and prevention of complications.

Causes

• Acute transverse myelitis often follows acute infectious diseases, such as measles or pneumonia (the inflammation occurs after the infection has subsided), and primary infections of the spinal cord itself, such as syphilis or acute disseminated encephalomyelitis.

• Acute transverse myelitis can accompany demyelinating diseases, such as acute multiple sclerosis, and inflammatory and necrotizing disorders of the spinal cord, such as hematomyelia.

• Certain toxic agents (carbon monoxide, lead, and arsenic) can cause a type of myelitis in which acute inflammation (followed by hemorrhage and possible necrosis) destroys the entire circumference (myelin, axis cylinders, and neurons) of the spinal cord.

• Other forms of myelitis may result from poliovirus, herpes zoster, herpesvirus B, or rabies virus; disorders that cause meningeal inflammation, such as syphilis, abscesses and other suppurative conditions, and tuberculosis; smallpox or polio vaccination; parasitic and fungal infections; and chronic adhesive arachnoiditis.

Signs and symptoms

• Patients with acute transverse myelitis develop flaccid paralysis of the legs (sometimes beginning in just one leg) with loss of sensory and sphincter functions. Such sensory loss may follow pain in the legs or trunk.

• Reflexes disappear in the early stages but may reappear later.

• The extent of damage depends on the level of the spinal cord affected; transverse myelitis rarely involves the arms.

• If spinal cord damage is severe, it may cause shock (hypotension and hypothermia).

Diagnostic tests

• CSF may be normal or show increased lymphocytes or elevated protein levels.

• Diagnostic evaluation must rule out spinal cord tumor and identify the cause of any underlying infection.

Treatment

No effective treatment exists for acute transverse myelitis. However, this condition requires appropriate treatment of any underlying infection. Some patients with postinfectious or multiple sclerosis-induced myelitis have received steroid therapy, but its benefits are not clear.

Clinical implications

• Frequently assess vital signs. Watch carefully for signs of spinal shock (hypotension and excessive sweating).

• Prevent contractures with range-of-motion exercises and proper alignment.

• Watch for signs of urinary tract infection from Foley catheters.

• Prevent skin infections and decubitus ulcers with meticulous skin care. Check pressure points often and keep skin clean and dry. Use a water bed or other pressure-relieving device.

• Initiate rehabilitation immediately. Assist the patient with physical therapy, bowel and bladder training, and life-style changes his condition requires.

Myocardial infarction
(Heart attack)

Description

Myocardial infarction is an area of necrotic myocardium, resulting from reduced or occluded blood flow through one of the coronary arteries. As a result of oxygen deprivation, the myocardium suffers progressive ischemia,

---

MI Sites

The site of the myocardial infarction (MI) depends on the vessels involved. Occlusion of the circumflex branch of the left coronary artery causes a lateral wall infarction; occlusion of the anterior descending branch of the left coronary artery, an anterior wall infarction. True posterior or inferior wall infarctions generally result from occlusion of the right coronary artery or one of its branches. Right ventricular infarctions can also result from right coronary artery occlusion, can accompany inferior infarctions, and may cause right heart failure. In transmural MI, tissue damage extends through all myocardial layers. In subendocardial MI, damage occurs only in the innermost layer.

---

leading to injury and finally necrosis. The extent of functional impairment and the patient's prognosis depend on the size and location of the infarct, the condition of the uninvolved myocardium, the potential for collateral circulation, and the effectiveness of compensatory mechanisms. (See *MI Sites*.) In the United States, MI is the leading cause of death.

Causes

An MI can arise from any condition in which myocardial oxygen supply cannot keep pace with demand.

Coronary artery disease (CAD)
—Atherosclerosis (the leading cause)
—Arteritis
—Trauma to coronary arteries
—Coronary mural thickening in metabolic diseases or intimal proliferative disease
—Luminal narrowing by other mechanisms, such as spasm of coronary arteries (Prinzmetal's angina), spasm after nitroglycerin withdrawal, aortic dissection, and coronary artery dissection

Coronary artery emboli
—Infective endocarditis
—Cardiac myxoma
—Cardiopulmonary bypass surgery and coronary arteriography
Myocardial oxygen supply-demand imbalance
—Aortic stenosis
—Aortic insufficiency
—Carbon monoxide poisoning
—Thyrotoxicosis
—Prolonged hypotension
Hematologic causes
—Polycythemia vera
—Thrombocytosis
—Disseminated intravascular coagulation
—Hypercoagulability
—Thrombosis
—Thrombocytopenic purpura
Miscellaneous causes
—Myocardial contusion
—Congenital coronary artery anomalies

Risk factors
• Positive family history
• Hypertension
• Smoking
• Elevated serum triglyceride and cholesterol levels
• Diabetes mellitus
• Obesity or excessive intake of saturated fats, carbohydrates, or salt
• Sedentary life-style
• Aging
• Stress or Type A personality (aggressive, ambitious, competitive attitude, addiction to work, chronic impatience)
• Oral contraceptive use

Signs and symptoms
• Chest pain (typically severe, persistent, unrelieved by rest or nitroglycerin; typically described as crushing or squeezing; usually substernal, but may radiate to left arm, jaw, neck or shoulder blades)
• Feeling of impending doom
• Fatigue
• Nausea, vomiting
• Shortness of breath

• Coolness of extremities
• Perspiration
• Anxiety
• Hypo- or hypertension
• Palpable precordial pulse
• Possibly, muffled heart sounds

Diagnostic tests
• Serial 12-lead EKG may show no abnormalities or may be inconclusive during the first few hours following an MI. When present, characteristic abnormalities show serial ST-T changes in subendocardial MI, and Q waves representing transmural MI.
• Serial serum enzymes measurements show elevated creatine phosphokinase (CPK), especially the CPK-MB isoenzyme, the cardiac muscle fraction of CPK.
• Echocardiography shows ventricular wall dyskinesia with a transmural MI.
• Thallium scans, 99^m technetium pyrophosphate scans, or radionuclide ventriculography evaluate MI effects. Radioimmunoassay (RIA), which detects cardiac myosin light chains (CM-LC), can also reveal early- and late-stage cardiac necrosis.

Treatment
The goals of treatment are to relieve chest pain, to stabilize heart rhythm, and to reduce cardiac workload. Therapy includes the following.
• Lidocaine for ventricular dysrhythmias or, if lidocaine is ineffective, other drugs, such as procainamide, quinidine, bretylium, or disopyramide
• Atropine I.V. or a temporary pacemaker to treat heart block or bradycardia
• Nitroglycerin (sublingual, topical, transdermal, or I.V.); calcium channel blockers, such as nifedipine, verapamil, and diltiazem (sublingual, P.O., or I.V.); or isosorbide dinitrate (sublingual, P.O., or I.V.) to relieve pain by redistributing blood to the ischemic area of the myocardium, increasing

Treating Acute MI with Streptokinase

In the early stages of acute myocardial infarction (MI), therapy with the thrombolytic drug streptokinase can dissolve the clot in an occluded artery, restoring perfusion and limiting the size of an infarction.

The physician threads an arterial catheter through the major blood vessels to the patient's heart, and dye is injected to locate the clot. Then streptokinase infusion begins with a bolus dose of 10,000 to 20,000 units. Infusion may continue for several hours at a dosage ranging from 2,000 to 6,000 units/minute. During this time, angiography assesses the treatment's effectiveness.

Streptokinase works by hastening fibrinolysis. It joins with plasminogen to form a complex that then reacts with additional plasminogen to form plasmin, a proteolytic enzyme that dissolves the clot and relieves the occlusion. (See below.)

Because streptokinase alters the natural clotting mechanisms, it can produce hemorrhage, especially at the site of recent surgery, needle puncture, or trauma. Special considerations after streptokinase therapy include:
• avoiding I.M. or I.V. injections for 24 hours
• maintaining alignment and immobility of the involved extremity: do not raise the head of the bed more than 15°
• checking the infusion site for bleeding every 15 minutes for 1 hour, every 30 minutes for the next 2 hours, then once every hour until the catheter is removed
• documenting pulse, color, temperature, and sensitivity of both extremities when checking the site for bleeding
• applying direct pressure to the infusion site for at least 30 minutes after catheter removal. Assess the involved extremity distal to the pressure point, and keep the patient on bed rest for at least 6 hours with his leg straight and the head of the bed no higher than 15 degrees
• watching for signs and symptoms of GI bleeding.

cardiac output, and reducing myocardial workload
• Morphine or meperidine I.V. for pain and sedation
• Bed rest with bedside commode to decrease cardiac workload
• Oxygen administration (by face mask or nasal cannula) at a modest flow rate for 24 to 48 hours, or a lower concentration if the patient has chronic obstructive pulmonary disease
• Pulmonary artery catheterization to detect left ventricular failure and to monitor response to treatment
• Drugs that increase contractility or blood pressure, or an intraaortic balloon pump for cardiogenic shock
• Thrombolytic therapy up to 6 hours after infarction, using intracoronary or systemic (I.V.) streptokinase. (See *Treating Acute MI with Streptokinase*.)
• Beta-adrenergic blockers, such as propranolol and timolol, after acute MI to help prevent reinfarction
• An inotropic drug, dobutamine, which is used to treat reduced myocardial contractility

Clinical implications

Care for patients who have suffered MI is directed toward detecting complications, preventing further myocardial damage, and promoting comfort, rest, and emotional well-being. Most patients with MI receive treatment in the critical care unit (CCU), under constant observation for complications.
• On admission to the CCU, monitor

Complications of Myocardial Infarction

COMPLICATION	DIAGNOSIS	TREATMENT
Dysrhythmias	• EKG shows premature ventricular contractions, ventricular tachycardia, or ventricular fibrillation; in inferior wall MI, bradycardia and junctional rhythms or AV block; in anterior wall MI, tachycardia or heart block.	• Antiarrhythmics • Atropine • Cardioversion • Pacemaker
Congestive heart failure	• In left heart failure, chest X-rays show venous congestion and cardiomegaly. • Catheterization shows increased pulmonary artery, pulmonary capillary wedge, and central venous pressures.	• Diuretics • Vasodilators • Inotropics • Cardiac glycosides
Cardiogenic shock	• Catheterization shows decreased cardiac output and increased pulmonary artery and pulmonary capillary wedge pressures. • Signs are hypotension, tachycardia, decreased level of consciousness, decreased urinary output, neck vein distention, and cool, pale skin.	• I.V. Fluids • Vasodilators • Cardiotonics • Cardiac glycosides • Intraaortic balloon pump (IABP) • Beta-adrenergic stimulants
Mitral regurgitation	• Auscultation reveals crackles and apical holosystolic murmur. • Catheterization shows increased pulmonary artery and pulmonary capillary wedge pressures. • Dyspnea is prominent. • Echocardiogram shows valve dysfunction.	• Nitroglycerin • Nitroprusside • IABP • Surgical replacement of the mitral valve and concomitant myocardial revascularization
Ventricular septal rupture	• In left-to-right shunt, auscultation reveals a harsh holosystolic murmur and thrill. • Catheterization shows increased pulmonary artery and pulmonary capillary wedge pressures. • Confirmation by increased oxygen saturation of right ventricle and pulmonary artery	• Surgical correction (may be postponed several weeks) • IABP • Nitroglycerin • Nitroprusside

Complications of Myocardial Infarction *(continued)*

COMPLICATION	DIAGNOSIS	TREATMENT
Pericarditis or Dressler's syndrome	• Auscultation reveals a friction rub. • Chest pain is relieved by sitting up.	• Anti-inflammatory agents, such as aspirin or corticosteroids
Ventricular aneurysm	• Chest X-ray may show cardiomegaly. • EKG may show dysrhythmias and persistent ST segment elevation. • Left ventriculography shows altered or paradoxical left ventricular motion.	• Cardioversion • Antiarrhythmics • Vasodilators • Anticoagulants • Cardiac glycosides • Diuretics • Surgical resection, if necessary
Thromboembolism	• Severe dyspnea and chest pain or neurologic changes • Nuclear scan shows ventilation/perfusion mismatch. • Angiography shows arterial blockage.	• Oxygen • Heparin • Endarterectomy

and record EKG, blood pressure, temperature, and heart and breath sounds.
• Assess pain, and administer analgesics, as ordered. Always record the severity and duration of pain. Avoid giving I.M. injections since absorption from the muscle is unpredictable.
• Check the patient's blood pressure after giving nitroglycerin, especially the first dose.
• Frequently monitor EKG to detect rate changes or dysrhythmias. Place rhythm strips in the patient's chart periodically for evaluation.
• During episodes of chest pain, obtain EKG, blood pressure, and pulmonary artery catheter measurements to determine changes.
• Watch for signs and symptoms of fluid retention (crackles, cough, tachypnea, edema), which may indicate impending heart failure. Carefully monitor daily weight, intake and output, respirations, serum enzyme levels, and blood pressure. Auscultate for adventitious breath sounds periodi-

cally (patients on bed rest frequently have atelectatic crackles, which may disappear after coughing) and for S_3 or S_4 gallops.
• Organize patient care and activities to maximize his periods of uninterrupted rest.
• Ask the dietary department to provide a clear liquid diet until nausea subsides. A low-cholesterol, low-sodium diet, without caffeine-containing beverages, may be ordered.
• Provide a stool softener to prevent straining at stool, which causes vagal stimulation and may slow heart rate. Allow the patient to use a bedside commode, and provide as much privacy as possible.
• Assist with range-of-motion exercises. If the patient is completely immobilized by a severe MI, turn him often. Antiembolism stockings help prevent venostasis and thrombophlebitis.
• Provide emotional support, and help reduce stress and anxiety; administer

---

Teaching Topics in MI

- An explanation of how atherosclerosis, thromboembolism, or coronary artery spasm occludes cardiac blood flow
- The area of infarction
- The importance of following the prescribed treatment plan to aid recovery and forestall complications
- Preparation for serial EKGs, blood enzyme studies, and other scheduled tests
- Importance of bed rest
- Exercise program and precautions
- Dietary restrictions
- Drugs and their administration
- Preparation for percutaneous transluminal coronary angioplasty, pulmonary artery catheterization, or other necessary procedures
- Preparation for open-heart surgery, if scheduled
- Other measures to reduce long-term complications, such as controlling weight, quitting smoking, and reducing stress
- Availability of support groups, such as the American Heart Association

---

tranquilizers, as needed. Explain procedures and answer questions. An explanation of the CCU environment and routine can lessen the patient's anxiety. Involve his family as much as possible in his care.

- Carefully prepare the MI patient for discharge. To promote compliance with prescribed medication regimen and other treatment measures, thoroughly explain dosages and therapy. Warn about drug side effects, and advise the patient to watch for and report signs of toxicity (anorexia, nausea, vomiting, and yellow vision, for example, if the patient is receiving digitalis).
- Review dietary restrictions with the patient. If he must follow a low-sodium or low-fat and low-cholesterol diet, provide a list of undesirable foods. Ask the dietitian to speak to the patient and his family.
- Counsel the patient to resume sexual activity progressively.
- Advise the patient about appropriate responses to new or recurrent symptoms.
- Advise the patient to report typical or atypical chest pain. Postinfarction syndrome may develop, producing chest pain that must be differentiated from recurrent MI, pulmonary infarct, or congestive heart failure.

- If the patient has a Holter monitor in place, explain its purpose and use.
- Stress the need to stop smoking. If necessary, refer the patient to a smoking cessation group. (See *Teaching Topics in MI*.)

Complications

See *Complications of Myocardial Infarction*, pp. 494 and 495.

Myocarditis

Description

Myocarditis is focal or diffuse inflammation of the cardiac muscle (myocardium). It may be acute or chronic and can occur at any age. Frequently, myocarditis fails to produce specific cardiovascular symptoms or EKG abnormalities, and recovery is usually spontaneous, without residual defects. Occasionally, myocarditis is complicated by congestive heart failure and, rarely, leads to cardiomyopathy.

Causes

- Viral infections (most common cause in the United States) such as coxsackievirus A and B strains and, possibly, poliomyelitis, influenza, rubeola, rubella, and adeno- and echoviruses
- Bacterial infections such as diphtheria, tuberculosis, typhoid fever, tetanus, and staphylococcal, pneumococcal, and gonococcal infections
- Hypersensitivity reactions such as acute rheumatic fever and postcardiotomy syndrome
- Radiation therapy to the chest in treating lung or breast cancer
- Chemical poisoning such as chronic alcoholism
- Parasitic infections, especially South American trypanosomiasis (Chagas' disease) in infants and immunosuppressed adults; also toxoplasmosis
- Helminthic infections such as trichinosis

Signs and symptoms

- Fatigue
- Dyspnea
- Palpitations
- Fever
- Occasionally, mild continuous pressure or soreness in the chest
- On examination, supraventricular and ventricular dysrhythmias, S_3 and S_4 gallops, a faint S_1, possibly a murmur of mitral regurgitation (from papillary muscle dysfunction), and, if pericarditis is present, a pericardial friction rub

Diagnostic tests

Laboratory tests cannot unequivocally confirm myocarditis.
- Cardiac enzymes (CPK, CPK_2, SGOT, and LDH) are elevated.
- WBC count and ESR are increased.
- Antibody titers (such as antistreptolysin O [ASO] titer in rheumatic fever) are elevated.
- EKG changes are the most reliable diagnostic aid. Typically, there are diffuse ST segment and T wave abnormalities as in pericarditis, conduction defects (prolonged P-R interval), and other supraventricular ectopic dysrhythmias.
- Stool and throat cultures may identify bacteria.
- Endomyocardial biopsy provides a definitive diagnosis.

Treatment

Treatment includes antibiotics for bacterial infection, modified bed rest to decrease heart workload, and careful management of complications.

Clinical implications

- Assess cardiovascular status frequently, watching for signs of congestive heart failure, such as dyspnea, hypotension, and tachycardia. Check for changes in cardiac rhythm or conduction.
- Stress the importance of bed rest. Assist with bathing, as necessary. Provide a bedside commode, since this stresses the heart less than using a bedpan. Give reassurance that activity limitations are temporary. Offer diversional activities that are physically undemanding.
- During recovery, recommend that the patient resume normal activities slowly and avoid competitive sports.

Complications

Although myocarditis is generally uncomplicated and self-limiting, it may induce myofibril degeneration that results in right and left heart failure and supraventricular and ventricular dysrhythmias. Sometimes myocarditis recurs or produces chronic valvulitis (when it results from rheumatic fever), cardiomyopathy, dysrhythmias, and thromboembolism.

Myringitis, infectious

Description

Acute infectious myringitis is characterized by inflammation, hemorrhage, and effusion of fluid into the tissue at the end of the external ear canal and the tympanic membrane. This self-limiting disorder (resolving spontaneously within 3 days to 2 weeks) often follows acute otitis media or upper respiratory tract infection and frequently occurs epidemically in children.

Chronic granular myringitis, a rare inflammation of the squamous layer of the tympanic membrane, causes gradual hearing loss. Without specific treatment, this condition can lead to stenosis of the ear canal, as granulation extends from the tympanic membrane to the external ear.

Causes
Acute infectious myringitis
—Usually follows viral infection or infection of any organism causing acute otitis media
—Rarely, follows atypical pneumonia caused by *Mycoplasma pneumoniae*
Chronic granular myringitis
—Unknown

Signs and symptoms
Acute infectious myringitis
—Severe ear pain. This is the initial symptom, commonly accompanied by tenderness over the mastoid process.
—Small, reddened, inflamed blebs. These form in the canal, on the tympanic membrane, and with bacterial invasion, in the middle ear.
—Hearing loss. This is rare unless fluid accumulates in the middle ear or a large bleb totally obstructs the external auditory meatus.
—Possible bloody discharge. This follows spontaneous rupture of these blebs.
—Fever (rare)
Chronic granular myringitis
—Pruritus
—Purulent discharge
—Gradual hearing loss

Diagnostic tests
Culture and sensitivity testing of exudate identifies any secondary infec-

tion present; however, physical examination establishes the diagnosis.

Treatment and clinical implications
Hospitalization is usually not required for acute infectious myringitis. Treatment consists of measures to relieve pain. Analgesics, such as aspirin or acetaminophen, and application of heat to the external ear are usually sufficient, but severe pain may necessitate use of codeine. Systemic or topical antibiotics prevent or treat secondary infection. Incision of blebs and evacuation of serum and blood may relieve pressure and help drain exudate but do not speed recovery.

Treatment of chronic granular myringitis consists of systemic antibiotics or local anti-inflammatory antibiotic combination eardrops, and surgical excision and cautery. If stenosis is present, surgical reconstruction is necessary.
• Stress the importance of completing prescribed antibiotic therapy.
• Teach the patient how to instill topical antibiotics (eardrops). When necessary, explain incision of blebs.
• To help prevent acute infectious myringitis, advise early treatment of acute otitis media.

N

Nasal papillomas

Description
A papilloma is a benign epithelial tissue overgrowth within the intranasal mucosa. Inverted papillomas grow into the underlying tissue, usually at the junction of the antrum and the ethmoidal sinus. They generally occur singly but sometimes are associated with a squamous cell cancer. Exophytic papillomas, which also tend to occur singly, arise from epithelial tissue, commonly on the surface of the nasal septum. Both types of papillomas are most prevalent in males. Recurrence is likely, even after surgical excision.

Cause
A papilloma may arise as a benign precursor of a neoplasm or as a response to tissue injury or viral infection, but its cause is unknown.

Signs and symptoms
On examination, inverted papillomas usually appear large, bulky, highly vascular, and edematous. Color varies from dark red to gray; consistency, from firm to friable. Exophytic papillomas are commonly raised, firm, and rubbery; pink to gray; and securely attached by a broad or pedunculated base to the mucous membrane. Symptoms include the following:
- Stuffiness
- Postnasal drip
- Headache
- Shortness of breath
- Rarely, severe respiratory distress and nasal drainage
- Epistaxis (most likely with exophytic papillomas)

Diagnostic tests
Histologic examination of excised tissue confirms the diagnosis.

Treatment
The most effective treatment is wide surgical excision or diathermy, with careful inspection of adjacent tissues and sinuses to rule out extension. Aspirin or acetaminophen, and decongestants may relieve symptoms.

Clinical implications
- If bleeding occurs, raise the head of the bed, and instruct the patient to expectorate blood into an emesis basin. Compress the sides of the nose against the septum for 10 to 15 minutes, and, if necessary, apply ice compresses to the nose. If bleeding does not stop, notify the physician.
- Check for airway obstruction. Place your hand under the patient's nostrils to assess air exchange, and watch for signs of mild shortness of breath.
- If surgery is scheduled, tell the patient what to expect postoperatively: that his nostrils will probably be packed and that he will have to breathe through his mouth. Instruct him not to blow his nose. (Packing is usually removed 12 to 24 hours after surgery.)
- Postoperatively, monitor vital signs and respiratory status. As needed, administer analgesics and facilitate breathing with a cool-mist vaporizer.

Provide good mouth care.
• Frequently change the mustache dressing or drop pad, to ensure proper absorption of drainage. Record type and amount of drainage. While the nasal packing is in place, expect scant, usually bright red, clotted drainage. Remember that the amount of drainage often increases for a few hours after the packing is removed.
• Because papillomas tend to recur, tell the patient to seek medical attention at the first sign of nasal discomfort, discharge, or congestion that does not subside with conservative treatment.
• Encourage regular follow-up visits to detect early signs of recurrence.

Nasal polyps

Description
Benign and edematous growths, nasal polyps are usually multiple, mobile, and bilateral. They may become large and numerous enough to cause nasal distention and enlargement of the bony framework, possibly occluding the airway. Associated clinical features are usually symptomatic of allergic rhinitis. They are more common in adults than in children and tend to recur. Nasal polyps occurring in children require testing to rule out cystic fibrosis.

Cause
Usually, continuous pressure resulting from a chronic allergy that causes pro-

longed mucous membrane edema in the nose and sinuses

Risk factors
• Chronic allergy
• Chronic sinusitis
• Chronic rhinitis
• Recurrent nasal infections

Signs and symptoms
• Nasal obstruction (primary indication)
• Anosmia
• Sensation of fullness in the face
• Nasal discharge
• Shortness of breath

Diagnostic tests
• X-rays of sinuses and nasal passages reveal soft tissue shadows over the affected areas.
• Examination with a nasal speculum shows a dry, red surface, with clear or gray growths. Large growths may resemble tumors.

Treatment
Generally, treatment consists of corticosteroids (either by direct injection into the polyps or by local spray) to temporarily reduce the polyp. Treatment of the underlying cause may include antihistamines to control allergy, and antibiotic therapy if infection is present. Local application of an astringent shrinks hypertrophied tissue. Medical management alone is rarely effective, however. For this reason, the treatment of choice is polypectomy (intranasal removal of the nasal polyp with a wire snare), usually performed under local anesthesia. Continued recurrence may require surgical opening of the ethmoidal and the maxillary sinuses, and evacuation of diseased tissue.

Preventing Nasal Polyps

• Instruct patients with allergies to avoid exposure to allergens and to take antihistamines at the first sign of an allergic reaction.
• Advise them to avoid overuse of nose drops and sprays.

Clinical implications
• Administer antihistamines, as ordered, for the patient with allergies. Prepare the patient for scheduled surgery by telling him what to expect

postoperatively, such as nasal packing for 1 to 2 days after surgery.

• After surgery, monitor for excessive bleeding or other drainage, and promote patient comfort.

• Elevate the head of the bed to facilitate breathing, reduce swelling, and promote adequate drainage. Change the mustache dressing or drip pad, as needed, and record the consistency, amount, and color of nasal drainage.

• Intermittently apply ice compresses over the nostrils to lessen swelling, prevent bleeding, and relieve pain.

• If nasal bleeding occurs—most likely after packing is removed—elevate the head of the bed, monitor vital signs, and advise the patient not to swallow blood. Compress the outside of the nose against the septum for 10 to 15 minutes. If bleeding persists, notify the physician immediately. Nasal packing may be necessary. (Also see *Preventing Nasal Polyps*.)

Near-drowning

Description

Near-drowning refers to surviving—temporarily, at least—the physiologic effects of hypoxemia and acidosis that result from submersion in fluid. Near-drowning occurs in three forms: (1) "dry"—the victim does not aspirate fluid but suffers respiratory obstruction or asphyxia (10% to 15% of patients); (2) "wet"—the victim aspirates fluid and suffers from asphyxia or secondary changes due to fluid aspiration (about 85% of patients); (3) secondary—the victim suffers recurrence of respiratory distress (usually aspiration pneumonia or pulmonary edema) within minutes or 1 to 2 days after a near-drowning incident.

Hypoxemia and metabolic acidosis are the most serious consequences of near-drowning. The consequences of aspiration depend on the fluid aspirated. After fresh-water aspiration, changes in the character of lung surfactant result in exudation of protein-rich plasma into the alveoli. This, plus increased capillary permeability, leads to pulmonary edema and hypoxemia. After salt-water aspiration, the hypertonicity of sea water exerts an osmotic force, which pulls fluid from pulmonary capillaries into the alveoli. The resulting intrapulmonary shunt causes hypoxemia. In addition, injury to the pulmonary capillary membrane may induce pulmonary edema.

Causes

• Inability to swim
• Panic, in swimmers
• Boating accident
• Heart attack while in water
• Blow to the head while in water
• Drinking heavily before swimming
• Suicide attempt

Signs and symptoms

• Apnea
• Shallow or gasping respirations
• Substernal chest pain
• Asystole
• Tachycardia
• Bradycardia
• Restlessness
• Irritability
• Lethargy
• Fever
• Confusion
• Unconsciousness
• Vomiting
• Abdominal distention
• Cough that produces a pink, frothy fluid
• Crackles and rhonchi heard on auscultation

Diagnostic tests

Diagnosis is based on a history of near-drowning and characteristic clinical features. Supportive diagnostic test results include the following.

• Arterial blood gas levels show decreased oxygen content, low HCO_3^-, and low pH.
• Blood tests may show leukocytosis.

Preventing Near-Drowning

Advise swimmers to do the following:
• Avoid drinking alcohol before swimming.
• Observe water safety measures.
• Take a water safety course such as those sponsored by the Red Cross, YMCA, or YWCA.

• EKG may reveal supraventricular tachycardia and occasional premature contractions as well as nonspecific ST segment abnormalities and T wave abnormalities.

Treatment and clinical implications

Emergency treatment begins with immediate CPR and administration of oxygen (100%).

• When the patient arrives at the hospital, assess for a patent airway. Establish one, if necessary. Continue CPR, intubate the patient, and provide respiratory assistance, such as mechanical ventilation with positive end expiratory pressure, if needed.

• Assess arterial blood gases.

• If the patient's abdomen is distended, insert a nasogastric tube. (Intubate the patient first if he is unconscious.)

• Start I.V. lines; insert a Foley catheter.

• Give medications, as ordered. Much controversy exists about the benefits of drug treatment of near-drowning victims. However, such treatment may include sodium bicarbonate for acidosis, corticosteroids for cerebral edema, antibiotics to prevent infections, and bronchodilators to ease bronchospasms.

• Remember, all near-drowning victims should be admitted for an observation period of 24 to 48 hours because of the possibility of secondary (delayed) drowning.

• Observe for pulmonary complications and signs of delayed drowning (confusion, substernal pain, adventitious breath sounds). Suction often. Pulmonary artery catheters may be useful in assessing cardiopulmonary status. Monitor vital signs, intake and output, and peripheral pulses. Check for skin perfusion. Watch for signs of infection.

• To facilitate breathing, raise the head of the bed slightly. (Also see *Preventing Near-Drowning*.)

Necrotizing enterocolitis

Description

Necrotizing enterocolitis (NEC) is characterized by diffuse or patchy intestinal necrosis, accompanied by sepsis in about one third of cases. Sepsis usually involves *Escherichia coli*, *Clostridia*, *Salmonella*, *Pseudomonas*, or *Klebsiella*. Initially, necrosis is localized, occurring anywhere along the intestine, but most often it is right-sided (in the ileum, ascending colon, or rectosigmoid). NEC occurs most often among premature infants (less than 34 weeks' gestation) and those of low birth weight (less than 5 lb [2.26 kg]). With early detection, the survival rate is 60% to 80%. If diffuse bleeding occurs, NEC usually results in disseminated intravascular coagulation (DIC).

Cause

• Unknown

Risk factors

Any infant who has suffered from perinatal hypoxemia has the potential for developing NEC. Risk factors include the following:

• Birth asphyxia
• Postnatal hypotension
• Respiratory distress
• Hypothermia

- Umbilical vessel catheterization
- Patent ductus arteriosus
- Significant prenatal stress such as premature rupture of membranes, placenta previa, maternal sepsis, toxemia of pregnancy, or breech or cesarean birth

Signs and symptoms

Distended (especially tense or rigid) abdomen, with gastric retention, is the earliest and most common sign of oncoming NEC, usually appearing from 1 to 10 days after birth. Other signs include the following:

- Increasing residual gastric contents
- Bile-stained vomitus
- Occult blood in the stool. One fourth of patients have bloody diarrhea.
- Taut abdomen. This may indicate peritonitis; skin over the abdomen may be red or shiny.
- Nonspecific signs and symptoms: thermal instability, lethargy, metabolic acidosis, jaundice, and DIC

Diagnostic tests

- Anteroposterior and lateral abdominal X-rays confirm the diagnosis. These X-rays show nonspecific intestinal dilation and, in later stages of NEC, pneumatosis cystoides intestinalis (gas or air in the intestinal wall).
- Platelet count may fall below 50,000/mm³.
- Serum sodium levels are decreased.
- Arterial blood gas studies show metabolic acidosis (a result of sepsis).
- Bilirubin levels are elevated as a result of infection-induced red blood cell breakdown.
- Blood and stool cultures identify the infecting organism.
- Clotting studies and hemoglobin levels identify associated DIC.
- Guaiac test detects occult blood in the stool.

Treatment

Successful treatment of NEC relies on early recognition. The first signs of NEC necessitate removal of the umbilical catheter (arterial or venous) if present and discontinuation of oral intake for 7 to 10 days to rest the injured bowel. I.V. fluids, including hyperalimentation, maintain fluid and electrolyte balance and nutrition during this time. Passage of a nasogastric (NG) tube aids bowel decompression. If coagulation studies indicate a need for transfusion, the infant usually receives dextran to promote hemodilution, increase mesenteric blood flow, and reduce platelet aggregation. Antibiotic therapy consists of parenteral administration of an aminoglycoside or ampicillin to suppress bacterial flora and prevent bowel perforation. (These drugs can also be administered through an NG tube, if necessary.) Anteroposterior and lateral X-rays every 4 to 6 hours monitor disease progression.

Surgery is indicated if the patient shows any of the following symptoms: signs of perforation (free intraperitoneal air on X-ray or symptoms of peritonitis), respiratory insufficiency (caused by severe abdominal distention), progressive and intractable acidosis, or DIC. Surgery removes all necrotic and acutely inflamed bowel and creates a temporary colostomy or ileostomy. Such surgery must leave at least 12″ (30 cm) of bowel, or the infant may suffer from malabsorption or chronic vitamin B_{12} deficiency.

Clinical implications

- Be alert for signs of gastric distention and perforation: apnea, cardiovascular shock, sudden drop in temperature, bradycardia, sudden listlessness, rag-doll limpness, increasing abdominal tenderness, edema, erythema, or involuntary rigidity of the abdomen. Take axillary temperatures to avoid perforating the bowel.
- Prevent cross-contamination by disposing of soiled diapers properly and washing hands with povidone-iodine after diaper changes.
- Try to prepare parents for potential

Preventing Necrotizing Enterocolitis (NEC)

• Encourage mothers to breast-feed, since breast milk contains live macrophages that fight infection and has a low pH that inhibits the growth of many organisms. Also, colostrum—fluid secreted before the milk—contains high concentrations of IgA, which directly protects the gut from infection and which the newborn lacks for several days postpartum.
• Tell mothers that they may refrigerate their milk for 48 hours but should neither freeze nor heat it, since extreme temperature changes destroy antibodies.
• Tell patients to use plastic—not glass—containers because leukocytes adhere to glass.

deterioration in their infant's condition. Be honest and explain all treatments, including why feedings are withheld.
• After surgery, the infant needs mechanical ventilation. Gently suction secretions, and assess respiration often.
• Replace fluids (lost through NG tube and stoma drainage). Include drainage losses in output records. Weigh the infant daily. Daily weight gain of 0.35 to 0.7 oz (9.9 to 19.8 g) indicates a good response to therapy.
• An infant with a temporary colostomy or ileostomy needs special care. Explain to the parents what a colostomy or ileostomy is and why it is necessary. Encourage them to participate in their infant's physical care after his condition is no longer critical.
• Provide good skin care. Because the infant's abdomen is small, the suture line is near the stoma; therefore, keeping the suture line clean can be a problem. Good skin care is essential, since the immature infant's skin is fragile and vulnerable to excoriation and the active enzymes in bowel secretions are corrosive.
• Improvise premature-sized colostomy bags from urine collection bags, medicine cups, or condoms. Karaya gum is helpful in making a seal. Watch for wound disruption, infection, and excoriation—potential dangers because of severe catabolism.

• Watch for intestinal malfunction from stricture or short-gut syndrome. Such complications usually develop 1 month after the infant resumes normal feedings.
• You may develop surrogate attachment to infants who require intensive care, but avoid unconscious exclusion of the parents. Encourage parental visits. (See also *Preventing Necrotizing Enterocolitis.*)

Complications
• Perforation (the major complication of NEC)
• Peritonitis

Nephrotic syndrome

Description
Nephrotic syndrome (NS) is a condition characterized by marked proteinuria, hypoalbuminemia, hyperlipemia, and edema. Although NS is not a disease itself, it results from a specific glomerular defect and indicates renal damage. Prognosis is highly variable, depending on the underlying cause. Some forms may progress to end-stage renal failure. About 75% of NS results from inflammation of the capillary loops in the glomeruli (primary glomerulonephritis). Classifi-

cations include lipid nephrosis (nil lesions), the main cause of NS in children; membranous glomerulonephritis, the most common lesions in adult idiopathic NS; focal glomerulosclerosis, which can develop spontaneously at any age, follow renal transplantation or result from heroin abuse; and membranoproliferative glomerulonephritis, which occurs primarily in children. (Also see *Pathophysiology of Nephrotic Syndrome,* p. 506.)

Causes
• Primary (idiopathic) glomerulonephritis
• Metabolic diseases such as diabetes mellitus
• Collagen vascular disorders such as systemic lupus erythematosus and periarteritis nodosa
• Circulatory diseases, such as congestive heart failure, sickle cell anemia, and renal vein thrombosis
• Nephrotoxins such as mercury, gold, and bismuth
• Allergic reactions
• Infections such as tuberculosis or enteritis
• Possibly, pregnancy, hereditary nephritis, multiple myeloma, and other neoplastic diseases

Signs and symptoms
• Mild to severe dependent edema of the ankles or sacrum or periorbital edema, especially in children. This is the dominant clinical feature of NS. It may lead to ascites, pleural effusion, and swollen external genitalia.
• Orthostatic hypotension
• Lethargy
• Anorexia
• Depression
• Pallor

Diagnostic tests
• Urine testing that reveals consistent proteinuria in excess of 3.5 g/24 hours, increased number of hyaline, granular, and waxy, fatty casts, and oval fat bodies strongly suggests NS.

• Blood values that support the diagnosis are increased cholesterol, phospholipids, and triglycerides and decreased albumin levels.
• Histologic identification of the lesion requires kidney biopsy.

Treatment
Effective treatment of NS necessitates correction of the underlying cause, if possible. Supportive treatment consists of protein replacement with a nutritional diet of 1.5 g protein/kg of body weight, with restricted sodium intake; diuretics for edema; and antibiotics for infection.

Some patients respond to an 8-week course of corticosteroid therapy (such as prednisone), followed by a maintenance dose. Others respond better to a combination course of prednisone and azathioprine, or cyclophosphamide.

Clinical implications
• Frequently check urine protein. (Urine containing protein appears frothy.)
• Measure blood pressure while patient is supine and also while he is standing; immediately report a drop in blood pressure that exceeds 20 mm Hg.
• After kidney biopsy, watch for bleeding and shock.
• Monitor intake and output and check weight at the same time each morning—after the patient voids and before he eats—and while he is wearing the same kind of clothing. Ask the dietitian to plan a high-protein, low-sodium diet.
• Give good skin care, since the patient with NS usually has edema.
• To avoid thrombophlebitis, encourage activity and exercise, and provide antiembolism stockings, as ordered.
• Watch for and teach the patient and family how to recognize drug therapy side effects, such as bone marrow toxicity from cytotoxic immunosuppres-

Pathophysiology of Nephrotic Syndrome

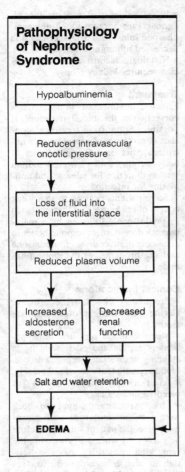

Hypoalbuminemia

↓

Reduced intravascular oncotic pressure

↓

Loss of fluid into the interstitial space

↓

Reduced plasma volume

↓

| Increased aldosterone secretion | Decreased renal function |

↓

Salt and water retention

↓

EDEMA

sives and cushingoid symptoms (muscle weakness, mental changes, acne, moon face, hirsutism, girdle obesity, purple striae, amenorrhea) from long-term steroid therapy. Other steroid-related complications include masked infections, increased susceptibility to infections, ulcers, GI bleeding, and steroid-induced diabetes; a steroid crisis may occur if the drug is discontinued abruptly. To prevent GI complications, administer steroids with an antacid or with cimetidine or ranitidine. Explain that steroid-related side effects will subside when therapy stops.

• Offer the patient and family reassurance and support, especially during the acute phase, when edema is severe and the patient's body image changes.

Neurofibromatosis
(Von Recklinghausen's disease)

Description
Neurofibromatosis is an inherited developmental disorder of the nervous system, muscles, bones, and skin. About 80,000 Americans are known to have neurofibromatosis; in others, this disorder is overlooked because symptoms are mild. The disease occurs in about 1 in 3,000 births. There is a 50% risk that the offspring of persons with neurofibromatosis will have this disease.

Diagnosis rests on typical clinical findings. Prognosis varies, but spinal or intracranial tumors can shorten life span. The disease is associated with meningiomas, suprarenal medullary secreting tumors, kyphoscoliosis, vascular and lymphatic nevi, and ocular and renal anomalies.

Causes
In some patients, the disease is transmitted as an autosomal dominant trait; in others, it occurs as a new mutation.

Signs and symptoms
Neurofibromatosis is present at birth, but symptoms generally appear during childhood or adolescence. Sometimes progression stops as the patient matures, but it may accelerate at puberty, during pregnancy, or after menopause. Clinical effects vary with the size and location of tumors.

• Multiple neurofibromas (pedunculated nodules) of varying sizes on the nerve trunks of extremities and on the nerves of head, neck, and body

- Café-au-lait spots
- Neurologic impairment from intracranial, spinal, and orbital tumors—and in 10% of patients, seizures, blindness, deafness, developmental delay, and mental deficiency
- Skeletal involvement—scoliosis, severe kyphoscoliosis, macrocephaly, and short stature
- Endocrine abnormalities
- Hypertension

Diagnostic tests

X-rays showing a widening internal auditory meatus and intervertebral foramen support this diagnosis, which rarely requires a tumor biopsy.

Treatment

Treatment consists of surgical removal of intracerebral or intraspinal tumors, when possible; correction of kyphoscoliosis; and, if necessary, cosmetic surgery for disfiguring or disabling growths.

Clinical implications

- Disfigurement may cause overwhelming social embarrassment and regression. Showing acceptance of the patient helps him adjust to his condition.
- Advise the patient to choose attractive clothing that covers unsightly nodules; suggest special cosmetics to cover skin lesions.
- Refer the patient for genetic counseling to discuss the 50% risk of transmitting this disorder to offspring. Refer him to the National Neurofibromatosis Foundation for more information.

Complications

- Congenital tibial pseudarthrosis
- Cancer of the nerve sheath
- Neurofibrosarcoma (in up to 8% of patients)
- Malignant changes in the tumors themselves

Neurogenic bladder
(Neuromuscular dysfunction of the lower urinary tract, neurologic bladder dysfunction, neuropathic bladder)

Description

Neurogenic bladder refers to all types of bladder dysfunction caused by an interruption of normal bladder innervation. (Subsequent complications include incontinence, residual urine retention, urinary infection, stone formation, and renal failure.) A neurogenic bladder can be spastic (hypertonic, reflex, or automatic), which is caused by an upper motor neuron lesion (above S2 to S4), or flaccid (hypotonic, atonic, nonreflex, or autonomous), which is caused by a lower motor neuron lesion (below S2 to S4).

Causes

At one time, neurogenic bladder was thought to result primarily from spinal cord injury; now, it appears to stem from a host of underlying conditions.

- Cerebral disorders, such as cerebrovascular accident, brain tumor (meningioma and glioma), Parkinson's disease, multiple sclerosis, dementia, and incontinence caused by aging
- Spinal cord disease or trauma, such as spinal stenosis (causing cord compression) or arachnoiditis (causing adhesions between the membranes covering the cord), cervical spondylosis, myelopathies from hereditary disorders or nutritional deficiencies, and, rarely, tabes dorsalis
- Disorders of peripheral innervation, including autonomic neuropathies resulting from endocrine disturbances, such as diabetes mellitus (most common)
- Metabolic disturbances, such as hypothyroidism, porphyria, or uremia (infrequent)
- Acute infectious diseases, such as

Guillain-Barré syndrome
• Heavy metal toxicity
• Chronic alcoholism
• Collagen disease, such as systemic lupus erythematosus
• Vascular diseases, such as atherosclerosis
• Distant effects of cancer, such as primary oat cell carcinoma of the lung
• Herpes zoster

Signs and symptoms

Neurogenic bladder produces a wide range of clinical effects, depending on the underlying cause and its effect on the structural integrity of the bladder.

All types of neurogenic bladder are associated with the following:
• Some degree of incontinence
• Changes in initiation or interruption of micturition
• Inability to empty bladder completely
• Possible vesicoureteral reflux, deterioration or infection in the upper urinary tract, and hydroureteral nephrosis

Spastic neurogenic bladder
Symptoms depend on the site and extent of the spinal cord lesion and may include the following:
—Involuntary or frequent scant urination, without a feeling of bladder fullness
—Spontaneous spasms of the arms and legs
—Increased anal sphincter tone
—Possible voiding and spontaneous contractions of the arms and legs with tactile stimulation of the abdomen, thighs, or genitalia
—Possible severe hypertension, bradycardia, and headaches, with bladder distention if cord lesions are in the upper thoracic (cervical) level

Flaccid neurogenic bladder
—Overflow incontinence
—Diminished anal sphincter tone
—Greatly distended bladder (evident on percussion or palpation) but without the accompanying feeling of bladder fullness because of sensory impairment

Diagnostic tests

Physical examination includes a complete assessment for overt neurologic disease.
• Spinal fluid analysis, showing increased protein level, may indicate cord tumor; increased gamma globulin level may indicate multiple sclerosis.
• Skull and vertebral column X-rays show fracture, dislocation, congenital anomalies, or metastasis.
• Myelography shows spinal cord compression (from tumor, spondylosis, or arachnoiditis).
• EEG may be abnormal if a brain tumor exists.
• Electromyelography confirms peripheral neuropathy.
• Brain and CT scans localize and identify brain masses.

Other tests, including the following, assess bladder function:
• Cystometry evaluates bladder nerve supply and detrusor muscle tone.
• Urethral pressure profile determines urethral function.
• Urinary flow study (uroflow) shows diminished or impaired urinary flow.
• Retrograde urethrography reveals presence of strictures and diverticula.
• Voiding cystography evaluates bladder neck function and continence.

Treatment

Treatment goals are to maintain the integrity of the upper urinary tract, control infection, and prevent urinary incontinence by evacuation of the bladder, drug therapy, surgery, or, less often, neural blocks and electrical stimulation. Techniques of bladder evacuation include Credé's method, Valsalva's maneuver, and intermittent self-catheterization. Credé's method, application of manual pressure over the lower abdomen, promotes complete emptying of the bladder. After appropriate instruction, most patients can perform this maneuver themselves. Even when performed properly, however, Credé's method is not always successful and may not eliminate the need for catheterization.

Intermittent self-catheterization—more effective than either Credé's method or Valsalva's maneuver—has proven to be a major advance in the treatment of neurogenic bladder because it allows complete emptying of the bladder without the risks of a Foley catheter. Intermittent self-catheterization and a bladder-retraining program is useful in patients with flaccid neurogenic bladder.

Drug therapy for neurogenic bladder may include bethanechol and phenoxybenzamine to facilitate bladder emptying and propantheline, methantheline, flavoxate, dicyclomine, and imipramine to facilitate urine storage. When conservative treatment fails, surgery may correct the structural impairment through transurethral resection of the bladder neck, a Y-V plasty, urethral dilation, external sphincterotomy, or urinary diversion procedures. Implantation of an artificial urinary sphincter may be necessary if permanent incontinence follows surgery.

Clinical implications

Care for patients with neurogenic bladder varies according to the underlying cause and the method of treatment.

• Assure the patient that the lengthy diagnostic process is necessary to identify the most effective treatment plan. After the treatment plan is chosen, explain it to the patient in detail.

• Use strict aseptic technique during insertion of a Foley catheter (a temporary measure to drain the incontinent patient's bladder). Do not interrupt the closed drainage system for any reason. Obtain urine specimens with a syringe and small-bore needle inserted through the aspirating port of the catheter itself (below the junction of the balloon instillation site). Irrigate in the same manner, if ordered.

• Clean the catheter insertion site with soap and water at least twice a day. Do not allow the catheter to become encrusted. Use a sterile applicator to apply antibiotic ointment around the meatus after catheter care. To prevent accidental urine reflux, clamp the tubing or empty the urinary drainage bag before transferring the patient to a wheelchair or stretcher.

• Watch for signs of infection (fever, cloudy or foul-smelling urine). Encourage the patient to drink plenty of fluids to prevent calculus formation and infection from urinary stasis. Try to keep the patient as mobile as possible. Perform passive range-of-motion exercises, if necessary.

• If a urinary diversion procedure is to be performed, arrange for consultation with an enterostomal therapist, and coordinate the care plans.

• Before discharge, teach the patient and his family evacuation techniques, as necessary (Credé's method, intermittent catheterization). Counsel him regarding sexual activities. Remember, the incontinent patient feels embarrassed and distressed. Provide emotional support.

Complications

• Incontinence
• Residual urine retention
• Urinary tract infection
• Stone formation
• Renal failure

Nezelof's syndrome

Description

Nezelof's syndrome is a primary immunodeficiency disease characterized by absent T cell function and variable B cell function, with fairly normal immunoglobulin levels and little or no specific antibody production. The degree of B cell deficiency varies. Nezelof's syndrome causes early onset of recurrent, progressively severe, and eventually fatal infections. A tendency toward cancer is common.

Causes
The causes are unknown, but theories include the following:
• An autosomal recessive trait
• A stem cell deficiency that causes T cell and B cell deficiencies
• An underdeveloped thymus gland that inhibits T lymphocyte development
• Failure to produce or secrete thymic humoral factors, particularly thymosin

Signs and symptoms
Clinical signs of Nezelof's syndrome may appear in infants or in toddlers up to 4 years and usually include the following:
• Recurrent pneumonia
• Otitis media
• Chronic fungal infections
• Upper respiratory tract infections
• Hepatosplenomegaly
• Diarrhea
• Poor eating habits
• Failure to thrive
• Weight loss
• Possibly, absent or enlarged lymph nodes and tonsils

Diagnostic tests
• Evidence of defective T cell immunity and moderate-to-marked decrease in T cell count provide a definitive diagnosis.
• B cell count and function vary; 50% of patients have normal B cells.
• Immunoglobulin levels vary.
• Isohemagglutinins are absent or normal.
• Eosinophilia may be present.

Treatment
Initial treatment is primarily supportive and includes use of antibiotics to fight infection and monthly immune globulin or fresh frozen plasma infusions (or, rarely, immune globulin injections), especially if the patient cannot produce specific antibodies.

Fetal thymus transplant can fully restore T cell immunity within weeks, but its effect is transient, necessitating repeated transplants. Both transfer-factor therapy and repeated injections of thymosin are only partially effective in restoring T cell immunity. Although difficult and somewhat risky, histocompatible bone marrow transplants have proved effective in restoring immunity.

Clinical implications
• When administering immune globulin I.V., infuse the first 50 ml very slowly, observing the patient for signs of hypersensitivity reaction.
• When giving immune globulin injections, prevent tissue damage by rotating injection sites and by injecting immune globulin deeply into a large muscle mass. If the child is to receive more than 1.5 ml of immune globulin, divide the dose and use more than one injection site.
• When caring for a patient with Nezelof's syndrome, continuously monitor for signs of infection.
• Teach the parents of a child with Nezelof's syndrome to recognize signs of infection, and warn them that their child must avoid crowds and persons who have active infections.

Complications
Sepsis may eventually occur as a result of infection. It is the usual cause of death in patients with this disorder.

Nocardiosis

Description
Nocardiosis is an acute, subacute, or chronic bacterial infection. It is most common in men, especially those with compromised immune defense mech-

anisms. Its mortality in brain infection exceeds 80%. In other forms, mortality is 50%, even with appropriate therapy.

Cause
An aerobic, weakly gram-positive species of the genus *Nocardia*—usually *Nocardia asteroides*, which is normally found in the soil and causes occasional sporadic disease in humans and animals worldwide

Mode of transmission
• Inhalation of organisms suspended in dust (usual mode)
• Direct inoculation through puncture wounds or abrasions

Signs and symptoms
The exact incubation period is unknown but is probably several weeks.
Pulmonary infection
Nocardiosis originates as a pulmonary infection and can cause the following symptoms:
—Cough (typically produces a thick, tenacious, purulent, mucopurulent, and possibly blood-tinged sputum)
—Fever (may be as high as 105° F. [40.6° C.])
—Chills
—Night sweats
—Anorexia
—Malaise
—Weight loss
Brain infection
If infection spreads through the blood to the brain, abscesses form and cause the following symptoms:
—Confusion
—Nausea
—Disorientation
—Dizziness
—Headache
—Seizures
—Purulent meningitis (can occur if a brain abscess ruptures)
Other effects
—Tracheitis
—Bronchitis
—Pericarditis
—Endocarditis
—Peritonitis
—Mediastinitis
—Septic arthritis
—Keratoconjunctivitis
—Extrapulmonary, hematogenous spread may cause lesions of kidneys, liver, subcutaneous tissue, and bone.

Diagnostic tests
Diagnosis is made with a typical clinical picture. Unfortunately, up to 40% of nocardial infections elude diagnosis until postmortem examination.
• Special staining techniques are often used to make the diagnosis because identification of *Nocardia* by culture of sputum or discharge is difficult.
• Biopsy of lung or other tissue is occasionally necessary for diagnosis.
• Chest X-rays vary and may show fluffy or interstitial infiltrates, nodules, or abscesses.
• Lumbar puncture shows nonspecific changes, such as increased opening pressure, in brain infection with meningitis.
• CSF shows increased WBC count and protein level and decreased glucose level compared with serum glucose in brain infection with meningitis.

Treatment
Nocardiosis requires 12 to 18 months of treatment, preferably with trimethoprim-sulfamethoxazole or high doses of sulfonamides. In patients who do not respond to sulfonamide treatment, other drugs, such as ampicillin or erythromycin, may be added. Treatment also includes surgical drainage of abscesses and excision of necrotic tissue. The acute phase requires complete bed rest. As the patient improves, activity can increase.

Clinical implications
Nocardiosis requires no isolation. It is not transmitted from person to person.
• Provide adequate nourishment

through total parenteral nutrition, nasogastric tube feedings, or a balanced diet.
• Give tepid sponge baths and antipyretics, as ordered, to reduce fever.
• Monitor for allergic reactions to antibiotics.
• High-dose sulfonamide therapy (especially sulfadiazine) predisposes the patient to crystalluria and oliguria. So assess frequently, force fluids, and alkalinize the urine with sodium bicarbonate, as ordered, to prevent these complications.
• In patients with pulmonary infection, administer intermittent positive-pressure breathing (IPPB), as ordered, with chest physiotherapy. Auscultate the lungs daily, checking for increased crackles or consolidation. Note and record amount, color, and thickness of sputum.
• In brain infection, regularly assess neurologic function. Watch for signs of increased intracranial pressure, such as decreased level of consciousness, and respiratory abnormalities.
• In long-term hospitalization, turn the patient often, and assist with range-of-motion exercises.
• Before the patient is discharged, stress the need to continue taking medication as scheduled, to maintain therapeutic blood levels even after symptoms subside. Explain the importance of frequent follow-up examinations. Provide support and encouragement to help the patient and his family cope with this long-term illness.

Nonspecific genitourinary infections

Description
Nonspecific genitourinary infections, including nongonococcal urethritis (NGU) in males and mild vaginitis or cervicitis in females, comprise a group of infections with similar manifestations that are not linked to a single organism. Such infections have become more prevalent since the mid-1960s and may be more widespread than gonorrhea. Prognosis is good if sexual partners are treated simultaneously.

Causes
Males
—*Chlamydia trachomatis* and *Urea plasma urealyticum* are often the cause.
—Bacteria such as staphylococci, diphtheroids, coliform organisms, and *Corynebacterium vaginale (Hemophilus vaginalis)* may also cause these infections.
—Less frequently, infection may be related to preexisting strictures, neoplasms, and chemical or traumatic inflammation.
Females
Less is known about these infections in females, but the following organisms may cause them:
—Chlamydial organisms
—Corynebacterial organisms

Mode of transmission
Primarily, through sexual intercourse

Signs and symptoms
Symptoms may be absent or may occur 1 week to 1 month after coitus.
Males
—Scant or moderate urethral discharge
—Variable dysuria
—Occasional hematuria
—Subclinical urethritis (may be found on physical examination, especially if the sex partner has a positive diagnosis)
Females
—Possibly, persistent vaginal discharge
—Possibly, acute or recurrent cystitis for which no underlying cause can be found
—Possibly, cervicitis with inflammatory erosion

Diagnostic tests

In males, microscopic examination of smears of prostatic or urethral secretions shows excess polymorphonuclear leukocytes but few, if any, specific organisms. In females, examination of cervical or urethral smears also reveals excess leukocytes and no specific organisms.

Treatment

Therapy for both sexes consists of oral tetracycline or erythromycin or of streptomycin followed by a sulfonamide. (Tetracycline is contraindicated in pregnant females.) For females, treatment may also include application of a sulfa vaginal cream. Cervicitis occasionally necessitates cryosurgery.

Clinical implications

• Tell female patients to clean the pubic area before applying vaginal medication and to avoid using tampons during treatment.
• Make sure the patient clearly understands and strictly follows the dosage schedule for all prescribed medications.

To prevent nonspecific genitourinary infections, follow these guidelines:

• Tell patients to abstain from sexual contact with infected partners, to use condoms during sexual activity and follow appropriate hygienic measures afterward, and to void before and after intercourse.
• Encourage patients to maintain adequate fluid intake.
• Advise female patients to avoid routine use of douches and feminine hygiene sprays, tight-fitting pants or panty hose, insertion of foreign objects into the vagina, and deodorant tampons.
• Suggest that female patients wear cotton underpants and remove them before going to bed.

O

Obesity

Description

Obesity is an excess of body fat, usually 20% above ideal body weight. Observation and comparison of height and weight to a standard height-weight table indicate obesity.

Cause

Obesity results from excessive calorie intake and inadequate expenditure of energy. Theories to explain this condition include hypothalamic dysfunction of hunger and satiety centers, genetic predisposition, abnormal absorption of nutrients, and impaired action of gastrointestinal and growth hormones and of hormonal regulators, such as insulin. Psychological factors may also contribute to obesity.

Risk factors

Obesity in parents increases the probability of obesity in children, based on genetic or environmental factors, such as activity levels and learned patterns of eating.

Diagnostic tests

Measurement of the thickness of subcutaneous fat folds with calipers provides an approximation of total body fat. Although this measurement is reliable and is not subject to daily fluctuations, it has little meaning for the patient in monitoring subsequent weight loss.

Treatment

Successful management of obesity must decrease the patient's daily calorie intake while increasing his activity level. Effective treatment must be based on a balanced, low-calorie diet that eliminates foods high in fat or sugar content. To achieve long-term benefits, lifelong maintenance of improved eating and exercise patterns is necessary.

The popular low-carbohydrate diets offer no long-term advantage; rapid early weight reduction is from loss of water, not fat.

Total fasting is an effective way to lose weight fast, but it requires close monitoring and supervision to minimize risks of ketonemia, electrolyte imbalance, hypotension, and loss of lean body mass. Prolonged fasting or very low-calorie diets have been associated with sudden death, possibly resulting from cardiac dysrhythmias caused by electrolyte abnormalities.

These methods have the overwhelming drawback of not teaching the patient long-term modification of eating patterns. They often lead to the "yo-yo syndrome"—repeated episodes of weight loss followed by weight gain.

Treatment may also include hypnosis and behavior modification techniques, which promote fundamental changes in eating habits and activity patterns. Besides, psychotherapy may be beneficial for some patients, because weight reduction may lead to depression or even psychosis.

Amphetamines and amphetamine congeners are used to enhance compliance with a prescribed diet by temporarily suppressing the appetite and creating a feeling of well-being. Their value in long-term weight control is questionable, however. Because of the potential for dependence and abuse, their use is usually avoided. If these drugs are used at all, they should be prescribed only for short-term therapy and should be monitored carefully.

Morbid obesity (body weight of 200% or more of standard) may be treated surgically with gastroplasty (gastric stapling) as a last resort. Gastroplasty decreases the volume of food that the stomach can hold and thereby produces satiety with small intake. This technique causes fewer complications than jejunoileal bypass, which induces a permanent malabsorption syndrome.

Clinical implications

• Obtain an accurate diet history to identify the patient's eating patterns and the importance of food to his lifestyle. Ask the patient to keep a careful record of what, where, and when he eats to help identify situations that normally provoke overeating.
• Explain the prescribed diet carefully, and encourage compliance to improve health status.
• To increase calorie expenditure, promote increased physical activity, including an exercise program. Recommended activity levels vary according to the patient's general condition and cardiovascular status.
• If the patient is taking appetite-suppressing drugs, watch carefully for signs of dependence or abuse and for side effects, such as insomnia, excitability, dry mouth, and gastrointestinal disturbances.
• Teach the patient who is grossly obese the importance of good skin care to prevent breakdown in moist skin folds. Regular use of powder to keep skin dry is recommended.

• To help prevent obesity in children, teach parents to avoid overfeeding their infants and to familiarize themselves with actual nutritional needs and optimum growth rates. Discourage parents from using food to reward or console their children, from emphasizing the importance of "clean plates," and from allowing eating to prevent hunger rather than to satisfy it.
• Encourage physical activity and exercise, especially in children and young adults, to establish lifelong patterns. Suggest low-calorie snacks, such as raw vegetables.

Complications

Obesity may lead to serious complications, which include the following:
• Respiratory difficulties
• Hypertension
• Cardiovascular disease
• Diabetes mellitus
• Renal disease
• Gallbladder disease
• Psychosocial difficulties

Obsessive-compulsive disorder

Description

Obsessive thoughts and compulsive behaviors represent recurring efforts to control overwhelming anxiety, guilt, or unacceptable impulses that persistently and involuntarily enter the consciousness (*DSM-III* classifies this as an anxiety disorder). Obsession refers to a recurrent idea, thought, or image. Compulsion, the action component, refers to a ritualistic, repetitive, and involuntary defensive behavior as an expression of anxiety. This disorder is relatively rare in the general population (0.05%). It occurs in both sexes, with typical onset in adolescents or young adults. Recent studies indicate a higher incidence in upper-class persons with higher intelligence. Major depression, organic brain syndrome,

Causes of Obsessive-Compulsive Disorder

PSYCHOANA-LYTIC THEORY	LEARNING THEORY	INTERPERSONAL THEORY	EXISTENTIAL-IST THEORY
Psychodynamic factors (ego defenses) • Isolation • Undoing • Reaction formation **Psychogenic factors** • Preoccupation with aggression • Preoccupation with dirt • Disturbed growth/development pattern related to anal/sadistic phase **Regression** • Fixation at earlier level of development (anal stage) • Ambivalence • Magical thinking	• Obsession—conditioned stimulus to anxiety • Compulsion—reduced anxiety reinforces behavior • Approach avoidance—reduces conflict • Emphasis on cognitive change to alter behavior	• Irrational inflexible coping strategies to handle intense anxiety or guilt • Unrealistic (rigid) view of self (self-hate, self-contempt—"bad me") • Avoidance of anxiety-laden relationships (withdrawal) • Defenses (sublimation, selective inattention, substitution, dissociation) • Inferiority feelings (to gain control of others) • Threat to autonomy and loss of individuality • Family patterns and coping styles that reinforce obsessions • Inability to enjoy life	• Inability to live with uncertainty or ambiguity • Wish to flee situation of great anxiety • Threat of nonexistence • Religious rituals • Excessively high morals

and schizophrenia may contribute to the onset of obsessive-compulsive disorder.

Obsessions and compulsions cause significant distress and may severely impair occupational and social functioning. Generally, an obsessive-compulsive disorder is chronic, often with remissions and flare-ups. Diagnosis rests on evidence of compulsively repetitive patterns of thought or behavior. A careful history may identify previous obsessive-compulsive personality traits. Often, the patient's description of his own behavior offers the best clues to this diagnosis. However, the patient also needs evaluation for other physical or psychiatric disorders. One telling difference between obsessive-compulsive states and schizophrenia, which may produce similar behavioral patterns, is that schizophrenics have lower visible levels of anxiety. The prognosis is better than average when symptoms are quickly identified, diagnosed, and treated, and when environmental stress is recognized and adjusted.

Cause

The cause of obsessive-compulsive disorder is unknown. Some studies suggest the possibility of brain lesions, but the most useful research and clinical studies lead to an explanation based on psychological theories. (See *Causes of Obsessive-Compulsive Disorder*.)

Signs and symptoms

This disorder may be manifested physically or behaviorally as ideas or impulses that refer either to actions completed or to future, anticipated events. These actions or events may be simple, mild, and uncomplicated or dramatic, elaborately complex, and ritualized. Their meanings may be obvious or may reflect inner psychological distortions that are unraveled only through intensive psychotherapy.

When the obsessive-compulsive phenomena are mental, no one knows that anything unusual is happening unless the patient talks about these private experiences. (See *Personality Types Susceptible to Obsessive-Compulsive Behavior*.)

Obsessive symptoms
—Thoughts of violence
—Thoughts of contamination
—Repetitive doubts and worry about a tragic event

Compulsive symptoms
Often, the patient's anxiety is so strong that he will avoid the situation or the object that evokes the impulse. For example, a patient with a recurring urge to push people down long flights of stairs may avoid climbing stairs in any building, live in a one-story house, and thereby control his behavior so he will not be tempted to act on this compulsion. Common compulsions include the following:
—Repetitive touching
—Doing and undoing (opening and closing doors, rearranging things)
—Washing (especially hands)
—Checking (to be sure no tragedy has occurred)

Treatment

Treatment of obsessive-compulsive states aims to reduce anxiety, resolve inner conflicts, relieve depression, and teach more effective ways of dealing with stress. Such treatment (especially during an acute episode) may include tranquilizing and antidepressant drugs. Intensive long-term psychotherapy, brief supportive psychotherapy, or group therapy are the preferred treatments.

Personality Types Susceptible to Obsessive-Compulsive Behavior

Obsessive-compulsive states seem to develop in certain personality types and under certain conditions. The obsessional person is usually rigid and conscientious and has great aspirations. He has a formal, reserved manner, with precise and careful movements and posture; he takes responsibility seriously and finds decision making difficult. He lacks creativity and the ability to find alternate solutions to his problems. Such a person has a tendency to be painfully accurate and complete—carefully qualifying his statements to avoid making a mistake and anticipating every move and gesture of the person to whom he speaks. His affect is flat and unemotional except for controlled anxiety. Self-awareness is totally intellectual, without accompanying emotion or feeling.

Behavorial Therapies

- **Aversion therapy**—application of a painful stimulus to create an aversion to the obsession that leads to undesirable behavior (compulsion).

- **Thought stopping**—a technique to break the habit of fear-inducing anticipatory thoughts. The patient is taught to stop unwanted thoughts by saying the word "stop" and then to focus his attention on achieving calmness and muscle relaxation.

- **Thought switching**—a technique to replace fear-inducing self-instructions with competent self-instructions. The patient is taught to replace negative thoughts with positive ones until the positive thoughts become strong enough to overcome the anxiety-provoking ones.

- **Flooding**—frequent full-intensity exposure (through use of imagery) to an object that triggers a symptom. Used with caution because it produces extreme discomfort.

- **Implosion therapy**—a form of desensitization through repeated exposure to a highly feared object.

- **Response prevention**—prevention of compulsive behavior by distraction, persuasion, or redirection of activity; may require hospitalization or involvement of family to be effective.

Behavioral therapies—aversion therapy, thought stopping, thought switching, flooding, implosion therapy, and response prevention—have also been effective. (See *Behavioral Therapies.*)

Clinical implications
Patient care should focus on reducing the associated anxiety, fears, and guilt; building the patient's self-esteem; and helping him understand why he needs the compulsive behavior.

- Approach the patient unhurriedly.
- Provide an accepting atmosphere; do not show shock, amusement, or criticism of the ritualistic behavior.
- Allow the patient time to carry out the ritualistic behavior (unless it is dangerous) until he can be distracted into some other activity. Blocking this behavior raises the patient's anxiety to an intolerable level.
- Encourage the patient to express his feelings about the anxiety that causes the compulsive behavior, especially when he seems fearful.
- Explore the patterns leading to the behavior or recurring problems.
- Listen attentively, offering feedback.
- Encourage use of appropriate defense mechanisms to relieve loneliness and isolation.
- Engage the patient in activities to create positive accomplishments and raise his self-esteem and confidence.
- Encourage active diversional resources, such as whistling or humming a tune, to divert attention from the unwanted thoughts and to promote a pleasurable experience.
- Assist the patient with new ways to solve problems and to develop more effective coping skills by setting limits on unacceptable behavior (for example, limit the number of times per day he may indulge in obsessive behavior). Gradually shorten the time allowed. Help him focus on other feelings or problems for the rest of the time.
- Help the patient identify progress and set realistic expectations of himself and others.
- Explain how to channel emotional

energy to relieve stress (through such activities as sports and creative endeavors).

• Identify insight and improved behavior (reduced compulsive behavior and/or fewer obsessive thoughts). Evaluate behavioral changes by your own and the patient's self-reports.

• Identify disturbing topics of conversation that reflect underlying anxiety or terror.

• Observe for interventions that do not work; reevaluate and recommend alternative strategies.

• Find ways to deal with the anger and frustration that the patient often arouses in you.

• Keep the patient's physical health in mind. For example, compulsive hand washing may cause skin breakdown, and rituals or preoccupations may cause inadequate food and fluid intake and exhaustion.

• Make reasonable demands and set reasonable limits; make their purpose clear. Avoid creating situations that increase frustration and provoke anger, which may interfere with treatment.

Orbital cellulitis

Description

Orbital cellulitis is an acute infection of the orbital tissues and eyelids that does not involve the eyeball. It may be primary or secondary. Primary orbital cellulitis is most common in young children. Typical clinical features establish the diagnosis. With treatment, prognosis is good. If cellulitis is not treated, infection may spread to the cavernous sinus or the meninges.

Causes

• Trauma, such as an insect bite, usually causes primary orbital cellulitis.

• Streptococcal, staphylococcal or pneumococcal infections of nearby structures can cause secondary orbital cellulitis.

Mode of transmission

• Bacteria enters directly into the orbital tissues and eyelids as a result of trauma in primary orbital cellulitis.

• Organisms from nearby infected structures invade the orbit, frequently by direct extension through the sinuses (especially the ethmoidal sinus), the bloodstream, or the lymphatic ducts in secondary orbital cellulitis.

Signs and symptoms

• Unilateral eyelid edema

• Hyperemia of the orbital tissue

• Reddened eyelids

• Matted eyelashes

• Proptosis that develops later in the infection (because of edematous tissues within the bony confines of the orbit). Initially, the eyeball is unaffected.

• Other indications: extreme orbital pain, impaired eye movement, chemosis, and purulent discharge from indurated areas

Diagnostic tests

• Wound culture and sensitivity testing determine the causative organism and specific antibiotic therapy.

• WBC count is elevated from orbital tissue infection.

• Ophthalmologic examination rules out cavernous sinus thrombosis.

Treatment

Prompt treatment prevents complications. Primary treatment consists of antibiotic therapy, depending on the results of culture and sensitivity tests. Systemic antibiotics (I.V., P.O.) and eye drops or ointment will be ordered. Supportive therapy consists of fluids; warm, moist compresses; and bed rest. If antibiotics fail, incision and drainage may be necessary.

Clinical implications

• Monitor vital signs, and maintain fluid and electrolyte balance.

• Apply compresses every 3 to 4 hours to localize inflammation and relieve discomfort. Teach the patient to apply these compresses. Give pain medication, as ordered, after assessing pain level.

• Before the patient's discharge, stress the importance of completing prescribed antibiotic therapy. Tell the patient to prevent orbital cellulitis by maintaining good general hygiene and carefully cleaning abrasions and cuts that occur near the orbit. Urge early treatment of orbital cellulitis to prevent infection from spreading.

Ornithosis
(Psittacosis, parrot fever)

Description
Ornithosis is an infectious disease occurring worldwide. It is mainly associated with occupational exposure to birds (for example, as poultry farming). Its incidence is higher in women and in persons aged 20 to 50 years. Classic symptoms and recent exposure to birds suggest the diagnosis. With adequate antimicrobial therapy, ornithosis is fatal in fewer than 4% of patients.

Cause
Chlamydia psittaci, a gram-negative, intracellular parasite

Mode of transmission
Psittacine birds (parrots, parakeets, cockatoos), pigeons, and turkeys may harbor *C. psittaci* in their blood, feathers, tissues, nasal secretions, liver, spleen, and feces. Transmission to humans occurs in the following ways.
• Primarily, inhalation of dust containing *C. psittaci* from bird droppings
• Direct contact with infected secretions or body tissues, as in laboratory personnel who work with birds
• Rarely, person-to-person transmission

Signs and symptoms
After an incubation period of 4 to 15 days, onset of symptoms may be insidious or sudden. Clinical effects include the following:
• Chills
• Low-grade fever. This increases to 103° to 105° F. (39.4° to 40.6° C.) for 7 to 10 days. With treatment, it declines during the second or third week.
• Headache
• Myalgia
• Sore throat
• Cough. This may be dry, hacking, and nonproductive, or may produce blood-tinged sputum.
• Abdominal distention and tenderness
• Nausea
• Vomiting
• Photophobia
• Decreased pulse rate
• Slightly increased respirations
• Secondary purulent lung infection
• Faint macular rash
• In severe infection, delirium, stupor, and in extensive pulmonary infiltration, cyanosis

Diagnostic tests
• Recovery of *C. psittaci* from mice, eggs, or tissue culture inoculated with the patient's blood or sputum is required for firm diagnosis.
• Comparison of acute and convalescent serum shows a fourfold rise in *Chlamydia* antibody titers.
• Chest X-rays during the first week of illness show a patchy lobar infiltrate.

Treatment
Ornithosis calls for treatment with tetracycline. If the infection is severe, tetracycline may be given I.V. until the fever subsides. Fever and other symptoms should begin to subside 48 to 72 hours after antibiotic treatment begins; but treatment must continue for 2 weeks after temperature returns to normal. If the patient cannot tolerate tetracycline, penicillin G procaine or chloramphenicol is an alternative.

Clinical implications

• Reduce fever with tepid alcohol or sponge baths and a cooling blanket.

• Reposition the patient often.

• Observe secretion precautions. During the acute, febrile stage, if the patient has a cough, wear a face mask and wash your hands carefully. Instruct him to use tissues when he coughs and to dispose of them in a closed plastic bag.

• To prevent ornithosis, those who raise birds for sale should feed them tetracycline-treated birdseed and follow regulations on bird importation. They should segregate infected or possibly infected birds from healthy birds, and disinfect structures that housed infected ones.

• Report all cases of ornithosis to public health authorities.

Osgood-Schlatter disease
(Osteochondrosis)

Description

Osgood-Schlatter disease is a painful, incomplete separation of the epiphysis of the tibial tubercle from the tibial shaft. It is most common in active adolescent boys. It frequently affects one or both knees. Severe disease may cause permanent tubercle enlargement.

Causes

Trauma, occurring before the complete fusion of the epiphysis to the main bone (between ages 10 and 15), is the usual cause. This may be a single violent action or repeated knee flexion against a tight quadriceps muscle. Other causes include locally deficient blood supply and genetic factors.

Signs and symptoms

• Constant aching, pain, and tenderness below the kneecap. This worsens during any activity that causes forceful contraction of the patellar tendon on the tubercle, such as ascending or descending stairs.

• Possibly, obvious soft-tissue swelling of the area

• Localized heat

Diagnostic tests

• Forcing the tibia into internal rotation while slowly extending the patient's knee from 90 degrees of flexion to about 30 degrees produces pain that subsides immediately with external rotation of the tibia.

• X-rays may be normal or show epiphyseal separation and soft-tissue swelling for up to 6 months after onset; eventually, they may show bone fragmentation.

Treatment

Treatment usually consists of immobilization for 6 to 8 weeks and supportive measures. Leg immobilization through reinforced elastic knee support, plaster cast, or splint allows revascularization and reossification of the tubercle and minimizes the pull of the quadriceps. Supportive measures include activity restrictions and, possibly, cortisone injections into the knee joint to relieve tenderness. In very mild cases, simple restriction of predisposing activities (bicycling, running) may be adequate.

Rarely, conservative measures fail, and surgery may be necessary. Such surgery includes removing or fixing the epiphysis or drilling holes through the tubercle to the main bone to form channels for rapid revascularization.

Clinical implications

• Monitor the patient's circulation, sensation, and pain, and watch for excessive bleeding after surgery.

• Assess motion daily for signs of limitation. Administer analgesics, as needed.

• Make sure the knee support or splint is not too tight. Keep the cast dry and clean, and "petal" it around the top and bottom margins to avoid skin irritation. Teach proper use of crutches. Tell the patient to protect the injured knee with padding and to avoid trauma and repeated flexion (running, contact sports).

• Monitor for muscle atrophy.

• Give reassurance and emotional support because disruption of normal activities is difficult for an active teenager. Emphasize that restrictions are temporary.

Osteoarthritis

Description

The most common form of arthritis, osteoarthritis is chronic, causing deterioration of the joint cartilage and formation of reactive new bone at the margins and subchondral areas of the joints. This degeneration results from a breakdown of chondrocytes, most often in the hips and knees. Earliest symptoms generally begin in middle age and may progress with advancing age. A thorough physical examination confirms typical symptoms, and lack of systemic symptoms rules out an inflammatory joint disorder, such as rheumatoid arthritis.

Disability depends on the site and severity of involvement and can range from minor limitation of the fingers to severe disability in persons with hip or knee involvement. The rate of progression varies, and joints may remain stable for years in an early stage of deterioration.

Causes

The exact cause of osteoarthritis is unknown. Primary osteoarthritis, a normal part of aging, results from many things, including metabolic, genetic, chemical, and mechanical factors. Secondary osteoarthritis usually follows an identifiable predisposing event—most commonly trauma or congenital deformity—and leads to degenerative changes.

Signs and symptoms

The severity of the following signs and symptoms increases with poor posture, obesity, and occupational stress:

• Joint pain that occurs particularly after exercise or weight bearing and that is usually relieved by rest is the most common symptom.

• Stiffness in the morning and after exercise (relieved by rest)

• Aching during changes in weather

• "Grating" of the joint during motion

• Limited movement

• Irreversible changes in the distal joints (Heberden's nodes) and proximal joints (Bouchard's nodes) occur in osteoarthritis of the interphalangeal joints. Nodes may be painless at first but eventually become red, swollen, and tender, causing numbness and loss of dexterity.

Diagnostic tests

X-rays of the affected joint help confirm diagnosis of osteoarthritis. X-rays may include posterior, anterior, lateral, and oblique views (with spinal involvement) and typically show narrowing of joint space or margin, cystlike bony deposits in joint space and margins, joint deformity from degeneration or articular damage, and bony growths at weight-bearing areas (hips, knees).

Treatment

Treatment is primarily palliative, through medication and surgery. Medications for relief of pain and joint inflammation include aspirin (or other nonnarcotic analgesics), phenylbutazone, indomethacin, fenoprofen, ibuprofen, propoxyphene, and in some cases, intraarticular injections of corticosteroids. Such injections may delay the development of nodes in the hands.

Effective treatment also reduces stress by supporting or stabilizing the joint with crutches, braces, cane, walker, cervical collar, or traction. Other supportive measures include massage, moist heat, paraffin dips for

Teaching Topics in Osteoarthritis

- An explanation of the disease process: primary or secondary osteoarthritis
- Importance of exercise to prevent loss of joint function and deformity
- Range-of-motion, extension, flexion, and isometric exercises
- Use of protective and assistive devices to avoid joint fatigue
- Medications and their administration
- Surgery: debridement, osteotomy, arthrodesis, or joint replacement
- Postoperative exercises and activity restrictions, if appropriate
- Other pain-relief measures: heat or cold therapy, massage

hands, protective techniques for preventing undue stress on the joints, adequate rest (particularly after activity), and occasionally exercise when the knees are affected.

The following surgical procedures are reserved for patients who have severe osteoarthritis with disability or uncontrollable pain:

- Arthroplasty (partial or total): replacement of a deteriorated joint or part with a prosthetic appliance
- Arthrodesis: surgical fusion of bones; used primarily in the spine (laminectomy)
- Osteoplasty: scraping of deteriorated bone from a joint
- Osteotomy: excision of bone to change alignment and relieve stress

Clinical implications

- Promote adequate rest, particularly after activity. Plan rest periods during the day, and provide for adequate sleep at night. Moderation is the key; teach the patient to "pace" daily activities.
- Assist with "physical therapy, and encourage the patient to perform gentle range-of-motion exercises.
- If the patient needs surgery, provide appropriate preoperative and postoperative care.
- Provide emotional support and reassurance to help the patient cope with limited mobility. Explain that osteoarthritis is *not* a systemic disease.

Specific patient care depends on the affected joint.

- Hand: Apply hot soaks and paraffin dips to relieve pain, as ordered.
- Spine (lumbar and sacral): Recommend a firm mattress (or bed board) to decrease morning pain.
- Spine (cervical): Check cervical collar for constriction; watch for redness with prolonged use.
- Hip: Use moist heat pads to relieve pain and administer antispasmodic drugs, as ordered. Assist with range-of-motion and strengthening exercises, always making sure the patient gets the proper rest afterward. Check crutches, cane, braces, and walker for proper fit, and teach the patient to use them correctly. For example, the patient with unilateral joint involvement should use an orthopedic appliance (such as a cane or walker) on the normal side. Advise use of cushions when sitting, and suggest an elevated toilet seat.
- Knee: Twice daily, assist with prescribed range-of-motion exercises, exercises to maintain muscle tone, and progressive resistance exercises to increase muscle strength. Provide elastic supports or braces if needed.

To minimize the long-term effects of osteoarthritis, teach the patient to follow these guidelines:

- Plan for adequate rest during the day, after exertion, and at night.
- Take medication exactly as prescribed, and report side effects immediately.
- Avoid overexertion. Take care to

stand and walk correctly, to minimize weight-bearing activities, and to be especially careful when stooping or picking up objects.

• Always wear well-fitting supportive shoes; do not allow the heels to become too worn down.

• Install safety devices at home, such as guard rails in the bathroom.

• Do range-of-motion exercises as gently as possible.

• Maintain proper body weight to lessen strain on joints. (Also see *Teaching Topics in Osteoarthritis,* p. 523.)

Osteogenesis imperfecta

Description

Osteogenesis imperfecta (brittle bones) is a hereditary disease of bone and connective tissue. This disease occurs in two forms. In the rare congenital form, hundreds of fractures may occur before birth and birth itself may cause fractures; other skeletal deformities reflect fractures that occurred in utero and healed in abnormal positions. This form is usually fatal within the first few days or weeks of life. In the late-appearing form (osteogenesis imperfecta tarda), the child appears normal at birth but recurring fractures (mostly of the extremities) develop after the first year of life. The incidence of such fractures decreases after puberty. Family history and characteristic features, such as blue sclera or deafness, establish the diagnosis.

Cause

Inherited as an autosomal dominant or recessive trait

Signs and symptoms

Fractures that occur with even slight trauma are the hallmark of this disease. In both forms, incomplete and relatively painless fractures that occur after birth and that receive no treat-

ment can produce deformities from bones healing in poor alignment. Other signs and symptoms include the following:

• Bilateral bulging skull

• Triangular-shaped head and face

• Prominent eyes

• Blue sclera

• Deafness, which occurs in one third of patients between ages 30 and 40

• Thin, translucent skin

• Subcutaneous hemorrhages

• Discolored teeth (blue-gray or yellow-brown) that break easily and are cavity-prone

• Poorly developed skeletal muscles

• Hypermobility of joints

• In osteogenesis imperfecta tarda, possible stunted growth or short stature

Diagnostic tests

• X-rays showing evidence of multiple, healed fractures and skeletal deformities and skull X-rays showing wide sutures with small, irregularly shaped islands of bone (wormian bones) between them support the diagnosis.

• Serum calcium and serum phosphorus levels are normal.

Treatment

Treatment aims to prevent deformities by traction, immobilization, or both, and to aid normal development and rehabilitation. Support includes the following:

• Checking the patient's circulatory, motor, and sensory abilities

• Encouraging the patient to walk when possible (these children develop a fear of walking)

• Teaching preventive measures (for example, the child must avoid contact sports or strenuous activity or must wear knee pads, helmets, or other protective devices when he engages in activities)

• Assessing for and treating scoliosis, a common complication

• Promoting preventive dental care and repair of dental caries

Clinical implications

• Educate the family. Teach the parents and child how to recognize fractures and how to correctly splint a fracture.

• Advise parents to encourage the child to develop interests that do not require strenuous physical activity and to develop his fine motor skills. These will promote the child's self-esteem.

• Help parents make arrangements for tutoring.

• Teach the child to assume responsibility for precautions during physical activity to help foster his independence.

• Stress good nutrition to heal bones.

• Refer the parents and child for genetic counseling.

• Administer analgesics, as ordered.

• Monitor dental and hearing needs. Stress nutrition, dental care, and immunizations in well-child visits.

Osteomyelitis

Description

Osteomyelitis is a pyogenic bone infection that may be chronic or acute. Although osteomyelitis often remains localized, it can spread through the bone to the marrow, cortex, and periosteum. Acute osteomyelitis is usually a blood-borne disease that most often affects rapidly growing children. Chronic osteomyelitis (rare) is characterized by multiple draining sinus tracts and metastatic lesions.

Osteomyelitis occurs more often in children than in adults—and particularly in boys. The most common sites of infection in children are the lower end of the femur and the upper end of the tibia, humerus, and radius. In adults, the most common sites are the pelvis and vertebrae, usually the result of contamination associated with surgery or trauma. Patient history, physical examination, and blood tests help

to confirm osteomyelitis. With prompt treatment, the prognosis for acute osteomyelitis is good. For chronic osteomyelitis, which is more prevalent in adults, the prognosis is still poor.

Cause

Osteomyelitis commonly results from a combination of local trauma—usually quite trivial but resulting in hematoma formation—and an acute infection originating elsewhere in the body.

The most common pyogenic organism in osteomyelitis is *Staphylococcus aureus;* others include *Streptococcus pyogenes, Pneumococcus, Pseudomonas aeruginosa, Escherichia coli,* and *Proteus vulgaris.* Typically, these organisms find a culture site in a hematoma from recent trauma or in a weakened area, such as the site of local infection (for example, furunculosis), and spread directly to bone.

Signs and symptoms

Usually, the clinical features of both chronic and acute osteomyelitis are the same, except that chronic infection can persist intermittently for years, flaring up spontaneously after minor trauma. Persistent drainage of pus from an old pocket in a sinus tract is sometimes the only symptom of chronic infection. Onset of acute osteomyelitis is usually rapid.

Local signs and symptoms
—Sudden pain in the affected bone
—Tenderness, heat, and swelling over the affected bone
—Restricted movement
Systemic signs and symptoms
—Tachycardia
—Sudden fever
—Nausea
—Malaise

Diagnostic tests

• WBC count shows leukocytosis.

• Erythrocyte sedimentation rate is elevated.

• Blood culture results identify causative organism.

• X-rays may not show bone involvement until the disease has been active for some time, usually 2 to 3 weeks.
• Bone scans can detect early infection.

Treatment

To prevent further bone damage, treatment for acute osteomyelitis should begin before definitive diagnosis. Treatment includes administration of large doses of antibiotics I.V. (usually a penicillinase-resistant penicillin, such as nafcillin or oxacillin) after blood cultures are taken; early surgical drainage to relieve pressure buildup and sequestrum formation; immobilization of the affected bone by plaster cast, traction, or bed rest; and supportive measures, such as analgesics and I.V. fluids.

If an abscess forms, treatment includes incision and drainage, followed by a culture of the drainage matter. Antibiotic therapy to control infection may include administration of systemic antibiotics; intracavitary instillation of antibiotics through closed-system continuous irrigation with low intermittent suction; limited irrigation with blood drainage system with suction (Hemovac); or local application of packed, wet, antibiotic-soaked dressings.

Besides needing antibiotic and immobilization therapy, chronic osteomyelitis usually requires surgery to remove dead bone (sequestrectomy) and to promote drainage (saucerization). Prognosis is poor even after surgery. Patients are often in great pain and require prolonged hospitalization. Therapy-resistant chronic osteomyelitis in an arm or leg may necessitate amputation.

Clinical implications

Major nursing concerns are to control infection, protect the bone from injury, and offer meticulous supportive care.

• Use strict aseptic technique when changing dressings and irrigating wounds. If the patient is in skeletal traction for compound fractures, cover insertion points of pin tracks with small, dry dressings, and tell him not to touch the skin around the pins and wires.
• Administer I.V. fluids to maintain adequate hydration, as necessary. Provide a diet high in protein and vitamin C.
• Assess vital signs, wound appearance, and new pain, which may indicate secondary infection, daily.
• Carefully monitor suctioning equipment. Do not let containers of solution being instilled become empty, allowing air into the system. Monitor the amount of solution instilled and suctioned.
• Support the affected limb with firm pillows. Keep the limb level with the body. Do not let it sag. Provide good skin care. Turn the patient gently every 2 hours and watch for signs of developing decubitus ulcers.
• Provide good cast care. Support the cast with firm pillows and "petal" the edges with pieces of adhesive tape or moleskin to smooth rough edges. Check circulation and drainage; if a wet spot appears on the cast, circle it with a marking pen and note the time of appearance (on the cast). Be aware of how much drainage is expected. Check the circled spot at least every 4 hours. Report any enlargement immediately.
• Protect the patient from mishaps, such as jerky movements and falls that may threaten bone integrity. Report sudden pain, crepitus, or deformity immediately. Watch for any sudden malposition of the limb, which may indicate fracture.
• Provide emotional support and appropriate diversions. Before discharge, the patient should learn how to protect and clean the wound and, most important, how to recognize signs of recurring infection (increased body temperature, redness, localized

heat, and swelling). Stress the need for follow-up examinations. Instruct the patient to seek prompt treatment for possible sources of recurrence—blisters, boils, styes, and impetigo.

Osteoporosis

Description

Osteoporosis is a metabolic bone disorder in which the rate of bone resorption accelerates while the rate of bone formation slows down, causing a loss of bone mass. Bones affected by this disease lose calcium and phosphate salts and, thus, become porous, brittle, and abnormally vulnerable to fracture. Osteoporosis may be primary or secondary to an underlying disease. Primary osteoporosis is often called senile or postmenopausal osteoporosis because it most commonly develops in elderly, postmenopausal women.

Osteoporosis primarily affects the weight-bearing vertebrae. Only when the condition is advanced or severe, as in Cushing's syndrome or hyperthyroidism, do comparable changes occur in the skull, ribs, and long bones.

Causes

Primary osteoporosis
—Unknown
Secondary osteoporosis
—Prolonged therapy with steroids or heparin
—Total immobilization or disuse of a bone (as with hemiplegia, for example)
—Alcoholism
—Malnutrition
—Malabsorption
—Scurvy
—Lactose intolerance
—Hyperthyroidism
—Osteogenesis imperfecta
—Sudeck's atrophy (localized to hands and feet, with recurring attacks)

Risk factors

• Inadequate dietary intake of calcium
• Declining gonadal adrenal function
• Estrogen deficiency
• Sedentary life-style

Signs and symptoms

Discovery of the disease may occur suddenly, but osteoporosis develops insidiously. Osteoporosis is usually discovered when an elderly person bends to lift something, hears a snapping sound, then feels a sudden pain in the lower back. Any movement or jarring aggravates the backache. Other symptoms include the following:
• Pain in the lower back that radiates around the trunk
• Various deformities
• Kyphosis
• Loss of height
• Markedly aged appearance

Diagnostic tests

• X-rays show typical degeneration in the lower thoracic and lumbar vertebrae. The vertebral bodies may appear flattened, with varying degrees of collapse and wedging, and may look denser than normal. Loss of bone mineral becomes evident in later stages.
• Serum calcium, phosphorus, and alkaline phosphatase levels are all within normal limits, but the parathyroid hormone level may be elevated.
• Bone biopsy specimens show thin, porous, but otherwise normal-looking bone tissue.

Treatment

Treatment is basically symptomatic and aims to prevent additional fractures and control pain. A physical therapy program, emphasizing gentle exercise and activity, is an important part of the treatment. Estrogen may be given to decrease the rate of bone resorption; fluoride, to stimulate bone formation; and calcium and vitamin D, to support normal bone metabolism. However, drug therapy merely arrests osteoporosis and does not cure it. Weakened vertebrae should be supported, usually with a back brace. Sur-

Teaching Topics in Osteoporosis

- An explanation of the disease process
- Risk factors for developing osteoporosis
- Importance of safety measures and proper body mechanics to prevent fractures
- Preparation for blood and urine studies, X-rays, and bone biopsy, if necessary
- Bone-strengthening exercises
- Importance of dietary calcium and sources of this mineral
- Vitamin and mineral supplements

gery can correct pathologic fractures of the femur by open reduction and internal fixation. Colles' fracture requires reduction with plaster-cast immobilization for 4 to 10 weeks.

The incidence of senile osteoporosis may be reduced through adequate intake of dietary calcium and regular exercise. Hormone and fluoride treatments may also offer some preventive benefit and are sometimes used this way. Secondary osteoporosis can be prevented through effective treatment of the underlying disease and by judicious use of steroid therapy, early mobilization after surgery or trauma, decreased alcohol consumption, careful observation for signs of malabsorption, and prompt treatment of hyperthyroidism.

Clinical Implications

The care plan should focus on the patient's fragility, stressing careful positioning, ambulation, and prescribed exercises.

- Check the patient's skin daily for redness, warmth, and new sites of pain, which may indicate new fractures. Encourage activity; help the patient walk several times daily. As appropriate, perform passive range-of-motion exercises or encourage the patient to perform active exercises. Make sure the patient regularly attends scheduled physical therapy sessions.
- Impose safety precautions.
- Explain to the patient's family and ancillary hospital personnel how easily an osteoporotic patient's bones can fracture.
- Provide a balanced diet high in nutrients that support skeletal metabolism: vitamin D, calcium, and protein. Administer analgesics, as needed. Apply heat to relieve pain.
- Before discharge, make sure the patient and his family clearly understand the prescribed drug regimen. The patient should also report any new pain sites immediately, especially after trauma, no matter how slight. Advise the patient to sleep on a firm mattress and avoid excessive bed rest. Make sure he knows how to wear his back brace.
- If a female patient is taking estrogen, emphasize the need for routine gynecologic checkups, including Pap tests, and tell her to report any abnormal bleeding.
- Thoroughly explain osteoporosis to the patient and his family. If the patient and family do not understand the nature of this disease, they may feel the fractures could have been prevented if they had been more careful.
- Teach the patient good body mechanics—to stoop before lifting anything and to avoid twisting movements and prolonged bending.
- Instruct the female patient taking estrogen in the proper technique for self-examination of the breasts. Tell her to perform this examination at least once a month and to report any lumps immediately. (See *Teaching Topics in Osteoporosis*.)

Complications

Fractures are the most common complication. As vertebral bodies weaken, spontaneous wedge fractures, pathologic fractures of the neck and femur, Colles' fractures after a minor fall, and hip fractures are all common.

Otitis externa
(External otitis, swimmer's ear)

Description
Otitis externa, inflammation of the skin of the external ear canal and auricle, may be acute or chronic. It is most common in the summer. With treatment, acute otitis externa usually subsides within 7 days—although it may become chronic—and tends to recur. Physical examination confirms otitis externa. Severe chronic otitis externa may reflect underlying diabetes mellitus, hypothyroidism, or nephritis.

Causes
- Usually, bacteria such as *Pseudomonas, Proteus vulgaris,* streptococci, and *Staphylococcus aureus*
- Fungi, such as *Aspergillus niger* and *Candida albicans*
- Dermatologic conditions, such as seborrhea or psoriasis

Risk factors
- Swimming in contaminated water; cerumen creates a culture medium for the water-borne organism.
- Cleaning the ear canal with a cotton swab, bobby pin, finger, or other foreign object irritates the ear canal and possibly introduces the infectious microorganism.
- Exposure to dust, hair care products, or other irritants causes the patient to scratch his ear, excoriating the auricle and canal.
- Regular use of earphones, earplugs, or earmuffs traps moisture in the ear canal, creating a culture medium for infection.
- Chronic drainage from a perforated tympanic membrane

Signs and symptoms
Acute otitis externa
The characteristic symptom is moderate to severe pain that is exacerbated by manipulating the auricle or tragus, clenching the teeth, opening the mouth, or chewing. Pain on palpation of the tragus or auricle distinguishes acute otitis externa from otitis media. Other symptoms of acute infection include the following:
- Fever
- Foul-smelling aural discharge
- Regional cellulitis
- Partial hearing loss
- A swollen external ear canal, seen on otoscopy
- Periauricular lymphadenopathy (tender nodes in front of the tragus, behind the ear, or in the upper neck)
- Occasionally, regional cellulitis

Fungal otitis externa
- May be asymptomatic. *A. niger* produces a black or gray, blotting paper-like growth in the ear canal, however.
- Thick, red epithelium. This is seen when fungal growth is removed.

Chronic otitis externa
- Pruritus (may lead to scaling and skin thickening)
- Possible aural discharge
- Thick, red epithelium in the ear canal (seen on physical examination)

Diagnostic tests
Microscopic examination or culture and sensitivity tests can identify the causative organism and determine appropriate antibiotic treatment.

Treatment
To relieve the pain of acute otitis externa, treatment includes heat application to the periauricular region (heat lamp; hot, damp compresses; heating pad), aspirin or acetaminophen, and codeine. Instillation of antibiotic eardrops (with or without hydrocortisone) follows cleansing of the ear and removal of debris. If fever persists or regional cellulitis develops, a systemic antibiotic is necessary.

Preventing Otitis Externa

• Suggest using lamb's wool earplugs coated with petrolatum to keep water out of the ears when showering or shampooing.
• Tell the patient to wear earplugs or to keep his head above water when swimming; to instill two or three drops of 3% boric acid solution in 70% alcohol before and after swimming, to toughen the skin of the external ear canal.
• Warn against cleaning the ears with cotton swabs or other objects.
• Urge prompt treatment of otitis media to prevent perforation of the tympanic membrane (otitis media may also lead to the more benign otitis externa).

As do other forms of this disorder, fungal otitis externa necessitates careful cleansing of the ear. Application of a keratolytic or 2% salicylic acid in cream containing nystatin may help treat otitis externa resulting from candidal organisms. Instillation of slightly acidic eardrops creates an unfavorable environment in the ear canal for most fungi and for *Pseudomonas* organisms. No specific treatment exists for otitis externa caused by *A. niger*, except repeated cleansing of the ear canal with baby oil.

In chronic otitis externa, primary treatment consists of cleansing the ear and removing debris. Supplemental therapy includes instillation of antibiotic eardrops or application of antibiotic ointment or cream (neomycin, bacitracin, or polymyxin, possibly combined with hydrocortisone). Another ointment contains phenol, salicylic acid, precipitated sulfur, and petrolatum and produces exfoliative and antipruritic effects.

For mild chronic otitis externa, treatment may include instilling antibiotic eardrops once or twice weekly and wearing specially fitted earplugs while showering, shampooing, or swimming.

Clinical implications

If the patient has acute otitis externa, follow these guidelines:
• Monitor vital signs, particularly temperature. Watch for and record the type and amount of aural drainage.
• Remove debris and gently cleanse the ear canal with mild Burow's solution (aluminum acetate). Place a wisp of cotton soaked with solution into the ear, and apply a saturated compress directly to the auricle. Afterward, dry the ear gently but thoroughly. (In severe otitis externa, such cleansing may be delayed until after initial treatment with antibiotic eardrops.)
• To instill eardrops in an adult, pull the pinna upward and backward to straighten the canal. To ensure that the drops reach the epithelium, insert a wisp of cotton moistened with eardrops.
• If the patient has chronic otitis externa, cleanse the ear thoroughly. Use wet soaks intermittently on oozing or infected skin. If the patient has a chronic fungal infection, cleanse the ear canal well, then apply an exfoliative ointment. (See also *Preventing Otitis Externa*.)

Otitis media

Description

Otitis media, inflammation of the middle ear, may be suppurative or secretory, acute or chronic. Acute otitis media is common in children. Its incidence rises during the winter months, paralleling the seasonal rise in non-bacterial respiratory tract infections. It results from disruption of eustachian tube patency. In the suppurative form, respiratory tract infection, allergic reaction, or positional changes (such as holding an infant supine during feeding) allow reflux of nasopharyngeal flora through the eustachian tube and colonization in the middle ear. In secretory otitis media, obstruction of the eustachian tube results in negative pressure in the middle ear that promotes transudation of sterile serous fluid from blood vessels in the membrane of the middle ear. With prompt treatment, prognosis for acute otitis media is excellent; however, prolonged accumulation of fluid within the middle ear cavity causes chronic otitis media.

Causes
Suppurative otitis media
—Pneumococci

—*Hemophilus influenzae*, the most common cause in children under age 6

—Beta hemolytic streptococci

—Staphylococci, the most common cause in children age 6 and over

—Gram-negative bacteria

Chronic suppurative otitis media
—Inadequate treatment of acute infection

—Infection by resistant strains of bacteria

Secretory otitis media
—Viral infection

—Allergy

—Barotrauma (pressure injury caused by inability to equalize pressures between the environment and the middle ear)

Chronic secretory otitis media
—Adenoidal tissue overgrowth that obstructs the eustachian tube

—Edema resulting from allergic rhinitis or chronic sinus infection

—Inadequate treatment of acute suppurative otitis media

Signs and symptoms
Acute suppurative otitis media
The patient may be asymptomatic, but usual clinical features include the following:

—Severe, deep, throbbing pain

—Signs of upper respiratory tract infection

—Mild to high fever

—Hearing loss, usually mild and conductive

—Dizziness

—Obscured or distorted bony landmarks of the tympanic membrane (evident on otoscopy)

—Nausea

—Vomiting

—Other possible effects: bulging of the tympanic membrane, with concomitant erythema, and purulent drainage in the ear canal from tympanic membrane rupture

Acute secretory otitis media
Frequently, the patient is asymptomatic, but signs and symptoms may include the following:

—Severe conductive hearing loss. This varies from 15 to 35 dB, depending on the thickness and amount of fluid in the middle ear cavity.

—Sensation of fullness in the ear

—Popping, crackling, or clicking sounds with swallowing or jaw movement

—Possibly, hearing an echo when speaking

—Possibly, a vague feeling of top-heaviness

—Tympanic membrane retraction. This causes the bony landmarks to appear more prominent (seen on otoscopy).

—Clear or amber fluid behind tympanic membrane. This is seen on otoscopy—possibly with meniscus and bubbles.

—Blue-black tympanic membrane. This is seen on otoscopy if hemorrhage into middle ear has occurred.

Chronic otitis media
This usually begins in childhood and persists into adulthood. Its effects include the following:

Preventing Otitis Media

- Teach recognition of upper respiratory tract infections and encourage early treatment.
- Instruct parents not to feed their infant in a supine position or put him to bed with a bottle. This prevents reflux of nasopharyngeal flora.
- To promote eustachian tube patency, instruct the patient to perform Valsalva's maneuver several times daily.

—Decreased or absent tympanic membrane motility
—Cholesteatoma (a cystlike mass in the middle ear)
—Painless, purulent discharge. This occurs in chronic suppurative otitis media.
—Conductive hearing loss. This varies with the size and type of tympanic membrane perforation and ossicular destruction.
—Thickening and sometimes scarring of the tympanic membrane. This is evident on otoscopy.

Diagnostic tests

Pneumatoscopy can show decreased tympanic membrane mobility, but this procedure is painful with the obviously bulging, erythematous tympanic membrane that occurs in acute suppurative otitis media.

Treatment

In acute suppurative otitis media, antibiotic therapy includes ampicillin or amoxicillin for infants, children, and adults. For those who are allergic to penicillin derivatives, therapy may include cefaclor or co-trimoxazole. Aspirin or acetaminophen are given to control pain and fever. Severe, painful bulging of the tympanic membrane usually necessitates myringotomy. Broad-spectrum antibiotics can help prevent acute suppurative otitis media in high-risk patients, such as children with recurring episodes of otitis. However, in patients with recurring otitis, antibiotics must be used sparingly and with discretion to prevent development of resistant strains of bacteria.

In acute secretory otitis media, inflation of the eustachian tube by performing Valsalva's maneuver several times a day may be the only treatment required. Otherwise, nasopharyngeal decongestant therapy may be helpful. It should continue for at least 2 weeks and, sometimes, indefinitely, with periodic evaluation. If decongestant therapy fails, myringotomy and aspiration of middle ear fluid, followed by insertion of a polyethylene tube into the tympanic membrane, are necessary for immediate and prolonged equalization of pressure. The tube falls out spontaneously after 9 to 12 months. Concomitant treatment of the underlying cause (such as elimination of allergens, or adenoidectomy for hypertrophied adenoids) may also be helpful in correcting this disorder.

Treatment of chronic otitis media includes antibiotics for exacerbations of acute infection, elimination of eustachian tube obstruction, treatment of otitis externa (when present), myringoplasty (tympanic membrane graft) and tympanoplasty to reconstruct middle ear structures when thickening and scarring are present, and, possibly, mastoidectomy. When present, cholesteatoma requires excision.

Clinical implications

- After myringotomy, maintain drainage flow. Do not place cotton or plugs deep in the ear canal; however, sterile cotton may be placed loosely in the external ear to absorb drainage. To prevent infection, change the cotton whenever it gets damp, and wash hands before and after giving ear care. Watch for and report headache, fever, severe pain, or disorientation.

• After tympanoplasty, reinforce dressings, and observe for excessive bleeding from the ear canal. Administer analgesics, as needed. Warn the patient against blowing his nose or getting the ear wet when bathing.

• Encourage the patient to complete the prescribed course of antibiotic treatment. If nasopharyngeal decongestants are ordered, teach correct instillation.

• Suggest application of heat to the ear to relieve pain.

• Advise the patient with acute secretory otitis media to watch for and immediately report pain and fever—signs of secondary infection. (See also *Preventing Otitis Media*.)

Complications

• Abscesses (brain, subperiosteal, and epidural)
• Sigmoid sinus or jugular vein thrombosis
• Septicemia
• Meningitis
• Suppurative labyrinthitis
• Facial paralysis
• Otitis externa

Otosclerosis

Description

The most common cause of conductive deafness, otosclerosis is the slow formation of spongy bone in the otic capsule, particularly at the oval window. It occurs in at least 10% of Caucasians and is twice as prevalent in females as in males, usually between ages 15 and 30. With surgery, prognosis is good.

Causes

Otosclerosis appears to result from a genetic factor transmitted as an autosomal dominant trait. Many patients with this disorder report family histories of hearing loss (excluding presbycusis). Pregnancy may trigger onset.

Signs and symptoms

• Slowly progressive unilateral hearing loss. This may advance to bilateral deafness.
• Tinnitus (low and medium pitch)
• Paracusis of Willis (hearing conversation better in a noisy environment than in a quiet one)

Diagnostic tests

• Rinne test that shows bone conduction lasting longer than air conduction (normally, the reverse is true) is diagnostic of otosclerosis. As otosclerosis progresses, bone conduction also deteriorates.

• Audiometric testing reveals hearing loss ranging from 60 dB in early stages to total loss as the disease advances.

• Weber's test detects sound lateralizing to the more affected ear.

Treatment

Generally, treatment consists of stapedectomy (removal of the stapes) and insertion of a prosthesis to restore partial or total hearing. This procedure is performed on only one ear at a time, beginning with the ear that has suffered greater damage. Postoperative treatment includes hospitalization for 2 to 3 days and antibiotics to prevent infection. If stapedectomy is not possible, a hearing aid (air conduction aid with molded ear insert receiver) enables the patient to hear conversation in normal surroundings. Use of a hearing aid is not as effective as stapedectomy.

Clinical implications

• During the first 24 hours after surgery, keep the patient lying flat, with his head turned so that the affected ear faces upward (to maintain the position of the graft). Enforce bed rest for 48 hours.

• Because the patient may be dizzy, keep the bed side rails up, and gradually assist him with ambulation.

• Assess for pain and vertigo, which may be relieved with repositioning or prescribed medication.

- Before the patient's discharge, instruct him to avoid loud noises and sudden pressure changes (such as those which occur while diving or flying) until healing is complete (usually 6 months).
- Advise the patient not to blow his nose for at least 1 week, to prevent contaminated air and bacteria from entering the eustachian tube.
- Stress the importance of protecting the ears against cold; avoiding any activities that provoke dizziness, such as straining, bending, or heavy lifting; and if possible, avoiding contact with anyone who has an upper respiratory tract infection.
- Teach the patient and family how to change the external ear dressing (eye or gauze pad) and care for the incision.
- Emphasize the need to complete the prescribed antibiotic regimen and to return for scheduled follow-up care.

Ovarian cancer

Description

After cancer of the breast, the colon, or the lung, primary ovarian cancer ranks as the most common cause of cancer deaths among American women. In women with previously treated breast cancer, metastatic ovarian cancer is more common than cancer at any other site. Incidence is noticeably higher in women of upper socioeconomic level between ages 40 and 65 and in single women. The disease may occur any time, including during childhood or pregnancy. Three main types of ovarian cancer exist: primary epithelial tumors (these account for 90% of all ovarian cancers), germ cell tumors, and sex cord (stromal) tumors. Ovarian tumors spread rapidly intraperitoneally by local extension or surface seeding and occasionally, through the lymphatic system and the bloodstream. Generally, extraperitoneal spread is through the diaphragm into the chest cavity, which may cause pleural effusions. Other metastasis is rare. Diagnosis of ovarian cancer requires clinical evaluation, complete patient history, surgical exploration, and histologic studies.

Prognosis varies with the histologic type and staging of the disease but is generally poor because ovarian tumors tend to progress rapidly. About 25% of women with ovarian cancer survive for 5 years, but prognosis may be improving because of recent advances in chemotherapy.

Cause

Unknown

Signs and symptoms

Typically, symptoms vary with the size of the tumor.

- Occasionally, in early stages, vague abdominal discomfort, dyspepsia, and other mild gastrointestinal disturbances
- Urinary frequency
- Constipation
- Pelvic discomfort
- Distention
- Weight loss
- Pain. This can mimic appendicitis in young patients. It results from tumor rupture, torsion, or infection.
- In some types of tumors, feminizing effects (such as bleeding between periods in premenopausal women) or virilizing effects
- In advanced ovarian cancer, ascites, postmenopausal bleeding (rarely), pain and symptoms related to metastatic sites (most often pleural effusion)

Diagnostic tests

Despite extensive testing, accurate diagnosis and staging are impossible without exploratory laparotomy, including lymph node evaluation and tumor resection. Preoperative evaluation involves the following tests:

- Pap smear (an inconclusive test that is positive in only a small number of

Staging Ovarian Cancer

Stage I: Growth limited to the ovaries
Stage Ia: Growth limited to one ovary; no ascites*
Stage Iai: No tumor on the external surface; capsule intact
Stage Iaii: Tumor on the external surface, or capsule(s) ruptured, or both
Stage Ib: Growth limited to both ovaries; no ascites
Stage Ibi: No tumor on the external surface; capsule intact
Stage Ibii: Tumor on the external surface, or capsule(s) ruptured, or both
Stage Ic: Tumor either Stage 1a or 1b, but with ascites present or with positive peritoneal washings
Stage II: Growth involving one or both ovaries with pelvic extension
Stage IIa: Extension and/or metastases to the uterus and/or tubes
Stage IIb: Extension to other pelvic tissues
Stage IIc: Tumor either Stage IIa or Stage IIb, but with ascites present or with positive peritoneal washings
Stage III: Growth involving one or both ovaries with intraperitoneal metastases outside the pelvis, or positive retroperitoneal nodes, or both. Tumor limited to the true pelvis with histologically proven malignant extension to small bowel or omentum.
Stage IV: Growth involving one or both ovaries with distant metastasis. If pleural effusion is present, there must be positive cytology to allot a case to Stage IV. Parenchymal liver metastasis signifies Stage IV.
Special Category: Unexplored cases that are thought to be ovarian carcinoma

*Ascites is peritoneal effusion that, in the opinion of the surgeon, is pathologic, clearly exceeds normal amounts, or both.

Reprinted from *Manual for Staging of Cancer* (Chicago: American Joint Committee for Cancer Staging and End Results Reporting, 1983). Used with permission.

women with ovarian cancer)
• Abdominal ultrasonography, CT scan, or X-ray (may delineate tumor size)
• Complete blood count, blood chemistries, and electrocardiography
• Intravenous pyelography to assess renal function and possible urinary tract anomalies or obstruction
• Chest X-ray to detect distant metastasis and pleural effusion
• Barium enema (especially in patients with gastrointestinal symptoms) to reveal obstruction and show its size
• Lymphangiography to show lymph node involvement
• Mammography to rule out primary breast cancer

• Liver function studies or a liver scan in patients with ascites
• Ascites fluid aspiration for cytologic identification of typical cells

Treatment

According to the staging of the disease (see *Staging Ovarian Cancer*) and the patient's age, treatment of ovarian cancer requires varying combinations of surgery, chemotherapy, and in some cases, radiation. Occasionally, in girls or young women with a unilateral encapsulated tumor who wish to maintain fertility, the following conservative approaches may be appropriate:
• Resection of the involved ovary
• Biopsies of the omentum and the uninvolved ovary

• Peritoneal washings for cytologic examination of pelvic fluid
• Careful follow-up, including periodic chest X-rays to rule out lung metastasis

Ovarian cancer usually requires more aggressive treatment, including total abdominal hysterectomy and bilateral salpingo-oophorectomy with tumor resection, omentectomy, appendectomy, lymph node palpation with probable lymphadenectomy, tissue biopsies, and peritoneal washings. Complete tumor resection is impossible if the tumor has matted around other organs or if it involves organs that cannot be resected. Bilateral salpingo-oophorectomy in a girl who has not reached puberty necessitates hormone replacement therapy, beginning at the age of puberty, to induce the development of secondary sex characteristics.

Chemotherapy extends the length of survival time in most ovarian cancer patients but is largely palliative in advanced disease. However, prolonged remissions are being achieved in some patients. Chemotherapeutic drugs useful in ovarian cancer include melphalan, chlorambucil, thiotepa, methotrexate, cyclophosphamide, doxorubicin, vincristine, vinblastine, actinomycin D, bleomycin, and cisplatin. These drugs are usually given in combination.

In early stage ovarian cancer, instillation of a radioisotope, such as ^{32}P, is occasionally useful when peritoneal washings are positive. Radiation treatment is likely to be more than merely palliative only if residual tumor size is ¾" (2 cm) or less; if there is no evidence of ascites or no metastatic deposits on the peritoneum, the liver, or kidneys; and if there are no distant metastases and no history of abdominal radiation. Immunotherapy is controversial and consists of I.V. or, in chronic ascites, intraperitoneal injection of *Corynebacterium parvulum* or Bacille Calmette-Guérin (BCG) vaccine.

Clinical implications

Because treatment for ovarian cancer varies widely, so must the patient care plan.

Before surgery, follow these guidelines:
• Thoroughly explain all preoperative tests, the expected course of treatment, and surgical and postoperative procedures.
• Reinforce what the surgeon has told the patient about the surgical procedures listed in the surgical consent form. Explain that this form lists multiple procedures because the extent of the surgery can be determined only after surgery has begun.
• If the patient is premenopausal, explain that bilateral oophorectomy artificially induces early menopause and she may experience hot flashes, headaches, palpitations, insomnia, depression, and excessive perspiration.

After surgery, follow these guidelines:
• Monitor vital signs frequently, and check I.V. fluids often. Monitor intake and output, and maintain good catheter care. Check the dressing regularly for excessive drainage or bleeding, and watch for signs of infection.
• Provide abdominal support, and watch for abdominal distention. Encourage coughing and deep breathing. Reposition the patient often, and encourage her to walk soon after surgery.
• Monitor and treat side effects of radiation and chemotherapy.
• If the patient is receiving immunotherapy, watch for flulike symptoms that may last 12 to 24 hours after drug administration. Give aspirin or acetaminophen for fever. Keep the patient well covered with blankets, and provide warm liquids to relieve chills. Administer an antiemetic, as needed.
• Provide psychological support for the patient and her family. Encourage

open communication among family members, but discourage overcompensation or "smothering" of the patient by her family. If the patient is a young woman who grieves for her lost fertility, help her (and her family) overcome possible feelings that "there's nothing else to live for." If the patient is a child, find out whether or not her parents have told her she has cancer, and deal with her questions accordingly. Also, enlist the help of a social worker, chaplain, and other members of the health care team for additional supportive care.

Ovarian cysts

Description

Ovarian cysts are usually nonneoplastic sacs on an ovary that contain fluid or semisolid material. Although these cysts are usually small and produce no symptoms, they require thorough investigation as possible sites of malignant change. Common types include follicular cysts, which are usually very small, semitransparent, and fluid filled; lutein cysts, including granulosa-lutein (corpus luteum) cysts, which are functional, nonneoplastic enlargements of the ovaries; and theca-lutein cysts, which are commonly bilateral and filled with clear, straw-colored fluid. Polycystic (or sclerocystic) ovarian disease is part of the Stein-Leventhal syndrome.

Ovarian cysts can develop any time between puberty and menopause, including during pregnancy. Granulosa-lutein cysts occur infrequently, usually during early pregnancy. Prognosis for nonneoplastic ovarian cysts is excellent.

Causes

Follicular cysts

These arise from follicles that over-

distend instead of going through the atretic stage of the menstrual cycle.

Granulosa-lutein cysts

These are caused by excessive accumulation of blood during the hemorrhagic phase of the menstrual cycle.

Theca-lutein cysts

These are often associated with hydatidiform mole, choriocarcinoma, or hormone therapy (with human chorionic gonadotropin [HCG] or clomiphene citrate).

Polycystic ovarian disease

This stems from endocrine abnormalities.

Signs and symptoms

General signs and symptoms

Cysts are usually asymptomatic, if small, unless torsion or rupture causes signs of acute abdomen.

—Mild pelvic discomfort
—Low back pain
—Dyspareunia
—Abnormal uterine bleeding (secondary to a disturbed ovulatory pattern)
—Acute abdominal pain (similar to that of appendicitis; occurs in ovarian cysts with torsion)

Specific signs and symptoms

—Unilateral pelvic discomfort and, with rupture, massive intraperitoneal hemorrhage occur in granulosa-lutein cysts that appear early in pregnancy.
—Amenorrhea, oligomenorrhea, or infertility may occur secondary to polycystic ovarian disease.
—Bilaterally enlarged ovaries are found on physical examination in polycystic ovarian disease.

Diagnostic tests

• Visualization of the ovary through ultrasound, laparoscopy, or surgery (often for another condition) confirms ovarian cysts.
• Extremely elevated HCG titers strongly suggest theca-lutein cysts.
• Urinary 17-ketosteroid concentrations are slightly elevated.
• Basal body temperature graphs and endometrial biopsy results show anovulation.

Treatment

Follicular cysts usually do not require treatment, because they tend to disappear spontaneously within 60 days. However, if they interfere with daily activities, clomiphene citrate P.O. for 5 days or progesterone I.M. (also for 5 days) reestablishes the ovarian hormonal cycle and induces ovulation. Oral contraceptives may also accelerate involution of functional cysts (including both types of lutein cysts and follicular cysts).

Treatment for granulosa-lutein cysts that occur during pregnancy is symptomatic because these cysts diminish during the third trimester and rarely require surgery. Theca-lutein cysts disappear spontaneously after elimination of hydatidiform mole, destruction of choriocarcinoma, or discontinuation of HCG or clomiphene citrate therapy.

Treatment for polycystic ovarian disease may include drugs, such as hydrocortisone or clomiphene citrate, to induce ovulation or, if drug therapy fails to induce ovulation, surgical wedge resection of one half to one-third of the ovary.

Surgery frequently becomes necessary both for diagnosis and treatment. For example, a cyst that remains after one menstrual period should be removed. Pathologic studies confirm diagnosis.

Clinical implications

Thorough patient teaching is a primary consideration. Carefully explain the nature of the particular cyst, the type of discomfort—if any—the patient is likely to experience, and how long the condition is expected to last.

• Preoperatively, watch for signs of cyst rupture, such as increasing abdominal pain, distention, and rigidity. Monitor vital signs for fever, tachypnea, or hypotension, a sign of possible peritonitis or intraperitoneal hemorrhage. Administer sedatives, as ordered, to ensure adequate preoperative rest.

• Postoperatively, encourage frequent movement in bed and early ambulation, as ordered. Early ambulation effectively prevents pulmonary embolism.

• Provide emotional support. Offer appropriate reassurance if the patient fears cancer or infertility.

• The patient may be worried about the possibility of recurrence, but assure her that recurrence is unlikely.

• Before the patient's discharge, advise her to increase her at-home activity gradually—preferably over 4 to 6 weeks. Tell her to abstain from intercourse, using tampons, and douching during this time.

Paget's disease
(Osteitis deformans)

Description

Paget's disease is a slowly progressive metabolic bone disease characterized by an initial phase of excessive bone resorption (osteoclastic phase), followed by a reactive phase of excessive abnormal bone formation (osteoblastic phase). The new bone structure, which is chaotic, fragile, and weak, causes painful deformities of both external contour and internal structure. Paget's disease usually localizes in one or several areas of the skeleton (most frequently the lower torso), but occasionally, skeletal deformity is widely distributed. It can be fatal, particularly when it is associated with congestive heart failure (widespread disease creates a continuous need for high cardiac output), bone sarcoma, or giant cell tumors.

Causes

The exact cause is unknown, but one theory holds that early viral infection (possibly with mumps virus) causes a dormant skeletal infection that erupts many years later as Paget's disease.

Signs and symptoms

• Asymptomatic in early stages
• Eventually, severe, persistent pain. This intensifies with weight bearing.
• Impaired movement. This may coexist with pain.
• Characteristic cranial enlargement. This occurs over frontal and occipital areas (hat size may increase).
• Headaches. These occur with skull involvement.
• Kyphosis
• Barrel-shaped chest. This may accompany kyphosis.
• Asymmetric bowing of the tibia and femur
• Warm and tender pagetic sites
• Increased susceptibility to pathologic fractures
• Slow and incomplete healing of pagetic fractures
• Waddling gait. This accompanies softening of the pelvic bones.

Diagnostic tests

• X-rays taken before overt symptoms develop show increased bone expansion and density.
• A bone scan, which is more sensitive than X-rays, clearly shows early pagetic lesions (radioisotope concentrates in areas of active disease).
• Bone biopsy reveals the characteristic mosaic pattern.
• Blood tests reveal anemia.
• Serum alkaline phosphatase is elevated. (Routine biochemical screens—which include serum alkaline phosphatase—make early diagnosis more common.)
• In 24-hour urine test, hydroxyproline (amino acid excreted by kidneys and index of osteoclastic hyperactivity) is elevated.

Treatment

Primary treatment consists of drug therapy and includes one of the following:

• Calcitonin (a hormone, given subcutaneously or I.M.) and etidronate (P.O.) retard bone resorption and reduce serum alkaline phosphate and urinary hydroxyproline secretion. Although calcitonin requires long-term maintenance therapy, improvement is noticeable after the first few weeks of treatment. Etidronate produces improvement after 1 to 3 months.

• Mithramycin, a cytotoxic antibiotic, decreases calcium, urinary hydroxyproline, and serum alkaline phosphatase. This medication produces remission of symptoms within 2 weeks and biochemical improvement in 1 to 2 months; however, it may destroy platelets or compromise renal function.

Self-administration of calcitonin and etidronate helps patients with Paget's disease lead near-normal lives. Nevertheless, these patients may need surgery to reduce or prevent pathologic fractures, correct secondary deformities, and relieve neurologic impairment. To decrease the risk of excessive bleeding due to hypervascular bone, drug therapy with calcitonin and etidronate or mithramycin must precede surgery. Joint replacement is difficult because bonding material (methyl methacrylate) does not set properly on pagetic bone.

Other treatment is symptomatic and supportive and varies according to symptoms. Aspirin, indomethacin, or ibuprofen usually controls pain.

Clinical implications
• To evaluate the effectiveness of analgesics, assess level of pain daily. Watch for new areas of pain or restricted movement—which may indicate new fracture sites—and sensory or motor disturbances, such as difficulty in hearing, seeing, or walking.

• Monitor serum calcium and alkaline phosphatase levels.

• If the patient is confined to prolonged bed rest, prevent decubitus ulcers by providing good skin care.

Reposition the patient frequently, and use a flotation mattress. Provide high-topped sneakers to prevent footdrop.

• Monitor intake and output. Encourage adequate fluid intake to minimize renal calculi formation.

• Demonstrate how to inject calcitonin and rotate injection sites. Warn the patient that side effects may occur (nausea, vomiting, local inflammation at injection site, facial flushing, itching of hands, and fever). Give reassurance that these side effects are usually mild and infrequent. Warn against imprudent use of analgesics.

• To help the patient adjust to the changes in life-style imposed by this disease, teach him how to pace activities and, if necessary, how to use assistive devices. Encourage him to follow a recommended exercise program—avoiding both immobility and excessive activity.

• Suggest a firm mattress or a bed board to minimize spinal deformities. To prevent falls at home, advise removing throw rugs and other small obstacles.

• Emphasize the importance of regular checkups, including the eyes and ears.

• Tell the patient receiving etidronate to take this medication with fruit juice 2 hours before or after meals (milk or other high-calcium fluids impair absorption), to divide daily dosage to minimize side effects, and to watch for and report stomach cramps, diarrhea, fractures, and increasing or new bone pain.

• Tell the patient receiving mithramycin to watch for signs of infection, easy bruising, bleeding, and temperature elevation and to report for regular follow-up laboratory tests.

• Help the patient and family make use of community support resources, such as a visiting nurse or home health agency. For more information, refer them to the Paget's Disease Foundation.

Complications

These include the following:
- Blindness caused by bony impingement on the cranial nerves
- Hearing loss with tinnitus and vertigo caused by bony impingement on the cranial nerves
- Hypertension
- Renal calculi
- Hypercalcemia
- Gout
- Congestive heart failure

Pancreatic cancer

Description

Second only to cancer of the colon, which is the deadliest GI cancer, pancreatic cancer now ranks fourth among all fatal carcinomas. Prognosis is poor, and most patients die within a year after diagnosis. Tumors of the pancreas are almost always adenocarcinomas. They arise most frequently (67% of the time) in the head of the pancreas. Rarer tumors are those of the body and tail of the pancreas and islet cell tumor. (Also see *Islet Cell Tumors.*) The two main tissue types of pancreatic cancer, both of which form fibrotic nodes, are cylinder cell (which arises in ducts and degenerates into cysts) and large, fatty, granular cell (which arises in parenchyma). See *Types of Pancreatic Cancer*, p. 543.

Causes

Unknown

Risk factors

- Cigarette smoking
- Diets high in fat and protein
- Food additives
- Exposure to industrial chemicals, such as beta-naphthalene, benzidine, and urea

Possible predisposing factors include the following:
- Chronic pancreatitis
- Diabetes mellitus
- Chronic alcohol abuse

Signs and symptoms

Most common features
—Weight loss
—Abdominal or low back pain
—Jaundice
—Diarrhea
Other generalized effects
—Fever
—Skin lesions (usually on legs)
—Emotional disturbances such as depression, anxiety, and premonition of fatal illness

---

Islet Cell Tumors

Relatively uncommon, islet cell tumors (insulinomas) may be benign or malignant. They produce symptoms in three stages.
1. *Slight hypoglycemia* —fatigue, restlessness, malaise, and excessive weight gain.
2. *Compensatory secretion of epinephrine* —pallor, clamminess, perspiration, palpitations, finger tremors, hunger, decreased temperature, increased pulse and blood pressure.
3. *Severe hypoglycemia* —ataxia, clouded sensorium, diplopia, episodes of violence and hysteria.
Usually, insulinomas metastasize to the liver alone but may metastasize to bone, brain, and lungs. Death results from a combination of hypoglycemic reactions and widespread metastasis. Treatment consists of enucleation of tumor (if benign) and chemotherapy with streptozocin or resection to include pancreatic tissue (if malignant).

Diagnostic tests

• Laparotomy with biopsy is necessary for definitive diagnosis; however, a biopsy may miss relatively small or deep-seated cancerous tissue or create a pancreatic fistula.

• X-rays, retroperitoneal insufflation, cholangiography, scintigraphy, and, particularly, barium swallow locate neoplasm and detect changes in the duodenum or stomach relating to carcinoma of the head of the pancreas.

• Ultrasound can identify a mass but not its histologic composition.

• CT scan is similar to ultrasound but shows greater detail.

• Angiography shows the tumor's vascular supply.

• Endoscopic retrograde cannulation of the pancreas or endoscopic pancreatography allows visualization, instillation of contrast medium, and, possibly, removal of a tissue specimen.

• Secretin test shows absence of pancreatic enzymes and suggests pancreatic duct obstruction and tumors of the pancreatic body and tail.

• Laboratory values supporting this diagnosis include increased serum bilirubin; occasionally, elevated serum amylase-lipase; prolonged prothrombin time; elevated SGOT and SGPT, indicating necrosis of the liver; elevated alkaline phosphatase (marked elevation occurs with biliary obstruction).

• Besides, plasma insulin immunoassay shows measurable serum insulin with islet cell tumors; hemoglobin and hematocrit values may show mild anemia; fasting blood sugar test results may indicate hypoglycemia or hyperglycemia; and occult blood in the stool may point to ulceration in the GI tract or ampulla of Vater.

Treatment

Treatment of pancreatic cancer is rarely successful because the tumor is often widely metastasized at diagnosis. Therapy consists of surgery and, possibly, radiation and chemotherapy. Small improvements have been made in the survival rate with surgery.

• Total pancreatectomy has perhaps increased survival time by removing a localized tumor or by controlling postoperative gastric ulceration.

• Cholecystojejunostomy, choledochoduodenostomy, and choledochojejunostomy have partially replaced radical resection to bypass obstructing common bile duct extensions and thereby ease jaundice and pruritus.

• Whipple's operation, or pancreatoduodenectomy, has a high mortality rate but can obtain wide lymphatic clearance, except with tumors located near the portal vein, superior mesenteric vein and artery, and celiac axis. This rarely used procedure removes the head of the pancreas, duodenum, portions of the body and tail of the pancreas, stomach, jejunum, pancreatic duct, and distal portion of the bile duct.

• Gastrojejunostomy is performed if radical resection is not indicated and duodenal obstruction is expected to develop later.

Although pancreatic carcinoma generally responds poorly to chemotherapy, recent studies using combinations of carmustine (BCNU), 5-fluorouracil, and doxorubicin show a trend toward longer survival time. Other medications used in pancreatic cancer include the following:

• Antibiotics (oral, I.V., or I.M.) to prevent infection and relieve symptoms

• Anticholinergics, particularly propantheline, to decrease GI tract spasm and motility and reduce pain and secretions

• Antacids (P.O. or by nasogastric tube) to decrease secretion of pancreatic enzymes and also to suppress peptic activity and thereby reduce stress-induced damage to gastric mucosa

• Diuretics to mobilize extracellular fluid from ascites

Types of Pancreatic Cancer

PATHOLOGY	CLINICAL FEATURES
Head of pancreas • Often obstructs ampulla of Vater and common bile duct • Directly metastasizes to duodenum • Adhesions anchor tumor to spine, stomach, and intestines.	• Jaundice (predominant symptom)—slowly progressive, unremitting; may cause skin (especially of the face and genitals) to turn olive green or black • Pruritus—often severe • Weight loss—rapid and severe (as great as 30 lbs [13.6 kg]); may lead to emaciation, weakness, and muscle atrophy • Slowed digestion, gastric distention, nausea, diarrhea, and steatorrhea with clay-colored stools • Liver and gallbladder enlargement from lymph node metastasis to biliary tract and duct wall results in compression and obstruction; gallbladder may be palpable (Courvoisier's sign). • Dull, nondescript, continuous abdominal pain radiating to upper right quadrant; relieved by bending forward • GI hemorrhage and biliary infection common
Body and tail of pancreas • Large nodular masses become fixed to retropancreatic tissues and spine. • Direct invasion of spleen, left kidney, suprarenal gland, diaphragm • Involvement of celiac plexus results in thrombosis of splenic vein and spleen infarction.	**Body** • Pain (predominant symptom)—usually epigastric—develops slowly and radiates to back; relieved by bending forward or sitting up; intensified by lying supine; most intense 3 to 4 hours after eating; when celiac plexus is involved, pain is more intense and lasts longer • Venous thrombosis and thrombophlebitis—frequent; may precede other symptoms by months • Splenomegaly (from infarction), hepatomegaly (occasionally), and jaundice (rarely) **Tail** Symptoms result from metastasis: • Abdominal tumor (most common finding) produces a palpable abdominal mass; abdominal pain radiates to left hypochondrium and left chest. • Anorexia leads to weight loss, emaciation, and weakness. • Splenomegaly and upper GI bleeding

• Insulin to provide adequate exogenous insulin after pancreatic resection
• Narcotics to relieve pain (used only after other analgesics fail, because morphine, meperidine, and codeine use can lead to biliary tract spasm and increase common bile duct pressure)

• Pancreatic enzymes (average dose 0.5 to 1 mg with meals) to assist digestion of proteins, carbohydrates, and fats when pancreatic juices are insufficient because of surgery or obstruction

Radiation therapy is usually ineffective except when used as an adjunct to 5-fluorouracil chemotherapy; then it may prolong survival time from 4 to 9 months. It can also ease the pain associated with nonresectable tumors.

Clinical implications

Comprehensive supportive care can prevent surgical complications, increase patient comfort, and help the patient and his family cope with inevitable death.

Before surgery, follow these guidelines:
• Ensure that the patient is medically stable and adequately nourished (this may take 4 to 5 days). If the patient cannot tolerate oral feedings, provide total parenteral nutrition and I.V. fat emulsions to correct deficiencies and maintain positive nitrogen balance.
• Give blood transfusions (to combat anemia), vitamin K (to overcome prothrombin deficiency), antibiotics (to prevent postoperative complications), and gastric lavage (to maintain gastric decompression), as ordered.
• Tell the patient about expected postoperative procedures and expected side effects of radiation and chemotherapy.

After surgery, follow these guidelines:
• Watch for and report complications, such as fistula, pancreatitis, fluid and electrolyte imbalance, infection, hemorrhage, skin breakdown, nutritional deficiency, hepatic failure, renal insufficiency, and diabetes.
• If the patient is receiving chemotherapy, watch for and symptomatically treat its toxic effects.

Throughout this illness, provide meticulous supportive care.
• Monitor fluid balance, abdominal girth, metabolic state, and weight daily. With weight loss, replace nutrients I.V., P.O., or by nasogastric tube. With weight gain (due to ascites), impose dietary restrictions, such as a low-sodium diet, as ordered. Maintain a 2,500-calorie-per-day diet.

• Serve small, frequent meals. Administer an oral pancreatic enzyme at mealtimes, if needed. As ordered, give an antacid to prevent stress ulcers.
• To prevent constipation, administer laxatives, stool softeners, and cathartics, as ordered; modify diet; and increase fluid intake. To increase GI motility, position the patient properly during and after meals, and assist him with walking when he is able.
• Ensure adequate rest and sleep (with a sedative, if warranted). Assist with range-of-motion exercises and isometrics, as appropriate.
• Administer analgesics for pain, and antibiotics and antipyretics for fever, as ordered. Note time, site (if injected), and response.
• Observe closely for signs of hypoglycemia or hyperglycemia; administer glucose or a hypoglycemic agent, such as tolbutamide, as ordered. Monitor blood glucose concentration, urine sugar, acetone, and response to treatment. Document progression of jaundice.
• Provide scrupulous skin care to avoid pruritus and necrosis. If the patient has overwhelming pruritus, prevent excoriation by clipping his nails and persuading him to wear light cotton gloves.
• Watch for signs of upper GI bleeding. Test stools and emesis for blood, and maintain a flow sheet of frequent hemoglobin and hematocrit determinations. To control active bleeding, promote gastric vasoconstriction with medication and iced saline lavage through a nasogastric or duodenal tube. Replace any fluid loss. Ease discomfort from pyloric obstruction with a nasogastric tube.
• To prevent thrombosis, apply antiembolism stockings and assist in range-of-motion exercises. If thrombosis occurs, elevate the patient's legs, apply moist heat to thrombus site and give an anticoagulant or aspirin, as ordered, to prevent further clot formation and pulmonary embolus.
• Encourage the patient to verbalize

his fears, which are valid. Promote family involvement, and offer the assistance of a chaplain or psychologist. Help the patient and his family deal with the impending reality of death.

Pancreatitis

Description
Pancreatitis, or inflammation of the pancreas, occurs in acute and chronic forms and may be due to edema, necrosis, or hemorrhage. Pancreatitis involves autodigestion: the enzymes normally excreted by the pancreas digest pancreatic tissue. Prognosis is good when pancreatitis follows biliary tract disease but poor when it follows alcoholism. Mortality rises as high as 60% when pancreatitis is associated with necrosis and hemorrhage. (Also see *Chronic Pancreatitis*.)

Causes
• Biliary tract disease, one of the most common causes
• Alcoholism, one of the most common causes
• Pancreatic carcinoma

• Certain drugs such as glucocorticoids, sulfonamides, chlorothiazide, and azathioprine
• Possibly, peptic ulcer, mumps, or hypothermia
• Less commonly, stenosis or obstruction of the sphincter of Oddi, hyperlipemia, metabolic endocrine disorders (hyperparathyroidism, hemochromatosis), vasculitis or vascular disease, viral infections, mycoplasmal pneumonia, and pregnancy

Signs and symptoms
• Steady epigastric pain centered close to the umbilicus, radiating between the tenth thoracic and sixth lumbar vertebrae, and unrelieved by vomiting may be the first and only symptom of mild pancreatitis.

A severe attack may cause the following:
• Extreme pain
• Persistent vomiting
• Abdominal rigidity
• Diminished bowel activity (suggesting peritonitis)
• Crackles at lung bases
• Left pleural effusion
• Extreme malaise
• Restlessness

Chronic Pancreatitis

Chronic pancreatitis is usually associated with alcoholism (in over half of all patients), but can also follow hyperparathyroidism, hyperlipemia, or, infrequently, gallstones, trauma, or peptic ulcer. Inflammation and fibrosis cause progressive pancreatic insufficiency and eventually destroy the pancreas. Symptoms of chronic pancreatitis include constant dull pain with occasional exacerbations, malabsorption, severe weight loss, and hyperglycemia (leading to diabetic symptoms). Relevant diagnostic measures include patient history, X-rays showing pancreatic calcification, elevated ESR, and examination of stool for steatorrhea.

The severe pain of chronic pancreatitis often requires large doses of analgesics or narcotics, making addiction a serious risk. Treatment also includes a low-fat diet and oral administration of pancreatic enzymes, such as pancreatin or pancrelipase to control steatorrhea, insulin or oral hypoglycemics to curb hyperglycemia, and, occasionally, surgical repair of biliary or pancreatic ducts, or the sphincter of Oddi to reduce pressure and promote the flow of pancreatic juice. Prognosis is good if the patient can avoid alcohol, poor if he cannot.

- Mottled skin
- Tachycardia
- Low-grade fever (100° to 102° F. [37.7° to 38.8° C.])
- Cold, sweaty extremities
- Possible ileus

Diagnostic tests

- Dramatically elevated serum amylase levels—frequently more than 500 units—confirm pancreatitis and rule out perforated peptic ulcer, acute cholecystitis, appendicitis, and bowel infarction or obstruction. Similarly dramatic elevations of amylase also occur in urine, ascites, or pleural fluid. Characteristically, amylase levels return to normal 48 hours after onset of pancreatitis, despite continuing symptoms.
- Serum lipase levels are increased and rise more slowly than serum amylase levels.
- Serum calcium levels are low from fat necrosis and formation of calcium soaps.
- WBC counts range from 8,000 to 20,000/mm³, with increased polymorphonuclear leukocytes.
- Glucose levels are elevated and may be as high as 900 mg/dl, indicating hyperglycemia.
- Hematocrit occasionally exceeds 50% concentrations.
- EKG changes (prolonged Q-T segment but normal T wave) help diagnose hypocalcemia.
- Abdominal X-rays may show dilation of the small or large bowel or calcification of the pancreas.
- GI series indicate extrinsic pressure on the duodenum or stomach due to edema of the pancreas head.
- Chest X-rays show left-sided pleural effusion.
- I.V. cholangiography helps distinguish acute cholecystitis from acute pancreatitis.
- Analysis of abdominal fluid detects amylase levels as high as 7,000 units. In the patient with a perforated bowel, it may also detect bacteria or bile.

Treatment

Treatment must maintain circulation and fluid volume, relieve pain, and decrease pancreatic secretions. Emergency treatment for shock (the most common cause of death in early-stage pancreatitis) consists of vigorous I.V. replacement of electrolytes and proteins. Metabolic acidosis secondary to hypovolemia and impaired cellular perfusion requires vigorous fluid volume replacement.

Treatment may also include meperidine for pain (although it may cause spasm of the sphincter of Oddi); diazepam for restlessness and agitation; and antibiotics, such as gentamicin, clindamycin, or chloramphenicol, for bacterial infections. Hypocalcemia requires infusion of 10% calcium gluconate; serum glucose levels greater than 300 mg/dl require insulin therapy.

After the emergency phase, continuing I.V. therapy should provide adequate electrolytes and protein solutions that do not stimulate the pancreas (glucose or free amino acids) for 5 to 7 days. If the patient is not ready to resume oral feedings by then, hyperalimentation may be necessary. Nonstimulating elemental gavage feedings may be safer because of the decreased risk of infection and overinfusion. In extreme cases, laparotomy to drain the pancreatic bed, 95% pancreatectomy, or a combination of cholecystostomy-gastrostomy, feeding jejunostomy, and drainage may be necessary.

Clinical implications

Acute pancreatitis is a life-threatening emergency. Design your care plan to provide meticulous supportive care and continuous monitoring of vital systems.

- Monitor vital signs and pulmonary artery pressure closely. If the patient has a central venous pressure line instead of a pulmonary artery catheter, monitor it closely for volume expan-

Teaching Topics in Chronic Pancreatitis

- An explanation of the cause of chronic pancreatitis
- Complications, such as diabetes and GI bleeding, and their warning signs
- Preparation for diagnostic tests, including endoscopic retrograde cholangiopancreatography (ERCP), biopsy, ultrasonography, and collection of stool specimens
- Dietary measures to decrease the demand for pancreatic enzymes
- Drug therapy to reduce gastric acidity, replace pancreatic enzymes, relieve pain, and control hyperglycemia
- Preparation for surgery, if necessary
- Measures to relieve symptoms and prevent complications, such as cessation of smoking and avoiding infection
- Availability of support groups

sion (it should not rise above 10 cm H_2O).

- Give plasma or albumin, if ordered, to maintain blood pressure. Record fluid intake and output, check urine output hourly, and monitor electrolyte levels.
- Assess for crackles, rhonchi, or decreased breath sounds.
- For bowel decompression, maintain constant nasogastric suctioning, and give nothing by mouth. Perform good mouth and nose care.
- Watch for signs of calcium deficiency—tetany, cramps, carpopedal spasm, and convulsions. If you suspect hypocalcemia, keep airway and suction apparatus handy and pad side rails.
- Administer analgesics as needed to relieve the patient's pain and anxiety. Remember that anticholinergics reduce salivary and sweat gland secretions. Warn the patient that he may experience dry mouth and facial flushing. *Caution:* Narrow-angle glaucoma contraindicates the use of atropine or its derivatives.
- Watch for adverse reactions to antibiotics: nephrotoxicity with aminoglycosides; pseudomembranous enterocolitis with clindamycin; and blood dyscrasias with chloramphenicol.
- Do not confuse thirst due to hyperglycemia (indicated by serum glucose

levels of up to 350 mg/dl and sugar and acetone in urine) with dry mouth due to nasogastric intubation and anticholinergics.
- Watch for complications due to hyperalimentation, such as sepsis, hypokalemia, overhydration, and metabolic acidosis. Watch for fever, cardiac irregularities, changes in arterial blood gas measurements, and deep respirations. Use strict aseptic technique when caring for the catheter insertion site. (See *Teaching Topics in Chronic Pancreatitis*.)

Complications
- Diabetes mellitus
- Pseudocyst
- Abscess

Parainfluenza

Description
Parainfluenza is a group of respiratory illnesses that affect both the upper and lower respiratory tracts. These self-limiting diseases resemble influenza but are milder and seldom fatal. Parainfluenza is rare among adults, but it is widespread among children because adults develop antibodies to the causes of these illnesses during childhood. By age 8, most children demonstrate an-

tibodies to some causes. Incidence of parainfluenza in children rises in the winter and spring.

Causes
Paramyxoviruses, a subgroup of myxoviruses, cause parainfluenza. Paramyxoviruses occur in four forms—Para 1 to 4—that are linked to several diseases: croup (Para 1, 2, 3), acute febrile respiratory illnesses (1, 2, 3), the common cold (1, 3, 4), pharyngitis (1, 3, 4), bronchitis (1, 3), and bronchopneumonia (1, 3). Para 3 ranks second to respiratory syncytial viruses (RSV) as the most common infecting organism in lower respiratory tract infections in children. Para 4 rarely causes symptomatic infections in humans.

Mode of transmission
- Direct contact
- Inhalation of contaminated airborne droplets

Signs and symptoms
After a short incubation period (usually 3 to 6 days), symptoms emerge that are similar to those of other respiratory diseases.
- Sudden fever
- Nasal discharge
- Reddened throat (with little or no exudate)
- Chills
- Muscle pain

Diagnostic tests
Isolation of the virus and serum antibody titers differentiate parainfluenza from other respiratory illnesses but are rarely performed.

Treatment and clinical implications
Parainfluenza may require no treatment or may require bed rest, antipyretics, analgesics, and antitussives, depending on the severity of the symptoms. Complications, such as croup and pneumonia, require appropriate treatment. No vaccine is effective against parainfluenza. Throughout this illness, monitor respiratory status and temperature, and ensure adequate fluid intake and rest.

Complications
In infants and very young children, parainfluenza may lead to croup or laryngotracheobronchitis.

Paranoid disorders

Description
Paranoid disorders are a group of mental disorders characterized by an impaired sense of reality and persistent delusions. These delusions are less bizarre than those in schizophrenic disorders and usually develop in logical progression. The patient maintains appropriate emotional responses and social behavior, with minimal personality deterioration. Generally, paranoid disorders have better prognoses than schizophrenic disorders.

Causes
- A hereditary predisposition is strongly suggested in paranoid disorders of later life.
- Inferiority feelings in the family have been linked to the development of paranoia by at least one study.

Risk factors
- Sensitive personality is particularly vulnerable to paranoia.
- Medical conditions are also known to exaggerate the risks of paranoid disorders. Among them are head injury and chronic alcoholism.
- Predisposing factors linked to aging include isolation, lack of stimulating interpersonal relationships, physical illness, and diminished hearing and vision.

Signs and symptoms
Symptoms, which must persist for at least 1 week to meet *DSM-III* criteria

Paranoid State or Paranoid Schizophrenia? Differential Diagnosis

Paranoid state	Paranoid schizophrenia
• Delusional system reflects reality; well systematized • Based on misinterpretations or elaborations of reality • No hallucinations • Affect and behavior normal	• Delusional system scattered, illogical, and poorly systematized • No relationship to reality or real events • Hallucinations possible • Inconsistent and inappropriate affect • Bizarre behavior

for paranoid illness, include the following:
• Persistent persecutory delusions or delusional jealousy. The patient's emotions and other behavior are congruent with the delusional content. These delusions are not accompanied by hallucinations, and the rest of the personality remains intact.
• Feelings of inadequacy
• Feelings of inferiority
• Criticizing and belittling others
• Commonly, resorting to denial and projection
• In elderly patients, possible sexual delusions. These include bizarre ideas of sexual abuse and irrational accusations of a spouse's infidelity or of ill-defined criminal and assaultive activity against them. Late-life delusional symptoms also commonly focus on domestic issues, such as marriage, food, or the home.

Diagnostic tests
• Psychological testing and thorough neurologic evaluation rules out delusional syndromes such as amphetamine-induced psychoses and dementia (also see *Paranoid State or Paranoid Schizophrenia? Differential Diagnosis*).
• Endocrine function tests identify thyroid disorders such as "myxedemic madness." Such tests may also point to hyperadrenalism, another medical source of paranoid ideation.
• Blood studies may show altered physiologic states, such as pernicious anemia, that may induce paranoia.

Treatment
Effective treatment of paranoia must correct the behavior and mood disturbances that result from the patient's mistaken belief system. Drug treatment with carefully selected neuroleptic medication is similar to that used in schizophrenic disorders. Since paranoia tends to develop in later life, dosage levels must take into account the physiologic changes associated with aging. Treatment may have to include mobilizing a support system for the isolated, aged patient.

Clinical implications
• Initially, limit the patient's contact with staff; designate a few staff members to develop relationships with him.
• Respect the patient's space and privacy. Observe how much physical closeness the patient can tolerate. Do not touch him without first telling him you are going to do so.
• Be aware of the potential for impulsive behavior related to fear of closeness and distorted perception of reality. Prevent self-destructive behavior.
• Notice what events tend to upset the patient.

• Watch for refusal of medications due to suspicion. Explore the patient's reasons for refusing them.
• Enhance the patient's confidence and self-esteem through participation in satisfying activities. Assess his hobbies and refer him to occupational therapy, if appropriate.
• In dealing with the patient, be honest, direct, straightforward, trustworthy, and dependable.
• Establish a caring relationship with the patient to reduce his feelings of loneliness. Move slowly, with a matter-of-fact manner. Be patient and persistent. Respond without anger or defensiveness to hostile remarks.
• Meet the patient's physical needs and monitor his mental status. Remember, neuroleptic drugs tend to cause more side effects in the older patient.
• Focus on reality. Provide feedback to correct distorted perceptions.
• Allow compulsive rituals unless they are physically harmful.
• Help the patient learn to feel comfortable in social interaction. Gradually increase social contacts after the patient has become comfortable with the staff.
• Provide the patient with a structured, moderately stimulating environment. Modify the environment to accommodate any physical deficits the patient may have, and keep it predictable. Tell the patient what to expect and when. Introduce change slowly.
• Limit intrusive diagnostic studies. Too many tests in too short a time tend to increase the patient's confusion.
• Assess recent life stressors.
• Mobilize resources to reduce the patient's loneliness and isolation. Explore the possibility of his involvement in a volunteer program or self-help group after discharge.
• Be aware of your own responses to the patient; his critical and belittling attitudes can be distressing.

Parkinson's disease
(Parkinsonism, paralysis agitans, shaking palsy)

Description
Parkinson's disease is a slowly progressive, degenerative, neurologic disorder. Laboratory data usually are of little value in identifying Parkinson's disease. Consequently, diagnosis is based on the patient's age and history and the characteristic clinical picture. Conclusive diagnosis is possible only after ruling out other causes of tremor, involutional depression, cerebral arteriosclerosis, and, in patients under age 30, intracranial tumors, Wilson's disease, or phenothiazine or other drug toxicity. Deterioration progresses for an average of 10 years, at which time death usually results from aspiration pneumonia or some other infection. Parkinson's disease, one of the most common crippling diseases in the United States, affects men more often than women. According to current statistics, Parkinson's strikes 1 in every 100 people over age 60.

Causes
Although the cause of Parkinson's disease is unknown, study of the extrapyramidal brain nuclei (corpus striatum, globus pallidus, substantia nigra) has established that a dopamine deficiency prevents affected brain cells from performing their normal inhibitory function within the central nervous system.

Signs and symptoms
• Insidious tremor that begins in the fingers (unilateral pill-roll tremor). Tremor increases during stress or anxiety and decreases with purposeful movement and sleep.
• Muscle rigidity. This causes resistance to passive muscle stretching, which may be uniform (lead-pipe rigidity) or jerky (cogwheel rigidity).
• Difficulty walking. Gait lacks nor-

mal parallel motion and may be retropulsive or propulsive.

* High-pitched monotone voice
* Drooling
* Masklike facial expression
* Loss of positive control (the patient walks with body bent forward)
* Dysarthria
* Dysphagia
* Oculogyric crises. Eyes are fixed upward, with involuntary tonic movements. Occasionally, blepharospasm.

Diagnostic tests
Urinalysis may support the diagnosis by revealing decreased dopamine levels.

Treatment
Because there is no cure for Parkinson's disease, the primary aim of treatment is to relieve symptoms and keep the patient functional as long as possible. Treatment consists of drugs, physical therapy, and, in severe disease states unresponsive to drugs, stereotactic neurosurgery.

Drug therapy usually includes levodopa, a dopamine replacement that is most effective during early stages. This drug is given in increasing doses until symptoms are relieved or side effects appear. Because these side effects can be serious, levodopa is now frequently given in combination with carbidopa to halt peripheral dopamine synthesis. When levodopa proves ineffective or too toxic, alternative drug therapy includes anticholinergics, such as trihexyphenidyl; antihistamines, such as diphenhydramine; and amantadine, an antiviral agent.

When drug therapy fails, stereotactic neurosurgery is sometimes an effective alternative. In this procedure, electrical coagulation, freezing, radioactivity, or ultrasound destroys the ventrolateral nucleus of the thalamus to prevent involuntary movement. Such neurosurgery is most effective in comparatively young, otherwise healthy persons with unilateral tremor or muscle rigidity. Like drug therapy,

---

Teaching Topics in Parkinson's Disease

* An explanation of the progressive course of Parkinson's disease
* Preparation for tests, such as positron emission tomography (to rule out structural abnormalities) and cerebrospinal fluid analysis (to determine dopamine levels)
* Dietary modifications
* Exercise program and precautions
* Techniques for unlocking a position
* Medications, their effects, and their administration
* Stereotaxic thalamotomy, if appropriate
* Self-help aids for dressing and walking
* Measures for preventing orthostatic hypotension
* Modification of the home for safety
* Availability of information and support groups

---

neurosurgery is a palliative measure that can only relieve symptoms.

Individually planned physical therapy complements drug treatment and neurosurgery to maintain normal muscle tone and function. Appropriate physical therapy includes both active and passive range-of-motion exercises, routine daily activities, walking, and baths and massage to help relax muscles.

Clinical implications
Effectively caring for the patient with Parkinson's disease requires careful monitoring of drug treatment, emphasis on teaching self-reliance, and generous psychological support.

* If the patient has had surgery, watch for signs of hemorrhage and increased intracranial pressure by frequently checking level of consciousness and vital signs.

• Encourage independence. The patient with excessive tremor may achieve partial control of his body by sitting on a chair and using its arms to steady himself. Remember that fatigue may cause him to depend more on others.

• Help the patient overcome problems. Help establish a regular bowel routine by encouraging him to drink at least 2,000 ml of liquids daily and eat high-bulk foods. He may need an elevated toilet seat to assist him from a standing to a sitting position.

• Give the patient and family emotional support. Teach them about the disease, its progressive stages, and drug side effects. Show the family how to prevent decubitus ulcers and contractures by proper positioning. Inform them of the dietary restrictions levodopa imposes, and explain household safety measures to prevent accidents. Help the patient and family express their feelings and frustrations about the progressively debilitating effects of the disease.

• Establish long- and short-term treatment goals, and be aware of the patient's need for intellectual stimulation and diversion.

• To obtain more information, refer the patient and family to the National Parkinson Foundation or the United Parkinson Foundation. (Also see *Teaching Topics in Parkinson's Disease*, p. 551.)

Patent ductus arteriosus

Description
Patent ductus arteriosus (PDA) is an abnormal opening between the pulmonary artery and the aorta. This defect creates a left-to-right shunt of blood from the aorta to the pulmonary artery and results in recirculation of arterial blood through the lungs. Relative resistances in pulmonary and systemic vasculature and the size of the ductus determine the amount of left-to-right shunting. Initially, PDA may produce no clinical effects, but in time it can precipitate pulmonary vascular disease, causing symptoms to appear by age 40. Prognosis is good if the shunt is small or surgical repair is effective. Otherwise, PDA may advance to intractable congestive heart failure, which may be fatal. This problem is most prevalent in premature infants. PDA often accompanies rubella syndrome and may be associated with other congenital defects, such as coarctation of the aorta, ventricular septal defect, and pulmonary and aortic stenoses.

Causes
Failure of the fetal ductus arteriosus (a fetal blood vessel that connects the pulmonary artery to the descending aorta) to close within days to weeks after birth

Signs and symptoms
Most children with PDA have only cardiac symptoms. Others may exhibit signs of heart disease.

• Respiratory distress with signs of congestive heart failure usually occurs in infants, especially those who are premature, with a large PDA.

• Frequent respiratory infections
• Slow motor development
• Failure to thrive
• Physical underdevelopment
• Fatigability
• Classic machinery murmur (Gibson murmur). Revealed on auscultation, this is a continuous murmur (during both systole and diastole) best heard at the base of the heart, at the second left intercostal space under the left clavicle in 85% of children with PDA. The murmur may obscure S_2. With a right-to-left shunt, however, the murmur may be absent.

• A thrill at the left sternal border and a prominent left ventricular impulse
• Cardiomegaly, especially of the left atrium and left ventricle

- Dilated ascending aorta
- Tachycardia
- Bounding peripheral arterial pulses (Corrigan's pulse)
- Widened pulse pressure
- By age 40, possible fatigability and dyspnea on exertion
- In the final stages of untreated PDA, cyanosis

Diagnostic tests
- Chest X-ray shows increased pulmonary vascular markings, prominent pulmonary arteries, and enlargement of the left ventricle and aorta.
- EKG may be normal or may indicate left ventricular hypertrophy and, in pulmonary vascular disease, biventricular hypertrophy.
- Echocardiography detects and helps estimate the size of a PDA. It also reveals an enlarged left atrium and left ventricle, or right ventricular hypertrophy from pulmonary vascular disease.
- Cardiac catheterization shows pulmonary arterial oxygen content higher than right ventricular content because of the influx of aortic blood. Increased pulmonary artery pressure indicates a large shunt or, if it exceeds systemic arterial pressure, severe pulmonary vascular disease.
- Catheterization allows calculation of blood volume crossing the ductus and can rule out associated cardiac defects. Dye injection definitively demonstrates PDA.

Treatment
Asymptomatic infants with PDA require no immediate treatment. Those with congestive heart failure require fluid restriction, diuretics, and digitalis to minimize or control symptoms. If these measures cannot control congestive heart failure, surgery is necessary to ligate the ductus. If symptoms are mild, surgical correction is usually delayed until age 1. Before surgery, children with PDA require antibiotics to protect against infective endocarditis.

Other forms of therapy include cardiac catheterization to deposit a plug in the ductus to stop shunting, or administration of indomethacin I.V. (a prostaglandin inhibitor that is an alternative to surgery in premature infants) to induce ductus spasm and closure.

Clinical implications
PDA necessitates careful monitoring, patient and family teaching, and emotional support.
- Watch carefully for signs of PDA in all premature infants.
- Be alert for respiratory distress symptoms resulting from congestive heart failure, which may develop rapidly in a premature infant. Frequently assess vital signs, EKG, electrolytes, and intake and output. Record response to diuretics and other therapy. Watch for signs of digitalis toxicity (poor feeding, vomiting).
- If the infant receives indomethacin for ductus closure, watch for possible side effects, such as diarrhea, jaundice, bleeding, and renal dysfunction.
- Before surgery, carefully explain all treatments and tests to parents. Include the child in your explanations. Arrange for the child and parents to meet the ICU staff.
- Immediately after surgery, the child may have a central venous pressure catheter and an arterial line in place. Carefully assess vital signs, intake and output, and arterial and venous pressures. Provide pain relief, as needed.
- Before discharge, review instructions to the parents about activity restrictions based on the child's tolerance and energy levels. Advise parents not to become overprotective as their child's tolerance for physical activity increases.
- Stress the need for regular medical follow-up. Advise parents to inform any physician who treats their child about his history of surgery for PDA—

even if the child is being treated for an unrelated medical problem.

Complications

- Congestive heart failure
- Pulmonary vascular disease
- Calcification of the ductal site
- Infective endocarditis

Pediculosis

Description

Pediculosis is infestation with blood-sucking lice. These lice feed on human blood and lay their eggs (nits) in body hairs or clothing fibers. After the nits hatch, the lice must feed within 24 hours or die. They mature in about 2 to 3 weeks. When a louse bites, it injects a toxin into the skin that produces mild irritation and a purpuric spot. Repeated bites cause sensitization to the toxin, leading to more serious inflammation. Treatment can eliminate lice.

Causes

See *Types of Pediculosis.*

Mode of transmission

See *Types of Pediculosis.*

Signs and symptoms

Pediculosis capitis
—Itching
—Excoriation with severe itching
—Matted, foul-smelling, lusterless hair (in severe cases)
—Occipital and cervical lymphadenopathy
—Oval, gray-white nits on hair shafts. These cannot be shaken loose like dandruff. The closer the nits are to the end of the hair shaft, the longer the infection has been present, since the ova are laid close to the scalp.

Pediculosis corporis
—Small, red papules. These usually occur on the shoulders, trunk, or buttocks and change to urticaria from scratching.
—Possible rashes or wheals. This is probably a sensitivity reaction.
—Dry, discolored, thickly encrusted skin. This can result, along with bacterial infection and scarring, if this condition is not treated.
—Possibly, headache, fever, and malaise in severe cases

Pediculosis pubis
—Skin irritation from scratching
—Possibly, small gray-blue spots on the thighs or upper body

Types of Pediculosis

TYPE	CAUSE	MODE OF TRANSMISSION
Pediculosis capitis (infestation with head lice)	*Pediculus humanus* var. *capitis*	Shared clothing, hats, combs, and hairbrushes
Pediculosis corporis (infestation with body lice)	*Pediculus humanus* var. *corporis*	Shared clothing and bedsheets
Pediculosis pubis (infestation with crab lice)	*Phthirus pubis*	• Sexual intercourse • Contact with clothes, bedsheets, or towels harboring lice

—Nits on pubic hairs, which feel coarse and grainy to touch

Treatment

For pediculosis capitis, treatment consists of lindane cream rubbed into the scalp at night, then rinsed out in the morning with lindane shampoo (this treatment should be repeated the following night). A fine-tooth comb dipped in vinegar removes nits from hair; washing hair with ordinary shampoo removes crustations.

Pediculosis corporis requires bathing with soap and water to remove lice from the body; in severe infestation, treatment with lindane may be necessary. Lice may be removed from clothes by washing, ironing, or dry cleaning. Storing clothes for more than 30 days or placing them in dry heat of 140° F. (60° C.) kills lice. If clothes cannot be washed or changed, application of 10% DDT or 10% lindane powder is effective.

Treatment of pediculosis pubis includes application of lindane cream or lotion (which is then left on for 24 hours), or shampooing with lindane shampoo. Treatment should be repeated in 1 week. Clothes and bedsheets must be laundered to prevent reinfestation.

Clinical implications

• Instruct patients how to use the creams, ointments, powders, and shampoos that can eliminate lice. To prevent self-infestation, avoid prolonged contact with the patient's hair, clothing, and bedsheets.
• Ask the patient with pediculosis pubis for a history of recent sexual contacts, so that they can be examined and treated.
• To prevent the spread of pediculosis to other hospitalized persons, examine all high-risk patients on admission, especially the elderly who depend on others for care, those admitted from nursing homes, or persons living in crowded conditions.

Pelvic inflammatory disease

Description

Pelvic inflammatory disease (PID) is any acute, subacute, recurrent, or chronic infection of the oviducts and ovaries, with adjacent tissue involve-

---

DESCRIPTION

• Most common species
• Feeds on the scalp; rarely in the eyebrows, eyelashes, and beard
• Commonly affects children, especially girls
• May be associated with overcrowded conditions and poor personal hygiene

• Lives in seams of clothing, next to skin; leaves only to feed on blood
• Associated with prolonged wearing of the same clothes, overcrowding, and poor personal hygiene

• Primarily found in pubic hairs but may extend to the eyebrows, eyelashes, and axillary body hair

Forms of Pelvic Inflammatory Disease

CAUSE AND CLINICAL FEATURES	DIAGNOSTIC FINDINGS
Salpingo-oophoritis • *Acute:* sudden onset of lower abdominal and pelvic pain, usually following menses; increased vaginal discharge; fever; malaise; lower abdominal pressure and tenderness; tachycardia; pelvic peritonitis • *Chronic:* recurring acute episodes	• Blood studies show leukocytosis or normal WBC count. • X-ray may show ileus. • Pelvic exam reveals extreme tenderness. • Smear of cervical or periurethral gland exudate shows gram-negative intracellular diplococci.
Cervicitis • *Acute:* purulent, foul-smelling vaginal discharge; vulvovaginitis, with itching or burning; red, edematous cervix; pelvic discomfort; sexual dysfunction; metrorrhagia; infertility; spontaneous abortion • *Chronic:* cervical dystocia, laceration or eversion of the cervix, ulcerative vesicular lesion (when cervicitis results from herpes simplex virus II)	• Cultures for *N. gonorrhoeae* are positive (>90% of patients). • Cytologic smears may reveal severe inflammation. • If cervicitis is not complicated by salpingitis, WBC count is normal or slightly elevated; ESR elevated. • In *acute cervicitis,* cervical palpation reveals tenderness. • In *chronic cervicitis,* causative organisms are usually staphylococcus or streptococcus.
Endometritis (generally postpartum or postabortion) • *Acute:* mucopurulent or purulent vaginal discharge oozing from the cervix; edematous, hyperemic endometrium, possibly leading to ulceration and necrosis (with virulent organisms); lower abdominal pain and tenderness; fever; rebound pain; abdominal muscle spasm; thrombophlebitis of uterine and pelvic vessels (in severe forms) • *Chronic:* recurring acute episodes (increasingly common because of widespread use of IUDs)	• In severe infection, palpation may reveal boggy uterus. • Uterine and blood samples are positive for causative organism, usually staphylococcus. • WBC count and ESR are elevated.

ment. It includes inflammation of the cervix (cervicitis), uterus (endometritis), fallopian tubes (salpingitis), and ovaries (oophoritis), which can extend to the connective tissue lying between the broad ligaments (parametritis). Early diagnosis and treatment prevents damage to the reproductive system.

Untreated PID may be fatal. (Also see *Forms of Pelvic Inflammatory Disease.*)

Causes
PID can result from infection with the following aerobic or anaerobic organisms:

• *Neisseria gonorrhoeae*, an aerobic organism—most common because it most readily penetrates the bacteriostatic barrier of cervical mucus
• One or several of the common bacteria found in cervical mucus, including staphylococci, streptococci, diphtheroids, chlamydiae, and coliforms such as *Pseudomonas* and *Escherichia coli*
• Multiplication of normally nonpathogenic bacteria in an altered endometrial environment (most commonly during parturition)

Risk factors
• Conditions or procedures such as conization or cauterization of the cervix, which alter or destroy cervical mucus, allowing bacteria to ascend into the uterine cavity
• Any procedure that can allow transfer of contaminated cervical mucus into the endometrial cavity by instrumentation, such as use of a biopsy curet, an irrigation catheter, tubal insufflation, abortion, or pelvic surgery
• Infection during or after pregnancy
• Infectious foci within the body, such as drainage from a chronically infected fallopian tube, a pelvic abscess, a ruptured appendix, or diverticulitis of the sigmoid colon

Signs and symptoms
Clinical features vary with the affected area but usually include the following:
• Profuse, purulent vaginal discharge
• Possible low-grade fever and malaise, especially if *N. gonorrhoeae* is the cause
• Lower abdominal pain
• Extreme pain on movement of the cervix or palpation of the adnexa

Diagnostic tests
• Gram stain of secretions from the endocervix or cul-de-sac identifies the infecting organism. Culture and sensitivity testing aid selection of the ap-propriate antibiotic. Urethral and rectal secretions may also be cultured.
• Ultrasonography identifies an adnexal or uterine mass.
• Culdocentesis obtains peritoneal fluid or pus for culture and sensitivity testing.

Treatment
To prevent progression of PID, antibiotic therapy begins immediately after culture specimens are obtained. Such therapy can be reevaluated as soon as laboratory results are available (usually after 24 to 48 hours). Infection may become chronic if treated inadequately.

The preferred antibiotic therapy for PID resulting from gonorrhea is penicillin G procaine I.M. in two injection sites, combined with probenecid P.O. If the patient is allergic to penicillin, tetracycline may be used. (A patient with gonorrhea may also require therapy for syphilis.) Supplemental treatment of PID may include bed rest, analgesics, and I.V. therapy.

Development of pelvic abscess necessitates adequate drainage. A ruptured pelvic abscess is a life-threatening condition. If this complication develops, the patient may need a total abdominal hysterectomy, with bilateral salpingo-oophorectomy.

Clinical implications
• After establishing that the patient has no drug allergies, administer antibiotics and analgesics, as ordered.
• Check for elevated temperature.
• Watch for abdominal rigidity and distention, possible signs of developing peritonitis. Provide frequent perineal care if vaginal drainage occurs.
• To prevent recurrence, encourage compliance with treatment, and explain the nature and seriousness of PID.
• Stress the need for the patient's sexual partner to be examined and, if necessary, treated for infection.
• Since PID may cause painful intercourse, advise the patient to consult with

her physician about sexual activity.
• To prevent infection after minor gynecologic procedures, such as dilatation and curettage, tell the patient to immediately report any fever, increased vaginal discharge, or pain. After such procedures, instruct her to avoid douching or intercourse for at least 7 days.

Complications
• Potentially fatal septicemia
• Pulmonary emboli
• Infertility
• Shock

Penile cancer

Description
Penile carcinoma rarely affects circumcised men in modern cultures; when it does occur, it is usually in men over age 50. The most common form, epidermoid squamous cell carcinoma, is usually found in the glans but may also occur on the corona glandis, and, rarely, in the preputial cavity. Early circumcision seems to prevent penile cancer by allowing for better personal hygiene and minimizing inflammatory (and often premalignant) lesions of the glans and prepuce. Incidence is not decreased in cultures that practice circumcision at a later date. Prognosis varies according to staging at time of diagnosis. If begun early enough, radiation therapy increases the 5-year survival rate to over 60%; surgery only, to over 55%. Unfortunately, many men delay treatment of penile cancer because they fear disfigurement and loss of sexual function.

Causes
The exact cause of penile cancer is unknown; however, it is usually associated with poor personal hygiene, and phimosis in uncircumcised men.

Signs and symptoms
Early signs
—Small, circumscribed lesion, a pimple, or a sore on the penis, which may go unnoticed in uncircumcised men
Late-stage signs
—Pain
—Hemorrhage
—Dysuria
—Purulent discharge
—Obstruction of the urinary meatus

Diagnostic tests
• Tissue biopsy is necessary for diagnosis.
• Preoperative baseline studies include complete blood count, urinalysis, electrocardiogram, and chest X-ray.
• Lymphangiographic preoperative evaluation of lymph node metastasis is difficult because of enlargement of inguinal lymph nodes due to infection of the primary lesion.

Treatment
Depending on the stage, treatment includes surgical resection of the primary tumor and possibly chemotherapy and radiation. Local tumors of the prepuce require only circumcision. Invasive tumors, however, require partial penectomy (unless contraindicated because of the patient's young age); tumors of the base of the penile shaft require total penectomy and inguinal node dissection (done less often in the United States than in other countries where incidence is higher). Radiation therapy may improve treatment effectiveness after resection of localized lesions without metastasis. It may also reduce the size of lymph nodes before nodal resection. It is not adequate primary treatment for groin metastasis, however. Bleomycin and methotrexate are usually used in chemotherapy but are not very effective.

Clinical implications
Penile cancer calls for good patient teaching, psychological support, and comprehensive postoperative care.

The patient with penile cancer fears disfigurement, pain, and loss of sexual function.

Before penile surgery, follow these guidelines:

• Spend time with the patient, and encourage him to talk about his fears.

• Supplement and reinforce what the physician has told the patient about the surgery and other treatment measures, and explain expected postoperative procedures, such as dressing changes and catheterization. Show him diagrams of the surgical procedure and pictures of the results of similar surgery to help him adapt to an altered body image.

• If the patient needs urinary diversion, refer him to the enterostomal therapist.

Although postpenectomy care varies with the procedure used and the treatment protocol, certain procedures are always applicable.

• Constantly monitor the patient's vital signs and record his intake and output accurately.

• Provide comprehensive skin care to prevent skin breakdown from urinary diversion or suprapubic catheterization. Keep the skin dry and free from urine. If the patient has a suprapubic catheter, make sure the catheter is patent at all times.

• Administer analgesics, as ordered. Elevate the penile stump with a small towel or pillow to minimize edema.

• Check the surgical site often for signs of infection, such as foul odor or excessive drainage on dressing.

• If the patient has had inguinal node dissection, watch for and immediately report signs of lymphedema, such as decreased circulation or disproportionate swelling of a leg.

• After partial penectomy, reassure the patient that the penile stump should be sufficient for urination and sexual function. Refer him for psychological or sexual counseling if necessary.

Peptic ulcers

Description

Peptic ulcers—circumscribed lesions in the gastric mucosal membrane—can develop in the lower esophagus, stomach, pylorus, duodenum, or jejunum from contact with gastric juice (especially hydrochloric acid and pepsin). About 80% of all peptic ulcers are duodenal ulcers, which affect the proximal part of the small intestine. These ulcers tend to afflict people with type O blood, perhaps because such people do not secrete blood group antigens (mucopolysaccharides, which may serve to protect the mucosa) in their saliva and other body fluids.

Duodenal ulcers may persist for life. When they heal, they usually leave scars that can later break down and ulcerate again under hyperacidic conditions. Thus, they often follow a chronic course, with remissions and exacerbations, and 5% to 10% of patients develop complications that necessitate surgery. Gastric ulcers, which affect the stomach mucosa, are most common in both middle-aged and elderly men, especially among the poor and undernourished and in chronic users of aspirin or alcohol. Benign gastric ulcers tend to recur. For unknown reasons, these ulcers often strike people with type A blood and may become malignant more often than duodenal ulcers.

Causes

The precise cause is unknown, but possibilities include the following:

• Decreased mucosal resistance
• Inadequate mucosal blood flow
• Defective mucus
• Psychogenic factors, which may stimulate long-term overproduction of gastric secretions that can erode the stomach, duodenum, or esophagus
• Back diffusion of acid through mucosa damaged by chronic gastritis or irritants, such as aspirin or alcohol

• Deterioration of the pylorus (this occurs in the elderly person), permitting reflux of bile into the stomach

• In duodenal ulcers, acid hypersecretion, possibly caused by an overactive vagus nerve

Signs and symptoms

Both kinds of ulcers may be asymptomatic.

Gastric ulcers
—Heartburn
—Indigestion
—Pain in the left epigastrium and a feeling of fullness and distention after eating a large meal
—Weight loss
—Repeated episodes of GI bleeding

Duodenal ulcers
Attacks usually occur about 2 hours after meals, whenever the stomach is empty, or after consumption of orange juice, coffee, aspirin, or alcohol. Exacerbations tend to recur several times a year, then fade into remission.
—Heartburn
—Well-localized midepigastric pain, which is relieved by eating food
—Weight gain. The patient eats to relieve discomfort.
—Sensation of hot water bubbling in the back of the throat

Diagnostic tests

• Upper GI tract X-rays show abnormalities in mucosa.

• Gastric secretory studies show hyperchlorhydria.

• Upper GI endoscopy or esophagogastroduodenoscopy confirms the presence of an ulcer.

• Biopsy rules out cancer.

• Stools may test positive for occult blood.

Treatment

Treatment is essentially symptomatic and emphasizes drug therapy and rest.

• Antacids reduce gastric acidity.

• Cimetidine or ranitidine, histamine-receptor antagonists, reduce gastric secretion in short-term therapy (up to 8 weeks).

• Anticholinergics, such as propantheline, inhibit the vagus nerve effect on the parietal cells and reduce gastrin production and excessive gastric activity in duodenal ulcers. These drugs are usually contraindicated in gastric ulcers, because they prolong gastric emptying and can aggravate the ulcer.

• Physical rest and, for gastric ulcers only, sedatives and tranquilizers, such as chlordiazepoxide and phenobarbital, promote healing.

• If GI bleeding occurs, emergency treatment begins with passage of a nasogastric tube to allow for iced saline lavage, possibly containing norepinephrine. Angiography facilitates placement of an intraarterial catheter, followed by infusion of vasopressin to constrict blood vessels and control bleeding. This type of therapy allows postponement of surgery until the patient's condition stabilizes. Surgery is indicated for perforation, unresponsiveness to conservative treatment, and suspected cancer. Surgical procedures for peptic ulcers include vagotomy and pyloroplasty and/or distal subtotal gastrectomy.

Clinical implications

Managing peptic ulcers requires careful administration of medications, thorough patient teaching, and skillful postoperative care.

• Administer medications, as ordered, and watch for cimetidine and anticholinergic side effects: dizziness, rash, mild diarrhea, muscle pain, leukopenia, and gynecomastia; and dry mouth, blurred vision, headache, constipation, and urinary retention, respectively. Anticholinergics are usually most effective when given 30 minutes before meals. Give sedatives and tranquilizers, as needed.

• Instruct the patient to take antacids 1 hour after meals. Advise the patient who has a history of cardiac disease or who is on a sodium-restricted diet to take only low-sodium antacids.

Teaching Topics in Ulcer Disease

• An explanation of the type of ulcer disease: duodenal or gastric
• Warning signs of hemorrhage, obstruction, and perforation
• Preparation for diagnostic tests, such as upper GI endoscopy and upper GI series, to confirm and evaluate ulcer disease
• Dietary modifications to neutralize acid and reduce gastric motility and secretions
• Medications to relieve symptoms: antacids, anticholinergics, and tranquilizers
• If necessary, preparation for surgery, such as gastroenterostomy and vagotomy
• Other measures: adequate rest, stress management, and cessation of smoking

Warn that antacids may cause changes in bowel habits (diarrhea with magnesium-containing antacids, constipation with aluminum-containing antacids).
• Warn the patient to avoid aspirin-containing drugs, reserpine, indomethacin, and phenylbutazone, because they irritate the gastric mucosa. For the same reason, warn against excessive intake of coffee, exposure to stressful situations, and consumption of alcoholic beverages during exacerbations (although alcohol may be consumed in moderation during remission). Advise the patient to stop smoking, because it stimulates gastric secretion.

After gastric surgery:
• Keep nasogastric tube patent. If the tube is not functioning, do not reposition it; you may damage the suture line or anastomosis. Notify the surgeon promptly.
• Monitor intake and output, including nasogastric tube drainage. Check bowel sounds, and allow the patient nothing by mouth until peristalsis resumes and the nasogastric tube is removed or clamped.
• Replace fluids and electrolytes. Assess for signs of dehydration, sodium deficiency, and metabolic alkalosis, which may occur secondary to gastric suction.
• Control postoperative pain with nar-

cotics and analgesics, as ordered.
• Watch for complications: hemorrhage; shock; iron, folate, or vitamin B_{12} deficiency anemia (from malabsorption or continued blood loss); and dumping syndrome (weakness, nausea, flatulence, diarrhea, distention, and palpitations within 30 minutes after a meal).
• To avoid dumping syndrome, advise the patient to lie down after meals; to drink fluids *between* meals rather than with meals; to avoid eating large amounts of carbohydrates; and to eat four to six small, high-protein, low-carbohydrate meals during the day. (Also see *Teaching Topics in Ulcer Disease*.)

Complications
• Penetration of pancreas
• Severe back pain
• Perforation
• Hemorrhage
• Pyloric obstruction

Pericarditis

Description
Pericarditis is an acute or chronic inflammation of the pericardium, the fibroserous sac that envelops, supports,

and protects the heart. Acute pericarditis can be fibrinous or effusive, with purulent serous or hemorrhagic exudate. Chronic constrictive pericarditis is characterized by dense fibrous pericardial thickening. Because pericarditis often coexists with other conditions, diagnosis of acute pericarditis depends on typical clinical features and the elimination of other possible causes. Prognosis depends on the underlying cause but is usually good in acute pericarditis, unless constriction occurs.

Causes
Common causes of this disease include the following:
• Bacterial, fungal, or viral infection (infectious pericarditis)
• Neoplasms (primary or metastatic from lungs, breasts, or other organs)
• High-dose radiation to the chest
• Uremia
• Hypersensitivity or autoimmune diseases such as rheumatic fever (the most common cause of pericarditis in children), systemic lupus erythematosus, and rheumatoid arthritis
• Postcardiac injury, such as myocardial infarction (which later causes an autoimmune reaction [Dressler's syndrome] in the pericardium), trauma, or surgery that leaves the pericardium intact but causes blood to leak into the pericardial cavity
• Drugs, such as hydralazine or procainamide
• Idiopathic factors (most common in acute pericarditis)
• Less commonly, aortic aneurysm with pericardial leakage, and myxedema with cholesterol deposits in the pericardium

Signs and symptoms
Acute pericarditis
—Typically, sharp and often sudden pain that usually starts over the sternum and radiates to the neck, shoulders, back, and arms. Unlike the pain of myocardial infarction, pericardial pain is often pleuritic, increasing with deep inspiration and decreasing when the patient sits up and leans forward.
—Pericardial friction rub. A classic symptom, this grating sound is heard as the heart moves. It can usually be heard best during forced expiration while the patient leans forward or is on his hands and knees in bed. It may have up to three components, corresponding to the timing of atrial systole, ventricular systole, and the rapid-filling phase of ventricular diastole. Occasionally, friction rub is heard only briefly or not at all.
Chronic constrictive pericarditis
—Gradual increase in systemic venous pressure
—Fluid retention, ascites, hepatomegaly (symptoms similar to those of chronic right heart failure)

Diagnostic tests
Laboratory results are not diagnostic. They reflect inflammation and may identify its cause.
• WBC count is normal or elevated, especially in infectious pericarditis.
• ESR is elevated.
• Cardiac enzymes are slightly elevated, with associated myocarditis.
• Culture of pericardial fluid obtained by open surgical drainage or cardiocentesis sometimes identifies a causative organism in bacterial or fungal pericarditis.
• EKG shows the following changes in acute pericarditis: elevation of ST segments in the standard limb leads and most precordial leads without significant changes in QRS morphology that occur with myocardial infarction; atrial ectopic rhythms, such as atrial fibrillation; and in pericardial effusion, diminished QRS voltage.
• Other pertinent laboratory data include BUN to check for uremia, antistreptolysin O titers to detect rheumatic fever, and a purified protein derivative skin test to check for tuberculosis.
• In pericardial effusion, echocar-

diography is diagnostic when it shows an echo-free space between the ventricular wall and the pericardium.

Treatment

The goal of treatment is to relieve symptoms and manage underlying systemic disease. In acute idiopathic pericarditis, postmyocardial infarction pericarditis, and post thoracotomy pericarditis, treatment consists of bed rest as long as fever and pain persist, and nonsteroidal drugs, such as aspirin and indomethacin, to relieve pain and reduce inflammation. If these drugs fail to relieve symptoms, corticosteroids may be used. Although corticosteroids produce rapid and effective relief, they must be used cautiously because episodes may recur when therapy is discontinued.

Infectious pericarditis that results from disease of the left pleural space, mediastinal abscesses, or septicemia requires antibiotics, surgical drainage, or both. If cardiac tamponade develops, the physician may perform emergency pericardiocentesis. Signs of cardiac tamponade include pulsus paradoxus, neck vein distention, dyspnea, and shock.

Recurrent pericarditis may necessitate partial pericardectomy, which creates a "window" that allows fluid to drain into the pleural space. In constrictive pericarditis, total pericardectomy to permit adequate filling and contraction of the heart may be necessary. Treatment must also include management of rheumatic fever, uremia, tuberculosis, and other underlying disorders.

Clinical implications

A patient with pericarditis needs complete bed rest. In addition, follow these guidelines:
• Assess pain in relation to respiration and body position to distinguish pericardial pain from myocardial ischemic pain.
• Place the patient in an upright position to relieve dyspnea and chest pain, provide analgesics and oxygen, and reassure the patient with acute pericarditis that his condition is temporary and treatable.
• Monitor for signs of cardiac compression or cardiac tamponade, which are possible complications of pericardial effusion. Signs include decreased blood pressure, increased central venous pressure, and pulsus paradoxus. Since cardiac tamponade requires immediate treatment, keep a pericardiocentesis set at bedside whenever pericardial effusion is suspected.
• Explain tests and treatments to the patient. If surgery is necessary, he should learn deep-breathing and coughing exercises beforehand. Postoperative care is similar to that given following cardiothoracic surgery.

Complications

Pericardial effusion, the major complication of acute pericarditis, may produce effects of heart failure (such as dyspnea, orthopnea, and tachycardia), ill-defined substernal chest pain, and a feeling of fullness in the chest. In very large pericardial effusions, cardiac dullness, diminished or absent apical impulse, and distant heart sounds are found on physical examination. If fluid accumulates rapidly, cardiac tamponade may occur, eventually leading to cardiovascular collapse and death.

Peripheral neuritis
(Multiple neuritis, peripheral neuropathy, polyneuritis)

Description

Peripheral neuritis is the degeneration of peripheral nerves that supply mainly the distal muscles of the extremities. This syndrome is associated with noninflammatory degeneration of the axon and myelin sheaths. Although peripheral neuritis can occur at any age, incidence is highest in men between ages 30 and 50. Onset is usually insidious, and patients may compensate by overusing unaffected muscles. Thus, patients often have a history of clumsiness and may complain of frequent vague sensations. Onset is rapid in severe infection and chronic alcohol intoxication. Patient history and physical examination delineate characteristic distribution of motor and sensory deficits. If the cause can be identified and corrected, prognosis is good.

Causes

Causes of peripheral neuritis include:
- Chronic intoxication (with ethyl alcohol, arsenic, lead, carbon disulfide, benzene, phosphorus, and sulfonamides)
- Infectious diseases (meningitis, diphtheria, syphilis, tuberculosis, pneumonia, mumps, and Guillain-Barré syndrome)
- Metabolic and inflammatory disorders (gout, diabetes mellitus, rheumatoid arthritis, polyarteritis nodosa, systemic lupus erythematosus)
- Nutritional disorders (beriberi and other vitamin deficiencies, and cachectic states)

Signs and symptoms

The clinical effects of peripheral neuritis develop slowly.
- Muscle weakness
- Flaccid paralysis
- Muscle wasting
- Loss of reflexes
- Pain of varying intensity
- Loss of ability to perceive vibratory sensations
- Paresthesia, hyperesthesia, or anesthesia in the hands and feet
- Absent or diminished deep-tendon reflexes
- Atrophied muscles, which are tender or hypersensitive to pressure or palpation
- Possible footdrop
- Cutaneous manifestations, including glossy, red skin and decreased sweating

Diagnostic tests

Electromyography may show delayed action potential if this condition impairs motor nerve function.

Treatment

Effective treatment of peripheral neuritis consists of supportive measures to relieve pain, adequate bed rest, and physical therapy, as needed. Most important, however, the underlying cause must be identified and corrected. For instance, it is essential to identify and remove the toxic agent, correct nutritional and vitamin deficiencies (the patient needs a high-calorie diet rich in vitamins, especially B-complex), or counsel the patient to avoid alcohol.

Clinical implications

- Relieve pain with correct positioning, analgesics, or possibly phenytoin, which has been used experimentally for neuritic pain, especially if associated with diabetic neuropathy.
- Instruct the patient to rest and refrain from using the affected extremity. To prevent pressure sores, apply a foot cradle. To prevent contractures, arrange for the patient to obtain splints, boards, braces, or other orthopedic appliances.
- After pain subsides, passive range-of-motion exercises or massage may be beneficial. Electrotherapy is used for nerve and muscle stimulation.

Peritonitis

Description

Peritonitis is an acute or chronic inflammation of the peritoneum, the membrane that lines the abdominal cavity and covers the visceral organs. Such inflammation may extend throughout the peritoneum or may be localized as an abscess. Peritonitis commonly decreases intestinal motility and causes intestinal distention, with gas. Mortality is 10%. Death usually results from bowel obstruction. The introduction of antibiotics has lowered mortality.

Causes

Bacterial invasion of the sterile peritoneum results in infection, inflammation, and perforation of the GI tract. Usually, this is a complication of appendicitis, diverticulitis, peptic ulcer, ulcerative colitis, volvulus, strangulated obstruction, abdominal neoplasm, or a stab wound. Peritonitis may also result from chemical inflammation, as in rupture of fallopian tubes or the bladder, perforation of a gastric ulcer, or released pancreatic enzymes.

Signs and symptoms

• Sudden, severe, diffuse abdominal pain (tends to intensify and localize in the area of the underlying disorder)
• Weakness
• Pallor
• Excessive sweating
• Cold skin
• Decreased intestinal motility and paralytic ileus
• Abdominal distention
• Acutely tender abdomen associated with rebound tenderness
• Shallow breathing
• Diminished movement by the patient to minimize pain
• Hypotension
• Tachycardia
• Signs of dehydration
• Fever of 103° F. (39.4° C.) or higher
• Possible shoulder pain and hiccups

Diagnostic tests

• Abdominal X-rays showing edematous and gaseous distention of the small and large bowel support the diagnosis. With perforation of a visceral organ, the X-ray shows air in the abdominal cavity.
• Chest X-ray may show elevation of the diaphragm.
• Blood studies show leukocytosis (more than 20,000 leukocytes/mm³).
• Paracentesis reveals bacteria, exudate, blood, pus, or urine.
• Laparotomy may be necessary to identify the underlying cause.

Treatment

Early treatment of GI inflammatory conditions and preoperative and postoperative antibiotic therapy help prevent peritonitis. Once peritonitis develops, emergency treatment is needed to combat infection, restore intestinal motility, and replace fluids and electrolytes.

Massive antibiotic therapy usually includes administration of cefoxitin with an aminoglycoside or penicillin G and clindamycin with an aminoglycoside, depending on the infecting organisms. To decrease peristalsis and prevent perforation, the patient should receive nothing by mouth; he should receive supportive fluids and electrolytes parenterally.

Other supplementary treatment measures include preoperative and postoperative administration of an analgesic, such as meperidine; nasogastric intubation to decompress the bowel; and possible use of a rectal tube to facilitate passage of flatus.

When peritonitis results from perforation, surgery is necessary as soon as the patient's condition is stable enough to tolerate it. The aim of surgery is to eliminate the source of infection by evacuating the spilled contents and inserting drains. Occasionally, abdominocentesis may be necessary to remove accumulated fluid. Irrigation of the abdominal cavity with antibiotic solutions during surgery may be appropriate.

Clinical implications

• Regularly monitor vital signs, fluid intake and output, and amount of nasogastric drainage or vomitus.

• Place the patient in semi-Fowler's position to help him deep-breathe with less pain and thus prevent pulmonary complications.

• Counteract mouth and nose dryness due to fever and nasogastric intubation with regular cleansing and lubrication.

After surgery to evacuate the peritoneum, follow these guidelines:

• Maintain parenteral fluid and electrolyte administration, as ordered. Record fluid intake and output, including nasogastric and incisional drainage.

• Place the patient in Fowler's position to promote drainage (through drainage tube) by gravity. Move him carefully, since the slightest movement will intensify the pain.

• Encourage and assist ambulation, as ordered, usually on the first postoperative day.

• Watch for signs of dehiscence (the patient may complain that "something gave way") and abscess formation (continued abdominal tenderness and fever).

• Frequently assess peristaltic activity by listening for bowel sounds and checking for gas, bowel movements, and soft abdomen. When peristalsis returns, and temperature and pulse rate are normal, gradually decrease parenteral fluids and increase oral fluids. If the patient has a nasogastric tube in place, clamp it for short intervals. If nausea or vomiting does not result, begin oral fluids, as ordered and tolerated.

Pernicious anemia
(Addison's anemia)

Description

Pernicious anemia is a progressive, megaloblastic, macrocytic anemia primarily affecting persons of northern European ancestry. Onset is typically between ages 50 and 60; incidence rises with increasing age. This disease causes serious neurologic, gastric, and intestinal abnormalities. Untreated pernicious anemia may lead to permanent neurologic disability and death.

Causes

This disorder is caused by a deficiency of vitamin B_{12}, which may result from a genetic predisposition or an inherited autoimmune response.

Signs and symptoms

Characteristic symptoms

Characteristically, pernicious anemia has an insidious onset but eventually causes an unmistakable triad of symptoms.

—Weakness
—Sore tongue
—Numbness and tingling in the extremities

The following symptoms also occur:

—Pale lips, gums, and tongue
—Faintly jaundiced sclerae

Systemic symptoms

—Possibly, pale to bright yellow skin
—Possibly, infection, especially of the genitourinary tract
—GI: nausea, vomiting, anorexia, weight loss, flatulence, diarrhea, and constipation. Gingival bleeding and tongue inflammation may hinder eating and intensify anorexia.
—CNS: neuritis; weakness in extremities; peripheral numbness and paresthesias; disturbed position sense; lack of coordination; ataxia; impaired fine finger movement; positive Babinski's and Romberg's signs; light-headedness; altered vision (diplopia, blurred vision), taste, and hearing (tinnitus); optic muscle atrophy; loss of bowel and bladder control; and in males, impotence, irritability, poor memory, headache, depression, and delirium. Although some of these symptoms are temporary, irreversible CNS changes may have occurred before treatment.
—Cardiovascular: weakness, fatigue,

light-headedness, palpitations, wide pulse pressure, dyspnea, orthopnea, tachycardia, premature beats, and, eventually, congestive heart failure.

Diagnostic tests
• The Schilling test is the definitive diagnostic test for pernicious anemia.
• Hemoglobin and RBC count are decreased.
• Mean corpuscular volume is increased (MCV>120), and because larger-than-normal RBCs contain increased amounts of hemoglobin, mean corpuscular hemoglobin concentration is also increased.
• WBC and platelet counts are often low, and large, malformed platelets may be present.
• Serum vitamin B_{12} assay levels may be less than 0.1 mcg/ml.
• Serum LDH is elevated.
• Bone marrow aspiration reveals erythroid hyperplasia (crowded red bone marrow), with increased numbers of megaloblasts but few normally developing RBCs.
• Gastric secretion analysis shows absence of free hydrochloric acid after histamine or pentagastrin injection.

Treatment
Early parenteral vitamin B_{12} replacement can reverse pernicious anemia and minimize complications and may prevent permanent neurologic damage. These injections rarely cause side effects or induce an allergic response. An initial high dose of parenteral vitamin B_{12} stimulates rapid RBC regeneration. Within 2 weeks, hemoglobin should rise to normal, and the patient's condition should improve markedly. Since rapid cell regeneration increases the patient's iron requirements, concomitant iron replacement is necessary to prevent iron deficiency anemia. After the patient's condition improves, vitamin B_{12} doses can be decreased to maintenance levels and given monthly. Such injections must be continued for life, and patients should learn self-administration.

If anemia causes extreme fatigue, the patient may require bed rest until hemoglobin rises. If hemoglobin is dangerously low, he may need blood transfusions, digitalis, a diuretic, and a low-sodium diet for congestive heart failure. Most important is the replacement of vitamin B_{12} to control the condition that led to this failure. Antibiotics help combat accompanying infections.

Clinical implications
Supportive measures minimize the risk of complications and speed recovery. Patient and family teaching can promote compliance with lifelong vitamin B_{12} replacement.
• If the patient has severe anemia, plan activities, rest periods, and necessary diagnostic tests to conserve his energy. Monitor pulse rate often; tachycardia is a sign that his activities are too strenuous.
• To ensure accurate Schilling test results, make sure that all urine over a 24-hour period is collected and that the specimens are uncontaminated.
• Warn the patient to guard against infections, since his weakened condition may increase susceptibility. Tell him to report signs of infection promptly, especially of pulmonary and urinary tract infections.
• Provide a well-balanced diet, including foods high in vitamin B_{12} (meat, liver, fish, eggs, and milk). Offer between-meal snacks, and encourage the family to bring favorite foods from home.
• Since a sore mouth and tongue make eating painful, ask the dietitian to avoid giving the patient irritating foods. If these symptoms make talking difficult, supply a pad and pencil or some other aid to facilitate nonverbal communication. Explain this problem to the family. Provide diluted mouthwash or, with severe conditions, swab the patient's mouth with tap water or warm saline solution.

• Warn the patient with a sensory deficit not to use a heating pad, since it may cause burns.

• If the patient is incontinent, establish a regular bowel and bladder routine. After the patient is discharged, a visiting nurse should follow up on this schedule and make adjustments, as needed.

• If neurologic damage causes behavioral problems, assess mental and neurologic status often. If necessary, give tranquilizers, as ordered, and apply a jacket restraint at night.

• Stress that vitamin B_{12} replacement is not a permanent cure and that these injections must be continued for life, even after symptoms subside.

• To prevent pernicious anemia, emphasize the importance of vitamin B_{12} supplements for patients who have had extensive gastric resections or who follow strict vegetarian diets.

Personality disorders

Description
Personality disorders are individual traits that reflect chronic, inflexible, and maladaptive patterns of behavior that cause discomfort and impair social and occupational function. Personality disorders fall on Axis II of the *DSM-III* classifications. They are widespread, but no statistics exist to reflect incidence. Patients with personality disorders do not usually receive treatment. When they do, they are usually managed on an outpatient basis.

Personality notations are appropriate and useful for all patients and help give a fuller picture of the patient and a more accurate diagnosis. For example, many features characteristic of personality disorders are apparent during an episode of another mental disorder (such as a major depressive episode in a patient with compulsive personality features). Central and essential to diagnosis is a history that shows maladaptive personality traits as characteristic of lifelong behavior, and not just occurring during the course of an illness.

Prognosis is variable. Personality disorders are self-limiting, in that most appear at adolescence and wane during middle age.

Causes
Only recently have personality disorders been categorized in detail, and research continues to identify their causes. Various theories attempt to explain their origin.

• Biological theories hold that these disorders may stem from chromosomal and neuronal abnormalities.

• Social theories hold that the disorders reflect learned responses, reinforcement, modeling, and aversive stimuli.

• Psychodynamic theories hold that personality disorders reflect deficiencies in ego and superego development and are related to mother-child relationships involving unresponsiveness, overprotectiveness, or early separation.

Signs and symptoms
Signs and symptoms of personality disorders differ according to the diagnosis. (See *Characteristics of Personality Disorders*.) They differ among individuals and within the same individual at different times.

Diagnostic tests
Psychological evaluation must rule out similar personality or psychiatric disorders.

Treatment
Treatment depends on the patient's symptoms but requires a trusting relationship in which the therapist can

Characteristics of Personality Disorders

PARANOID

Suspicion; concern with hidden motives
Inability to relax (hypervigilance), anxiety
Fault-finding with resultant anger
Inability to collaborate
Social isolation
Poor self-image
Coldness, detachment, absence of tender feelings
Need to feel in control
Odd or eccentric appearance to others
Hostility
Argumentativeness, overt antagonism
Conflict with authority
Hypersensitivity
Jealousy
Poor sense of humor

AVOIDANT

Devastated by separation and loss
Somatic symptoms
Anxiety and fearfulness
Low self-esteem
Dependence in relationships
Social withdrawal: mistrust, fear of rejection, but desire for close relationships
Depression (loneliness)

COMPULSIVE

Perfectionism
Physical symptoms usually due to overwork
Confident attitude with others
Rigid, cold, businesslike attitude; inability to express affection
Need for control
Depression (worthlessness and low self-esteem)
Procrastination, indecision

SCHIZOID AND SCHIZOTYPAL

Suspicion
Inability to relax
Passive antagonism
Hypersensitivity to criticism
Social withdrawal
Poor self-image
Coldness, absence of warm feelings, detachment, indifference to others' feelings
Odd or eccentric appearance to others
Elaborative, detailed speech
Ideas of reference
Depersonalization
Dependency
Flat or depressed affect

DEPENDENT

Devastated by separation and loss
Somatic symptoms
Desire for human contact
Self-consciousness and feelings of inadequacy
Overly compliant, clinging behavior; avoids independence, leaves major decisions to others
Depression (inadequacy and helplessness)

PASSIVE-AGGRESSIVE

Intentional inefficiency (social and occupational), nonadherence to etiquette, forgetfulness; falls asleep at unsuitable times
Complaining and blaming behavior; feelings of confusion and mistreatment
Fear of authority
Chronic lateness, procrastination, dawdling
Resentment, sullenness, stubbornness
No overt hostility or anger

(continued)

Characteristics of Personality Disorders *(continued)*

HISTRIONIC

Craving for stimulation and attention
Intolerance of being alone
Manipulative, divisive behavior
Depression (emptiness, loneliness)
Inability to put others' needs first
Attention-getting via dependency,
  helplessness, obnoxious behav-
  ior, or seductive or charming
  behavior; affect may be very in-
  tense
Multiple physical complaints
Tantrums and angry outbursts
Superficial attachments
Dramatic, emotional, or erratic
  behavior

ANTISOCIAL

Superficial charm, wit, and intelligence, often with manipulative
  and seductive behavior; inability
  or refusal to accept guilt for
  self-serving, destructive behavior
Failure at school and work: school
  grades markedly below expectations, truancy, delinquency,
  chronic violations of rules, suspension or expulsion from school,
  running away from home;
  inability to keep a job
Promiscuity, casual sexual relationships, desertion, two or more
  divorces or separations
Repeated substance abuse
Thefts, illegal occupations, multiple
  arrests, vandalism
Inability to function as a responsible
  parent (child abuse or neglect)
Fights, assaults, abuse of others
Impulsiveness, recklessness,
  inability to plan ahead

NARCISSISTIC

Craving for stimulation and attention
Intolerance of being alone
Manipulative behavior
Depression (humiliation, anger)
No capacity for empathy
Exaggeration of achievements and
  talents: attitude self-centeredness;
  arrogant behavior ensuring his
  needs take priority
Grandiosity; preoccupation with
  fantasies of unlimited success,
  power, or beauty

BORDERLINE

Impulsive and unpredictable
  behavior in self-damaging areas:
  spending, sex, gambling, substance abuse, shoplifting,
  and overeating
Unstable and intense interpersonal
  relationships: attitude shifts
  within days or hours; idealization,
  devaluation, or manipulation
Inappropriate, intense anger
Identity disturbance with uncertain
  self-image, uncertain gender
  identity, uncertain relationship
  commitments, and behavior
  based on imitation
Unstable affect with mood swings
  within hours or days
Intolerance of being alone, a sense
  of emptiness or boredom
Self-destructive behavior: suicidal
  gestures, self-mutilation, recurrent
  accidents and physical fights
Fear of abandonment displayed in
  clinging and distancing maneuvers
Projection
Evaluation of things and people at
  extremes of good or bad with
  no gray areas between
Acting out of feelings instead of
  expressing feelings verbally or
  appropriately
Manipulation: pitting others (including staff) against each other

use a directive approach. Drug therapy is usually ineffective but may be used to relieve severe distress, such as acute anxiety or depression. Family and group therapy are effective. Hospital inpatient milieu therapy in crisis situations and possibly for long-term treatment of borderline personality disorders can sometimes be effective. Inpatient treatment is controversial, however, since patients with personality disorders tend to be noncompliant with extended therapeutic regimes. For such patients, outpatient therapy may be more useful.

Clinical implications

First, know your own feelings and reactions as the basis for assessing the patient's overt responses. Keep in mind

---

Disorders of Impulse Control

Disorders of impulse control fall into three categories, as outlined below. The three types share these essential features: failure to resist an impulse to perform an act that is harmful to self or others; rising intrapsychic tension before committing the act; and feelings of pleasure, gratification, or release of tension upon committing the act, possibly (but not always) followed by regret or guilt. Patient management is also the same for all three types. When caring for a patient with a disorder of impulse control, remember to: set clear, fair, firm limits on behavior; encourage therapeutic interpersonal relationships with staff; and, as appropriate, refer the patient for psychotherapy and/or to self-help organizations, such as Gamblers' Anonymous.

TYPES	MECHANISMS
• Pathological gambling • Kleptomania	• Functions at id level (immediate gratification) • Has limited superego strength; ineffective conscience • Lives for the here and now without thought of the future • Is unable to plan or work toward realistic, long-range goals
• Pyromania	• Inconsistent parenting • Fire experienced as punishment, becomes acceptable mode of retaliation • Anger and rage that build up and then are released • A hypnotic and anxiety-reducing effect from watching fire
• Intermittent explosive disorder • Isolated explosive disorder	• Difficulty in sharing feelings and in intrapersonal relationships • Acting-out behavior (screaming, breaking objects, physical abuse) that occurs intermittently or rarely (isolated) when rising intrapsychic tension becomes intolerable because of problems with job, family, finances, intrapsychic conflict; when desires and conscience conflict, severe tension is released in an explosive way • Impulsive behavior releases tension temporarily but (guilt vs. pleasure causes conflict) an intrapsychic conflict again develops, causing recurring need for release of tension

that many of these patients do not respond well to interviewing, whereas others are charming masters of deceit. Offer patient, persistent, consistent, and flexible care. Take a direct, involved approach to ensure the patient's trust.

Nursing goals for the patient with a personality disorder include teaching social skills; reinforcing appropriate behavior; setting limits on inappropriate behavior; encouraging expression of feelings, self-analysis of behavior, and accountability for actions; and finally, helping the patient seek appropriate employment.

Pharyngitis

Description
The most common throat disorder, pharyngitis is an acute or chronic inflammation of the pharynx. It is widespread among adults who live or work in dusty or very dry environments, use their voices excessively, use tobacco or alcohol habitually, or suffer from chronic sinusitis, persistent coughs, or allergies. Acute pharyngitis may precede the common cold or other communicable diseases. Chronic pharyngitis is often an extension of nasopharyngeal obstruction or inflammation. Uncomplicated pharyngitis usually subsides in 3 to 10 days.

Causes
• Virus, in 90% of patients
• Bacteria, most often streptococci, especially in children

Signs and symptoms
• Sore throat
• Slight difficulty swallowing. Swallowing saliva is usually more painful than swallowing food.
• Possible sensation of a lump in the throat

• Possible constant, aggravating urge to swallow
• Reddened, inflamed posterior pharyngeal wall
• Red, edematous mucous membranes studded with white and yellow follicles
• Exudate (usually confined to the lymphoid areas of the throat, sparing the tonsillar pillars)
• Associated features: possible mild fever, headache, and muscle and joint pain (especially in bacterial pharyngitis)

Diagnostic tests
Throat culture may identify bacterial organisms if they are the cause of inflammation.

Treatment
Treatment of acute viral pharyngitis is usually symptomatic, consisting mainly of rest, warm saline gargles, throat lozenges containing a mild anesthetic, plenty of fluids, and analgesics, as needed. If the patient cannot swallow fluids, hospitalization may be required for I.V. hydration.

Bacterial pharyngitis necessitates rigorous treatment with penicillin—or another broad-spectrum antibiotic if the patient is allergic to penicillin—because streptococci are the chief infecting organisms. Antibiotic therapy should continue for 48 hours after visible signs of infection have disappeared, or for at least 7 to 10 days.

Chronic pharyngitis requires the same supportive measures as acute pharyngitis but with greater emphasis on eliminating the underlying cause, such as an allergen. Preventive measures include adequate humidification and avoiding excessive exposure to air conditioning. In addition, the patient who smokes should be urged to stop smoking.

Clinical implications
• Administer analgesics and warm saline gargles, as ordered and as appropriate. Encourage the patient to drink plenty of fluids (up to 2,500 ml/day).

- Monitor intake and output scrupulously, and watch for signs of dehydration (cracked lips, dry mucous membranes, low urinary output). Provide meticulous mouth care to prevent dry lips and oral pyoderma, and maintain a restful environment.
- Obtain throat cultures, and administer antibiotics, as ordered. If the patient has acute bacterial pharyngitis, emphasize the importance of completing the full course of antibiotic therapy. Teach the patient with chronic pharyngitis how to minimize sources of throat irritation in the environment, such as by using a bedside humidifier. Refer the patient to a smoking cessation program, if appropriate.

Phenylketonuria
(Phenylalaninemia, phenylpyruvic oligophrenia)

Description
Phenylketonuria (PKU) is an inborn error of phenylalanine metabolism. In the United States, this disorder occurs once in approximately 14,000 births. About 1 person in 60 is an asymptomatic carrier.

Causes
This disorder is caused by the absence or deficiency of phenylalanine hydroxylase, the enzyme responsible for converting the amino acid phenylalanine into tyrosine. Accumulation of phenylalanine is toxic to brain tissue. PKU is transmitted by an autosomal recessive gene.

Signs and symptoms
An infant with PKU appears normal at birth but by 4 months of age begins to show signs of arrested brain development.

- Mental retardation (can be minimized by early detection and treatment)
- Personality disturbances (schizoid and antisocial personality patterns and uncontrollable temper)
- Lighter complexion than unaffected sibling
- Often, blue eyes
- Macrocephaly
- Eczematous skin lesions or dry, rough skin
- Musty (mousy) odor
- Seizures (usually begin 6 to 12 months after birth in about one-third of patients)
- Hyperactivity
- Irritability
- Purposeless, repetitive motions
- Increased muscle tone
- Awkward gait

Diagnostic tests
Most states require screening for PKU at birth.

- The Guthrie screening test on a capillary blood sample (bacterial inhibition assay) reliably detects PKU. Since phenylalanine levels may be normal at birth, however, the infant should be reevaluated after he has received dietary protein for 24 to 48 hours.
- Adding a few drops of 10% ferric chloride solution to a wet diaper is another method of detecting PKU. If the area turns a deep, bluish-green color, phenylpyruvic acid is present in the urine.
- Phenylalanine blood levels are elevated. This test plus the presence of phenylpyruvic acid in the infant's urine confirm the diagnosis. (Urine should also be tested 4 to 6 weeks after birth, because urinary levels of phenylpyruvic acid vary with the amount of protein ingested.)

Treatment
Treatment consists of restricting dietary intake of the amino acid phenylalanine to keep phenylalanine blood levels between 3 and 9 mg/dl. Since most natural proteins contain 5% phe-

nylalanine, they must be limited in the child's diet. An enzymatic hydrolysate of casein, such as Lofenalac powder or Progestimil powder, is substituted for milk in the diets of affected infants. This milk substitute contains a minimal amount of phenylalanine, normal amounts of other amino acids, and added amounts of carbohydrate and fat. When blood and urine tests are acceptable, phenylalanine restrictions may be relaxed.

Such a diet calls for careful monitoring. Since the body does not make phenylalanine, overzealous dietary restriction can induce phenylalanine deficiency, producing lethargy, anorexia, anemia, skin rashes, and diarrhea.

Clinical implications

In caring for a phenylketonuric child, it is especially important to teach both the parents and child about this disease and to provide emotional support and counseling. (Psychological and emotional problems may result from the difficult dietary restrictions.) Teach the child and his parents about the critical importance of adhering to his diet. The child must avoid breads, cheese, eggs, flour, meat, poultry, fish, nuts, milk, legumes, and Nutrasweet. He will need frequent tests for urine phenylpyruvic and blood phenylalanine levels to evaluate the diet's effectiveness.

As the child grows older and is supervised less closely, his parents have less control over what he eats. As a result, deviation from the restricted diet becomes more likely, and so does the risk of further brain damage. Encourage parents to allow the child some choices in the kinds of low-protein foods he wants to eat so that he will feel trusted and more responsible. Teach parents about normal physical and mental growth and development so that they can recognize developmental delays that may point to excessive phenylalanine intake.

To prevent this disorder, infants should be routinely screened for PKU, since detection and control of phenyl-

alanine intake soon after birth can prevent severe mental retardation. Refer phenylketonuric females who reach reproductive age for genetic counseling, since recent research indicates that their offspring may have a higher than normal incidence of brain damage; microcephaly; and major congenital malformations, especially of the heart and central nervous system. Such damage may be prevented with a low-phenylalanine diet during pregnancy.

Pheochromocytoma

Description

Pheochromocytoma is a chromaffin-cell tumor of the adrenal medulla that secretes an excess of the catecholamines epinephrine and norepinephrine. According to some estimates, about 0.5% of newly diagnosed patients with hypertension have pheochromocytoma. A history of acute episodes of hypertension strongly suggests pheochromocytoma. This tumor is usually benign, but it may be malignant in as many as 10% of patients. It affects all races and both sexes, occurring primarily between ages 30 and 40.

Often, pheochromocytoma is diagnosed during pregnancy, when uterine pressure on the tumor induces more frequent attacks. Such attacks can prove fatal for both mother and fetus as a result of cerebrovascular accident, acute pulmonary edema, cardiac dysrhythmias, or hypoxia.

This disorder is potentially fatal, but prognosis is generally good with treatment. Pheochromocytoma-induced kidney damage is irreversible, however.

Causes

Pheochromocytoma may result from an inherited autosomal dominant trait.

Signs and symptoms

Symptomatic episodes may recur as seldom as once every 2 months or as often as 25 times a day. They may occur spontaneously or may follow certain precipitating events, such as postural change, exercise, laughter, smoking, induction of anesthesia, urination, or a change in environmental or body temperature.

- Persistent or paroxysmal hypertension (the cardinal sign)
- Palpitations
- Tachycardia
- Headache
- Diaphoresis
- Pallor
- Warmth or flushing
- Paresthesia
- Tremor
- Excitation
- Fright
- Nervousness
- Feelings of impending doom
- Abdominal pain
- Tachypnea
- Nausea and vomiting
- Postural hypotension
- Paradoxical response to antihypertensive drugs (common)
- Glycosuria
- Hyperglycemia
- Hypermetabolism

Diagnostic tests

- Increased urinary excretion of total free catecholamine and its metabolites, vanillylmandelic acid (VMA) and metanephrine, as measured by analysis of a 2- to 4-hour or a 24-hour urine collection, confirms pheochromocytoma. Labile blood pressure necessitates urine collection during a hypertensive episode and comparison of this specimen to a baseline specimen.
- Direct assay of total plasma catecholamines may show levels 10 to 50 times higher than normal.
- Provocative tests with tyramine or glucagon and depressor tests (phentolamine) suggest the diagnosis. However, because they may precipitate a hypertensive crisis or result in a false positive or negative, they are rarely used.
- Angiography demonstrates an adrenal medullary tumor; intravenous pyelography with nephrotomography, adrenal venography, or CT scan helps locate the tumor.
- Palpation of the area surrounding the tumor may induce a typical acute attack and help confirm the diagnosis if the tumor is palpable.

Treatment

Surgical removal of the tumor is the treatment of choice. To decrease blood pressure, an alpha-adrenergic blocking agent (phentolamine or phenoxybenzamine) or, more recently, metyrosine (which blocks catecholamine synthesis) is administered from 1 day to 2 weeks before surgery. A beta-adrenergic blocking agent (propranolol) may also be used after achieving alpha blockade. Postoperatively, I.V. fluids, plasma volume expanders, vasopressors, and transfusions may be required if marked hypotension occurs. However, persistent hypertension in the immediate postoperative period is more common.

If surgery is not feasible, alpha- and beta-adrenergic blocking agents—such as phenoxybenzamine and propranolol, respectively—are beneficial in controlling catecholamine effects and preventing attacks. Acute attack or hypertensive crisis requires I.V. administration of phentolamine (push or drip) or nitroprusside to normalize blood pressure.

Clinical implications

- To ensure the reliability of urine catecholamine measurements, make sure the patient avoids foods high in vanillin (such as coffee, nuts, chocolate, and bananas) for 2 days before urine collection for VMA measurements. Also, be aware of possible drug therapy that may interfere with the accurate determination of VMA (such as guaifenesin and salicylates). Collect the urine in a special container, with hydrochloric acid, that has been prepared by the laboratory.

• Obtain blood pressure readings often, since transient hypertensive attacks are possible. Tell the patient to report headaches, palpitations, nervousness, or other symptoms of an acute attack. If hypertensive crisis develops, monitor blood pressure and heart rate every 2 to 5 minutes until blood pressure stabilizes at an acceptable level.

• Check urine for glucose, and watch for weight loss from hypermetabolism.

• After surgery, blood pressure may rise or fall sharply. Keep the patient quiet. Provide a private room, if possible, since excitement may trigger a hypertensive episode. Postoperative hypertension is common, because the stress of surgery and manipulation of the adrenal gland stimulate secretion of catecholamines. Since this excess secretion causes profuse sweating, keep the room cool, and change the patient's clothing and bedding often. If the patient receives phentolamine, monitor blood pressure closely. Observe and record side effects: dizziness, hypotension, tachycardia. The first 24 to 48 hours immediately after surgery are the most critical, since blood pressure can drop drastically.

• If the patient is receiving vasopressors I.V., check blood pressure every 3 to 5 minutes, and regulate the drip to maintain a safe pressure. Arterial pressure lines facilitate constant monitoring.

• Watch for abdominal distention and return of bowel sounds.

• Check dressings and vital signs for indications of hemorrhage (increased pulse rate, decreased blood pressure, cold and clammy skin, pallor, unresponsiveness).

• Give analgesics for pain, as ordered, but monitor blood pressure carefully, since many analgesics, especially meperidine, can cause hypotension.

• If autosomal dominant transmission of pheochromocytoma is suspected, the patient's family should also be evaluated for this condition.

Phobias
(Phobic disorder, phobic neurosis)

Description
Classified as a form of anxiety disorder, a phobia is a persistent, irrational fear of places or things that compels the patient to avoid them. Although he knows that his fear is out of proportion to any actual danger, the patient cannot control it or explain it away. Many people harbor irrational fears, such as the fear of harmless insects, which have no major impact on their lives. In contrast, the phobic patient's irrational fear causes severe distress and impairment of function. These patients usually have no family history of psychiatric illness or of the same phobia. Most often, diagnosis of a phobia is based on careful history taking, observation of the patient, and a description of his behavior by the patient, his family, and friends. Patient interviews and a mental status examination help to confirm the diagnosis of a phobic disorder. Because phobias tend to be chronic and resistant to treatment, the prognosis is only fair.

Three types of phobia exist: agoraphobia, social phobia, and simple phobia. (See *Identifying Phobic Disorders.*) Of the milder forms of mental illness, phobias are among the most persistent.

Causes
• Drug withdrawal
• Drug abuse
• Anxiety-related behavior, such as the inability to cope with anger and dependence

Identifying Phobic Disorders

Phobic disorders can take three forms and can even coexist in some patients. To help identify phobias, review the following information.

Agoraphobia affects 60% of all phobic patients who seek help. This severe phobia commonly affects women and tends to be chronic, with occasional remissions and flare-ups. Patients with agoraphobia fear being alone and losing control in public places where escape is difficult or where help is not available. Typically, they fear *situations*, such as being in crowds, tunnels, or elevators. These fears can dominate their lives, restricting their normal activities and even confining them to their homes.

Social phobias are similar to agoraphobia. The central fear is one of self-embarrassment, which compels the patient to avoid the scrutiny of others. But most of these fears involve specific *functions*, such as using public lavatories or speaking in public. Characteristically, social phobias affect adolescents.

Simple phobias are the most common, easiest to identify, and most thematic. The patient fears certain objects or situations, such as animals, lightning, or high places. Usually, these fears begin in childhood and follow a chronic course with no remissions. They almost always stem from an actual or anticipated confrontation with the feared object or situation.

Signs and symptoms

All types of phobias
—Severe anxiety, often panic
—Discomfort that is out of proportion to the threat of the feared object or situation
—Profuse sweating
—Poor motor control
—Tachycardia
—Elevated blood pressure

Simple phobias
—If the patient suddenly confronts the feared object or situation, he may suffer a panic attack.

Social phobias
—The patient feels shameful, inept, or stupid in social interaction and expects others to criticize or laugh at him. His anxiety is not focused.

Agoraphobia
—Anxiety causes the patient to restrict his movements to an increasingly smaller area, leading to the inability to leave home without suffering a panic attack. To avoid leaving the familiar setting of his home, he may become pleading, demanding, manipulative, or even infantile. A feeling of helplessness predominates, and obsessive behavior often occurs.

Treatment

The effectiveness of treatment depends on the severity of the patient's phobia. Because phobic behavior may never be completely cured, the goal of treatment is to help the patient function effectively. Although antianxiety drugs may help control phobia, they must be prescribed with caution to prevent addiction. Antidepressants may help relieve symptoms in patients with agoraphobia, but they cannot cure it completely.

Systematic desensitization, a behavioral therapy, may be more effective than drugs, especially if it includes encouragement, instruction, and suggestion. Such therapy should help the patient understand that his phobia is symbolic of a more fundamental anxiety and that he must deal with it directly.

In some cities, phobia clinics and

Mechanisms of Anxiety Disorders

In generalized anxiety disorder or panic disorder, anxiety is the primary feature.

In phobic disorder, anxiety results when the patient *confronts* a threatening situation.

In obsessive-compulsive disorder, anxiety results when the patient *resists* threatening thoughts and feelings.

In posttraumatic stress disorder, the patient *reexperiences* anxiety related to an exceptionally traumatic event.

---

group therapy are available. People who have recovered from phobias can often help other phobic patients.

Clinical implications

• Stay with the patient until he feels comfortable alone.

• Work in an unhurried, reassuring manner. To make the atmosphere conducive to expression of feelings, intervene calmly, listen actively, and reinforce and encourage the patient constantly. Provide privacy, if needed.

• Give feedback and reliable information about the feared object or situation. Support a realistic view of the situation to reduce fear.

• Ask the patient how he normally copes with the fear. When he is able to face the fear, encourage him to verbalize and explore his personal strengths and resources with you.

• Prevent unpleasant surprises that could intensify the patient's fear.

• Avoid enforcing inactivity, which can actually increase fear.

• Reduce demands on the patient so that he has more energy available for coping.

• Teach the patient to use a systematic desensitization technique, such as deep-breathing or relaxation exercises. Then bring the feared object closer until he can tolerate it with less anxiety.

• Explain how fatigue can increase stress and fear.

• Suggest ways to channel the patient's energy and relieve stress (such as running and creative activities).

• Recommend relaxation methods, such as listening to music and meditating.

• Educate the patient's family and friends about the phobia and help them become a support system.

• Refer the patient to a physician for medical intervention, if necessary.

(Also see *Mechanisms of Anxiety Disorders*.)

Pilonidal disease

Description

In pilonidal disease, a coccygeal cyst—which usually contains hair—becomes infected and produces an abscess, a draining sinus, or a fistula.

Causes

Congenital

—Tendency to hirsutism

Acquired

—Stretching or irritation of the sacrococcygeal area (intergluteal fold) from prolonged rough exercise (such as horseback riding), heat, excessive perspiration, or constricting clothing

Signs and symptoms

Usually, a pilonidal cyst produces no symptoms until it becomes infected.

• Local pain

• Tenderness

• Swelling

- Heat
- Continuous or intermittent purulent drainage
- Chills
- Fever
- Headache
- Malaise
- On physical examination, a possible series of openings along the midline, with thin, brown, foul-smelling drainage or a protruding tuft of hair; possible purulent drainage with pressure on the sinus tract

Diagnostic tests
Cultures of discharge from the infected sinus may show staphylococci or skin bacteria but do not usually contain bowel bacteria.

Treatment
Conservative treatment of pilonidal disease consists of incision and drainage of abscesses, regular extraction of protruding hairs, and sitz baths (four to six times daily). However, persistent infections may necessitate surgical excision of the entire affected area. After excision of a pilonidal abscess, the patient requires regular follow-up care to monitor wound healing. The surgeon may periodically palpate the wound during healing with a cotton-tipped applicator, curette excess granulation tissue, and extract loose hairs to promote wound healing from the inside out and to prevent dead cells from collecting in the wound. Complete healing may take several months.

Clinical implications
- Before incision and drainage of pilonidal abscess, assure the patient he will receive adequate pain relief.
- After surgery, check the compression dressing for signs of excessive bleeding, and change the dressing, as directed. Encourage the patient to walk within 24 hours.
- Tell the patient to wear a gauze sponge over the wound site after the dressing is removed, to allow ventilation and prevent friction from clothing. Recommend correction of the underlying inflammatory process, as necessary.
- Prepare the patient for digital examination and testing by explaining procedures thoroughly.
- After surgery, check vital signs often until the patient is stable. Watch for signs of hemorrhage (excessive blood on rectal dressing).
- If surgery was performed under spinal anesthesia, record first leg motion, and keep the patient lying flat for 6 to 8 hours after surgery.
- When the patient's condition is stable, resume normal diet, and record time of first bowel movement. Administer stool softeners, as ordered. Give analgesics, provide sitz baths, and change perianal dressing, as ordered.

Pituitary tumors

Description
Pituitary tumors, which constitute 10% of intracranial neoplasms, originate most often in the anterior pituitary (adenohypophysis). Pituitary tumors are not malignant in the strict sense, but because their growth is invasive, they are considered neoplastic. They occur in adults of both sexes, usually during the third and fourth decades of life. The three tissue types of pituitary tumors include chromophobe adenoma (90%), basophil adenoma, and eosinophil adenoma. Prognosis is fair to good, depending on the extent to which the tumor spreads beyond the sella turcica.

Causes
Unknown

Risk factors
- A predisposition to pituitary tumors may be inherited through an autosomal dominant trait.

- Chromophobe adenoma may be associated with production of adrenocorticotropic hormone (ACTH), melanocyte-stimulating hormone, growth hormone, and prolactin.
- Basophil adenoma may be associated with evidence of excessive ACTH production and consequently with signs of Cushing's syndrome.
- Eosinophil adenoma may be associated with excessive growth hormone.

Signs and symptoms
Neurologic
—Frontal headache
—Visual symptoms (beginning with blurring and progressing to field cuts [hemianopias] and then unilateral blindness)
—Cranial nerve involvement (III, IV, VI) resulting in strabismus; double vision, with compensating head tilting and dizziness; conjugate deviation of gaze; nystagmus; lid ptosis; and limited eye movements
—Increased intracranial pressure
—Possible personality changes or dementia
—Seizures
—Rhinorrhea
Endocrine
—Symptoms of hypopituitarism (for example, amenorrhea, decreased libido and impotence in men, skin changes [waxy appearance, decreased wrinkles, and pigmentation], loss of axillary and pubic hair, lethargy, weakness, increased fatigability, intolerance to cold, and constipation)
—Addisonian crisis (nausea, vomiting, hypoglycemia, hypotension, and circulatory collapse)
—Possible signs of diabetes insipidus
—Amenorrhea and galactorrhea, with prolactin-secreting adenomas
—Acromegaly, with growth hormone–secreting adenomas
—Cushing's syndrome, with ACTH-secreting adenomas

Diagnostic tests
- Skull X-rays and CT scans show enlargement of the sella turcica or erosion of its floor. If growth hormone secretion predominates, X-rays show enlarged paranasal sinuses and mandible, thickened cranial bones, and separated teeth.
- Carotid angiogram shows displacement of the anterior cerebral and internal carotid arteries if the tumor mass is enlarging; it also rules out intracerebral aneurysm.
- CT scan may confirm the existence of the adenoma and accurately depict its size.
- Cerebrospinal fluid analysis may show increased protein levels.
- Endocrine function tests may contribute helpful information, but results are often ambiguous and inconclusive.

Treatment
Surgical options include transfrontal removal of large tumors impinging on the optic apparatus and transsphenoidal resection for smaller tumors confined to the pituitary fossa. Radiation is the primary treatment for small, nonsecretory tumors that do not extend beyond the sella turcica or for patients who may be poor postoperative risks; otherwise, it is an adjunct to surgery.

Postoperative treatment includes hormone replacement with cortisone, thyroid, and sex hormones; correction of electrolyte imbalance; and insulin therapy as necessary.

Drug therapy may include bromocriptine, an ergot derivative that shrinks prolactin-secreting and growth hormone–secreting tumors. Cyproheptadine, an antiserotonin drug, can reduce increased corticosteroid levels in the patient with Cushing's syndrome.

Adjuvant radiotherapy is used when only partial removal of the tumor is possible. Cryohypophysectomy (the freezing of the area with a probe inserted by transsphenoidal route) is a promising alternative to surgical dissection of the tumor.

Clinical implications

• Conduct a comprehensive health history and physical assessment to establish the time of onset of neurologic and endocrine dysfunction and to provide baseline data for later comparison.

• Establish a supportive, trusting relationship with the patient and family to assist them in coping with the diagnosis, treatment, and potential long-term changes. Make sure they understand that the patient needs lifelong evaluations and possibly hormone replacement.

• Reassure the patient that some of the distressing physical and behavioral signs and symptoms caused by pituitary dysfunction (for example, altered sexual drive, impotence, infertility, loss of hair, and emotional lability) will disappear with treatment.

• Maintain a safe, clutter-free environment for the visually impaired or acromegalic patient. Reassure him that he will probably recover his sight.

• Position patients who have undergone supratentorial or transphenoidal hypophysectomy with the head of the bed elevated about 30 degrees, to promote venous drainage from the head and reduce cerebral edema. Place the patient on his side to allow drainage of secretions and prevent aspiration.

• Withhold oral fluids, which can cause vomiting and subsequent increased intracranial pressure. Do not allow a patient who has had transsphenoidal surgery to blow his nose. Watch for cerebrospinal fluid drainage from the nose. Also check for symptoms of cerebral edema and bleeding. Monitor for signs of infection from the contaminated upper respiratory tract. Make sure the patient understands that he will lose his sense of smell.

• Regularly compare the patient's

postoperative neurologic status (especially level of consciousness) with your baseline assessment.

• Monitor intake and output to detect fluid and electrolyte imbalances.

• Before discharge, encourage the patient to purchase and wear a Medic Alert bracelet or necklace that identifies his hormone deficiencies and their proper treatment.

Pityriasis rosea

Description

Pityriasis rosea is an acute, inflammatory, self-limiting skin disease that is not contagious.

Causes

Unknown

Signs and symptoms

• An erythematous, oval "herald" patch that is slightly raised and often goes undetected

• Later, a generalized eruption of papulosquamous lesions

• Characteristic arrangement of lesions along body cleavage lines, producing a pattern similar to that of a pine tree

• Pruritus—usually mild but possibly severe

Treatment and clinical implications

Treatment focuses on relief of pruritus, with emollients, oatmeal baths, antihistamines, and, occasionally, exposure to ultraviolet light or sunlight. Topical steroids in a hydrophilic cream base may be beneficial. Rarely, if inflammation is severe, systemic corticosteroids may be required.

• Reassure the patient that pityriasis rosea is noncontagious, that spontaneous remission usually occurs in 2 to 6 weeks, and that lesions usually do not recur.

• Urge the patient not to scratch. Advise him that hot baths may intensify itching. Encourage the use of antipruritics.

Placenta previa

Description

In placenta previa, the placenta is implanted in the lower uterine segment, where it encroaches on the internal cervical os. This lower segment of the uterus fails to provide as much nourishment as the fundus. The placenta tends to spread out, seeking the blood supply it needs, and becomes larger and thinner than normal. Hemorrhage occurs as the internal cervical os effaces and dilates, tearing the uterine vessels. This disorder, one of the most common causes of bleeding during the second half of pregnancy, occurs more commonly in multigravidas than in primigravidas. Generally, termination of pregnancy is necessary when placenta previa is diagnosed in the presence of heavy maternal bleeding. Maternal prognosis is good if hemorrhage can be controlled. Fetal prognosis depends on gestational age and amount of blood lost. (See *Three Types of Placenta Previa*.)

Causes
Unknown

Risk factors
Factors that may affect the site of placental attachment to the uterine wall include the following:
• Early or late fertilization
• Receptivity and adequacy of the uterine lining
• Multiple pregnancy (the placenta requires a larger surface for attachment) and multiparity
• Previous uterine surgery
• Advanced maternal age

Signs and symptoms
• Painless third-trimester bleeding
• Various fetal malpresentations

Diagnostic tests
• Ultrasound scanning for placental position confirms the diagnosis, along with the pelvic examination.
• Hemoglobin is decreased.
• Soft-tissue X-rays, femoral arteriography, retrograde catheterization, or radioisotope scanning or localization locate the placenta. However, these tests are usually performed only when ultrasound is unavailable. They have limited value and are risky.

Treatment
Treatment of placenta previa is designed to assess, control, and restore blood loss; to deliver a viable infant; and to prevent coagulation disorders. Immediate therapy includes starting an I.V. line (using a large-bore catheter) for fluid and blood replacement; drawing blood for hemoglobin, hematocrit studies, and typing and cross matching; initiating external electronic fetal monitoring; monitoring maternal blood pressure, pulse rate, and respirations; and assessing the amount of vaginal bleeding.

If the fetus is premature, treatment consists of careful observation after determination of the degree of placenta previa and necessary fluid and blood replacement. If clinical evaluation confirms complete placenta previa, the patient is usually hospitalized because the risk of hemorrhage increases. As soon as the fetus is sufficiently mature, or with intervening severe hemorrhage, immediate delivery by cesarean section may be necessary. Vaginal delivery is considered only when the bleeding is minimal and placenta previa is marginal or when the labor is rapid. Because of the possibility of fetal blood loss through the placenta, a pediatric team should be on hand during delivery to immediately assess and treat neonatal shock, blood loss, and hypoxia.

Clinical implications
• If the patient shows active bleeding because of placenta previa, a primary

Three Types of Placenta Previa

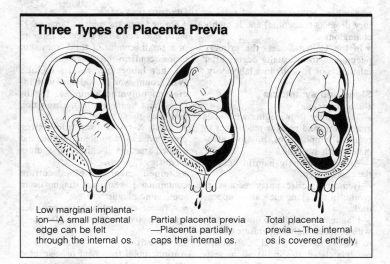

Low marginal implantation—A small placental edge can be felt through the internal os.

Partial placenta previa —Placenta partially caps the internal os.

Total placenta previa —The internal os is covered entirely.

nurse should be assigned for continuous monitoring.

• Prepare the patient and her family for a possible cesarean section and the birth of a premature infant. Thoroughly explain postpartum care, so the patient and her family know what measures to expect.

• Provide emotional support during labor. Because of the infant's prematurity, the patient may not be given analgesics: labor pain may be intense. Reassure her of her progress throughout labor, and keep her informed of fetal condition. Although neonatal death is a possibility, continued monitoring and prompt management reduce this prospect.

Complications
Maternal and neonatal shock

Plague
(Black death)

Description
Plague is an acute infection that occurs in several forms: bubonic plague, the

most common; septicemic plague, a severe, rapid, systemic form; and pneumonic plague, which can be an acutely fulminant primary form or can be secondary to bubonic plague. Without treatment, mortality is about 60% in bubonic plague and approaches 100% in both septicemic and pneumonic plague. With treatment, reported mortality is approximately 18%. Prognosis is related to the delay between onset and treatment and to the patient's age and physical condition.

Causes
The gram-negative, nonmotile, nonsporulating bacillus *Yersinia pestis* (formerly called *Pasteurella pestis*)

Mode of transmission
• Plague is usually transmitted to a human through the bite of a flea from an infected rodent host, such as a rat, squirrel, prairie dog, or hare.

• Occasionally, transmission occurs when infected animals or their tissues are handled.

• A secondary pneumonic form is

transmitted by contaminated respiratory droplets (coughing) and is highly contagious.
• In the United States, the primary pneumonic form usually occurs after inhalation of *Y. pestis* in a laboratory.

Signs and symptoms
Bubonic plague
—The milder form begins with malaise, fever, and pain or tenderness in regional lymph nodes, possibly associated with swelling.
—An excruciatingly painful bubo is the classic sign.
—Hemorrhagic areas may become necrotic; in the skin, such areas appear dark.
—Plague may also begin dramatically, with a sudden high temperature of 103° to 106° F. (39.5° to 41.1° C.), chills, myalgia, headache, prostration, restlessness, disorientation, delirium, toxemia, and staggering gait.
—Occasional symptoms include abdominal pain, nausea, vomiting, and constipation, followed by diarrhea (frequently bloody), skin mottling, petechiae, and circulatory collapse.
Primary pneumonic plague
—High fever
—Chills
—Severe headache
—Tachycardia
—Tachypnea
—Dyspnea
—Productive cough (first, mucoid sputum; later, frothy pink or red sputum)
Secondary pneumonic plague
—Cough, producing bloody sputum
—Severe prostration
—Respiratory distress
Septicemic plague
—Typically, no overt lymph node enlargement
—Hyperpyrexia
—Convulsions
—Prostration
—Shock and disseminated intravascular coagulation (DIC)

Diagnostic tests
• Stained smears and cultures of *Y. pestis* obtained from a needle aspirate of a small amount of fluid from skin lesions confirm this diagnosis.
• Other laboratory results include WBC count over 20,000/mm³ with increased polymorphonuclear leukocytes, and hemagglutination reaction (antibody titer).
• Chest X-ray shows fulminating pneumonia in pneumonic plague, and stained smear and culture of sputum identifies *Y. pestis*.
• Stained smear and blood culture containing *Y. pestis* are diagnostic in septicemic plague.
• A fluorescent antibody test provides a presumptive diagnosis of plague.

Treatment
Antimicrobial treatment of suspected plague must begin immediately after blood specimens have been taken for culture. Usually, treatment consists of large doses of streptomycin, the drug proven most effective against *Y. pestis*. Other effective drugs include tetracycline, chloramphenicol, kanamycin, and possibly trimethoprimsulfamethoxazole. Penicillins are ineffective against plague.

In both septicemic and pneumonic plagues, lifesaving antimicrobial treatment must begin within 18 hours of onset. Supportive management aims to control fever, shock, and convulsions and to maintain fluid balance.

After antimicrobial therapy has begun, glucocorticoids can combat life-threatening toxemia and shock. Diazepam relieves restlessness. If the patient develops DIC, treatment may include heparin.

Clinical implications
Patients with plague infections require strict isolation, which may be discontinued 48 hours after antimicrobial therapy begins unless respiratory symptoms develop.
• Carefully dispose of soiled dressings, feces, and sputum, and launder

soiled linens. When caring for a patient with pneumonic plague, always wear a gown, mask, and gloves. Handle all exudates, purulent discharge, and laboratory specimens with rubber gloves. For further information on precautions, consult your infection control officer.

• Treat buboes with hot, moist compresses. Never excise or drain them, since this may spread the infection.

• When septicemic plague causes peripheral tissue necrosis, prevent further injury to necrotic tissue. Avoid using restraints or armboards, and pad the side rails.

• Obtain a history of patient contacts. They should be quarantined for 6 days of observation. Administer prophylactic tetracycline, as ordered.

• Report suspected cases to local public health officials so they can identify the source of infection.

• To help prevent plague, discourage contact with wild animals (especially those that are sick or dead), and support programs to reduce insect and rodent populations. Recommend immunization with plague vaccine to travelers to or residents of endemic areas, even though the effect of immunization is transient.

Complications
Septicemic plague causes widespread nonspecific tissue damage—such as peritoneal or pleural effusions, pericarditis, and meningitis—and is rapidly fatal unless promptly and correctly treated. DIC and shock may also occur.

Platelet function disorders

Description
Platelet function disorders are similar to thrombocytopenia but result from platelet dysfunction rather than platelet deficiency. They characteristically cause defects in platelet adhesion or procoagulation activity (ability to bind coagulation factors to form a stable fibrin clot). Such disorders may also create defects in platelet aggregation and thromboxane A_2 and may produce abnormalities by preventing the release of adenosine diphosphate (defective platelet release reaction). Prognosis varies widely.

Causes
• Inheritance (autosomal recessive)
• Drugs such as aspirin or carbenicillin
• Systemic diseases such as uremia
• Other hematologic disorders

Signs and symptoms
First overt signs
—Petechiae or purpura
—Excessive bruising
—Bleeding of the nose and gums
More serious signs
—External hemorrhage
—Internal hemorrhage into the muscles and visceral organs
—Excessive bleeding during surgery

Diagnostic tests
Prolonged bleeding time in a patient with both a normal platelet count and normal clotting factors suggests this diagnosis.

• Determination of the defective mechanism requires a blood film and a platelet function test to measure platelet release reaction and aggregation. Depending on the type of platelet dysfunction, some or all of the test results may be abnormal.

• Poor clot retraction and decreased prothrombin conversion are typical findings.

• Baseline testing includes CBC and differential and appropriate tests to determine hemorrhage sites.

• Plasma clotting factors, platelet counts, and prothrombin, activated partial thromboplastin, and thrombin times are usually normal.

Treatment

Platelet replacement is the only satisfactory treatment for inherited platelet dysfunction. However, acquired platelet function disorders respond to adequate treatment of the underlying disease or discontinuation of damaging drug therapy. Plasmapheresis effectively controls bleeding caused by a plasma element that is inhibiting platelet function. During this procedure, one or more units of whole blood are removed from the patient; the plasma is removed from the whole blood, and the remaining packed RBCs are reinfused.

Clinical implications

• Obtain an accurate patient history, including onset of bleeding, use of drugs (especially aspirin), and family history of bleeding disorders.
• Watch closely for bleeding from skin, nose, gums, GI tract, or an injury site.
• Help the patient avoid unnecessary trauma. Advise him to tell his dentist about this condition before undergoing oral surgery. (Also stress the need for good oral hygiene to help prevent such surgery.)
• Alert other health care team members to the patient's hemorrhagic potential, especially before he undergoes diagnostic tests that may cause trauma and bleeding.
• Observe the patient undergoing plasmapheresis for hypovolemia, hypotension, tachycardia, vasoconstriction, and other signs of volume depletion.
• If platelet dysfunction is inherited, help the patient and family understand and accept the nature of this disorder. Teach them how to manage potential bleeding episodes. Warn them that petechiae, ecchymoses, and bleeding from the nose, gums, and GI tract signal abnormal bleeding and should be reported immediately.
• Tell the patient with a known coagulopathy or hepatic disease to avoid aspirin, aspirin compounds, and other agents that impair coagulation.

• Instruct the patient to take measures to prevent bleeding, such as using an electric razor and soft-bristled toothbrush and not using power tools or drinking alcohol excessively.
• Advise the patient to wear a medical identification bracelet or to carry a card identifying him as a potential bleeder.

Pleural effusion and empyema

Description

Pleural effusion is an excess of fluid in the pleural space. Normally, this space contains a small amount of extracellular fluid that lubricates the pleural surfaces. Transudative pleural effusion results when excessive hydrostatic pressure or decreased osmotic pressure causes excessive amounts of fluid to pass across intact capillaries. Exudative pleural effusions result when capillaries exhibit increased permeability with or without changes in hydrostatic and colloid osmotic pressures, allowing protein-rich fluid to leak into the pleural space.

Empyema is the accumulation of pus and necrotic tissue in the pleural space. It is usually associated with infection. Blood (hemothorax) and chyle (chylothorax) may also collect in this space.

Causes

Transudative pleural effusion
—Congestive heart failure
—Hepatic disease with ascites
—Peritoneal dialysis
—Hypoalbuminemia
—Disorders resulting in overexpanded intravascular volume
Exudative pleural effusion
—Tuberculosis
—Subphrenic abscess
—Pancreatitis

—Bacterial or fungal pneumonitis or empyema
—Malignancy
—Pulmonary embolism with or without infarction
—Collagen disorders (lupus erythematosus and rheumatoid arthritis)
—Myxedema
—Chest trauma

Empyema
—May be idiopathic
—Possibly associated with pneumonitis, carcinoma, perforation, or esophageal rupture

Signs and symptoms

Pleural effusion
—Dyspnea
—Pleural friction rub
—Possible pleuritic pain that worsens with coughing or deep breathing
—Dry cough
—Dullness on percussion
—Tachycardia
—Tachypnea
—Decreased chest motion and breath sounds

Empyema
—Fever
—Malaise
—Night sweats
—Chest pain
—Cough
—Weight loss
—Absent or distant breath sounds
—Decreased respiratory excursion on the affected side

Diagnostic tests

• Chest X-ray shows radiopaque fluid in dependent regions.
• Pleural biopsy may be particularly useful for confirming tuberculosis or malignancy.
• The most useful test is thoracentesis, in which analysis of aspirated pleural fluid shows the following:
—In transudative effusions, specific gravity is usually < 1.015 and protein < 3 g/dl.
—In exudative effusions, ratio of protein in pleural fluid to serum is ≥ 0.5, pleural fluid LDH is ≥ 200 IU, and ratio of LDH in pleural fluid to LDH in serum is ≥ 0.6.
—In empyema, acute inflammatory WBCs and microorganisms are present.
—In empyema or rheumatoid arthritis, extremely decreased pleural fluid glucose levels occur.
—If a pleural effusion results from esophageal rupture or pancreatitis, amylase levels in aspirated fluid are usually higher than serum levels.
—In empyema, cell analysis shows leukocytosis.
—Aspirated fluid also may be tested for LE cells, antinuclear antibodies, and neoplastic cells. It may be analyzed for color and consistency; acid-fast bacillus, fungal, and bacterial cultures; and triglycerides (in chylothorax).

Treatment

Depending on the amount of fluid present, symptomatic effusion may require either thoracentesis to remove fluid or careful monitoring of the patient's own reabsorption of the fluid. Hemothorax requires drainage to prevent fibrothorax formation. Treatment of empyema requires insertion of one or more chest tubes after thoracentesis to allow drainage of purulent material and, possibly, decortication (surgical removal of the thick coating over the lung) or rib resection to allow open drainage and lung expansion. Empyema also requires parenteral antibiotics. Associated hypoxia requires oxygen administration.

Clinical implications

• Explain thoracentesis to the patient.
• Give reassurance during thoracentesis and observe for complications during and after the procedure.
• Administer oxygen and, in empyema, antibiotics, as ordered.
• Encourage the patient to do deep-breathing exercises to promote lung

expansion. Use an incentive spirometer to promote deep breathing.

• Provide meticulous chest tube care, and use aseptic technique for changing dressings around the tube insertion site in empyema. Record the amount, color, and consistency of any tube drainage.

• If the patient has open drainage through a rib resection or intercostal tube, use hand and dressing precautions. Since weeks of such drainage are usually necessary to obliterate the space, make visiting nurse referrals for patients who will be discharged with the tube in place.

• If pleural effusion was a complication of pneumonia or influenza, advise prompt medical attention for chest colds.

Pleurisy
(Pleuritis)

Description
Pleurisy is inflammation of the visceral and parietal pleurae that line the inside of the thoracic cage and envelop the lungs.

Causes
Pleurisy develops as a complication of the following:
• Pneumonia
• Tuberculosis
• Viruses
• Systemic lupus erythematosus
• Rheumatoid arthritis
• Uremia
• Dressler's syndrome
• Cancer
• Pulmonary infarction
• Chest trauma

Signs and symptoms
• Sharp, stabbing pain that increases with respiration may be so severe that it limits movement on the affected side during breathing.

• Dyspnea also occurs.
• Auscultation reveals a characteristic pleural friction rub—a coarse, creaky sound heard during late inspiration and early expiration, directly over the area of pleural inflammation.
• Palpation over the affected area may reveal coarse vibration.
• Other symptoms vary according to the underlying pathologic process.

Treatment
Treatment is generally symptomatic and it includes anti-inflammatory agents, analgesics, and bed rest. Severe pain may require intercostal nerve block. Pleurisy with pleural effusion calls for therapeutic and diagnostic thoracentesis.

Clinical implications
• Stress the importance of bed rest and plan your care to allow the patient as much uninterrupted rest as possible.
• Administer antitussives and pain medication, as ordered, but be careful not to overmedicate. If the pain requires a narcotic analgesic, warn the patient about to be discharged to avoid overuse because such medication depresses coughing and respiration.
• Encourage the patient to cough. To minimize pain, apply firm pressure at the site of the pain during coughing exercises.

Pneumonia

Description
Pneumonia is an acute infection of the lung parenchyma that often impairs gas exchange. Prognosis is usually good for people who have normal lungs and adequate host defenses before the onset of pneumonia; however, bacterial pneumonia is the fifth leading cause of death in debilitated patients.

Causes
• Primary pneumonia results from the inhalation or aspiration of a viral, bac-

terial, fungal, protozoal, mycobacterial, mycoplasmal, or rickettsial pathogen.

• Secondary pneumonia may follow initial lung damage from a noxious chemical or other insult (superinfection) or may result from hematogenous spread of bacteria from a distant focus. (See *Types of Pneumonia*, pp. 590 to 593.)

Risk factors
Bacterial and viral pneumonia
—Chronic illness and debilitation
—Cancer (particularly lung cancer)
—Abdominal and thoracic surgery
—Atelectasis
—Common colds or other viral respiratory infections
—Chronic respiratory disease
—Influenza
—Smoking
—Malnutrition
—Alcoholism
—Sickle cell disease
—Tracheostomy
—Exposure to noxious gases
—Aspiration
—Immunosuppressive therapy
Aspiration pneumonia
—Old age
—Debilitation
—Nasogastric tube feedings
—Impaired gag reflex
—Poor oral hygiene
—Decreased level of consciousness

Signs and symptoms
• The five cardinal symptoms of early bacterial pneumonia are coughing, sputum production, pleuritic chest pain, shaking chills, and fever.
• Physical signs vary widely, ranging from diffuse, fine rales to signs of localized or extensive consolidation and pleural effusion.

Diagnostic tests
• Chest X-ray showing infiltrates and sputum smear demonstrating acute inflammatory cells support the diagnosis.

• Positive blood cultures in patients with pulmonary infiltrates strongly suggest pneumonia produced by the organisms isolated from the blood cultures.
• Occasionally, a transtracheal aspirate of tracheobronchial secretions or bronchoscopy with brushings may be done to obtain material for smear and culture.

Treatment
Antimicrobial therapy varies with the infecting agent. Therapy should be re-evaluated early in the course of treatment. Supportive measures include humidified oxygen therapy for hypoxia, mechanical ventilation for respiratory failure, a high-calorie diet and adequate fluid intake, bed rest, and an analgesic to relieve pleuritic chest pain. Patients with severe pneumonia who are mechanically ventilated may require positive end-expiratory pressure to facilitate adequate oxygenation.

Clinical implications
Correct supportive care can increase patient comfort, avoid complications, and speed recovery.
• Maintain patent airway and adequate oxygenation. Measure arterial blood gases, especially in hypoxic patients. Administer supplemental oxygen as ordered. (Usually oxygen is administered if PO_2 is less than 60 mm Hg.) Patients with underlying chronic lung disease should be given oxygen cautiously.
• Teach the patient how to cough and perform deep-breathing exercises to clear secretions, and encourage him to do so often. In severe pneumonia that requires endotracheal intubation or tracheostomy with or without mechanical ventilation, provide thorough respiratory care and suction often, using sterile technique, to remove secretions.
• Administer antibiotics, as ordered, and pain medication, as needed. Fever and dehydration may require I.V. fluids

Types of Pneumonia

TYPE	SIGNS AND SYMPTOMS
VIRAL **Influenza** (prognosis poor even with treatment; 50% mortality)	• Cough (initially nonproductive; later, purulent sputum), marked cyanosis, dyspnea, high fever, chills, substernal pain and discomfort, moist rales, frontal headache, myalgia • Death results from cardiopulmonary collapse
Adenovirus (insidious onset; usually affects young adults)	• Sore throat, fever, cough, chills, malaise, small amounts of mucoid sputum, retrosternal chest pain, anorexia, rhinitis, adenopathy, scattered rales, and rhonchi
Respiratory syncytial virus (most prevalent in infants and children)	• Listlessness, irritability, tachypnea with retraction of intercostal muscles, slight sputum production, fine moist rales, fever, severe malaise, and possibly cough or croup
Measles/rubeola	• Fever, dyspnea, cough, small amounts of sputum, coryza, skin rash, and cervical adenopathy
Chicken pox/varicella (uncommon in children, but present in 30% of adults with varicella)	• Cough, dyspnea, cyanosis, tachypnea, pleuritic chest pain, hemoptysis and rhonchi 1 to 6 days after onset of rash
Cytomegalovirus	• Difficult to distinguish from other nonbacterial pneumonias • Fever, cough, shaking chills, dyspnea, cyanosis, weakness, and diffuse rales • Occurs in neonates as devastating multisystemic infection; in normal adults resembles mononucleosis; in immunocompromised hosts, varies from clinically inapparent to devastating infection

DIAGNOSIS	TREATMENT
• *Chest X-ray:* diffuse bilateral bronchopneumonia radiating from hilus • *WBC count:* normal to slightly elevated • *Sputum smears:* no specific organisms	*Supportive:* for respiratory failure, endotracheal intubation and ventilator assistance; for fever, hypothermia blanket or antipyretics; for influenza A, amantadine
• *Chest X-ray:* patchy distribution of pneumonia, more severe than indicated by physical examination • *WBC count:* normal to slightly elevated	• Symptoms only treated • Mortality low; usually clears with no residual effects
• *Chest X-ray:* patchy bilateral consolidation • *WBC count:* normal to slightly elevated	• *Supportive:* humidified air, oxygen, antimicrobials often given until viral etiology confirmed • Complete recovery in 1 to 3 weeks
• *Chest X-ray:* reticular infiltrates, sometimes with hilar lymph node enlargement • *Lung tissue specimen:* characteristic giant cells	• *Supportive:* bed rest, adequate hydration, antimicrobials; assisted ventilation, if necessary
• *Chest X-ray:* shows more extensive pneumonia than indicated by physical examination, and bilateral, patchy, diffuse, nodular infiltrates • *Sputum analysis:* predominant mononuclear cells and characteristic intranuclear inclusion bodies, with characteristic skin rash, confirm diagnosis	• *Supportive:* adequate hydration, oxygen therapy in critically ill patients
• *Chest X-ray:* in early stages, variable patchy infiltrates; later, bilateral, nodular, and more predominant in lower lobes • *Percutaneous aspiration of lung tissue, transbronchial biopsy or open lung biopsy:* microscopic examination shows typical intranuclear and cytoplasmic inclusions; the virus can be cultured from lung tissue	• Usually, benign and self-limiting in mononucleosislike form • *Supportive:* adequate hydration and nutrition, oxygen therapy, bed rest • In immunosuppressed patients, disease more severe and possibly fatal

(continued)

Types of Pneumonia (continued)

TYPE	SIGNS AND SYMPTOMS
BACTERIAL **Streptococcus** **(Diplococcus pneu-** **moniae)**	• Sudden onset of a single, shaking chill, and sustained temperature of 102° to 104° F. (38.9° to 40° C.); often preceded by upper respiratory tract infection
Klebsiella	• Fever and recurrent chills; cough producing rusty, bloody, viscous sputum (currant jelly); cyanosis of lips and nail beds due to hypoxemia; shallow, grunting respirations • Likely in patients with chronic alcoholism, pulmonary disease, and diabetes
Staphylococcus	• Temperature of 102° to 104° F. (38.9° to 40° C.), recurrent shaking chills, bloody sputum, dyspnea, tachypnea, and hypoxemia • Should be suspected with viral illness, such as influenza or measles, and in patients with cystic fibrosis
ASPIRATION Results from vomiting and aspiration of gastric or oropharyngeal contents into trachea and lungs	• Noncardiogenic pulmonary edema that may follow damage to respiratory epithelium from contact with stomach acid • Rales, dyspnea, cyanosis, hypotension, and tachycardia • May be subacute pneumonia with cavity formation, or lung abscess may occur if foreign body is present

and electrolyte replacement.

• Maintain adequate nutrition to offset high caloric utilization secondary to infection. Ask the dietary department to provide a high-calorie, high-protein diet consisting of soft, easy-to-eat foods. Encourage the patient to eat. As necessary, supplement oral feedings with nasogastric tube feedings or parenteral nutrition. Monitor fluid intake and output.

• Provide a quiet, calm environment for the patient, with frequent rest periods.

• Give emotional support by explaining all procedures (especially intuba-tion and suctioning) to the patient and his family. Encourage family visits.

• To control the spread of infection, dispose of secretions properly. Tell the patient to sneeze and cough into a disposable tissue; tape a waxed bag to the side of the bed for used tissues. To prevent pneumonia, advise the patient to avoid using antibiotics indiscriminately during minor viral infections, because this may result in upper air-

DIAGNOSIS	TREATMENT
• *Chest X-ray:* areas of consolidation, often lobar • *WBC count:* elevated • *Sputum culture:* may show gram-positive *S. pneumoniae;* this organism not always recovered	• *Antimicrobial therapy:* penicillin G (or erythromycin, in patients allergic to penicillin) for 7 to 10 days after obtaining culture specimen but without waiting for results
• *Chest X-ray:* typically, but not always, consolidation in the upper lobe that causes bulging of fissures • *WBC count:* elevated • *Sputum culture and Gram stain:* may show gram-positive cocci *Klebsiella*	• *Antimicrobial therapy:* aminoglycoside plus, in serious infections, a cephalosporin
• *Chest X-ray:* multiple abscesses and infiltrates; high incidence of empyema • *WBC count:* elevated • *Sputum culture and Gram stain:* may show gram-positive staphylococci	• *Antimicrobial therapy:* nafcillin or oxacillin for 14 days if staphylococci are penicillinase producing • Chest tube drainage of empyema
• *Chest X-ray:* locates areas of infiltrates, which suggest diagnosis	• *Antimicrobial therapy:* penicillin G or clindamycin • *Supportive:* oxygen therapy, suctioning, coughing, deep breathing, adequate hydration, and I.V. steroids

way colonization with antibiotic-resistant bacteria. If the patient then develops pneumonia, the infecting organisms may require treatment with more toxic antibiotics.

• Encourage annual influenza vaccination and Pneumovax for high-risk patients such as those with COPD, chronic heart disease, and sickle cell disease.

• Urge all bedridden and postoperative patients to perform deep-breathing and coughing exercises frequently. Position such patients properly to promote full aeration and drainage of secretions.

• To prevent aspiration during nasogastric tube feedings, elevate the patient's head, check the position of the tube, and administer feedings slowly. Do not give large volumes at one time, because this could cause vomiting. If the patient has an endotracheal tube, inflate the tube cuff. Keep his head elevated for at least half an hour after feeding.

Complications

• Hypoxemia
• Respiratory failure
• Pleural effusion
• Empyema
• Lung abscess
• Bacteremia, with spread of infection to other parts of the body, resulting in meningitis, endocarditis, and pericarditis

Pneumothorax

Description

Pneumothorax is an accumulation of air or gas between the parietal and visceral pleurae. The amount of air or gas trapped in the intrapleural space determines the degree of lung collapse. In tension pneumothorax, air in the pleural space is under higher pressure than air in adjacent lung and vascular structures. Without prompt treatment, tension or large-volume pneumothorax results in fatal pulmonary and circulatory impairment.

Causes

Spontaneous pneumothorax
—Ruptured congenital blebs
—Ruptured emphysematous bullae
—Tubercular or malignant lesions that erode into the pleural space
—Interstitial lung disease, such as eosinophilic granuloma
Traumatic pneumothorax
—Insertion of a central venous pressure line
—Thoracic surgery
—Penetrating chest injury
—Transbronchial biopsy
—Thoracentesis or closed pleural biopsy
Tension pneumothorax
—Positive pleural pressure, which develops as a result of any of the causes of traumatic pneumothorax

Signs and symptoms

Spontaneous pneumothorax may be asymptomatic. Profound respiratory distress occurs in moderate-to-severe pneumothorax. Weak and rapid pulse, pallor, neck vein distention, and anxiety accompany tension pneumothorax. In general, however, symptoms of pneumothorax include the following:
• Sudden, sharp, pleuritic pain
• Asymmetric chest wall movement
• Shortness of breath
• Cyanosis
• Decreased or absent breath sounds over the collapsed lung
• Hyperresonance on the affected side
• Crackling beneath the skin, on palpation

Diagnostic tests

• Chest X-ray showing air in the pleural space and possibly mediastinal shift confirms the diagnosis.
• Arterial blood gas findings include pH less than 7.35, PO_2 less than 80 mm Hg, and PCO_2 above 45 mm Hg, if the pneumothorax is significant.

Treatment

Treatment is conservative for spontaneous pneumothorax in which no signs of increased pleural pressure (indicating tension pneumothorax) appear, lung collapse is less than 30%, and the patient shows no signs of dyspnea or other indications of physiologic compromise. Such treatment consists of bed rest; careful monitoring of blood pressure, pulse rate, and respirations; oxygen administration; and, possibly, needle aspiration of air with a large-bore needle attached to a syringe. If more than 30% of the lung is collapsed, treatment to reexpand lung includes placing a thoracostomy tube, connected to an underwater seal or suction at low pressures, in the second or third intercostal space in the midclavicular line.

Recurring spontaneous pneumothorax requires thoracotomy and pleurectomy. These procedures prevent recurrence by causing the lung to adhere to the parietal pleura. Traumatic or tension pneumothorax requires chest tube drainage. Traumatic pneumothorax may also require surgical repair.

Clinical implications

• Watch for pallor, gasping respirations, and sudden chest pain. Carefully monitor vital signs at least every hour for indications of shock, increasing respiratory distress, or mediastinal shift. Listen for breath sounds over both lungs. Falling blood pressure and rising pulse and respiration rates may indicate tension pneumothorax, which could be fatal without prompt treatment.

• Urge the patient to control coughing and gasping during thoracostomy. However, after the chest tube is in place, encourage him to cough and breathe deeply (at least once an hour) to facilitate lung expansion.

• In the patient undergoing chest tube drainage, watch for continuing air leakage (bubbling), indicating the lung defect has failed to close; this may require surgery. Also, watch for increasing subcutaneous emphysema by checking around the neck or at the tube insertion site for crackling beneath the skin. If the patient is on a ventilator, watch for difficulty in breathing in time with the ventilator, as well as pressure changes on ventilator gauges.

• Change dressings around the chest tube insertion site, as necessary. Be careful not to reposition or dislodge the tube. If the tube dislodges, place a petrolatum gauze dressing over the opening immediately to prevent rapid lung collapse.

• Monitor vital signs frequently after thoracotomy. Also, for the first 24 hours, assess respiratory status by checking breath sounds hourly. Observe the chest tube site for leakage, and note the amount and color of drainage. Walk the patient, as ordered (usually on the first postoperative day), to facilitate deep inspiration and lung expansion.

• Reassure the patient, and explain what pneumothorax is, what causes it, and all diagnostic tests and procedures. Make him as comfortable as possible. (The patient with pneumothorax is usually most comfortable sitting upright.)

Poisoning

Description

Inhalation, ingestion, or injection of or skin contamination with any toxic substance is a common problem. In fact, in the United States, approximately 10 million persons are poisoned annually, 4,000 of them fatally. In children, accidental poisoning is the fourth leading cause of death. Prognosis depends on the amount of poison absorbed, its toxicity, and the time interval between poisoning and treatment.

Causes

Poisoning in children
—Most commonly results from ingestion of salicylates, cleaning agents, insecticides, paints, cosmetics
Poisoning in adults
—Chemicals in the workplace, such as chlorine, carbon dioxide, hydrogen sulfide, and ammonia
—Improper cooking, canning, or storage of food
—Ingestion of or skin contamination from plants
—Accidental or intentional drug overdose

Signs and symptoms

Symptoms vary according to the poison, but may include the following:
• Decreased level of consciousness
• Headache
• Hypotension
• Cardiac dysrhythmias

Initial Assessment Checklist

Assess the ABCs first and intervene appropriately.

Check for:
- hypoactivity, decreased level of consciousness, bradycardia, or decreased respiratory rate, suggesting central nervous system (CNS) depression
- hyperactivity, tachycardia, tachypnea, or hyperventilation, suggesting CNS stimulation
- needle tracks, possibly indicating drug injection
- circumoral blisters or crystal residue, possibly indicating corrosive substance ingestion; blisters or erythema on the skin, possibly indicating barbiturate, carbon monoxide, or glutethimide poisoning; or powdered residue on the patient's skin or clothing, possibly from an insecticide

Intervene by:
- inducing vomiting with syrup of ipecac or performing gastric lavage
- starting an I.V. and giving dextrose 50% in water, thiamine, and naloxone (Narcan), as ordered, if the patient is unresponsive
- administering activated charcoal and cathartics, as ordered
- forcing diuresis and altering the patient's urine pH

Prepare for:
- advanced life support
- intubation and mechanically assisted ventilation
- administration of an antidote based on toxicology screening results
- hemodialysis, peritoneal dialysis, or hemoperfusion

- Dyspnea
- Seizures
- Blisters or erythema
- Burning sensation in mouth or throat

Diagnostic tests
- Toxicologic studies (including drug screens) of poison levels in the mouth, vomitus, urine, feces, or blood or on the victim's hands or clothing confirm the diagnosis.
- Chest X-rays may show pulmonary infiltrates or edema in inhalation poisoning.
- X-rays may show aspiration pneumonia in petroleum distillate inhalation.

Treatment
Treatment includes emergency resuscitation and support, prevention of further absorption of poison, continuing supportive or symptomatic care, and, when possible, a specific antidote. If barbiturate, glutethimide, or tranquil-

izer poisoning causes hypothermia, use a hyperthermia blanket to control the patient's temperature.

Clinical implications
- Assess cardiopulmonary and respiratory function. If necessary, begin CPR. Carefully monitor vital signs and level of consciousness.
- Depending on the poison, prevent further absorption of ingested poison by inducing emesis using syrup of ipecac or by administering gastric lavage and cathartics (magnesium sulfate). The effectiveness of treatment depends on the speed of absorption and the time elapsed between ingestion and removal. With syrup of ipecac, give warm water (usually less than 1 quart [less than 1 liter]) until vomiting occurs, or give another dose of ipecac, as ordered.

• Never induce emesis if you suspect corrosive acid poisoning, if the patient is unconscious or has convulsions, or if the gag reflex is impaired in a conscious patient. Instead, neutralize the poison by instilling the appropriate antidote by nasogastric tube. Common antidotes include milk, magnesium salts (milk of magnesia), activated charcoal, or other chelating agents (deferoxamine, edetate disodium [EDTA]). When possible, add the antidote to water or juice. (Note: The removal of hydrocarbon poisoning is controversial. In the conscious patient, because there is a lower risk of aspiration with ipecac-induced emesis than with lavage, emesis is becoming the preferred treatment, but some physicians still use lavage. Moreover, some believe that because of poor absorption, kerosene [a hydrocarbon] does not require removal from the GI tract; others believe removal depends on the amount ingested.)

• When you do want to induce emesis and the patient has already taken syrup of ipecac, do not give activated charcoal to neutralize the poison after emesis. Activated charcoal absorbs ipecac.

• To perform gastric lavage, instill 30 ml of fluid by nasogastric tube; then aspirate the liquid. Repeat until aspirate is clear. Save vomitus and aspirate for analysis. (To prevent aspiration in the unconscious patient, an endotracheal tube should be in place before lavage.)

• If several hours have passed since the patient ingested the poison, use large quantities of I.V. fluids to increase diuresis. The fluid used depends on the patient's acid-base balance and cardiovascular status, and on the flow rate.

• Severe poisoning by ingestion may call for peritoneal dialysis or hemodialysis.

• To prevent further absorption of inhaled poison, remove the patient to fresh or uncontaminated air. Alert the anesthesia department and provide supplemental oxygen. Some patients may require intubation.

• To prevent further absorption from skin contamination, remove the clothing covering the contaminated skin, and immediately flush the area with large amounts of water.

• If the patient is in severe pain, give analgesics, as ordered. Frequently monitor fluid intake and output, vital signs, and level of consciousness.

• Keep the patient warm, and provide support in a quiet environment.

• If the poison was ingested intentionally, refer the patient for counseling to prevent future suicide attempts.

• For more specific treatment, contact the local poison control center.

(See *Initial Assessment Checklist* and *Preventing Accidental Poisoning*.)

Preventing Accidental Poisoning

To prevent accidental poisoning, instruct patients to read the label before they take medicine. Tell them to store all medications and household chemicals properly, keep them out of reach of children, and discard old medications. Warn them not to take medicines prescribed for someone else, not to transfer medicines from their original bottles to other containers without labeling them properly, and never to transfer poisons to food containers. Parents should not take medicine in front of their young children or call medicine "candy" to get children to take it. Stress the importance of using toxic sprays only in well-ventilated areas and of following instructions carefully. Tell patients to use pesticides carefully and to keep the number of the nearest poison control center handy.

Poliomyelitis
(Polio, infantile paralysis)

Description

Poliomyelitis is an acute communicable disease ranging in severity from inapparent infection to fatal paralytic illness. Inapparent (subclinical) infections constitute 95% of all poliovirus infections. Abortive poliomyelitis is a minor illness. Major poliomyelitis involves the CNS and takes two forms: nonparalytic and paralytic. Children often show a biphasic course, in which the onset of major illness occurs after recovery from the minor illness stage.

When the disease affects the medulla of the brain, it is called bulbar paralytic poliomyelitis, which is the most perilous type. Incidence peaked during the 1940s and early 1950s, and led to the development of the Salk vaccine.

Minor polio outbreaks still occur, usually among nonimmunized groups, as among the Amish of Pennsylvania in 1979. The disease strikes most often during the summer and fall. Once confined mainly to infants and children, poliomyelitis occurs more often today in people over age 15.

Prognosis depends largely on the site affected. If the CNS is spared, prognosis is excellent. CNS infection can cause paralysis and death, however.

Causes

Poliovirus, which has three antigenically distinct serotypes—types I, II, and III

Mode of transmission

From person to person by direct contact with infected oropharyngeal secretions or feces

Signs and symptoms

Abortive poliomyelitis
This is a minor illness.
—Slight fever
—Malaise
—Headache
—Sore throat
—Inflamed pharynx
—Vomiting

Nonparalytic poliomyelitis
—Moderate fever
—Headache
—Vomiting
—Lethargy
—Irritability
—Pains in the neck, back, arms, legs, and abdomen
—Muscle tenderness and spasms in the extensors of the neck and back, and sometimes in the hamstring
—Resistance to neck flexion
—Hoyne's sign

Paralytic poliomyelitis
—Moderate fever
—Headache
—Vomiting
—Lethargy
—Irritability
—Widespread pain
—Rapidly developing asymmetrical muscle weakness, progressing to flaccid paralysis
—Loss of superficial and deep reflexes
—Paresthesias
—Urine retention
—Constipation
—Abdominal distention
—Nuchal rigidity
—Hoyne's, Kernig's, and Brudzinski's signs

Bulbar paralytic poliomyelitis
—Symptoms of encephalitis
—Facial weakness
—Dysphasia
—Difficulty in chewing
—Inability to swallow or expel saliva
—Respiratory distress

Diagnostic tests

• Isolation of the poliovirus from throat washings early in the disease, from stools throughout the disease, and from CSF cultures in CNS infection confirms the diagnosis.
• Convalescent serum antibody titers

Polio Protection

Dr. Jonas Salk's poliomyelitis vaccine, which became available in 1955, has been rightly called one of the miracle drugs of modern medicine. The vaccine contains dead (formalin-inactivated) polioviruses that stimulate production of circulating antibodies in the human body. This vaccine so effectively eliminated poliomyelitis that today it is hard to appreciate how feared the disease once was.

However, even miracle drugs can be improved. Today, the Sabin vaccine, which can be taken orally and is more than 90% effective, is the vaccine of choice in preventing poliomyelitis. The Sabin vaccine is available in trivalent and monovalent forms. The trivalent form (TOPV) contains live but weakened organisms of all three poliovirus serotypes in one solution. TOPV is generally preferred to the monovalent form (MOPV), which contains only one viral type and is useful only when the particular serotype is known.

All infants should be immunized with the Sabin vaccine; pregnant women may be vaccinated without risk. However, because of the risk of contracting poliomyelitis from the vaccine, it is contraindicated in patients with immunodeficiency diseases, leukemia, or lymphoma, and in those receiving corticosteroids, antimetabolites, other immunosuppressants, or radiation therapy. These patients are usually immunized with the Salk vaccine. When possible, immunodeficient patients should avoid contact with family members who are receiving the Sabin vaccine for at least 2 weeks after vaccination. Sabin vaccine is no longer routinely advised for adults unless they are likely to be exposed to this disease or plan travel to endemic areas.

---

four times greater than acute titers support the diagnosis.
• CSF pressure and protein levels may be slightly increased.

Treatment

Treatment is supportive and includes analgesics to ease headache, back pain, and leg spasms. Morphine is contraindicated because of the danger of additional respiratory suppression. Moist heat applications may also reduce muscle spasm and pain.

Bed rest is necessary only until extreme discomfort subsides. In paralytic poliomyelitis, this may take many months. Paralytic polio also requires long-term rehabilitation using physical therapy, braces, corrective shoes, and, in some cases, orthopedic surgery.

Clinical implications

Your patient care plan must be comprehensive to help prevent complica-

tions and to assist polio patients—physically and emotionally—during their prolonged convalescence.
• Observe the patient carefully for signs of paralysis and other neurologic damage, which can occur rapidly. Maintain a patent airway, and watch for respiratory weakness and difficulty in swallowing. A tracheotomy is often done at the first sign of respiratory distress. Following this, the patient is then placed on a mechanical ventilator. Remember to reassure the patient that his breathing is being supported.
• Practice strict aseptic technique during suctioning. Be sure to use only sterile solutions to nebulize medications.
• Perform a brief neurologic assessment at least once a day, but do not demand any vigorous muscle activity. Encourage a return to mild activity as soon as the patient is able.
• Check blood pressure frequently, especially with bulbar poliomyelitis,

which can cause hypertension or shock because of its effect on the brain stem.

• Watch for signs of fecal impaction (due to dehydration and intestinal inactivity). To prevent this, give sufficient fluids to ensure an adequate daily output of urine of low specific gravity (1.5 to 2 liters/day for adults).

• Monitor the bedridden patient's food intake to ensure an adequate, well-balanced diet. If tube feedings are required, give liquid baby foods, juices, lactose, and vitamins.

• To prevent pressure sores, give good skin care.

• Provide high-topped sneakers or use a footboard to prevent footdrop. To alleviate discomfort, use foam rubber pads and sandbags, as needed, and light splints, as ordered.

• To control the spread of poliomyelitis, wash your hands thoroughly after contact with the patient, especially after contact with excretions. Instruct the ambulatory patient to do the same. (Only hospital personnel who have been vaccinated against poliomyelitis may have direct contact with the patient.)

• Provide emotional support to the patient and his family. Reassure the nonparalytic patient that his chances for recovery are good. Long-term support and encouragement are essential for maximum rehabilitation.

• When caring for a paralytic patient, help set up an interdisciplinary rehabilitation program. Such a program should include physical and occupational therapists, physicians, and, if necessary, a psychiatrist to help manage the emotional problems that develop in a patient suddenly facing severe physical disabilities.

Complications
• Hypertension
• Urinary tract infection
• Urolithiasis
• Atelectasis
• Pneumonia
• Myocarditis
• Cor pulmonale

• Skeletal and soft-tissue deformities
• Paralytic ileus
(See *Polio Protection,* p. 599.)

Polycystic kidney disease

Description
An inherited disorder, polycystic kidney disease is characterized by multiple, bilateral, grapelike clusters of fluid-filled cysts that grossly enlarge the kidneys, compressing and eventually replacing functioning renal tissue. This disease appears in two distinct forms. The infantile form causes stillbirth or early neonatal death. A few infants with this disease survive for 2 years and then develop fatal renal, congestive heart, or respiratory failure. Onset of the adult form is insidious but usually becomes obvious between ages 30 and 50. Rarely, it may not cause symptoms until the patient is in his seventies. In the adult form, renal deterioration is more gradual, but it progresses relentlessly to uremia, just as it does in the infantile form.

Causes
• The infantile form appears to be inherited as an autosomal recessive trait.
• The adult form appears to be inherited as an autosomal dominant trait.

Signs and symptoms
Infantile polycystic disease
—Pronounced epicanthal folds
—Pointed nose
—Small chin
—Floppy, low-set ears (Potter facies)
—Huge bilateral masses on the flanks.
These are symmetrical and tense.
Adult polycystic disease
—Nonspecific early effects include hypertension, polyuria, and symptoms of urinary tract infection.
—Later symptoms include lumbar

pain, widening girth, and swollen or tender abdomen.

—Advanced problems may include recurrent hematuria, life-threatening retroperitoneal bleeding, proteinuria, and colicky abdominal pain. Both kidneys are grossly enlarged and palpable.

Diagnostic tests

• Intravenous or retrograde pyelography reveals enlarged kidneys, with elongation of the pelvis, flattening of the calyces, and indentations caused by cysts. Excretory urography of the newborn shows poor excretion of contrast medium.

• Ultrasound and CT scans show kidney enlargement and presence of cysts; CT scan demonstrates multiple areas of cystic damage.

• Urinalysis and creatinine clearance tests—nonspecific tests that evaluate renal function—indicate abnormalities.

Treatment

Polycystic kidney disease cannot be cured, but careful management of associated urinary tract infections and secondary hypertension may prolong life. Progressive renal failure requires treatment similar to that for other types of renal disease, including dialysis or, rarely, kidney transplant.

When adult polycystic kidney disease is discovered in the asymptomatic stage, careful monitoring is required, including urine cultures and creatinine clearance tests repeated at 6-month intervals. When urine culture detects infection, prompt and vigorous antibiotic treatment is necessary even for asymptomatic infection. As renal impairment progresses, selected patients may undergo dialysis, transplantation, or both. Cystic abscess or retroperitoneal bleeding may require surgical drainage; intractable pain (a rare symptom) may also require surgery. However, since this disease is bilateral, nephrectomy usually is not recommended, because it aggravates the risk of infection in the remaining kidney.

Clinical implications

• Refer the young adult patient or parents of infants with polycystic kidney disease for genetic counseling. Such parents will probably have many questions about the risk to other offspring.

• Provide supportive care to minimize any associated symptoms. Carefully assess the patient's life-style and his physical and mental state; determine how rapidly the disease is progressing. Use this information to plan individualized patient care.

• Acquaint yourself with all aspects of end-stage renal disease, including dialysis and transplantation, so you can provide appropriate care and patient teaching as the disease progresses.

• Explain all diagnostic procedures to the patient or his family.

• Administer antibiotics, as ordered, for urinary tract infection. Stress to the patient the need to take medication exactly as prescribed, even if symptoms are minimal or absent.

Complications

The infant with polycystic kidney disease characteristically shows signs of respiratory distress and congestive heart failure. Eventually, he develops uremia and renal failure. Accompanying hepatic fibrosis may cause portal hypertension and bleeding varices to develop as well.

About 10 years after symptoms appear in affected adults, progressive compression of kidney structures by the enlarging mass produces renal failure.

Polycythemia vera
(Primary polycythemia, erythremia, polycythemia rubra vera, splenomegalic polycythemia, Vasquez-Osler disease)

Description

Polycythemia vera is a chronic, myeloproliferative disorder characterized by increased RBC mass, leukocytosis, thrombocytosis, and increased hemoglobin concentration, with normal or decreased plasma volume. It usually occurs between ages 40 and 60. Prognosis depends on age at diagnosis, treatment used, and complications. Mortality is high if polycythemia is untreated or is associated with leukemia or myeloid metaplasia.

Causes
In polycythemia vera, uncontrolled and rapid cellular reproduction and maturation cause proliferation or hyperplasia of all bone marrow cells (panmyelosis). The cause of such uncontrolled cellular activity is unknown, but it is probably due to a multipotential stem cell defect.

Signs and symptoms
(See *Clinical Features of Polycythemia Vera.*)

Diagnostic tests
• Laboratory studies confirm polycythemia vera by showing increased RBC mass and normal arterial oxygen saturation in association with splenomegaly or two of the following:
—Thrombocytosis
—Leukocytosis
—Elevated leukocyte alkaline phosphatase level
—Elevated serum vitamin B_{12} or unbound B_{12}-binding capacity
• Serum uric acid is increased.
• Blood histamine is increased.
• Serum iron concentration is decreased.
• Urinary erythropoietin is decreased or absent.
• Bone marrow biopsy reveals panmyelosis.

Treatment
Phlebotomy, the primary treatment, can reduce red cell mass promptly. The frequency of phlebotomy and the amount of blood removed with each treatment depends on the patient's condition. Typically, 350 to 500 ml of blood can be removed every other day until the patient's hematocrit is reduced to the low normal range. After repeated phlebotomies, the patient develops iron deficiency, which stabilizes red cell production and reduces the need for phlebotomy.

Phlebotomy does not reduce the white cell or platelet count and will not control the hyperuricemia associated with marrow cell proliferation. For severe symptoms related to these manifestations, myelosuppressive therapy may be used. Radioactive phosphorus (^{32}P) or chemotherapeutic agents such as melphalan, busulfan, or chlorambucil can satisfactorily control the disease in most cases. These agents may cause leukemia, however. They should be reserved for older patients and those with serious problems not controlled by phlebotomy. Patients of any age who have had previous thrombotic problems should be considered for myelosuppressive therapy.

Clinical implications
If the patient requires phlebotomy, explain the procedure, and reassure the patient that it will relieve distressing symptoms.
• Tell the patient to watch for and report any symptoms of iron deficiency (pallor, weight loss, asthenia, and glossitis).
• Keep the patient active and ambulatory to prevent thrombosis. If bed rest is necessary, prescribe a daily program of both active and passive range-of-motion exercises.
• Watch for complications: hypervolemia, thrombocytosis, and signs of an impending cerebrovascular accident.
• Regularly examine the patient closely for bleeding. Tell him which are the most common bleeding sites (nose, gingiva, and skin), so he can check for bleeding. Advise him to report any abnormal bleeding promptly.

Clinical Features of Polycythemia Vera

SYMPTOMS	CAUSES
Eye, ear, nose, and throat • Visual disturbances (blurring, diplopia, scotoma, engorged veins of fundus and retina) and congestion of conjunctiva, retina, retinal veins, oral mucous membrane	• Hypervolemia and hyperviscosity
• Epistaxis or gingival bleeding	• Engorgement of capillary beds
CNS • Headache or fullness in the head, lethargy, weakness, fatigue, syncope, tinnitus, paresthesia of digits, and impaired mentation	• Hypervolemia and hyperviscosity
Cardiovascular • Hypertension	• Hypervolemia and hyperviscosity
• Intermittent claudication, thrombosis and emboli, angina, thrombophlebitis	• Hypervolemia, thrombocytosis, and vascular disease
• Hemorrhage	• Engorgement of capillary beds
Skin • Pruritus (especially after hot bath)	• Basophilia (secondary histamine release)
• Urticaria	• Altered histamine metabolism
• Ruddy cyanosis	• Hypervolemia and hyperviscosity due to congested vessels, increased oxyhemoglobin, and reduced hemoglobin
• Night sweats	• Hypermetabolism
• Ecchymosis	• Hemorrhage
GI and hepatic • Epigastric distress	• Hypervolemia and hyperviscosity
• Early satiety and fullness	• Hepatosplenomegaly
• Peptic ulcer pain	• Gastric thrombosis and hemorrhage
• Hepatosplenomegaly	• Congestion, extramedullary hemopoiesis, and myeloid metaplasia
• Weight loss	• Hypermetabolism
Respiratory • Dyspnea	• Hypervolemia and hyperviscosity
Musculoskeletal • Joint symptoms	• Increased urate production secondary to nucleoprotein turnover

- To compensate for increased uric acid production, give the patient additional fluids, administer allopurinol, as ordered, and alkalinize the urine to prevent uric acid calculi.
- If the patient has symptomatic splenomegaly, suggest or provide small, frequent meals, followed by a rest period, to prevent nausea and vomiting.
- Report acute abdominal pain immediately; it may signal splenic infarction, renal calculi, or abdominal organ thrombosis.

During myelosuppressive chemotherapy, follow these guidelines:

- Monitor CBC and platelet count before and during therapy. If leukopenia develops in an outpatient, warn him that his resistance to infection is low. Advise him to avoid crowds, and make sure he knows the symptoms of infection. If leukopenia develops in a hospitalized patient who needs reverse isolation, follow institutional guidelines.
- Tell the patient about possible side effects, such as nausea and vomiting, and measures to prevent or manage them.

During treatment with ^{32}P, follow these guidelines:

- Explain the procedure to relieve anxiety. Tell the patient he may require repeated phlebotomies until ^{32}P takes effect. Make sure you have a blood sample for CBC and platelet count before beginning treatment. (Note: The health care professional who administers ^{32}P should take radiation precautions to prevent contamination.)
- Have the patient lie down during I.V. administration (to facilitate the procedure and prevent extravasation) and for 15 to 20 minutes afterward.

Complications
- Hemorrhage
- Thrombosis

Polymyositis and dermatomyositis

Description
Diffuse, inflammatory myopathies of unknown cause, polymyositis and dermatomyositis produce symmetrical weakness of striated muscle—primarily proximal muscles of the shoulder and pelvic girdles, neck, and pharynx. In dermatomyositis, such muscle weakness is accompanied by cutaneous involvement. These diseases usually progress slowly, with frequent exacerbations and remissions.

Usually, prognosis worsens with age. The 7-year survival rate for adults is approximately 60%, with death often occurring from associated cancer, respiratory disease, heart failure, or side effects of therapy (corticosteroids and immunosuppressants). On the other hand, 80% to 90% of affected children regain normal function if properly treated; if untreated, however, childhood dermatomyositis may progress rapidly to disabling contractures and muscular atrophy.

Causes
Although the cause of polymyositis remains puzzling, it may result from autoimmunity, perhaps combined with defective T-cell function.

Signs and symptoms
Polymyositis
—Muscle weakness, tenderness, and discomfort (affects proximal muscles [shoulder, pelvic girdle] more often than distal muscles)
—Inability to move against resistance
—Proximal dysphagia
—Dysphonia
Dermatomyositis
—Erythematous rash (usually erupts on the face, neck, upper back, chest, and arms and around the nail beds)
—Characteristic heliotropic rash (appears on the eyelids, accompanied by periorbital edema)

—Grotton's papules (violet, flat-topped lesions; may appear on the interphalangeal joints)

Diagnostic tests

• Muscle biopsy that shows necrosis, degeneration, regeneration, and interstitial chronic lymphocytic infiltration confirms the diagnosis.
• Erythrocyte sedimentation rate is increased.
• WBC count is increased.
• Muscle enzymes (creatine phosphokinase, aldolase, and SGOT) are increased.
• Urine creatine is increased.
• Urine creatinine is decreased.
• Electromyography shows polyphasic short-duration potentials, fibrillation (positive-spike waves), and bizarre, high-frequency, repetitive changes.
• Antinuclear antibodies are present.

Treatment

High-dose corticosteroid therapy relieves inflammation and lowers muscle enzyme levels. Within 2 to 6 weeks after treatment, serum muscle enzyme levels usually return to normal and muscle strength improves, permitting a gradual tapering down of corticosteroid dosage. If the patient responds poorly to corticosteroids, treatment may include cytotoxic or immunosuppressive drugs, such as cyclophosphamide, intermittent I.V. or daily P.O. Supportive therapy includes bed rest during the acute phase, range-of-motion exercises to prevent contractures, analgesics and application of heat to relieve painful muscle spasms, and diphenhydramine to relieve itching. Patients over age 40 need thorough assessment for coexisting cancer.

Clinical implications

• Assess level of pain, muscular weakness, and range of motion daily. Administer analgesics, as needed.
• If the patient is confined to bed, prevent decubitus ulcers by giving good skin care. To prevent footdrop and con-tractures, provide high-topped sneakers, and assist with passive range-of-motion exercises at least four times daily. Teach the patient's family how to perform these exercises with the patient.
• When you assist with muscle biopsy, make sure the biopsy is not taken from an area of recent needle insertion, such as an injection or electromyography site.
• If the patient has a skin rash, warn him against scratching, which may cause infection. If antipruritic medication does not relieve severe itching, apply tepid sponges or compresses.
• Encourage the patient to feed and dress himself to the best of his ability but to ask for help when needed. Advise him to pace his activities to counteract muscle weakness. Encourage him to express his anxiety. Ease his fear or dependence by giving reassurance that muscle weakness is probably temporary.
• Explain the disease to the patient and his family. Prepare them for diagnostic procedures and possible side effects of corticosteroid therapy (weight gain, hirsutism, hypertension, edema, amenorrhea, purplish striae, glycosuria, acne, easy bruising). Advise a low-sodium diet to prevent fluid retention. Emphatically warn against abruptly discontinuing corticosteroids. Reassure the patient that steroid-induced weight gain will diminish when the drug is discontinued.

Porphyrias

Description

Porphyrias are metabolic disorders that affect the biosynthesis of heme (a component of hemoglobin) and cause

Clinical Variants of Porphyria

PORPHYRIA	SIGNS AND SYMPTOMS	TREATMENT
ERYTHROPOIETIC PORPHYRIA **Günther's disease** • Usual onset before age 5	• Red urine (earliest, most characteristic sign); severe cutaneous photosensitivity, leading to vesicular or bullous eruptions on exposed areas, and eventual scarring and ulceration • Hypertrichosis • Brown- or red-stained teeth • Splenomegaly, hemolytic anemia	• Anti-inflammatory ointments, such as 1% hydrocortisone, for dermatitis • Prednisone to reverse anemia • Transfusion of packed red cells to inhibit erythropoiesis and reduce level of excreted porphyrins • Hemin for recurrent attacks • Splenectomy for hemolytic anemia
ERYTHROHEPATIC PORPHYRIA **Protoporphyria** • Usually affects children • Occurs most often in males	• Photosensitive dermatitis • Hemolytic anemia • Chronic hepatic disease	• Avoidance of causative factors • Beta-carotene to reduce photosensitivity
Toxic-acquired porphyria • Usually affects children • Significant mortality	• Acute colicky pain • Anorexia, nausea, vomiting • Behavioral changes • Convulsions, coma	• Chlorpromazine I.V. (25 mg every 4 to 6 hours during an acute attack) to relieve pain and GI symptoms • Avoidance of lead exposure
HEPATIC PORPHYRIA **Acute intermittent porphyria** • Most common form • Affects females most often, usually between ages 15 and 40	• Colicky abdominal pain with fever, general malaise, and hypertension • Peripheral neuritis, behavioral changes, possibly leading to frank psychosis • Respiratory paralysis can occur	• Chlorpromazine I.V. (25 mg every 4 to 6 hours) to relieve abdominal pain and control psychic abnormalities • Avoidance of barbiturates, infections, alcohol, and fasting • Hemin for recurrent attacks

Clinical Variants of Porphyria *(continued)*		
PORPHYRIA	**SIGNS AND SYMPTOMS**	**TREATMENT**
HEPATIC PORPHYRIA *(continued)*		
Variegate porphyria • Usual onset between ages 30 and 50 • Occurs almost exclusively among South African whites • Affects males and females equally	• Skin lesions, extremely fragile skin in exposed areas • Hypertrichosis • Hyperpigmentation • Abdominal pain during acute attack • Neuropsychiatric manifestations	• High-carbohydrate diet • Avoidance of sunlight, or wearing of protective clothing when avoidance is not possible • Hemin for recurrent attacks
Porphyria cutanea tarda • Most frequent in men aged 40 to 60 • Highest incidence in South Africans	• Facial pigmentation • Red-brown urine • Photosensitive dermatitis • Hypertrichosis	• Avoidance of precipitating factors, such as alcohol and estrogens • Phlebotomy at 2-week intervals to lower serum iron level
Hereditary coproporphyria • Rare • Affects males and females equally	• Asymptomatic or mild neurologic, abdominal, or psychiatric symptoms	• High-carbohydrate diet • Avoidance of barbiturates • Hemin for recurrent attacks

excessive production and excretion of porphyrins or their precursors. Porphyrins, which are present in all protoplasm, figure prominently in energy storage and utilization. Classification of porphyrias depends on the site of excessive porphyrin production. They may be erythropoietic (erythroid cells in bone marrow), hepatic (in the liver), or erythrohepatic (in bone marrow and liver). An acute episode of intermittent hepatic porphyria may cause fatal respiratory paralysis. In the other forms of porphyrias, prognosis is good with proper treatment.

Causes
Porphyrias are inherited as autosomal dominant traits, except for Günther's disease (autosomal recessive trait) and toxic-acquired porphyria (usually from ingestion of or exposure to lead).

Signs and symptoms
• Photosensitivity
• Acute abdominal pain
• Neuropathy
(For specific signs and symptoms and treatment, see *Clinical Variants of Porphyria*.)

Diagnostic tests
• Screening tests for porphyrins or their precursors (such as aminolevu-

linic acid [ALA] and porphobilinogen [PBG]) in urine, stool, or blood are usually required for diagnosis. Skin biopsy may be performed.

• Urinary lead level of 0.2 mg/liter confirms toxic porphyria.

• Serum iron levels may be increased in porphyria cutanea tarda.

• WBC count, bilirubin, and alkaline phosphatase are increased in acute intermittent porphyria.

Treatment and clinical implications

• Warn the patient against excessive sun exposure. Administer beta-carotene to reduce photosensitivity.

• Administer hemin (an enzyme inhibitor derived from processed red blood cells) to control recurrent attacks of acute intermittent porphyria, Günther's disease, variegate porphyria, and hereditary coproporphyria.

• Encourage a high-carbohydrate diet to decrease urinary excretion of ALA and PBG, with restricted fluid intake to inhibit release of antidiuretic hormone.

• Warn the patient to avoid precipitating factors, especially alcohol, barbiturates, estrogens, and fasting.

Posttraumatic stress disorder

Description

The psychological consequences of a traumatic event that occurs outside the range of usual human experience are identified as posttraumatic stress disorder (PTSD). This is classified in *DSM-III* as an anxiety disorder. Such a disorder can be acute, chronic, or delayed and can follow a natural disaster (flood, tornado), a manmade disaster (war, imprisonment, torture, car accidents, large fires), or an assault or rape.

Causes

In most persons with PTSD, the stressor is a necessary but insufficient cause of the persisting symptoms. Even the most severe stressors do not produce PTSD in everyone, so psychological, physical, genetic, and social factors may also contribute to it.

Risk factors

• The very young and very old have more difficulty coping with unusual stressors.

• Preexisting psychopathology can also predispose to this disorder.

Signs and symptoms

Characteristic symptoms that persist after unusual trauma confirm this diagnosis. Symptoms may include any of the following:

• Recurrent, intrusive recollections or nightmares

• Sleep disturbances

• Chronic anxiety or panic attacks

• Memory impairment

• Difficulty in concentrating

• Feelings of detachment or estrangement that destroy interpersonal relationships

• Headaches

• Depression and suicidal thoughts

• Rage and use of violence to solve problems

Diagnostic tests

A psychiatric examination should include a mental status assessment and tests for organic impairment and should focus on other psychiatric syndromes that accompany PTSD, such as depression, generalized anxiety, and phobia.

Treatment

Goals of treatment include reducing the target symptoms, preventing chronic disability, and promoting occupational and social rehabilitation. Specific treatment may emphasize behavioral techniques (relaxation therapy to decrease anxiety and induce sleep, or progressive desensitization);

antianxiety and antidepressant drugs, prescribed with caution to avoid possible dependence; or brief psychotherapy (supportive, insight, or cathartic) to minimize the risks of dependency and chronicity.

Support groups are highly effective and are provided through many Veterans Administration centers and crisis clinics. These groups provide a forum in which victims of PTSD can work through their feelings with others who have had similar conflicts. Group settings are appropriate for most degrees of symptoms presented. Some group programs include spouses and families in their treatment process. Rehabilitation in physical, social, and occupational areas is also available for victims of chronic PTSD. Many patients need treatment for depression, alcohol and/or drug abuse, or medical conditions before psychological healing can take place.

Clinical implications

The goal of intervention is to encourage the victim of PTSD to express his grief and complete the mourning process so he can go on with his life. Keep in mind that such a patient tends to sharply test your commitment and interest. First examine your feelings about the event (war or other trauma) so that you will not react with disdain and shock. This hampers the working relationship and reinforces the patient's poor self-image and sense of guilt.

To develop an effective therapeutic relationship, follow these guidelines:
• Know and practice crisis intervention techniques as appropriate.
• Establish trust by accepting the patient's current level of functioning and by assuming a positive, consistent, honest, and nonjudgmental attitude.
• Help the patient to regain control over angry impulses by identifying situations in which he lost control and by talking about past and precipitating events (conceptual labeling) to help with later problem-solving skills.
• Give approval as the patient shows a commitment to work on his problem.
• Deal constructively with anger. Encourage joint assessment of angry outbursts (identify how anger escalates, explore preventive measures that family members can take to regain control). Provide a safe, staff-monitored room in which the patient can safely deal with urges to commit physical violence or self-abuse by displacement (such as pounding and throwing clay or destroying selected items). Encourage him to move from physical to verbal expressions of anger.
• Relieve shame and guilt precipitated by real actions—such as killing and mutilation—that violated a consciously held moral code through clarification (putting behavior into perspective), atonement (helping the patient see that he has atoned by social isolation and by engaging in self-destructive behavior), and restitution (having clergy help him conquer guilt, once authority and trust in others is accepted).
• Provide for or refer the patient to group therapy with other victims for peer support and forgiveness.
• Refer the patient to appropriate community resources.

Potassium imbalance

Description

Potassium, a cation that is the dominant cellular electrolyte, facilitates contraction of both skeletal and smooth muscles—including myocardial contraction—and figures prominently in nerve impulse conduction, acid-base balance, enzyme action, and cell membrane function. Because serum potassium level has such a narrow normal range (3.5 to 5 mEq/liter), a slight deviation in either direction can produce profound clinical consequences. Paradoxically, both hypokalemia (po-

Clinical Features of Potassium Imbalance

DYSFUNCTION	HYPOKALEMIA	HYPERKALEMIA
Cardiovascular	• Dizziness, hypotension, dysrhythmias, EKG changes (flattened T waves, elevated U waves, depressed ST segment), cardiac arrest (with serum potassium levels < 2.5 mEq/liter)	• Tachycardia and later bradycardia, EKG changes (tented and elevated T waves, widened QRS, prolonged PR interval, flattened or absent P waves, depressed ST segment), cardiac arrest (with levels > 7.0 mEq/liter)
GI	• Nausea and vomiting, anorexia, diarrhea, abdominal distention, paralytic ileus or decreased peristalsis	• Nausea, diarrhea, abdominal cramps
Musculoskeletal	• Muscle weakness and fatigue, leg cramps	• Muscle weakness, flaccid paralysis
Genitourinary	• Polyuria	• Oliguria, anuria
CNS	• Malaise, irritability, confusion, mental depression, speech changes, decreased reflexes, respiratory paralysis	• Hyperreflexia progressing to weakness, numbness, tingling, and flaccid paralysis
Acid-base balance	• Metabolic alkalosis	• Metabolic acidosis

tassium deficiency) and hyperkalemia (potassium excess) can lead to muscle weakness and flaccid paralysis, because both create an ionic imbalance that diminishes neuromuscular tissue excitability. Both conditions also diminish excitability and conduction rate of the heart muscle, which may lead to cardiac arrest.

Causes
Hypokalemia
—Excessive GI or urinary losses because of vomiting, gastric suction, diarrhea, dehydration, anorexia, or chronic laxative abuse
—Trauma (injury, burns, or surgery)

in which damaged cells release potassium, which enters serum or extracellular fluid, to be excreted in the urine
—Chronic renal disease, with tubular potassium wasting
—Certain drugs, especially potassium-wasting diuretics, steroids, and certain sodium-containing antibiotics (carbenicillin)
—Acid-base imbalances, which cause a shift of potassium into cells without true depletion
—Prolonged potassium-free I.V. therapy
—Hyperglycemia, which causes osmotic diuresis and glycosuria

—Cushing's syndrome, primary hyperaldosteronism, excessive ingestion of licorice, and severe serum magnesium deficiency

Hyperkalemia
—Excessive amounts of potassium infused intravenously or administered orally
—Decreased urine output
—Renal dysfunction or failure
—Use of potassium-sparing diuretics, such as triamterene, by patients with renal disease
—Many injuries or conditions that release cellular potassium or favor its retention, such as burns, crushing injuries, diminished renal function, adrenal gland insufficiency, dehydration, or diabetic acidosis

Signs and symptoms
(See *Clinical Features of Potassium Imbalance*.)

Diagnostic tests
• Serum potassium levels < 3.5 mEq/liter confirm hypokalemia.
• Serum potassium levels > 5 mEq/liter confirm hyperkalemia.
• EKG changes occur. (See *EKG Changes in Potassium Imbalance*, p. 612.)
• Additional tests may be necessary to determine the underlying cause of the imbalance.

Treatment
For hypokalemia, replacement therapy with potassium chloride (I.V. or P.O.) is the primary treatment. When diuresis is necessary, spironolactone, a potassium-sparing diuretic, may be administered concurrently with a potassium-wasting diuretic to minimize potassium loss. Hypokalemia can be prevented by giving a maintenance dose of potassium I.V. to patients who may not take anything by mouth and to others predisposed to potassium loss.

For hyperkalemia, rapid infusion of 10% calcium gluconate decreases myocardial irritability and temporarily prevents cardiac arrest but does not correct serum potassium excess. It is also contraindicated in patients receiving digitalis. As an emergency measure, sodium bicarbonate I.V. increases pH and causes potassium to shift back into the cells. Insulin and 10% to 50% glucose I.V. also move potassium back into cells, but their effect lasts only 6 hours. Repeated use is less effective. Sodium polystyrene sulfonate (Kayexalate) with 70% sorbitol produces exchange of sodium ions for potassium ions in the intestine. Hemodialysis or peritoneal dialysis also aids in removal of excess potassium.

Clinical implications
For the patient with hypokalemia, follow these guidelines:
• Check serum potassium and other electrolyte levels often.
• Assess intake and output carefully. Remember, the kidneys excrete 80% to 90% of ingested potassium. Never give supplementary potassium to a patient whose urinary output is below 600 ml/day. Also, measure gastrointestinal loss from suctioning or vomiting.
• Administer slow-release potassium or dilute oral potassium supplements in 4 oz (120 ml) or more of water or fluid to reduce irritation of gastric and small-bowel mucosa. Determine the patient's serum chloride level. If it is low, give a potassium chloride supplement, as ordered. If it is normal, administer potassium gluconate, as ordered.
• Give potassium I.V. only after it is diluted in solution; potassium is very irritating to vascular, subcutaneous, and fatty tissues and may cause phlebitis or tissue necrosis if it infiltrates. Infuse slowly (no more than 20 mEq/liter/hour) to prevent hyperkalemia. *Never* administer by I.V. push or bolus; it may cause cardiac arrest.
• Carefully monitor patients receiving

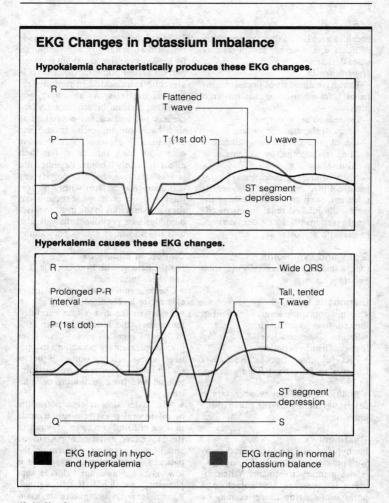

EKG Changes in Potassium Imbalance

Hypokalemia characteristically produces these EKG changes.

R

Flattened
T wave

P

T (1st dot)

U wave

Q

ST segment
depression

S

Hyperkalemia causes these EKG changes.

R

Wide QRS

Prolonged P-R
interval

Tall, tented
T wave

P (1st dot)

T

ST segment
depression

Q

S

■ EKG tracing in hypo-
and hyperkalemia

■ EKG tracing in normal
potassium balance

digitalis, because hypokalemia enhances its action and may produce signs of digitalis toxicity.

• To prevent hypokalemia, instruct patients (especially those predisposed to hypokalemia by long-term diuretic therapy) to include potassium-rich foods in their diet—oranges, bananas, tomatoes, dark green leafy vegetables, milk, dried fruits, apricots, and peanuts.

• Monitor cardiac rhythm, and report any irregularities immediately.

To manage the patient with hyperkalemia, follow these guidelines:

• As in hypokalemia, frequently monitor serum potassium and other electrolyte levels, and carefully record intake and output.

• Administer sodium polystyrene sulfonate orally or rectally (by retention enema). Watch for signs of hypoka-

lemia with prolonged use and for clinical effects of hypoglycemia with repeated insulin and glucose treatment.
• Watch for signs of hyperkalemia in predisposed patients, especially those with poor urinary output or those receiving potassium supplements P.O. or I.V.
• Before giving a blood transfusion, check to see how long ago the blood was donated.
• Blood cell hemolysis releases potassium. Infuse only *fresh* blood for patients with average-to-high serum potassium levels.
• Monitor for and report cardiac dysrhythmias.

Precocious puberty in females

Description
In females, precocious puberty is the onset of pubertal changes (breast development, appearance of pubic and axillary hair, and menarche) before age 9 (normally, the mean age for menarche is 13). In true precocious puberty, the ovaries mature and pubertal changes progress in an orderly manner. In pseudoprecocious puberty, pubertal changes occur without corresponding ovarian maturation.

Causes
True precocious puberty
—Primarily, early development and activation of the endocrine glands without corresponding abnormality
—CNS disorders resulting from tumors, trauma, infection, or other lesions

Pseudoprecocious puberty
—Increased levels of sex hormones

due to ovarian and adrenocortical tumors, adrenal cortical virilizing hyperplasia, and ingestion of estrogens or androgens
—Increased end-organ sensitivity to low levels of circulating sex hormones

Signs and symptoms
All changes occur before age 9 and may occur independently or simultaneously.
• Rapid growth spurt
• Thelarche (breast development)
• Pubarche (pubic hair development)
• Menarche

Diagnostic tests
• X-rays of hands, wrists, knees, and hips determine bone age and possible premature epiphyseal closure.
• Vaginal smear detects estrogen secretion, urinary tests determine gonadotropic activity and excretion of 17-ketosteroids, and radioimmunoassay reveals both luteinizing and follicle-stimulating hormones.
• Laparoscopy or exploratory laparotomy may verify a suspected abdominal lesion.
• EEG, ventriculography, pneumoencephalography, CT scan, or angiography can detect CNS disorders.

Treatment
In precocious thelarche and pubarche, no treatment is necessary. Although still controversial, treatment of constitutional true precocious puberty may include medroxyprogesterone to reduce secretion of gonadotropins and prevent menstruation. Other therapy depends on the cause of precocious puberty and its stage of development.
• Adrenogenital syndrome necessitates cortical or adrenocortical steroid replacement.
• Abdominal tumors necessitate surgery to remove ovarian and adrenal tumors. Regression of secondary sex characteristics may follow such sur-

gery, especially in young children.
• Choriocarcinomas require surgery and chemotherapy.
• Hypothyroidism requires thyroid extract or levothyroxine to decrease gonadotropic secretions.
• Drug ingestion requires that the medication be discontinued.

Clinical implications

The dramatic physical changes produced by precocious puberty can be upsetting and alarming for the child and her family. Provide a calm, supportive atmosphere, and encourage the patient and family to express their feelings about these changes. Explain all diagnostic procedures, and tell the patient and family that surgery may be necessary.
• Explain the condition to the child in terms she can understand to prevent feelings of shame and loss of self-esteem. Provide appropriate sex education, including information on menstruation and related hygiene.
• Tell parents that although their daughter seems physically mature, she is not psychologically mature, and the discrepancy between physical appearance and psychological and psychosexual maturation may create problems. Warn them against expecting more maturity of her than they would expect of other children her age.
• Suggest that parents continue to dress their daughter in clothes that are appropriate for her age and styles that do not call attention to her physical development.
• Reassure parents that precocious puberty does not usually precipitate precocious sexual behavior.

Precocious puberty in males

Description

In precocious puberty, boys begin to mature sexually before age 10. It can occur as true precocious puberty, the most common form, with early maturation of the hypothalamic-pituitary-gonadal axis, development of secondary sexual characteristics, gonadal development, and spermatogenesis. It can also occur as pseudoprecocious puberty, with development of secondary sexual characteristics without gonadal development. Boys with true precocious puberty reportedly have fathered children at an age as young as 7 years.

In most boys with precocious puberty, sexual characteristics develop in essentially normal sequence. These children function normally when they reach adulthood.

Causes

True precocious puberty
—Idiopathic; may be transmitted as a dominant trait in some patients
—Pituitary or hypothalamic lesions that cause excessive secretion of gonadotropin
Pseudoprecocious puberty
—Testicular tumors
—Congenital adrenogenital syndrome

Signs and symptoms

Precocious puberty (all forms)
—Early bone development, initial growth spurt, early muscle development, and premature closure of the epiphyses, which results in stunted adult stature
—Adult hair pattern
—Penile growth
—Bilateral enlarged testes
Precocious puberty resulting from cerebral lesions
—Nausea
—Vomiting
—Headache
—Visual disturbances
—Symptoms of internal hydrocephalus
Pseudoprecocity resulting from testicular tumors
—Adult hair patterns and acne
—Discrepancy in testes size. The en-

larged testis may be hard or may contain a palpable, isolated nodule.
Pseudoprecocity resulting from adrenogenital syndrome
—Adult skin tone
—Excessive hair (including beard)
—Deepened voice
—Stocky and muscular appearance
—Enlarged penis, scrotal sac, and prostate (but not testes)

Diagnostic tests
True precocity
—Serum levels of luteinizing hormone, follicle-stimulating hormone, and ACTH are elevated.
—Plasma tests for testosterone demonstrate elevated levels (equal to those of an adult male).
—Evaluation of ejaculate reveals presence of live spermatozoa.
—Brain scan, skull X-rays, and EEG can detect possible CNS tumors.
—Skull and hand X-rays reveal advanced bone age.

A child with an initial diagnosis of idiopathic precocious puberty should be reassessed regularly for possible tumors.
Pseudoprecocity
• Chromosomal karyotype analysis demonstrates abnormal pattern of autosomes and sex chromosomes.
• The patient's 24-hour urinary 17-ketosteroids and other steroid excretion levels are increased.

Treatment
Boys with idiopathic precocious puberty usually require no medical treatment and, except for stunted growth, suffer no physical complications in adulthood. Supportive psychological counseling is the most important therapy.

When precocious puberty is caused by tumors, the outlook is less encouraging. Brain tumors necessitate neurosurgery but commonly resist treatment and may prove fatal. Testicular tumors may be treated by removing the affected testis (orchiectomy). Cancerous tumors additionally require chemotherapy and lymphatic radiation therapy, and have a poor prognosis.

Adrenogenital syndrome, which causes precocious puberty, may respond to lifelong therapy with glucocorticoids (cortisol) to inhibit corticotropin production.

Clinical implications
• Emphasize to parents that social and emotional development should remain consistent with the child's chronologic age, not with his physical development. Advise parents not to place unrealistic demands on the child or to expect him to act older than his age.
• Reassure the child that although his body is changing more rapidly than those of other boys, eventually they will experience the same changes. Help him feel less self-conscious about his differences. Suggest clothing that deemphasizes sexual development.
• Provide sex education for the child with true precocity.
• If appropriate, explain side effects of glucocorticoids (cushingoid symptoms) to the child and parents.

Pregnancy-induced hypertension
(Toxemia of pregnancy)

Description
Pregnancy-induced hypertension (PIH), a potentially life-threatening disorder, usually develops late in the second trimester or in the third trimester. Preeclampsia, the nonconvulsive form of toxemia, develops in about 7% of pregnancies. It can be mild or severe, and the incidence is significantly higher in low socioeconomic groups. Eclampsia is the convulsive form of toxemia. About 5% of females with preeclampsia develop eclampsia. Of these, about 15% die from toxemia itself or its complications.

Fetal mortality is high due to the increased incidence of premature delivery.

Causes
Unknown

Signs and symptoms
Mild preeclampsia
—Hypertension (140 mm Hg systolic pressure, or a rise of 30 mm Hg or greater above the patient's normal systolic pressure, measured on two occasions, 6 hours apart; 90 mm Hg diastolic pressure, or a rise of 15 mm Hg or greater above the patient's normal diastolic pressure, measured on two occasions, 6 hours apart)
—Proteinuria (more than 500 mg/24 hours)
—Generalized edema (especially of the hands, face, and feet)
—Sudden weight gain (more than 3 lb [1.36 kg] a week during the second trimester or more than 1 lb [0.45 kg] a week during the third trimester)
Severe preeclampsia
—Increased hypertension (150/110 mm Hg or higher on two occasions, 6 hours apart, at bed rest)
—Increased proteinuria (5 g/24 hours or more, eventually leading to the development of oliguria)
—Blurred vision
—Epigastric pain or heartburn
—Irritability
—Emotional tension
—Severe frontal headache
—Possible hyperactive deep-tendon reflexes
Eclampsia
—Magnified symptoms of preeclampsia
—Convulsions
—Possible coma

Diagnostic tests
• Ophthalmoscopic examination may reveal vascular spasm, papilledema, retinal edema or detachment, and arteriovenous nicking or hemorrhage in eclampsia.

• Real-time ultrasonography and stress and nonstress tests evaluate fetal well-being.

Treatment
Therapy for preeclampsia is designed to halt the disorder's progress—specifically, the early effects of eclampsia, such as convulsions, residual hypertension, and renal shutdown—and to ensure fetal survival. Some physicians advocate the prompt induction of labor, especially if the patient is near term; others follow a more conservative approach. Therapy may include sedatives, such as phenobarbital, along with complete bed rest, to relieve anxiety, reduce hypertension, and evaluate response to therapy. If renal function remains adequate, a high-protein, low-sodium, low-carbohydrate diet with increased fluid intake is recommended.

If the patient's blood pressure fails to respond to bed rest and sedation and persistently rises above 160/110 mm Hg, or if CNS irritability increases, magnesium sulfate may produce general sedation, promote diuresis, reduce blood pressure, and prevent convulsions. If these measures fail to improve the patient's condition, or if fetal life is endangered (as determined by stress or nonstress tests), cesarean section or oxytocin induction may be required to terminate the pregnancy.

Emergency treatment of eclamptic convulsions consists of immediate administration of diazepam I.V., followed by magnesium sulfate via I.V. drip, oxygen administration, and electronic fetal monitoring. After the patient's condition stabilizes, a cesarean section may be performed.

Adequate nutrition, good prenatal care, and control of preexisting hypertension during pregnancy decrease the incidence and severity of preeclampsia.

Clinical implications
• Monitor regularly for changes in blood pressure, pulse rate, respiration,

Teaching Topics in PIH

- An explanation of the classic signs of PIH and how the disorder compromises maternal and fetal blood flow
- Importance of treatment to preserve maternal and fetal health—and life
- How to collect urine for laboratory tests (a clean-catch midstream specimen and a 24-hour specimen)
- Preparation for amniocentesis and fetal monitoring, if appropriate
- Activity restrictions
- Importance of a nutritious, high-protein diet
- Drugs and their administration
- How to monitor PIH at home by measuring daily weight, blood pressure, and urine protein level
- Symptoms of worsening PIH
- Preparation for emergency delivery by induced labor or cesarean section, if indicated

fetal heart tones, vision, level of consciousness, and deep-tendon reflexes and for headache unrelieved by medication. Report changes immediately. Assess these signs before administering medications. Absence of patellar reflexes may indicate magnesium sulfate toxicity.

- Assess fluid balance by measuring intake and output and by checking daily weight.

- Observe for signs of fetal distress by closely monitoring the results of stress and nonstress tests.

- Instruct the patient to lie in a left lateral position to increase venous return, cardiac output, and renal blood flow.

- Keep emergency resuscitative equipment and drugs (including diazepam and magnesium sulfate) available in case of convulsions and cardiac or respiratory arrest. Also keep calcium gluconate at the bedside, since it counteracts the toxic effects of magnesium sulfate.

- To protect the patient from injury, maintain seizure precautions. Do not leave an unstable patient unattended.

- Assist with emergency medical treatment for the convulsive patient. Provide a quiet, darkened room until

the patient's condition stabilizes, and enforce absolute bed rest. Carefully monitor administration of magnesium sulfate. Give oxygen, as ordered. Do not administer anything by mouth. Insert an indwelling (Foley) catheter for accurate measurement of intake and output.

- Provide emotional support for the patient and family. If the patient's condition necessitates premature delivery, point out that infants of mothers with toxemia are usually small for gestational age but sometimes fare better than other premature babies of the same weight, possibly because they have developed adaptive responses to stress in utero.

(See *Teaching Topics in PIH*.)

Complications

Complications of persistent convulsions include cerebral hemorrhage, blindness, abruptio placentae, premature labor, stillbirth, renal failure, and hepatic damage.

Premenstrual syndrome

Description

Premenstrual syndrome (PMS) is characterized by varying symptoms that appear 7 to 14 days before menses and usually subside with its onset. The effects of PMS range from minimal discomfort to severe, disruptive symptoms. Incidence seems to rise with age and parity.

Causes

Although the direct cause of PMS is unknown, it is believed to result from a progesterone deficiency in the luteal phase of the menstrual cycle or from an increased estrogen-progesterone ratio. About 10% of patients with PMS have elevated prolactin levels.

Signs and symptoms

Behavioral
—Mild-to-severe personality changes
—Nervousness
—Hostility
—Irritability
—Agitation
—Sleep disturbances
—Fatigue
—Lethargy
—Depression

Somatic
—Breast tenderness or swelling
—Abdominal tenderness or bloating
—Joint pain
—Headache
—Edema
—Diarrhea or constipation
—Exacerbations of skin problems, such as acne or skin rash
—Respiratory problems such as asthma
—Neurologic problems such as seizures

Diagnostic tests

• Estrogen and progesterone blood levels may be evaluated to help rule out hormonal imbalance.
• Psychological evaluation is also recommended to rule out or detect an underlying psychiatric disorder.

Treatment

Treatment is primarily symptomatic and may include tranquilizers, sedatives, antidepressants, vitamins, and progestins. Effective treatment may require a diet that is low in simple sugars, caffeine, and salt, with adequate amounts of protein and complex carbohydrates and, possibly, vitamin supplements. (Salt restriction or the use of diuretics may be unnecessary.)

Clinical implications

• Inform the patient that self-help groups exist for women with PMS. If appropriate, help her contact such a group.
• Obtain a complete patient history to help identify any emotional problems that may contribute to PMS. If necessary, refer the patient for psychological counseling.
• If possible, discuss life-style changes—such as avoiding stimulants—that might help alleviate symptoms by reducing stress and anxiety.
• Advise further medical consultation if severe symptoms disrupt the patient's normal life-style.

Proctitis

Description

Proctitis is acute or chronic inflammation of the rectal mucosa. Prognosis is good unless massive bleeding occurs.

Causes

Contributing factors include the following:
• Chronic constipation
• Habitual laxative use
• Emotional upset
• Radiation, especially for cancer of the cervix and of the uterus
• Endocrine dysfunction
• Rectal injury
• Rectal medications
• Bacterial infections
• Allergies (especially to milk)
• Vasomotor disturbance that interferes with normal muscle control
• Food poisoning

Signs and symptoms
- Tenesmus
- Constipation
- A feeling of rectal fullness
- Left abdominal cramps
- An intense urge to defecate, which produces a small amount of stool that may contain blood and mucus

Diagnostic tests
- Sigmoidoscopy shows edematous, bright red or pink rectal mucosa that is thick, shiny, friable, and possibly ulcerated. In chronic proctitis, sigmoidoscopy shows thickened mucosa, loss of vascular pattern, and stricture of the rectal lumen.
- Biopsy to rule out carcinoma may be performed.
- A bacteriologic examination may be necessary.

Treatment and clinical implications
Primary treatment eliminates the underlying cause (fecal impaction, laxatives, or other medications). Soothing enemas, or steroid (hydrocortisone) suppositories or enemas may be helpful if proctitis is due to radiation. Tranquilizers may be appropriate for the patient with emotional stress.

Tell the patient to watch for and report bleeding and other persistent symptoms. Fully explain proctitis and its treatment to help him understand the disorder and prevent its recurrence. As appropriate, offer emotional support and reassurance during rectal examinations and treatment.

Progressive systemic sclerosis
(CREST syndrome, scleroderma)

Description
Progressive systemic sclerosis (PSS) is a diffuse connective tissue disease characterized by fibrotic, degenerative, and occasionally inflammatory changes in skin, blood vessels, synovial membranes, skeletal muscles, and internal organs (especially the esophagus, intestinal tract, thyroid, heart, lungs, and kidneys). It affects women more frequently than men, especially between ages 30 and 50. Approximately 30% of patients with PSS die within 5 years of onset.

Causes
Unknown

Signs and symptoms
- Raynaud's phenomenon—blanching, cyanosis, and erythema of the fingers and toes—usually the earliest symptom
- Possible ulcers on the tips of the fingers and toes
- Pain, stiffness, and swelling of fingers and joints
- Skin thickening, causing a masklike facial appearance
- Heartburn, dysphagia
- Abdominal distention
- Diarrhea, constipation
- Malodorous, floating stools
- Weight loss
- Dysrhythmias
- Dyspnea
- Malignant hypertension

Diagnostic tests
- Blood studies: slightly elevated erythrocyte sedimentation rate, positive rheumatoid factor in 25% to 35% of patients, and positive antinuclear antibody (low titer, speckled pattern)
- Urinalysis: proteinuria, microscopic hematuria, and casts (with renal involvement)
- Hand X-rays: terminal phalangeal tuft resorption, subcutaneous calcification, and joint space narrowing and erosion
- Chest X-rays: bilateral basilar pulmonary fibrosis
- GI X-rays: distal esophageal hypomotility and stricture, duodenal loop di-

lation, small-bowel malabsorption pattern, and large diverticula
• Pulmonary function studies: decreased diffusion and vital capacity
• EKG: possible nonspecific abnormalities related to myocardial fibrosis
• Skin biopsy: possible changes consistent with the progress of the disease, such as marked thickening of the dermis and occlusive vessel changes

Treatment
Currently, no cure exists for PSS. Treatment aims to preserve normal body functions and minimize complications. Use of immunosuppressants, such as chlorambucil, is a common palliative measure. Corticosteroids and colchicine have been used experimentally and seem to stabilize symptoms; D-penicillamine may be helpful. Blood platelet levels need to be monitored throughout drug and immunosuppressive therapy. Other treatment varies according to symptoms.
• Raynaud's phenomenon: various vasodilators and antihypertensive agents (such as methyldopa and reserpine), intermittent cervical sympathetic blockade, or, rarely, thoracic sympathectomy
• Chronic digital ulcerations: a digital plaster cast to immobilize the affected area, minimize trauma, and maintain cleanliness; possibly, surgical debridement
• Esophagitis with stricture: antacids; cimetidine; a soft, bland diet; and periodic esophageal dilation
• Small-bowel involvement (diarrhea, pain, malabsorption, weight loss): broad-spectrum antibiotics, such as erythromycin or tetracycline, to counteract bacterial overgrowth in the duodenum and jejunum related to hypomotility
• Scleroderma kidney (with malignant hypertension and impending renal failure): dialysis, antihypertensive agents, and calcium channel blockers

• Hand debilitation: physical therapy to maintain function and promote muscle strength, heat therapy to relieve joint stiffness, and patient teaching to ease performance of daily activities

Clinical implications
• Assess motion restrictions, pain, vital signs, intake and output, respiratory function, and daily weight.
• Because of compromised circulation, warn against finger-stick blood tests.
• Remember that air conditioning may aggravate Raynaud's phenomenon.
• Help the patient and family adjust to the patient's new body image and to the limitations and dependency these changes cause. Teach the patient to avoid fatigue by pacing activities and organizing schedules to include necessary rest. The patient and family need to accept that this condition is incurable.
• Encourage them to express their feelings, and help them cope with their fears and frustrations by offering information about the disease, its treatment, and relevant diagnostic tests.
• Whenever possible, let the patient participate in treatment by measuring his own intake and output, planning his own diet, assisting in dialysis, giving himself heat therapy, and doing prescribed exercises.

Prostatic cancer

Description
Prostatic cancer is the second most common neoplasm found in men over age 50 and the third leading cause of cancer death among males. Incidence is highest among blacks and in men with blood type A; it is lowest in Orientals. Its occurrence is unaffected by socioeconomic status or fertility. All males over age 40 should receive a rectal examination as part of their physical examination.

Staging Prostatic Cancer

Staging procedures for prostatic cancer include X-rays and laboratory and radioisotopic studies for clinical diagnosis; laparotomy, bone marrow aspiration, open or needle biopsy; and surgical resection and histologic examination of the prostate gland and possibly the regional lymph nodes.

Stage A: Incidental finding without symptoms
• Stage A1: Three or fewer well-differentiated foci
• Stage A2: More than three foci, poorly differentiated and more extensive than in Stage A1

Stage B: Palpable prostatic lesion
• Stage B1: Lesion less than 2 cm in diameter involving one lobe
• Stage B2: Lesion greater than 2 cm in diameter with diffuse involvement

Stage C: Extension of lesion beyond the prostatic capsule, but with no signs of metastasis

Stage D: Metastatic carcinoma
• Stage D1: Involvement of pelvic lymph nodes below the aortic bifurcation
• Stage D2: Lymph node involvement above the aortic bifurcation or metastasis to other distant sites

---

When prostatic cancer is treated in its localized form, the 5-year survival rate is 70%. After metastasis, the rate is under 35%. When prostatic cancer is fatal, death is usually the result of widespread bone metastases.

Causes
Unknown

Signs and symptoms
Signs and symptoms of prostatic cancer appear only in the advanced stages of the disease. Clinical effects include the following:
• Difficulty initiating a urinary stream
• Dribbling
• Urine retention
• Unexplained cystitis
• Rarely, hematuria
• On rectal examination, a hard nodule. This may be felt before symptoms develop, except in Stage A.

Diagnostic tests
• Biopsy confirms this diagnosis.
• Serum acid phosphatase is elevated in two-thirds of patients with metas-

tasized prostatic cancer. Successful therapy returns the serum acid phosphatase level to normal. A subsequent rise points to recurrence.
• Alkaline phosphatase levels that are increased and a positive bone scan point to bone metastasis.
• Routine bone X-rays do not always show evidence of metastasis.
(See *Staging Prostatic Cancer*.)

Treatment
Correct management of prostatic cancer depends on clinical assessment, tolerance to therapy, expected life span, and the stage of the disease. Treatment must be chosen carefully since prostatic cancer usually affects older men, who frequently have serious coexisting disorders such as hypertension, diabetes, or cardiac disease.

Therapy varies with each stage of the disease and generally includes radiation, prostatectomy, orchiectomy (removal of the testes) to decrease androgen production, and hormone therapy with synthetic estrogen (diethylstilbestrol [DES]). Radical prostatectomy is usually effective for localized lesions with no evidence of metastasis.

Radiation therapy is used for Stage B and C prostatic cancer and locally invasive lesions in Stage A, and also to relieve bone pain from metastatic skeletal involvement.

If hormone therapy, surgery, or radiation therapy are not feasible or successful, chemotherapy may be tried. Chemotherapy for prostatic cancer employs various combinations of cyclophosphamide, vinblastine, doxorubicin, bleomycin, cisplatin, and vindesine.

Clinical implications

The patient care plan should emphasize psychological support of patients facing prostatectomy, good postoperative care, and symptomatic treatment of radiation side effects.

• Before prostatectomy, follow these guidelines:
—Explain the expected effects of surgery (such as impotence and possible incontinence), as well as the side effects of radiation.
—Encourage the patient to express his fears.
—Instruct the patient about postoperative procedures.
—Teach the patient perineal exercises (done either sitting or standing) to minimize incontinence.
• After prostatectomy, follow these guidelines:
—Regularly check dressing, incision, and drainage systems for excessive bleeding; watch for signs of bleeding (cold, clammy skin, pallor, restlessness, falling blood pressure, and rising pulse rate).
—Watch for signs of infection. Maintain adequate fluid intake (at least 2,000 ml daily).
—Give antispasmodics, as ordered, to control postoperative bladder spasms. Give analgesics, as needed.

—Because urinary incontinence is a common problem after prostatectomy, keep the patient's skin clean and dry.
—When a patient receives radiation or hormonal therapy, watch for and treat nausea, vomiting, dry skin, and alopecia. Also watch for side effects of DES (gynecomastia, fluid retention, nausea, and vomiting). Watch for thrombophlebitis (pain, tenderness, swelling, warmth, and redness in calf), which is always a possibility in patients receiving DES.
• After a suprapubic prostatectomy, follow these guidelines:
—Keep the skin around the suprapubic drain dry and free from drainage and urine leakage.
—Allow the patient's family to assist in his care, and encourage their psychological support.
—Give meticulous catheter care.
• After transurethral resection:
—Watch for signs of urethral stricture and for abdominal distention (a result of urethral stricture or catheter blockage by a blood clot).
—Irrigate the catheter, as ordered.
• After a perineal prostatectomy:
—Avoid taking rectal temperature or inserting enema tubes or other rectal tubes.
—Provide pads to absorb urinary drainage and a rubber ring for the patient to sit on. Frequent sitz baths relieve pain and inflammation.
• After perineal and retropubic prostatectomy, give reassurance that urine leakage after catheter removal is normal and will disappear in time.

Prostatitis

Description

Prostatitis, inflammation of the prostate gland, may be acute or chronic. Acute prostatitis most often results from gram-negative bacteria and is easy to recognize and treat. However, chronic prostatitis, the most common cause of recurrent urinary tract infection in men, is less easy to recognize. As many as 35% of men over age 50 have chronic prostatitis.

Causes
• Primarily, infection by *Escherichia coli*
• Infection by *Klebsiella, Enterobacter, Proteus, Pseudomonas, Streptococcus*, or *Staphylococcus*

Signs and symptoms
Acute prostatitis
—Sudden fever
—Chills
—Low back pain
—Myalgia
—Perineal fullness
—Arthralgia
—Urinary urgency
—Possible dysuria, nocturia, some degree of urinary obstruction, and cloudy urine
—On rectal palpation of the prostate, marked tenderness, induration, swelling, firmness, and warmth
Chronic prostatitis
—May be asymptomatic
—Usually, same symptoms as acute prostatitis, but less severe
—Other possible signs: painful ejaculation, hemospermia, persistent urethral discharge, and sexual dysfunction

Diagnostic tests
• Urine culture can often identify the infecting organism.
• Comparison of urine cultures of samples obtained by the Meares and Stamey technique confirms the diagnosis. This test requires four specimens: one collected when the patient starts voiding (voided bladder one— VB1), another midstream (VB2), another after the patient stops voiding and the physician massages the prostate to produce secretions (EPS), and a final voided specimen (VB3). A significant increase in colony count of the prostatic specimens (EPS and VB3) confirms prostatitis.

Treatment
Systemic antibiotic therapy, based on sensitivity studies, is the treatment of choice for acute prostatitis. Aminoglycosides, such as gentamicin or tobramycin, may be the most effective drugs for severe cases. Co-trimoxazole is widely used to treat chronic prostatitis, which usually requires a long-term course of treatment (at least 6 weeks).

Supportive therapy includes bed rest, adequate hydration, and administration of analgesics, antipyretics, and stool softeners, as necessary.

If drug therapy is unsuccessful in treating chronic prostatitis, treatment may include transurethral resection of the prostate. To be effective, this procedure requires removal of all infected tissue. The procedure is usually not performed on young adults, because it usually leads to retrograde ejaculation and sterility. Total prostatectomy is curative but may cause sexual impotence and incontinence.

Clinical implications
• Ensure bed rest and adequate hydration. Provide stool softeners and administer sitz baths, as ordered.
• As necessary, prepare to assist with suprapubic needle aspiration of the bladder or a suprapubic cystostomy.
• Administer prescribed medications, as ordered. Emphasize to the patient the need for strict adherence to the prescribed drug treatment regimen. Instruct the patient to drink at least eight glasses of water a day.

Protein-calorie malnutrition

Description
One of the most prevalent and serious depletion disorders, protein-calorie malnutrition (PCM) occurs as maras-

mus (protein-calorie deficiency), characterized by growth failure and wasting, and as kwashiorkor (protein deficiency), characterized by tissue edema and damage. Both forms vary from mild to severe and may be fatal, depending on accompanying stress (particularly sepsis or injury) and duration of deprivation.

Causes
• Insufficient dietary intake because of excessive dieting, N.P.O. restrictions for an extended period, poor food choices, and lack of adequate food supply (mostly in underdeveloped countries)
• Increased energy demands because of extensive burns, traumatic injuries, systemic infection, and cancer
• Defective utilization of nutrients because of malabsorption syndrome, short bowel syndrome, and Crohn's disease
• Impaired digestion, absorption, or use of nutrients because of metabolic or endocrine diseases, such as juvenile diabetes

Signs and symptoms
Marasmus
—Small size for chronological age
—Sparse, dull hair
—Inactivity
—Mental apathy
—Dry, flaky skin
—Frequent infections
—Possible anorexia and diarrhea
—Irritability
—Swollen thyroid gland
—Spoon-shaped, brittle nails
—Red, swollen lips
—Decreased libido; amenorrhea
—Paresthesias
—Knock-kneed or bowed legs
—Possible dysrhythmias
Kwashiorkor
—Diminished adipose tissue (children may continue to grow in height)
—Edema (may mask muscle wasting)
—Dry, peeling skin
—Hepatomegaly

Diagnostic tests
• Height and weight are less than 80% of standard for the patient's age and sex, and arm circumference and triceps skinfold are below standard.
• Serum albumin concentration is less than 2.8 g/100 ml (normal is 3.3 to 4.3 g/100 ml).
• Urinary creatinine (24-hour) shows lean body mass status after creatinine excretion is related to height and ideal body weight to yield creatinine-height index.
• Skin tests with standard antigens (streptokinase-streptodornase) to indicate degree of immune compromise by determining reactivity expressed as a percentage of normal reaction.
• CBC reveals moderate anemia.

Treatment
The aim of treatment is to provide sufficient proteins, calories, and other nutrients for nutritional rehabilitation and maintenance. When treating severe PCM, restoring fluid and electrolyte balance parentally is the initial concern. A patient who shows normal absorption may receive enteral nutrition after anorexia has subsided. When possible, the preferred treatment is oral feeding of high-quality protein foods, especially milk, and protein-calorie supplements. A patient who is unwilling or unable to eat may require supplementary feedings through a nasogastric tube or total parenteral nutrition (TPN) through a central venous catheter. Accompanying infection must also be treated, preferably with antibiotics that do not inhibit protein synthesis. Cautious realimentation is essential to prevent complications from overloading the compromised metabolic system.

Clinical implications
• Encourage the patient with PCM to consume as many nutritious foods and beverages as possible (it is often helpful to "cheer him on" as he eats). As-

sist the patient to eat, if necessary. Cooperate closely with the dietitian to monitor intake and to provide acceptable meals and snacks.

• If TPN is necessary, observe strict aseptic technique when handling catheters, tubes, and solutions when changing dressings.

• Watch for PCM in patients who have been hospitalized for a prolonged period, have had no oral intake for several days, or are cachectic.

• To help eradicate PCM in developing countries, encourage prolonged breast-feeding, educate mothers about their children's needs, and provide supplementary foods, as needed.

Pseudomembranous enterocolitis

Description
Pseudomembranous enterocolitis is an acute inflammation and necrosis of the small and large intestines, which usually affects the mucosa but may extend into submucosa and, rarely, other layers. This disorder has occurred postoperatively in debilitated patients who have undergone abdominal surgery or patients who have been treated with broad-spectrum antibiotics. Marked by severe diarrhea, this rare condition is usually fatal in 1 to 7 days because of severe dehydration and toxicity, peritonitis, or perforation.

Causes
The exact cause is unknown; however, *Clostridium difficile* is thought to produce a toxin that may play a role in its development.

Signs and symptoms
• Sudden onset of copious watery or bloody diarrhea
• Abdominal pain
• Fever

Diagnostic tests
• A rectal biopsy through sigmoidoscopy confirms pseudomembranous enterocolitis.
• Stool cultures can identify *C. difficile*.

Treatment
A patient receiving broad-spectrum antibiotic therapy requires immediate discontinuation of the antibiotics. Effective treatment includes antibiotics such as vancomycin, metronidazole, or bacitracin. A patient with mild pseudomembranous enterocolitis may receive anion exchange resins, such as cholestyramine, to bind the toxin produced by *C. difficile*. Supportive treatment must maintain fluid and electrolyte balance and combat hypotension and shock with pressors, such as dopamine and levarterenol.

Clinical implications
• Monitor vital signs, skin color, and level of consciousness. Immediately report signs of shock.
• Record fluid intake and output, including fluid lost in stools. Watch for dehydration (poor skin turgor, sunken eyes, and decreased urine output).
• Check serum electrolytes daily, and watch for clinical signs of hypokalemia, especially malaise, and weak, rapid, irregular pulse.

Complications
• Severe dehydration
• Electrolyte imbalance
• Hypotension
• Shock
• Colonic perforation

Psoriasis

Description
Psoriasis is a chronic, recurrent disease marked by epidermal proliferation. Its lesions, which appear as erythematous papules and plaques

covered with silvery scales, vary widely in severity and distribution. Although this disorder is most common in adults, it may strike at any age, including infancy. Psoriasis is characterized by recurring remissions and exacerbations. Flare-ups are often related to specific systemic and environmental factors such as pregnancy, cold weather, and emotional stress, but they may be unpredictable. They can usually be controlled with therapy.

Causes
The tendency to develop psoriasis is genetically determined. Researchers have discovered significantly higher than normal incidence of certain histocompatibility antigens (HLA) in patients with psoriasis, suggesting a possible autoimmune deficiency.

Signs and symptoms
• Usually, small erythematous papules (initial symptom). These enlarge or coalesce to form red, elevated plaques with silver scabs on the scalp, chest, elbows, knees, back, buttocks, and genitals.
• Pruritus
• Pain (common)
• Possible nail pitting and joint stiffness

Diagnostic tests
• Skin biopsy may be needed to establish the diagnosis; however, patient history and appearance of the lesions may permit diagnosis.
• Serum uric acid is typically elevated.
• HLA antigens 13 and 17 may be present.

Treatment
Treatment depends on the type of psoriasis, the extent of the disease and the patient's response to it, and what effect the disease has on the patient's lifestyle. No permanent cure exists, and all methods of treatment are merely palliative.

Removal of psoriatic scales necessitates application of occlusive ointment bases, such as petrolatum, salicylic acid preparations, or preparations containing urea. These medications soften the scales, which can then be removed by scrubbing carefully with a soft brush in an oatmeal or salt bath.

Methods to retard rapid cell production include exposure to ultraviolet light (wavelength B [UVB] or natural sunlight) to the point of minimal erythema. Tar preparations or crude coal tar itself may be applied to affected areas about 15 minutes before exposure or may be left on overnight and wiped off the next morning. A thin layer of petrolatum may be applied before UVB exposure.

Steroid creams are useful to control psoriasis. A potent fluorinated steroid works well, except on the face and intertriginous areas. Small, stubborn plaques that resist local treatment may require intralesional steroid injections. Anthralin, combined with a paste mixture, may be used for well-defined plaques but must not be applied to unaffected areas, because it may cause an allergic reaction. It also stains the skin.

In a patient with severe chronic psoriasis, the Goeckerman regimen—which combines tar baths and UVB treatments—may help achieve remission and clear the skin in 3 to 5 weeks. The Ingram technique is a variation of this treatment, using anthralin instead of tar. A program called PUVA combines administration of methoxsalen with exposure to ultraviolet light, wavelength A (UVA). As a last resort, a cytotoxin, usually methotrexate, may help severe, refractory psoriasis.

Low-dosage antihistamines, oatmeal baths, emollients (perhaps with phenol and methol), and open wet dressings may help relieve pruritus. Aspirin and local heat help alleviate the pain of psoriatic arthritis; severe cases may require nonsteroidal anti-inflammatory drugs, such as indomethacin.

Therapy for psoriasis of the scalp often consists of a tar shampoo, followed by application of a steroid lotion while the hair is still wet. No effective treatment exists for psoriasis of the nails. The nails usually improve as skin lesions improve.

Clinical implications

Design the patient's care plan to include patient teaching, careful monitoring for side effects of therapy, and sympathetic support.
• Make sure the patient understands his prescribed therapy; provide written instructions to avoid confusion. Teach application of prescribed creams and lotions. A steroid cream, for example, should be applied in a thin film and rubbed into the skin until the cream disappears. Steroid creams are usually covered with an occlusive dressing and left on overnight. Anthralin and tar should be applied with a downward motion to avoid rubbing them into the follicles. Gloves should be worn, because anthralin stains the skin. After application, the patient may dust himself with powder to prevent anthralin from rubbing off on his clothes. Warn the patient never to put an occlusive dressing over anthralin. Suggest use of mineral oil, then soap and water, to remove anthralin. Caution the patient to avoid scrubbing his skin vigorously. If a medication has been applied to the scales to soften them, suggest the patient use a soft brush to remove them.
• Watch for side effects, especially allergic reactions to anthralin, atrophy and acne from steroids, and burning, itching, nausea, and squamous cell epitheliomas from PUVA. Evaluate the patient on methotrexate weekly for RBC, WBC, and platelet counts, because cytotoxins may cause hepatic or bone marrow toxicity. Liver biopsy may be performed to assess the effects of methotrexate.

• Caution the patient receiving PUVA therapy to stay out of the sun on the day of treatment and to protect his eyes with sunglasses that screen UVA for 24 hours after treatment. Tell him to wear goggles during exposure to this light.
• Be aware that psoriasis can cause psychological problems. Assure the patient that psoriasis is not contagious, and although exacerbations and remissions occur, they are controllable with treatment. However, be sure he understands there is no cure. Also, since stressful situations tend to exacerbate psoriasis, help the patient learn to cope with these situations. Explain the relationship between psoriasis and arthritis, but point out that psoriasis causes no other systemic disturbances. Refer patients to the National Psoriasis Foundation, which provides information and directs patients to local chapters.

Psychogenic pain disorder

Description

The striking feature of psychogenic pain disorder is a persistent complaint of pain without appropriate physical findings. Although psychogenic pain has no physical cause, it is as real to the patient as organic pain. An important feature in psychogenic pain disorder is secondary gain. The pain may allow the patient to avoid a stressful situation or receive attention not otherwise available. This secondary gain is essential to the persistence of the pain. Unfortunately, the patient does not usually acknowledge any psychological basis for his pain. Such pain is usually chronic, with exacerbations at times of stress. Its complications, including loss of work, interference with interpersonal relationships, drug dependence, extensive evaluations, and surgical procedures, can make prognosis grim.

Causes

Psychogenic pain disorder has no specific cause. Severe psychological stress or conflict is evident, but may not be as clearly time-related to the pain as in conversion disorders.

Signs and symptoms

The cardinal feature is chronic, consistent complaints of pain without confirming physical disease. Such pain does not follow anatomic pathways.

Diagnostic tests

• A complete medical evaluation is needed to rule out organic diseases, such as multiple sclerosis, neuropathy, or tension headaches.

• A psychiatric evaluation must rule out malingering, use of the complaint to receive narcotics, depressive disorder, somatization disorder, hypochondriasis, schizophrenia, or a personality disorder.

Treatment

The goal of treatment is not necessarily to eradicate the pain, but rather to ease it and help the patient live with it. Treatment should avoid long, invasive evaluations and surgical interventions. Treatment at a comprehensive pain center may be helpful. Supportive measures for pain relief may include hot or cold packs, physical therapy, distraction techniques, or cutaneous stimulation with massage or transcutaneous electrical nerve stimulation (TENS). Measures to reduce the patient's anxiety may also be helpful. A continuing supportive relationship with an understanding health care professional is essential for effective management. Regularly scheduled follow-up appointments are helpful.

Analgesics usually become an issue because the patient believes, "I have to fight for everything I get." The patient should clearly be told what medication he will receive and should receive other supportive pain relief measures as well. Regularly scheduled analgesic doses can be more effective than as-needed scheduling; regular doses reduce pain by reducing anxiety about asking for medication. The use of placebos will destroy trust when the patient discovers the deceit.

Clinical implications

• Provide a caring, accepting atmosphere where the patient's complaints are taken seriously and every effort is made to provide relief. This does not mean providing increasing amounts of narcotics on demand; rather, it means communicating to the patient that you will collaborate in a treatment plan, and clearly stating the limitations. For example, you might say, "I can stay with you now for 15 minutes, but you cannot receive another dose until 2 p.m."

• Do not tell the patient he is imagining the pain or can wait longer for medication that is due. Assess his complaints and help him understand what is contributing to the pain. You might ask, "I've noticed you complain of more pain after your doctor visits. What are his visits like for you?" to elicit contributing perceptions and fears.

• Teach the patient noninvasive, drug-free methods of pain control, such as guided imagery, relaxation techniques, or distraction through reading or writing.

• Encourage the patient to maintain independence despite his pain.

• Offer attention at times other than during the patient's complaints of pain, to weaken the link to secondary gain.

• Avoid confronting the patient with the psychogenic nature of his pain. This is rarely helpful because such pain is his means of avoiding psychological conflict. Psychiatric care can be useful, so consider psychiatric referrals. Realize, however, that such patients usually resist psychiatric intervention and do not expect it to replace analgesic measures.

Psychosexual dysfunction

Description
Psychosexual dysfunction is evident by impairment of one or more of the four physiologic phases of the sexual response cycle, also termed the stages of orgasm: 1) appetitive—desire for and fantasies about sexual activity; 2) excitement—the physiologic changes associated with sexual arousal; 3) orgasm—the peak of sexual pleasure, with psychological and physiologic effects; and 4) resolution—recovery and relaxation after orgasm.

Psychosexual dysfunction may be lifelong or may develop after a period of normal function, generalized or limited to certain situations or partners, and total or partial. The most common age at onset is early adult life; the common age of clinical presentation is the late twenties and early thirties. The course is variable.

Causes
Psychological factors, such as fear of pain, pregnancy, or inadequacy; guilt associated with sexual pleasure; or conflict with a partner

Signs and symptoms
Any of the following may occur:
Females
—Delay or absence of orgasm despite sexual stimulation of adequate duration and intensity
—Functional dyspareunia
—Functional vaginismus
Males
—Delay or absence of ejaculation during adequate sexual stimulation
—Premature ejaculation, which occurs before or immediately after penetration or before the wishes of his partner

Diagnostic tests
• Diagnosis of psychosexual disorders rests on the patient's subjective report of problems of frequency, chronicity, stress, and quality. No true norms exist to define minimum activity and type or quality of sexual function. Great variations are characteristic.
• Medical evaluation must rule out physical causes of sexual impairment: diabetes, syphilis, multiple sclerosis, and other disorders of the sacral segments of the spinal cord or lumbar innervation of the spine and certain drugs.
• Psychiatric testing may be necessary to rule out psychiatric illnesses, such as depression, which may cause sexual impairment.

Treatment
Psychosexual disorders can be mild or transient. They are sometimes quite challenging. Treatment has become increasingly sophisticated. Sex education may be used to correct erroneous sexual notions, to change problematic attitudes, and to impart new information. Topics may include anatomic data and coital and pleasure-enhancing techniques.

Psychotherapy may include behavioral, supportive, and insight-oriented techniques. These are aimed at encouraging expression of feelings, reducing and controlling anxiety, weakening inhibitions, undoing faulty learning, and promoting assertiveness.

Marital counseling supplements sexual information and advice with an examination of the couple's relationship. Their sexual difficulties may be secondary to other conflicts that, when resolved, lead to improved sexual relations.

Physical therapies and mechanical aids may be of assistance in some cases. Females may be helped by exercises (Kegel exercises) that tone and strengthen the vaginal muscles.

Clinical implications
Through meticulous interviewing techniques that follow up on leads from

the patient; thorough, nonjudgmental assessments; and expert teaching and counseling techniques, you can influence the patient's improvement. To contribute significantly, you must understand the theory of normal sexual development and function so you can dispel myths and misconceptions of sexual function. Counsel to help overcome guilt, shame, and body image disturbances. As needed, refer the patient for special treatment and counseling.

Pulmonary edema

Description
Pulmonary edema is the accumulation of fluid in the extravascular spaces of the lung. In cardiogenic pulmonary edema, fluid accumulation results from elevations in pulmonary venous and capillary hydrostatic pressures. A common complication of cardiac disorders, pulmonary edema can occur as a chronic condition or develop quickly and rapidly become fatal.

Causes
• Congestive heart failure (most common)
• Barbiturate and opiate poisoning
• Hodgkin's disease
• Obliterative lymphangitis after radiation
• Extensive burns
• Nephrosis
• Hepatic disease
• Nutritional deficiency
• Protein-losing enteropathy
• Pulmonary veno-occlusive disease
• Mitral stenosis and left atrial myxoma
• Infusion of excessive volumes of I.V. fluids
• Hemorrhagic pancreatitis
• Near drowning and inhalation of irritating gases

Signs and symptoms
Clinical features of pulmonary edema permit a working diagnosis. (See *Staging Pulmonary Edema*.)

Diagnostic tests
• Arterial blood gases usually show hypoxia; PCO_2 is variable. Both profound respiratory alkalosis and acidosis may occur. Metabolic acidosis occurs when cardiac output is low.
• Chest X-ray shows diffuse haziness of the lung fields and, often, cardiomegaly and pleural effusions.
• Pulmonary artery catheterization helps identify left ventricular failure by showing elevated pulmonary wedge pressures. This helps to rule out adult respiratory distress syndrome in which pulmonary wedge pressure is usually normal.

Treatment
Treatment of pulmonary edema is designed to reduce extravascular fluid, to improve gas exchange and myocardial function, and, if possible, to correct the underlying pathology. Administration of high concentrations of oxygen by cannula, mask, and, if necessary, assisted ventilation improves oxygen delivery to the tissues and often improves acid-base disturbances. A bronchodilator, such as aminophylline, may decrease bronchospasm and enhance myocardial contractility. Diuretics, such as furosemide and ethacrynic acid, promote diuresis, thereby assisting in the mobilization of extravascular fluid.

Treatment of myocardial dysfunction includes digitalis or pressor agents to increase cardiac contractility, antiarrhythmics (particularly when dysrhythmias are associated with decreased cardiac output), and, occasionally, arterial vasodilators, such as nitroprusside, which decrease peripheral vascular resistance and thereby decrease left ventricular workload. Other treatment includes morphine to reduce anxiety and dyspnea and to dilate the systemic venous bed.

Staging Pulmonary Edema

STAGE	PATHOPHYSIOLOGY	SIGNS AND SYMPTOMS
Initial	• Usually, left ventricular failure increases pulmonary vascular bed pressure, forcing fluid and solutes from the intravascular compartment into the interstitium of the lungs. As the interstitium overloads with fluid, fluid enters the peripheral alveoli, impairing adequate gas exchange.	• Persistent cough—patient feels like he has "a cold coming on" • Slight dyspnea/orthopnea • Exercise intolerance • Restlessness • Anxiety • Crepitant rales may be heard over the dependent portion of the lungs • Diastolic gallop
Acute	• Fluid accumulation throughout pulmonary vasculature and further filling of the alveoli	• Acute shortness of breath • Respirations—rapid, noisy (audible wheeze, rales) • Cough more intense, producing frothy, blood-tinged sputum • Cyanosis • Diaphoresis, cold and clammy skin • Tachycardia, dysrhythmias • Hypotension
Advanced	• Patient's condition rapidly deteriorates as the bronchial tree fills with fluid.	• Decreased level of consciousness • Ventricular dysrhythmias • Shock • Diminished breath sounds

Rotating tourniquets may be used as an emergency measure to reduce venous return to the heart from the extremities.

Clinical implications

• Carefully monitor the vulnerable patient for early signs of pulmonary edema, especially tachypnea, tachycardia, and abnormal breath sounds.

Report any abnormalities. Check for peripheral edema, which may also indicate that fluid is accumulating in pulmonary tissue.

• Administer oxygen, as ordered.

• Monitor vital signs every 15 to 30 minutes while administering nitroprusside in 5% dextrose in water by I.V. drip. Discard unused nitroprusside solution after 4 hours, and protect it from light by wrapping the bottle or bag with aluminum foil. Watch for dysrhythmias in patients receiving digitalis and for marked respiratory depression in those receiving morphine.

• Assess the patient's condition frequently, and record response to treatment. Monitor arterial blood gas measurements, oral and I.V. fluid intake, urinary output, and, in the patient with a pulmonary artery catheter, pulmonary end diastolic and wedge pressures. Check the cardiac monitor often. Report changes immediately.

• Record the sequence and time of rotating tourniquets.

• Reassure the patient, who may be frightened by decreased respiratory capability, in a calm voice, and explain all procedures to him. Provide emotional support to his family as well.

Pulmonary embolism and infarction

Description

The most common pulmonary complication in hospitalized patients, pulmonary embolism is an obstruction of the pulmonary arterial bed by a dislodged thrombus or foreign substance. Although pulmonary infarction may be so mild as to be asymptomatic, massive embolism (more than 50% obstruction of pulmonary arterial circulation) and infarction can be rapidly fatal.

Causes

Pulmonary embolism
—Usually, this results from dislodged thrombi originating in the leg veins. Other less common sources of thrombi are the pelvic veins, renal veins, hepatic vein, right heart, and upper extremities.

—Rarely, the emboli contain air, fat, amniotic fluid, or talc (from drugs intended for oral administration that are injected intravenously by addicts), or tumor cells.

Pulmonary infarction
—This may evolve from pulmonary embolism, especially in patients with chronic cardiac or pulmonary disease.

Risk factors

• Long-term immobility
• Chronic pulmonary disease
• Congestive heart failure or atrial fibrillation
• Thrombophlebitis
• Polycythemia vera
• Thrombocytosis
• Autoimmune hemolytic anemia
• Sickle cell disease
• Varicose veins
• Recent surgery
• Advanced age
• Pregnancy
• Lower extremity fractures or surgery
• Burns
• Obesity
• Vascular injury
• Cancer
• Oral contraceptive use

Signs and symptoms

Total occlusion of the main pulmonary artery is rapidly fatal; smaller or fragmented emboli produce symptoms that vary with the size, number, and location of the emboli.

• Usually, the first symptom of pulmonary embolism is dyspnea, which may be accompanied by anginal or pleuritic chest pain.

• Other clinical features include tachycardia, productive cough (sputum may be blood-tinged), and low-grade fever.

• Less common signs include massive hemoptysis, splinting of the chest, leg edema, and, with a large embolus, cyanosis, syncope, and distended neck veins.

• Signs of circulatory collapse (weak, rapid pulse; hypotension) and signs of hypoxia (restlessness) may occur.

- Auscultation occasionally reveals a right ventricular (S_3) gallop and increased intensity of a pulmonic component of S_2. Crackles and a pleural rub also may be heard at the site of embolism.

Diagnostic tests

- Chest X-ray helps to rule out other pulmonary diseases; it shows areas of atelectasis, elevated diaphragm and pleural effusion, prominent pulmonary artery, and, occasionally, the characteristic wedge-shaped infiltrate suggestive of pulmonary embolism.
- Lung scan shows perfusion defects in areas beyond occluded vessels; normal lung scan rules out pulmonary embolism.
- Pulmonary angiography is the most definitive test. It poses some risk to the patient, and its use depends on the uncertainty of the diagnosis and the need to avoid unnecessary anticoagulant therapy in high-risk patients.
- EKG is inconclusive but helps distinguish pulmonary embolism from myocardial infarction. In extensive embolism, EKG may show right axis deviation, right bundle branch block, tall peaked P waves, depression of ST segments and T-wave inversions (indicative of right heart strain), and supraventricular tachydysrhythmias.
- Arterial blood gas measurements showing decreased PO_2 and PCO_2 are characteristic but do not always occur.
- Thoracentesis may rule out empyema, which indicates pneumonia, if pleural effusion is present.

Treatment

Treatment is designed to maintain adequate cardiovascular and pulmonary function during resolution of the obstruction and to prevent recurrence of emboli. Since most emboli largely resolve within 10 to 14 days, treatment consists of oxygen therapy, as needed, and anticoagulation with heparin to inhibit new thrombus formation. Patients with massive pulmonary embolism and shock may require fibrinolytic therapy with urokinase or streptokinase to enhance fibrinolysis of the pulmonary emboli and remaining thrombi. Emboli that cause hypotension may require the use of vasopressors. Treatment for septic emboli requires antibiotic therapy, not anticoagulants, and evaluation of the source of infection, particularly endocarditis.

Surgery to interrupt the inferior vena cava is reserved for patients who cannot take anticoagulants or who have recurrent emboli during anticoagulant therapy. It should not be performed without angiographic demonstration of pulmonary embolism. Surgery consists of vena caval ligation, plication, or insertion of a device (umbrella filter) to filter blood returning to the heart and lungs.

To prevent postoperative venous thromboembolism, a combination of heparin and dihydroergotamine (Embolex) may be administered. Embolex is more effective than heparin alone.

Clinical implications

- Give oxygen by nasal cannula or mask. Check arterial blood gases in the presence of fresh emboli or worsening dyspnea. Be prepared to provide endotracheal intubation with assisted ventilation if breathing is severely compromised.
- Administer heparin, as ordered, through I.V. push or continuous drip. Monitor coagulation studies daily.
- After the patient is stable, encourage him to move about often, and assist with isometric and range-of-motion exercises. Check pedal pulses, temperature, and color of feet to detect venostasis. *Never* vigorously massage the patient's legs.
- Walk the patient as soon as possible after surgery to prevent venostasis.
- Report frequent pleuritic chest pain, so analgesics can be prescribed. Also,

incentive spirometry can assist in deep breathing.

• Warn the patient not to cross his legs. This promotes thrombus formation.

• To relieve anxiety, explain procedures and treatments. Encourage the patient's family to participate in his care.

• Most patients need treatment with an oral anticoagulant (warfarin) for 4 to 6 months after a pulmonary embolism. Advise the patient to watch for signs of bleeding (bloody stools, blood in urine, large ecchymoses), to take the prescribed medication exactly as ordered, and to avoid taking any additional medication (even for headaches or colds) or changing doses of medication without consulting the physician. Stress the importance of follow-up laboratory tests to monitor anticoagulant therapy.

• To prevent pulmonary emboli, encourage early ambulation in patients predisposed to this condition. With close medical supervision, low-dose heparin may be useful prophylactically.

Pulmonary hypertension

Description
In adults, pulmonary hypertension is indicated by resting systolic pulmonary artery pressure above 30 mm Hg and mean pulmonary artery pressure above 18 mm Hg. It may be primary (rare) or secondary (far more common). Primary, or idiopathic, pulmonary hypertension occurs most often in women between ages 20 and 40, usually is fatal within 3 to 4 years, and shows the highest mortality among pregnant women. Secondary pulmonary hypertension results from existing cardiac and/or pulmonary disease.

Prognosis depends on the severity of the underlying disorder.

Causes
Primary pulmonary hypertension
—Thought to result from altered immune mechanisms because this form of pulmonary hypertension occurs in association with collagen diseases
Secondary pulmonary hypertension
—Alveolar hypoventilation in chronic obstructive pulmonary disease (most common cause in the United States), sarcoidosis, diffuse interstitial pneumonia, malignant metastases, and scleroderma
—Vascular obstruction from pulmonary embolism, vasculitis, and disorders that cause obstructions of small or large pulmonary veins, such as left atrial myxoma, idiopathic veno-occlusive disease, fibrosing mediastinitis, and mediastinal neoplasm
—Primary cardiac disease, which may be congenital (such as patent ductus arteriosus, or atrial or ventricular septal defect) or acquired (such as rheumatic valvular disease and mitral stenosis)

Signs and symptoms
• Increasing dyspnea on exertion
• Weakness
• Syncope
• Fatigability
• Possible signs of right heart failure, including peripheral edema, ascites, neck vein distention, and hepatomegaly

Diagnostic tests
• Arterial blood gases show hypoxemia (decreased PO_2).
• EKG shows right axis deviation and tall or peaked P waves in inferior leads in right ventricular hypertrophy.
• Cardiac catheterization shows increased pulmonary artery pressures (PAP)—pulmonary systolic pressure is above 30 mm Hg; pulmonary capillary wedge pressure (PCWP) is increased if the underlying cause is left atrial

myxoma, mitral stenosis, or left ventricular failure.

• Pulmonary angiography detects filling defects in pulmonary vasculature, such as those that develop in patients with pulmonary emboli.

• Pulmonary function tests in underlying obstructive disease may show decreased flow rates and increased residual volume; in underlying restrictive disease, total lung capacity may decrease.

Treatment

Treatment usually includes oxygen therapy to decrease hypoxemia and resulting pulmonary vascular resistance. For patients with right ventricular failure, treatment also includes fluid restriction, digitalis to increase cardiac output, and diuretics to decrease intravascular volume and extravascular fluid accumulation. Of course, an important goal of treatment is correction of the underlying cause.

Clinical implications

• Administer oxygen therapy, as ordered, and observe the response. Report any signs of increasing dyspnea so that the physician can adjust treatment accordingly.

• Monitor arterial blood gases for acidosis and hypoxemia. Report any change in level of consciousness immediately.

• When caring for a patient with right heart failure, especially one receiving diuretics, record weight daily, carefully measure intake and output, and explain all medications and diet restrictions. Check for increasing neck vein distention, which may indicate fluid overload.

• Monitor vital signs, especially blood pressure and heart rate. Watch for hypotension and tachycardia. If the patient has a pulmonary artery catheter, check PAP and PCWP, as ordered, and report any changes.

• Before discharge, help the patient adjust to the limitations imposed by this disorder. Advise against overexertion and suggest frequent rest periods between activities. Refer the patient to the social services department if special equipment, such as oxygen equipment, is needed for home use. Make sure he understands the prescribed diet and medications.

Pyelonephritis

Description

One of the most common renal diseases, acute pyelonephritis is a sudden inflammation caused by bacteria. It primarily affects the interstitial area and the renal pelvis or, less often, the renal tubules. With treatment and continued follow-up, prognosis is good. Extensive permanent damage is rare. (Also see *Chronic Pyelonephritis,* p. 636.)

Causes

• Bacterial infection of the kidney, most commonly resulting from an ascending infection, less commonly from hematogenous or lymphatic spread

• Infecting organisms: *Escherichia coli* (most common), *Proteus, Pseudomonas, Staphylococcus aureus,* and *Streptococcus faecalis* (enterococcus)

Risk factors

• Diagnostic and therapeutic use of instruments, as in catheterization, cystoscopy, or urologic surgery

• Inability to empty the bladder (for example, in patients with neurogenic bladder), urinary stasis, or urinary obstruction due to tumors, strictures, or benign prostatic hypertrophy

• Sexual activity in women (intercourse increases the risk of bacterial contamination)

• Pregnancy (about 5% of pregnant

Chronic Pyelonephritis

Chronic pyelonephritis is a persistent kidney inflammation that can scar the kidneys and may lead to chronic renal failure. Its etiology may be bacterial, metastatic, or urogenous. This disease is most common in patients who are predisposed to recurrent acute pyelonephritis, such as those with urinary obstructions or vesicoureteral reflux.

Patients with chronic pyelonephritis may have a childhood history of unexplained fevers or bed-wetting. Clinical effects may include flank pain, anemia, low urine specific gravity, proteinuria, leukocytes in urine, and, especially in late stages, hypertension. Uremia rarely develops from chronic pyelonephritis unless structural abnormalities exist in the excretory system. Bacteriuria may be intermittent. When no bacteria are found in the urine, diagnosis depends on intravenous pyelography (renal pelvis may appear small and flattened) and renal biopsy.

Effective treatment of chronic pyelonephritis requires control of hypertension, elimination of the existing obstruction (when possible), and long-term antimicrobial therapy.

women develop asymptomatic bacteriuria; if untreated, about 40% develop pyelonephritis)
• Diabetes (glycosuria may support bacterial growth in the urine)
• Other renal diseases

Signs and symptoms
• Urinary urgency
• Urinary frequency
• Burning during urination
• Dysuria
• Nocturia
• Hematuria (usually microscopic but may be gross)
• Possibly cloudy urine with an ammoniacal or fishy odor
• Temperature of 102° F. (38.9° C.) or higher
• Shaking chills
• Flank pain
• Anorexia
• General fatigue

Diagnostic tests
• Urinalysis reveals pyuria and possibly a few RBCs; low specific gravity and osmolality; slightly alkaline pH; and possible proteinuria, glycosuria, and ketonuria.
• Urine culture reveals more than 100,000 organisms/mm³ of urine.

• Plain film of the kidneys-ureters-bladder may reveal calculi, tumors, or cysts in the kidneys and the urinary tract.
• Intravenous pyelography may show asymmetrical kidneys.

Treatment
Treatment centers on antibiotic therapy appropriate to the specific infecting organism, after identification by urine culture and sensitivity studies. When the infecting organism cannot be identified, therapy usually consists of a broad-spectrum antibiotic. If the patient is pregnant, antibiotics must be prescribed cautiously. Urinary analgesics, such as phenazopyridine, are also appropriate.

Symptoms may disappear after several days of antibiotic therapy. Although urine usually becomes sterile within 48 to 72 hours, the course of such therapy is 10 to 14 days. Follow-up treatment includes reculturing urine 1 week after drug therapy stops, then periodically for the next year to detect residual or recurring infection. Most patients with uncomplicated infections respond well to therapy and do not suffer reinfection.

In infection from obstruction or vesicoureteral reflux, antibiotics may be less effective. Treatment may then necessitate surgery to relieve the obstruction or correct the anomaly. Patients at high risk of recurring urinary tract and kidney infections—such as those with prolonged use of an indwelling (Foley) catheter or maintenance antibiotic therapy—require long-term follow-up.

Clinical implications
• Administer antipyretics for fever.
• Force fluids to achieve urinary output of more than 2,000 ml/day. Do not encourage intake of more than 2 to 3 liters, because this may decrease the effectiveness of the antibiotics.
• Provide an acid-ash diet to prevent stone formation.
• Teach proper technique for collecting a clean-catch urine specimen. Be sure to refrigerate or culture a urine specimen within 30 minutes of collection to prevent overgrowth of bacteria.
• Stress the need to complete prescribed antibiotic therapy, even after symptoms subside. Encourage long-term follow-up care for high-risk patients.

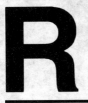

Rabies
(Hydrophobia)

Description
Rabies is an acute CNS infection caused by a virus. If symptoms occur, rabies is almost always fatal. Treatment soon after a bite, however, may prevent fatal CNS invasion.

Causes
An RNA virus

Mode of transmission
Bite of an infected animal

Signs and symptoms
Prodromal phase
—Slight fever
—Malaise
—Headache
—Sore throat
—Persistent loose cough
Acute phase
—Anxiety
—Photophobia
—Irritability
—Weakness of facial muscles
—Marked restlessness
—Ocular palsies
—In severe cases, tachycardia or bradycardia, cyclic respirations, urinary retention, and temperature of 103° F. (39.4° C.)
—Possible painful pharyngeal muscle spasms with difficulty swallowing and expulsion of frothy saliva from the mouth
Terminal phase
—Progressive, generalized, flaccid paralysis that ultimately leads to peripheral vascular collapse, coma, and death

Diagnostic tests
• Virus isolation from the patient's saliva or throat and examination of his blood for fluorescent rabies antibody (FRA) are considered the most definitive diagnostic tests.
• WBC count and polymorphonuclear and large mononuclear cell counts are increased.
• Urinalysis shows elevated glucose, acetone, and protein levels.
• Confinement of the suspected animal for 10 days of observation by a veterinarian also helps support this diagnosis. If the animal appears rabid, it should be killed and its brain tissue tested for FRA and Negri bodies (oval or round masses that conclusively confirm rabies).

Treatment
Treatment consists of wound treatment and immunization as soon as possible after exposure. Thoroughly wash all bite wounds and scratches with soap and water for at least 10 minutes. (See *First Aid in Animal Bites.*) Check the patient's immunization status, and administer tetanus-diphtheria prophylaxis, if needed. Take measures to control bacterial infection, as ordered. If the wound requires suturing, special treatment and suturing techniques must be used to allow proper wound drainage.

First Aid in Animal Bites

Immediately wash the bite vigorously with soap and water for at least 10 minutes to remove the animal's saliva. Flush the wound with a viricidal agent, followed by a clear-water rinse. Then apply a sterile dressing. If possible, do not suture the wound, and do not immediately stop the bleeding (unless it is massive), since blood flow helps to cleanse the wound.

Question the patient about the bite. Ask if he provoked the animal (if so, chances are it is not rabid) and if he can identify it or its owner (the animal may be confined for observation). Consult local health authorities for treatment information.

Clinical implications

• When injecting rabies vaccine, rotate injection sites on the upper arm or thigh. Watch for and symptomatically treat redness, itching, pain, and tenderness at the injection site.

• Cooperate with public health authorities to determine the vaccination status of the animal. If the animal is proven rabid, help identify others at risk.

If rabies develops, aggressive supportive care (even after onset of coma) can make probable death less agonizing.

• Monitor cardiac and pulmonary function continuously.

• Isolate the patient. Wear a gown, gloves, and protection for the eyes and mouth when handling saliva and articles contaminated with saliva. Take precautions to avoid being bitten by the patient during the excitation phase.

• Keep the room dark and quiet.

• Establish communication with the patient and his family. Provide psychological support to help them cope with the patient's symptoms and probable death.

• To help prevent this dreaded disease, stress the need for vaccination of household pets that may be exposed to rabid wild animals. Warn persons not to try to touch wild animals, especially if they appear ill or overly docile (a possible sign of rabies). Assist in the prophylactic administration of rabies vaccine to high-risk persons, such as farm workers, forest rangers, spelunkers (cave explorers), and veterinarians.

Radiation exposure

Description

Expanded use of ionized radiation has vastly increased the incidence of radiation exposure. The amount of radiation absorbed by a human body is measured in radiation absorbed doses (rads), not to be confused with roentgens, which are used to measure radiation emissions. Ionized radiation (X-rays, protons, neutrons, and alpha, beta, and gamma rays) may cause immediate cell necrosis or disturbed DNA synthesis, which impairs cell function and division. Rapidly dividing cells—bone marrow, hair follicles, gonads lymph tissue—are most susceptible to radiation damage. The existence and severity of tissue damage depend on the amount of body area exposed (the smaller, the better), length of exposure, dosage absorbed, distance from the source, and presence of protective shielding. Cancer patients receiving radiation therapy and nuclear power plant workers are the most likely victims. More than 600 rad is nearly always fatal. However, when radiation is focused on a small area, the body can absorb and survive many thousands of rads, if they are administered in carefully controlled doses over a long period of time. This basic principle is the key to safe and successful radiation therapy.

Causes
Exposure to radiation can occur by inhalation, ingestion, or direct contact.

Signs and symptoms
Acute hematopoietic radiation exposure (200 to 500 rad)
—Initially, nausea, vomiting, diarrhea and anorexia
—During latent period, nosebleeds, hemorrhage, petechiae, pallor, weakness, oropharyngeal abscesses, increased susceptibility to infection
Acute GI radiation exposure (400 rad or more)
—Initially, ulceration, infection, and intractable nausea, vomiting, and diarrhea, resulting in severe fluid and electrolyte imbalance
—Later, symptoms of circulatory collapse and death
Acute cerebral radiation poisoning (1,000 rad or more)
—Nausea, vomiting, diarrhea within hours
—Lethargy, tremors, convulsions, confusion, coma, and possibly death within hours or days
Delayed or chronic effects
—Repeated, prolonged exposure to small doses over a long time can lead to skin damage, causing dryness, erythema, atrophy, and malignant lesions. (Such damage can also follow acute exposure.)
—Other delayed effects include alopecia, brittle nails, hypothyroidism, amenorrhea, cataracts, decreased fertility, and symptoms of anemia, leukopenia, thrombocytopenia, malignant neoplasms, bone necrosis and fractures, and, finally, a shortened life span.

—Long-term exposure to radiation may retard fetal growth or may cause genetic defects.

Diagnostic tests
• CBC reveals decreased hematocrit and hemoglobin values, and WBC, platelet, and lymphocyte counts.
• Serum electrolyte analysis reveals decreased potassium and chloride from vomiting.
• Bone marrow studies show blood dyscrasia.
• X-rays may reveal bone necrosis.
• A Geiger counter may help determine the amount of radiation in open wounds.

Treatment
Treatment is essentially symptomatic and includes antiemetics to counter nausea and vomiting, fluid and electrolyte replacement, antibiotics, and possibly sedatives, if convulsions occur. Transfusions of plasma, platelets, and red blood cells may be necessary. Bone marrow transplant is a controversial treatment but may be the only recourse in extreme cases. When radiation exposure results from inhalation or ingestion of large amounts of radioiodine, potassium iodide or a strong iodine solution may be given to block thyroid uptake.

Clinical implications
• To minimize radiation exposure, dispose of all contaminated clothing properly. If the patient's skin is contaminated, wash his body thoroughly with a chelating solution (calcium trisodium pentetate or calcium disodium edetate) and water. Debride and irrigate open wounds. If he recently ingested radioactive material, induce vomiting and start lavage.
• Monitor intake and output, and maintain fluid and electrolyte balance. Give I.V. fluids and electrolytes, as ordered. If the patient can take oral feedings, encourage a high-protein, high-calorie diet. Tell him to use a soft toothbrush to minimize gum bleeding.

Offer lidocaine to soothe painful mouth ulcers.
• To prevent skin breakdown, make sure the patient avoids extreme temperatures, tight clothing, and drying soaps. Use rigid aseptic technique.
• Prevent complications. Monitor vital signs and watch for signs of hemorrhage.
• Provide emotional support for the patient and his family, especially after severe exposure. Suggest genetic counseling and screening, as needed.

Hospital personnel can avoid exposure to radiation by wearing proper shielding devices when supervising X-ray and radiation treatments. If you work in these vulnerable areas, wear a radiation detection badge and turn it in periodically for readings.

Rape trauma syndrome

Description

The term *rape* refers to illicit sexual intercourse without consent. It is a violent assault, in which sex is used as a weapon. Rape inflicts varying degrees of physical and psychological trauma. Rape trauma syndrome occurs during the period following the rape or attempted rape. It refers to the victim's short-term and long-term reactions and to the methods used to cope with this trauma.

Known victims of rape range in age from 2 months to 97 years. The age group most affected is 10- to 19-year-olds. The average age of the victim is 13½. More than 50% of rapes occur in the home. About one-third of these involve a male intruder who forces his way into a home. Approximately half the time, the victim has some casual acquaintance with the attacker. Most rapists are 15 to 24 years old. Usually, the attack is planned.

In most cases, the rapist is a man and the victim is a woman. However, rapes do occur between persons of the same sex, especially in prisons,

If the Rape Victim is a Child

Carefully interview the child to assess how well he or she will be able to deal with the situation after going home. Interview the child alone, away from the parents. Tell parents this is being done for the child's comfort, not to keep secrets from them. Ask them what words the child is comfortable with when referring to parts of the anatomy. A young child will place only as much importance on an experience as others do unless there is physical pain. A good question to ask is, "Did someone touch you when you didn't want to be touched?" As with other rape victims, record information in the child's own words. A complete pelvic examination is necessary only if penetration has occurred; such an examination requires parental consent and an analgesic or local anesthetic.

The child and the parents need counseling to minimize possible emotional disturbances. Encourage the child to talk about the experience, and try to alleviate any confusion. A young victim may regress; an older child may become fearful about being left alone. The child's behavior may change at school or at home.

Help parents understand that it is normal for them to feel angry and guilty, but warn them against displacing or projecting these feelings onto the child. Instruct them to assure the child that they are not angry with her or him; that the child is good and did not cause the incident; that they are sorry it happened but glad the child is all right; and that the family will work the problems out together.

Assessing a Rape Victim

When a rape victim arrives in the emergency department, assess her physical injuries. If she is not *seriously* injured, allow her to remain clothed and take her to a private room, where she can talk with you or a counselor before the necessary physical examination. Remember, immediate reactions to rape differ and include crying, laughing, hostility, confusion, withdrawal, or outward calm; often anger and rage do not surface until later. During the assault, the victim may have felt demeaned, helpless, and afraid for her life; afterward, she may feel ashamed, guilty, shocked, and vulnerable, and have a sense of disbelief and lowered self-esteem. Offer support and reassurance. Help her explore her feelings; listen, convey trust and respect, and remain nonjudgmental. Do not leave her alone unless she asks you to.

Obtain an accurate history of the rape, pertinent to physical assessment. (Remember: Your notes may be used as evidence if the rapist is tried.) Record the victim's statements in the first person, using quotation marks. Also document objective information provided by others. Never speculate as to what may have happened or record subjective impressions or thoughts. Include in your notes the time the victim arrived at the hospital, the date and time of the alleged rape, and the time the victim was examined. Obtain a past medical history.

Thoroughly explain the physical examination, and tell her why it is necessary (to rule out internal injuries and obtain a specimen for venereal disease testing). Obtain her informed consent for treatment and for the police report. Allow her some control, if possible; for instance, ask her if she is ready to be examined or if she would rather wait a bit.

Before the examination, ask the victim whether she douched, bathed, or washed before coming to the hospital. Note this on her chart. Have her change into a hospital gown, and place her clothing in *paper bags*. (*Never* use plastic bags, because secretions and seminal stains will mold, destroying

---

schools, hospitals, and other institutions. Also, children are often the victims of rape; most of these cases involve manual, oral, or genital contact with the child's genitals. Usually, the rapist is a member of the child's family. In rare instances, a man or child is sexually abused by a woman.

Prognosis is good if the rape victim receives physical and emotional support and counseling to help her deal with her feelings. Victims who articulate their feelings are able to cope with fears, interact with others, and return to normal routines faster than those who do not.

Causes
Various cultural, sociological, and psychological factors may contribute to rape.

- Increasing exposure to sex
- Permissiveness
- Cynicism about relationships
- Feelings of anger, and powerlessness amid social pressures
- Feelings of violence or hatred toward women
- Sexual problems, such as impotence or premature ejaculation
- Feelings of social isolation and inability to form warm, loving relationships
- Psychopathic need for violence for physical pleasure or to satisfy a need for power

Signs and symptoms
See *If the Rape Victim is a Child*, p. 641, and *Assessing a Rape Victim*.

valuable evidence.) Label each bag and its contents.

Tell the victim she may urinate, but warn her not to wipe or otherwise cleanse the perineal area. Stay with her, or ask a counselor to stay with her, throughout the examination.

Even if the victim was not beaten, physical examination (including a pelvic examination by a gynecologist) will probably show signs of physical trauma, especially if the assault was prolonged. Depending on specific body areas attacked, a patient may have a sore throat, mouth irritation, difficulty swallowing, ecchymoses, or rectal pain and bleeding.

If additional physical violence accompanied the rape, the victim may have hematomas, lacerations, bleeding, severe internal injuries, and hemorrhage; and if the rape occurred outdoors, she may suffer from exposure. X-rays may reveal fractures.

Assist throughout the examination, providing support and reassurance. During the exam, assist in specimen collection, including those for semen and gonorrhea. Carefully label all specimens with the patient's name, the physician's name, and the location from which the specimen was obtained. List all specimens in your notes. If the case comes to trial, specimens will be used for evidence. Accuracy is vital.

Carefully collect and label fingernail scrapings and foreign material obtained by combing the victim's pubic hair; these also provide valuable evidence. Note to whom these specimens are given.

For a male victim, be especially alert for injury to the mouth, perineum, and anus. As ordered, obtain a pharyngeal sample for a gonorrhea culture and rectal aspirate for acid phosphatase or sperm analysis.

Most states require the hospital to report all incidents of rape. The patient may elect not to press charges and not to assist the police investigation. Refer the patient to a support group.

Diagnostic tests

See *If the Rape Victim is a Child*, p. 641, and *Assessing a Rape Victim*.

Treatment and clinical implications

Treatment consists of supportive measures and protection against venereal disease and, if the patient wishes, against pregnancy. Give probenecid P.O., with penicillin G procaine I.M., as ordered, to prevent venereal disease.

Since cultures cannot detect gonorrhea for 5 to 6 days after the rape, or syphilis for 6 weeks, stress the importance of returning for follow-up venereal disease testing. If the victim wishes to prevent possible pregnancy as a result of the rape, she may be given large doses of oral diethylstilbestrol

(DES) for 5 consecutive days. Immediately inserting an intrauterine device (IUD) may prevent pregnancy but may also cause an infection. Adverse effects of DES usage and IUD insertion should be explained. The victim may wait 3 to 4 weeks and have a dilatation and curettage or a vacuum aspiration to abort a pregnancy.

If the patient has vulvar lacerations and hair cuts, the doctor will clean the area and repair the lacerations after all the evidence is obtained. Topical use of ice packs may reduce vulvar swelling.

Recovery from rape, which may be prolonged, consists of the acute phase (immediate reaction) and the reorganization phase. During the acute phase, physical aspects include pain, loss of appetite, and wound healing; emotional reactions typically include shaking, crying, and mood swings. Feelings of grief, anger, fear, or revenge may color the victim's social interactions. Counseling helps the victim identify her coping mechanisms. She may relate more easily to a counselor of the same sex.

During the reorganization phase, which usually begins a week after the rape and may last months or years, the victim is concerned with restructuring her life. Initially, she often has nightmares in which she is powerless. Later dreams show her gradually gaining more control. When she is alone, she may also suffer from "daymares"—frightening thoughts about the rape. She may have reduced sexual desire or may develop fear of intercourse or mistrust of men.

Legal proceedings during this time force the victim to relive the trauma, leaving her feeling lonely and isolated, perhaps even temporarily halting her emotional recovery. To help her cope, encourage her to write her thoughts, feelings, and reactions in a daily diary, and refer her to organizations such as Women Organized Against Rape or a local rape crisis center for empathy and advice.

Raynaud's disease

Description
Raynaud's disease is one of several primary arteriospastic disorders characterized by episodic vasospasm in the small peripheral arteries and arterioles, precipitated by exposure to cold or stress. This condition occurs bilaterally and usually affects the hands or, less often, the feet. Clinical criteria that establish Raynaud's disease include skin color changes induced by cold or stress; bilateral involvement;

absence of gangrene or, if present, minimal cutaneous gangrene; normal arterial pulses; and patient history of clinical symptoms of longer than 2 years' duration. It is a benign condition, requiring no specific treatment and with no serious sequelae.

Raynaud's phenomenon, however, a condition often associated with several connective tissue disorders—such as scleroderma, systemic lupus erythematosus, or polymyositis—has a progressive course, leading to ischemia, gangrene, and amputation. Distinction between the two disorders is difficult, because some patients who experience mild symptoms of Raynaud's disease for several years may later develop overt connective tissue disease—especially scleroderma.

Causes
Although the cause is unknown, several theories account for reduced digital blood flow:
• Intrinsic vascular wall hyperactivity to cold
• Increased vasomotor tone due to sympathetic stimulation
• Antigen-antibody immune response (the most probable theory, since abnormal immunologic test results accompany Raynaud's phenomenon)

Signs and symptoms
• After exposure to cold or stress, the skin on the fingers typically blanches, then becomes cyanotic before changing to red and before changing from cold to normal temperature.
• Numbness and tingling may also occur.
• Symptoms are relieved by warmth.
• In long-standing disease, trophic changes, such as sclerodactyly, ulcerations, or chronic paronychia, may result.

Diagnostic tests
Tests may be performed to rule out secondary disease processes, such as chronic arterial occlusive or connective tissue disease.

Treatment
Initially, treatment consists of avoidance of cold, mechanical, or chemical injury; cessation of smoking; and reassurance that symptoms are benign. Since drug side effects, especially from vasodilators, may be more bothersome than the disease itself, drug therapy is reserved for unusually severe symptoms. Such therapy may include use of phenoxybenzamine or reserpine. Sympathectomy may be helpful when conservative modalities fail to prevent ischemic ulcers.

Clinical implications
• Warn against exposure to the cold. Tell the patient to wear mittens or gloves in cold weather or when handling cold items or defrosting the freezer.
• Advise the patient to avoid stressful situations and to stop smoking.
• Instruct the patient to inspect the skin frequently and to seek immediate care for signs of skin breakdown or infection.
• Teach the patient about drugs, their use, and their side effects.
• Provide psychological support and reassurance to allay the patient's fear of amputation and disfigurement.

Rectal polyps

Description
Rectal polyps are masses of tissue that rise above the mucosal membrane and protrude into the GI tract. Types of polyps include common polypoid adenomas, villous adenomas, hereditary polyposis, focal polypoid hyperplasia, and juvenile polyps (hamartomas). Most rectal polyps are benign. However, villous and hereditary polyps show a marked inclination to become malignant. Indeed, a striking feature of familial polyposis is its frequent association with rectosigmoid adenocarcinoma.

Causes
Unrestrained cell growth in the upper epithelium

Risk factors
• Heredity
• Age (incidence rises after age 70)
• Infection
• Diet

Signs and symptoms
• Generally asymptomatic
• Rectal bleeding (most common sign)

Diagnostic tests
• Proctosigmoidoscopy or colonoscopy with rectal biopsy confirms the diagnosis.
• Stool may be positive for occult blood.
• Hemoglobin and hematocrit levels are low because of bleeding.

Treatment
Treatment varies according to the type and size of polyps, and their location within the colon. Common polypoid adenomas less than 1 cm require polypectomy, commonly by fulguration (destruction by high-frequency electricity) during endoscopy. For common polypoid adenomas over 4 cm and all invasive villous adenomas, treatment usually consists of abdominoperineal resection. Focal polypoid hyperplasia necessitates local fulguration. Depending upon GI involvement, hereditary polyps necessitate total abdominoperineal resection with a permanent ileostomy, subtotal colectomy with ileoproctostomy, or ileal anal anastomosis. Juvenile polyps are prone to autoamputation; if this does not occur, snare removal during colonoscopy is the treatment of choice.

Clinical implications
During diagnostic evaluation, follow these guidelines:
• Check sodium, potassium, and chloride levels daily in the patient with fluid imbalance. Adjust fluid and elec-

trolytes, as necessary. Administer normal saline solution with potassium I.V., as ordered. Weigh the patient daily, and record the amount of diarrhea. Watch for signs of dehydration (decreased urine, increased BUN levels).

• Tell the patient to watch for and report evidence of rectal bleeding.

After biopsy and fulguration, follow these guidelines:

• Check for signs of perforation and hemorrhage, such as sudden hypotension, decrease in hemoglobin or hematocrit, shock, abdominal pain, and passage of red blood through the rectum.

• Watch for and record the first bowel movement, which may not occur for 2 to 3 days.

• Walk the patient within 24 hours of the procedure.

• Provide sitz baths for 3 days.

• If the patient has benign polyps, stress the need for routine follow-up studies to check the polypoid growth rate.

• Prepare the patient with precancerous or familial lesions for abdominoperineal resection. Provide emotional support and preoperative instruction.

• After ileostomy or subtotal colectomy with ileoproctostomy, care for abdominal dressings, I.V. lines, and indwelling (Foley) catheter. Record intake and output, and check vital signs for hypotension and surgical complications. Administer pain medication, as ordered. To prevent embolism, walk the patient as soon as possible, and apply antiembolism stockings. Encourage the patient to perform range-of-motion exercises. Provide enterostomal therapy and teach stoma care.

Complications

• Fluid and electrolyte depletion associated with diarrhea and bloody stools

• Secondary anemia

Rectal prolapse

Description

Rectal prolapse is the circumferential protrusion of one or more layers of the mucous membrane through the anus. Prolapse may be complete (with displacement of the anal sphincter or bowel herniation) or partial (displacement of the mucosal layer).

Causes

Weakened sphincters or weakened longitudinal, rectal, or levator ani muscles

Risk factors

Conditions that affect the pelvic floor or rectum, including neurologic disorders, injury, tumor, aging, chronic wasting diseases, and nutritional disorders

Signs and symptoms

Typical clinical features and visual examination confirm the diagnosis.

• Protrusion of tissue from the rectum, which may occur during defecation or walking

• Persistent sensation of rectal fullness

• Bloody diarrhea

• Pain in the lower abdomen

• In complete prolapse, protrusion of the full thickness of the bowel wall and, possibly, the sphincter muscle; and mucosa falling into bulky, concentric folds

• In partial prolapse, only partially protruding mucosa and a smaller mass of radial mucosal folds; straining during examination may disclose the full extent of prolapse

Treatment and clinical implications

Treatment varies according to the underlying cause. Sometimes eliminating this cause (straining, coughing, nutritional disorders) is the only treatment necessary. In a child, prolapsed tissue usually diminishes as the child grows. In an older patient, injection of a sclerosing agent to cause a fibrotic reaction fixes the rectum in place. Severe or chronic prolapse requires surgical repair by strengthening or tightening the sphincters with wire or by anterior or rectal resection of prolapsed tissue.

• Help the patient prevent constipation by teaching correct diet and stool-softening regimen. Advise the patient with severe prolapse and incontinence to wear a perineal pad.

• Before surgery, explain possible complications, including permanent rectal incontinence.

• After surgery, watch for immediate complications (hemorrhage) and later ones (pelvic abscess, fever, pus drainage, pain, rectal stenosis, constipation, or pain on defecation). Teach perineal strengthening exercises: Have the patient lie down, with his back flat on the mattress; then ask him to pull in his abdomen and squeeze while taking a deep breath. Or have the patient repeatedly squeeze and relax his buttocks while sitting on a chair.

Reiter's syndrome

Description

A self-limiting syndrome associated with polyarthritis (dominant feature), urethritis, balanitis, conjunctivitis, and mucocutaneous lesions. This disease usually affects young men aged 20 to 40. It is rare in women and children.

Causes

• While the exact cause of Reiter's syndrome is unknown, most cases follow venereal or enteric infection.

• Genetic susceptibility is likely.

Signs and symptoms

Genitourinary symptoms
—Dysuria
—Hematuria
—Urgency and frequency
—Mucopurulent penile discharge
—Swelling and redness of the urethral meatus
—Suprapubic pain

Musculoskeletal symptoms
—Asymmetric and extremely variable polyarticular arthritis is the most common symptom and tends to develop in weight-bearing joints of the legs and sometimes in the low back or sacroiliac joints.
—Muscle wasting near affected joints

Ocular symptoms
—Redness associated with mild conjunctivitis
—In severe cases, possible burning, itching, and profuse mucopurulent discharge

Dermatological symptoms
—Possible macular to hyperkeratotic lesions

Diagnostic tests

• HLA-B27 antigen testing proves positive for most patients.

• CBC shows increased WBC count and decreased RBC count.

• Urethral discharge and synovial fluid contain many WBCs, mostly polymorphonuclear leukocytes; synovial fluid is high in complement and protein and is grossly purulent.

• Cultures of discharge and synovial fluid rule out other causes such as gonococci.

• X-rays are normal during the first few weeks and may remain so, but some patients may show osteoporosis in inflamed areas. If inflammation persists, X-rays may show erosions of the small joints, periosteal proliferation (new bone formation) of involved joints, and calcaneal spurs.

Treatment

No specific treatment exists for Reiter's syndrome. Most patients recover in 2 to 16 weeks. About 50% of patients have recurring acute attacks, while the rest follow a chronic course, experiencing continued synovitis and sacroiliitis. In acute stages, limited weight bearing or complete bed rest may be necessary.

Anti-inflammatory agents can be given for relief of discomfort and fever. Steroids may be used for persistent skin lesions; gold therapy, for bony erosion. Physical therapy includes range-of-motion and strengthening exercises and the use of padded or supportive shoes to prevent contractures and deformities of the feet.

Clinical implications
• Communicate an accepting, nonjudgmental attitude, since the patient may be embarrassed if attacks are associated with sexual activity.
• Explain Reiter's syndrome to the patient. Discuss the recommended medications and their possible side effects. Warn the patient to take medications with meals or milk to prevent GI bleeding.
• Encourage normal daily activity and moderate exercise. Suggest a firm mattress and encourage good posture and body mechanics.
• Arrange for occupational counseling if the patient has severe or chronic joint impairment.

Complications
• Prostatitis
• Hemorrhagic cystitis
• Keratitis
• Iritis
• Retinitis
• Optic neuritis

Relapsing fever
(Tick, fowl-nest, cabin, or vagabond fever; or bilious typhoid)

Description
Relapsing fever refers to any one of several acute infectious diseases marked by recurrent febrile episodes. Untreated louse-borne relapsing fever normally carries a mortality rate of more than 10%. However, during an epidemic, the mortality rate may rise as high as 50%. The victims are usually indigent people who are already suffering from other infections and malnutrition. With treatment, however, prognosis for both louse- and tick-borne relapsing fevers is excellent.

Causes
Spirochetes of the genus *Borrelia*

Mode of transmission
• Relapsing fever is transmitted to humans by lice or ticks.
• Rodents and other wild animals serve as the primary reservoirs for the *Borrelia* spirochetes.
• Humans can become secondary reservoirs but cannot transmit this infection by ordinary contagion; however, congenital infection and transmission by contaminated blood are possible.

Signs and symptoms
• Sudden increase in temperature approaching 105° F. (40.5° C.)
• Prostration
• Headache
• Severe myalgia
• Arthralgia
• Diarrhea
• Vomiting
• Coughing
• Eye or chest pain
• Possible splenomegaly, hepatomegaly, and lymphadenopathy
• Tachycardia and tachypnea
• Possible transient, macular rash over the torso
• After 3 to 6 days, quick drop in temperature accompanied by profuse sweating

Diagnostic tests
• Blood smears during febrile periods, using Wright's or Giemsa stain, demonstrate the spirochetes and confirm

the diagnosis. *Borrelia* spirochetes may be harder to detect in later relapses, because their number in the blood declines. In such cases, injecting the patient's blood or tissue into a young rat and incubating the organism in the rat's blood for 1 to 10 days often facilitates spirochete identification.

• Urine and cerebrospinal fluid demonstrate the spirochetes in severe infection.

• WBC count is often increased as high as 25,000/mm³; however, it may be normal.

• Erythrocyte sedimentation rate is increased.

Treatment

Oral tetracycline is the treatment of choice; it may be given I.V., if necessary, and should continue for 4 to 5 days. In cases of tetracycline allergy or resistance, penicillin G may be administered as an alternative. However, neither drug should be given at the height of a severe febrile attack. If they are given, Jarisch-Herxheimer reaction may occur, causing malaise, rigors, leukopenia, flushing, fever, tachycardia, rising respiration rate, and hypotension. This reaction, which is caused by toxic by-products from massive spirochete destruction, can mimic septic shock and may prove fatal. Antimicrobial therapy should be postponed until the fever subsides. Until then, supportive therapy (consisting of parenteral fluids and electrolytes) should be given instead.

When neither tetracycline nor penicillin G controls relapsing fever, chloramphenicol may be given with caution. Complete blood count should be performed regularly during treatment with chloramphenicol because a fatal granulocytopenia, thrombocytopenia, or even aplastic anemia may develop.

Clinical implications

• During the initial evaluation period, obtain a complete history of the patient's travels.

• Throughout febrile periods, monitor vital signs, level of consciousness, and temperature every 4 hours. Watch for and immediately report any signs of neurologic complications, such as decreasing level of consciousness or seizures. To reduce fever, give tepid sponge baths and antipyretics, as ordered.

• Maintain adequate fluid intake to prevent dehydration.

• Treat flushing, hypotension, or tachycardia with vasopressors or fluids, as ordered.

• Look for symptoms of relapsing fever in family members and in others who may have been exposed to ticks or lice along with the victim.

• Use proper handwashing technique, and teach it to the patient. Isolation is unnecessary because the disease is not transmitted from person to person.

• Report all cases of louse- or tick-borne relapsing fever to local public health authorities, as required by law.

Complications

• Nephritis
• Bronchitis
• Pneumonia
• Endocarditis
• Seizures
• Cranial nerve lesions
• Paralysis
• Coma
• Massive bleeding
• Splenic rupture
• Circulatory failure

Renal calculi
(Kidney stones)

Description

Renal calculi may form anywhere in the urinary tract but usually develop in the renal pelvis or the calyces of the kidneys. Such formation follows precipitation of substances normally dissolved in the urine (calcium oxalate, calcium phosphate, magnesium ammonium phosphate, or occasionally urate or cystine). Renal calculi vary in size and may be solitary or multiple. They may remain in the renal pelvis or enter the ureter and may damage renal parenchyma. Large calculi cause pressure necrosis. In certain locations, calculi cause obstruction, with resultant hydronephrosis, and tend to recur.

Causes
Unknown.

Risk factors
• Dehydration: Decreased urine production concentrates calculus-forming substances.
• Infection: Infected, damaged tissue serves as a site for calculus development; pH changes provide a favorable medium for calculus formation (especially for magnesium ammonium phosphate or calcium phosphate calculi); or infected calculi (usually magnesium ammonium phosphate or staghorn calculi) may develop if bacteria serve as the nucleus in calculus formation. Such infections may promote destruction of renal parenchyma.
• Obstruction: Urinary stasis (as in immobility from spinal cord injury) allows calculus constituents to collect and adhere, forming calculi. Obstruction also promotes infection, which, in turn, compounds the obstruction.
• Metabolic factors: Hyperparathyroidism, renal tubular acidosis, elevated uric acid (usually with gout), defective metabolism of oxalate, genetically defective metabolism of cystine, and excessive intake of vitamin D or dietary calcium may predispose to renal calculi.

Signs and symptoms
Clinical effects vary with size, location, and etiology of the calculus.
• Pain is the key symptom.

• The pain of classic renal colic travels from the costovertebral angle to the flank, to the suprapubic region and external genitalia. The pain fluctuates in intensity and may be excruciating at its peak.
• If calculi are in the renal pelvis and calyces, pain may be more constant and dull.
• Back pain occurs from calculi that produce an obstruction within a kidney.
• Nausea and vomiting usually accompany severe pain.
• Other symptoms include abdominal distention, fever and chills, possible hematuria, pyuria, and, rarely, anuria.

Diagnostic tests
• Kidney-ureter-bladder X-rays reveal most renal calculi.
• Stone analysis shows mineral content.
• Intravenous pyelography confirms the diagnosis and determines the size and location of calculi.
• Kidney ultrasonography is an easily performed, noninvasive, nontoxic test to detect obstructive changes, such as hydronephrosis.
• Urine culture of midstream sample may indicate urinary tract infection.
• Urinalysis may be normal or may show increased specific gravity and acid or alkaline pH suitable for different types of stone formation. Other urinalysis findings include hematuria (gross or microscopic), crystals (urate, calcium, or cystine), casts, and pyuria with or without bacteria and WBCs.
• A 24-hour urine collection is evaluated for calcium oxalate, phosphorus, and uric acid excretion levels.

Other laboratory results support the diagnosis:
• Serial blood calcium and phosphorus levels detect hyperparathyroidism and show increased calcium level in proportion to normal serum protein.
• Blood protein level determines free calcium unbound to protein.
• Blood chloride and bicarbonate levels may show renal tubular acidosis.

Teaching Topics in Renal Calculi

- An explanation of how calculi precipitate from urine, including factors that influence their formation
- The importance of treatment to prevent urinary tract obstruction, which may lead to kidney infection, hydronephrosis, and renal insufficiency
- Preparation for blood and urine tests to determine the cause and composition of calculi and for radiography or ultrasonography to pinpoint their location
- Importance of prescribed dietary restrictions and adequate hydration to prevent recurrence of calculi
- Drugs to adjust urine pH, if appropriate
- Preparation for surgery or extracorporeal shock wave lithotripsy, as indicated
- Home care of percutaneous nephrostomy tube, if appropriate
- How to strain urine for calculi and test urine pH
- Signs and symptoms of infection

- Increased blood uric acid levels may indicate gout as the cause.

Treatment

Since 90% of renal calculi are smaller than 5 mm in diameter, treatment usually consists of measures to promote their natural passage. Along with vigorous hydration, such treatment includes antimicrobial therapy (varying with the cultured organism) for infection; analgesics, such as meperidine, for pain; and diuretics to prevent urinary stasis and further calculus formation (thiazides decrease calcium excretion into the urine). Prophylaxis to prevent calculus formation includes a low-calcium diet for absorptive hypercalciuria, parathyroidectomy for hyperparathyroidism, allopurinol for uric acid calculi, and daily administration of ascorbic acid P.O. to acidify the urine.

Calculi too large for natural passage may require surgical removal. When a calculus is in the ureter, a cystoscope may be inserted through the urethra and the calculus manipulated with catheters or retrieval instruments. Extraction of calculi from other areas (kidney, calyx, renal pelvis) may necessitate a flank or lower abdominal approach. Percutaneous ultrasonic lithotripsy and extracorporeal shock wave lithotripsy shatter the calculus into fragments for removal by suction or natural passage.

Clinical implications

- To aid diagnosis, maintain a 24- to 48-hour record of urine pH, with nitrazine pH paper; strain all urine through gauze or a tea strainer, and save all solid material recovered for analysis.
- To facilitate spontaneous passage, encourage the patient to walk, if possible. Also promote sufficient intake of fluids to maintain a urinary output of 3 to 4 liters/day (urine should be very dilute and colorless). To help acidify urine, offer fruit juices, particularly cranberry juice. If the patient cannot drink the required amount of fluid, supplemental I.V. fluids may be given. Record intake and output and daily weight to assess fluid status and renal function.
- Stress the importance of proper diet and compliance with drug therapy.
- If surgery is necessary, give reassurance by supplementing and reinforcing what the surgeon has told the patient about the procedure. Explain

preoperative and postoperative care. (See *Teaching Topics in Renal Calculi*, p. 651.)

• After surgery, the patient will probably have an indwelling catheter or a nephrostomy tube. Unless one of his kidneys was removed, expect bloody drainage from the catheter. Never irrigate the catheter without a physician's order. Check dressings regularly for bloody drainage. Immediately report suspected hemorrhage. Use sterile technique when changing dressings or providing catheter care.

• Watch for signs of infection, and give antibiotics, as ordered. To prevent pneumonia, encourage frequent position changes, and walk the patient as soon as possible. Have him hold a small pillow over the operative site to splint the incision and facilitate deep-breathing and coughing exercises.

• Before discharge, teach the patient and family the importance of following the prescribed dietary and medication regimens to prevent recurrence of calculi. Encourage increased fluid intake. If appropriate, show the patient how to check his urine pH, and instruct him to keep a daily record. Tell him to immediately report symptoms of acute obstruction (pain, inability to void).

Renal failure, acute

Description

Acute renal failure is the sudden interruption of kidney function due to obstruction, reduced circulation, or renal parenchymal disease. It is usually reversible with medical treatment; otherwise, it may progress to end-stage renal disease, uremic syndrome, and death.

Causes

Prerenal failure

This is associated with diminished blood flow to the kidneys.

—Hypovolemia
—Shock
—Embolism
—Blood loss
—Sepsis
—Pooling of fluid in ascites or burns
—Cardiovascular disorders, such as congestive heart failure, dysrhythmias, and tamponade

Intrinsic renal failure

—Acute tubular necrosis (the most common cause)
—Acute poststreptococcal glomerulonephritis
—Systemic lupus erythematosus
—Periarteritis nodosa
—Vasculitis
—Sickle cell disease
—Bilateral renal vein thrombosis
—Nephrotoxins
—Ischemia
—Renal myeloma
—Acute pyelonephritis

Postrenal failure

This is associated with bilateral obstruction of urinary outflow.

—Kidney stones
—Blood clots
—Tumors
—Benign prostatic hypertrophy
—Strictures
—Urethral edema from catheterization
—Papillae from papillary necrosis

Signs and symptoms

• Urinary: oliguria or, rarely, anuria, usually the earliest symptom
• GI: anorexia, nausea, vomiting, diarrhea or constipation, stomatitis, bleeding, hematemesis, dry mucous membranes, uremic breath
• CNS: headache, drowsiness, irritability, confusion, peripheral neuropathy, convulsions, coma
• Cutaneous: dryness, pruritus, pallor, purpura, and, rarely, uremic frost
• Cardiovascular: early in the disease, hypotension; later, hypertension, dysrhythmias, symptoms of fluid over-

Teaching Topics in Acute Renal Failure

• An explanation of ARF, including its cause (prerenal, intrarenal, or postrenal) and phase (oliguric or diuretic)
• The importance of treatment to prevent complications, most notably chronic renal failure
• Signs and symptoms of uremia, hypervolemia, hypovolemia, and hyperkalemia
• Preparation for laboratory tests, such as serum electrolytes and urinalysis
• Preparation for kidney-ureter-bladder radiography, renal ultrasonography, or other scheduled imaging studies
• Dietary restrictions, such as avoidance or limited intake of potassium, sodium, and protein
• Instructions to restrict or increase fluids, as indicated
• Drugs and their administration
• An explanation of hemodialysis or peritoneal dialysis, if appropriate
• How to monitor fluid balance

load, congestive heart failure, systemic edema, anemia, altered clotting mechanisms
• Respiratory: pulmonary edema, Kussmaul respiration

Diagnostic tests
• Blood tests show elevated BUN, serum creatinine, and potassium and low blood pH, bicarbonate, hematocrit, and hemoglobin.
• Urine samples show casts, cellular debris, decreased specific gravity, and, in glomerular diseases, proteinuria and urine osmolality close to serum osmolality.
• Urine sodium level is < 20 mEq/liter if oliguria results from decreased perfusion; > 40 mEq/liter if it results from an intrinsic problem.
• Other studies include ultrasound of the kidneys, plain films of the abdomen and the kidneys, ureters, and bladder, intravenous pyelography, renal scan, retrograde pyelography, and nephrotomography.

Treatment
Supportive measures include a diet high in calories and low in protein, sodium, and potassium, with supplemental vitamins and restricted fluids. Meticulous electrolyte monitoring is essential to detect hyperkalemia. If hyperkalemia occurs, acute therapy may include dialysis, hypertonic glucose and insulin infusions, and sodium bicarbonate—all administered I.V.—and sodium polystyrene sulfonate, P.O. or by enema, to remove potassium from the body.

If theses measures fail to control uremic symptoms, hemodialysis or peritoneal dialysis may be necessary.

Clinical implications
• Measure and record intake and output, including all body fluids, such as wound drainage, nasogastric output, and diarrhea. Weigh the patient daily.
• Assess hematocrit and hemoglobin levels and replace blood components, as ordered. *Do not* use whole blood if the patient is prone to congestive heart failure and cannot tolerate extra fluid volume.
• Monitor vital signs. Watch for and report any signs of pericarditis (pleuritic chest pain, tachycardia, pericardial friction rub), inadequate renal perfusion (hypotension), and acidosis.
• Maintain electrolyte balance. Strictly monitor potassium levels. Watch for symptoms of hyperkalemia

(malaise, anorexia, paresthesia, or muscle weakness) and EKG changes (tall, peaked T waves, widening QRS segment, and disappearing P waves), and report them immediately. Avoid administering medications containing potassium.

• Maintain nutritional status. Provide a high-calorie, low-protein, low-sodium, and low-potassium diet, with vitamin supplements. Give the anorectic patient small, frequent meals.

• Use aseptic technique, since the patient is highly susceptible to infection.

• Prevent complications of immobility.

• Provide good mouth care frequently, since mucous membranes are dry.

• Monitor for GI bleeding by guaiac testing all stools for blood.

• Use appropriate safety measures, such as side rails and restraints, since the patient with CNS involvement may be dizzy or confused.

• Provide emotional support to the patient and his family. Reassure them by clearly and fully explaining all procedures.

• Assist with peritoneal dialysis or hemodialysis, as needed. (See *Teaching Topics in Acute Renal Failure*, p. 653.)

Complications
• Metabolic acidosis
• Electrolyte imbalances
• Infection

Renal failure, chronic

Description
Chronic renal failure is usually the end result of a gradually progressive loss of renal function. Occasionally, it is the result of a rapidly progressive disease of sudden onset. Few symptoms develop until after more than 75% of glomerular filtration is lost. Then the remaining normal parenchyma deteriorate progressively, and symptoms worsen as renal function decreases. If

this condition continues unchecked, uremic toxins accumulate and produce potentially fatal physiologic changes in all major organ systems. If the patient can tolerate it, maintenance dialysis or kidney transplant can sustain life.

Causes
• Chronic glomerular disease, such as glomerulonephritis
• Chronic infections, such as chronic pyelonephritis or tuberculosis
• Congenital anomalies, such as polycystic kidneys
• Vascular diseases, such as renal nephrosclerosis or hypertension
• Obstructive processes, such as calculi
• Collagen diseases, such as systemic lupus erythematosus
• Nephrotoxic agents, such as longterm aminoglycoside therapy
• Endocrine diseases, such as diabetic neuropathy
• Acute renal failure that fails to respond to treatment

Signs and symptoms; complications
See *Chronic Renal Failure—Effect on Body Systems*.

Diagnostic tests
• Creatinine clearance tests can identify the stage of chronic renal failure.
—Reduced renal reserve (creatinine clearance glomerular filtration rate [GFR] is 40 to 70 ml/minute)
—Renal insufficiency (GFR 20 to 40 ml/minute)
—Renal failure (GFR 10 to 20 ml/minute)
—End-stage renal disease (GFR less than 10 ml/minute)
• Blood studies show elevated BUN, serum creatinine, and potassium levels; decreased arterial pH and bicarbonate; and low hemoglobin and hematocrit.
• Urine specific gravity becomes fixed

Chronic Renal Failure—Effect on Body Systems

• *Renal and urologic:* Initially, salt-wasting and consequent hyponatremia produce hypotension, dry mouth, loss of skin turgor, listlessness, fatigue, and nausea. Later, somnolence and confusion develop. As the number of functioning nephrons decreases, so does the kidneys' capacity to excrete sodium, resulting in salt retention and overload. Accumulation of potassium causes muscle irritability, then muscle weakness as the potassium level continues to rise. Fluid overload and metabolic acidosis also occur. Urinary output decreases; urine is very dilute and contains casts and crystals.
• *Cardiovascular:* Renal failure leads to hypertension, dysrhythmias (including life-threatening ventricular tachycardia or fibrillation), cardiomyopathy, uremic pericarditis, pericardial effusion with possible cardiac tamponade, congestive heart failure, and peripheral edema.
• *Respiratory:* Pulmonary changes include reduced pulmonary macrophage activity with increased susceptibility to infection, pulmonary edema, pleuritic pain, pleural friction rub and effusions, uremic pleuritis and uremic lung (or uremic pneumonitis), dyspnea due to congestive heart failure, and Kussmaul's respirations as a result of acidosis.
• *GI:* Inflammation and ulceration of GI mucosa cause stomatitis, gum ulceration and bleeding, and possibly parotitis, esophagitis, gastritis, duodenal ulcers, lesions on the small and large bowel, uremic colitis, pancreatitis, and proctitis. Other GI symptoms include a metallic taste in the mouth, uremic fetor (ammonia smell on breath), anorexia, nausea, and vomiting.
• *Cutaneous:* Typically, the skin is pallid, yellowish bronze, dry, and scaly. Other cutaneous symptoms include severe itching, purpura, ecchymoses, petechiae, uremic frost (most often in critically ill or terminal patients), thin brittle fingernails with characteristic lines, and dry, brittle hair that may change color and fall out easily.
• *Neurologic:* Restless leg syndrome, one of the first signs of peripheral neuropathy, causes pain, burning, and itching in the legs and feet, which may be relieved by voluntarily shaking, moving, or rocking them. Eventually, this condition progresses to paresthesia and motor nerve dysfunction (usually bilateral footdrop) unless dialysis is initiated. Other signs and symptoms include muscle cramping and twitching, shortened memory and attention span, apathy, drowsiness, irritability, confusion, coma, and convulsions. EEG changes indicate metabolic encephalopathy.
• *Endocrine:* Common endocrine abnormalities include stunted growth patterns in children (even with elevated growth hormone levels), infertility and decreased libido in both sexes, amenorrhea and cessation of menses in women, impotence and decreased sperm production in men, increased aldosterone secretion and impaired carbohydrate metabolism (increased blood glucose levels similar to diabetes mellitus).
• *Hematopoietic:* Anemia, decreased RBC survival time, blood loss from dialysis and GI bleeding, mild thrombocytopenia, and platelet defects occur. Other problems include increased bleeding and clotting disorders, demonstrated by purpura, hemorrhage from body orifices, easy bruising, ecchymoses, and petechiae.
• *Skeletal:* Calcium-phosphorus imbalance and consequent parathyroid hormone imbalances cause muscle and bone pain, skeletal demineralization, pathologic fractures, and calcifications in the brain, eyes, gums, joints, myocardium, and blood vessels. Arterial calcification may produce coronary artery disease. In children, renal osteodystrophy may develop.

at 1.010; urinalysis may show proteinuria, glycosuria, erythrocytes, leukocytes, and casts, depending on the etiology.

• X-ray studies include kidney-ureter-bladder films, intravenous pyelography, nephrotomography, renal scan, and renal arteriography.

• Kidney biopsy allows histologic identification of underlying pathology.

Treatment

Hemodialysis or peritoneal dialysis (particularly newer techniques—continuous ambulatory peritoneal dialysis [CAPD] and continuous cyclic peritoneal dialysis [CCPD]) can help control most manifestations of end-stage renal disease; altering dialyzing bath fluids can correct fluid and electrolyte disturbances. However, anemia, peripheral neuropathy, cardiopulmonary and GI complications, sexual dysfunction, and skeletal defects may persist. In addition, maintenance dialysis itself may produce complications, including serum hepatitis (hepatitis B) due to numerous blood transfusions, protein wasting, refractory ascites, and dialysis dementia.

Conservative treatment aims to correct specific symptoms. A low-protein diet reduces the production of end products of protein metabolism that the kidneys cannot excrete. (A patient receiving continuous peritoneal dialysis should have a high-protein diet.) A high-calorie diet prevents ketoacidosis and the negative nitrogen balance that results in catabolism and tissue atrophy. Such a diet also restricts sodium and potassium.

Maintaining fluid balance requires careful monitoring of vital signs, weight changes, and urine volume (if present). Loop diuretics, such as Lasix (if some renal function remains), and fluid restriction can reduce fluid retention. Digitalis may be used to mobilize edema fluids; antihypertensives, to control blood pressure and associated edema. Antiemetics taken before meals may relieve nausea and vomiting; cimetidine or ranitidine may decrease gastric irritation. Methylcellulose or docusate can help prevent constipation.

Treatment may also include regular stool analysis (guaiac test) to detect occult blood and, as needed, cleansing enemas to remove blood from the GI tract. Anemia necessitates iron and folate supplements; severe anemia requires infusion of fresh-frozen packed cells or washed packed cells. However, transfusions relieve anemia only temporarily. Androgen therapy (with testosterone or nandrolone) may increase RBC production.

Drug therapy often relieves associated symptoms: an antipruritic such as trimeprazine or diphenhydramine for itching, and aluminum hydroxide gel to lower serum phosphate levels. The patient may also benefit from supplementary vitamins (particularly B vitamins and vitamin D) and essential amino acids.

Careful monitoring of serum potassium levels is necessary to detect hyperkalemia. Emergency treatment for severe hyperkalemia includes dialysis therapy and administration of 50% hypertonic glucose I.V., regular insulin, calcium gluconate I.V., sodium bicarbonate I.V., and cation-exchange resins, such as sodium polystyrene sulfonate. Cardiac tamponade resulting from pericardial effusion may require emergency pericardial tap or surgery.

Blood gas measurements may indicate acidosis; intensive dialysis and thoracentesis can relieve pulmonary edema and pleural effusions. (See *Continuous Ambulatory Peritoneal Dialysis*.)

Clinical implications

Since chronic renal failure has such widespread clinical effects, it requires meticulous and carefully coordinated supportive care.

Continuous Ambulatory Peritoneal Dialysis

Continuous ambulatory peritoneal dialysis (CAPD) is a relatively new, increasingly useful alternative to hemodialysis in patients with renal failure. Using the peritoneum as a dialysis membrane, it allows almost uninterrupted exchange of dialysis solution. With this method, four to six exchanges of fresh dialysis solution are infused each day. The approximate dwell-time for the daytime exchanges is 5 hours; for the overnight exchange, the dwell-time is 8 to 10 hours. After each dwell-time, the patient removes the dialyzing solution by gravity drainage. This form of dialysis offers the unique advantages of a simple, easily taught procedure and patient independence from a special treatment center.

A. In this procedure, a Tenchkoff catheter is surgically implanted in the abdomen, just below the umbilicus. A bag of dialysis solution is aseptically attached to the tube, and the fluid allowed to flow into the peritoneal cavity (this takes about 10 minutes).

B. The dialyzing fluid remains in the peritoneal cavity for about 4 to 6 hours. During this time, the bag may be rolled up and placed under a shirt or blouse, and the patient can go about normal activities while dialysis takes place.

C. The fluid is then drained out of the peritoneal cavity through gravity flow by unrolling the bag and suspending it below the pelvis (drainage takes about 20 minutes). After it drains, the patient aseptically connects a new bag of dialyzing solution and fills the peritoneal cavity again. He repeats this procedure four to six times a day.

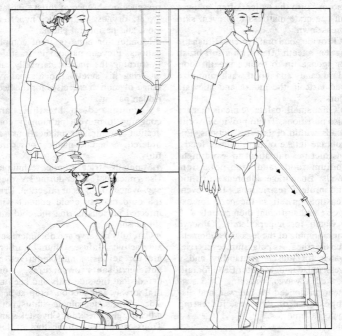

Teaching Topics in Chronic Renal Failure

• An explanation of nephron damage in CRF, including its stage of progression
• Importance of treatment to delay onset of end-stage renal disease and prevent complications, such as uremia
• Preparation for blood and urine tests and for other scheduled diagnostic studies, such as kidney-ureter-bladder radiography and renal ultrasonography
• Prescribed diet and fluid restrictions
• Drugs and their administration
• An explanation of hemodialysis or peritoneal dialysis
• Preparation for renal transplantation or nephrectomy, if indicated
• How to prevent peritonitis at home
• How to monitor fluid balance at home

• Good skin care is important. Bathe the patient daily, using superfatted soaps, oatmeal baths, and skin lotion to ease pruritus. Give good perineal care, using mild soap and water. Pad the side rails to guard against ecchymoses. Turn the patient often, and use an egg-crate mattress to prevent skin breakdown.

• Provide good oral hygiene. Brush the patient's teeth often with a soft brush or sponge tip to reduce breath odor. Hard candy and mouthwash minimize bad taste in the mouth and alleviate thirst.

• Offer small, palatable meals that are also nutritious. Try to provide favorite foods within dietary restrictions. Encourage intake of high-calorie foods. Instruct the outpatient to avoid high-sodium foods and high-potassium foods. Encourage adherence to fluid and protein restrictions. To prevent constipation, stress the need for exercise and sufficient dietary bulk.

• Watch for hyperkalemia. Observe for cramping of the legs and abdomen, and diarrhea. As potassium levels rise, watch for muscle irritability and a weak pulse rate. Monitor EKG for tall, peaked T waves, widening QRS segment, prolonged PR interval, and disappearance of P waves, indicating hyperkalemia.

• Assess hydration status carefully. Check for jugular vein distention, and auscultate the lungs for rales. Measure daily intake and output carefully, including all drainage, emesis, diarrhea, and blood loss. Record daily weight, presence or absence of thirst, axillary sweat, dryness of tongue, hypertension, and peripheral edema.

• Monitor for bone or joint complications. Prevent pathologic fractures by turning the patient carefully and ensuring his safety. Provide passive range-of-motion exercises for the bedridden patient.

• Encourage deep breathing and coughing to prevent pulmonary congestion. Administer medications, as ordered. Schedule medications carefully.

• Maintain strict aseptic technique. Use a micropore filter during I.V. therapy. Watch for signs of infection. Urge the outpatient to avoid contact with infected persons during the cold and flu season.

• Carefully observe and document seizure activity. Infuse sodium bicarbonate for acidosis, and sedatives or anticonvulsants for seizures, as ordered. Pad the side rails and keep an oral airway and suction setup at bedside. Assess neurologic status periodically, and check for Chvostek's and Trousseau's signs, indicators of low serum calcium levels.

- Observe for signs of bleeding.
- Report signs of pericarditis, such as a pericardial friction rub and chest pain. Also, watch for the disappearance of friction rub, with a drop of 15 to 20 mm Hg in blood pressure during inspiration (paradoxical pulse)—an early sign of pericardial tamponade.
- If the patient requires dialysis, explain the procedure fully and check for complications during and after the procedure.
- Refer the patient and his family to appropriate counseling agencies for assistance in coping with chronic renal failure. (See *Teaching Topics in Chronic Renal Failure*.)

Renal infarction

Description
Renal infarction is the formation of a coagulated, necrotic area in one or both kidneys that results from renal blood vessel occlusion. The location and size of the infarct depend on the site of vascular occlusion. Most often, infarction affects the renal cortex, but it can extend into the medulla. Residual renal function after infarction depends on the extent of the damage.

Causes
- Most commonly, renal artery embolism secondary to mitral stenosis, infective endocarditis, atrial fibrillation, microthrombi in the left ventricle, rheumatic valvular disease, or recent myocardial infarction
- Atherosclerosis, with or without thrombus formation
- Thrombus from flank trauma, sickle cell anemia, scleroderma, and arterionephrosclerosis

Signs and symptoms
- May be asymptomatic
- Severe upper abdominal pain or gnawing flank pain and tenderness

- Costovertebral tenderness
- Fever
- Anorexia
- Nausea and vomiting

Diagnostic tests
- Urinalysis reveals proteinuria and microscopic hematuria.
- Urine enzyme levels, especially of LDH and alkaline phosphatase, are often elevated as a result of tissue destruction.
- Serum enzyme levels—especially of SGOT, alkaline phosphatase, and LDH—are elevated.
- Blood studies may also reveal leukocytosis and increased erythrocyte sedimentation rate.
- Intravenous pyelography (IVP) shows diminished or absent excretion of contrast dye, indicating vascular occlusion or urethral obstruction.
- Isotopic renal scan, a benign, noninvasive technique, demonstrates absent or reduced blood flow to the kidneys.
- Renal arteriography provides proof of existing infarction but is used as a last resort, because it is a high-risk procedure.

Treatment
Infection in the infarcted area or significant hypertension may require surgical repair of the occlusion or nephrectomy. Surgery to establish collateral circulation to the area can relieve renovascular hypertension. Persistent hypertension may respond to antihypertensives and a low-sodium diet. Additional treatments may include administration of intraarterial streptokinase (to lyse blood clots) and catheter embolectomy.

Clinical implications
Assess the degree of renal function and offer supportive care to maintain homeostasis.
- Monitor intake and output, vital signs (particularly blood pressure), electrolytes, and daily weight. Watch for signs of fluid overload, such as

dyspnea, tachycardia, pulmonary edema, and electrolyte imbalances.
• Carefully explain all diagnostic procedures.
• Provide reassurance and emotional support for the patient and family.
• Encourage the patient to return for follow-up examination, which usually includes IVP or a renal scan to assess regained renal function.

Complications
Renovascular hypertension

Renal tubular acidosis

Description
Renal tubular acidosis (RTA)—a syndrome of persistent dehydration, hyperchloremia, hypokalemia, metabolic acidosis, and nephrocalcinosis—results from the kidneys' inability to conserve bicarbonate. This disorder occurs as distal RTA (Type I, classic RTA) or proximal RTA (Type II). Distal RTA results from an inability of the distal tubule to secrete hydrogen ions against established gradients across the tubular membrane. This results in decreased excretion of titratable acids and ammonium, and increased loss of potassium and bicarbonate in the urine. Proximal RTA results from defective reabsorption of bicarbonate in the proximal tubule. This causes bicarbonate to flood the distal tubule, which normally secretes hydrogen ions, and leads to impaired formation of titratable acids and ammonium for excretion. Prognosis is usually good but depends on the severity of renal damage that precedes treatment.

Causes
Primary distal RTA
—Possibly, a hereditary defect
Secondary distal RTA
—Starvation
—Malnutrition
—Hepatic cirrhosis
—Several genetically transmitted disorders
—Possibly other renal or systemic disorders
Primary proximal RTA
—Idiopathic
Secondary proximal RTA
—Proximal tubular cell damage in disease

Signs and symptoms
These occur especially in children:
• Anorexia
• Vomiting
• Occasional fever
• Polyuria
• Dehydration
• Growth retardation
• Apathy and weakness
• Tissue wasting
• Constipation

Diagnostic tests
• Serum bicarbonate, pH, potassium, and phosphorus are decreased.
• Serum chloride and alkaline phosphatase are increased.
• Urine tests show alkalinity with low titratable acids and ammonium content, increased bicarbonate and potassium, and low specific gravity.
• X-rays may show nephrocalcinosis in later states.

Treatment
Supportive treatment for patients with RTA requires replacement of those substances being abnormally excreted, especially bicarbonate, and may include sodium bicarbonate tablets or Shohl's solution to control acidosis, potassium P.O. for dangerously low potassium levels, and vitamin D for bone disease. If pyelonephritis occurs, treatment may include antibiotics as well.

Clinical implications
• Urge compliance with all medication instructions. Inform the patient and his family that the prognosis for RTA and

bone lesion healing is directly related to the adequacy of treatment.

• Monitor laboratory values, especially potassium, for hypokalemia.

• Test urine for pH, and strain it for calculi.

• If rickets develops, explain the condition and its treatment to the patient and his family.

• Teach the patient how to recognize signs and symptoms of calculi (hematuria, low abdominal or flank pain). Advise him to immediately report any such signs and symptoms.

• Instruct the patient with low potassium levels to eat foods with a high potassium content, such as bananas and baked potatoes. Orange juice is also high in potassium.

• Since RTA may be caused by a genetic defect, encourage family members to seek genetic counseling or screening for this disorder.

Complications
• Nephrocalcinosis
• Pyelonephritis
• Rickets

Renovascular hypertension

Description
Renovascular hypertension is a rise in systemic blood pressure resulting from stenosis of the major renal arteries or their branches or from intrarenal atherosclerosis. This narrowing or sclerosis may be partial or complete, and the resulting blood pressure elevation, benign or malignant. Stenosis or occlusion of the renal artery stimulates the affected kidney to release the enzyme renin, which converts angiotensinogen—a plasma protein—to angiotensin I. As angiotensin I circulates through the lungs and liver, it converts to angiotensin II, which causes peripheral vasoconstriction, increased arterial pressure and aldosterone secretion, and, eventually, hypertension.

Causes
• Atherosclerosis and fibromuscular diseases of the renal artery wall layers (primary causes in 95% of patients)
• Arteritis
• Anomalies of the renal arteries
• Embolism
• Trauma
• Tumor
• Dissecting aneurysm

Signs and symptoms
• Elevated systemic blood pressure
• Headache
• Palpitations
• Tachycardia
• Anxiety
• Light-headedness
• Decreased tolerance of temperature extremes
• Retinopathy
• Mental sluggishness

Diagnostic tests
• Isotopic renal blood flow scan and rapid-sequence intravenous pyelography identify abnormalities of renal blood flow and discrepancies of kidney size and shape.

• Renal arteriography reveals the actual arterial stenosis or obstruction.

• Plasma renin levels in blood samples from both the right and left renal veins are compared with the level in a sample from the inferior vena cava. Increased renin level implicates the affected kidney and determines whether surgical correction can reverse hypertension.

Treatment
Surgery, the treatment of choice, is performed to restore adequate circulation and to control severe hypertension or severely impaired renal function by renal artery bypass, endarterectomy, arterioplasty, or, as a last

resort, nephrectomy. Balloon catheter renal artery dilatation is used in selected cases to correct renal artery stenosis without the risks and morbidity of surgery. Symptomatic measures include antihypertensives, diuretics, and a sodium-restricted diet.

Clinical implications

The care plan must emphasize helping the patient and family understand renovascular hypertension and the importance of following prescribed treatment.

• Monitor intake and output and daily weight. Check blood pressure in both arms regularly, with the patient lying down and standing. A drop of 20 mm Hg or more on arising may necessitate an adjustment in antihypertensive medications. Assess renal function daily.

• Administer drugs, as ordered. Maintain fluid and sodium restrictions. Explain the purpose of a low-sodium diet.

• Explain the diagnostic tests, and prepare the patient appropriately; for example, adequately hydrate the patient before tests that use contrast media. After intravenous pyelography or arteriography, watch for complications.

• If a nephrectomy is necessary, reassure the patient that the remaining kidney is adequate for renal function.

• Postoperatively, watch for bleeding and hypotension. If the sutures around the renal vessels slip, the patient can quickly go into shock, since kidneys receive 25% of cardiac output.

• Provide a quiet, stress-free environment, if possible. Urge the patient and family members to have regular blood pressure screenings.

Complications

• Congestive heart failure
• Myocardial infarction
• Cerebrovascular accident
• Occasionally, renal failure

Respiratory acidosis

Description

An acid-base disturbance characterized by reduced alveolar ventilation and manifested by hypercapnia (PCO_2 greater than 45 mm Hg), respiratory acidosis can be acute (due to a sudden failure in ventilation) or chronic (as in long-term pulmonary disease). Prognosis depends on the severity of the underlying disturbance, as well as the patient's general clinical condition.

Causes

• Drugs such as narcotics, anesthetics, hypnotics, and sedatives
• CNS trauma
• Chronic metabolic alkalosis with respiratory compensatory mechanisms
• Neuromuscular disease such as myasthenia gravis, Guillain-Barré syndrome, and poliomyelitis
• Airway obstruction
• Parenchymal lung disease that interferes with alveolar ventilation
• Chronic obstructive pulmonary disease (COPD)
• Asthma
• Severe adult respiratory distress syndrome
• Large pneumothorax
• Extensive pneumonia
• Pulmonary edema

Signs and symptoms

CNS effects
—Range from restlessness, confusion, and apprehension to somnolence, with a fine or flapping tremor (asterixis), or coma
—Possible headaches, dyspnea and tachypnea with papilledema and depressed reflexes

Cardiovascular effects
—Possible tachycardia, hypertension, atrial and ventricular dysrhythmias
—In severe acidosis, possible hypotension with vasodilation (bounding pulses and warm periphery)

Diagnostic tests
Arterial blood gas measurements confirm respiratory acidosis: PCO_2 over the normal 45 mm Hg; pH usually below the normal range of 7.35 to 7.45; and HCO_3 normal in the acute stage, but elevated in the chronic stage.

Treatment
Effective treatment for respiratory acidosis is designed to correct the underlying source of alveolar hypoventilation.

Significantly reduced alveolar ventilation may require mechanical ventilation until the underlying condition can be effectively treated. In COPD this includes bronchodilators, oxygen, and antibiotics; drug therapy for conditions such as myasthenia gravis; removal of foreign bodies from the airway; antibiotics for pneumonia; dialysis to remove toxic drugs; and correction of metabolic alkalosis.

Dangerously low blood pH levels (less than 7.15) can produce profound CNS and cardiovascular deterioration and may require administration of sodium bicarbonate I.V. In chronic lung disease, elevated carbon dioxide levels may persist despite optimal treatment.

Clinical implications
• Be alert for critical changes in the patient's respiratory, CNS, and cardiovascular functions. Report any such changes immediately, as well as any variations in arterial blood gas measurements and electrolyte status. Maintain adequate hydration.

• Maintain a patent airway and provide adequate humidification if acidosis requires mechanical ventilation. Perform tracheal suctioning regularly and vigorous chest physiotherapy, if ordered. Continuously monitor ventilator settings and respiratory status.

• To prevent respiratory acidosis, closely monitor patients with COPD and chronic carbon dioxide retention for signs of acidosis. Also, administer oxygen at low flow rates and closely monitor all patients who receive narcotics and sedatives. Instruct the patient who has received a general anesthetic to turn, cough, and perform deep-breathing exercises frequently to prevent the onset of respiratory acidosis.

Respiratory alkalosis

Description
Respiratory alkalosis is a condition marked by a decrease in PCO_2 to less than 35 mm Hg, which is due to alveolar hyperventilation. Uncomplicated respiratory alkalosis leads to a decrease in hydrogen ion concentration, which causes elevated blood pH. Hypocapnia occurs when the elimination of carbon dioxide by the lungs exceeds the production of carbon dioxide at the cellular level.

Causes
Pulmonary
—Pneumonia
—Interstitial lung disease
—Pulmonary vascular disease
—Acute asthma
Nonpulmonary
—Anxiety
—Fever
—Aspirin toxicity
—Metabolic acidosis
—CNS disease (inflammation or tumor)
—Gram-negative septicemia
—Hepatic failure

Signs and symptoms
• Deep, rapid breathing, possibly above 40 respirations a minute and much like the Kussmaul breathing of diabetic acidosis (the cardinal symptom)
• Light-headedness or dizziness
• Agitation

- Circumoral and peripheral paresthesias
- Carpopedal spasms
- Twitching (possibly progressing to tetany)
- Muscle weakness
- Hyperpnea and cardiac dysrhythmias in severe respiratory alkalosis

Diagnostic tests

Arterial blood gas measurements confirm respiratory alkalosis and rule out respiratory compensation for metabolic acidosis: PCO_2 below 35 mm Hg; pH elevated in proportion to fall in PCO_2 in the acute stage, but falling toward normal in the chronic stage; HCO_3 normal in the acute stage, but below normal in the chronic stage.

Treatment

Treatment is designed to eradicate the underlying condition—for example, removal of ingested toxins, treatment of fever or sepsis, and treatment of CNS disease. In severe respiratory alkalosis, the patient may be instructed to breathe into a paper bag, which helps relieve acute anxiety and increases carbon dioxide levels.

Prevention of hyperventilation in patients receiving mechanical ventilation requires monitoring arterial blood gases and adjusting dead space or minute ventilation volume.

Clinical implications

- Watch for and report any changes in neurologic, neuromuscular, or cardiovascular functions.
- Remember that twitching and cardiac dysrhythmias may be associated with alkalemia and electrolyte imbalances. Monitor arterial blood gas and serum electrolyte levels closely, reporting any variations immediately.
- Explain all diagnostic tests and procedures to reduce anxiety.

Retinal detachment

Description

Retinal detachment occurs when the layers of the retina become separated, creating a subretinal space. This space then fills with fluid, called subretinal fluid. Retinal detachment usually involves only one eye, but may involve the other eye later. Surgical reattachment is often successful. However, prognosis for good vision depends on the area of the eye that has been affected.

Causes

- Degenerative changes of aging (the most common cause)
- Trauma
- Inflammation
- Tumors
- Systemic diseases, such as accelerated hypertension
- Rarely, retinopathy of prematurity

Risk factors

- Myopia
- Cataract surgery

Signs and symptoms

- Visual floaters
- Light flashes
- Gradual, painless vision loss (may be described as a curtain that eliminates a portion of the visual field)

Diagnostic tests

- Ophthalmoscopy after full pupil dilation confirms the diagnosis. Examination shows the usually transparent retina as gray and opaque. In severe detachment, examination reveals folds in the retina and a ballooning out of the area.
- Indirect ophthalmoscopy is also used to search the retina for tears and holes.

Treatment

Treatment depends on the location and severity of the detachment. It may include restricting eye movements

---

Teaching Topics in Retinal Tear and Detachment

- An explanation of the disease process: retinal tear or detachment
- Risk of vision loss without treatment
- Preparation for indirect ophthalmoscopy with scleral depression, slit-lamp examination, or other nonroutine eye tests
- Cryotherapy, photocoagulation, or diathermy for retinal tear or detachment
- Surgical scleral buckling for retinal detachment
- Posttherapy activity restrictions
- Eye drops and their administration

(through bed rest, sedation, and, if the patient's macula is threatened, a pressure patch) and positioning the head so the tear or hole is below the rest of the eye. A hole in the peripheral retina can be treated with cryotherapy; a hole in the posterior portion, with laser therapy. Retinal detachment rarely heals spontaneously; surgery, consisting of scleral buckling, is necessary to reattach the retina.

Clinical implications
- Provide emotional support, since the patient may be understandably distraught because of his loss of vision.
- To prepare the patient for surgery, wash his face with no-tears shampoo. Give antibiotics and cycloplegic/mydriatic eye drops, as ordered.
- Postoperatively, position the patient on his back or on his unoperated side. Elevating the head of the bed may make him feel more comfortable. Allow him to use the bathroom after complete recovery from anesthesia. But discourage him from straining at stool or bending down unnecessarily; these actions can raise intraocular pressure. Tell him to avoid activities that may cause him to bump his eye.
- After removing the pressure patch, gently cleanse the eye with cycloplegic eye drops and steroid/antibiotic eye drops, as ordered. Use cold compresses to decrease swelling and pain.
- Administer medications for pain, as needed. Notify the patient's physician

if pain persists. Teach the patient and his family how to properly instill eye drops, and stress the importance of compliance and follow-up care. Suggest dark glasses to compensate for light sensitivity. (See *Teaching Topics in Retinal Tear and Detachment*.)

Retinitis pigmentosa

Description
Retinitis pigmentosa is a genetically induced, progressive destruction of the retinal rods, resulting in atrophy of the pigment epithelium and eventual blindness. Retinitis pigmentosa often accompanies other hereditary disorders in several distinct syndromes. The most common is Laurence-Moon-Biedl syndrome, typified by visual destruction from retinitis pigmentosa, obesity, mental retardation, polydactyly, and hypogenitalism.

Causes
- May be inherited as an autosomal recessive trait
- May be transmitted as an X-linked trait (more severe form)

Signs and symptoms
- Night blindness, typically occurring in adolescence
- Gradual development of tunnel or "gun-barrel" vision
- Eventually, blindness

Diagnostic tests
• Electroretinography shows absent retinal response or response time slower than normal.
• Visual field testing (using a tangent screen) detects ring scotomata.
• Fluorescein angiography visualizes white dots (areas of dyspigmentation) in the epithelium.
• Ophthalmoscopy may initially show normal fundi but later reveals a characteristic black pigmentary disturbance.

Treatment
Although extensive research continues, no cure exists for retinitis pigmentosa.

Clinical implications
• Teach the patient and family what they need to know about retinitis pigmentosa. Explain that it is hereditary, and suggest genetic counseling for adults who risk transmitting it to their children.
• Tell the patient to wear dark glasses in bright sunlight. Warn him that he might not be able to drive a car at night. (Special new glasses can help patients with retinitis pigmentosa see at night but are experimental and expensive.)
• Refer the patient to a social service agency or to the National Retinitis Pigmentosa Foundation for information and for counseling to prepare him for eventual blindness. If the patient is willing, arrange for him to learn braille.
• Since the prospect of blindness is frightening, your emotional support and guidance are indispensable.

Reye's syndrome

Description
Reye's syndrome is an acute childhood illness that causes fatty infiltration of the liver with concurrent hyperammonemia, encephalopathy, and increased intracranial pressure (ICP). In addition, fatty infiltration of the kidneys, brain, and myocardium may occur. Reye's syndrome affects children from infancy to adolescence and occurs equally in boys and girls.

Prognosis depends on the severity of CNS depression. ICP monitoring and consequent early treatment of increased ICP, along with other treatment measures, have cut mortality to about 20%. Previously, it was as high as 90%. Death is usually a result of cerebral edema or respiratory arrest. Comatose patients who survive may have residual brain damage.

Causes
• Almost always follows within 1 to 3 days of an acute viral infection, such as an upper respiratory infection, type B influenza, or varicella (chicken pox)
• May be linked to aspirin use

Signs and symptoms
The severity of the child's signs and symptoms varies with the degree of encephalopathy and cerebral edema.
• Recurrent vomiting
• Progressive changes in level of consciousness, from drowsiness and lethargy to stupor and coma
• Fever, diaphoresis
• Signs of dehydration
• Hyperactive reflexes
• Respiratory distress (progressing from hyperventilation to Cheyne-Stokes and apneic respirations)
• Unilateral or bilateral fixed and dilated pupils with severe encephalopathy
• Seizures
• Decorticate or decerebrate posturing

Diagnostic tests
• Liver function studies show SGOT and SGPT elevated to twice normal levels; bilirubin is usually normal.

Stages of Treatment for Reye's Syndrome

SIGNS AND SYMPTOMS	BASELINE TREATMENT	BASELINE INTERVENTION
Stage I: vomiting, lethargy, hepatic dysfunction	• To decrease intracranial pressure and brain edema, give I.V. fluids at ⅔ maintenance. Also give an osmotic diuretic or furosemide. • To treat hypoprothrombinemia, give vitamin K; if vitamin K is unsuccessful, give fresh-frozen plasma. • Monitor serum ammonia, blood glucose, plasma osmolality every 4 to 8 hours to check progress.	• Monitor vital signs and check level of consciousness for increasing lethargy. Take vital signs more often as the patient's condition deteriorates. • Monitor fluid intake and output to prevent fluid overload. Maintain urine output at 1.0 ml/kg/hr; plasma osmolality, 290 mOsm; and blood glucose, 150 mg/ml. (*Goal:* Keep glucose high, osmolality normal to high, and ammonia low.) Also, restrict protein.
Stage II: hyperventilation, delirium, hepatic dysfunction, hyperactive reflexes	• Continue baseline treatment.	• Maintain seizure precautions. • Immediately report any signs of coma that require invasive, supportive therapy, such as intubation. • Keep head of bed at 30-degree angle.
Stage III: coma, hyperventilation, decorticate rigidity, hepatic dysfunction	• Continue baseline and seizure treatment. • Monitor ICP with a subarachnoid screw or other invasive device. • Provide endotracheal intubation and mechanical ventilation to control Pco_2 levels. A paralyzing agent, such as pancuronium I.V., may help maintain ventilation. • Give mannitol I.V. or glycerol by nasogastric tube.	• Monitor ICP (should be <20 mm Hg before suctioning) or give thiopental I.V., as ordered; as necessary, hyperventilate the patient. • When ventilating the patient, maintain Pco_2 between 20 and 30 torr and Po_2 between 80 and 100 torr. • Closely monitor cardiovascular status with a pulmonary artery catheter or central venous pressure line. • Give good skin and mouth care, and perform range-of-motion exercises. *(continued)*

Stages of Treatment for Reye's Syndrome *(continued)*

SIGNS AND SYMPTOMS	BASELINE TREATMENT	BASELINE INTERVENTION
Stage IV: deepening coma; decerebrate rigidity; large, fixed pupils; minimal hepatic dysfunction	• Continue baseline and supportive care. • If all previous measures fail, some pediatric centers use barbiturate coma, decompressive craniotomy, hypothermia, or exchange transfusion.	• Check patient for loss of reflexes and signs of flaccidity. • Give the family the extra support they need, considering their child's poor prognosis.
Stage V: seizures, loss of deeptendon reflexes, flaccidity, respiratory arrest, ammonia level above 300 mg/100 ml	• Continue baseline and supportive care.	• Help the family to face the patient's impending death.

• Liver biopsy reveals fatty droplets uniformly distributed throughout cells.
• CSF analysis yields WBC count less than 10/mm³; with coma, CSF pressure is increased.
• Coagulation studies show prolonged PT and PTT.
• Blood studies show serum ammonia levels are elevated; serum glucose levels, normal or, in 15% of cases, low; and serum fatty acid and lactate levels, increased. (For treatment and clinical implications, see *Stages of Treatment for Reye's Syndrome*, p. 667.)

Rheumatic fever and rheumatic heart disease

Description

Acute rheumatic fever is a systemic inflammatory disease of childhood, often recurrent, that follows a Group A beta-hemolytic streptococcal infec-

tion. Rheumatic heart disease refers to the cardiac manifestations of rheumatic fever. It includes pancarditis (myocarditis, pericarditis, and endocarditis) during the early acute phase and chronic valvular disease in the later phases. Long-term antibiotic therapy can minimize recurrence of rheumatic fever, reducing the risk of permanent cardiac damage and eventual valvular deformity. However, severe pancarditis occasionally produces fatal congestive heart failure during the acute phase.

Causes
Rheumatic fever
—Appears to be a hypersensitivity reaction to a Group A beta-hemolytic streptococcal infection
Rheumatic heart disease
—Episodes of rheumatic fever

Signs and symptoms
• Fever
• Migratory joint pain
• Occasionally, skin lesions
• Possible firm, movable, nontender subcutaneous nodules near tendons or bony prominences of joints
• Possible chorea (later symptom)
• Possible pleural friction rub and pain
• Possible heart murmur
—A systolic murmur of mitral regurgitation (high-pitched, blowing, holosystolic, loudest at apex, possibly radiating to the anterior axillary line)
—A midsystolic murmur due to stiffening and swelling of the mitral leaflet
—Occasionally, a diastolic murmur of aortic regurgitation (low-pitched, rumbling, almost inaudible)

Diagnostic tests
WBC count and ESR may be elevated (especially during the acute phase); blood studies show slight anemia due to suppressed erythropoiesis during inflammation.
• C-reactive protein is positive (especially during acute phase).
• Cardiac enzymes may be increased in severe carditis.
• Antistreptolysin O titer is elevated in 95% of patients within 2 months of onset.
• EKG changes are not diagnostic; however, 20% of patients show a prolonged PR interval.
• Chest X-rays show normal heart size, except with myocarditis, congestive heart failure, or pericardial effusion.
• Echocardiography helps evaluate valvular damage, chamber size, and ventricular function.
• Cardiac catheterization evaluates valvular damage and left ventricular function in severe cardiac dysfunction.

Treatment
Effective management eradicates the streptococcal infection, relieves symptoms, and prevents recurrence, reducing the chance of permanent cardiac damage. During the acute phase, treatment includes penicillin or (for patients with penicillin hypersensitivity) erythromycin. Salicylates, such as aspirin, relieve fever and minimize joint swelling and pain; if carditis is present or salicylates fail to relieve pain and inflammation, corticosteroids may be used. Supportive treatment requires strict bed rest for about 5 weeks during the acute phase with active carditis, followed by a progressive increase in physical activity, depending on clinical and laboratory findings and the response to treatment.

After the acute phase subsides, a monthly I.M. injection of penicillin G benzathine or daily doses of oral sulfadiazine or penicillin G may be used to prevent recurrence. Such preventive treatment usually continues for at least 5 years or until age 25. Congestive heart failure necessitates continued bed rest and diuretics. Severe mitral or aortic valvular dysfunction causing persistent congestive heart failure requires corrective valvular surgery, including commissurotomy (separation of the adherent, thickened leaflets of the mitral valve), valvuloplasty (repair of valve), or valve replacement (with prosthetic valve). Corrective valvular surgery is rarely necessary before late adolescence.

Clinical implications
Because rheumatic fever and rheumatic heart disease require prolonged treatment, your care plan should include comprehensive patient teaching to promote compliance with the prescribed therapy.
• Before giving penicillin, ask the patient or (if the patient is a child) his parents if he has ever had a hypersensitive reaction to it. Tell them to stop the drug and call the physician immediately if the patient develops a rash, fever, chills, or other signs of allergy at any time during penicillin therapy.

• Instruct the patient and his family to watch for and report early signs of congestive heart failure such as dyspnea and a hacking, nonproductive cough.

• Stress the need for bed rest during the acute phase and suggest appropriate, physically undemanding diversions. After the acute phase, encourage the family and friends to spend as much time as possible with the patient to minimize boredom. Advise parents to secure tutorial services to help the child keep up with schoolwork during the long convalescence.

• Help parents overcome any guilt feelings they may have about their child's illness. Tell them that failure to seek treatment for streptococcal infection is common, since this illness often seems no worse than a cold. Encourage the parents and the child to vent their frustrations during the long, tedious recovery. If the child has severe carditis, help them prepare for permanent changes in the child's lifestyle.

• Teach the patient and family about this disease and its treatment. Warn parents to watch for and immediately report signs of recurrent streptococcal infection—sudden sore throat, diffuse throat redness and oropharyngeal exudate, swollen and tender cervical lymph glands, pain on swallowing, temperature of 101° to 104° F. (38.3° to 40° C.), headache, and nausea. Urge them to keep the child away from persons with respiratory tract infections.

• Promote good dental hygiene to prevent gingival infection. Make sure the patient and his family understand the need to comply with prolonged antibiotic therapy and follow-up care, and the need for additional antibiotics during dental surgery. Arrange for a visiting nurse to oversee home care, if necessary.

Complications
Congestive heart failure

Rheumatoid arthritis

Description
A chronic, systemic, inflammatory disease, rheumatoid arthritis (RA) primarily attacks peripheral joints and surrounding muscles, tendons, ligaments, and blood vessels. Spontaneous remissions and unpredictable exacerbations mark the course of this potentially crippling disease. Rheumatoid arthritis usually requires lifelong treatment and sometimes surgery. In most patients, the disease follows an intermittent course and allows normal activity, although 10% suffer total disability from severe articular deformity or associated extraarticular symptoms, or both. Prognosis worsens with the development of nodules, vasculitis, and high titers of rheumatoid factor (RF).

Causes
The causes are unknown, but RA is currently believed to have an autoimmune basis.

Signs and symptoms
Initial symptoms
—Fatigue
—Malaise
—Anorexia
—Persistent low-grade fever
—Weight loss
—Lymphadenopathy
—Vague articular symptoms
Later symptoms
—Joint pain, tenderness, warmth, and swelling (typical joint symptoms occur bilaterally and symmetrically)
—Morning stiffness
—Possible paresthesias in hands and feet
—Possible stiff, weak, or painful muscles
—Rheumatoid nodules (subcutaneous, round or oval, nontender masses, usually on pressure areas, such as the elbow)

When Arthritis Requires Surgery

Arthritis severe enough to necessitate total knee or total hip arthroplasty calls for comprehensive preoperative teaching and postoperative care.

Before surgery:
• Explain surgical procedures and show the patient the prosthesis to be used, if available. Also, explain preoperative procedures (skin scrubs, prophylactic antibiotics).
• Teach the patient postoperative exercises (such as isometrics), and supervise his practice. Also, teach deep-breathing and coughing exercises.
• Explain that total hip or knee arthroplasty requires frequent range-of-motion exercises of the leg after surgery; total knee arthroplasty requires frequent leg-lift exercises.
• Show the patient how to use a trapeze to move himself about in bed after surgery, and make sure he has a fracture bedpan handy.
• Tell the patient what kind of dressings to expect after surgery. After total knee arthroplasty, he may have a cast, compression dressing, or dressing with a posterior splint. After total hip arthroplasty, he will have an abduction pillow between the legs to help keep the hip prosthesis in place.

After surgery:
• Closely monitor and record vital signs. Watch for complications, such as steroid crisis and shock in patients receiving steroids. Measure distal leg pulses often, marking them with a waterproof marker to make them easier to find.
• As soon as the patient awakens, have him do active dorsiflexion; if he cannot do this, report it immediately. Supervise isometrics every 2 hours. After total hip arthroplasty, check traction for pressure areas and keep the head of the bed raised between 30 and 45 degrees.
• Change or reinforce dressings, as needed, using aseptic technique. Check wounds for hematoma, excessive drainage, color changes, or foul odor—all possible signs of infection. (Wounds on RA patients may heal slowly.) Avoid contaminating dressings while helping the patient use the urinal or bedpan.
• Administer blood replacement products, antibiotics, and pain medication, as ordered. Monitor serum electrolytes, hemoglobin, and hematocrit.
• Have the patient turn, cough, and deep breathe every 2 hours; then percuss his chest.
• After total knee arthroplasty, keep the patient's leg extended and slightly elevated.
• After total hip arthroplasty, keep the patient's hip in abduction to prevent dislocation. Watch for and immediately report any inability to rotate the hip or bear weight on it, increased pain, or a leg that appears shorter—all may indicate dislocation.
• As soon as allowed, help the patient get out of bed and sit in a chair, keeping his weight on the unaffected side. When he is ready to walk, consult the physical therapist for walking instruction and aids.

Advanced symptoms
—Joint deformities
—Diminished joint function

Diagnostic tests
• X-rays, in early stages, show bone demineralization and soft-tissue swelling; later, loss of cartilage and narrowing of joint spaces; finally, cartilage and bone destruction, and erosion, subluxations, and deformities.

• RF test is positive in 75% to 80% of patients, as indicated by a titer of 1:160 or higher.

• Synovial fluid analysis shows increased volume and turbidity, but decreased viscosity and complement (C3 and C4) levels; WBC count is often more than $10,000/mm^3$.

• Serum protein electrophoresis may show elevated serum globulins.

• Erythrocyte sedimentation rate is elevated in 85% to 90% of patients (may be useful to monitor response to therapy, since elevation commonly parallels disease activity).

• CBC usually shows moderate anemia and slight leukocytosis.

Treatment

Salicylates, particularly aspirin, are the mainstay of RA therapy, since they decrease inflammation and relieve joint pain. Other useful medications include nonsteroidal anti-inflammatory agents (such as indomethacin, fenoprofen, and ibuprofen), antimalarials (chloroquine and hydroxychloroquine), gold salts, penicillamine, and corticosteroids (prednisone). Immunosuppressives, such as cyclophosphamide and azathioprine, are also therapeutic.

Supportive measures include 8 to 10 hours of sleep every night, frequent rest periods between daily activities, and splinting to rest inflamed joints. A physical therapy program including range-of-motion exercises and carefully individualized therapeutic exercises forestalls loss of joint function. Application of heat relaxes muscles and relieves pain. Moist heat (hot soaks, paraffin baths, whirlpool) usually works best for patients with chronic disease. Ice packs are effective during acute episodes.

Advanced disease may require synovectomy, joint reconstruction, or total joint arthroplasty.

Clinical implications

• Assess all joints carefully. Look for deformities, contractures, immobility, and inability to perform everyday activities.

• Monitor vital signs, and note weight changes, sensory disturbances, and level of pain. Administer analgesics, as ordered, and watch for side effects.

• Give meticulous skin care. Use lotion or cleansing oil, not soap, for dry skin.

• Explain all diagnostic tests and procedures. Tell the patient to expect multiple blood samples to allow firm diagnosis and accurate monitoring of therapy.

• Monitor the duration, not the intensity, of morning stiffness, because duration more accurately reflects the severity of the disease. Encourage the patient to take hot showers or baths at bedtime or in the morning to reduce the need for pain medication.

• Apply splints carefully. Observe for pressure sores if the patient is in traction or wearing splints.

• Explain the nature of RA. Make sure the patient and his family understand that RA is a chronic disease that requires major changes in life-style. Emphasize that no miracle cures exist, despite claims to the contrary.

• Encourage a balanced diet, but make sure the patient understands that special diets will not cure RA. Stress the need for weight control, since obesity adds further stress to joints.

• Urge the patient to perform activities of daily living such as dressing and feeding himself (supply easy-to-open cartons, lightweight cups, and unpackaged silverware).

• Provide emotional support. Encourage the patient with RA to discuss his fears concerning dependency, sexuality, body image, and self-esteem. Refer him to an appropriate social service agency, as needed.

• Discuss sexual aids: alternative positions, pain medication, and moist heat to increase mobility.

Teaching Topics in Rheumatoid Arthritis

• Explanation of the chronicity and variable symptoms of rheumatoid arthritis
• Importance of strict compliance with treatment to prevent complications, such as worsening pain and deformity
• Preparation for blood tests and, if ordered, synovial fluid analysis
• Administration of salicylates or other medication, such as nonsteroidal anti-inflammatory drugs
• A balanced program of rest and activity
• An exercise program to reduce stiffness and promote mobility
• Importance of joint protection, including the need for good body mechanics and use of assistive devices
• Dietary considerations, including devices to ease meal preparation
• Application of heat or cold to reduce stiffness, swelling, or pain
• Sexual activity
• Sources of information and support

• Before discharge, make sure the patient knows how and when to take prescribed medication and how to recognize possible side effects.
• Teach the patient how to stand, walk, and sit correctly: upright and erect. Tell him to sit in chairs with high seats and armrests. He will find it easier to get up from a chair if his knees are lower than his hips. Suggest an elevated toilet seat.
• Instruct the patient to pace daily activities, resting for 5 to 10 minutes out of each hour and alternating sitting and standing tasks. Adequate sleep is important, and so is correct sleeping posture. He should sleep on his back on a firm mattress and should avoid placing a pillow under his knees, which encourages flexion deformity.
• Teach him to avoid putting undue stress on joints and to use the largest joint available for a given task. Enlist the aid of the occupational therapist to teach how to simplify activities and protect arthritic joints.
• Suggest dressing aids—a long-handled shoehorn, a reacher, elastic shoelaces, a zipper-pull, and a button-hook—and helpful household items,

such as easy-to-open drawers, a hand-held shower nozzle, handrails, and grab bars.
• For more information on coping with RA, refer the patient to the Arthritis Foundation. (See *When Arthritis Requires Surgery*, p. 671, and *Teaching Topics in Rheumatoid Arthritis*.)

Complications
Extraarticular effects may include the following:
• Vasculitis
• Pericarditis
• Pleuritis
• Scleritis
• Episcleritis
• Pulmonary nodules or fibrosis
• Infection
• Osteoporosis
• Myositis
• Lymphadenopathy
• Peripheral neuritis

Rocky Mountain spotted fever

Description
Rocky Mountain spotted fever (RMSF) is a tick-borne, febrile, rash-producing illness that is endemic throughout the

Preventing Rocky Mountain Spotted Fever

• Avoid tick-infested areas, if possible. If you must go to a tick-infested area, check your entire body, including scalp, every 3 to 4 hours for attached ticks. Wear protective clothing, such as a long-sleeved shirt and slacks tucked into firmly laced boots.
• Apply insect repellent to clothes and exposed skin.
• If you find a tick attached to your body, do not crush it, as this may contaminate the bite wound. To detach the tick, place a drop of oil, alcohol, gasoline, or kerosene on it or hold a lighted cigarette near it.
• If you are at high risk (for instance, if you work in a laboratory with rickettsiae, or if you are planning an extended camping trip and will be far from adequate medical facilities), you should receive vaccination against this disease.

continental United States. It is particularly prevalent in the Southeast and Southwest and is becoming more common because of the increasing popularity of outdoor activities such as camping and backpacking. Eruptions begin about the wrists, ankles, or forehead; within 2 days, they cover the entire body, including the scalp, palms, and soles. The rash consists of erythematous macules 1 to 5 mm in diameter that blanch on pressure and may become petechial and maculopapular if untreated. By the 3rd week, the skin peels off and may become gangrenous over the elbows, fingers, and toes.

RMSF is fatal in about 5% of patients. Mortality rises when treatment is delayed; it is also greater in older patients.

Causes
Rickettsia rickettsii

Mode of transmission
• *R. rickettsii* is transmitted by the wood tick (*Dermacentor andersoni*) in the West and by the dog tick (*Dermacentor variabilis*) in the East.
• RMSF is transmitted to a human or small animal by the prolonged bite (4 to 6 hours) of an adult tick.
• Occasionally, this disease is acquired through inhalation or through contact of abraded skin with tick excreta or tissue fluids.

Signs and symptoms
• Persistent temperature of 102° to 104° F. (38.9° to 40° C.)
• Generalized, excruciating headache
• Aching in the bones, muscles, joints, and back
• Thick white lingual coating that gradually turns brown
• Rash
• Gradually increasing pulse rate (possibly reaching 150 beats/minute)
• Thready, rapid pulse and hypotension (less than 90 mm Hg systolic pressure). These signs herald imminent death from vascular collapse.
• Other clinical signs and symptoms: bronchial cough, rapid respirations (as many as 60 breaths/minute), anorexia, nausea, vomiting, constipation, abdominal pain, hepatomegaly, splenomegaly, insomnia, restlessness, and, in extreme cases, delirium

Diagnostic tests
• A positive complement fixation test (which shows a fourfold increase in convalescent antibody titer compared with acute titers) and a history of tick bite or travel to a tick-infested area usually establish the diagnosis.
• Blood cultures should be performed to isolate the organism and confirm the diagnosis.
• Another common but less reliable

antibody test is the Weil-Felix reaction, which also shows a fourfold increase between the acute and convalescent sera titer levels. Increased titers usually develop after 10 to 14 days and persist for several months.

• Platelet count shows thrombocytopenia (12,000 to 150,000/mm³).

• WBC count is increased (11,000 to 33,000/mm³) during the 2nd week of illness. (See *Preventing Rocky Mountain Spotted Fever*.)

Treatment

Treatment requires careful removal of the tick and administration of antibiotics, such as chloramphenicol or tetracycline, until 3 days after the fever subsides. Treatment also includes symptomatic measures and, in disseminated intravascular coagulation (DIC), heparin and platelet transfusion.

Special considerations

• Carefully monitor intake and output. Watch closely for decreased urinary output—a possible indicator of renal failure. Also watch for signs of dehydration, such as poor skin turgor and dry mouth. Give antipyretics, as ordered, and tepid sponge baths to reduce fever.

• Monitor vital signs, and watch for profound hypotension and shock. Also, be prepared to give oxygen therapy and assisted ventilation for pulmonary complications.

• Turn the patient frequently to prevent decubitus ulcers and pneumonia.

• Pay attention to the patient's nutritional needs: vomiting may necessitate intravenous nutrition or frequent small meals.

• Give meticulous mouth care.

Complications

• Lobar pneumonia
• Otitis media
• Parotitis
• DIC
• Renal failure

Rosacea

Description

A chronic skin eruption, rosacea produces flushing and dilation of the small blood vessels in the face, especially the nose and cheeks. Papules and pustules may also occur but without the characteristic comedones of acne vulgaris. Rosacea is most common in white women between ages 30 and 50. When it occurs in men, however, it is usually more severe and often associated with rhinophyma, which is characterized by dilated follicles and thickened, bulbous skin on the nose. Ocular involvement may result in blepharitis, conjunctivitis, uveitis, or keratitis. Rosacea usually spreads slowly and rarely subsides spontaneously.

Causes

The causes are unknown, but aggravating factors include the following:
• Stress
• Infection
• Vitamin deficiency
• Endocrine abnormalities
• Anything that produces flushing—for example, hot beverages such as tea or coffee, tobacco, alcohol, spicy foods, physical activity, sunlight, and extreme heat or cold

Signs and symptoms

• Rosacea generally begins with periodic flushing across the central oval of the face, accompanied later by telangiectasias, papules, pustules, and nodules.

• Rhinophyma is commonly associated with severe rosacea but may occur alone; it usually appears first on the lower half of the nose and produces red, thickened skin and follicular enlargement.

• Related ocular lesions are uncommon.

Treatment and clinical implications

Treatment of the acneiform component of rosacea consists of tetracycline P.O. in gradually decreasing doses as symptoms subside. Topical application of hydrocortisone ointment reduces erythema and inflammation. Other treatment may include electrolysis to destroy large, dilated blood vessels and removal of excess tissue in patients with rhinophyma.

• Instruct the patient to avoid hot beverages, alcohol, and other possible causes of flushing.

• Assess the effect of rosacea on body image. Since it is always apparent on the face, your support and reassurance are essential.

Roseola infantum
(Exanthema subitum)

Description

Roseola infantum, an acute, benign infection, usually affects infants and young children (ages 6 months to 3 years). Characteristically, it first causes a high fever and then a rash that accompanies an abrupt drop to normal temperature.

Causes

Presumably, a virus

Signs and symptoms

• Abruptly rising, unexplainable fever and sometimes seizures occur. Temperature peaks at 103° to 105° F. (39.4° to 40.6° C.) for 3 to 5 days, then drops suddenly.

• In the early febrile period, the infant may be anorexic, irritable, and listless but does not seem particularly ill.

• Simultaneously with an abrupt drop in temperature, a maculopapular, nonpruritic rash develops, which blanches on pressure. The rash is profuse on the infant's trunk, arms, and neck, and is mild on the face and legs. It fades within 24 hours.

Treatment and clinical implications

Because roseola is self-limiting, treatment is supportive and symptomatic: antipyretics to lower fever and, if necessary, anticonvulsants to relieve seizures.

Teach parents how to lower their infant's fever by giving tepid baths, keeping him in lightweight clothes, and maintaining normal room temperature. Stress the need for adequate fluid intake. Strict bed rest and isolation are unnecessary. Tell parents that a short febrile convulsion will not cause brain damage. Explain that convulsions will cease after fever subsides and that phenobarbital is likely to cause drowsiness. If it causes stupor, parents should call their physician immediately.

Rubella
(German measles)

Description

Rubella is an acute, mildly contagious disease that produces a distinctive, 3-day rash and lymphadenopathy. It occurs most often among children aged 5 to 9, adolescents, and young adults. A maculopapular eruption begins on the face and spreads rapidly, often covering the trunk (may be confluent) and extremities within hours. The rash fades in the downward order in which it appeared and usually disappears on the third day. The period of communicability lasts from about 10 days before until 5 days after the rash appears. Worldwide in distribution, rubella flourishes during the spring (particularly in big cities), and epidemics occur sporadically. This disease is self-limiting, and the prognosis is excellent. (For information on congenital rubella, see *Expanded Rubella Syndrome*.)

Expanded Rubella Syndrome

Congenital rubella is by far the most serious form of the disease. Intrauterine rubella infection, especially during the first trimester, can lead to spontaneous abortion or stillbirth, as well as single or multiple birth defects. (As a rule, the earlier the infection occurs during pregnancy, the greater the damage to the fetus.) The combination of cataracts, deafness, and cardiac disease comprises the classic rubella syndrome. Low birth weight, microcephaly, and mental retardation are other common manifestations. However, researchers now believe that congenital rubella can cause several more disorders, many of which do not appear until later in life. These include dental abnormalities, thrombocytopenic purpura, hemolytic and hypoplastic anemia, encephalitis, giant-cell hepatitis, seborrheic dermatitis, and diabetes mellitus. Indeed, it now appears that congenital rubella may be a lifelong disease. This theory is supported by the fact that the rubella virus has been isolated from urine 15 years after its acquisition in the uterus.

Infants born with congenital rubella should be isolated immediately, because they excrete the virus for a period of from several months to a year after birth. Cataracts and cardiac defects may require surgery. Prognosis depends on the particular malformations that occur. The overall mortality for rubella infants is 6%, but it is higher for babies born with thrombocytopenic purpura, congenital cardiac disease, or encephalitis. Parents of affected children need emotional support and guidance in finding help from community resources and organizations.

Causes
Rubella virus

Mode of transmission
• The rubella virus is transmitted through contact with the blood, urine, stools, or nasopharyngeal secretions of infected persons, and possibly by contact with contaminated articles of clothing.
• It is transmitted across the placenta, and, especially in the first trimester of pregnancy, it can cause serious birth defects.

Signs and symptoms
• Rubella rash is usually the cardinal symptom.
• Small, red, petechial macules on the soft palate (Forschheimer spots) may precede or accompany the rash.
• Possible low-grade fever, mild coryza, and conjunctivitis may accompany the rash; in adults and adolescents, these signs may precede the rash.

• Suboccipital, postauricular, and postcervical lymph node enlargement is a hallmark of rubella.

Diagnostic tests
• Cell cultures of the throat, blood, urine, and cerebrospinal fluid can confirm the presence of the virus; however, the diagnosis is often based on the history and characteristic signs.
• Convalescent serum that shows a fourfold rise in antibody titers confirms the diagnosis.

Treatment
Since the rubella rash is self-limiting and only mildly pruritic, it does not require topical or systemic medication. Treatment consists of aspirin for fever and joint pain. Bed rest is not necessary, but the patient should be isolated until the rash disappears.

Immunization with live virus vaccine RA27/3, the only rubella vaccine available in the United States, is necessary for prevention and appears to be more immunogenic than previous vaccines. The rubella vaccine should be given with measles and mumps vaccines at age 15 months to decrease the cost and the number of injections needed.

Clinical implications
• Make the patient with active rubella as comfortable as possible. Give children books to read or games to play to keep them occupied.
• Explain why respiratory isolation is necessary. Make sure the patient or parents understand how important it is to avoid exposing pregnant women to this disease.
• Report confirmed cases of rubella to local public health officials.
• Know how to manage rubella immunization before giving the vaccine.
• Obtain a history of allergies, especially to neomycin. If the patient has this allergy or if he has had a reaction to immunization in the past, check with the physician before giving the vaccine.
• Ask women of childbearing age if they are pregnant. If they are or think they may be, *do not* give the vaccine. Warn women who receive rubella vaccine to use an effective means of birth control for at least 3 months after immunization.
• Give the vaccine at least 3 months after any administration of immune globulin or blood, which could have antibodies that neutralize the vaccine.
• Do not vaccinate any immunocompromised patients, patients with immunodeficiency diseases, or those receiving immunosuppressive, radiation, or corticosteroid therapy. Instead, administer immune serum globulin, as ordered, to prevent or reduce infection in susceptible patients.

• After giving the vaccine, observe for signs of anaphylaxis for at least 30 minutes. Keep epinephrine 1:1,000 handy.
• Warn about possible mild fever, slight rash, transient arthralgia (in adolescents), and arthritis (in elderly persons). Suggest aspirin or acetaminophen for fever.
• Advise the patient to apply warmth to the injection site for 24 hours after immunization (to help the body absorb the vaccine). If swelling persists after the initial 24 hours, suggest a cold compress to promote vasoconstriction and prevent antigenic cyst formation.

Complications
Complications are rare, but they include the following:
• Hemorrhagic problems, such as thrombocytopenia
• Transient arthritis in young women

Rubeola
(Measles, morbilli)

Description
Rubeola is an acute, highly contagious infection that may be one of the most common and most serious of all communicable childhood diseases. Vaccination has reduced the occurrence of measles during childhood; as a result, measles is becoming more prevalent in adolescents and adults. In the United States, prognosis is usually excellent. However, measles is a major cause of death in children in underdeveloped countries.

Causes
Paramyxovirus

Mode of transmission
Direct contact with contaminated respiratory droplets

Signs and symptoms
Prodromal stage
Symptoms during this stage of greatest

Administering Measles Vaccine

Warn the patient or his parents that possible side effects are anorexia, malaise, rash, mild thrombocytopenia or leukopenia, and fever. Advise them that the vaccine may produce slight reactions, usually within 7 to 10 days.
• Ask the patient about known allergies, especially to neomycin (each dose contains a small amount). However, a patient who is allergic to eggs may receive the vaccine, because it contains only minimal amounts of albumin and yolk components.
• Avoid giving the vaccine to a pregnant woman (ask for date of last menstrual period). Warn female patients to avoid pregnancy for at least 3 months after vaccination.
• Do not vaccinate children with untreated tuberculosis, immunodeficiencies, leukemia, or lymphoma, or those receiving immunosuppressants. If such children are exposed to the virus, recommend they receive gamma globulin (gamma globulin will not prevent measles but will lessen its severity). Older unimmunized children who have been exposed to measles for more than 5 days may also require gamma globulin. Be sure to immunize them 3 months later.
• Delay vaccination for 8 to 12 weeks after administration of whole blood, plasma, or gamma globulin, because measles antibodies in these components may neutralize the vaccine.
• Watch for signs of anaphylaxis for 30 minutes after vaccination. Keep epinephrine 1:1,000 handy.
• Advise application of a warm compress to the vaccination site to facilitate absorption of the vaccine. If swelling occurs within 24 hours after vaccination, tell the patient to apply cold compresses to promote vasoconstriction and to prevent antigenic cyst formation.

Usually, one bout of measles renders immunity (a second infection is extremely rare and may represent misdiagnosis); infants under age 4 months may be immune because of circulating maternal antibodies. Under normal conditions, measles vaccine is not administered to children younger than age 15 months. However, during an epidemic, infants as young as 6 months may receive the vaccine; they must be reimmunized at age 15 months. An alternate approach calls for administration of gamma globulin to infants between ages 6 and 15 months who are likely to be exposed to measles.

communicability include the following:
—Fever
—Malaise
—Coryza
—Cough
—Conjunctivitis
—Photophobia
—Hoarseness
—Koplik's spots. The hallmark of the disease, these tiny, bluish gray specks surrounded by a red halo appear on the oral mucosa at the end of the prodrome.

Next stage
The measles rash appears behind the ears and on the neck and cheeks as faint macules, which become papular and erythematous and spread downward rapidly, ending with the feet. This is accompanied by the following:
—Temperature of 103° to 105° F. (39.4° to 40.6° C.)
—Severe cough
—Rhinorrhea
—Puffy red eyes

Diagnostic tests
• Measles virus may be isolated from the blood, nasopharyngeal secretions, and urine during the febrile period; however, diagnosis is usually based on history and characteristic manifestations.
• Serum antibodies appear within 3 days after onset of the rash, and reach peak titers 2 to 4 weeks later.

Treatment and clinical implications
Treatment for measles requires bed rest, relief of symptoms, and respiratory isolation throughout the communicable period. Vaporizers and a warm environment help reduce respiratory irritation. Cough preparations and antibiotics are usually ineffective. Antipyretics can reduce fever. Therapy must also combat complications.
• Teach parents supportive measures, and stress the need for isolation, plenty of rest, and increased fluid intake. Advise them to cope with photophobia by darkening the room or providing sunglasses, and to reduce fever with antipyretics and tepid sponge baths.
• Warn parents to watch for and report the early signs and symptoms of complications. (See *Administering Measles Vaccine*, p. 679.)

Complications
• Encephalitis
• Otitis media
• Pneumonia
• Secondary bacterial infection
• Subacute sclerosing panencephalitis is rare and usually fatal.

Salmonellosis

Description
One of the most common infections in the United States (over 2 million new cases appear annually), salmonellosis is a form of gastroenteritis. It occurs as enterocolitis, bacteremia, localized infection, typhoid, or paratyphoid fever. Nontyphoidal forms of salmonellosis usually produce mild-to-moderate illness, with low mortality.

Typhoid, the most severe form of salmonellosis, usually lasts from 1 to 4 weeks. Mortality is about 3% of persons who are treated and 10% of those untreated. Death usually results from complications. An attack of typhoid confers lifelong immunity, although 3% of patients become carriers.

Causes
Gram-negative bacilli of the genus *Salmonella*, a member of the Enterobacteriaceae family

Mode of transmission
Nontyphoidal salmonellosis
—Usually through the ingestion of contaminated or inadequately processed foods, especially eggs, chicken, turkey, and duck
—Contact with infected persons or animals
—Ingestion of contaminated dry milk, chocolate bars, or pharmaceuticals of animal origin
—Fecal-oral spread in children under age 5

Typhoid
—Most frequently from drinking water contaminated by excretions of a carrier

Signs and symptoms
Clinical manifestations vary. (See *Clinical Variants of Salmonellosis,* pp. 682-683.)

Diagnostic tests
• Isolation of the organism in a culture, particularly blood (in typhoid, paratyphoid, and bacteremia) or feces (in enterocolitis, paratyphoid, and typhoid) usually establishes the diagnosis.
• Other appropriate culture specimens include urine, bone marrow, pus, and vomitus. In endemic areas, clinical symptoms of enterocolitis allow a working diagnosis before the cultures are found to be positive.
• Presence of *S. typhi* in stool 1 or more years after treatment indicates that the patient is a carrier.
• Widal's test, an agglutination reaction against somatic and flagellar antigens, may suggest typhoid with a fourfold rise in titer. However, drug use or hepatic disease can also increase these titers and invalidate test results.
• Other supportive laboratory values may include transient leukocytosis during the 1st week of typhoidal salmonellosis, leukopenia during the 3rd week, and leukocytosis in local infection.

Clinical Variants of Salmonellosis

VARIANT	CAUSE	CLINICAL FEATURES
Enterocolitis	Any species of nontyphoidal *Salmonella,* but usually *S. enteritidis.* Incubation period, 6 to 48 hours.	Mild-to-severe abdominal pain, diarrhea, sudden fever to 102° F. (38.8° C.), nausea, vomiting; usually self-limiting, but may progress to enteric fever (resembling typhoid), local abscesses (usually abdominal), dehydration, septicemia
Paratyphoid	*S. paratyphi* and *S. schottmülleri* (formerly *S. paratyphi B*). Incubation period, 3 weeks or more.	Fever and transient diarrhea; generally resembles typhoid but less severe
Bacteremia	Any *Salmonella* species, but most commonly *S. choleraesuis.* Incubation period varies.	Fever, chills, anorexia, weight loss (without GI symptoms), joint pains
Typhoid fever	*S. typhi* enters GI tract and invades the bloodstream via the lymphatics, setting up intracellular sites. During this phase, infection of biliary tract leads to intestinal seeding with millions of bacilli. Involved lymphoid tissues (especially Peyer's patches in ileum) enlarge, ulcerate, and necrose, resulting in hemorrhage. Incubation period, usually 1 to 2 weeks.	Symptoms of enterocolitis may develop within hours of ingestion of *S. typhi*; they usually subside before onset of typhoid fever symptoms **1st week:** gradually increasing fever, anorexia, myalgia, malaise, headache **2nd week:** remittent fever up to 104° F. (40° C.) usually in the evening, chills, diaphoresis, weakness, delirium, increasing abdominal pain and distention, diarrhea or constipation, cough, moist rales, tender abdomen with enlarged spleen, maculopapular rash (especially on abdomen) **3rd week:** persistent fever, increasing fatigue and weakness; usually subsides end of third week, although relapses may occur **Complications:** intestinal perforation or hemorrhage, abscesses, thrombophlebitis, cerebral thrombosis, pneumonia, osteomyelitis, myocarditis, acute circulatory failure, chronic carrier state

Clinical Variants of Salmonellosis (continued)		
VARIANT	CAUSE	CLINICAL FEATURES
Localized infections	Usually follow bacteremia caused by *Salmonella* species.	Symptoms determined by site of localization; localized abscesses may cause osteomyelitis, endocarditis, bronchopneumonia, pyelonephritis, and arthritis

Treatment

Antimicrobial therapy for typhoid, paratyphoid, and bacteremia depends on organism sensitivity. It may include ampicillin, amoxicillin, chloramphenicol, and, in the severely toxemic patient, trimethoprim-sulfamethoxazole. Localized abscesses may also need surgical drainage. Enterocolitis requires a short course of antibiotics only if it causes septicemia or prolonged fever. Symptomatic treatment includes bed rest and, most important, replacement of fluids and electrolytes. Camphorated opium tincture, kaolin with pectin, diphenoxylate hydrochloride, codeine, or small doses of morphine may be necessary to relieve diarrhea and control cramps for patients who must remain active.

Clinical implications

• Follow enteric precautions. Teach the patient to use proper handwashing technique, especially after defecating and before eating or handling food. Wear gloves and a gown when disposing of feces or fecally contaminated objects. Continue enteric precautions until three consecutive stool cultures are negative—the first one 48 hours after antibiotic treatment ends, followed by two more at 24-hour intervals.

• Observe the patient closely for signs of bowel perforation: sudden pain in the lower right abdomen, possibly after one or more rectal bleeding episodes; sudden fall in temperature or blood pressure; and rising pulse rate.

• During acute infection, plan your care and other activities to allow the patient as much rest as possible. Raise the side rails and use other safety measures because the patient may become delirious.

• Accurately record intake and output. Maintain adequate I.V. hydration. When the patient can tolerate oral feedings, encourage high-calorie fluids, such as milkshakes. Watch for constipation.

• Provide good skin and mouth care.

• *Do not* administer antipyretics. These mask fever and lead to possible hypothermia. Instead, to promote heat loss through the skin without causing shivering (which keeps fever high by vasoconstriction), apply tepid, wet towels (do not use alcohol or ice) to the patient's groin and axillae. To promote heat loss by vasodilation of peripheral blood vessels, use additional wet towels on the arms and legs, wiping with long, vigorous strokes.

• After draining the abscesses of a joint, provide heat, elevation, and passive range-of-motion exercises to decrease swelling and maintain mobility.

• If the patient has positive stool cultures on discharge, tell him to use a different bathroom than other family members, if possible (while he is on antibiotics), and to avoid preparing

uncooked foods, such as salads, for family members.
• To prevent salmonellosis, advise prompt refrigeration of meat and cooked foods (avoid keeping them at room temperature for any prolonged period), and teach the importance of proper hand washing. Advise those at high risk of contracting typhoid (lab workers, travelers) to seek vaccination.

Sarcoidosis

Description
Sarcoidosis is a multisystemic, granulomatous disorder that characteristically produces lymphadenopathy, pulmonary infiltration, and skeletal, liver, eye, or skin lesions. Acute sarcoidosis usually resolves within 2 years. Chronic, progressive sarcoidosis, which is uncommon, is associated with pulmonary fibrosis and progressive pulmonary disability.

Causes
The cause of sarcoidosis is unknown, but the following possible causes have been considered:
• Hypersensitivity response (possibly from T-cell imbalance) to such agents as atypical mycobacteria, fungi, and pine pollen
• Genetic predisposition, suggested by a slightly higher incidence of sarcoidosis within the same family
• Chemicals

Signs and symptoms
Initial symptoms include arthralgia (in the wrists, ankles, and elbows), fatigue, malaise, and weight loss.
  The following clinical features vary according to the extent and location of the fibrosis:
• Respiratory—breathlessness, cough (usually nonproductive), substernal pain
• Cutaneous—erythema nodosum,

cutaneous skin nodules with maculopapular eruptions, extensive nasal mucosal lesions
• Ophthalmic—anterior uveitis (common); blindness (rare)
• Lymphatic—bilateral hilar and right paratracheal lymphadenopathy, and splenomegaly
• Musculoskeletal—muscle weakness, polyarthralgia, pain, punched-out lesions on phalanges
• Genitourinary—symptoms of hypercalciuria
• Cardiovascular—dysrhythmias (premature beats, bundle branch or complete heart block)
• CNS—cranial or peripheral nerve palsies, convulsions

Diagnostic tests
• A positive Kveim-Siltzbach skin test supports the diagnosis.
• Chest X-ray shows bilateral hilar and right paratracheal adenopathy with or without diffuse interstitial infiltrates; occasionally, large nodular lesions are present in lung parenchyma.
• Lymph node, skin, or lung biopsy shows noncaseating granulomas; cultures for mycobacteria and fungi are negative.
• Other laboratory data may include increased serum calcium, mild anemia, leukocytosis, and hyperglobulinemia.
• Pulmonary function tests reveal decreased total lung capacity and compliance and decreased diffusing capacity.
• Arterial oxygen tension is decreased.

Treatment
Asymptomatic sarcoidosis requires no treatment. However, sarcoidosis that causes ocular, respiratory, CNS, cardiac, or systemic symptoms (such as fever and weight loss) requires treatment with systemic or topical steroids, as does sarcoidosis that produces hypercalcemia or destructive skin lesions. Such therapy is usually continued for 1 to 2 years, but some

patients may need lifelong therapy. Other treatment includes a low-calcium diet and avoidance of direct exposure to sunlight in patients with hypercalcemia.

Clinical implications
• Watch for and report any complications.
• For the patient with arthralgia, administer analgesics, as ordered. Record signs of progressive muscle weakness.
• Provide a nutritious, high-calorie diet and plenty of fluids. If the patient has hypercalcemia, suggest a low-calcium diet. Weigh the patient regularly to detect weight loss.
• Monitor respiratory function. Check chest X-rays for extent of lung involvement. Note and record any bloody sputum or increase in sputum. If the patient has pulmonary hypertension or end-stage cor pulmonale, check arterial blood gas measurements, watch for dysrhythmias, and administer oxygen, as needed.
• Since steroids may induce or worsen diabetes mellitus, test urine for glucose and acetone at least every 12 hours at the beginning of steroid therapy. Also, watch for other steroid side effects.
• When preparing the patient for discharge, stress the need for compliance with prescribed steroid therapy and regular, careful follow-up examinations and treatment.
• Refer the patient with failing vision to community support and resource groups and the American Foundation for the Blind, if necessary.

Complications
• Pulmonary hypertension
• Cor pulmonale
• Granulomatous hepatitis (usually asymptomatic)
• Hypercalciuria
• Rarely, cardiomyopathy
• Glaucoma
• Basilar meningitis
• Diabetes insipidus

Scabies

Description
Scabies is a contagious skin infection that occurs worldwide.

Causes
Infestation with *Sarcoptes scabiei* var. *hominis* (itch mite)

Mode of transmission
• Skin contact
• Sexual contact

Risk factors
• Overcrowded conditions
• Poor hygiene

Signs and symptoms
• Itching that intensifies at night
• Characteristic lesions (usually excoriated [may appear as erythematous nodules], approximately ⅜″ long; and usually between fingers, on flexor surfaces of the wrists, on elbows, in axillary folds, at the waistline; on nipples in females, on genitalia in males, and possibly on head and neck in infants)

Diagnostic tests
• Visual examination of the contents of the scabietic burrow may reveal the itch mite.
• A drop of mineral oil placed over the burrow, followed by superficial scraping and examination of expressed material under a low-power microscope, may reveal ova or mite feces.
• Skin clearing with a therapeutic trial of a pediculicide confirms the diagnosis if scabies is strongly suspected but diagnostic tests offer no positive identification of the mite.

Treatment
Usually, treatment of scabies consists of bathing with soap and water, followed by application of a pediculicide.

Lindane cream should be applied in a thin layer over the entire skin surface and left on for 8 to 12 hours. Because this cream is not ovicidal, application must be repeated in 1 week. Another pediculicide, crotamiton cream, may be applied twice in 48 hours.

Approximately 10% of a pediculicide is absorbed systemically. A less toxic alternative therapy for infants and pregnant females is a 6% to 10% solution of sulfur, applied for 3 consecutive days.

Persistent pruritus is usually due to mite sensitization or contact dermatitis, which may develop from repeated use of pediculicides. An antipruritic emollient or topical steroid can reduce itching. Intralesional steroids may resolve erythematous nodules.

Clinical implications
• Instruct the patient to apply lindane cream from the neck down, covering his entire body. (He may need assistance to reach all body areas.) Afterward, he must wait about 15 minutes before dressing and must avoid bathing for 24 hours. Contaminated clothing and linens must be washed or dry-cleaned.
• Tell the patient not to apply lindane cream if his skin is raw or inflamed. Advise him that if skin irritation or hypersensitivity reaction develops, he should notify the physician immediately, discontinue using the drug, and wash it off his skin thoroughly.
• Suggest that family members and other close contacts of the patient be checked for possible symptoms.
• If a hospitalized patient has scabies, prevent transmission to other patients. Practice good hand washing technique or wear gloves when touching the patient; observe wound and skin precautions for 24 hours after treatment with a pediculicide; sterilize blood pressure cuffs (by gas autoclave) before using

them on other patients; isolate linens until the patient is noninfectious; and thoroughly disinfect the patient's room after discharge.

Complications
Secondary bacterial infection

Schistosomiasis
(Bilharziasis)

Description
Schistosomiasis is a slowly progressive disease caused by blood flukes. The degree of infection determines the intensity of illness. Complications can be fatal.

Causes
Blood flukes of the class Trematoda: *Schistosoma mansoni* and *S. japonicum*, which infect the intestinal tract; *S. haematobium*, which infects the urinary tract (See *Types of Schistosomes*.)

Mode of transmission
Bathing, swimming, wading, or working in water contaminated with *Schistosoma* larvae, which penetrate the skin or mucous membranes

Signs and symptoms
Signs and symptoms of schistosomiasis depend on the site of infection and the stage of the disease.
• Transient pruritic rash (develops at the site of cercariae penetration)
• Fever
• Myalgia
• Cough
• Possible flaccid paralysis, seizures, and skin abscesses

Diagnostic tests
• Ova in the urine or stool or a mucosal lesion biopsy confirms the diagnosis.
• WBC count shows eosinophilia.

Types of Schistosomes

Species	S. mansoni	S. japonicum	S. haematobium
Incidence	Western hemisphere, particularly Puerto Rico, Lesser Antilles, Brazil, and Venezuela; also Nile delta, Sudan, and central Africa	Affects men more than women; particularly prevalent among farmers in Japan, China, and the Philippines	Africa, Cyprus, Greece, India
Signs and symptoms	Irregular fever, malaise, weakness, abdominal distress, weight loss, diarrhea, ascites, hepatosplenomegaly, portal hypertension, fistulas, intestinal stricture	Irregular fever, malaise, weakness, abdominal distress, weight loss, diarrhea, ascites, hepatosplenomegaly, portal hypertension, fistulas, intestinal stricture	Terminal hematuria, dysuria, ureteral colic; with secondary infection, colicky pain, intermittent flank pain, vague GI complaints, total renal failure
Treatment	Praziquantel; oxamniquine P.O.	Praziquantel; niridazole P.O.; stibocaptate (rare)	Praziquantel; metrifonate P.O.; niridazole P.O.
Side effects	Headache, abdominal pain, drowsiness, nausea, vomiting, anorexia, weakness, diarrhea, lassitude, myalgia	Headache, abdominal pain, drowsiness, nausea, thrombocytopenia, hypotension, syncope, bradycardia, EKG changes, vomiting, diarrhea, colic, hepatic necrosis, dyspnea, severe arthralgia, albuminuria, fever, dermatitis	Headache, abdominal pain, drowsiness, nausea, vomiting, diarrhea, anorexia, dizziness, insomnia, cardiac dysrhythmia, anxiety, confusion, hallucinations, convulsions

Treatment

The treatment of choice is the anthelmintic drug praziquantel. The patient will need to be examined again 3 to 6 months after treatment. If this checkup detects any living ova, treatment may be resumed.

Clinical implications

To help prevent schistosomiasis, teach those in endemic areas to work for a pure water supply and to avoid contaminated water. If they must enter this water, tell them to wear protective clothing and to dry themselves afterward.

Complications
- Portal hypertension
- Pulmonary hypertension
- Heart failure
- Ascites
- Hematemesis from ruptured esophageal varices
- Renal failure

Schizophrenic disorders

Description
This group of disorders is marked mainly by withdrawal into self and failure to distinguish reality from fantasy. *DSM-III* recognizes five types of schizophrenia: catatonic, paranoid, disorganized, undifferentiated, and residual. According to the *DSM-III* classification, schizophrenic disorders have these essential features: presence of psychotic features during the acute phase; deterioration from a previous level of functioning; onset before age 45; and presence of symptoms for at least 6 months, with deterioration in occupational functioning, social relations, or self-care. According to current statistics, an estimated 2 million Americans may suffer from this disease.

Schizophrenic disorders produce varying degrees of impairment. As many as a third of such patients have just one psychotic episode and no more. Some patients have no disability between periods of exacerbation; others need continuous institutional care. Prognosis worsens with each acute episode.

Causes
The causes are unknown, but various theories—both biological and psychological—have been proposed.
- Genetic predisposition
- Hyperdopaminergic condition
- Deficiency or disturbance of beta-endorphins
- Disturbed family and interpersonal patterns

Signs and symptoms
No single symptom or characteristic is present in all schizophrenic disorders. The five subtypes differ markedly.
Catatonic schizophrenia
—Possible inability to take care of personal needs
—Diminished sensitivity to painful stimuli
—Negativism
—Rigidity
—Posturing
—Possible rapid swings between excitement and stupor
—Possible extreme psychomotor agitation with excessive, senseless, or incoherent shouting or talking
—Possible increased potential for destructive, violent behavior
Paranoid schizophrenia
—Characteristic persecutory or grandiose delusional thought content and possible delusional jealousy
—Possible minimal impairment of function if the patient does not act upon delusional thoughts
—Commonly, stilted formality or intensity in interactions with others
—Possible unfocused anxiety, anger, argumentativeness, and violence
—Possible gender-identity problems
(See *Other Subtypes of Schizophrenia*, p. 689, and *Childhood Schizophrenia*, p. 690.)

Diagnostic tests
Diagnosis of schizophrenic disorders remains difficult and controversial. Psychiatrists consider the following features important: developmental background, genetic and family history, current environmental stressors, relationship of patient to interviewer, level of patient's premorbid adjustment, course of illness, and response to treatment.

Psychological tests may help, although none clearly confirms this diagnosis.
- The dexamethasone suppression test

Other Subtypes of Schizophrenia

Besides catatonic and paranoid schizophrenia, *DSM-III* lists three other subtypes of schizophrenia: disorganized, undifferentiated, and residual. This table lists characteristics of these other subtypes and special considerations for all three.

TYPE OF SCHIZO-PHRENIA	SPECIAL CONSIDERATIONS FOR ALL TYPES
Disorganized • Marked incoherence; regressive, chaotic speech • Flat, incongruous, or silly affect • Delusions not systematized into coherent theme • Hallucinations fragmented • Unpredictable laughter • Grimaces • Mannerisms • Hypochondriacal complaints • Extreme social withdrawal • Oddities of behavior • Regressive behavior **Undifferentiated** • Prominent psychotic symptoms that meet criteria for more than one subtype **Residual** • Previous history of episode of schizophrenia with prominent psychotic symptoms • Present clinical picture without prominent psychotic symptoms • Continuing evidence of illness, such as inappropriate affect, social withdrawal, eccentric behavior, illogical thinking, or loosening of associations	• Distinguish adult behavior from regressed behavior; reward adult behavior. Work with patient to increase sense of his own responsibility to improve level of functioning. • Engage patient in reality-oriented activities that involve human contact: inpatient social skills training groups; outpatient day-care, sheltered workshops. Provide reality-based explanations for distorted body images or hypochondriacal complaints. • Avoid promoting dependence. Meet patient's needs, but only do for patient what he cannot do for himself. • Remember, institutionalization may produce symptoms and handicaps that are not part of illness, so evaluate symptoms carefully. • Clarify private language, autistic inventions, or neologisms. Give patient feedback that what he says is not understood. • Assist patient to engage in meaningful interpersonal relationships; do not avoid patient; maintain sense of hope for possible improvement and convey this to patient. • Expect patient to put nurse through rigorous period of testing before he shows evidence of trust. • Mobilize all resources to provide support system for patient to reduce his vulnerability to stress. • Encourage compliance with neuroleptic medication regimen. Patients relapse when medication is discontinued. • Involve family in treatment; teach them symptoms associated with relapse and suggest ways to manage symptoms. These include tension, nervousness, insomnia, decreased concentration ability, and loss of interest. • Provide continued support in assisting patient to learn social skills.

Childhood Schizophrenia

Schizophrenic reactions that occur before puberty (age 12) are included in this group; some children have these reactions as early as age 2.

Schizophrenic children may be confused and anxious but may be responsive to those who are taking care of them and to their environment. Usually, they have learned to talk but do not always feel the need to communicate. When they do speak, their language is not always meaningful. These children are not able to differentiate between what is real and what is not. Those who become ill when very young are not able to distinguish themselves from others around them (autistic tendency) and are usually hospitalized.

The nurse must work to establish a loving, secure, accepting relationship with the schizophrenic child. She can help him distinguish his own body from those of others. Only after he begins to improve or to develop *some* concept of himself is it advisable to involve him in a daily routine. One goal is to provide regular intervals for the child to rest, work, or play. Another important goal is to have such a child learn to eat, dress, and bathe himself. If his family's life-style has been upset, all members may need psychotherapy as a unit.

may be used to aid diagnosis, but some psychiatrists question its accuracy.

• CT scans have shown enlarged ventricles in schizophrenics.

• The ventricular brain ratio (VBR) determination may also support diagnosis; some studies have reported an elevated VBR ratio in schizophrenics.

• Other tests may be performed to rule out drug abuse or other organic disorders.

Treatment

The goals of treatment for patients with schizophrenic disorders include equipping them with the skills they need to live in an unrestrictive environmental setting that offers opportunity for meaningful interpersonal relationships. Another major aim of treatment is control of this illness through continuous administration of carefully selected neuroleptic drugs. Drug treatment should be continuous because schizophrenic patients relapse when it is discontinued.

Clinicians disagree about the effectiveness of psychotherapy in schizophrenics. Some consider it a useful adjunct to reduce loneliness, isolation, and withdrawal and to enhance productivity.

Clinical implications

Patient management varies according to the patient's symptoms and the type of schizophrenia.

For catatonic schizophrenia, follow these guidelines:

• Assess for physical illness. Remember that the mute patient will not complain of pain or physical symptoms. If he is in a bizarre posture, he is consequently at risk for pressure sores or decreased circulation to a body area.

• Meet physical needs for adequate food, fluid, exercise, and elimination. Follow orders with respect to nutrition, urinary catheterization, and enema.

• Provide range-of-motion exercises or walk the patient every 2 hours.

• Prevent physical exhaustion and injury during periods of hyperactivity.

• Tell the patient directly, specifically, and concisely what needs to be done.

• Spend some time with the patient even if he is mute and unresponsive.

The patient is acutely aware of his environment even though he seems not to be. Your presence can be reassuring and supportive. Avoid mutual withdrawal.

• Verbalize for the patient the message his nonverbal behavior seems to convey; encourage him to do so as well.

• Emphasize reality in all contacts to reduce distorted perceptions.

• Stay alert for violent outbursts; get help promptly to intervene safely for yourself and the patient.

For paranoid schizophrenia, follow these guidelines:

• When the patient is newly admitted, minimize contact with staff.

• Do not crowd the patient physically or psychologically. He may strike out to protect himself.

• Be flexible. Allow the patient some control. Approach him in a calm and unhurried manner.

• Respond to the patient's condescending attitudes with neutral remarks. Do not let the patient put you on the defensive and do not take his remarks personally.

• Do not try to combat the patient's delusions with logic.

• Build trust; be honest and dependable. Do not threaten or make promises you cannot fulfill.

• Make sure the patient's nutritional needs are met. If he thinks food is poisoned, let him fix his own food when possible, or offer foods in closed containers he can open.

• Monitor the patient carefully for side effects of neuroleptic drugs: drug-induced parkinsonism, acute dystonia, akathisia, tardive dyskinesia, and malignant neuroleptic syndrome. Document and report adverse effects promptly.

• If the patient is hallucinating, explore the content of the hallucinations. If he hears voices, find out if he thinks he must do what they command. Tell the patient you do not hear the voices but you know they are real to him.

• If the patient is expressing suicidal thoughts, institute suicide precautions. Document his behavior and your precautions.

• If he is expressing homicidal thoughts, institute homicidal precautions. Notify the physician and the potential victim. Document the patient's comments and who was notified.

• Decode autistic inventions and other private language. Let the patient know when you do not understand what he is saying.

• Do not touch the patient without telling him first exactly what you are going to do.

• Postpone procedures that require physical contact with hospital personnel until the patient is less suspicious or agitated.

Scoliosis

Description

Scoliosis is a lateral curvature of the spine that may be found in the thoracic, lumbar, or thoracolumbar spinal segment. The curve may be convex to the right (more common in thoracic curves) or to the left (more common in lumbar curves). Rotation of the vertebral column around its axis occurs and may cause rib cage deformity. Scoliosis is often associated with kyphosis (humpback) and lordosis (swayback).

Causes

Functional (postural) scoliosis
This is not a fixed deformity of the spinal column.
—Poor posture
—Discrepancy in leg lengths
Structural scoliosis
This type involves deformity of the vertebral bodies.
—Congenital: usually related to a congenital defect, such as wedge vertebrae, fused ribs or vertebrae, or hemivertebrae
—Paralytic or musculoskeletal: devel-

ops several months after asymmetric paralysis of the trunk muscles due to polio, cerebral palsy, or muscular dystrophy

—Idiopathic (the most common form): may be transmitted as an autosomal dominant or multifactorial trait; appears in a previously straight spine during the growing years

Signs and symptoms

• The most common curve in functional or structural scoliosis arises in the thoracic segment, with convexity to the right, and compensatory curves (S curves) in the cervical segment above and the lumbar segment below, both with convexity to the left.

• Backache, fatigue, and dyspnea may occur when the disease is well established.

• Physical examination reveals unequal shoulder heights, elbow levels, and heights of the iliac crests.

• Muscles on the convex side of the curve may be rounded; those on the concave side, flattened, producing asymmetry of paraspinal muscles.

Diagnostic tests

Anterior, posterior, and lateral spinal X-rays, taken with the patient standing upright and bending, confirm scoliosis and determine the degree of curvature and flexibility of the spine.

Treatment

The severity of the deformity and potential spine growth determine appropriate treatment, which may include close observation, exercise, a brace (for example, a Milwaukee brace), surgery, or a combination of these. To be most effective, treatment should begin early, when spinal deformity is still subtle.

A curve of less than 25° is mild and can be monitored by X-rays and an examination every 3 months. An exercise program may strengthen torso muscles and prevent curve progression. A heel lift may help.

A curve of 30° to 50° requires spinal

exercises and a brace. (Transcutaneous electrical stimulation may be used as an alternative.) Usually, a brace halts progression in most patients but does not reverse established curvature.

A curve of 40° or more requires surgery (spinal fusion), since a lateral curve progresses at the rate of 1° a year even after skeletal maturity.

Some surgeons prescribe Cotrel dynamic traction for 7 to 10 days for preoperative preparation.

Most spinal fusions require postoperative immobilization in a localizer cast (Risser cast) for 3 to 6 months. Postoperatively, periodic checkups are required for several months to monitor stability of the correction.

Clinical implications

Scoliosis often affects adolescent girls, who are likely to find limitations on their activities and treatment with orthopedic appliances distressing. Therefore, provide emotional support, along with meticulous skin and cast care, and patient teaching.

If the patient needs a brace, follow these guidelines:

• Enlist the help of a physical therapist, a social worker, and an orthotist (orthopedic appliance specialist). Before the patient goes home, explain what the brace does and how to care for it.

• Tell the patient to wear the brace 23 hours a day and to remove it only for bathing and exercise. While she is still adjusting to the brace, tell her to lie down and rest several times a day.

• To prevent skin breakdown, advise the patient not to use lotions, ointments, or powders on areas where the brace contacts the skin. Instead, suggest she use rubbing alcohol or tincture of benzoin to toughen the skin. Tell her to keep the skin dry and clean and to wear a snug T-shirt under the brace.

• Advise the patient to increase activities gradually and avoid vigorous

Cast Syndrome

Cast syndrome is a serious complication that sometimes follows spinal surgery and application of a body cast. Characterized by nausea, abdominal pressure, and vague abdominal pain, cast syndrome probably results from hyperextension of the spine. Hyperextension of the spine accentuates lumbar lordosis, with compression of the third portion of the duodenum between the superior mesenteric artery anteriorly, and the aorta and vertebral column posteriorly. High intestinal obstruction produces nausea, vomiting, and ischemic infarction of the mesentery.

After removal of the cast, treatment includes decompression and removal of gastric contents with a nasogastric tube and suction. The patient is given I.V. fluids and nothing by mouth. Antiemetics should be given sparingly, since they may mask symptoms of cast syndrome. Surgery may be required to release the ligament of Treitz, which attaches to the fourth portion of the duodenum. Untreated cast syndrome may be fatal.

Teach patients who are discharged in body jackets, localizer casts, or high hip spica casts how to recognize cast syndrome, which may develop as late as several weeks or months after application of the cast.

sports. Emphasize the importance of conscientiously performing prescribed exercises. Recommend swimming during the hour out of the brace, but strongly warn against diving.

• Instruct the patient to turn her whole body, instead of just her head, when looking to the side.

If the patient needs traction or a cast before surgery, follow these guidelines:

• Explain these procedures to the patient and family. Remember that application of a body cast can be traumatic, since it is done on a special frame and the patient's head and face are covered throughout the procedure.

• Check the skin around the cast edge daily. Keep the cast clean and dry, and edges of the cast "petaled" (padded). Warn the patient not to insert anything or let anything get under the cast and to immediately report cracks in the cast, pain, burning, skin breakdown, numbness, or odor.

• Before surgery, assure the patient and family that she will have adequate pain control postoperatively.

After corrective surgery, follow these guidelines:

• Check neurovascular status in all extremities every 2 to 4 hours for the first 48 hours, then several times a day. Logroll the patient often.

• Measure intake, output, and urine specific gravity to monitor effects of blood loss, which is often substantial.

• Monitor abdominal distention and bowel sounds.

• Encourage deep-breathing exercises to avoid pulmonary complications.

• Medicate for pain, especially before any activity.

• Promote active range-of-motion exercises to help maintain muscle strength.

• Watch for skin breakdown and signs of cast syndrome (see *Cast Syndrome*). Teach the patient how to recognize these signs.

• Remove antiembolism stockings for at least 30 minutes daily.

• Offer emotional support to help prevent depression that may result from altered body image and immobility. Encourage the patient to wear her own clothes, wash her hair, and use makeup.

• If the patient is being discharged with a Harrington rod and cast and must have bed rest, arrange for a social worker and a visiting nurse to provide home care. Before discharge, check with the surgeon about activity limitations, and make sure the patient understands them.

• If you work in a school, screen children routinely for scoliosis during physical examination.

Complications

Untreated scoliosis may result in the following:

• Pulmonary insufficiency
• Degenerative arthritis of the spine
• Disk disease
• Sciatica

Seizure disorder

Description

A seizure disorder is a condition of the brain characterized by recurrent paroxysmal events resulting from the rapid, uncontrolled discharge of central nervous system neurons. Seizures may be classified as partial or generalized (some patients may be affected by more than one type). Partial seizures arise from a localized area of the brain and include jacksonian and complex partial seizures (psychomotor or temporal lobe). Generalized seizures cause a generalized electrical abnormality within the brain and include absence (petit mal) and generalized tonic-clonic (grand mal) seizures. Status epilepticus is a continuous seizure state, which can occur in all seizure types. Seizure disorder probably affects 1% to 2% of the population. However, the prognosis is good if the patient adheres strictly to prescribed treatment.

Causes

• Unknown in about half of cases
• Birth trauma (inadequate oxygen supply to the brain, blood imcompatibility, or hemorrhage)

• Perinatal infection
• Anoxia
• Infectious diseases (meningitis, encephalitis, or brain abscess)
• Ingestion of toxins (mercury, lead, or carbon monoxide)
• Tumors of the brain
• Inherited disorders or degenerative disease, such as phenylketonuria or tuberous sclerosis
• Head injury or trauma
• Metabolic disorders, such as hypoglycemia or hypoparathyroidism
• Cerebrovascular accident (hemorrhage, thrombosis, or embolism)

Signs and symptoms

Jacksonian seizure
—This begins as a localized motor seizure characterized by a spread of abnormal activity to adjacent areas of the brain.
—It typically produces a stiffening or jerking in one extremity, accompanied by a tingling sensation in the same area.

Complex partial seizure
—This may begin with an aura, such as a visual disturbance.
—Purposeless behavior, such as aimless wandering, occurs.
—Temporary mental confusion follows.

Absence (petit mal) seizure
—This usually begins with a brief change in level of consciousness, indicated by blinking or rolling of the eyes, a blank stare, and slight mouth movements.
—Posture and preseizure activity are maintained without difficulty.
—Typically, each seizure lasts from 1 to 10 seconds.
—If not properly treated, seizures can recur as often as 100 times a day.

Generalized tonic-clonic (grand mal) seizure
—This typically begins with a loud cry, precipitated by air rushing from the lungs through the vocal cords.
—The patient then falls to the ground, losing consciousness.
—The body stiffens (tonic phase), then

Teaching Topics in Seizures

- Explanation of how the brain's abnormal electrical activity leads to seizures
- The patient's type of seizure
- Preparation for diagnostic tests, such as EEG and a CT scan, to help determine the seizure's cause
- Drugs and their administration, including the risks of overmedication and undermedication
- Trigger factors, including fatigue and hypoglycemia
- Importance of a normal diet to provide energy for normal neuron function
- Preparation for craniotomy, if necessary
- Measures, such as wearing a medical identification bracelet, to alert others to the patient's condition
- Precautions for an imminent seizure
- How the family or other caregivers should manage a seizure
- Sources of additional information and support

alternates between episodes of muscular spasm and relaxation (clonic phase).
—Tongue biting, incontinence, labored breathing, apnea, and subsequent cyanosis may also occur.
—The seizure stops in 2 to 5 minutes.
—The patient then regains consciousness but is somewhat confused and may complain of drowsiness, fatigue, headache, muscle soreness, and arm or leg weakness. He may fall into deep sleep following the seizure.

Diagnostic tests
- CT scan offers density readings of the brain and may indicate abnormalities in internal structures.
- EEG showing paroxysmal abnormalities confirms the diagnosis by providing evidence of the continuing tendency to have seizures. (A normal EEG does not rule out seizure disorder because the paroxysmal abnormalities occur intermittently.)
- Other helpful tests may include serum glucose and calcium studies, skull X-rays, lumbar puncture, brain scan, and cerebral angiography.

Treatment
Usually, treatment consists of drug therapy specific to the type of seizure.

The most commonly prescribed drugs include phenytoin, carbamazepine, phenobarbital, or primidone administered individually for generalized tonic-clonic seizures and complex partial seizures. Valproic acid, clonazepam, and ethosuximide are commonly prescribed for absence seizures.

A patient taking antiepileptic medications requires constant monitoring for toxic signs, such as nystagmus, ataxia, lethargy, dizziness, drowsiness, slurred speech, irritability, nausea, and vomiting.

If drug therapy fails, treatment may include surgical removal of a demonstrated focal lesion to attempt to bring an end to seizures. Emergency treatment for status epilepticus usually consists of diazepam, phenytoin, or phenobarbital; 50% dextrose I.V. (when seizures are secondary to hypoglycemia); and thiamine I.V. (in chronic alcoholism or withdrawal).

Clinical implications
- Encourage the patient and family to express their feelings about the patient's condition. Answer their questions, and help them cope by dispelling

myths; for example, the myth that a seizure disorder is contagious.

• Assure them that the condition is controllable for most patients who follow a prescribed regimen of medication, and that most patients maintain a normal life-style.

• Stress the need for compliance with the prescribed drug schedule. Assure the patient that antiepileptic drugs are safe when taken as ordered. Reinforce dosage instructions, and find methods to help the patient remember to take medications. Caution him to monitor the amount of medication left so he does not run out of it.

• Warn against possible side effects—drowsiness, lethargy, hyperactivity, confusion, visual and sleep disturbances—all of which indicate the need for dosage adjustment. Phenytoin therapy may lead to hyperplasia of the gums, which may be relieved by conscientious oral hygiene. Instruct the patient to report side effects immediately.

• Emphasize the importance of having antiepileptic drug blood levels checked at regular intervals, even if the seizures are under control.

• Warn the patient against drinking alcoholic beverages.

• Know which social agencies in your community can help. Refer the patient to the Epilepsy Foundation of America for general information and to the state motor vehicle department for information about a driver's license.

• Because generalized tonic-clonic seizures may necessitate first aid, instruct the patient's family to give such aid correctly.

• Avoid restraining the patient during a seizure. Help the patient to a lying position, loosen any tight clothing, and place something flat and soft, such as a pillow, jacket, or hand, under his head.

• Clear the area of hard objects. *Do not* force anything into the patient's mouth if his teeth are clenched. A tongue blade or spoon could lacerate

mouth and lips or displace teeth, precipitating respiratory distress. However, if the patient's mouth is open, protect his tongue by placing a soft object (such as a folded cloth) between his teeth. Turn his head to provide an open airway.

• After the seizure subsides, reassure the patient that he is all right, orient him to time and place, and inform him that he has had a seizure.

• If the patient has a complex partial seizure, *do not* restrain him during the seizure. Clear the area of any hard objects. Protect him from injury by gently calling his name and directing him away from the source of danger. After the seizure passes, reassure him and tell him that he has just had a seizure.

(See *Teaching Topics in Seizures,* p. 695.)

Septal perforation and deviation

Description
Perforated septum, a hole in the nasal septum between the two air passages, usually occurs in the anterior cartilaginous septum but may occur in the bony septum. Deviated septum, a shift from the midline that commonly occurs in normal growth, is present in most adults. This condition may be severe enough to obstruct the passage of air through the nostrils. With surgical correction, prognosis for either perforated or deviated septum is good.

Causes
Septal perforation
—Traumatic irritation (most common)
—Perichondritis
—Syphilis
—Tuberculosis
—Untreated septal hematoma
—Inhalation of irritating chemicals
—Cocaine snorting

—Chronic nasal infections
—Nasal carcinoma
—Granuloma
—Chronic sinusitis
Deviated septum
—Nasal trauma resulting from a fall, a blow to the nose, or surgery that further exaggerates deviation commonly occuring during normal growth

Signs and symptoms
Septal perforation
—Usually asymptomatic if small, but may produce a whistle on inspiration
—If large, causes rhinitis, epistaxis, nasal crusting, and watery discharge
Deviated septum
—Crooked nose
—Nasal obstruction, with severe deviation
—Sensation of fullness in the face
—Shortness of breath
—Nasal discharge
—Recurring epistaxis
—Headache
—Symptoms of infection and sinusitis

Diagnostic tests
Inspection of the nasal mucosa with bright light and a nasal speculum confirms the diagnosis.

Treatment
Symptomatic treatment of perforated septum includes decongestants to reduce nasal congestion by local vasoconstriction, local application of lanolin or petrolatum to prevent ulceration and crusting, and antibiotics to combat infection. Surgery may be necessary to graft part of the perichondrial layer over the perforation. Also, a plastic or Silastic "button" prosthesis may be used to close the perforation.

Symptomatic treatment of deviated septum usually includes analgesics to relieve headache, decongestants to minimize secretions, and vasoconstrictors, nasal packing, or cautery as needed to control hemorrhage. Manipulation of the nasal septum at birth can correct congenital deviated septum.

Corrective surgical procedures include the following:

• Reconstruction of the nasal septum by submucous resection repositions the nasal septal cartilage and relieves nasal obstruction.

• Rhinoplasty corrects nasal structure deformity.

• Septoplasty relieves nasal obstruction and enhances cosmetic appearance.

Clinical implications
• Warn the patient with perforation or severe deviation against blowing his nose. To relieve nasal congestion, instill saline nose drops and suggest use of a humidifier. Give decongestants, as ordered.

• To treat epistaxis, elevate the head of the bed, provide an emesis basin, and instruct the patient to expectorate any blood. Compress the outer portion of the nose against the septum for 10 to 15 minutes, and apply ice packs. If bleeding persists, notify the physician.

• If corrective surgery is scheduled, prepare the patient to expect postoperative facial edema, periorbital bruising, and nasal packing, which remains in place for 12 to 24 hours. The patient must breathe through his mouth. After surgery for deviated septum, the patient may also have a splint on his nose.

• To reduce or prevent edema and promote drainage, place the patient in semi-Fowler's position, and use a cool-mist vaporizer to liquefy secretions and facilitate normal breathing. To lessen facial edema and pain, place crushed ice in a rubber glove or a small ice bag, and apply the glove or ice bag intermittently over the eyes and nose for 24 hours.

• Because the patient is breathing through his mouth, provide frequent and meticulous mouth care.

• Change the mustache dressing or drip pad, as needed. Record the color, consistency, and amount of drainage.

While nasal packing is in place, expect slight, bright red drainage with clots. After packing is removed, watch for purulent discharge, an indication of infection.

• Watch for and report excessive swallowing, hematoma, or a falling or flapping septum (depressed or soft and unstable septum). Intranasal examination is necessary to detect hematoma formation. Any of these complications requires surgical correction.

• Administer sedatives and analgesics, as ordered. Because of its anticoagulant properties, aspirin is contraindicated after surgery for septal deviation or perforation.

• Noseblowing may cause bruising and swelling even after nasal packing is removed. After surgery, the patient must limit physical activity for 2 or 3 days and must stop smoking for at least 2 days.

Septic arthritis
(Infectious arthritis)

Description
A medical emergency, septic arthritis is caused by bacterial invasion of a joint, resulting in inflammation of the synovial lining. If the organisms enter the joint cavity, effusion and pyogenesis follow, with eventual destruction of bone and cartilage. Septic arthritis can lead to ankylosis and even fatal septicemia. Prompt antibiotic therapy and joint aspiration or drainage cure most patients, however.

Causes
Bacteria that usually spread from a primary site of infection, usually in adjacent bone or soft tissue, through the bloodstream to the joint

Risk factors
• Any concurrent bacterial infection
• ~~rious~~ chronic illness
• ~~holism~~

• Age
• Immunosuppression
• Intravenous drug abuse
• Recent articular trauma
• Joint surgery
• Intraarticular injections
• Local joint abnormalities

Signs and symptoms
• Abrupt onset, with intense pain, inflammation, and swelling of the affected joint
• Low-grade fever
• Possibly, migratory polyarthritis preceding localization of infection
• If bacteria invade the hip, possible pain in the groin, upper thigh, buttock, or knee

Diagnostic tests
• Identification of the infecting organism by Gram stain or culture of synovial fluid or biopsy of synovial membrane confirms septic arthritis.
• Joint fluid analysis shows gross pus or watery, cloudy fluid of decreased viscosity usually with 50,000 or more white cells/mm^3, containing primarily neutrophils.
• Synovial fluid glucose is often low, compared with simultaneous 6-hour postprandial blood glucose.
• When synovial fluid culture is negative, positive blood culture may confirm the diagnosis.
• X-rays can show typical changes as early as 1 week after initial infection— distention of joint capsules, for example, followed by narrowing of joint space (indicating cartilage damage) and erosions of bone (joint destruction).
• Radioisotope joint scan for less accessible joints (such as spinal articulations) may help detect infection or inflammation but is not itself diagnostic.
• WBC count may be elevated, with many polymorphonuclear cells.
• Erythrocyte sedimentation rate is increased.
• Two sets of positive culture and Gram stain smears of skin exudates,

Other Types of Arthritis

• *Intermittent hydrarthrosis*—a rare, benign condition characterized by regular, recurrent joint effusions—most commonly affects the knee. The patient may have difficulty moving the affected joint but have no other arthritic symptoms. The cause of intermittent hydrarthrosis is unknown; onset is usually at or soon after puberty and may be linked to familial tendencies, allergies, or menstruation. No effective treatment exists.

• *Traumatic arthritis* results from blunt, penetrating, or repeated trauma or from forced inappropriate motion of a joint or ligament. Clinical effects may include swelling, pain, tenderness, joint instability, and internal bleeding. Treatment includes analgesics, anti-inflammatories, application of cold followed by heat, and, if needed, compression dressings, splinting, joint aspiration, casting, or possibly surgery.

• *Schönlein-Henoch purpura*, a vasculitic syndrome, is marked by palpable purpura, abdominal pain, and arthralgia that most commonly affects the knees and ankles, producing swollen, warm, and tender joints without joint erosion or deformity. Most patients have microscopic hematuria and proteinuria 4 to 8 weeks after onset. Renal involvement is also common. Incidence is highest in children and young adults, occurring most often in the spring after a respiratory infection. Treatment may include corticosteroids.

• *Hemophilic arthrosis* produces transient or permanent joint changes. Often precipitated by trauma, hemophilic arthrosis usually arises between ages 1 and 5 and tends to recur until about age 10. It usually affects only one joint at a time—most commonly the knee, elbow, or ankle—and tends to recur in the same joint. Initially, the patient may feel only mild discomfort; later, he may experience warmth, swelling, tenderness, and severe pain with adjacent muscle spasm that leads to flexion of the extremity. Mild hemophilic arthrosis may cause only limited stiffness that subsides within a few days. In prolonged bleeding, however, symptoms may subside after weeks or months or not at all. Severe hemophilic arthrosis may be accompanied by fever and leukocytosis; severe, prolonged, or repeated bleeding may lead to chronic hemophilic joint disease. Effective treatment includes I.V. infusion of the deficient clotting factor, bed rest with the affected extremity elevated, application of ice packs, analgesics, and joint aspiration. Physical therapy includes progressive range-of-motion and muscle-strengthening exercises to restore motion and to prevent contractures and muscle atrophy.

---

sputum, urethral discharge, stools, urine, or nasopharyngeal smear confirm septic arthritis.

• Lactic assay can distinguish septic from nonseptic arthritis.

Treatment
Antibiotic therapy should begin promptly. It may be modified when sensitivity results become available. Bioassays or bactericidal assays of synovial fluid and bioassays of blood may confirm clearing of the infection.

Treatment of septic arthritis re-

quires monitoring of progress through frequent analysis of joint fluid cultures, synovial fluid leukocyte counts, and glucose determinations. Codeine or propoxyphene can be given for pain, if needed. (Aspirin causes a misleading reduction in swelling, hindering accurate monitoring of progress.) The affected joint can be immobilized with a splint or put into traction until movement can be tolerated.

Needle aspiration (arthrocentesis) to remove grossly purulent joint fluid should be repeated daily until fluid appears normal. If excessive fluid is aspirated or the leukocyte count remains elevated, open surgical drainage (usually arthrotomy with lavage of the joint) may be necessary for resistant infection or chronic septic arthritis.

Late reconstructive surgery is warranted only for severe joint damage and only after all signs of active infection have disappeared, which usually takes several months. In some cases, the recommended procedure may be arthroplasty or joint fusion. Prosthetic replacement remains controversial because it may exacerbate the infection, but it has helped patients with damaged femoral heads or acetabula.

Clinical implications
• Practice strict aseptic technique with all procedures. Wash hands carefully before and after giving care. Dispose of soiled linens and dressings properly. Prevent contact between immunosuppressed patients and infected patients.
• Watch for signs of joint inflammation. Monitor vital signs and fever pattern. Remember that corticosteroids mask signs of infection.
• Check splints or traction regularly. Keep the joint in proper alignment, but avoid prolonged immobilization. Start passive range-of-motion exercises immediately, and progress to active exercises as soon as the patient can move the affected joint and put weight on it.
• Monitor pain levels and medicate accordingly, especially before exercise, remembering that the pain of septic arthritis is easy to underestimate. Administer analgesics and narcotics for acute pain, and heat or ice packs for moderate pain.
• Carefully evaluate the patient's condition after joint aspiration. Provide emotional support throughout the diagnostic tests and procedures, which should be previously explained to the patient. Warn the patient before the first aspiration that it will be *extremely* painful.

• Discuss all prescribed medications with the patient. Explain why therapy must be carefully monitored. (See *Other Types of Arthritis,* p. 699.)

Septic shock

Description
Second only to cardiogenic shock as the leading cause of shock death, septic shock (usually a result of bacterial infection) causes inadequate blood perfusion and circulatory collapse. It occurs most often among hospitalized patients. About 25% of patients who develop gram-negative bacteremia go into shock. Unless vigorous treatment begins promptly, preferably before symptoms fully develop, septic shock rapidly progresses to death (often within a few hours) in up to 80% of these patients.

Causes
In two-thirds of patients, infection with gram-negative bacteria; in others, gram-positive bacteria

Risk factors
• Primary infection of the genitourinary, biliary, GI, and gynecologic tracts in hospitalized patients
• Surgery
• I.V. therapy
• Catheterization
• Immunodeficiency
• Advanced age
• Trauma
• Burns
• Diabetes mellitus
• Cirrhosis
• Disseminated cancer

Signs and symptoms
The symptoms of septic shock vary according to the stage of the shock, the organism causing it, and the age of the patient.
Early stage
—Oliguria

—Sudden fever (over 101° F. [38.3° C.])
—Chills
—Nausea and vomiting
—Diarrhea
—Prostration

Late stage
—Restlessness and apprehension
—Irritability
—Thirst
—Tachycardia
—Tachypnea
—Hypotension, altered consciousness, and hyperventilation (may be the only signs in infants and the elderly)
—Hypothermia and anuria (late signs)

Diagnostic tests

• In early stages, arterial blood gas measurements indicate respiratory alkalosis (low PCO_2, low or normal bicarbonate, high pH); as shock progresses, metabolic acidosis develops with hypoxemia indicated by decreasing PCO_2 (may increase as respiratory failure ensues), PO_2, HCO_3^-, and pH.
• Blood cultures isolate the infecting organism.
• Platelet count is decreased and leukocyte count is increased (15,000 to 30,000/mm³).
• BUN and creatinine are increased; creatinine clearance is decreased.
• Prothrombin consumption and partial thromboplastin time are abnormal.
• Simultaneous measurement of urine and plasma osmolalities for renal failure shows urine osmolality below 400 mOsm, with a ratio of urine to plasma below 1.5.
• Central venous pressure (CVP) is decreased.
• Pulmonary artery and wedge pressures are decreased.
• Cardiac output is decreased (in early septic shock, cardiac output increases).
• EKG shows ST segment depression and inverted T waves and dysrhythmias resembling myocardial infarction.

Treatment

The first goal of treatment is to monitor and reverse shock through volume expansion with I.V. fluids and insertion of a pulmonary artery catheter to check pulmonary circulation and pulmonary wedge pressure (PWP). Administration of whole blood or plasma can then raise the PWP to a satisfactory level of 14 to 18 mm Hg. A respirator may be necessary for proper ventilation to overcome hypoxia. Urinary catheterization allows accurate measurement of hourly urine output.

Treatment also requires immediate administration of I.V. antibiotics to control the infection. Other measures to combat infection include surgery to drain and excise abscesses, and debridement.

If shock persists after fluid infusion, treatment with vasopressors, such as dopamine, maintains adequate blood perfusion in the brain, liver, digestive tract, kidneys, and skin. Other treatment includes I.V. bicarbonate to correct acidosis and I.V. corticosteroids, which may improve blood perfusion and increase cardiac output.

Clinical implications

Determine which of your patients are at high risk of developing septic shock. Know the signs of impending septic shock, but do not rely solely on technical aids to judge the patient's status. Consider any change in mental status and urinary output as significant as a change in CVP. Report such changes promptly.
• Carefully maintain the pulmonary artery catheter. Check blood gas measurements for adequate oxygenation or gas exchange, and report any changes immediately.
• Keep accurate intake and output records. Maintain urine output (0.5 to 1 ml/kg/hour) and adequate systolic pressure. Be careful to avoid fluid overload.
• Administer drugs, as ordered.

Complications
- Disseminated intravascular coagulation
- Renal failure
- Heart failure
- GI ulcers
- Hepatic abnormality

Severe combined immunodeficiency disease (SCID)

Description
In severe combined immunodeficiency disease (SCID), both cell-mediated (T cell) and humoral (B cell) immunity are deficient or absent in infancy, resulting in susceptibility to infection from all classes of microorganisms. At least three types of SCID exist: reticular dysgenesis, the most severe type, in which the hematopoietic stem cell fails to differentiate into lymphocytes and granulocytes; Swiss-type agammaglobulinemia, in which the hematopoietic stem cell fails to differentiate into lymphocytes alone; and enzyme deficiency, such as adenosine deaminase deficiency, in which the buildup of toxic products in the lymphoid tissue causes damage and subsequent dysfunction. Most untreated patients die from infection within 1 year of birth.

Causes
- SCID is usually transmitted as an autosomal recessive trait, although it may be X-linked.
- In most cases, the genetic defect seems associated with failure of the stem cell to differentiate into T and B lymphocytes; less commonly, it results from enzyme deficiency.

Signs and symptoms
- Recurrent, overwhelming infections within 1 year of birth in most infants
- Failure to thrive

Diagnostic tests
Diagnosis is often made clinically, but severely diminished, absent, or nonfunctioning T cells and lymph node biopsy showing absence of lymphocytes can confirm diagnosis of SCID.

Treatment
Treatment aims to restore immune response and prevent infection. Histocompatible bone marrow transplant is the only satisfactory treatment available to correct immunodeficiency. Since bone marrow cells must be HLA- (human leukocyte antigen) and MLC- (mixed leukocyte culture) matched, the most common donors are histocompatible siblings. But because bone marrow transplant can produce a potentially fatal graft-versus-host (GVH) reaction, newer methods of bone marrow transplant that eliminate GVH reaction (such as lectin separation and the use of monoclonal antibodies) are being evaluated.

Fetal thymus and liver transplants have achieved limited success. Administration of immune globulin may also play a role in treatment. Some SCID infants have received long-term protection by being isolated in a completely sterile environment. However, this approach is not effective if the infant already has had recurring infections.

Clinical implications
Patient care is primarily preventive and supportive.
- Constantly monitor the infant for early signs of infection. If infection develops, provide prompt and aggressive drug therapy, as ordered. Also watch for side effects of any medications given.
- Avoid vaccinations, and give only irradiated blood products if transfusion is ordered.
- Although SCID infants must remain in strict protective isolation, try to provide a stimulating atmosphere to promote growth and development.
- Encourage parents to visit their child

often, to hold him, and to bring him toys that can be easily sterilized.

• Explain all procedures, medications, and precautions to them.

• Maintain a normal day/night routine, and talk to the child as much as possible. If parents cannot visit, call them often to report on the infant's condition.

• Since parents will have questions about the vulnerability of future offspring, refer them for genetic counseling. Parents and siblings need psychological and spiritual support to help them cope with the child's inevitable long-term illness and early death. They may also need a social service referral for assistance in coping with the financial burden of the child's long-term hospitalization.

Shigellosis
(Bacillary dysentery)

Description

Shigellosis is an acute bacterial intestinal infection. It is most common in children ages 1 to 4; however, adults often acquire the illness from children. Prognosis is good. Usually, mild infections subside within 10 days. Severe infections may persist for 2 to 6 weeks.

Causes

The bacterium *Shigella*, a short, nonmotile, gram-negative rod, which can be classified into four groups, all of which may cause shigellosis: Group A *(Shigella dysenteriae)*, which is most common in Central America and causes particularly severe infection and septicemia; Group B *(Shigella flexneri)*; Group C *(Shigella boydii)*; and Group D *(Shigella sonnei)*

Mode of transmission

• Fecal-oral route
• Direct contact with contaminated objects

• Ingestion of contaminated food or water

Signs and symptoms

Children
—High fever
—Diarrhea with tenesmus
—Nausea
—Vomiting
—Irritability
—Drowsiness
—Abdominal pain and distention
—Possible pus, mucus, and blood in the stool
—Without treatment, rapid and overwhelming dehydration and weight loss

Adults
—Sporadic, intense abdominal pain. This may be relieved at first by passing formed stools.
—Eventually, rectal irritability
—Tenesmus
—In severe infection, headache and prostration
—Possible pus, mucus, and blood in the stool
—Usually, no fever

Diagnostic tests

• Microscopic examination of a fresh stool may reveal mucus, RBCs, and polymorphonuclear leukocytes; direct immunofluorescence with specific antisera may detect *Shigella*.

• Sigmoidoscopy/proctoscopy may reveal typical superficial ulcerations.

Treatment

Treatment of shigellosis includes enteric precautions, low-residue diet, and, most important, replacement of fluids and electrolytes with I.V. infusions of normal saline solution (with electrolytes) in sufficient quantities to maintain urine output of 40 to 50 ml/hour. Antibiotics are of questionable value but may be used in an attempt to eliminate the pathogen and thereby prevent further spread. Ampicillin, tetracycline, or sulfamethoxazole with trimethoprim may be useful in severe cases, especially in children with overwhelming fluid and electrolyte loss.

Antidiarrheals that slow intestinal motility are contraindicated in shigellosis, since they delay fecal excretion of *Shigella* and prolong fever and diarrhea. An investigational vaccine containing attenuated strains of *Shigella* appears promising in preventing shigellosis.

Clinical implications

- To prevent dehydration, administer I.V. fluids, as ordered. Measure intake and output (including stools) carefully.
- Because correct identification of *Shigella* requires examination and culture of fresh stool specimens, hand carry stool specimens directly to the laboratory. Because shigellosis is suspected, include this information on the lab slip.
- Use a disposable hot-water bottle to relieve abdominal discomfort, and schedule care to conserve patient strength.
- To help prevent spread of this disease, maintain enteric precautions until the stool specimen is negative. Before entering the patient's room, wash your hands and put on a gown and gloves. Also, wash your hands after removing the gown and gloves. Keep the patient's (and your own) nails short to avoid harboring organisms. Change soiled linen promptly and store it in an isolation container.
- During shigellosis outbreaks, obtain stool specimens from all potentially infected staff, and instruct those infected to remain away from work until two stool specimens are negative.

Complications

Complications of shigellosis are not common but may be fatal in children and debilitated patients. They include electrolyte imbalance (especially hypokalemia), metabolic acidosis, and shock. Less common complications include conjunctivitis, iritis, arthritis, rectal prolapse, secondary bacterial infection, acute blood loss from mucosal ulcers, and toxic neuritis.

Sickle cell anemia

Description

A congenital hemolytic anemia that occurs primarily but not exclusively in blacks, sickle cell anemia results from a defective hemoglobin molecule (hemoglobin S) that causes RBCs to roughen and become sickle-shaped. These cells impair circulation, resulting in chronic ill health, periodic crises, long-term complications, and premature death. At present, only symptomatic treatment is available. Half of affected patients die by their early 20s. Few live to middle age.

Causes

Sickle cell anemia

—Homozygous inheritance of the hemoglobin S–producing gene, which causes substitution of the amino acid valine for glutamic acid in the B hemoglobin chain (See also *Sickle Cell Trait*.)

Painful vasocclusive crisis (hallmark of the disease)

—Blood vessel obstruction by rigid, tangled cells, which causes tissue anoxia and possible necrosis

Aplastic (megaloblastic) crisis

—Bone marrow depression

Acute sequestration crisis (rare)

—Massive entrapment of red cells in the spleen and liver

Hemolytic crisis (rare)

—Probably results from complications of sickle cell anemia, such as infection, rather than the disorder itself

Signs and symptoms

Sickle cell anemia

—Tachycardia

—Cardiomegaly

—Systolic and diastolic murmurs

Sickle Cell Trait

This relatively benign condition results from heterozygous inheritance of the abnormal hemoglobin-S–producing gene. Like sickle cell anemia, this condition is most common in blacks. Sickle cell trait *never* progresses to sickle cell anemia.

In persons with sickle cell trait (also called carriers), 20% to 40% of their total hemoglobin is hemoglobin S; the rest is normal.

Such persons usually have no symptoms. They have normal hemoglobin and hematocrit values and can expect a normal life span. Nevertheless, they must avoid situations that provoke hypoxia, since these occasionally cause a sickling crisis similar to that in sickle cell anemia.

Genetic counseling is essential for sickle cell carriers. If two sickle cell carriers marry, each of their children has a 25% chance of inheriting sickle cell anemia.

—Chronic fatigue
—Unexplained dyspnea or dyspnea on exertion
—Hepatomegaly
—Splenomegaly during early childhood
—Jaundice
—Pallor
—Joint swelling
—Aching bones
—Chest pains
—Ischemic leg ulcers (especially around the ankles)
—Increased susceptibility to infection
Painful vasocclusive crisis
—Severe abdominal, thoracic, muscular, or bone pain
—Possible increased jaundice and dark urine
—Low-grade fever
—Spleen shrinkage in long-term disease
Aplastic crisis
—Pallor
—Lethargy
—Sleepiness
—Dyspnea
—Possible coma
Acute sequestration crisis
—Lethargy
—Pallor
—Symptoms of hypovolemic shock, if untreated

Hemolytic crisis
—Hepatomegaly
—Worsening of jaundice
—Pallor
—Listlessness

Diagnostic tests

• Stained blood smear showing sickle cells and hemoglobin electrophoresis showing hemoglobin S confirm the diagnosis. (Ideally, electrophoresis should be done on umbilical cord blood samples at birth, especially if the parents are known to carry the sickle cell trait.)
• CBC shows low RBC and elevated WBC and platelet counts; hemoglobin may be low or normal.
• Erythrocyte sedimentation rate is decreased.
• Serum iron is increased.
• RBC survival time is decreased.
• Reticulocyte count is increased.

Treatment

Treatment is primarily symptomatic and can usually take place at home. If the patient's hemoglobin drops suddenly or if his condition deteriorates rapidly, hospitalization is needed for transfusion of packed red cells. In a sequestration crisis, treatment may include sedation and administration of analgesics, blood transfusion, oxygen administration, and administration of

---

Teaching Topics in Sickle Cell Anemia

• Explanation of sickle cell anemia, including its inheritance pattern and possible complications
• Symptoms of sickle cell anemia requiring immediate medical attention
• Precipitating factors for vaso-occlusive crisis (VOC)
• Explanation of blood tests
• The importance of good nutrition, especially adequate intake of foods containing folic acid
• The importance of immunizations and of taking prescribed medication
• Home treatment of VOC
• The need for careful monitoring of the patient's condition
• Sources of help and information

---

large amounts of oral or I.V. fluids. A good antisickling agent is not yet available. The most commonly used drug, sodium cyanate, has many adverse effects.

Clinical implications

Suspect any of the sickle cell crises in a sickle cell anemia patient with pale lips, tongue, palms, or nail beds; lethargy; listlessness; sleepiness, with difficulty awakening; irritability; severe pain; temperature over 104°F. (40°C.) or a fever of 100° F. (37.8° C.) that persists for 2 days.

Actions to take during a painful crisis include the following:
• Apply warm compresses to painful areas, and cover the child with a blanket. (Never use cold compresses, since they aggravate the condition.)
• Administer an analgesic-antipyretic, such as aspirin or acetaminophen.
• Encourage bed rest, and place the patient in a sitting position. If dehydration or severe pain occurs, hospitalization may be necessary.
• When cultures indicate, give antibiotics as ordered.

During remission, help the patient prevent exacerbation by these measures:
• Advise him to avoid tight clothing that restricts circulation.
• Warn against strenuous exercise, vasoconstricting medications, cold tem-

peratures (including drinking large amounts of ice water and swimming), unpressurized aircraft, high altitudes, and other conditions that provoke hypoxia.
• Stress the importance of normal childhood immunizations, meticulous wound care, good oral hygiene, regular dental checkups, and a balanced diet as safeguards against infection.
• Emphasize the need for prompt treatment of infection.
• Make him aware of the need to increase fluid intake to prevent dehydration that results from impaired ability to concentrate urine properly.
• To encourage normal mental and social development, warn parents against being overprotective. Although the child must avoid strenuous exercise, he can enjoy most everyday activities.
• Refer parents of children with sickle cell anemia for genetic counseling to answer their questions about the risk to future offspring. Recommend screening of the family members to determine if they are heterozygote carriers. These parents may also need psychological counseling to cope with guilt feelings. In addition, suggest they join an appropriate community support group.

Sickle cell anemia calls for the following special precautions:
• Warn women with sickle cell anemia that they are poor obstetrical risks.

However, their use of oral contraceptives is also risky. Refer them for birth control counseling by a gynecologist. If such women *do* become pregnant, they should maintain a balanced diet during pregnancy and may benefit from a folic acid supplement.

• During general anesthesia, a patient with sickle cell anemia requires adequate ventilation to prevent hypoxic crisis. Therefore, make sure the surgeon and the anesthesiologist are aware that the patient has sickle cell anemia, and provide a preoperative transfusion of packed red cells, as needed.

• Men with sickle cell anemia may develop sudden, painful episodes of priapism. Reassure them that these episodes are common and have no permanent harmful effects. (See *Teaching Topics in Sickle Cell Anemia*.)

Complications

• Organ infarction problems, such as retinopathy and nephropathy
• Cerebrovascular accident
• Infection, especially meningitis, sepsis, and pneumonia

Sideroblastic anemias

Description

Sideroblastic anemias comprise a group of heterogenous disorders with a common defect—failure to use iron in hemoglobin synthesis, despite the availability of adequate iron stores. These anemias may be hereditary or acquired. The acquired form, in turn, can be primary or secondary. Hereditary sideroblastic anemia often responds to treatment with pyridoxine (vitamin B_6). Correction of the secondary acquired form depends on the causative disorder. The primary acquired (idiopathic) form, however, resists treatment and usually proves fatal within 10 years after onset of complications or a concomitant disease.

Causes

Hereditary form
—X-linked inheritance, occurring mostly in young males (females are carriers and usually show no signs of this disorder)

Primary acquired form
—Unknown

Secondary acquired form
—Ingestion of or exposure to toxins, such as alcohol and lead, or to drugs, such as isoniazid and chloramphenicol
—Complication of other diseases, such as rheumatoid arthritis, lupus erythematosus, multiple myeloma, tuberculosis, and severe infections

Signs and symptoms

Sideroblastic anemias usually produce the following nonspecific clinical effects, which may exist for several years before being identified:
• Anorexia
• Fatigue
• Weakness
• Dizziness
• Pale skin and mucous membranes
• Occasionally, enlarged lymph nodes
• Possible heart and liver failure, which causes dyspnea, exertional angina, slight jaundice, and hepatosplenomegaly

Diagnostic tests

• On microscopic examination of bone marrow aspirate, stained with Prussian blue or alizarin red dye, ringed sideroblasts confirm this diagnosis. Microscopic examination of blood shows erythrocytes to be hypochromic or normochromic and slightly macrocytic. Red cell precursors may be megaloblastic, with anisocytosis (abnormal variation in RBC size) and poikilocytosis (abnormal variation in RBC shape).
• Hemoglobin is decreased.
• Serum iron and transferrin are increased.
• Urobilinogen and bilirubin levels are increased.
• CBC typically shows normal levels of platelets and leukocytes, but occa-

sionally thrombocytopenia or leukopenia occurs.

Treatment

Treatment of sideroblastic anemias depends on the underlying cause. The hereditary form usually responds to several weeks of treatment with high doses of pyridoxine. The acquired secondary form usually subsides after the causative drug or toxin is removed or the underlying condition is adequately treated. Folic acid supplements may also be beneficial when concomitant megaloblastic nuclear changes in RBC precursors are present. Elderly patients with sideroblastic anemia—most commonly the primary acquired form—are less likely to improve quickly and are more likely to develop serious complications. Deferoxamine may be used to treat chronic iron overload in selected patients.

Carefully cross-matched transfusions (providing needed hemoglobin) or high doses of androgens are effective palliative measures for some patients with the primary acquired form of sideroblastic anemia. However, this form is essentially refractory to treatment and usually leads to death from acute leukemia or from respiratory or cardiac complications.

Some patients with sideroblastic anemia may benefit from phlebotomy to prevent hemochromatosis. Phlebotomy increases the rate of erythropoiesis and decreases excess iron stores; thus, it reduces serum and total-body iron levels.

Clinical implications

• Administer medications, as ordered. Teach the patient the importance of continuing prescribed therapy, even after he begins to feel better.
• Provide frequent rest periods if the patient becomes easily fatigued.
• If phlebotomy is scheduled, explain the procedure thoroughly to help reduce anxiety. If this procedure must be repeated frequently, provide a high-protein diet to help replace the protein lost during phlebotomy. Encourage the patient to follow a similar diet at home.
• Always inquire about the possibility of exposure to lead in the home (especially for children) or on the job.
• Identify patients who abuse alcohol; refer them for appropriate therapy.

Silicosis

Description

Silicosis is a progressive disease characterized by nodular lesions, which commonly progress to fibrosis. It is the most common form of pneumoconiosis. Silicosis can be classified according to the severity of pulmonary disease and the rapidity of its onset and progression; it usually occurs as a simple asymptomatic illness. Acute silicosis develops after 1 to 3 years in workers (sandblasters, tunnel workers) exposed to very high concentrations of respirable silica. Accelerated silicosis appears after an average of 10 years of exposure to lower concentrations of free silica. Chronic silicosis develops after 20 or more years of exposure to lower concentrations of free silica. Prognosis is good, unless the disease progresses into the complicated fibrotic form, which causes respiratory insufficiency and cor pulmonale and is associated with pulmonary tuberculosis.

Causes

Inhalation and pulmonary deposition of respirable crystalline silica dust, mostly from quartz

Risk factors

Occupational exposure to silica dust

Signs and symptoms

• May be asymptomatic in initial stages

• Dyspnea on exertion, which worsens if disease progresses
• Cough
• Tachypnea
• Weight loss
• Fatigue
• General weakness
• CNS changes, such as confusion, in advanced stage
• In chronic silicosis, possible decreased chest expansion, diminished intensity of breath sounds, and fine-to-medium rales

Diagnostic tests

• Chest X-rays show small, discrete, nodular lesions distributed throughout both lung fields but typically concentrated in the upper lung zones; the hilar lung nodes may be enlarged and exhibit "eggshell" calcification in simple silicosis. In complicated silicosis, X-rays show one or more conglomerate masses of dense tissue.
• Pulmonary function studies yield the following results:
—FVC is reduced in complicated silicosis.
—FEV is reduced in obstructive disease (emphysematous areas of silicosis); it is also reduced in complicated silicosis, but the ratio of FEV_1 to FVC is normal or high.
—MVV is reduced in both restrictive and obstructive diseases.
—DLCO is reduced when fibrosis destroys alveolar walls and obliterates pulmonary capillaries, or when fibrosis thickens the alveolar capillary membrane.
• Arterial blood gas studies show the following:
—PO_2 is normal in simple silicosis but may be significantly decreased in the late stages of chronic or complicated disease, when the patient breathes room air.
—PCO_2 is normal in early stages but may decrease due to hyperventilation; it may increase as a restrictive pattern develops, particularly if the patient is hypoxic and has severe impairment of alveolar ventilation.

Treatment and clinical implications

The goal of treatment is to relieve respiratory symptoms, to manage hypoxia and cor pulmonale, and to prevent respiratory tract irritation and infections. Treatment also includes careful observation for the development of tuberculosis. Respiratory symptoms may be relieved through daily use of bronchodilating aerosols and increased fluid intake (at least 3 liters daily). Steam inhalation and chest physical therapy techniques, such as controlled coughing and segmental bronchial drainage, with chest percussion and vibration, help clear secretions. In severe cases, it may be necessary to administer oxygen by cannula or mask (1 to 2 liters/minute) for the patient with chronic hypoxia, or by mechanical ventilation if arterial oxygen cannot be maintained above 40 mm Hg. Respiratory infections require prompt administration of antibiotics.

Teach the patient to prevent infections by avoiding crowds and persons with respiratory infections, and by receiving influenza and pneumococcal vaccines.

Increase exercise tolerance by encouraging regular activity. Advise the patient to plan his daily activities to decrease the work of breathing. He should pace himself, rest often, and generally move slowly through his daily routine.

Complications

• Right ventricular failure and cor pulmonale
• Tuberculosis

Sinusitis

Description

Sinusitis, inflammation of the paranasal sinuses, may be acute, subacute, chronic, allergic, or hyperplastic.

Surgery for Chronic and Hyperplastic Sinusitis

For maxillary sinusitis:
• *Nasal window procedure* creates an opening in the sinus, allowing secretions and pus to drain through the nose.
• *Caldwell-Luc procedure* removes diseased mucosa in the maxillary sinus through an incision under the upper lip.

For chronic ethmoid sinusitis:
• *Ethmoidectomy* removes all infected tissue through an external or intranasal incision into the ethmoidal sinus.

For sphenoid sinusitis:
• *External ethmoidectomy* removes infected ethmoidal sinus tissue through a crescent-shaped incision, beginning under the inner eyebrow and extending along the side of the nose.

For chronic frontal sinusitis:
• *Fronto-ethmoidectomy* removes infected frontal sinus tissue through an extended external ethmoidectomy.
• *Osteoplastic flap* drains the sinuses through an incision across the skull, behind the hairline.

Acute sinusitis usually results from the common cold and lingers in subacute form in only about 10% of patients. Chronic sinusitis follows persistent bacterial infection. Allergic sinusitis accompanies allergic rhinitis. Hyperplastic sinusitis is a combination of purulent acute sinusitis and allergic sinusitis or rhinitis. Prognosis is good for all types.

Causes
• Bacterial or viral infection
• Allergy

Signs and symptoms
• Nasal congestion
• Pressure
• Pain (maxillary sinusitis causes pain over the cheeks and upper teeth; ethmoid sinusitis, pain over the eyes; frontal sinusitis, pain over the eyebrows; and sphenoid sinusitis [rare], pain behind the eyes)
• Fever, in acute sinusitis
• Nasal discharge (may be purulent in the acute and subacute forms; continuous in the chronic form; watery in the allergic form)
• Nasal stuffiness
• Possible inflammation and pus on nasal examination

Diagnostic tests
• Sinus X-rays reveal cloudiness in the affected sinus, air-fluid levels, or thickened mucosal lining.
• Antral puncture promotes drainage and removal of purulent material. It may also provide a specimen for culture and sensitivity identification of the infecting organism, but this is rarely done.
• Transillumination allows inspection of the sinus cavities by passing a light through them; purulent drainage prevents passage of light.

Treatment
Antibiotics are the primary treatment for the patient with acute sinusitis. Analgesics may be prescribed to relieve pain. Other appropriate measures include vasoconstrictors, such as epinephrine or phenylephrine, to decrease nasal secretions. Steam inhalation also promotes vasoconstriction, in addition to encouraging drainage. Antibiotics are necessary to combat persistent in-

fection. Local applications of heat may help to relieve pain and congestion.

In subacute sinusitis, antibiotic therapy is also the primary treatment. As in acute sinusitis, vasoconstrictors may lessen nasal secretions.

Treatment of allergic sinusitis must include treatment of allergic rhinitis—administration of antihistamines, identification of allergens by skin testing, and desensitization by immunotherapy. Severe allergic symptoms may require treatment with corticosteroids and epinephrine.

In both chronic sinusitis and hyperplastic sinusitis, antihistamines, antibiotics, and a steroid nasal spray may relieve pain and congestion. If irrigation fails to relieve symptoms, one or more sinuses may require surgery. (See also *Surgery for Chronic and Hyperplastic Sinusitis.*)

Clinical implications

• Enforce bed rest, and encourage the patient to drink plenty of fluids to promote drainage in the acute form. Do not elevate the head of the bed more than 30°.

• To relieve pain and promote drainage, apply warm compresses continuously, or four times daily for 2-hour intervals. In addition, give analgesics and antihistamines, as needed.

• Tell the patient to finish the prescribed antibiotics, even if his symptoms disappear.

• Watch for and report complications, such as vomiting, chills, fever, edema of the forehead or eyelids, blurred or double vision, and personality changes.

• If surgery is necessary, tell the patient what to expect postoperatively. Nasal packing will be in place for 12 to 24 hours after surgery. He will have to breathe through his mouth and will not be able to blow his nose. After surgery, monitor for excessive drainage or bleeding, and watch for complications.

• To prevent edema and promote drainage, place the patient in semi-

Fowler's position. To relieve edema and pain and minimize bleeding, apply ice compresses or a rubber glove filled with ice chips over the nose and iced saline gauze over the eyes. Continue these measures for 24 hours.

• Frequently change the mustache dressing or drip pad, and record the consistency, amount, and color of drainage (expect scant, bright red, and clotty drainage).

• Because the patient will be breathing through his mouth, provide meticulous mouth care.

• Tell the patient that even after the packing is removed, nose blowing may cause bleeding and swelling. If the patient is a smoker, instruct him not to smoke for at least 2 to 3 days after surgery.

Sjögren's syndrome

Description

The second most common autoimmune rheumatic disorder after rheumatoid arthritis, Sjögren's syndrome (SS) is characterized by diminished lacrimal and salivary gland secretion (sicca complex). This syndrome occurs mainly in women (90% of patients). Mean age of occurrence is 50. SS may be a primary disorder or associated with connective tissue disorders such as rheumatoid arthritis, scleroderma, systemic lupus erythematosus, and polymyositis. In some patients, the disorder is limited to the exocrine glands (glandular SS); in others, it also involves other organs, such as the lung and kidney (extraglandular SS).

Causes

Unknown

Signs and symptoms

• Decreased or absent salivation
• Dry eyes with a persistent burning, gritty sensation

- Possible dryness of the vagina, causing dyspareunia
- Possible skin dryness
- Difficulty talking, chewing, and swallowing
- Ulcers and soreness of the lips and oral mucosa
- Possible enlargement of parotid and submaxillary glands
- Possible nasal crusting and epistaxis
- Fatigue
- Possible nonproductive cough and polyuria

Diagnostic tests

- Erythrocyte sedimentation rate is almost always increased.
- CBC shows mild anemia and leukopenia in 30% of patients.
- Hypergammaglobulinemia occurs in 50% of patients.
- Rheumatoid factor is positive in most patients.
- Antinuclear antibodies are positive in 50% to 80% of patients.
- Antisalivary duct antibodies are positive.
- Schirmer's tearing test and slit-lamp examination with rose bengal dye are used to measure eye involvement.
- Measuring the volume of parotid saliva and performing secretory sialography and salivary scintigraphy evaluate salivary gland involvement.
- Lower lip biopsy shows salivary gland infiltration by lymphocytes.

Treatment and clinical implications

Treatment is usually symptomatic and includes conservative measures to relieve ocular or oral dryness. Mouth dryness can be relieved by using a methylcellulose swab or spray and by drinking plenty of fluids, especially at mealtime. Meticulous oral hygiene is essential, including regular flossing, brushing, and fluoride treatment at home and frequent dental checkups. Advise the patient to avoid drugs that decrease saliva production, such as atropine derivatives, antihistamines,

anticholinergics, and antidepressants. If mouth lesions make eating painful, suggest high-protein, high-calorie liquid supplements to prevent malnutrition. Advise the patient to avoid sugar, which contributes to dental caries, and tobacco, alcohol, and spicy, salty, or highly acidic foods, which cause mouth irritation.

Instill artificial tears as often as every half hour to prevent eye damage (corneal ulcerations, corneal opacifications) from insufficient tear secretions. Some patients may also benefit from instillation of an eye ointment at bedtime, or from twice-a-day use of sustained-release cellulose capsules (Lacrisert). Suggest the use of sunglasses to protect the patient's eyes from dust, wind, and strong light. Moisture chamber spectacles may also be helpful. Because dry eyes are more susceptible to infection, advise the patient to keep her face clean and to avoid rubbing her eyes. If infection develops, antibiotics should be given immediately. Topical steroids should be avoided.

To help relieve respiratory dryness, stress the need to humidify home and work environments. Suggest normal saline solution drops or aerosolized spray for nasal dryness. Advise the patient to avoid prolonged hot showers and baths and to use moisturizing lotions to help ease dry skin. Suggest K-Y Lubricating Jelly as a vaginal lubricant.

Other treatment measures vary with associated extraglandular findings. Parotid gland enlargement requires local heat and analgesics; pulmonary and renal interstitial disease, corticosteroids; accompanying lymphoma, a combination of chemotherapy, surgery, or radiation.

Refer the patient to the Sjögren's Syndrome Foundation for additional information and support.

Snakebites, poisonous

Description

Each year, poisonous snakes bite about 7,000 persons in the United States. Such bites are most common during summer afternoons, in grassy or rocky habitats. Poisonous snakebites are medical emergencies. With prompt, correct treatment, they need not be fatal.

Causes

In the United States, poisonous snakes include the following:
• Pit vipers (Crotalidae), which include rattlesnakes, water moccasins, and copperheads
• Coral snakes

Signs and symptoms

Pit viper envenomation
—Immediate and progressively severe pain and edema (the entire extremity may swell within a few hours)
—Local elevation in skin temperature
—Fever
—Skin discoloration
—Petechiae
—Ecchymoses
—Blebs
—Blisters
—Bloody wound discharge
—Local necrosis
—Nausea and vomiting
—Diarrhea
—Tachycardia and hypotension
—Lymphadenopathy
—Possible neurotoxic effects, including local and facial numbness and tingling, fasciculation and twitching of skeletal muscles, convulsions (especially in children), extreme anxiety, difficulty in speaking, fainting, weakness, dizziness, excessive sweating, occasional paralysis, mild-to-severe respiratory distress, headache, blurred vision, marked thirst, and, in severe envenomation, coma and death

—Possible hematemesis, hematuria, melena, bleeding gums, and internal bleeding

Coral snakebite envenomation
Clinical effects are delayed.
—Little or no local tissue reaction
—Local paresthesia
—Weakness
—Euphoria
—Drowsiness
—Nausea and vomiting
—Difficulty swallowing and marked salivation; dysphonia
—Ptosis and blurred vision
—Miosis
—Respiratory distress and possible respiratory failure
—Loss of muscle coordination
—Abnormal reflexes
—Peripheral paralysis
—Bleeding

Diagnostic tests

• Blood tests may show prolonged bleeding time and partial thromboplastin time, decreased hemoglobin and hematocrit, and sharply decreased platelet count (less than 200,000/mm^3).
• Urinalysis may show hematuria, and, in infection (a snake's mouth contains gram-negative bacteria), increased WBC count.
• Chest X-ray may show pulmonary edema or emboli.
• EKG may show tachycardia and ectopic beats.
• EEG is abnormal in severe envenomation.

Treatment

Prompt, appropriate first aid can reduce venom absorption and prevent severe symptoms.
• If possible, identify the snake, but do not waste time trying to find it.
• Immediately immobilize the limb below heart level, and instruct the victim to remain as quiet as possible.
• Apply a slightly *constrictive tourniquet* (one that obstructs only lymphatic and superficial venous blood flow) about 4″ (10 cm) above the fang

marks, or just above the first joint proximal to the bite. Caution: Do not apply this constrictive tourniquet if more than 30 minutes has elapsed since the bite. Also, total constrictive tourniquet time should not exceed 2 hours, nor should it delay antivenin administration. Release the tourniquet for 60 to 90 seconds every 30 minutes, but consider that release may be necessary only if swelling progresses rapidly.

• Apply a *tight tourniquet* only for extremely severe envenomation by a coral snake. In this case, release the tourniquet every 10 minutes for 90 seconds until you can administer antivenin. Remember: Loss of limb is possible if a tourniquet is too tight or if tourniquet time is too long.

• Wash the skin over the fang marks. Within 30 minutes of pit viper bites, make an incision through the marks approximately ½″ (1.27 cm) long and ⅛″ (3 mm) deep. Be especially careful if the bite is on the hand, where blood vessels and tendons are close to the skin surface. Using a bulb syringe— or, if no other means is available, mouth suction—apply suction for 20 to 30 minutes and for up to 2 hours in the absence of antivenin administration. Remember: An incision and suction are effective only in pit viper bites and only within 30 minutes of the bite. Also, mouth suction is contraindicated if the rescuer has oral ulcers.

• Never give the victim alcoholic drinks or stimulants, since these speed venom absorption. Never apply ice to a snakebite: it increases tissue damage.

• Transport the victim as quickly as possible, keeping him warm and at rest. Record the signs and symptoms of progressive envenomation and when they develop. Most snakebite victims are hospitalized for only 24 to 48 hours, but some remain longer after severe envenomation. Usually, treatment consists of antivenin administration, though minor snakebites may not require antivenin. Other treatment includes tetanus toxoid or tetanus immune globulin (human); broad-spectrum antibiotics; and, depending on respiratory status, severity of pain, and type of snakebite (narcotics are contraindicated in coral snakebites), aspirin, codeine, morphine, or meperidine. Usually, necrotic snakebites need surgical debridement after 3 or 4 days. Intense, rapidly progressive edema requires fasciotomy within 2 or 3 hours of the bite. Extreme envenomation may require limb amputation and subsequent reconstructive surgery, rehabilitation, and physical therapy.

Clinical implications
When the patient arrives at the hospital, immobilize the extremity if this has not already been done. If a tight tourniquet has been applied within the past hour, apply a loose tourniquet proximally and remove the first tourniquet. Release the second tourniquet gradually during antivenin administration, as ordered. A sudden release of venom into the bloodstream can cause cardiorespiratory collapse, so keep emergency equipment handy.

• On a flow sheet, document vital signs, level of consciousness, skin color, swelling, respiratory status, and a description of the bite, surrounding area, and symptoms. Monitor vital signs every 15 minutes and check for a pulse in the affected limb.

• Start an I.V. with a large-bore needle for antivenin administration. Severe bites that result in coagulotoxic signs and symptoms may require two I.V. lines: one for antivenin, the second for blood products.

• Before antivenin administration, obtain a patient history of allergies (especially to horse serum) and other medical problems. Perform hypersensitivity tests, as ordered, and assist with desensitization, as needed. During antivenin administration, keep epinephrine, oxygen, and vasopressors available to combat anaphylaxis from horse serum.

• Give packed cells, whole blood, I.V. fluids, and possibly fresh-frozen plasma or platelets, as ordered, to counteract coagulotoxicity and maintain blood pressure. If the patient develops respiratory distress and requires endotracheal intubation or tracheotomy, give good tracheostomy care.

• Give analgesics, as needed. Do not give narcotics to victims of coral snakebites. Clean the snakebite using sterile technique. Open, debride, and drain any blebs and blisters, because they may contain venom. Be sure to change dressings daily.

• Encourage hikers and campers to carry a snakebite kit if they will be more than a half-hour from the nearest hospital.

Complications
• Coma
• Shock

Sodium imbalance

Description
Sodium is the major cation (90%) in extracellular fluid; potassium, the major cation in intracellular fluid. During repolarization, the sodium-potassium pump continually shifts sodium into the cells and potassium out of the cells. During depolarization, it does the reverse. Sodium cation functions include maintaining tonicity and concentration of extracellular fluid, acid-base balance (reabsorption of sodium ion and excretion of hydrogen ion), nerve conduction and neuromuscular function, glandular secretion, and water balance. Although the body requires only 2 to 4 g of sodium daily, most Americans consume 6 to 10 g daily (mostly sodium chloride, as table salt), excreting excess sodium through the kidneys and skin.

Causes
Hyponatremia (decreased serum sodium concentration)
—GI losses due to vomiting, suctioning, or diarrhea
—Excessive perspiration or fever
—Potent diuretics
—Tap water enemas
—Excessive drinking of water, infusion of I.V. dextrose in water without other solutes, malnutrition or starvation, and low-sodium diet, usually in combination with one of the other causes
—Trauma, surgery (wound drainage), or burns, which cause sodium to shift into damaged cells
—Adrenal gland insufficiency (Addison's disease) or hypoaldosteronism
—Cirrhosis of the liver with ascites
—Syndrome of inappropriate antidiuretic hormone secretion (SIADH)
Hypernatremia (increased serum sodium concentration)
—Decreased water intake
—Excess adrenocortical hormones, as in Cushing's syndrome
—ADH deficiency (diabetes insipidus)
—Salt intoxication (less common), which may be produced by excessive ingestion of table salt

Signs and symptoms
Sodium imbalance has profound physiologic effects and can induce severe CNS, cardiovascular, and GI abnormalities. (See *Clinical Effects of Sodium Imbalance,* p. 716.)

Diagnostic tests
• Serum sodium level less than 135 mEq/liter is the definition of hyponatremia.
• Serum sodium level greater than 145 mEq/liter is the definition of hypernatremia. (Additional laboratory studies are necessary to determine etiology and differentiate between a true deficit and an apparent deficit due to sodium shift or to hypervolemia or hypovolemia.)

Clinical Effects of Sodium Imbalance

DYSFUNCTION	HYPONATREMIA	HYPERNATREMIA
CNS	• Anxiety, headaches, muscle twitching and weakness, convulsions	• Fever, agitation, restlessness, convulsions
Cardiovascular	• Hypotension; tachycardia; with severe deficit, vasomotor collapse, thready pulse	• Hypertension, tachycardia, pitting edema, excessive weight gain
GI	• Nausea, vomiting, abdominal cramps	• Rough, dry tongue; intense thirst
Genitourinary	• Oliguria or anuria	• Oliguria
Respiratory	• Cyanosis with severe deficiency	• Dyspnea, respiratory arrest, and death (from dramatic rise in osmotic pressure)
Cutaneous	• Cold, clammy skin; decreased skin turgor	• Flushed skin; dry, sticky mucous membranes

• Urine sodium greater than 100 mEq/ 24 hours, with low serum osmolality, supports a diagnosis of true hyponatremia.
• Urine sodium less than 40 mEq/24 hours, with high serum osmolality, supports a diagnosis of true hypernatremia.

Treatment

Therapy for mild hyponatremia usually consists of restricted free-water intake when it is due to hemodilution, SIADH, or conditions such as congestive heart failure, cirrhosis of the liver, and renal failure. If fluid restriction alone fails to normalize serum sodium levels, demeclocycline or lithium, which block ADH action in the renal tubules, can be used to promote water excretion. In extremely rare instances of severe symptomatic hyponatremia, when serum sodium levels fall below 110 mEq/liter, treatment may include infusion of 3% or 5% saline solution.

Treatment with saline infusion requires careful monitoring of venous pressure to prevent potentially fatal circulatory overload. The aim of treatment of secondary hyponatremia is to correct the underlying disorder.

Primary treatment of hypernatremia is administration of salt-free solutions (such as dextrose in water) to return serum sodium levels to normal, followed by infusion of 0.45% sodium chloride to prevent hyponatremia. Other measures include a sodium-restricted diet and discontinuation of drugs that promote sodium retention.

Clinical implications

When managing the patient with hyponatremia, follow these guidelines:
• Watch for and report extremely low serum sodium and accompanying

serum chloride levels. Monitor urine specific gravity and other laboratory results. Record fluid intake and output accurately, and weigh the patient daily.
• During administration of isosmolar or hyperosmolar saline solution, watch closely for signs of hypervolemia (dyspnea, rales, engorged neck or hand veins). Report conditions that may cause excessive sodium loss—diaphoresis or prolonged diarrhea or vomiting, and severe burns.
• Refer the patient on maintenance dosage of diuretics to a dietitian for instruction about dietary sodium intake.
• To prevent hyponatremia, administer isosmolar solutions.

When managing the patient with hypernatremia, follow these guidelines:
• Measure serum sodium levels every 6 hours or at least daily. Monitor vital signs for changes, especially for rising pulse rate. Watch for signs of hypervolemia, especially in the patient receiving I.V. fluids.
• Record fluid intake and output accurately, checking for body fluid loss. Weigh the patient daily.
• Obtain a drug history to check for drugs that promote sodium retention.
• Explain the importance of sodium restriction, and teach the patient how to plan a low-sodium diet. Closely monitor the serum sodium levels of high-risk patients.

Somatization disorder

Description
Somatization disorder is present when multiple signs and symptoms that suggest physical disorders exist without a verifiable disease or pathophysiologic condition to account for them. Commonly, the patient with somatization disorder undergoes repeated medical evaluations, which—unlike the symptoms themselves—can be potentially damaging and debilitating. Such a patient can always find just one more hospital or physician to do another diagnostic workup. However, unlike the hypochondriac, he is not preoccupied with the belief that he has a specific disease. Exacerbations occur during times of stress.

Causes
This disorder has no specific cause. Its symptoms can begin or worsen after many kinds of losses (job security or personal relationship).

Signs and symptoms
The essential feature of this disorder is the pattern of recurrent, multiple symptoms and complaints. These complaints can involve any body system but most commonly involve the following:
• The GI tract, with nausea, vomiting, and abdominal pain
• The neurologic system, with weakness, paresthesias, and headaches
• The cardiopulmonary system, with dizziness, chest pain, and palpitations

Diagnostic tests
• No specific test or procedure verifies somatization disorder.
• Diagnostic evaluation should rule out physical causes that typically cause vague, confusing symptoms, such as multiple sclerosis, hypothyroidism, systemic lupus erythematosus, or porphyria.
• Psychological evaluation should rule out depression, schizophrenia with somatic delusions, hypochondriasis, psychogenic pain, and malingering.

Treatment
The goal of treatment is not to eradicate the patient's symptoms, but rather to help him learn to live with them. After diagnostic evaluation has ruled out organic causes, the patient should be told that he has no serious illness but will continue to receive care to ease his symptoms.

The most important aspect of treatment is a continuing, supportive relationship with a sympathetic health care provider who acknowledges the patient's symptoms and is willing to help him live with them. The patient should have regularly scheduled appointments for review of symptoms and basic physical evaluation, but the main aspect of follow-up is review of the patient's coping. Follow-up appointments should last approximately 20 to 30 minutes and should focus on new symptoms or any change in old symptoms to avoid missing a developing physical disease. As many as 30% of patients initially diagnosed with somatization disorder eventually develop an organic disease. Patients with somatization disorder rarely acknowledge any psychological aspect of their illness, and reject psychiatric treatment.

Clinical implications
• Acknowledge the patient's symptoms and support his efforts to function and cope despite distress. Under no circumstances should you tell the patient his symptoms are imaginary. But do tell him the results and meanings of tests.
• Emphasize the patient's strengths. ("It's good that you can still work with this pain.") Gently point out the time relationship between stress and physical symptoms.
• Help the patient to manage stress, not get rid of symptoms. Typically, his relationships are linked to his symptoms. Remedying the symptoms can impair his interactions with others.
• Develop a care plan with some input from the patient. The care plan should include participation of the patient's family. Encourage and help them to understand the patient's need for troublesome symptoms.

Spinal cord defects
(Spina bifida, meningocele, myelomeningocele)

Description
Spina bifida occulta is the most common and least severe spinal cord defect. It is characterized by incomplete closure of one or more vertebrae without protrusion of the spinal cord or meninges. However, in more severe forms of spina bifida, incomplete closure of one or more vertebrae causes protrusion of the spinal contents in an external sac or cystic lesion. In spina bifida with meningocele, this sac contains meninges and CSF. In spina bifida with myelomeningocele (meningomyelocele), this sac contains meninges, CSF, and a portion of the spinal cord or nerve roots distal to the conus medullaris.

Prognosis varies with the degree of accompanying neurologic deficit. It is worst in patients with large, open lesions, neurogenic bladders (which predispose to infection and renal failure), or total paralysis of the legs. Because such features are usually absent in spina bifida occulta and meningocele, prognosis is much better than in myelomeningocele, and many patients with these conditions can lead normal lives.

Spina bifida is relatively common. It affects about 5% of the population. (See *Encephalocele.*)

Causes
Defective embryonic neural tube closure during the first trimester of pregnancy

Signs and symptoms
Spina bifida occulta
—Often accompanied by a depression or dimple, tuft of hair, soft fatty deposits, port wine nevi, or a combination of these abnormalities on the

Encephalocele

An encephalocele is a congenital saclike protrusion of the meninges and brain through a defective opening in the skull. Usually, it is in the occipital area, but it may also occur in the parietal, nasopharyngeal, or frontal area.

Clinical effects of encephalocele vary with the degree of tissue involvement and location of the defect. Paralysis and hydrocephalus are common.

Symptoms vary with the degree of tissue involvement and the location of the defect. Often, paralysis and hydrocephalus are associated with encephalocele.

Treatment includes surgery during infancy to place protruding tissues back in the skull, excise the sac, and correct associated craniofacial abnormalities. Always handle an infant with encephalocele carefully and avoid pressure on the sac. Both before and after surgery, watch for signs of increased intracranial pressure (bulging fontanelles). As the child grows older, teach his parents to watch for developmental deficiencies that may signal mental retardation.

skin over the spinal defect
—Does not usually cause neurologic dysfunction but occasionally is associated with foot weakness or bowel and bladder disturbances
Meningocele
—A saclike structure protruding over the spine
—Rarely, neurologic dysfunction
Myelomeningocele
—A saclike structure protruding over the spine
—Permanent neurologic dysfunction, such as flaccid or spastic paralysis and bowel and bladder incontinence
—Associated disorders, including trophic skin disturbances (ulcerations, cyanosis), clubfoot, knee contractures, hydrocephalus (in about 90% of patients), and possible mental retardation, Arnold-Chiari syndrome (in which part of the brain protrudes into the spinal canal), and curvature of the spine

Diagnostic tests

• Spinal X-ray shows the bone defect in spina bifida occulta; myelography differentiates it from other spinal abnormalities, especially spinal cord tumors.

• Transillumination of the protruding sac can sometimes distinguish between meningocele and myelomenin-

gocele. (In meningocele, it typically transilluminates; in myelomeningocele, it does not.)

• Skull X-rays, cephalic measurements, and CT scan demonstrate associated hydrocephalus.

• Other appropriate laboratory tests in patients with myelomeningocele include urinalysis, urine cultures, and tests for renal function in older children and adults with urinary incontinence.

• Amniocentesis detects open neural tube defects, such as myelomeningocele and meningocele; alpha-fetoprotein level is increased by 14 weeks of gestation. (This procedure is recommended for all pregnant women who have previously had children with spinal cord defects, since these women are at an increased risk of having children with similar defects.)

Treatment

Spina bifida occulta usually requires no treatment. If neuromuscular problems occur during growth, surgery may be indicated, however.

Treatment for meningocele consists solely of surgical closure of the protruding sac and continual assessment of growth and development. Treatment of myelomeningocele requires surgical repair of the sac and supportive measures to promote independence and prevent further complications. Unfortunately, surgery cannot reverse neurologic deficit. Usually, a shunt is necessary to relieve associated hydrocephalus.

In older children or adults, rehabilitation measures include the following:
• Waist supports, long leg braces, walkers, crutches, and other orthopedic appliances
• Colostomy or diet and bowel training to manage fecal incontinence
• Neurogenic bladder management with a urinary antiseptic, regular application of Credé's method (manual compression of the bladder) to reduce urinary stasis, possibly intermittent catheterization, and antispasmodics such as bethanechol or propantheline; in severe cases, insertion of an artificial urinary sphincter or urinary diversion

Clinical implications

Care of the patient with a severe spinal defect requires a team approach by the neurosurgeon, orthopedist, urologist, nurse, social worker, occupational and physical therapists, and parents. Obviously, care is most complex when the neurologic deficit is severe. Immediate goals include psychological support to help parents accept the diagnosis, and pre- and postoperative care. Long-term goals include patient and family teaching and measures to prevent contractures, decubitus ulcers, urinary tract infections, and other complications.

Before surgery for meningocele or myelomeningocele, follow these guidelines:
• Prevent local infection by cleansing the defect gently with sterile saline solution or other solutions, as ordered. Inspect the defect often for signs of infection, and cover it with sterile dressings moistened with sterile saline solution. Prevent skin breakdown by placing sheepskin or a foam pad under the infant. Give antibiotics, as ordered.
• Handle the infant carefully, and do not apply pressure to the defect. Usually, he cannot wear a diaper or a shirt until after surgical correction, because it will irritate the sac, so keep him warm in an infant incubator (isolette). Position him on his abdomen to prevent contamination of the sac with urine or feces. Hold and cuddle the infant, but avoid placing pressure on the sac.
• Measure head circumference daily, and watch for signs of hydrocephalus and meningeal irritation, such as fever or nuchal rigidity.
• Minimize contractures by passive range-of-motion exercises. (Casting may also be used.)
• To prevent hip dislocation, moderately abduct hips with a pad between the knees, or with sandbags and ankle rolls.
• Monitor intake and output. Watch for decreased skin turgor, dryness, or other signs of dehydration. To prevent urinary tract infection, use Credé's method to empty the bladder every 2 hours during the day and once during the night. Provide meticulous skin care to genitals and buttocks to prevent infection.
• Ensure adequate nutrition.

After surgical repair of the defect, follow these guidelines:
• Watch for hydrocephalus, which often follows such surgery.
• Monitor vital signs often. Watch for signs of shock, infection, and increased intracranial pressure (projectile vomiting). Remember that before age 2, infants do not show typical signs of increased intracranial pressure, since suture lines are not fully closed. In infants, the most telling sign is bulging fontanelles.
• Change the dressing regularly, as ordered, and check for drainage, wound rupture, and infection.

• Refer parents for genetic counseling, and suggest that amniocentesis be performed in future pregnancies. For more information and names of support groups, refer parents to the Spina Bifida Association of America.

Teach parents how to cope with the infant's physical problems and successfully meet long-range treatment goals. They should be able to do the following:
• Recognize early signs of complications, such as hydrocephalus, decubitus ulcers, and urinary tract infection.
• Provide psychological support and encourage a positive attitude.
• Use Credé's method to empty the bladder regularly. (Encourage parents to begin training their child in a bladder routine by age 3. Emphasize the need for increased fluid intake to prevent urinary tract infection. Teach intermittent catheterization and conduit hygiene, as ordered. If the child has an artificial urinary sphincter, teach him how to use it.)
• Prevent bowel obstruction. (Stress the need for increased fluid intake, a high-bulk diet, exercise, and use of a stool softener, as ordered. Teach parents to empty their child's bowel by exerting slight pressure on his abdomen, telling him to bear down, and giving a glycerin suppository, as needed.)
• Recognize developmental lags early—a possible result of hydrocephalus. (If present, stress the importance of follow-up IQ assessment to help plan realistic educational goals. The child may need to attend a school with special facilities. Also, stress the need for stimulation to ensure maximum mental development. Help parents plan activities appropriate to their child's age and abilities.)

Spinal injuries without cord damage

Description
Spinal injuries include fractures, contusions, and compressions of the vertebral column. Usually, they are the result of trauma to the head or neck. The real danger lies in possible spinal cord damage. Spinal fractures most commonly occur in the fifth, sixth, and seventh cervical, twelfth thoracic, and first lumbar vertebrae.

Causes
• Most serious spinal injuries result from motor vehicle accidents, falls, dives into shallow water, and gunshot wounds.
• Less serious injuries result from lifting heavy objects and experiencing minor falls.

Signs and symptoms
• Muscle spasm and back pain that worsens with movement is the most obvious symptom.
• In cervical fractures, pain may produce point tenderness.
• In dorsal and lumbar fractures, pain may radiate to other body areas, such as the legs.
• If the injury damages the spinal cord, clinical effects range from mild paresthesia to quadriplegia and shock.

Diagnostic tests
• Spinal X-rays locate the fracture.
• Lumbar puncture may show increased CSF pressure from a lesion or trauma in spinal compression.
• Myelography locates the spinal mass.
• CT scan also provides valuable information.

Treatment
The primary treatment after spinal injury is immediate immobilization to stabilize the spine and prevent cord damage. Other treatment is supportive. Cervical injuries require immobilization, using sandbags on both sides of the patient's head, a plaster

cast, hard cervical collar, or skeletal traction with skull tongs (Crutchfield, Barton, Vinke) or a halo device.

Treatment of stable lumbar and dorsal fractures consists of bed rest on firm support (such as a bed board), analgesics, and muscle relaxants until the fracture stabilizes (usually 10 to 12 weeks). Later treatment includes exercises to strengthen the back muscles and a back brace or corset to provide support while walking.

An unstable dorsal or lumbar fracture requires a plaster cast, a turning frame, and, in severe fracture, a laminectomy and spinal fusion.

When the damage results in compression of the spinal column, neurosurgery may relieve the pressure. Surface wounds accompanying the spinal injury require tetanus prophylaxis unless the patient has had recent immunization.

Clinical implications

In all spinal injuries, suspect cord damage until proven otherwise.

• During initial assessment and during X-rays, immobilize the patient on a firm surface, with sandbags on both sides of his head. Tell him not to move. Avoid moving him, since hyperflexion can damage the cord. If you must move the patient, get at least one other member of the staff to help you logroll him, to avoid disturbing body alignment.

• Throughout assessment, offer comfort and reassurance. Remember, the fear of possible paralysis will be overwhelming. Allow a family member who is not too distraught to accompany him and talk to him quietly and calmly.

• If the injury necessitates surgery, administer prophylactic antibiotics, as ordered. Catheterize the patient, as ordered, to avoid urinary retention, and monitor defecation patterns to avoid impaction.

• Explain traction methods to the patient and his family, and reassure them that traction devices do not penetrate the brain.

• If the patient has a halo or skull-tong traction device, cleanse pin sites daily, trim hair short, and provide analgesics for persistent headaches.

• During traction, turn the patient often to prevent pneumonia, embolism, and skin breakdown. Perform passive range-of-motion exercises to maintain muscle tone. If available, use a CircOlectric bed or Stryker frame to facilitate turning and to avoid spinal cord injury.

• Turn the patient on his side during feedings to prevent aspiration. Create a relaxed atmosphere at mealtimes.

• Suggest appropriate diversionary activities to fill the hours of immobility. Offer prism glasses for reading.

• Watch closely for neurologic changes. Immediately report changes in skin sensation and loss of muscle strength; either could point to pressure on the spinal cord, possibly as a result of edema or shifting bone fragments.

• Help the patient walk as soon as the physician allows. He will probably have to wear a back brace.

• Before discharge, instruct the patient about continuing analgesics or other medication, and stress the importance of regular follow-up examinations.

• To help prevent spinal injury from becoming spinal *cord* injury, educate firefighters, police, paramedics, and the general public about the proper way to handle such injuries.

Spinal neoplasms

Description

Spinal neoplasms are of many tumor types. They involve the cord or its roots and, if untreated, can eventually cause paralysis. As primary tumors, they originate in the meningeal coverings, the parenchyma of the cord or its roots, the intraspinal vasculature, or the vertebrae. About 60% of all primary spinal cord neoplasms are intradural tumors (meningiomas and schwannomas), and 25% are extradural tumors that occur as metastatic foci from primary tumors found elsewhere in the body (breasts, lungs, prostate, bone marrow [leukemia], or lymphatics [lymphomas]). Neoplasms occurring within the cord itself (astrocytomas or ependymomas) are comparatively rare, accounting for only about 10%. Prognosis varies depending on tumor type and progression.

Causes
- Unknown for primary neoplasms
- Metastatic foci of primary tumors

Signs and symptoms
- Pain (most severe directly over the tumor, radiates around the trunk or down the limb on the affected side, and is unrelieved by bed rest)
- Motor symptoms, including asymmetric spastic muscle weakness, decreased muscle tone, exaggerated reflexes, and a positive Babinski's sign
- If the tumor is at the level of the cauda equina, muscle flaccidity, muscle wasting, weakness, and progressive diminution in tendon reflexes (characteristic)
- Sensory deficits, including contralateral loss of pain, temperature, and touch sensation (Brown-Séquard syndrome). These losses are less obvious to the patient than functional motor changes. Caudal lesions invariably produce paresthesias in the nerve distribution pathway of the involved roots.
- Urinary retention (an inevitable late sign with cord compression). Early signs include incomplete emptying or difficulty with the urinary stream, which is usually unnoticed or ignored.
- Bladder and bowel incontinence, with cauda equina tumors
- Constipation

Diagnostic tests
- A spinal tap shows clear yellow CSF as a result of increased protein levels if the flow is completely blocked. If the flow is partially blocked, protein levels rise, but the fluid is only slightly yellow in proportion to the CSF protein level. A Pap smear of the CSF may show malignant cells of metastatic carcinoma.
- X-rays show distortions of the intervertebral foramina; changes in the vertebrae or collapsed areas in the vertebral body; and localized enlargement of the spinal canal, indicating an adjacent block.
- Myelography identifies the level of the lesion by outlining it if the tumor is causing partial obstruction; it shows anatomic relationship to the cord and the dura. If obstruction is complete, the injected dye cannot flow past the tumor.
- A radioisotope bone scan demonstrates metastatic invasion of the vertebrae by showing a characteristic increase in osteoblastic activity.
- CT scan shows cord compression and tumor location.
- Frozen section biopsy at surgery identifies the tissue type.

Treatment
Treatment of spinal cord tumors usually includes decompression or radiation. Laminectomy is indicated for primary tumors that produce spinal cord or cauda equina compression. It is *not* usually indicated for metastatic tumors. If the patient has incomplete paraplegia or rapid onset, emergency surgical decompression may save cord function. Steroid therapy minimizes cord edema until surgery can be performed. Partial removal of intramedullary gliomas, followed by radiation, may alleviate symptoms for a short time. Metastatic extradural tumors can be controlled with radiation, analgesics, and, in the case of hormone-mediated tumors (breast and prostate),

appropriate hormone therapy. Transcutaneous electrical nerve stimulation (TENS) may control radicular pain from spinal cord tumors and is a useful alternative to narcotic analgesics.

Clinical implications
• On your first contact with the patient, perform a complete neurologic evaluation to obtain baseline data for planning future care and evaluating changes in clinical status.
• Care for the patient with a spinal cord tumor is basically the same as that for the patient with spinal cord injury. It requires psychological support, rehabilitation (including bowel and bladder retraining), and prevention of infection and skin breakdown. After laminectomy, care includes checking neurologic status frequently, changing position by logrolling, administering analgesics, monitoring frequently for infection, and aiding in early walking.
• Help the patient and his family to understand and cope with the diagnosis, treatment, potential disabilities, and necessary changes in life-style.
• Take safety precautions for the patient with impaired sensation and motor deficits. Use side rails if the patient is bedridden. If he is not, encourage him to wear flat shoes, and remove scatter rugs and clutter to prevent falls.
• Encourage the patient to be independent in performing daily activities. Avoid aggravating pain by moving the patient slowly and by making sure his body is well aligned when giving personal care. Advise him to use TENS to block radicular pain.
• Administer steroids and antacids, as ordered, for cord edema after radiation therapy. Monitor for sensory or motor dysfunction, which indicates the need for more steroids.
• Enforce bed rest for the patient with vertebral body involvement until the physician says he can safely walk, because body weight alone can cause cord collapse and cord laceration from bone fragments.

• Logroll and position the patient on his side every 2 hours to prevent decubitus ulcers and other complications of immobility.
• If the patient is to wear a back brace, make sure he does wear it whenever he gets out of bed.

Sporotrichosis

Description
Sporotrichosis is a chronic disease that occurs in three forms: cutaneous lymphatic, which produces nodular erythematous primary lesions and secondary lesions along lymphatic channels; pulmonary, a rare form that produces a productive cough and pulmonary lesions; and disseminated, another rare form, which may cause arthritis or osteomyelitis. The course of sporotrichosis is slow, with the typical incubation period lasting from 1 week to 3 months. The prognosis is good and fatalities are rare. However, untreated skin lesions may cause secondary bacterial infection.

Causes
The fungus *Sporothrix schenckii* found in soil, wood, sphagnum moss, and decaying vegetation throughout the world

Mode of transmission
• Direct contact of fungus with broken skin
• Inhalation of fungus, in pulmonary type

Risk factors
Occupational exposure for horticulturists, agricultural workers, and home gardeners

Signs and symptoms
Cutaneous lymphatic sporotrichosis
—Skin lesions, usually on the hands

or fingers. Typically, each lesion begins as a small, painless, movable subcutaneous nodule, but grows progressively larger, discolors, and eventually ulcerates.

—Subsequent formation of additional lesions along the adjacent lymph node chain

Pulmonary sporotrichosis
—Productive cough
—Lung cavities and nodules
—Hilar adenopathy
—Pleural effusion
—Fibrosis
—Formation of a fungus ball
—Sarcoidosis and tuberculosis (often present)

Disseminated sporotrichosis
—Multifocal spreading lesions in skin or lungs
—Weight loss
—Anorexia
—Synovial or bony lesions
—Possible arthritis or osteomyelitis

Diagnostic tests
Culture of *S. schenckii* in sputum, pus, or bone drainage

Treatment
The cutaneous lymphatic form usually responds to application of a saturated solution of potassium iodide, usually continued for 1 to 2 months after lesions heal. Occasionally, cutaneous lesions must be excised or drained. The disseminated form responds to I.V. amphotericin B but may require several weeks of treatment. Local heat application relieves pain. Cavitary pulmonary lesions may require surgery.

Clinical implications
• Sporotrichosis does not require isolation.
• Keep lesions clean, make the patient as comfortable as possible, and carefully dispose of contaminated dressings.

• Warn patients about possible adverse effects of drugs. Because amphotericin B may cause fever, chills, nausea, and vomiting, give antipyretics and antiemetics, as ordered.
• To help prevent sporotrichosis, advise horticulturists and home gardeners to wear gloves while working.

Sprains and strains

Description
A sprain is a complete or incomplete tear in the supporting ligaments surrounding a joint. A strain is an injury to a muscle or tendinous attachment. (See also *Muscle-Tendon Ruptures*, p. 726.) Both injuries usually heal without surgical repair.

Causes
• *Sprain* usually follows a sharp twist.
• *Strain* usually follows vigorous muscle overuse or overstress.

Signs and symptoms
Sprain
—Local pain (especially during joint movement)
—Swelling
—Loss of mobility (may not occur until several hours after the injury)
—Black and blue discoloration

Acute strain
—Sharp, transient pain
—Possible snapping noise at time of injury
—Rapid swelling
—Ecchymoses (appear after several days)
—Muscle tenderness when pain subsides

Chronic strain
—Stiffness
—Soreness
—Generalized tenderness

Treatment and clinical implications
Treatment of sprains consists of controlling pain and swelling, and im-

Muscle-Tendon Ruptures

Perhaps the most serious muscle-tendon injury is a rupture of the muscle-tendon junction. These ruptures may occur at any such junction, but they are most common at the Achilles' tendon, which extends from the posterior calf muscle to the foot. An Achilles' tendon rupture produces a sudden sharp pain and, until swelling begins, a palpable defect. Such ruptures typically occur in men between ages 35 and 40, especially during physical activities such as jogging or tennis.

To distinguish Achilles' tendon rupture from other ankle injuries, the physician performs this simple test: With the patient prone and his feet hanging off the foot of the table, the physician squeezes the calf muscle. If this causes plantar flexion, the tendon is intact; if ankle dorsiflexion, it is partially intact; if there is no flexion of any kind, the tendon is ruptured.

Usually an Achilles' tendon rupture requires surgical repair, followed first by a long leg cast for 4 weeks, and then by a short cast for an additional 4 weeks.

mobilizing the injured joint to promote healing. Immediately after the injury, control swelling by elevating the joint above the level of the heart, and by intermittently applying ice for 12 to 48 hours. To prevent cold injury, place a towel between the ice pack and the skin.

Immobilize the joint, using an elastic bandage or, if the sprain is severe, a soft cast. Depending on the severity of the injury, codeine or another analgesic may be necessary. If the patient has a sprained ankle, he may need crutches and crutch gait training. Because patients with sprains seldom require hospitalization, provide comprehensive patient teaching.

• Tell the patient to elevate the joint for 48 to 72 hours after the injury (while sleeping, joint can be elevated with pillows) and to apply ice intermittently for 12 to 48 hours.

• If an elastic bandage has been applied, teach the patient to reapply it by wrapping from below to above the injury, forming a figure eight. For a sprained ankle, apply the bandage from the toes to midcalf. Tell the patient to remove the bandage before going to sleep and to loosen it if it causes the leg to become pale, numb, or painful.

• Instruct the patient to call the physician if pain worsens or persists (if

so, an additional X-ray may detect a fracture originally missed).

An immobilized sprain usually heals in 2 to 3 weeks, and the patient can then gradually resume normal activities. Occasionally, however, torn ligaments do not heal properly and cause recurrent dislocation, necessitating surgical repair. Some athletes may request immediate surgical repair to hasten healing; to prevent sprains, they may tape their wrists and ankles before sports activities.

Acute strains require analgesics and immediate application of ice for up to 48 hours, followed by heat application. Complete muscle rupture may require surgical repair. Chronic strains usually do not require treatment, but local heat application, aspirin, or an analgesic-muscle relaxant relieves discomfort.

Spurious polycythemia
(Relative polycythemia, stress erythrocytosis, stress polycythemia, benign polycythemia, Gaisböck's syndrome, pseudopolycythemia)

Description
Spurious polycythemia is characterized by increased hematocrit and nor-

mal or decreased RBC total mass. It results from decreasing plasma volume and subsequent hemoconcentration. This decrease usually affects middle-aged persons and occurs more often in men than in women.

Causes
- Dehydration
- Hemoconcentration due to stress
- High normal red cell mass and low normal plasma volume

Risk factors
- Hypertension
- Thromboembolitic disease
- Elevated serum cholesterol and uric acid levels
- Familial tendency
- Type A personality
- Chronic smoking
- Middle age

Signs and symptoms
Characteristic signs and symptoms
—Ruddy appearance
—Short neck
—Slight hypertension
—Tendency to hypoventilate when recumbent
Other possible signs and symptoms
—Cardiac disease
—Pulmonary disease

Diagnostic tests
- Hemoglobin and hematocrit levels are elevated.
- RBC count is elevated.
- Plasma volume may be decreased or normal.
- Cholesterol and lipid levels may be elevated.
- Uric acid level may be elevated.

Treatment
Rehydration with appropriate fluids and electrolytes is the primary therapy for spurious polycythemia secondary to dehydration. Therapy must also include appropriate measures to prevent continuing fluid loss as well as measures to prevent thromboembolism.

Clinical implications
- During rehydration, carefully monitor intake and output to maintain fluid and electrolyte balance.
- To prevent thromboemboli in predisposed patients, suggest regular exercise and a low-cholesterol diet. Antilipemics may also be necessary. Reduced calorie intake may be required for the obese patient.
- Whenever appropriate, suggest counseling about the patient's work habits and lack of relaxation. If the patient is a smoker, make sure he understands how important it is that he stop smoking. Then, refer him to a smoking cessation program, if necessary.
- Emphasize the need for follow-up examinations every 3 to 4 months after leaving the hospital.
- Thoroughly explain spurious polycythemia, all diagnostic measures, and therapy. The hard-driving person predisposed to spurious polycythemia is likely to be more inquisitive and anxious than the average patient. Answer his questions honestly, but take care to reassure him that he can effectively control symptoms by complying with the prescribed treatment.

Squamous cell carcinoma

Description
Squamous cell carcinoma of the skin is an invasive tumor with metastatic potential that arises from the keratinizing epidermal cells. Squamous cell carcinoma commonly develops on sun-damaged areas of the skin. Lesions on sun-damaged skin tend not to be as invasive, with less tendency to metastasize than lesions on unexposed skin except for lesions on the lower lip and the ears. These are almost invariably markedly invasive metastatic lesions, usually with a poor prognosis. Oth-

erwise, prognosis is excellent with treatment, being better with a well-differentiated lesion than with a poorly differentiated one in an unusual location.

Causes
- Overexposure to sun's ultraviolet rays
- X-ray therapy
- Ingestion of herbicides containing arsenic
- Chronic skin irritation and inflammation
- Exposure to local carcinogens (such as tar and oil)

Risk factors
- Race (fair-skinned whites), sex (males), age (over 60)
- Outdoor employment and residence in a sunny, warm climate
- Presence of premalignant lesions
- Presence of hereditary diseases (such as xeroderma pigmentosum and albinism)
- Presence of smallpox vaccination site, psoriasis, or chronic discoid lupus erythematosus

Signs and symptoms
Characteristic findings in normal skin
—Nodule growing on a firm indurated base
—Possible ulceration at lesion site
Characteristic findings in transformation of a premalignant lesion
—Inflammation of preexisting lesion
—Induration of preexisting lesion
Other associated problems
If metastasis to regional lymph nodes occurs, the following symptoms are seen:
—Pain
—Malaise
—Fatigue
—Weakness
—Anorexia

Diagnostic tests
Excisional biopsy of the lesion confirms the diagnosis.

Treatment
The size, shape, location, and invasiveness of a squamous cell tumor and the condition of the underlying tissue determine the treatment method used. A deeply invasive tumor may require a combination of techniques. Depending on the lesion, treatment may consist of the following:
- Wide surgical excision
- Electrodesiccation and curettage. These offer good cosmetic results for smaller lesions.
- Radiation therapy. This is usually used for older or debilitated patients.
- Chemosurgery. This is reserved for resistant or recurrent lesions.

Clinical implications
The care plan for patients with squamous cell carcinoma should emphasize meticulous wound care, emotional support, and thorough patient instruction.
- Coordinate a consistent care plan for changing the patient's dressings. Establishing a standard routine helps the patient and family learn how to care for the wound.
- Keep the wound dry and clean.
- Try to control odor with balsam of Peru, yogurt flakes, oil of cloves, or other odor-masking substances, even though they are often ineffective for long-term use. Topical or systemic antibiotics also temporarily control odor and eventually alter the lesion's bacterial flora.
- Be prepared for other problems that accompany a metastatic disease (pain, fatigue, weakness, anorexia).
- Help the patient and family set realistic goals and expectations.
- Disfiguring lesions are distressing to both the patient and you. Try to accept the patient as he is and to increase his self-esteem and strengthen a caring relationship.

To prevent squamous cell carcinoma, tell patients to follow these guidelines:
- Avoid excessive sun exposure.

- Wear protective clothing (hats, long sleeves).
- Periodically examine the skin for precancerous lesions; have any removed promptly.
- Use strong sunscreening agents containing para-aminobenzoic acid (PABA), benzophenone, and zinc oxide. Apply these agents 30 to 60 minutes before sun exposure.
- Use lipscreens to protect the lips from sun damage.

Staphylococcal scalded skin syndrome

Description
A severe skin disorder, staphylococcal scalded skin syndrome (SSSS) is marked by epidermal erythema, peeling, and necrosis that give the skin a scalded appearance. SSSS is most prevalent in infants aged 1 to 3 months but may develop in children; it is uncommon in adults. This disease follows a consistent pattern of progression, and most patients recover fully. Mortality is 2% to 3%, with death usually resulting from complications.

Causes
Group 2 *Staphylococcus aureus,* primarily phage type 71

Mode of transmission
Direct contact of the *S. aureus* with cutaneous tissue

Risk factors
- Impaired immunity
- Renal insufficiency

Signs and symptoms
Cutaneous changes progress through three stages:
- Erythema. This becomes visible, usually around the mouth and other orifices, and may spread in widening circles over the entire body surface. The skin becomes tender; Nikolsky's sign (sloughing of the skin when friction is applied) may appear.
- Exfoliation (24 to 48 hours later). In the more common, localized form of this disease, superficial erosions and minimal crusting occur, usually around body orifices, and may spread to exposed areas of the skin. In the more severe forms, large, flaccid bullae erupt and may spread to cover extensive areas of the body. These bullae eventually rupture, revealing sections of denuded skin.
- Desquamation. In this final stage, affected areas dry up, and powdery scales form. Normal skin replaces these scales in 5 to 7 days.

Diagnostic tests
- Cultures of skin lesions revealing Group 2 *S. aureus* confirms the diagnosis.
- Exfoliative cytology and biopsy aid in differential diagnosis, ruling out erythema multiforme and drug-induced toxic epidermal necrolysis.

Treatment
Treatment includes systemic antibiotics—usually penicillinase-resistant penicillin—to prevent secondary infections, and replacement to maintain fluid and electrolyte balance.

Clinical implications
- Provide special care for the neonate, if required, including placement in a warming infant incubator to maintain body temperature and provide isolation.
- Carefully monitor intake and output to assess fluid and electrolyte balance. In severe cases, I.V. fluid replacement may be necessary.
- Check vital signs. Be especially alert for a sudden rise in temperature, indicating sepsis, which requires prompt, aggressive treatment.
- Maintain skin integrity. Use strict aseptic technique to preclude secondary infection, especially during the ex-

foliative stage, because of open lesions. To prevent friction and sloughing of the skin, leave affected areas uncovered or loosely covered. Place cotton between severely affected fingers and toes to prevent webbing.

• Administer warm baths and soaks during the recovery period. Gently debride exfoliated areas.

• Reassure parents that complications are rare and residual scars are unlikely.

Stereotyped movement disorders
(Tics)

Description
These disorders are spasmodic, purposeless, and involuntary movements of isolated groups of muscles. (See also *Tourette's Syndrome*.) Tics occur most frequently between ages 5 and 12. They may be transient or chronic.

Prognosis is good when treatment corrects the underlying psychopathology.

Causes
Overwhelming anxiety, usually associated with normal maturation in which the ego can no longer balance conflicting influences from desires and environment

Signs and symptoms
Usually, tics involve the facial muscles, causing frequent eye blinking, twitching of the mouth, and wrinkling of the forehead. These movements are recurrent, involuntary, and repetitive. Tics may also involve coughing, sniffling, or jerking head movements. Tics become more pronounced when the patient is anxious or under stress. Most patients can, with conscious effort, control them for short periods.

Treatment
Effective treatment requires an at-

Tourette's Syndrome

This syndrome, the most severe of the stereotyped movement disorders, is now thought to have an organic origin (unlike the rest of these disorders). It is marked by violent twitching or convulsive movements of the face, arms, and other body parts. These movements may be associated with bizarre vocalizations—explosive sounds, a loud, barking cough, or compulsive shouting of obscene words.

Treatment
Because Tourette's syndrome may reflect a neurologic abnormality, its treatment now includes psychotropic drugs as well as psychotherapy. Haloperidol (Haldol) has proven effective in controlling the tics and vocalizations.

Special considerations
Patients with this disorder suffer overwhelming embarrassment and guilt, since their bizarre behavior is likely to provoke sharp criticism.

• Offer such patients reassurance and emotional support. Explain to their families that their abnormal behavior is involuntary.

• Encourage these patients to seek medical attention and to continue drug treatment, as prescribed. Encourage them to contact the Tourette's Syndrome Association in Bayside, N.Y., for more information.

tempt to correct the underlying psychopathology by identifying and resolving the sources of the patient's anxiety, stress, and intrapsychic conflict. Without such an attempt, the patient can control tics only briefly—and then only with intense effort.

Clinical implications
Help the patient to identify and eliminate any avoidable stress and to learn positive new ways to deal with anxiety.

Stomatitis and other oral infections

Description
Stomatitis is an inflammation of the oral mucosa that may also extend to the buccal mucosa, lips, and palate. There are two main types: acute herpetic stomatitis and aphthous stomatitis. Acute herpetic stomatitis is usually self-limiting; however, it may be severe and, in newborns, may be generalized and potentially fatal. Aphthous stomatitis usually heals spontaneously in 10 to 14 days. Other oral infections include gingivitis, periodontitis, and Vincent's angina (see *Oral Infections,* p. 732.)

Causes
Acute herpetic stomatitis
—Herpesvirus
Aphthous stomatitis
Many predisposing factors can lead to this type of stomatitis:
—Stress
—Fatigue
—Anxiety
—Febrile states
—Trauma
—Solar overexposure

Signs and symptoms
Acute herpetic stomatitis
—Mouth pain
—Malaise
—Lethargy
—Anorexia
—Irritability
—Fever
—Swollen gums that bleed easily
—Tender mucous membranes
—Papulovesicular ulcers in mouth or throat that eventually become punched-out lesions with reddened areolae
—Possible submaxillary lymphadenitis
Aphthous stomatitis
—Burning of mucous membranes
—Tingling of mucous membranes
—Slight swelling of mucous membranes
—Single or multiple shallow ulcers (whitish centers and red borders) that heal at one site but then appear at another

Diagnostic tests
Smear of ulcer exudate identifies the causative organism in Vincent's angina.

Treatment and clinical implications
For acute herpetic stomatitis, treatment is conservative. For local symptoms, management includes warm-water mouth rinses (antiseptic mouthwashes are contraindicated because they are irritating) and a topical anesthetic to relieve mouth ulcer pain. Supplementary treatment includes bland or liquid diet and, in severe cases, I.V. fluids and bed rest.

For aphthous stomatitis, primary treatment is application of a topical anesthetic. Effective long-term treatment requires alleviation or prevention of precipitating factors.

Strabismus
(Squint, heterotropia, cross-eye, wall eye)

Description
In strabismus, the absence of normal, parallel, or coordinated eye movement results in eye malalignment. Strabis-

Oral Infections

DISEASE AND CAUSES	SIGNS AND SYMPTOMS
Gingivitis (inflammation of the gingiva) • Early sign of hypovitaminosis, diabetes, blood dyscrasias • Occasionally related to use of oral contraceptives	• Inflammation with painless swelling, redness, change of normal contours, bleeding, and periodontal pocket (gum detachment from teeth)
Periodontitis (progression of gingivitis; inflammation of the oral mucosa) • Early sign of hypovitaminosis, diabetes, blood dyscrasias • Occasionally related to use of oral contraceptives • Dental factors: calculus, poor oral hygiene, malocclusion. Major cause of tooth loss after middle age	• Acute onset of bright red gum inflammation, painless swelling of interdental papillae, easy bleeding • Loosening of teeth, typically without inflammatory symptoms, progressing to loss of teeth and alveolar bone • Acute systemic infection (fever, chills)
Vincent's angina (trench mouth, necrotizing ulcerative gingivitis) • Fusiform bacillus or spirochete infection • Predisposing factors: stress, poor oral hygiene, insufficient rest, nutritional deficiency, smoking	• Sudden onset: painful, superficial bleeding gingival ulcers (rarely, on buccal mucosa) covered with a gray-white membrane • Ulcers become punched out lesions after slight pressure or irritation. • Malaise, mild fever, excessive salivation, bad breath, pain on swallowing or talking, enlarged submaxillary lymph nodes
Glossitis (inflammation of the tongue) • Streptococcal infection • Irritation or injury; jagged teeth; illfitting dentures; biting during convulsions; alcohol; spicy foods; smoking; sensitivity to toothpaste or mouthwash • Vitamin B deficiency; anemia • Skin conditions: lichen planus, erythema multiforme, pemphigus vulgaris	• Reddened ulcerated or swollen tongue (may obstruct airway) • Painful chewing and swallowing • Speech difficulty • Painful tongue without inflammation

mus affects about 2% of the population, primarily children, and incidence is higher in persons with CNS disorders, such as cerebral palsy, mental retardation, and Down's syndrome. Prognosis for correction varies with the timing of treatment and the onset of the disease.

Causes
Unknown but may include congenital defect, trauma, or amblyopia (lazy eye) caused by hyperopia (farsightedness) or anisometropia (unequal refractive power)

TREATMENT

- Removal of irritating factors (calculus, faulty dentures)
- Good oral hygiene; regular dental checkups; vigorous chewing
- Oral or topical corticosteroids

- Scaling, root planing, and curettage for infection control
- Periodontal surgery to prevent recurrence
- Good oral hygiene, regular dental checkups, vigorous chewing

---

- Removal of devitalized tissue with ultrasonic cavitron
- Antibiotics (penicillin or erythromycin P.O.) for infection
- Analgesics, as needed
- Hourly mouth rinses (with equal amounts of hydrogen peroxide and warm water)
- Soft, nonirritating diet; rest; no smoking
- With treatment, improvement common within 24 hours

- Treatment of underlying cause
- Topical anesthetic mouthwash or systemic analgesics (aspirin and acetaminophen) for painful lesions
- Good oral hygiene; regular dental checkups; vigorous chewing
- Avoidance of hot, cold, or spicy foods, and alcohol

Signs and symptoms

- Malalignment of the eyes (esotropia [eyes deviate inward], exotropia [eyes deviate outward], hypertropia (eyes deviate upward), or hypotropia [eyes deviate downward])
- Diplopia
- Other visual disturbances

Diagnostic tests

- Visual acuity test evaluates the degree of visual defect.
- Hirschberg's method detects malalignment.
- Retinoscopy determines refractive error.
- Maddox rods test assesses specific muscle involvement.
- Convergence test shows distance at which convergence is sustained.
- Duction test reveals limitation of eye movement.
- Cover-uncover test demonstrates eye deviation and the rate of recovery to original alignment.
- Alternate-cover test shows intermittent or latent deviation.
- Neurologic examination determines whether condition is muscular or neurologic in origin and should be performed if the onset of strabismus is sudden or if the CNS is involved.

Treatment

Initial treatment depends on the type of strabismus. For strabismic amblyopia, therapy includes patching the normal eye and prescribing corrective glasses to keep the eye straight and to counteract farsightedness (especially in accommodative esotropia). Surgery is often necessary for cosmetic and psychological reasons to correct strabismus due to basic esotropia, or residual accommodative esotropia after correction with glasses. Timing of surgery varies with individual circumstances. For example, a 6-month-old infant with equal visual acuity and a large esotropia will have the deviation corrected surgically. But a child with unequal visual acuity and an acquired deviation will have the affected eye patched until visual acuity is equal, and then will undergo surgery.

Surgical correction includes recession (moving the muscle posteriorly from its original insertion) or resection (shortening the muscle). Postoperative therapy may include patching the

Teaching Topics in Strabismus

- Explanation of type and cause of strabismus
- Preparation for diagnostic tests such as eye examination, retinoscopy, and other scheduled tests
- Application of patch, if indicated
- Administration of eye drops/ointments, if indicated
- Pre- and postoperative instruction specific to recession or resection, if indicated
- Eye exercises, if indicated
- Follow-up care required

affected eye and applying combination antibiotic/steroid eye drops. Eye exercises and corrective glasses may still be necessary. Surgery may have to be repeated.

Clinical implications
- Postoperatively, discourage a child from rubbing his eyes.
- Gently wipe the child's tears, which will be serosanguineous. Parents may become upset by this aspect of surgery. Reassure them that this is normal.
- Administer antiemetics, if necessary.
- Apply antibiotic ointment to the affected eye.
- Because this surgery is usually a one-day procedure, most children are discharged after they recover from anesthesia. Encourage compliance with recommended follow-up care.

Complications
- Amblyopia occurs if strabismus develops early in life before bifocal fixation is established.
- Possible postoperative surgical complications include overcorrection or undercorrection, slipped muscle, and perforation of the globe. (See also *Teaching Topics in Strabismus*.)

Strongyloidiasis
(Threadworm infection)

Description
Strongyloidiasis is a parasitic intestinal infection occurring worldwide. It is endemic in the tropics and subtropics. Infection does not confer immunity, and, without treatment, autoinfection often occurs. Most patients with strongyloidiasis recover completely, but debilitation from protein loss is occasionally fatal.

Causes
The helminth *Strongyloides stercoralis*

Mode of transmission
- Skin contact (usually feet) with soil containing infective *S. stercoralis* filariform larvae
- In autoinfection, rhabdoid larvae mature within the intestine to become infective filariform larvae.

Signs and symptoms
The patient's resistance and the extent of infection determine the severity of symptoms.
- Erythematous maculopapular rash at the penetration site, with subsequent swelling and pruritus
- Typically, minor hemorrhages, pneumonitis, and pneumonia
- Frequent, watery, and bloody diarrhea, accompanied by intermittent abdominal pain

Diagnostic tests
- Stool specimen (fresh) revealing *S. stercoralis* larvae confirms the diagnosis.
- Sputum specimen during pulmonary phase may show many eosinophils and larvae.

- Serum eosinophils are increased in disseminated strongyloidiasis.
- Chest X-ray is positive during the pulmonary phase of infection.
- Hemoglobin is as low as 6 g.
- WBC count with differential shows eosinophils numbering 450 to 700/mm³.

Treatment
Because of potential autoinfection, treatment with thiabendazole is required for 2 to 3 days (total dose not to exceed 3 g). Patients also need protein replacement, blood transfusions, and I.V. fluids. Retreatment is necessary if *S. stercoralis* remains in stools after therapy. Glucocorticoids are contraindicated because they increase the risk of autoinfection and dissemination.

Clinical implications
- Keep accurate intake and output records, especially if treatment includes blood transfusions and I.V. fluids. Ask the dietary department to provide a high-protein diet. The patient may need tube feedings to increase caloric intake.
- Wear gloves when handling bedpans or giving perineal care, and dispose of feces promptly.
- Since direct person-to-person transmission does not occur, isolation is not required. Label stool specimens for laboratory as contaminated.
- Warn the patient that thiabendazole may cause mild nausea, vomiting, drowsiness, and giddiness.
- In pulmonary infection, reposition the patient frequently, encourage coughing and deep breathing, and administer oxygen, as ordered.
- To prevent reinfection, teach the patient proper hand-washing technique. Stress the importance of washing hands before eating and after defecating, and of wearing shoes when in endemic areas. Check the patient's family and close contacts for signs of infection. Emphasize the need for follow-up stool examination, continuing several weeks after treatment.

Complications
- Malnutrition
- Anemia
- Intestinal lesions resembling ulcerated colitis
- Intestinal perforation
- Possible potentially fatal dissemination
- Possible secondary bacterial infections

Stye
(Hordeolum)

Description
A localized, purulent staphylococcal infection, a stye can occur externally (in the lumen of the smaller glands of Zeis or in Moll's glands) or internally (in the larger meibomian gland). Usually, this infection responds well to treatment but tends to recur. If untreated, a stye can eventually lead to cellulitis of the eyelid.

Cause
Staphylococci

Mode of transmission
Direct contact of a staphylococcal organism with the lid glands of the eyes

Signs and symptoms
- Redness
- Swelling
- Pain
- Possible abscess formation (typically forms at the lid margin, with an eyelash pointing outward from its center)

Diagnostic tests
Culture of purulent material from the abscess revealing a staphylococcal organism confirms the diagnosis.

Treatment

Treatment consists of warm compresses applied for 10 to 15 minutes, 4 times a day for 3 to 4 days, to facilitate drainage of the abscess, to relieve pain and inflammation, and to promote suppuration. Drug therapy includes a topical sulfonamide or antibiotic eye drops or ointment and, occasionally, a systemic antibiotic. If conservative treatment fails, incision and drainage may be necessary.

Clinical implications

• Instruct the patient to use a clean cloth for each application of warm compresses and to dispose of it or launder it separately to prevent spreading this infection to family members. For the same reason, the patient should avoid sharing towels and washcloths.
• Warn against squeezing the stye. This spreads the infection and may cause cellulitis.
• Teach the patient or family members the proper technique for instilling eye drops or ointments into the cul-de-sac of the lower eyelid.

Sudden infant death syndrome
(Crib death)

Description

Sudden infant death syndrome (SIDS) is one of the leading causes of death in apparently healthy infants, usually between ages 4 weeks and 7 months, for unknown reasons. Typically, parents put the infant to bed and later find him dead, often with no indications of a struggle or distress of any kind. SIDS has occurred throughout history, all over the world, and in all climates.

Causes

Possibly an abnormality in the control of ventilation, which may be caused by undetected abnormalities such as an immature respiratory system and respiratory dysfunction

Risk factors

• Underweight
• Mother under age 20
• Poverty
• Seasonal (occurs most often in winter)
• History of apneic periods

Signs and symptoms

Depending upon how long the infant has been apneic, the following signs may be present:
• Mottled complexion, with extreme cyanosis of lips and fingertips
• Pooling of blood in legs and feet, which may be mistaken for bruises
• Absent pulse and respirations
• Diaper wet and full of stool
• Possibly frothy, blood-tinged sputum around mouth or on crib sheets
• Possible abnormal position or tangled blankets suggesting movement just before death

Treatment and clinical implications

If the parents bring the infant to the emergency room, the physician will decide whether to try to resuscitate him. Such an infant, successfully resuscitated, or any infant who had a sibling stricken by SIDS, should be tested for infantile apnea. If tests are positive, a home apnea monitor may be recommended. Since most infants cannot be resuscitated, however, treatment focuses on emotional support for the family.
• Make sure that both parents are present when the child's death is announced. The parents may lash out at emergency room personnel, the babysitter, or anyone else involved in the child's care—even at each other. Stay calm and let them express their feelings. Reassure them that they were not to blame.
• Let the parents see the baby in a private room. Allow them to express their grief in their own way. Stay in

the room with them, if appropriate. Offer to call clergy, friends, or relatives.

• After the parents and family have recovered from their initial shock, explain the necessity for an autopsy to confirm the diagnosis of SIDS (in some states, this is mandatory). At this time, provide the family with some basic facts about SIDS and encourage them to give their consent for the autopsy. Make sure they receive the autopsy report promptly.

• Find out whether there is a local counseling and information program for SIDS parents. Participants in such a program will contact the parents, ensure that they receive the autopsy report promptly, put them in touch with a professional counselor, and maintain supportive telephone contact. Also, find out whether there is a local SIDS parents' group. Such a group can provide significant emotional support. Contact the National Sudden Infant Death Foundation for information about such local groups.

• If your hospital's policy is to assign a public health nurse to the family, she will provide the continuing reassurance and assistance the parents will need.

• If the parents decide to have another child, they will need information and counseling to help them deal with the pregnancy and the first year of the new infant's life.

Syndrome of inappropriate antidiuretic hormone secretion (SIADH)

Description

Syndrome of Inappropriate Antidiuretic Hormone Secretion (SIADH) is a condition in which there is excessive release of ADH, which disturbs fluid and electrolyte balance. Such disturbances result from inability to excrete dilute urine, retention of free water, expansion of extracellular fluid volume, and hyponatremia. Prognosis depends on the underlying disorder and response to treatment.

Causes

SIADH occurs secondary to diseases that affect the osmoreceptors (supraoptic nucleus) of the hypothalamus.

Neoplastic diseases
—Oat cell carcinoma (the leading cause—80% of cases)
—Pancreatic cancer
—Prostatic cancer
—Hodgkin's disease
—Thymoma

CNS disorders
—Tumor or abscess
—Cerebrovascular accident
—Head injury
—Guillain-Barré syndrome
—Lupus erythematosus

Pulmonary disorders
—Pneumonia
—Tuberculosis
—Lung abscess
—Positive-pressure ventilation

Drugs
—Chlorpropamide
—Vincristine
—Cyclophosphamide
—Carbamazepine
—Clofibrate
—Morphine

Miscellaneous conditions
—Myxedema
—Psychosis

Signs and symptoms

• Weight gain
• Anorexia
• Nausea and vomiting
• Muscle weakness
• Restlessness
• Possible convulsions
• Possible coma
• Possible edema (rare—only if water overload exceeds 4 liters)

Diagnostic tests

Two tests are needed to confirm the diagnosis:

• Serum osmolality is less than 380 mOsm/kg of water.
• Serum sodium is less than 123 mEq/liter.

Treatment

Treatment for SIADH is symptomatic. It begins with restricted water intake (500 to 1,000 ml/day). With severe water intoxication, administration of 200 to 300 ml of 5% saline may be necessary to raise serum sodium level. When possible, treatment should include correction of the underlying cause of SIADH. If SIADH is due to cancer, success in alleviating water retention may be obtained by surgical resection, irradiation, or chemotherapy. If fluid restriction is ineffective, demeclocycline or lithium may help by blocking the renal response to ADH.

Clinical implications

• Closely monitor and record intake and output, vital signs, and daily weight. Watch for hyponatremia.
• Observe for restlessness, irritability, convulsions, congestive heart failure, and unresponsiveness due to hyponatremia and water intoxication.
• To prevent water intoxication, explain to the patient and his family why he *must* restrict his intake.

Syphilis

Description

Syphilis is a chronic, infectious, venereal disease that begins in the mucous membranes and quickly becomes systemic, spreading to nearby lymph nodes and the bloodstream. This disease, when untreated, is characterized by progressive stages: primary, secondary, latent, and late (formerly called tertiary). Syphilis is the third most prevalent reportable infectious disease in the United States. Incidence is highest among urban populations, especially in persons between ages 15 and 39. Untreated syphilis leads to crippling or death, but prognosis is excellent with early treatment.

Causes

The spirochete *Treponema pallidum*

Mode of transmission

• Sexual contact during the primary, secondary, and early latent stages of infection
• Prenatal transmission (see *Prenatal Syphilis.*)

Signs and symptoms

Primary syphilis
This applies to a period of 3 weeks following contact.
—Chancres (small, fluid-filled lesions on genitalia, anus, fingers, lips, tongue, nipples, tonsils, or eyelids that eventually erode and develop indurated, raised edges and clear bases)
—Possible regional lymphadenopathy (unilateral or bilateral)
Secondary syphilis
This applies to a period from a few days to 8 weeks after onset of initial chancres.
—Rash (macular, papular, pustular, or nodular)
—Symmetrical mucocutaneous lesions. Macules often erupt between rolls of fat on the trunk and, proximally, on the arms, palms, soles, face, and scalp. In warm, moist areas (perineum, scrotum, vulva, between rolls of fat), the lesions enlarge and erode, producing highly contagious, pink or grayish-white lesions (condylomata lata).
—General lymphadenopathy
—Mild constitutional symptoms such as headache, malaise, anorexia, weight loss, nausea, vomiting, and sore throat
—Brittle and pitted nails
—Possible low-grade fever
—Possible alopecia
Latent syphilis
This is characterized by an absence of clinical symptoms.

Prenatal Syphilis

A woman can transmit syphilis transplacentally to her unborn child throughout pregnancy. This type of syphilis is often called congenital, but prenatal is a more accurate term. Approximately 50% of infected fetuses die before or shortly after birth. Prognosis is better for infants who develop overt infection after age 2.

The infant with prenatal syphilis may appear healthy at birth, but usually develops characteristic lesions—vesicular, bullous eruptions, often on the palms and soles—3 weeks later. Shortly afterward, a maculopapular rash similar to that in secondary syphilis may erupt on the face, mouth, genitalia, palms, or soles. Condylomata lata often occur around the anus. Lesions may erupt on the mucous membranes of the mouth, pharynx, and nose. When the infant's larynx is affected, his cry becomes weak and forced. If the nasal mucous membranes are involved, he may also develop nasal discharge, which can be slight and mucopurulent or copious with blood-tinged pus. Visceral and bone lesions, liver or spleen enlargement with ascites, and nephrotic syndrome may also develop.

Late prenatal syphilis becomes apparent after age 2; it may be identifiable only through blood studies or may cause unmistakable syphilitic changes: screwdriver-shaped central incisors, deformed molars or cusps, thick clavicles, saber shins, bowed tibias, nasal septum perforation, eighth nerve deafness, and neurosyphilis.

In the infant with prenatal syphilis, VDRL titer, if reactive at birth, stays the same or rises, indicating active disease. The infant's titer drops in 3 months if the mother has received effective prenatal treatment. Absolute diagnosis necessitates dark-field examination of umbilical vein blood or lesion drainage.

An infant with abnormal CSF may be treated with aqueous crystalline penicillin G, I.M. or I.V., (50,000 units/kg of body weight/day divided in two doses for at least 10 days), or aqueous penicillin G procaine I.M. (50,000 units/kg of body weight/day for at least 10 days). An infant with normal CSF may be treated with a single injection of penicillin G benzathine (50,000 units/kg of body weight). When caring for a child with prenatal syphilis, record the extent of the rash, and watch for signs of systemic involvement, especially laryngeal swelling, jaundice, and decreasing urinary output.

Late syphilis

This applies to three subtypes: late benign syphilis, cardiovascular syphilis, and neurosyphilis. Any or all may be present. In late benign syphilis, the typical lesion is a gumma—a chronic superficial nodule or deep, granulomatous lesion that is solitary, asymmetric, painless, and indurated. Other symptoms of this subtype include the following:

—Possible liver involvement causing epigastric pain, tenderness, enlarged spleen, and anemia

—Possible upper respiratory involvement with potential perforation of the nasal septum or palate

In cardiovascular syphilis, symptoms may be absent, or the following may occur:

—Aortitis
—Aortic regurgitation
—Aortic aneurysm

In neurosyphilis, meningitis and widespread CNS damage typically occur. Symptoms of CNS damage include the following:

—General paresis
—Personality changes
—Arm and leg weakness

Diagnostic tests
• Culture of a lesion, identifying *T. pallidum*, provides immediate diagnosis in primary, secondary, and prenatal syphilis.
• The fluorescent treponemal antibody absorption (FTA-ABS) test identifies antigens of *T. pallidum* in tissue, ocular fluid, CSF, tracheobronchial secretions, and exudates from lesions in all stages of syphilis.
• Venereal Disease Research Laboratory (VDRL) slide test and rapid plasma reagin (RPR) test detect nonspecific antibodies.
• CSF examination identifies neurosyphilis when total protein level is above 40 mg/100 ml, VDRL slide test is reactive, and cell count exceeds five mononuclear cells/mm^3.

Treatment
Treatment of choice is administration of penicillin I.M. For early syphilis, treatment may consist of a single injection of penicillin G benzathine I.M. (2.4 million units). Syphilis of more than 1 year's duration should be treated with penicillin G benzathine I.M. (2.4 million units/week for 3 weeks).

Patients who are allergic to penicillin may be treated successfully with tetracycline or erythromycin (in either case, 500 mg P.O. four times a day for 15 days for early syphilis; 30 days, for late infections). Tetracycline is contraindicated in pregnant females.

Clinical implications
• Make sure the patient clearly understands the dosage schedule for medication.
• Stress the importance of completing the course of therapy even after symptoms subside.
• Check for history of drug sensitivity before administering the first dose. Promote rest and adequate nutrition.
• In secondary syphilis, keep lesions clean and dry. If they are draining, dispose of contaminated materials properly.

• In late syphilis, provide symptomatic care during prolonged treatment.
• In cardiovascular syphilis, check for signs of decreased cardiac output (decreased urinary output, hypoxia, decreased sensorium) and pulmonary congestion.
• In neurosyphilis, regularly check level of consciousness, mood, and coherence. Watch for signs of ataxia.
• Urge patients to seek VDRL testing after 3, 6, 12, and 24 months to detect possible relapse. Patients treated for latent or late syphilis should receive blood tests at 6-month intervals for 2 years.
• Be sure to report all cases of syphilis to local public health authorities. Urge the patient to inform sexual partners of his infection so they can receive treatment.

Systemic lupus erythematosus

Description
A chronic inflammatory disorder of the connective tissue, systemic lupus erythematosus (SLE) affects multiple organ systems (as well as the skin) and can be fatal. SLE is characterized by recurring remissions and exacerbations. Exacerbations are especially common during the spring and summer. The annual incidence of SLE averages 75 cases per 1 million people. It strikes women 8 times as often as men, increasing to 15 times as often during childbearing years. SLE occurs worldwide but is most prevalent among Asians and blacks. Prognosis improves with early detection and treatment but remains poor for patients who develop cardiovascular, renal, or neurologic complications or severe bacterial infections.

Cause
Evidence points to interrelated im-

munologic, environmental, hormonal, and genetic factors.

Risk factors
- Genetic predisposition
- Physical or mental stress
- Streptococcal or viral infections
- Exposure to sunlight or ultraviolet light
- Immunization
- Pregnancy
- Abnormal estrogen metabolism
- Medications such as procainamide, hydralazine, anticonvulsants, and, less frequently, penicillins, sulfa drugs, and oral contraceptives

Signs and symptoms
Characteristic findings
—Facial erythema (butterfly rash)
—Nonerosive arthritis
—Photosensitivity
Potential findings
—Discoid rash
—Oral or nasopharyngeal ulcerations
—Pleuritis
—Pericarditis
—Seizures
—Psychoses
—Patchy alopecia
Constitutional symptoms
—Aching
—Malaise
—Fatigue
—Low-grade or spiking fever
—Chills
—Anorexia
—Weight loss
—Lymph node enlargement
—Abdominal pain
—Nausea and vomiting
—Diarrhea or constipation
—Irregular menstrual periods or amenorrhea

Diagnostic tests
- Antinuclear antibody (ANA), anti-DNA, and lupus erythematosus (LE) cell tests are the most specific tests for SLE in most patients with active disease.

Teaching Topics in SLE

- Explanation of the disorder, including its unpredictable exacerbations and remissions
- Prevention of complications
- Need for repeated diagnostic tests
- Corticosteroids or other prescribed drugs
- Avoiding fatigue and balancing rest and activity
- Apheresis to treat life-threatening complications and acute flare-ups, if necessary
- Measures to prevent infection and skin breakdown
- Avoiding sun and cold exposure
- Stress-reduction techniques

- CBC with differential may show anemia and decreased WBC count.
- Platelet count may be decreased.
- Erythrocyte sedimentation rate may be elevated.
- Serum electrophoresis may show hypergammaglobulinemia.
- Urine studies may show RBCs and WBCs, urine casts and sediment, and significant protein loss (more than 3.5 g/24 hours).
- Blood studies showing decreased serum complement (C3 and C4) levels indicate active disease.
- Chest X-ray may show pleurisy or lupus pneumonitis.
- EKG may show conduction defect with cardiac involvement or pericarditis.
- Kidney biopsy determines disease stage and extent of renal involvement.

Treatment
Patients with mild disease require little or no medication. Nonsteroidal anti-inflammatory compounds, including aspirin, often control arthritis symp-

toms. Skin lesions need topical treatment. Corticosteroid creams, such as flurandrenolide, are recommended for acute lesions.

Refractory skin lesions are treated with intralesional corticosteroids or antimalarials, such as hydroxychloroquine and chloroquine. Because these two drugs can cause retinal damage, such treatment requires ophthalmologic examination every 6 months.

Corticosteroids remain the treatment of choice for systemic symptoms of SLE, for acute generalized exacerbations, or for serious disease related to vital organ systems, such as pleuritis, pericarditis, lupus nephritis, vasculitis, and CNS involvement. Initial doses equivalent to 60 mg or more of prednisone often bring noticeable improvement within 48 hours. As soon as symptoms are under control, steroid dosage is tapered slowly. Diffuse proliferative glomerulonephritis, a major complication of SLE, requires treatment with large doses of steroids. If renal failure occurs, dialysis or kidney transplant may be necessary. In some patients, cytotoxic drugs—such as azathioprine and cyclophosphamide—may delay or prevent deteriorating renal status. Antihypertensive drugs and dietary changes may also be warranted in renal disease.

The photosensitive patient should wear protective clothing (hat, sunglasses, long sleeves, slacks) and use a screening agent containing para-aminobenzoic acid when in the sun.

Clinical Implications

Careful assessment, supportive measures, emotional support, and patient teaching are all important parts of the care plan for patients with SLE.

• Watch for constitutional symptoms: joint pain or stiffness, weakness, fever, fatigue, and chills.

• Observe for dyspnea, chest pain, and edema of the extremities.

• Note the size, type, and location of skin lesions.

• Check urine for hematuria, scalp for hair loss, and skin and mucous membranes for petechiae, bleeding, ulceration, pallor, and bruising.

• Provide a balanced diet. Renal involvement may mandate a low-sodium, low-protein diet.

• Urge the patient to get plenty of rest. Schedule diagnostic tests and procedures to allow adequate rest. Explain all tests and procedures. Tell the patient that several blood samples are needed initially, then periodically, to monitor progress.

• Apply heat packs to relieve joint pain and stiffness. Encourage regular exercise to maintain full range of motion and prevent contractures. Teach range-of-motion exercises, as well as body alignment and postural techniques. Arrange for physical therapy and occupational counseling, as appropriate.

• Explain the expected benefit of prescribed medications, and watch for side effects, especially when the patient is taking high doses of corticosteroids.

• Monitor vital signs, intake and output, weight, and laboratory reports closely. Check pulse rates regularly, and observe for orthopnea. Check stools and GI secretions for blood.

• Observe for hypertension, weight gain, and other signs of renal involvement.

• Assess for signs of neurologic damage: personality change, paranoid or psychotic behavior, ptosis, or diplopia. Take seizure precautions. If Raynaud's phenomenon is present, warm and protect the patient's hands and feet.

• Support the female patient's self-image by offering helpful cosmetic tips, such as suggesting the use of hypoallergenic makeup, and by referring her to a hairdresser who specializes in scalp disorders. Encourage her to take an interest in her appearance.

• Advise the patient to purchase medications in quantity, if possible. Warn against "miracle" drugs for relief of arthritis symptoms.

• Refer the patient to the Lupus Foundation of America and the Arthritis Foundation, as necessary.

• Reassure a woman with SLE that she can have a safe, successful pregnancy if she has no serious renal or neurologic impairment.

Complications

• Vasculitis, possibly leading to infarctive lesions, necrotic leg ulcers, or digital gangrene

• Raynaud's phenomenon

• Cardiopulmonary abnormalities such as myocarditis, endocarditis, tachycardia, parenchymal infiltrates, and pneumonitis

• Renal abnormalities such as hematuria, urinary tract infections, and kidney failure

• CNS abnormalities such as emotional instability, organic brain syndrome, headache, irritability, and depression (See also *Teaching Topics in SLE*, p. 741.)

T

Taeniasis
(Tapeworm disease, cestodiasis)

Description
Taeniasis is a parasitic infestation. It is usually a chronic, benign intestinal disease; however, infestation with the parasite *Taenia solium* may cause dangerous systemic and CNS symptoms if larvae invade the brain and striated muscle of vital organs.

Causes
• *Taenia saginata* (beef tapeworm)
• *Taenia solium* (pork tapeworm)
• *Diphyllobothrium latum* (fish tapeworm)
• *Hymenolepis nana* (dwarf tapeworm)

Mode of transmission
• Ingestion of uncooked or undercooked beef, pork, or fish that contains tapeworm *T. saginata*, *T. solium*, or *D. latum* cysts
• Direct from person to person via *H. nana* ova passed in stool

Signs and symptoms
T. saginata
—Crawling sensation in the perianal area
—Intestinal obstruction
—Appendicitis
T. solium
—Seizures
—Headaches
—Personality changes
D. latum
—Anemia (hemoglobin as low as 6 g)
H. nana
Dependent on patient's nutritional status and number of parasites, mild infestation may cause no symptoms. Severe infestation causes the following symptoms:
—Anorexia
—Diarrhea
—Restlessness
—Dizziness
—Apathy

Diagnostic tests
Stool specimen containing tapeworm ova or body segments confirms the diagnosis.

Treatment
Treatment with niclosamide offers a cure in up to 95% of patients. In beef, pork, and fish tapeworm infestation, the drug is given once; in severe dwarf tapeworm infestation, twice (5 to 7 days each spaced 2 weeks apart).

In beef tapeworm disease, absence of strobilae (multiple tapeworm segments) in feces within 2 to 3 hours after such treatment necessitates administration of a laxative. During treatment for pork tapeworm, a laxative or induced vomiting is contraindicated because of the danger of autoinfection and systemic disease. After drug treatment, all types of tapeworm infestation require follow-up stool specimens during the next 3 to 5 weeks to check for remaining ova or worm segments. Persistent infestation often requires a second course of medication.

Clinical implications

• Obtain a complete history, including recent travel to endemic areas, dietary habits, and physical symptoms.
• Dispose of the patient's excretions carefully. Wear gloves when giving personal care and handling fecal excretions, bedpans, and bed linens. Wash your hands thoroughly and instruct the patient to do the same.
• Tell the patient not to consume anything after midnight on the day niclosamide therapy is to start. The drug must be given on an empty stomach. After administering the drug, document passage of strobilae.
• In pork tapeworm infestation, use enteric and secretion precautions. Avoid procedures and drugs that may cause vomiting or gagging. If the patient is a child or is incontinent, he requires a private room. Obtain a list of contacts.
• Document level of consciousness, and report any changes immediately. If CNS symptoms appear, keep an artificial airway or padded tongue blade close at hand, raise side rails, keep the bed low, and help with walking, as needed.
• To prevent reinfection, teach proper hand-washing technique and the need to cook meat and fish thoroughly. Stress the need for follow-up evaluations to monitor the success of therapy and to detect possible reinfection.

Tay-Sachs disease
(Amaurotic familial idiocy)

Description

The most common of the lipid storage diseases, Tay-Sachs disease produces progressive mental and motor deterioration. It is quite rare, although it strikes persons of Ashkenazic Jewish ancestry about 100 times more often than the general population. About 1 in 30 such persons are heterozygous carriers of this defective gene. If two such carriers have children, each of their offspring has a 25% chance of having Tay-Sachs disease. It is always fatal, usually before age 5.

Causes

Congenital deficiency of the enzyme hexosaminidase A

Risk factors

• Ashkenazic Jewish ancestry
• Familial history of the disease

Signs and symptoms

Newborn
—Possible exaggerated Moro reflex
3 to 6 months
—Apathy
—Responds to loud noises only
—Increasing physical and mental deterioration
—Progressive vision loss
6 to 18 months
—Deafness
—Blindness
—Seizures
—Generalized paralysis and spasticity
—Dilated pupils, unreactive to light
18 months to 2 years
—Decerebrate rigidity
—Complete vegetative state
2 years to death
—Recurrent bronchopneumonia
—Persistent complete vegetative state

Diagnostic tests

• Enzyme analysis showing deficient hexosaminidase A is the key to diagnosis.
• Ophthalmic examination showing optic nerve atrophy and a distinctive cherry-red spot on the retina further supports the diagnosis.

Treatment

Tay-Sachs disease has no known cure. Supportive treatment includes tube feedings using nutritional supplements, suctioning and postural drainage to remove pharyngeal secretions, skin care to prevent decubiti once the patient is bedridden, and mild laxatives to relieve neurogenic constipation. Unfortunately, anticonvulsants usually fail to prevent seizures. Because patients need round-the-clock physical care, parents often place them in long-term special-care facilities.

Clinical implications

The most important nursing action is to help the family deal with inevitably progressive illness and death.

• Refer parents for genetic counseling, and stress the importance of amniocentesis in future pregnancies. Refer siblings for screening to determine if they are carriers. If they are adult carriers, refer them for genetic counseling, but stress that there is no danger of transmitting the disease to offspring if they do not marry another carrier.

• Because parents may feel excessive stress or guilt due to their child's illness and the emotional and financial burden it places on them, refer them for psychological counseling if indicated.

• If parents care for their child at home, teach them how to do suctioning, postural drainage, and tube feeding. Also teach them how to give good skin care to prevent decubiti.

• For more information on this disease, refer parents to the National Tay-Sachs and Allied Diseases Association, Inc.

Tendinitis and bursitis

Description

Tendinitis is a painful inflammation of tendons and of tendon-muscle attachments to bone, usually in the shoulder rotator cuff, hip, Achilles' tendon, or hamstring. A form of tendinitis, calcific dendritis, produces proximal

weakness. Bursitis is a painful inflammation of one or more of the bursae—closed sacs that contain small amounts of synovial fluid and facilitate the motion of muscles and tendons over bony prominences. Bursitis usually occurs in the subdeltoid, olecranon, trochanteric, calcaneal, or prepatellar bursae. Bursitis may be septic, calcific, acute, or chronic.

Causes

Tendinitis
—Trauma
—Musculoskeletal disorders such as rheumatic diseases and congenital defects
—Postural misalignment
—Abnormal body development
—Hypermobility

Acute and chronic bursitis
—Recurring trauma that stresses or pressures a joint
—Inflammatory joint disease (rheumatoid arthritis, gout)

Septic bursitis
—Wound infection
—Bacterial invasion of skin over the bursa

Signs and symptoms

Tendinitis
—Restricted shoulder movement, especially abduction
—Localized pain. Typically this is most severe at night. It extends from the acromion to the deltoid muscle insertion when the arm is abducted between 50° and 130°.
—Swelling
—Adverse reaction to heat. Pain is intensified rather than relieved.

Calcific tendinitis
—Proximal weakness
—Possible acute calcific bursitis

Bursitis
—Irritation at site
—Inflammation at site
—Pain
—Limited movement

Diagnostic tests
Tendinitis
—X-rays may show bony fragments, osteophyte sclerosis, or calcium deposits.
—Arthrography may show occasional small irregularities on the undersurface of the tendon.
Bursitis
—X-rays may show calcium deposits in calcific bursitis.

Treatment
Treatment to relieve pain includes resting the joint (by immobilization with a sling, splint, or cast), systemic analgesics, application of cold or heat, ultrasound, or local injection of an anesthetic and corticosteroids to reduce inflammation. A mixture of a corticosteroid and an anesthetic, such as lidocaine, usually provides immediate pain relief. Extended-release injections of a corticosteroid, such as triamcinolone or prednisolone, offer longer pain relief. Until the patient is free of pain and able to perform range-of-motion exercises easily, treatment also includes oral anti-inflammatory agents, such as sulindac and indomethacin. Short-term analgesics include codeine, propoxyphene, acetaminophen with codeine, and, occasionally, oxycodone.

Supplementary treatment includes fluid removal by aspiration, physical therapy to preserve motion and prevent frozen joints (improvement usually follows in 1 to 4 weeks), and heat therapy (for calcific tendinitis, ice packs). Rarely, calcific tendinitis requires surgical removal of calcium deposits. Long-term control of chronic bursitis and tendinitis may require changes in life-style to prevent recurring joint irritation.

Clinical implications
• Assess the severity of pain and the range of motion to determine effectiveness of the treatment.

• Before injecting corticosteroids or local anesthetics, ask the patient about his drug allergies.
• Assist with intraarticular injection. Scrub the patient's skin thoroughly with povidone-iodine or a comparable solution, and shave the injection site, if necessary. After the injection, massage the area to ensure penetration through the tissue and joint space. Apply ice intermittently for about 4 hours to minimize pain. Avoid applying heat to the area for 2 days.

Because patient teaching is essential, tell the patient to follow these guidelines:
• Take anti-inflammatory agents with milk to minimize GI distress, and report any signs of distress immediately.
• Perform strengthening exercises and avoid activities that aggravate the joint.
• Wear a triangular sling during the first few days of an attack of subdeltoid bursitis or tendinitis to support the arm and protect the shoulder, particularly at night. (Demonstrate how to wear the sling so it will not put too much weight on the shoulder. Instruct the patient's family how to pin the sling or how to tie a square knot that will lie flat on the back of the patient's neck. To protect the shoulder during sleep, a splint may be worn instead of a sling. Instruct the patient to remove the splint during the day.)
• Maintain joint mobility and prevent muscle atrophy by performing exercises or physical therapy when he is free of pain.

Testicular cancer

Description
Malignant testicular tumors primarily affect young to middle-aged adults and are the leading cause of death from solid tumors in men between the ages of 15 and 34. In testicular tumors occurring in children (which are rare),

---

Staging Testicular Cancer

Staging work-up in testicular cancer combines surgical evaluation with pathologic staging. Usually, it includes testicular and tumor resection with lymph node dissection (especially inguinal exploration) to determine nodal involvement.

Stage I: Tumor confined to one testis, with no clinical or radiographic evidence of extratesticular spread

Stage II: Cancer metastasized to regional lymph nodes but not beyond

Stage III: Metastasis beyond regional nodes, usually to abdominal, mediastinal, supraclavicular, or pulmonary nodes

---

50% are detectable before age 5. With few exceptions, testicular tumors are of gonadal cell origin.

Prognosis varies with the cancer cell type and staging (see *Staging Testicular Cancer*). When treated with surgery and radiation, 100% of patients with Stage I or II seminomas and 90% of those with Stage I nonseminomas survive beyond 5 years. Prognosis is poor if this disease is advanced beyond Stage II at diagnosis.

Causes
Unknown

Risk factors
• History of cryptorchidism (even when this condition has been surgically corrected)
• Caucasian race

Signs and symptoms
• Firm, painless, smooth testicular mass
• Testicular heaviness
• Possible gynecomastia and nipple tenderness
• Possible ureteral obstruction, abdominal mass, cough, hemoptysis, shortness of breath, weight loss, fatigue, pallor, and lethargy in late stages—with lymph node involvement and distant metastases

Diagnostic tests
Several tests may be used together to confirm the diagnosis:

• Intravenous pyelography (detects ureteral deviation resulting from paraaortic node involvement)
• Urinary or serum luteinizing hormone levels
• Lymphangiography followed by ultrasound examination
• Hematologic workup, including CBC
• Testicular biopsy (verifies tumor cell type—essential for effective treatment)

Treatment
Treatment includes surgery, radiation, and chemotherapy. The intensity of therapy varies with tumor cell type and staging. Surgery includes orchiectomy and retroperitoneal node dissection to prevent extension of the disease and to aid in staging. Most surgeons remove just the testis, not the scrotum, which allows for a prosthetic testicular implant at a later date. Hormone replacement may be necessary to supplement depleted hormonal levels, especially after bilateral orchiectomy.

Treatment of seminomas involves postoperative radiation to the retroperitoneal and homolateral iliac nodes and, in patients with retroperitoneal extension, prophylactic radiation to the mediastinal and supraclavicular nodes. In nonseminomas, treatment includes radiation to all positive nodes.

Chemotherapy is essential in patients with large abdominal or mediastinal nodes and frank distant metastases or in others at high risk of developing metastases. Cyclophosphamide produces excellent results in seminomas. Combinations of vinblastine, doxorubicin, bleomycin, cisplatin, and vindesine are effective in nonseminomas.

Clinical implications

Begin to develop a care plan as soon as the diagnosis is made. Care should emphasize dealing with the patient's psychological response to the disease, preventing postoperative complications, and minimizing and controlling the side effects of radiation and chemotherapy. The young patient with testicular cancer faces difficult treatment and fears sexual impairment and disfigurement.

Before orchiectomy, follow these guidelines:
• Encourage the patient to talk about his fears. Try to establish a trusting relationship so that he feels comfortable asking questions.
• Give reassurance that sterility and impotence do not follow unilateral orchiectomy. Explain that synthetic hormones can supplement depleted hormonal levels. Inform the patient that most surgeons do not remove the scrotum, and that implant of a testicular prosthesis can correct disfigurement.

After orchiectomy, follow these guidelines:
• For the first day after surgery, apply an ice pack to the scrotum and provide analgesics, as ordered.
• Check for excessive bleeding, swelling, and signs of infection.
• Provide a scrotal athletic supporter to minimize pain during ambulation.
• During chemotherapy, know what side effects to expect and how to prevent or ease them. Give antiemetics, as needed, to prevent severe nausea and vomiting, and small, frequent feedings to maintain oral intake despite anorexia. Develop a good mouth care regimen, and check for stomatitis. Watch for signs of myelosuppression.
• If the patient receives vinblastine, assess for neurotoxicity (manifested by such symptoms as peripheral paresthesias, jaw pain, and muscle cramps).
• If he receives cisplatin, check for ototoxicity.
• To prevent renal damage, increase fluid intake, give I.V. hydration, as ordered, with a potassium supplement, and provide diuresis, as ordered, with furosemide or mannitol.

Testicular torsion

Description

Testicular torsion is an abnormal twisting of the spermatic cord. This condition is almost always (90%) unilateral. Testicular torsion is most common between ages 12 and 18, but it may occur at any age. Prognosis is good with early detection and prompt treatment. If untreated, eventual infarction of the testis will occur.

Causes

Intravaginal torsion
—Abnormality of the tunica in which the testis is abnormally positioned
—Narrowing of the mesentery support
Extravaginal torsion
—Loose attachment of the tunica vaginalis to the scrotal line, causing spermatic cord rotation
—Sudden forceful contraction of the cremaster muscle (possible precipitating factor)

Signs and symptoms

Excruciating pain in the affected testis or iliac fossa is the characteristic symptom.

Diagnostic tests

Doppler ultrasonography helps distinguish testicular torsion from strangulated hernia, undescended testes, or epididymitis.

Treatment
Treatment consists of immediate surgical repair by orchiopexy (fixation of a viable testis to the scrotum) or orchiectomy (excision of a nonviable testis).

Clinical implications
• Promote the patient's comfort before and after surgery.
• After surgery, administer pain medication, as ordered. Monitor voiding, and apply an ice bag with a cover, to reduce edema. Protect the wound from contamination. Otherwise, allow the patient to perform as many normal daily activities as possible.

Tetanus
(Lockjaw)

Description
Tetanus is an acute exotoxin-mediated infection. Usually, it is systemic; less often, localized. Tetanus is fatal in up to 60% of unimmunized persons, usually within 10 days of onset. When symptoms develop within 3 days after exposure, the prognosis is poor. Tetanus occurs worldwide, but it is more prevalent in agricultural regions and developing countries that lack mass immunization programs.

Causes
The anaerobic, spore-forming, gram-positive bacillus *Clostridium tetani*

Mode of transmission
• Puncture wound contaminated by soil, dust, or animal excreta containing *C. tetani*
• Burns and minor wounds
• Unhealed umbilical cord in an infant delivered under unsterile conditions when the mother is not immunized

Signs and symptoms
Localized tetanus
—Spasm
—Increased muscle tone near the wound
Generalized tetanus
—Marked muscle hypertonicity
—Hyperactive deep-tendon reflexes
—Tachycardia
—Profuse sweating
—Low-grade fever
—Painful, involuntary muscle contractions (may include neck, facial, and somatic muscles)
—Intermittent tonic convulsions
Neonatal tetanus
—Difficulty in sucking (progresses to inability to suck 3 to 10 days after birth)
—Excessive crying
—Irritability
—Nuchal rigidity

Diagnostic tests
Culture of wound identifies *C. tetani* in only one third of patients. Often, diagnosis must rest on clinical features, a history of trauma, and lack of tetanus immunization.

Treatment
Within 72 hours after a puncture wound, a patient who has not been immunized first requires tetanus immune globulin (TIG) or tetanus antitoxin to confer temporary protection. Next, he needs active immunization with tetanus toxoid. A patient who has not received tetanus immunization within 5 years needs a booster injection of tetanus toxoid.

If tetanus develops despite immediate postinjury treatment, the patient will require airway maintenance and a muscle relaxant, such as diazepam, to decrease muscle rigidity and spasm. If muscle contractions are not relieved by muscle relaxants, a neuromuscular blocker may be needed. The patient with tetanus needs high-dose antibiotics (penicillin administered I.V., if he is not allergic to it).

Clinical implications
When caring for the tetanus victim, follow these guidelines:
• Thoroughly debride and cleanse the injury site with 3% hydrogen peroxide, and check the patient's immunization history. Record the cause of injury. If it is a dog bite, report the case to local public health authorities.
• Before giving penicillin and TIG, antitoxin, or toxoid, obtain an accurate history of allergies to immunizations or penicillin. If the patient has a history of any allergies, keep epinephrine 1:1,000 and resuscitative equipment available.
• Stress the importance of maintaining active immunization with a booster dose of tetanus toxoid every 10 years.
    After tetanus develops, follow these guidelines:
• Maintain an adequate airway and ventilation to prevent pneumonia and atelectasis. Suction often and watch for signs of respiratory distress. Keep emergency airway equipment on hand, because the patient may require artificial ventilation or oxygen administration.
• Maintain an I.V. line for medications and emergency care, if necessary.
• Monitor EKG frequently for dysrhythmias. Accurately record intake and output, and check vital signs often.
• Turn the patient frequently to prevent bedsores and pulmonary stasis.
• Since even minimal external stimulation provokes muscle spasms, keep the patient's room dark and quiet. Warn visitors not to upset or overly stimulate the patient.
• If urinary retention develops, insert an indwelling (Foley) catheter.
• Give muscle relaxants and sedatives, as ordered, and schedule patient care to coincide with heaviest sedation.
• Insert an artificial airway, if necessary, to prevent tongue injury and maintain airway during spasms.
• Provide adequate nutrition to meet the patient's increased metabolic needs. The patient may need nasogastric feedings or hyperalimentation.

Complications
• Atelectasis
• Pneumonia
• Pulmonary emboli
• Acute gastric ulcers
• Flexion contractures
• Cardiac dysrhythmias

Tetralogy of Fallot

Description
Tetralogy of Fallot is a complex of four cardiac defects: ventricular septal defect (VSD), right ventricular outflow tract obstruction (pulmonary stenosis), right ventricular hypertrophy, and dextroposition of the aorta, with overriding of the VSD. Blood shunts right to left through the VSD, permitting unoxygenated blood to mix with oxygenated blood, resulting in cyanosis. Tetralogy of Fallot sometimes coexists with other congenital heart defects, such as patent ductus arteriosus or atrial septal defect. It accounts for about 10% of all congenital heart disease and occurs equally in boys and girls. Before surgical advances made correction possible, approximately one third of these children died in infancy.

Causes
Unknown, but the disorder results from embryologic hypoplasia of the outflow tract of the right ventricle.

Risk factors
• Fetal alcohol syndrome
• Ingestion of thalidomide by mother during pregnancy

Signs and symptoms
Symptoms vary with the degree of pulmonary stenosis, interacting with VSD size and location.
Characteristic symptoms in infants
—Cyanosis (the hallmark)
—Dyspnea

—Deep, sighing respirations
—Bradycardia
—Fainting
—Seizures
—Loss of consciousness

Possible symptoms in older children
—Clubbing
—Diminished exercise tolerance
—Increasing dyspnea on exertion
—Growth retardation
—Eating difficulties
—Squatting position when short of breath

Diagnostic tests

• Chest X-ray may demonstrate decreased pulmonary vascular marking and a boot-shaped cardiac silhouette.
• EKG shows right ventricular hypertrophy, right axis deviation, and possibly right atrial hypertrophy.
• Echocardiography identifies septal overriding of the aorta, the VSD, and pulmonary stenosis, and detects the hypertrophied walls of the right ventricle.
• Laboratory findings reveal diminished arterial oxygen saturation and polycythemia (hematocrit may be more than 60%) if the cyanosis is severe and long-standing.
• Cardiac catheterization confirms the diagnosis by visualizing pulmonary stenosis, VSD, and the overriding aorta and by ruling out other cyanotic heart defects. (Oxygen saturation in aortic blood can be measured during catheterization.)

Treatment

Effective management of tetralogy of Fallot necessitates prevention and treatment of complications, measures to relieve cyanosis, and palliative or corrective surgery. During cyanotic spells, the knee-chest position and administration of oxygen and morphine improve oxygenation. Propranolol (a beta-adrenergic blocking agent) may prevent hypoxic spells.

Palliative surgery is performed on infants with potentially fatal hypoxic spells. The goal of surgery is to enhance blood flow to the lungs to reduce hypoxia; this is often accomplished by joining the subclavian artery to the pulmonary artery (Blalock-Taussig procedure). Supportive measures include prophylactic antibiotics to prevent infective endocarditis or cerebral abscess administered before, during, and after bowel, bladder, or any other surgery or dental treatments. Management may also include phlebotomy in children with polycythemia.

Complete corrective surgery to relieve pulmonary stenosis and close the VSD, directing left ventricular outflow to the aorta, requires cardiopulmonary bypass with hypothermia to decrease oxygen utilization during surgery, especially in young children. An infant may have this corrective surgery without prior palliative surgery. It is usually done when progressive hypoxia and polycythemia impair the quality of his life, rather than at a specific age. However, most children require surgery before they reach school age.

Clinical implications

• Explain tetralogy of Fallot to the parents. Inform them that their child will set his own exercise limits and will know when to rest. Make sure they understand that their child can engage in physical activity, and advise them not to be overprotective.
• Teach parents to recognize serious hypoxic spells, which can cause such signs as dramatically increased cyanosis; deep, sighing respirations; and loss of consciousness. Tell them to place their child in the knee-chest position and to report such spells immediately. Emergency treatment may be necessary.
• To prevent infective endocarditis and other infections, warn parents to keep their child away from persons with infections. Urge them to encourage good dental hygiene, and tell them to watch for ear, nose, and throat infections and dental caries, all of which necessitate

immediate treatment. When dental care, infections, or surgery requires prophylactic antibiotics, tell parents to make sure the child completes the prescribed regimen.

• If the child requires medical attention for an unrelated problem, advise the parents to inform the physician immediately of the child's history of tetralogy of Fallot, since any treatment must take this serious heart defect into consideration.

• During hospitalization, alert the staff to the child's condition. Because of the right-to-left shunt through the VSD, treat I.V. lines like arterial lines. Remember, a clot dislodged from a catheter tip in a vein can cross the VSD and cause cerebral embolism. The same thing can happen if air enters the venous lines.

After palliative surgery, follow these guidelines:

• Monitor oxygenation and arterial blood gas (ABG) values closely in the ICU.

• If the child has undergone the Blalock-Taussig procedure, do not use the arm on the operative side for measuring blood pressure, inserting I.V. lines, or drawing blood samples, because blood perfusion on this side diminishes greatly until collateral circulation develops. Note this on the child's chart and at his bedside.

After corrective surgery, follow these guidelines:

• Watch for right bundle branch block or more serious disturbances of atrioventricular conduction and for ventricular ectopic beats.

• Be alert for other postoperative complications, such as bleeding, right ventricular failure, and respiratory failure. After surgery, transient congestive heart failure is common and may require treatment with digoxin and diuretics.

• Monitor left atrial pressure directly. A pulmonary artery catheter may also be used to check central venous and pulmonary artery pressures.

• Frequently check color and vital signs. Obtain ABG measurements regularly to assess oxygenation. As needed, suction to prevent atelectasis and pneumonia. Monitor mechanical ventilation.

• Monitor and record intake and output accurately.

• If atrioventricular block develops with a low heart rate, a temporary external pacemaker may be necessary.

• If blood pressure or cardiac output is inadequate, catecholamines may be ordered by continuous I.V. infusion. To decrease left ventricular workload, administer nitroprusside, if ordered. Provide analgesics, as needed.

• Keep the parents informed about their child's progress. After discharge, the child may require digoxin, diuretics, and other drugs. Stress the importance of complying with the prescribed regimen, and make sure the parents know how and when to administer these medications. Teach parents to watch for signs of digitalis toxicity (anorexia, nausea, vomiting). Prophylactic antibiotics to prevent infective endocarditis will still be required.

• Advise the parents to avoid becoming overprotective as the child's tolerance for physical activity rises.

Complications

• Cerebral abscesses
• Pulmonary thrombosis
• Venous thrombosis
• Cerebral embolism
• Infective endocarditis
• Increased incidence of spontaneous abortion and premature births in females reaching childbearing age, and low birth weight in their infants

Thalassemia

Description
Thalassemia is a group of hemolytic anemias characterized by defective synthesis in the polypeptide chains

necessary for hemoglobin production. β-thalassemia, the most common type (resulting from defective beta polypeptide chain synthesis), occurs in three forms: thalassemia major, intermedia, and minor. Prognosis for β-thalassemia varies. Patients with thalassemia major seldom survive to adulthood. Children with thalassemia intermedia develop normally into adulthood, although puberty is usually delayed; persons with thalassemia minor can expect a normal life span.

Causes

Causes vary, depending upon the type of thalassemia.

• Thalassemia major and intermedia result from homozygous inheritance of the partially dominant autosomal gene responsible for this trait.

• Thalassemia minor results from heterozygous inheritance of the same gene.

Risk factors

Ethnic origin is the major risk factor.

• Persons of Mediterranean ancestry, especially Italians and Greeks (highest risk)

• Blacks

• Chinese from southern China

• Southeastern Asians

• Persons from India

Signs and symptoms

The severity of the resulting anemia depends on whether the patient is homozygous or heterozygous for the thalassemic trait.

Thalassemia major

—First signs are pallor and yellow skin and sclerae in infants aged 3 to 6 months.

—Later signs include severe anemia, splenomegaly or hepatomegaly, with abdominal enlargement; frequent infections; bleeding tendencies (epistaxis); anorexia; altered appearance with small body, large head, and possible mongoloid features; and possible mental retardation.

Thalassemia intermedia

—Anemia

—Jaundice

—Splenomegaly

—Possible signs of hemosiderosis

Thalassemia minor

—Mild anemia

Diagnostic tests

Thalassemia major

—RBCs and hemoglobin are decreased.

—Reticulocytes, bilirubin, and urinary and fecal urobilinogen are elevated.

—Serum folate level is low, indicating increased folate utilization by the hypertrophied bone marrow.

—Peripheral blood smear reveals target cells (extremely thin and fragile RBCs), pale nucleated RBCs, and marked anisocytosis.

—Skull and skeletal X-rays show a thinning and widening of the marrow space in the skull and long bones, possible granular appearance in the bones of the skull and vertebrae, possible areas of osteoporosis in the long bones, and deformities (rectangular or biconvex) of the phalanges.

—Hemoglobin electrophoresis demonstrates a significant rise in HbF and slight increase in HbA_2.

Thalassemia intermedia

—RBCs are hypochromic and microcytic.

Thalassemia minor

—RBCs are slightly hypochromic and microcytic.

—Hemoglobin electrophoresis shows a significant increase in HgA_2 and a moderate rise in HbF.

Treatment

Treatment of thalassemia major is essentially supportive. For example, infections require prompt treatment with appropriate antibiotics. Folic acid supplements help maintain folic acid levels in the face of increased requirements. Transfusions of packed RBCs raise hemoglobin levels but must be used judiciously to minimize iron overload. Splenectomy and bone marrow transplantation have been tried, but their effectiveness has not been confirmed.

Thalassemia intermedia and thalassemia minor usually do not require treatment.

Iron supplements are contraindicated in all forms of thalassemia.

Clinical implications
• Be sure to tell persons with thalassemia minor that their condition is benign.
• During and after RBC transfusions for thalassemia major, watch for adverse reactions—chills, fever, rash, itching, and hives.
• Stress the importance of good nutrition, meticulous wound care, periodic dental checkups, and other measures to prevent infection.
• Discuss with the parents of a young patient various options for healthy physical and creative outlets. Such a child must avoid strenuous athletic activity because of increased oxygen demand and the tendency toward pathologic fractures, but he may participate in less stressful activities.
• Teach parents to watch for signs of hepatitis and iron overload—always possible with frequent transfusions.
• Since parents may have questions about the vulnerability of future offspring, refer them for genetic counseling. Also, refer adult patients with thalassemia minor and thalassemia intermedia for genetic counseling; they need to recognize the risk of transmitting thalassemia major to their children if they marry another person with thalassemia. If such persons choose to marry and have children, all their children should be evaluated for thalassemia by age 1.

Complications
Thalassemia major may cause a variety of complications before death.

• Pathologic fractures
• Cardiac dysrhythmias
• Heart failure
• Other complications caused by iron deposits from repeated blood transfusions

---

Thoracic aortic aneurysm

Description
Thoracic aortic aneurysm is an abnormal widening of the ascending, transverse, or descending part of the aorta. The aneurysm may be dissecting, a hemorrhagic separation in the aortic wall, usually within the medial layer; saccular, an outpouching of the arterial wall, with a narrow neck; or fusiform, a spindle-shaped enlargement encompassing the entire aortic circumference. Some aneurysms progress to serious and eventually lethal complications. Thoracic aortic aneurysms are most common in men between ages 50 and 70; dissecting aneurysms, in blacks.

Causes
• Atherosclerosis is the leading cause.
• Intimal tear in the ascending aorta can initiate a dissecting aneurysm.
• Other possible causes include infection of the aortic arch and descending segments, congenital defects, trauma, syphilis, and hypertension (in dissecting aneurysm).

Signs and symptoms
Characteristic effects
—Pain (most common). In dissecting aneurysm, pain is typically sudden in onset, with a tearing or ripping sensation in thorax or anterior chest, and may extend to neck, shoulder, lower back, or abdomen but rarely to jaw and arms.
—Syncope
—Pallor
—Sweating
—Shortness of breath
—Increased pulse rate

—Cyanosis
—Leg weakness
—Transient paralysis
—Diastolic murmur
—Abrupt loss of radial and femoral pulses or wide variations in pulses or blood pressure between arms and legs

Saccular or fusiform aneurysms
Effects vary according to size and location of aneurysm and degree of compression, distortion, or erosion of surrounding structures.
—Aortic valve insufficiency
—Diastolic murmur
—Substernal ache in shoulders, lower back, or abdomen
—Marked respiratory distress, with dyspnea, brassy cough, wheezing
—Hoarseness or loss of voice
—Dysphagia (rare)
—Possible paresthesias or neuralgia

Diagnostic tests
• Postero-anterior and oblique chest X-rays show widening of the aorta.
• Aortography, the most definitive test, shows the lumen of the aneurysm, its size and location, and the false lumen in dissecting aneurysm.
• EKG helps distinguish thoracic aneurysm from myocardial infarction.
• Echocardiography may help identify dissecting aneurysm of the aortic root.
• Hemoglobin may be normal or decreased due to blood loss from a leaking aneurysm.
• CT scan can confirm and locate the aneurysm and may be used to monitor its progression.
• Magnetic resonance imaging may aid diagnosis.

Treatment
Dissecting aortic aneurysm is an extreme emergency that requires prompt surgery and stabilizing measures: antihypertensives, such as nitroprusside; negative inotropic agents that decrease contractile force, such as propranolol; oxygen for respiratory distress; narcotics for pain; I.V. fluids; and, if necessary, whole blood transfusions.

Surgery consists of resecting the aneurysm, restoring normal blood flow through a Dacron or Teflon graft, and, with aortic valve insufficiency, replacing the aortic valve. Postoperative measures include careful monitoring and continuous assessment in the ICU, antibiotics, endotracheal and chest tubes, EKG monitoring, and pulmonary artery catheterization.

Clinical implications
• Monitor blood pressure, pulmonary capillary wedge pressure, and central venous pressure. Assess pain, breathing, and carotid, radial, and femoral pulses.
• Make sure laboratory tests include CBC, differential, electrolytes, typing and cross matching for whole blood, arterial blood gas studies, and urinalysis.
• Insert an indwelling (Foley) catheter. Administer dextrose 5% in water or lactated Ringer's solution, and antibiotics, as ordered.
• Carefully monitor nitroprusside I.V.; use a separate I.V. line for infusion. Adjust the dose by slowly increasing the infusion rate. Meanwhile, check blood pressure every 5 minutes until it stabilizes.
• With suspected bleeding from an aneurysm, transfuse whole blood, as ordered.
• Explain diagnostic tests. If surgery is scheduled, explain the procedure and expected postoperative care (I.V. lines, endotracheal and drainage tubes, cardiac monitoring, ventilation).

After repair of a thoracic aneurysm, follow these guidelines:
• Carefully assess level of consciousness. Monitor vital signs, pulmonary artery and capillary wedge and central venous pressures, pulse rate, urinary output, and pain.
• Check respiratory function. Carefully observe and record type and amount of chest tube drainage, and

frequently assess heart and lung sounds.
• Monitor I.V. therapy.
• Give medications, as ordered.
• Watch for signs of infection, especially fever, and excessive drainage on dressing.
• Assist with range-of-motion exercises of legs to prevent thromboembolic phenomenon due to venostasis during prolonged bed rest.
• After stabilization of vital signs and respiration, encourage and assist the patient in turning, coughing, and deep breathing. If necessary, provide intermittent positive-pressure breathing to promote lung expansion. Help the patient walk as soon as he can.
• Before discharge, ensure compliance with antihypertensive therapy by explaining the need for such drugs and the expected side effects. Teach the patient how to monitor his blood pressure. Refer him to community agencies for continued support and assistance, as needed.
• Throughout hospitalization, offer the patient and family psychological support. Answer all questions honestly, and provide reassurance.

Complications
Rupture of the aneurysm is the major complication.

Throat abscesses

Description
Throat abscesses may be peritonsillar (quinsy) or retropharyngeal. Peritonsillar abscess forms in the connective tissue between the tonsil capsule and constrictor muscle of the pharynx. It occurs most commonly in adolescents and young adults. Retropharyngeal abscess forms between the posterior pharyngeal wall and prevertebral fascia. Its acute form occurs most commonly in children under age 2. The chronic form may occur at any age.

Causes
Peritonsillar abscess
—Complication of acute tonsillitis, usually after streptococcal or staphylococcal infection
Acute retropharyngeal abscess
—Infection in the retropharyngeal lymph glands, which may follow an upper respiratory tract bacterial infection
Chronic retropharyngeal abscess
—Tuberculosis of the cervical spine

Signs and symptoms
Peritonsillar abscess
—Severe throat pain
—Occasional ear pain on the affected side
—Tenderness of the submandibular gland
—Dysphagia and drooling
—Trismus
—Other effects, including fever, chills, malaise, rancid breath, nausea, muffled speech, dehydration, cervical adenopathy, and localized or systemic sepsis
Retropharyngeal abscess
—Pain
—Dysphagia
—Fever
—Nasal obstruction with abscess in upper pharynx
—Dyspnea, progressive inspiratory stridor, and neck hyperextension with abscess in low position
—Drooling and muffled crying in children

Diagnostic tests
Peritonsillar abscess
—Culture may reveal streptococcal or staphylococcal infection.
Retropharyngeal abscess
—X-rays show the larynx pushed forward and a widened space between the posterior pharyngeal wall and vertebrae.
—Culture and sensitivity tests isolate the causative organism.

Treatment

For early-stage peritonsillar abscess, large doses of penicillin or another broad-spectrum antibiotic are necessary. For late-stage abscess, with cellulitis of the tonsillar space, primary treatment is usually incision and drainage under a local anesthetic, followed by antibiotic therapy for 7 to 10 days. Tonsillectomy, scheduled no sooner than 1 month after healing, prevents recurrence but is recommended only after several episodes.

In acute retropharyngeal abscess, the primary treatment is incision and drainage through the pharyngeal wall. In chronic retropharyngeal abscess, drainage is performed through an external incision behind the sternomastoid muscle. During incision and drainage, strong, continuous mouth suction is necessary to prevent aspiration of pus. Postoperative drug therapy includes antibiotics (usually penicillin) and analgesics.

Clinical Implications

• Be alert for signs of respiratory obstruction (inspiratory stridor, dyspnea, increasing restlessness, or cyanosis). Keep emergency airway equipment nearby.

• Explain the drainage procedure to the patient or his parents. Since the procedure is usually done under a local anesthetic, the patient may be apprehensive.

• Assist with incision and drainage. To allow easy expectoration and suction of pus and blood, place the patient in a semirecumbent or sitting position.

• After incision and drainage, give antibiotics, analgesics, and antipyretics, as ordered. Stress the importance of completing the full course of prescribed antibiotic therapy.

• Monitor vital signs, and report any significant changes or bleeding. Assess pain and treat accordingly.

• If the patient is unable to swallow, ensure adequate hydration with I.V. therapy. Monitor fluid intake and output, and watch for dehydration.

• Provide meticulous mouth care. Apply petrolatum to the patient's lips. Promote healing with warm saline gargles or throat irrigations for 24 to 36 hours after incision and drainage. Encourage adequate rest.

Complications

• Laryngeal edema
• Aspiration
• Asphyxia

Thrombocytopenia

Description

The most common cause of hemorrhagic disorders, thrombocytopenia is characterized by a deficient number of circulating platelets. Since platelets play a vital role in coagulation, this disease poses a serious threat to hemostasis. Thrombocytopenia may be congenital or acquired. Prognosis is excellent in drug-induced thrombocytopenia if the offending drug is withdrawn. In such cases, recovery may be immediate. Otherwise, prognosis depends on response to treatment of the underlying cause.

Causes

Diminished or defective platelet production

—Congenital causes include Wiskott-Aldrich syndrome, maternal ingestion of thiazides, neonatal rubella, and thrombopoietin deficiency.

—Acquired causes include aplastic anemia, marrow infiltration (acute and chronic leukemias, tumor), nutritional deficiency (B_{12}, folic acid), myelosuppressive agents, drugs that directly influence platelet production (thiazides, alcohol, hormones), radiation, and viral infections (measles, dengue).

Increased peripheral platelet destruction

—Congenital causes may be nonimmune (prematurity, erythroblastosis fetalis, infection) or immune (drug sensitivity, maternal idiopathic thrombocytopenia purpura [ITP]).

—Acquired causes may be nonimmune (infection, disseminated intravascular coagulation, thrombotic thrombocytopenic purpura) or immune (drug-induced, especially with quinine and quinidine; posttransfusion purpura; acute and chronic ITP; sepsis; alcohol).

Platelet sequestration
—Hypersplenism
—Hypothermia
Platelet loss
—Hemorrhage
—Extracorporeal perfusion

Signs and symptoms
• Abnormal bleeding (typically sudden onset; petechiae or ecchymoses in the skin or bleeding into any mucous membrane)
• Malaise
• Fatigue
• General weakness
• Lethargy
• Large blood-filled bullae in mouth (characteristic sign in adults)

Diagnostic tests
• Coagulation test shows diminished platelet count.
• Bleeding time is prolonged.
• Bone marrow studies may reveal a greater number of megakaryocytes and shortened platelet survival.

Treatment
Treatment varies with the underlying cause and may include corticosteroids to enhance vascular integrity. Removal of the offending agents in drug-induced thrombocytopenia or proper treatment of the underlying cause, when possible, is essential. Platelet transfusions are helpful only in treating complications of severe hemorrhage.

Clinical implications
When caring for the patient with

Teaching Topics in Thrombocytopenia

• Explanation of platelets' role in clotting
• Explanation of the possible causes of the patient's thrombocytopenia
• Severity of thrombocytopenia
• Signs and symptoms of serious bleeding
• Platelet counts and other diagnostic tests
• Activity restrictions
• Administration of corticosteroids
• Platelet infusions and possible reactions
• Explanation of splenectomy, if performed

---

thrombocytopenia, take every possible precaution against bleeding.
• Protect the patient from trauma. Keep the side rails up, and pad them, if possible. Promote the use of an electric razor and a soft toothbrush. Avoid all invasive procedures, such as venipuncture or urinary catheterization, if possible. When venipuncture is unavoidable, be sure to exert pressure on the puncture site for at least 20 minutes or until the bleeding stops.
• Monitor platelet count daily.
• Test stool for blood (guaiac); test urine and emesis for blood (dipstick).
• Watch for bleeding (petechiae, ecchymoses, surgical or GI bleeding, menorrhagia).
• Warn the patient to avoid taking aspirin in any form, as well as other drugs that impair coagulation. Teach him how to recognize aspirin compounds that are listed on labels of over-the-counter remedies.
• Advise the patient to avoid straining at stool or coughing, as both can lead to increased intracranial pressure, possibly causing cerebral hemorrhage in the patient with thrombocytopenia. Provide a stool softener, if necessary.

• During periods of active bleeding, maintain the patient on strict bed rest, if necessary.
• When administering platelet concentrate, remember that platelets are extremely fragile; infuse them quickly, using the administration set recommended by your blood bank.
• During platelet transfusion, monitor for febrile reaction (flushing, chills, fever, headache, tachycardia, hypertension). HLA-typed platelets may be ordered to prevent febrile reaction. If the patient has a history of minor reactions, he may benefit from acetaminophen and diphenhydramine before the transfusion.
• If thrombocytopenia is drug-induced, stress the importance of avoiding the offending drug.
• While the patient is receiving steroid therapy, monitor his fluid and electrolyte balance, and watch for infection, pathologic fractures, and mood changes.
• If the patient must receive long-term steroid therapy, teach him to watch for and report cushingoid symptoms (acne, moon face, hirsutism, buffalo hump, hypertension, girdle obesity, thinning arms and legs, glycosuria, and edema). Emphasize that steroid doses must be discontinued gradually.

Complications
Hemorrhage, which may lead to tachycardia, shortness of breath, loss of consciousness, and death (See also *Teaching Topics in Thrombocytopenia*, p. 759.)

Thrombophlebitis

Description
An acute condition characterized by inflammation and thrombus formation, thrombophlebitis may occur in deep (intermuscular or intramuscular) or superficial (subcutaneous) veins. Deep-vein thrombophlebitis affects small veins, such as the soleal venous

sinuses, or large veins, such as the vena cava, and the femoral, iliac, and subclavian veins. This disorder is frequently progressive, leading to pulmonary embolism. Superficial thrombophlebitis is usually self-limiting and rarely leads to pulmonary embolism.

Causes
Deep-vein thrombophlebitis
—Idiopathic
—Endothelial damage
—Accelerated blood clotting
—Reduced blood flow
Superficial thrombophlebitis
—Trauma
—Infection
—I.V. drug abuse
—Chemical irritation due to extensive use of the I.V. route for medications and diagnostic tests

Risk factors
• Prolonged bed rest
• Trauma
• Childbirth
• Use of oral contraceptives

Signs and symptoms
Clinical features vary with the site and length of the affected vein.
Deep-vein thrombophlebitis
—Severe pain
—Fever
—Chills
—Malaise
—Possible swelling and cyanosis of the affected arm or leg
Superficial thrombophlebitis
—Heat, pain, swelling, rubor, tenderness, and induration along length of affected vein
—Possible lymphadenitis with extensive vein involvement

Diagnostic tests
• Doppler ultrasonography identifies reduced blood flow to a specific area and any obstruction to venous flow,

Teaching Topics in DVT

- An explanation of how a thrombus occludes blood flow through a vein
- The importance of prompt treatment to prevent potentially fatal pulmonary embolism or debilitating chronic venous insufficiency
- Preparation for diagnostic tests, such as Doppler ultrasonography, impedance plethysmography, venography, and blood clotting studies
- The need for rest and limb elevation during the acute stage of DVT, and for regular exercise after the acute stage has passed
- Increased intake of protein and vitamins B_{12} and C to maintain skin integrity; other dietary modifications to improve overall cardiovascular health
- Anticoagulant drug use and precautions
- Application of antiembolism stockings to prevent venous stasis and embolism
- Skin care to prevent venous ulcers
- Care of existing ulcers
- Preparation for thrombectomy, if ordered
- Warning signs of pulmonary embolism and chronic venous insufficiency

particularly in iliofemoral deep-vein thrombophlebitis.

- Plethysmography shows decreased circulation distal to the affected area; it is more sensitive than ultrasound in detecting deep-vein thrombophlebitis.
- Phlebography (usually confirms diagnosis) shows filling defects and diverted blood flow.

Treatment

The goals of treatment are to control thrombus development, prevent complications, relieve pain, and prevent recurrence of the disorder. Symptomatic measures include bed rest, with elevation of the affected arm or leg; warm, moist soaks to the affected area; and analgesics, as ordered. After an acute episode of deep-vein thrombophlebitis subsides, the patient may begin to walk while wearing antiembolism stockings (applied before getting out of bed).

Treatment may also include anticoagulants (initially, heparin; later, warfarin) to prolong clotting time. Full anticoagulant dose must be discontinued before any surgical procedure, due to the risk of hemorrhage. After some types of surgery, especially major abdominal or pelvic operations, prophylactic doses of anticoagulants may

reduce the risk of deep-vein thrombophlebitis and pulmonary embolism.

For lysis of acute, extensive deep-vein thrombosis, treatment should include streptokinase. Rarely, deep-vein thrombophlebitis may cause complete venous occlusion, which necessitates venous interruption through simple ligation to vein plication, or clipping.

Therapy for severe superficial thrombophlebitis may include an anti-inflammatory drug, such as indomethacin, along with antiembolism stockings, warm soaks, and elevation of the patient's leg.

Clinical implications

Patient teaching, identification of high-risk patients, and measures to prevent venostasis can prevent deep-vein thrombophlebitis. Close monitoring of anticoagulant therapy can prevent serious complications, such as internal hemorrhage.

- Enforce bed rest, as ordered, and elevate the patient's affected arm or leg. If you plan to use pillows for elevating the leg, place them to support the entire length of the affected extremity and prevent possible compression of the popliteal space.

• Apply warm soaks to increase circulation to the affected area and to relieve pain and inflammation. Give analgesics to relieve pain, as ordered.

• Measure and record the circumference of the affected arm or leg daily, and compare this to the circumference of the other arm or leg. To ensure accuracy and consistency of serial measurements, mark the skin over the area and measure at the same spot daily.

• Administer heparin I.V., as ordered, with an infusion monitor or pump to control the flow rate, if necessary.

• Measure partial thromboplastin time regularly for the patient on heparin therapy; prothrombin time for the patient on warfarin (therapeutic anticoagulation values for both are 1.5 to 2 times control values). Watch for signs and symptoms of bleeding, such as dark, tarry stools; coffee-ground vomitus; and ecchymoses. Encourage the patient to use an electric razor and to avoid medications that contain aspirin.

• Be alert for signs of pulmonary emboli (rales, dyspnea, hemoptysis, sudden changes in mental status, restlessness, and hypotension).

• To prepare the patient with thrombophlebitis for discharge, emphasize the importance of follow-up blood studies to monitor anticoagulant therapy.

• If the patient is being discharged on heparin therapy, teach him or his family how to give subcutaneous injections. If he requires further assistance, arrange for a visiting nurse.

• Tell the patient to avoid prolonged sitting or standing to help prevent recurrence.

• Teach the patient how to apply and use antiembolism stockings properly. Tell him to report any complications, such as cold, blue toes.

• To prevent thrombophlebitis in high-risk patients, perform range-of-motion exercises while the patient is on bed rest, use intermittent pneumatic calf massage during lengthy surgical or diagnostic procedures, apply antiembolism stockings postoperatively, and encourage early ambulation.

Complications
Pulmonary embolus is a potentially lethal complication of deep-vein thrombosis. (See also *Teaching Topics in DVT,* p. 761.)

Thyroid cancer

Description
Thyroid carcinoma occurs in all age-groups, especially in persons who have had radiation treatment to the neck area. Papillary and follicular carcinomas are most common and are usually associated with prolonged survival. Medullary (solid) carcinoma is a rare form (5%) of thyroid cancer that is familial and is often associated with pheochromocytoma. It is completely curable when detected before it causes symptoms. Untreated, it grows rapidly, often metastasizing to bone, liver, and kidney. Giant and spindle cell cancer (anaplastic tumor) resists radiation and is almost never curable by resection. It metastasizes rapidly and causes death by tracheal invasion and compression of adjacent structures.

Causes
The exact cause of thyroid cancer is unknown. However, radiation therapy used to shrink enlarged thymus glands, tonsils, or adenoids, and to treat acne and other skin disorders in children in the 1950s have been known to cause thyroid cancer in some individuals.

Risk factors
• Radiation exposure
• Prolonged thyroid-stimulating hor-

mone (TSH) stimulation (through radiation or heredity)
- Familial predisposition
- Chronic goiter

Signs and symptoms
- Painless nodule
- Hard nodule in an enlarged thyroid gland or palpable lymph nodes with thyroid enlargement
- Hoarseness
- Dysphagia
- Dyspnea
- Pain on palpation (with progression)
- Possible hypothyroidism
- Possible hyperthyroidism
- Other associated findings: diarrhea, anorexia, irritability, vocal cord paralysis, and symptoms of distant metastases

Diagnostic tests
- Thyroid scan differentiates between functional nodes and hypofunctional nodes.
- Needle biopsy diagnoses medullary cancer.
- Ultrasound scan diagnoses medullary cancer.
- Serum calcitonin assay is a reliable clue to silent medullary carcinoma.

Treatment
Treatment varies and may include one or any combination of the following:
- Total or subtotal thyroidectomy, with modified node dissection (bilateral or hemolateral) on the side of the primary cancer (papillary or follicular cancer)
- Total thyroidectomy and radical neck excision (for medullary, or giant and spindle cell cancer)
- Radiation (^{131}I), with external radiation (for large inoperable cancer and sometimes postoperatively in lieu of radical neck excision) or by itself (for local or distant metastases)
- Adjunctive thyroid suppression, with exogenous thyroid hormones suppressing TSH production, and simultaneous administration of an adrenergic blocking agent, such as propranolol, increasing tolerance to surgery and radiation
- Chemotherapy, which is experimental. Doxorubicin is sometimes beneficial with metastasizing thyroid cancer.

Clinical implications
Care of the patient after extensive tumor and node excision is identical to other radical neck postoperative care.
- Before surgery, tell the patient to expect temporary voice loss or hoarseness lasting several days after surgery. Also, explain the operation and postoperative procedures and teach proper postoperative positioning. Ideally, the patient should be euthyroid before surgery, as demonstrated by a normal EEG, thyroid function tests, and pulse rate.

After surgery, follow these guidelines:
- When the patient regains consciousness, keep him in semi-Fowler's position, with his head neither hyperextended nor flexed, to avoid pressure on the suture line. Support his head and neck with sandbags and pillows. When you move him, continue this support with your hands.
- After monitoring vital signs, check the patient's dressing, neck, and back for bleeding. If he complains that the dressing feels tight, loosen the dressing and call the physician immediately.
- Check serum calcium levels daily, and watch for and report complications: hemorrhage and shock (elevated pulse and hypotension), tetany (carpopedal spasm, twitching, convulsions), thyroid storm (high fever, severe tachycardia, delirium, dehydration, and extreme irritability), and respiratory obstruction (dyspnea, crowing respirations, retraction of neck tissues).
- Keep a tracheotomy set and oxygen equipment handy in case of respiratory obstruction. Use continuous steam inhalation in the patient's room until his chest is clear.

• Administer I.V. fluids, as ordered, and provide a soft diet, as needed. Many patients can tolerate a regular diet within 24 hours of surgery, however.

Thyroiditis

Description

Inflammation of the thyroid gland occurs as autoimmune thyroiditis (long-term inflammatory disease), subacute granulomatous thyroiditis (self-limiting inflammation), Riedel's thyroiditis (rare, invasive fibrotic process), and miscellaneous thyroiditis (acute suppurative, chronic infective, and chronic noninfective). Thyroiditis is more common in women than in men.

Causes

Autoimmune thyroiditis
—Antibodies to thyroid antigens
Subacute granulomatous thyroiditis
—Mumps
—Influenza
—Coxsackieviral infection
—Adenoviral infection
Riedel's thyroiditis
—Possible autoimmune process
—Possible subacute process
Miscellaneous thyroiditis
—Bacterial invasion of the gland in suppurative thyroiditis
—Tuberculosis, syphilis, or actinomycosis in chronic infective form
—Sarcoidosis and amyloidosis in chronic noninfective thyroiditis

Signs and symptoms

Autoimmune thyroiditis
—Usually asymptomatic
Subacute granulomatous thyroiditis
—Possible painful and tender thyroid
—Possible dysphagia
Riedel's thyroiditis
—Possible compression of the trachea or esophagus
—Firm thyroid on palpation

Miscellaneous thyroiditis
—Fever
—Pain, tenderness, and reddened skin over the thyroid gland

Diagnostic tests

Precise diagnosis depends on the type of thyroiditis.
Autoimmune thyroiditis
—Precipitin test is positive.
—Thyroglobulin and microsomal antibody titers are high.
Subacute granulomatous thyroiditis
—Erythrocyte sedimentation rate is elevated.
—Thyroid hormone levels are increased.
—Thyroidal radioiodine uptake is decreased.
Chronic infective and noninfective thyroiditis
—Diagnostic tests vary, depending on underlying infection or other disease.

Treatment

Treatment varies with the type of thyroiditis. Drug therapy includes levothyroxine for accompanying hypothyroidism, analgesics and anti-inflammatory drugs for mild subacute granulomatous thyroiditis, propranolol for transient hyperthyroidism, and steroids for severe episodes of acute illness. Suppurative thyroiditis requires antibiotic therapy. A partial thyroidectomy may be necessary to relieve tracheal or esophageal compression in Riedel's thyroiditis.

Clinical implications

• Before treatment, obtain a patient history to identify underlying diseases that may cause thyroiditis, such as tuberculosis or a recent viral infection.
• Check vital signs, and examine the patient's neck for unusual swelling, enlargement, or redness. Provide a liquid diet if the patient has difficulty swallowing, especially when due to fibrosis. If the neck is swollen, measure and record the circumference daily to monitor progressive enlargement.
• Administer antibiotics, as ordered,

and report and record elevations in temperature, which may indicate developing resistance to the antibiotic.

• Instruct the patient to watch for and report signs of hypothyroidism (lethargy, restlessness, sensitivity to cold, forgetfulness, or dry skin), especially if he has Hashimoto's thyroiditis, which often causes hypothyroidism. Check for signs of hyperthyroidism (nervousness, tremor, weakness), which often occur in subacute thyroiditis.

• After thyroidectomy, check vital signs every 15 to 30 minutes until the patient's condition stabilizes.

• Stay alert for signs of tetany secondary to accidental parathyroid injury during surgery. Keep 10% calcium gluconate available for I.V. use, if needed.

• Assess dressings frequently for excessive bleeding.

• Watch for signs of airway obstruction, such as difficulty in talking or increased swallowing; keep tracheotomy equipment handy.

• Explain to the patient that lifelong thyroid hormone replacement therapy is necessary. Tell him to watch for signs of overdosage, such as nervousness and palpitations.

Tinea versicolor
(Pityriasis versicolor)

Description

A chronic, superficial, fungal infection, tinea versicolor may produce a multicolored rash, commonly on the upper trunk. This condition, primarily a cosmetic defect, usually affects young persons, especially during warm weather, and is most prevalent in tropical countries. Recurrence is common.

Causes

The fungus *Pityrosporon orbiculare (Microsporum furfur)*

Mode of transmission

Introduction of the fungus into the skin

Signs and symptoms

• Skin lesions (characteristic sign). Typically raised or macular, round or oval, slightly scaly, tawny (although may be white to brown); distributed on upper trunk and may extend to lower abdomen, neck, arms, and rarely face

• Patchy tanning on exposure to sunlight

• Possible inflammation, burning, and itching

Diagnostic tests

• Wood's light examination revealing lesions strongly suggests tinea versicolor.

• Microscopic examination of skin scrapings confirms it by showing hyphae and clusters of yeast.

Treatment

The most economical and effective treatment is selenium sulfide lotion 2.5% applied once a day for 7 days. It is left on the skin for 10 minutes, then rinsed off thoroughly. In persistent cases, therapy may require a single 12-hour application of this lotion followed by weekly cleansing with an antifungal soap (3% sulfur and 20% salicylic acid). Either treatment may cause temporary redness and irritation.

More expensive treatments include topical antifungals, such as tolnaftate, applied twice daily for a month; and oral antifungals, such as griseofulvin and ketoconazole.

Clinical implications

• Instruct the patient to apply selenium sulfide lotion, as ordered.

• Assure the patient that once his fungal infection is cured, discolored areas will gradually blend in after exposure to the sun or ultraviolet light.

• Since recurrence of tinea versicolor is common, advise the patient to watch for new areas of discoloration.

Tonsillitis

Description

Tonsillitis, or inflammation of the tonsils, can be acute or chronic. The uncomplicated acute form usually lasts 4 to 6 days and commonly affects children between ages 5 and 10. Tonsils tend to hypertrophy during childhood and atrophy after puberty.

Causes

- Beta-hemolytic streptococci (most common)
- Other types of bacteria
- Viruses

Signs and symptoms

Acute tonsillitis

Discomfort usually subsides after 72 hours.

—Mild to severe sore throat
—Dysphagia
—Fever
—Swelling and tenderness of lymph glands in submandibular area
—Muscle and joint pain
—Chills
—Malaise
—Headache
—Pain (often referred to ears)
—Possible urge to swallow constantly
—Constricted feeling in back of throat
—Possible cessation of eating in very young child

Chronic tonsillitis

—Recurrent sore throat
—Purulent drainage in tonsillar crypts
—Frequent attacks of acute tonsillitis

Diagnostic tests

- Culture may determine the infecting organism.
- WBC count may be elevated.

Treatment

Treatment of acute tonsillitis requires rest, adequate fluid intake, administration of aspirin or acetaminophen, and, for bacterial infection, antibiotics. When the causative organism is Group A beta-hemolytic streptococcus, penicillin is the drug of choice (erythromycin or another broad-spectrum antibiotic may be given if the patient is allergic to penicillin). To prevent complications, antibiotic therapy should continue for 10 days. Chronic tonsillitis or the development of complications (obstructions from tonsillar hypertrophy, peritonsillar abscess) may require a tonsillectomy, but only after the patient has been free of tonsillar or respiratory tract infections for 3 to 4 weeks.

Clinical implications

- Despite dysphagia, urge the patient to drink plenty of fluids, especially if he has a fever. Offer a child ice cream and flavored drinks and ices. Suggest gargling to soothe the throat, unless it exacerbates pain. Make sure the patient and parents understand the importance of completing the prescribed course of antibiotic therapy.
- Before tonsillectomy, explain to the adult patient that a local anesthetic prevents pain but allows a sensation of pressure during surgery. Warn the patient to expect considerable throat discomfort and some bleeding postoperatively.
- For the pediatric patient, keep your explanation simple and nonthreatening. Show the child the operating and recovery rooms, and briefly explain the hospital routine. Most hospitals allow one parent to stay with the child.
- Postoperatively, maintain a patent airway. To prevent aspiration, place the patient on his side. Monitor vital signs frequently, and check for bleeding. Immediately report excessive bleeding, increased pulse rate, or dropping blood pressure.
- After the patient is fully alert and the gag reflex has returned, allow him to drink water. Later, urge him to drink plenty of nonirritating fluids, to walk, and to take frequent deep breaths to

prevent pulmonary complications. Give pain medication, as needed.

• Before discharge, provide the patient or parents with written instructions on home care. Tell them to expect a white scab to form in the throat between 5 and 10 days postoperatively, and to report bleeding, ear discomfort, or a fever that lasts longer than 3 days.

Complications

• Obstruction from tonsillar hypertrophy
• Peritonsillar abscess

Torticollis
(Wryneck)

Description

This neck deformity, in which the sternocleidomastoid neck muscles are spastic or shortened, causes bending of the head to the affected side and rotation of the chin to the opposite side. This disorder may be congenital or acquired. Incidence of congenital (muscular) torticollis is highest in infants after difficult delivery (breech presentation), in firstborn infants, and in girls. Acquired torticollis usually develops during the first 10 years of life or after age 40.

Causes

Congenital torticollis
—Malposition of the head in utero
—Prenatal injury
—Fibroma
—Interruption of blood supply
—Fibrotic rupture of the sternocleidomastoid muscle, with hematoma and scar formation
Acquired torticollis
—Acute torticollis is due to muscular damage from inflammatory diseases, such as myositis, lymphadenitis, and tuberculosis or cervical spinal injuries that produce scar tissue contracture.
—Spasmodic torticollis results from rhythmic muscle spasms caused by an organic CNS disorder.

—Hysterical torticollis is due to a psychogenic inability to control neck muscles.

Signs and symptoms

Congenital torticollis
—Firm, nontender, palpable enlargement of the sternocleidomastoid muscle at birth and visible for several weeks after
—Possible flattening of the infant's head and face on affected side that gradually worsens
—Chin turned away from the side of the shortened muscle, and head tilted to shortened side
—Possible elevation of shoulder on affected side, restricting neck movement
Acquired torticollis
—Recurring unilateral stiffness of neck muscles
—Drawing sensation in neck
—Momentary twitching or contraction that pulls the head to the affected side
—Severe neuralgic pain throughout head and neck

Diagnostic tests

X-rays of the cervical spine may reveal an associated disorder (such as tuberculosis, scar tissue formation, or arthritis) in acquired torticollis.

Treatment

Treatment of congenital torticollis aims to stretch the shortened muscle. Nonsurgical treatment includes passive neck stretching and proper positioning during sleep for an infant and active stretching exercises for an older child—for example, touching the ear opposite the affected side to the shoulder and touching the chin to the same shoulder.

Surgical correction involves sectioning the sternocleidomastoid muscle. This should be done during preschool years and only if other therapies fail.

Treatment of acquired torticollis aims to correct the underlying cause of the disease. In the acute form, application of heat, cervical traction, and gentle massage may help relieve pain. Stretching exercises and a neck brace may relieve symptoms of the spasmodic and hysterical forms. Treatment of elderly patients with acquired torticollis may include drugs such as carbidopa, carbamazepine (Tegretol), and haloperidol (Haldol).

Clinical implications
• To aid early diagnosis of torticollis of the congenital type, observe the infant for limited neck movement, and thoroughly assess his degree of discomfort.
• Teach the parents of an affected child how to perform stretching exercises with the child. Suggest that they place toys or hanging mobiles on the side of the crib opposite the affected side of the child's neck, to encourage the child to move his head and stretch his neck.
• If surgery is necessary, prepare the patient by shaving the neck to the hairline on the affected side.

After corrective surgery, follow these guidelines:
• Monitor the patient closely for nausea or signs of respiratory complications, especially if he is in cervical traction. Keep suction equipment available to prevent aspiration.
• The patient may be in a cast or in traction day and night or at night only. Give meticulous cast care, including the monitoring of circulation, sensation, and color around the cast. Protect the cast around the patient's chin and mouth with waterproof material. Check for skin irritation, pressure areas, or softening of cast pad.
• Provide emotional support for the patient and family to relieve their anxiety due to fear, pain, limitations from the brace or traction, and an altered body image.
• Begin stretching exercises, such as those outlined above, as soon as the patient can tolerate them.

• Before discharge, explain to the patient or parents the importance of continuing daily heat applications, massages, and stretching exercises, as prescribed, and of keeping the cast clean and dry. Emphasize that physical therapy is essential for a successful rehabilitation after the cast is removed.

Toxic epidermal necrolysis
(Scalded skin syndrome)

Description
Toxic epidermal necrolysis (TEN) is a rare, severe skin disorder that causes epidermal erythema, superficial necrosis, and skin erosions. The skin appears to be scalded; hence the term scalded skin syndrome. Mortality is high (30%), especially among the debilitated and the elderly. Reepithelialization is slow, and residual scarring is common. TEN primarily affects adults.

Causes
The immediate cause is unknown. Possible causes include any of the following:
• Toxins such as carbon monoxide
• Allergens such as drugs—most commonly butazones, sulfonamides, penicillins, barbiturates, and hydantoins

Signs and symptoms
Early symptoms
—Inflammation of the mucous membranes
—Burning sensation in the conjunctivae
—Malaise
—Fever
—Generalized skin tenderness
Later symptoms
Eruptions occur in three phases:
—Diffuse, erythematous rash
—Vesication and blistering
—Large-scale epidermal necrolysis and desquamation

Diagnostic tests
• Culture and Gram stain of lesions determine whether infection is present.
• Exfoliative cytology and biopsy aid in ruling out erythema multiforme and exfoliative dermatitis.

Treatment and clinical implications
Treatment consists of high-dose systemic corticosteroids and maintenance of fluid and electrolyte balance with I.V. fluid replacement. Frequent determinations of hemoglobin and hematocrit, electrolytes, serum proteins, and blood gases are necessary.
• Monitor vital signs, central venous pressure, and urinary output. Watch for signs of renal failure (decreased urinary output) and bleeding. Report temperature elevations immediately, and obtain blood cultures and sensitivity tests promptly, as ordered, to detect and treat septic infection.
• Prevent secondary infection. Protective isolation and prophylactic antibiotic therapy may be necessary.
• Maintain skin integrity as much as possible. The patient should not wear clothing and should be covered loosely to prevent friction and sloughing of skin. A turning frame is helpful.
• Administer analgesics, as needed. Applying cool, sterile compresses may relieve some discomfort.
• Provide frequent eye care to remove exudate. Ocular lesions are common.
• Provide emotional support for the patient and family.

Complications
Systemic complications include the following:
• Bronchopneumonia
• Pulmonary edema
• GI and esophageal hemorrhage
• Shock
• Renal failure
• Sepsis
• Disseminated intravascular coagulation

Toxic shock syndrome

Description
Toxic shock syndrome (TSS) is an acute bacterial infection. It usually affects menstruating women under age 30. (Of the reported cases, 96% involve women, and 92% of these cases began during menstruation.) A strong correlation exists between TSS and use of superabsorbent tampons. Incidence is rising, and the recurrence rate is about 30%.

Causes
• Introduction of penicillin-resistant *Staphylococcus aureus* into body tissue through the continuous use of tampons during menstruation
• An existing *S. aureus* infection, such as abscess, osteomyelitis, and postsurgical infection

Signs and symptoms
• Intense myalgias
• Fever over 104° F. (40° C.)
• Vomiting
• Diarrhea
• Headache
• Decreased level of consciousness
• Rigors
• Conjunctival hyperemia
• Vaginal hyperemia and discharge
• Severe hypotension and hypovolemic shock
• Deep red rash, especially on palms and soles, that later desquamates

Diagnostic tests
• Culture of vaginal discharge revealing *S. aureus* helps support the diagnosis.
• Creatine phosphokinase shows a fivefold or greater increase.
• BUN and creatinine levels are elevated at least twice the normal level, showing renal involvement.
• Bilirubin and hepatic enzymes

(SGOT or SGPT) are elevated at least twice the normal levels, showing liver involvement.
• Thrombocytes are decreased and platelet count is less than 100,000/mm³, showing blood involvement.

Treatment
Treatment consists of I.V. antistaphylococcal antibiotics that are beta-lactamase–resistant, such as oxacillin, nafcillin, and methicillin. To reverse shock, expect to replace fluids with saline solution and colloids, as ordered.

Clinical implications
• Monitor the patient's vital signs frequently.
• Administer antibiotics slowly and strictly on time. Be sure to watch for signs of penicillin allergy.
• Check the patient's fluid and electrolyte balance.
• Obtain specimens of vaginal and cervical secretions for culture of *S. aureus*.
• Tell the patient to avoid tampons.
• Take secretion precautions for all vaginal and lesion drainage.

Complications
• Persistent neuropsychological abnormalities
• Mild renal failure
• Rash
• Cyanotic arms and legs

Toxoplasmosis

Description
Toxoplasmosis is one of the most common infectious diseases, occurring in two forms: congenital and acquired. Distributed worldwide, it is less common in cold or hot, arid climates and at high elevations. It usually causes localized infection but may produce significant generalized infection, especially in immunodeficient patients

or newborns. Congenital toxoplasmosis is characterized by lesions of the central nervous system.

Causes
The protozoan *Toxoplasma gondii*

Mode of transmission
• Ingestion of tissue cysts in raw or uncooked meat
• Fecal-oral contamination from infected cats
• Transplacental transmission from an infected mother

Signs and symptoms
Congenital toxoplasmosis
The later in pregnancy maternal infection occurs, the greater the risk of congenital infection in the infant. Obvious signs include the following:
—Retinochoroiditis
—Hydrocephalus or microcephalus
—Cerebral calcification
—Convulsions
—Lymphadenopathy
—Fever
—Hepatosplenomegaly
—Jaundice
—Rash
—Possible strabismus, blindness, epilepsy, and mental retardation months to years later
—Possible stillbirth if acquired in first trimester of pregnancy
Acquired toxoplasmosis
—In localized infection, fever, malaise, myalgia, headache, fatigue, sore throat, and lymphadenopathy
—In generalized infection, encephalitis, fever, headache, vomiting, delirium, convulsions, and a diffuse, maculopapular rash (except on palms, soles, and scalp)

Diagnostic tests
• Specimens of body fluids, blood, and tissue showing *T. gondii* antibodies confirm the diagnosis.
• Inoculation of mice with specimens of body fluids, blood, and tissues with subsequent isolation of *T. gondii* confirms the diagnosis.

Treatment

Treatment is most effective during the acute stage. It consists of drug therapy with sulfonamides and pyrimethamine for approximately 4 weeks, and possibly folinic acid to control pyrimethamine side effects. No safe, effective treatment exists for chronic toxoplasmosis or toxoplasmosis occurring during the first trimester of pregnancy.

Clinical implications

When caring for patients with toxoplasmosis, monitor drug therapy carefully and emphasize thorough patient teaching to prevent complications and control spread of the disease.

• Since sulfonamides cause blood dyscrasias and pyrimethamine depresses bone marrow, closely monitor results of blood studies. Also emphasize the importance of regularly scheduled follow-up care.

• Teach all persons to wash their hands after working with soil (since it may be contaminated with cat oocysts); to cook meat thoroughly and freeze it promptly if it is not for immediate use; to change cat litter daily (cat oocysts do not become infective until 1 to 4 days after excretion); to cover children's sandboxes; and to keep flies away from food (flies transport oocysts).

• Report all cases of toxoplasmosis to your local public health department.

Complications

Generalized infection may cause any of the following:

• Myocarditis
• Pneumonitis
• Hepatitis
• Polymyositis

Tracheoesophageal fistula and esophageal atresia

Description

Tracheoesophageal fistula is a developmental anomaly characterized by an abnormal connection between the trachea and the esophagus. It usually accompanies esophageal atresia, in which the esophagus is closed off at some point. (See *Types of Tracheoesophageal Anomalies*, p. 772.) These disorders require immediate diagnosis and correction. They may coexist with other serious anomalies, such as congenital heart disease, imperforate anus, genitourinary abnormalities, and intestinal atresia. Esophageal atresia occurs in about 1 of every 4,000 live births. About one third of these infants are born prematurely.

Causes

Failure of the embryonic esophagus and trachea to develop and separate correctly

Signs and symptoms

Type A esophageal atresia
—Excessive drooling
—Regurgitation, respiratory distress, and aspiration after feeding
Type B and Type D tracheoesophageal fistula
—Immediate aspiration of saliva
—Bacterial pneumonitis
Type C tracheoesophageal fistula
—Coughing, struggling, becoming cyanotic and apneic soon after swallowing fluids
—Possible respiratory distress and stomach distention
—Possible chemical pneumonitis
Type E (or H-type) tracheoesophageal fistula
—Recurrent pneumonitis, pulmonary infection, and abdominal distention
—Coughing, choking, and becoming cyanotic after drinking

Diagnostic tests

The following procedures confirm tracheoesophageal fistula:

• A #10 or #12 French catheter passed through the nose meets an ob-

Types of Tracheoesophageal Anomalies

Congenital malformations of the esophagus occur in about 1 in 4,000 live births. The American Academy of Pediatrics classification of the anatomic variations of tracheoesophageal anomalies is:

• **Type A** (7.7%): esophageal atresia without fistula

• **Type B** (0.8%): esophageal atresia with tracheoesophageal fistula to the proximal segment

• **Type C** (86.5%): esophageal atresia with fistula to the distal segment

• **Type D** (0.7%): esophageal atresia with fistula to both segments

• **Type E (or H-Type)** (4.2%): tracheoesophageal fistula without atresia

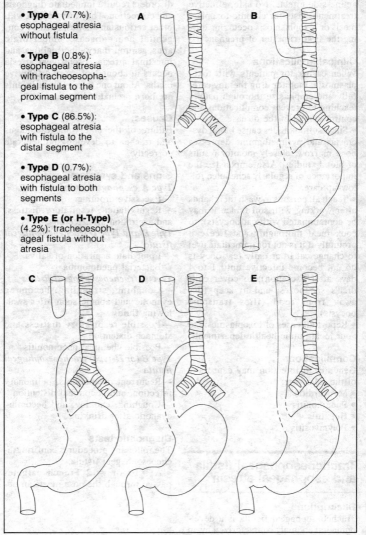

struction (esophageal atresia) approximately 4" to 5" (10 to 13 cm) distal to the nostrils. Aspirate of gastric contents is less acidic than normal.
• Chest X-ray demonstrates the position of the catheter and can also show a dilated, air-filled upper esophageal pouch; pneumonia in the right upper lobe; or bilateral pneumonitis. Both pneumonia and pneumonitis suggest aspiration.
• Abdominal X-ray shows gas in the bowel in a distal fistula (type C) but not in a proximal fistula (type B) or in atresia without fistula (type A).
• Cinefluorography visualizes the tip of the upper pouch and differentiates between overflow aspiration from a blind end (atresia) and aspiration due to passage of liquids through a tracheoesophageal fistula.

Treatment

Tracheoesophageal fistula and esophageal atresia require surgical correction and are usually surgical emergencies. The type of surgical procedure and when it is performed depend on the nature of the anomaly, the patient's general condition, and the presence of coexisting congenital defects.

Both before and after surgery, positioning varies with the physician's approach and the child's anatomy. The child may be placed supine, with his head low to facilitate drainage, or with his head elevated to prevent aspiration. Prior to surgery, the child should receive I.V. fluids, as necessary, and appropriate antibiotics for superimposed infection.

Correction of esophageal atresia alone requires anastomosis of the proximal and distal esophageal segments in one or two stages. End-to-end anastomosis often produces postoperative stricture; end-to-side anastomosis is less likely to do so. If the esophageal ends are widely separated, treatment may include a colonic interposition (grafting a piece of the colon) or elongation of the proximal segment of the esophagus by bougienage. About 10 days after surgery, and again 1 month and 3 months later, X-rays are required to evaluate the effectiveness of surgical repair.

Postoperative treatment includes placement of a suction catheter in the upper esophageal pouch to control secretions and prevent aspiration; maintaining the infant in an upright position to avoid reflux of gastric juices into the trachea; I.V. fluids and nothing by mouth; gastrostomy to prevent reflux and allow feeding; and appropriate antibiotics for pneumonia.

Clinical implications
• Monitor respiratory status. Administer oxygen and perform pulmonary physiotherapy and suctioning, as needed. Provide a humid environment.
• Administer antibiotics and parenteral fluids, as ordered. Keep accurate intake and output records.
• If the patient has chest tubes postoperatively, check them frequently for patency. Maintain proper suction, measure and mark drainage periodically, and milk tubing, as necessary.
• Observe carefully for signs of complications, such as abnormal esophageal motility, recurrent fistulas, pneumothorax, and esophageal stricture.
• Maintain gastrostomy tube feedings, as ordered. Such feedings initially consist of dextrose and water (not more than 5% solution); later, add a proprietary formula (first diluted and then full strength). If the infant develops gastric atony, use an isosmolar formula. Oral feedings can usually resume 8 to 10 days postoperatively. If gastrostomy feedings and oral feedings are impossible due to intolerance to them or decreased intestinal motility, the infant requires total parenteral nutrition.

• Give the infant a pacifier to satisfy his sucking needs but *only* when he can safely handle secretions, since sucking stimulates secretion of saliva.
• Offer the parents support and guidance in dealing with their infant's acute illness. Encourage them to participate in the infant's care and to hold and touch him as much as possible to facilitate bonding.

Complications
General postoperative complications include impaired esophageal motility, hiatal hernia, and reflux esophagitis. Other postoperative complications vary, depending on the underlying problem.
Tracheoesophageal fistula repair
—Recurrent fistulas
—Esophageal motility dysfunction
—Esophageal stricture
—Recurrent bronchitis
—Pneumothorax
—Failure to thrive
Esophageal atresia repair
—Esophageal motility dysfunction
—Hiatal hernia

Trachoma

Description
The most common cause of blindness in underdeveloped areas of the world, trachoma is a chronic form of keratoconjunctivitis. This infection is usually confined to the eye but can also localize in the urethra. Although trachoma itself is self-limiting, it causes permanent damage to the cornea and conjunctiva. Severe trachoma may lead to blindness, especially if a secondary bacterial infection develops. Trachoma is prevalent in Africa, Latin America, and Asia, particularly in children. In the United States, it is prevalent among American Indians of the Southwest.

Causes
Chlamydia trachomatis

Mode of transmission
• Direct contact between family members or schoolchildren
• Eye-to-eye transmission by flies and gnats in endemic areas

Risk factors
• Poverty
• Poor hygiene
• Exposure to an infected person

Signs and symptoms
Initial infection
—Visible conjunctival follicles
—Red, edematous eyelids
—Eye pain
—Photophobia
—Tearing
—Exudation
Untreated infection at 1 month
—Enlarged conjunctival follicles (inflamed papillae that later become yellow or gray)
—Vascularization of the cornea under the upper lid
Continued progression in untreated infection
—Corneal scarring
—Visual distortion
—Possible obstruction of the lacrimal ducts
—Possible dryness of the eyes
—Possible blindness

Diagnostic tests
Microscopic examination of Giemsa-stained conjunctival scraping confirms diagnosis by showing cytoplasmic inclusion bodies, some polymorphonuclear reaction, plasma cells, Leber's cells (large macrophages containing phagocytosed debris), and follicle cells.

Treatment and clinical implications
Primary treatment of trachoma consists of 3 to 4 weeks of topical or systemic antibiotic therapy with tetracycline, erythromycin, or sulfon-

amides. (Tetracycline is contraindicated in pregnant females because it may adversely affect the fetus, and in children under age 7, in whom it may discolor teeth permanently.) Severe entropion requires surgical correction.

Patient teaching is essential, especially the following:

• Emphasize the importance of hand washing and making the best use of available water supplies to maintain good personal hygiene. To prevent trachoma, warn patients not to allow flies or gnats to settle around the eyes.

• Because no definitive preventive measure exists (vaccines offer temporary and partial protection, at best), stress the need for strict compliance with the prescribed drug therapy.

• If ordered, teach the patient or family members how to instill eye drops correctly.

Transposition of the great arteries

Description

In this congenital heart defect, the great arteries are reversed. The aorta arises from the right ventricle and the pulmonary artery from the left ventricle, producing two noncommunicating circulatory systems (pulmonary and systemic). Transposition accounts for up to 5% of all congenital heart defects and often coexists with other congenital heart defects, such as ventricular septal defect (VSD), VSD with pulmonary stenosis (PS), atrial septal defect (ASD), and patent ductus arteriosus (PDA). It affects males two to three times more often than females.

Causes

Faulty embryonic development of unknown cause

Signs and symptoms
Newborns
—Cyanosis and tachypnea that worsen with crying
—Signs of congestive heart failure (typically gallop rhythm, tachycardia, dyspnea, hepatomegaly, and cardiomegaly)
—Loud S_2
—Possible murmurs and other associated signs if ASD, VSD, PDA, or PS is present
Older children
—Diminished exercise tolerance
—Fatigability
—Coughing
—Clubbing
—Possible murmurs (more pronounced than in newborns) if ASD, VSD, PDA, or PS is present

Diagnostic tests

• Chest X-rays are normal in the first days of life. Within days to weeks, right atrial and right ventricular enlargement characteristically cause the heart to appear oblong. X-rays also show increased pulmonary vascular markings, except when pulmonary stenosis coexists.

• EKG typically reveals right axis deviation and right ventricular hypertrophy but may be normal in a neonate.

• Echocardiography demonstrates the reversed position of the aorta and pulmonary artery, and records echoes from both semilunar valves simultaneously, due to aortic valve displacement. It also detects other cardiac defects.

• Cardiac catheterization reveals decreased oxygen saturation in left ventricular blood and aortic blood; increased right atrial, right ventricular, and pulmonary artery oxygen saturation; and right ventricular systolic pressure equal to systemic pressure. Dye injection reveals the transposed vessels and the presence of any other cardiac defects and confirms the diagnosis.

• Arterial blood gas measurements indicate hypoxia and secondary metabolic acidosis.

Treatment

An infant with transposition may have atrial balloon septostomy (Rashkind procedure) during cardiac catheterization. This procedure enlarges the patent foramen ovale, which improves oxygenation by allowing greater mixing of the pulmonary and systemic circulation. Atrial balloon septostomy requires passage of a balloon-tipped catheter through the foramen ovale, and subsequent inflation and withdrawal across the atrial septum. This procedure alleviates hypoxia to a certain degree. Afterward, digoxin and diuretics can lessen congestive heart failure until the infant is ready to withstand corrective surgery (usually before age 1).

One of three surgical procedures can correct transposition, depending on the defect's physiology. The Mustard procedure replaces the atrial septum with a Dacron or pericardial partition that allows systemic venous blood to be channeled to the pulmonary artery—which carries the blood to the lungs for oxygenation—and oxygenated blood returning to the heart to be channeled from the pulmonary veins into the aorta. The Senning procedure accomplishes the same result, using the atrial septum to create partitions to redirect blood flow. In the arterial switch, or Jantene procedure, transposed arteries are surgically anastomosed to the correct ventricle. For this procedure to be successful, the left ventricle must be used to pump at systemic pressure, as it does in neonates or in children with a left ventricular outflow obstruction or a large VSD. Surgery also corrects other heart defects.

Clinical Implications

• Explain cardiac catheterization and all necessary procedures to the parents. Offer emotional support.
• Monitor vital signs, arterial blood gas measurements, urinary output, and central venous pressure, watching for signs of congestive heart failure. Give digoxin and I.V. fluids, being careful to avoid fluid overload.
• Teach parents to recognize signs of congestive heart failure and digoxin toxicity (poor feeding, vomiting). Stress the importance of regular checkups to monitor cardiovascular status.
• Teach parents to protect their infant from infection and to give antibiotics.
• Tell the parents to let their child develop normally. They need not restrict activities. He will set his own limits.
• If the patient is scheduled for surgery, explain the procedure to the parents and child, if old enough. Teach them about the ICU, and introduce them to the staff. Also explain postoperative care.
• Preoperatively, monitor arterial blood gas measurements, acid-base balance, intake and output, and vital signs.

After corrective surgery, follow these guidelines:
• Monitor cardiac output by checking blood pressure, skin color, heart rate, urinary output, central venous and left atrial pressures, and level of consciousness. Report abnormalities or changes.
• Carefully measure arterial blood gases.
• To detect supraventricular conduction blocks and dysrhythmias, monitor the patient closely. Watch for signs of atrioventricular blocks, atrial dysrhythmias, and faulty sinoatrial function.
• After Mustard or Senning procedures, watch for signs of baffle obstruction, such as marked facial edema.
• Encourage parents to help their child assume new activity levels and independence. Teach them about postoperative antibiotic prophylaxis for endocarditis.

Trichinosis
(Trichiniasis, trichinellosis)

Description
Trichinosis is an infection that occurs worldwide, especially in populations that eat pork or bear meat. Trichinosis may produce multiple symptoms; respiratory, CNS, and cardiovascular complications; and rarely death.

Causes
Larvae of the roundworm *Trichinella spiralis*

Mode of transmission
Ingestion of uncooked or undercooked meat (primarily swine, less often in dogs, cats, bears, foxes, wolves, and marine animals) that contains *T. spiralis* cysts

Signs and symptoms
Symptoms vary with the stage and degree of infection.
Stage 1—Invasion (occurs 1 week after ingestion)
—Anorexia
—Nausea
—Vomiting
—Diarrhea
—Abdominal pain
—Cramps
Stage 2—Dissemination (occurs 7 to 10 days after ingestion)
—Edema, especially of the eyelids and face
—Muscle pain, particularly in extremities
—Possible itching and burning skin, sweating, skin lesions, fever (102° to 104° F. [38.9° to 40° C.]) and delirium
—Possible severe respiratory, cardiovascular, or CNS infections, palpitations, and lethargy
Stage 3—Encystment (occurs during convalescence, usually 1 week later)
—Encysted larvae in muscle fiber

Diagnostic tests
• Acute and convalescent antibody titers confirm the diagnosis if they are elevated.
• Stool specimen may contain mature worms and larvae during the invasion stage.
• Skin testing may show a positive histamine-like reactivity 15 minutes after intradermal injection of the antigen (within 17 to 20 days after ingestion).
• SGOT, SGPT, CPK, and LDH levels are elevated during acute stages.
• Eosinophil count may be elevated up to 15,000/mm³.
• CSF lymphocyte level may be normal or increased (to 300/mm³), indicating CNS involvement.
• CSF protein level may be increased, indicating CNS involvement.

Treatment and clinical implications
Thiabendazole effectively combats this parasite during the invasion stage. Severe infection (especially CNS invasion) may warrant glucocorticoids to fight against possible inflammation.
• Question the patient about recent ingestion of pork products and the methods used to store and cook them.
• Reduce fever with alcohol rubs, tepid baths, cooling blankets, or antipyretics. Relieve muscular pain with analgesics, enforced bed rest, and proper body alignment.
• Avoid touching painful muscle areas when giving patient care.
• To prevent decubitus ulcers, frequently reposition the patient, and gently massage bony prominences.
• Tell the patient that possible side effects of thiabendazole are nausea, vomiting, dizziness, dermatitis, and fever.
• Explain the importance of bed rest. Sudden death from cardiac involvement may occur in a patient with moderate to severe infection who has resumed activity too soon. Warn the patient to continue bed rest into the convalescent stage to avoid a serious relapse and possible death.

To help prevent trichinosis, follow these guidelines:
- Educate the public about proper cooking and storing methods not only for pork and pork products, but also for meat from carnivores. To kill trichinae, internal meat temperatures should reach 131° F. (55° C.) unless the meat has been cured or frozen.
- Warn travelers to foreign countries or to economically depressed areas in the United States to avoid eating pork. Swine in these areas are often fed raw garbage.
- Report all cases of trichinosis to local public health authorities.

Trichomoniasis

Description
A protozoal infection of the lower genitourinary tract, trichomoniasis affects about 15% of sexually active females and 10% of sexually active males. Incidence is worldwide. In females, the condition may be acute or chronic. Recurrence of trichomoniasis is minimized when sexual partners are treated concurrently.

Causes
Trichomonas vaginalis

Mode of transmission
- Intercourse (most common)
- Contaminated douche equipment or moist washcloths
- Vaginal delivery when the mother is infected

Risk factors
- Use of oral contraceptives
- Pregnancy
- Bacterial overgrowth
- Exudative vaginal or cervical lesions
- Frequent douching

Signs and symptoms
Approximately 70% of females—including those with chronic infections—and most males with trichomoniasis are asymptomatic. Acute infection may produce variable signs such as the following:
Females
—Vaginal discharge (gray or greenish-yellow and possibly profuse, frothy, and malodorous)
—Severe itching
—Redness
—Swelling
—Tenderness
—Dyspareunia
—Dysuria
—Urinary frequency
—Possible postcoital spotting, menorrhagia, or dysmenorrhea
Males
—Urethritis (mild to severe, transient)
—Possible dysuria
—Possible urinary frequency

Diagnostic tests
- Direct microscopic examination of vaginal or seminal discharge is decisive when it reveals *T. vaginalis*.
- Urine specimens that are clear may also reveal *T. vaginalis*.
- Cytologic smear of the cervix may be abnormal if trichomoniasis is untreated.

Treatment
Metronidazole P.O., given to both sexual partners, effectively cures trichomoniasis. Metronidazole may be given in small doses for 7 days, or in a single, large dose. For females, a mild douche with a vinegar and water solution may help acidify vaginal pH.

Acidifying or antiseptic douches are useful to relieve symptoms in pregnant females with trichomoniasis. Such douches may minimize the extent of infection if used promptly. Metronidazole P.O. has not proven safe during pregnancy, especially in the first trimester. Pregnant patients may insert clotrimazole vaginal tablets at bedtime for 7 days.

After treatment, both sexual partners require a follow-up examination to check for residual signs of infection.

Clinical implications

• Instruct the patient not to douche before being examined for trichomoniasis.

• To help prevent reinfection during treatment, urge abstinence from intercourse, or encourage the use of condoms. Tell the patient to use an acidic douche each day of treatment and to avoid using tampons.

• Warn the patient to abstain from alcoholic beverages while taking metronidazole, since alcohol consumption may provoke a disulfiram-type reaction (confusion, headache, cramps, vomiting, convulsions). Also, tell the patient that this drug may turn urine dark brown.

• Caution the patient to avoid over-the-counter douches and vaginal sprays, since chronic use can alter vaginal pH.

• Tell the patient she can reduce the risk of genitourinary bacterial growth by wearing loose-fitting, cotton underwear that allows ventilation; bacteria flourish in a warm, dark, moist environment.

• To prevent newborns from contracting trichomoniasis, make sure pregnant females with this infection receive adequate treatment before delivery.

Trigeminal neuralgia
(Tic douloureux)

Description

Trigeminal neuralgia is a painful disorder of one or more branches of the fifth cranial (trigeminal) nerve that produces paroxysmal attacks of excruciating facial pain precipitated by stimulation of a trigger zone. It occurs mostly in people over age 40, in women more often than men, and on the right side of the face more often than the left. Trigeminal neuralgia can subside spontaneously, with remissions lasting from several months to years.

Causes

Unknown

Signs and symptoms

Searing or burning pain is the characteristic sign—typically lightning jabs, lasting from 1 to 15 minutes (usually 1 to 2 minutes), localized in an area innervated by one of the divisions of the trigeminal nerve, and initiated by a light touch to a hypersensitive area such as the tip of the nose, cheeks, or gums.

Diagnostic tests

The patient's pain history is the basis for diagnosis. However, the following tests may be done to rule out sinus or tooth infections, and tumors:

• Skull X-rays
• CT scan

Treatment

Oral administration of carbamazepine or phenytoin may temporarily relieve or prevent pain. Narcotics may be helpful during the pain episode.

When these medical measures fail or attacks become increasingly frequent or severe, neurosurgical procedures may provide permanent relief. The preferred procedure is percutaneous electrocoagulation of nerve rootlets, under local anesthesia. New treatments include a percutaneous radiofrequency procedure, which causes partial root destruction and relieves pain, and microsurgery for vascular decompression of the trigeminal nerve.

Clinical implications

• Observe and record the characteristics of each attack, including the patient's protective mechanisms.

• Provide adequate nutrition in small, frequent meals at room temperature.

• If the patient is receiving carbamazepine, watch for cutaneous and hematologic reactions (erythematous and pruritic rashes, urticaria, photosensitivity, exfoliative dermatitis, leukopenia, agranulocytosis, eosinophilia, aplastic anemia, thrombocytopenia) and, possibly, urinary retention and transient drowsiness. For the first 3 months of carbamazepine therapy, CBC and liver function should be monitored weekly, then monthly thereafter. Warn the patient to report immediately fever, sore throat, mouth ulcers, easy bruising, or petechial or purpuric hemorrhage, since these may signal thrombocytopenia or aplastic anemia and may require discontinuation of drug therapy.

• If the patient is receiving phenytoin, also watch for side effects, including ataxia, skin eruptions, gingival hyperplasia, and nystagmus.

• After resection of the first branch of the trigeminal nerve, tell the patient to avoid rubbing his eyes and using aerosol spray. Advise him to wear glasses or goggles outdoors and to blink often.

• After surgery to sever the second or third branch, tell the patient to avoid hot foods and drinks, which could burn his mouth, and to chew carefully to avoid biting his mouth. Advise him to place food in the unaffected side of his mouth when chewing, to brush his teeth and rinse his mouth often, and to see the dentist twice a year to detect cavities. (Cavities in the area of the severed nerve will not cause pain.)

• After surgical decompression of the root or partial nerve dissection, check neurologic and vital signs frequently.

• Provide emotional support, and encourage the patient to express his fear and anxiety. Promote independence through self-care and maximum physical activity. Reinforce natural avoidance of stimulation (air, heat, cold) of trigger zones (lips, cheeks, gums).

Tuberculosis

Description

This acute or chronic infection is characterized by pulmonary infiltrates, formation of granulomas with caseation, fibrosis, and cavitation. The organism may disseminate through the lymph system to the circulatory system and then throughout the body. Sites of extrapulmonary tuberculosis include pleura, meninges, joints, lymph nodes, peritoneum, genitourinary tract, and bowel. The American Lung Association estimates that active disease afflicts nearly 14 out of every 100,000 people. Prognosis is excellent with correct treatment.

Causes
• *Mycobacterium tuberculosis* (the major cause)
• Other strains of mycobacteria

Mode of transmission
Inhalation of droplet nuclei when infected persons cough or sneeze

Risk factors
Primary infection
—Poverty
—Crowded, poorly ventilated living conditions
Reinfection
—Gastrectomy
—Uncontrolled diabetes mellitus
—Hodgkin's disease
—Leukemia
—Corticosteroid therapy
—Immunosuppressive therapy
—Silicosis

Signs and symptoms
Primary infection
This is usually asymptomatic but may produce any of the following nonspecific symptoms:
—Fatigue
—Weakness
—Anorexia
—Weight loss
—Night sweats
—Low-grade fever

Reinfection

Any of the following symptoms may occur:

—Cough
—Productive mucopurulent sputum
—Possible hemoptysis
—Chest pains

Diagnostic tests

• Chest X-ray shows nodular lesions, patchy infiltrates (many in upper lobes), cavity formation, scar tissue, and calcium deposits; however, it may not distinguish active from inactive tuberculosis.

• Tuberculin skin test detects infection with tuberculosis but does not distinguish the disease from uncomplicated infection.

• Stains and cultures (of sputum, CSF, urine, drainage from abscess, or pleural fluid) show heat-sensitive, nonmotile, aerobic, acid-fast bacilli and confirm the diagnosis.

Treatment

Antitubercular therapy with daily oral doses of isoniazid or rifampin (with ethambutol added in some cases) for at least 9 months usually cures tuberculosis. After 2 to 4 weeks, the disease is usually no longer infectious, and the patient can resume his normal lifestyle while continuing to take medication. Patients with atypical mycobacterial disease or drug-resistant tuberculosis may require second-line drugs, such as capreomycin, streptomycin, para-aminosalicylic acid, pyrazinamide, and cycloserine.

Clinical implications

• Isolate the infectious patient in a quiet, well-ventilated room until he is no longer contagious. Teach the patient to cough and sneeze into tissues and to dispose of all secretions properly. Place a covered trash can nearby or tape a waxed bag to the side of the bed for used tissues. Instruct the patient to wear a mask when outside of his room. Visitors and hospital personnel should also wear masks when they are in the patient's room.

• Remind the patient to get plenty of rest. Stress the importance of eating balanced meals to promote recovery. If the patient is anorexic, urge him to eat small meals throughout the day. Record weight weekly.

• Be alert for side effects of medications. Since isoniazid sometimes leads to hepatitis or peripheral neuritis, monitor SGOT and SGPT levels. To prevent or treat peripheral neuritis, give pyridoxine (vitamin B_6) as ordered. If the patient receives ethambutol, watch for optic neuritis; if it develops, discontinue the drug. If he receives rifampin, watch for hepatitis and purpura. Observe the patient for other complications, such as hemoptysis.

• Before discharge, teach the patient to watch for side effects from medication and warn him to report them immediately. Emphasize the importance of regular follow-up examinations, and instruct the patient and his family about the signs and symptoms of recurring tuberculosis. Stress the need to follow long-term treatment faithfully.

• Advise persons who have been exposed to infected patients to receive tuberculin tests and, if ordered, chest X-rays and prophylactic isoniazid.

Ulcerative colitis

Description
Ulcerative colitis is an inflammatory, often chronic disease that affects the mucosa and submucosa of the colon. It usually begins in the rectum and sigmoid colon, and often extends upward into the entire colon. It rarely affects the small intestine, except for the terminal ileum. Severity ranges from a mild, localized disorder to a fulminant disease that may cause a perforated colon, progressing to potentially fatal peritonitis and toxemia. It occurs primarily in young adults, especially women. It is also more prevalent among Jews and in higher socioeconomic groups.

Causes
Unknown

Risk factors
- Family history of the disease
- Bacterial infection
- Allergic reaction to food, milk, or other substances that release inflammatory histamine in the bowel
- Overproduction of enzymes that break down the mucous membranes
- Emotional stress
- Autoimmune reactions, such as arthritis, hemolytic anemia, erythema nodosum, and uveitis

Signs and symptoms
- Recurrent bloody diarrhea and asymptomatic remissions are the hallmark signs of ulcerative colitis. The stool typically contains pus and mucus.
- Spastic rectum and anus
- Abdominal pain
- Irritability
- Weight loss
- Weakness
- Anorexia
- Nausea and vomiting

Diagnostic tests
- Sigmoidoscopy showing increased mucosal friability, decreased mucosal detail, and thick inflammatory exudate suggests this diagnosis.
- Biopsy helps to confirm the diagnosis.
- Colonoscopy may be done to determine extent of the disease and evaluate strictured areas and pseudopolyps.
- Barium enema may be done to assess the extent of the disease and detect complications, such as strictures and carcinoma.
- Stool specimen may be cultured and analyzed for leukocytes, ova, and parasites.
- Erythrocyte sedimentation rate will be increased in relation to the severity of the attack.
- Other supportive laboratory values include decreased serum levels of potassium, magnesium, hemoglobin, and albumin as well as leukocytosis and increased prothrombin time.

Treatment
The goals of treatment are to control inflammation, replace nutritional losses and blood volume, and prevent

complications. Supportive treatment includes bed rest, I.V. fluid replacement, and a clear-liquid diet. For patients awaiting surgery or showing signs of dehydration and debilitation from excessive diarrhea, I.V. hyperalimentation rests the intestinal tract, decreases stool volume, and restores positive nitrogen balance. Blood transfusions or iron supplements may be needed to correct anemia.

Drug therapy to control inflammation includes adrenocorticotropic hormone and adrenal corticosteroids, such as prednisone, prednisolone, and hydrocortisone. Sulfasalazine, which has anti-inflammatory and antimicrobial properties, may also be used. Antispasmodics such as tincture of belladonna, and antidiarrheals such as diphenoxylate compound are used only for patients with frequent, troublesome diarrheal stools whose ulcerative colitis is under control. These drugs may precipitate massive dilation of the colon (toxic megacolon) and are usually contraindicated.

Surgery is the treatment of last resort if the patient has toxic megacolon, fails to respond to drugs and supportive measures, or finds symptoms unbearable. The most common surgical technique is proctocolectomy with ileostomy. Total colectomy and ileorectal anastomosis is done less often because of its associated mortality (2% to 5%). This procedure removes the entire colon and anastomoses the rectum and the terminal ileum. It requires observation of the remaining rectal stump for any signs of malignancy or colitis.

Pouch ileostomy, in which a pouch is created from a small loop of the terminal ileum and a nipple valve formed from the distal ileum, is gaining popularity in some areas. The resulting stoma opens just above the pubic hairline; the pouch empties through a catheter inserted in the stoma several times a day. In ulcerative colitis, colectomy to prevent colon cancer is controversial.

Clinical implications

● Accurately record intake and output, particularly the frequency and volume of stools. Watch for signs of dehydration (poor skin turgor, furrowed tongue) and electrolyte imbalances, especially signs of hypokalemia (muscle weakness, paresthesia) and hypernatremia (tachycardia, flushed skin, fever, dry tongue). Monitor hemoglobin and hematocrit, and give blood transfusions, as ordered. Provide good mouth care for the patient who is allowed nothing by mouth.

● After each bowel movement, thoroughly clean the skin around the rectum. Provide an air mattress or sheepskin to help prevent skin breakdown.

● Administer medication, as ordered. Watch for side effects of prolonged corticosteroid therapy (moonface, hirsutism, edema, gastric irritation). Be aware that such therapy may mask infection.

● If the patient needs hyperalimentation, change dressings, as ordered, assess for inflammation at the insertion site, and check urine every 6 hours for sugar and acetone.

● Take precautionary measures if the patient is prone to bleeding. Watch closely for signs of complications, such as a perforated colon and peritonitis (fever, severe abdominal pain, abdominal rigidity and tenderness, cool clammy skin), and toxic megacolon (abdominal distention, decreased bowel sounds).

Carefully prepare the patient for surgery, especially by informing him about ileostomy.

● Explain what a stoma is, what it looks like, and how it differs from normal anatomy. Provide information (available from the United Ostomy Association), and arrange for the patient to be visited by an enterostomal therapist and a recovered ileostomate, if possible.

• Encourage the patient to verbalize his feelings. Provide emotional support and a quiet environment.

• Do a bowel preparation, as ordered. This usually involves keeping the patient on a clear-liquid diet, using cleansing enemas, and administering antimicrobials, such as neomycin.

After surgery, give meticulous supportive care.

• Keep the nasogastric tube patent. After removal of the tube, provide a clear-liquid diet, and gradually advance to a low-residue diet, as tolerated.

• After a proctocolectomy and ileostomy, teach good stoma care. Wash the skin around the stoma with soapy water and dry thoroughly. Apply karaya gum around the stoma's base to avoid irritation and make a watertight seal. Attrach the pouch over the karaya ring. Cut an opening in the ring to fit over the stoma, and secure the pouch to the skin. Empty the pouch when it is one-third full. Encourage the patient to take over this care.

• After a pouch ileostomy, uncork the catheter every hour to allow contents to drain. After 10 to 14 days, gradually increase the length of time the catheter is left corked until it can be opened every 3 hours. Then, remove the catheter and reinsert it every 3 to 4 hours for drainage. Teach the patient how to insert the catheter and how to take care of the stoma.

• Encourage the patient to have regular physical examinations, since he is at risk of developing colorectal cancer.

Complications
Ulcerative colitis may lead to complications affecting many body systems.

• Blood: anemia from iron deficiency, coagulation defects due to vitamin K deficiency

• Skin: erythema nodosum on the face and arms, pyoderma gangrenosum on the legs and ankles

• Eye: uveitis

• Liver: pericholangitis, sclerosing cholangitis, cirrhosis, possible cholangiocarcinoma

• Musculoskeletal: arthritis, ankylosing spondylitis, loss of muscle mass

• GI: strictures, pseudopolyps, stenosis, and perforated colon, leading to peritonitis and toxemia

• Colorectal cancer: greater than normal risk, especially if onset of the disease occurs before age 15 or if it has persisted for longer than 10 years

Undescended testes
(Cryptorchidism)

Description
In this congenital disorder, one or both testes fail to descend into the scrotum, remaining in the abdomen, inguinal canal, or at the external ring. Although this condition may be bilateral, it more commonly affects the right testis. True undescended testes remain along the path of normal descent, while ectopic testes deviate from that path.

Causes
The causes of undescended testes are unknown; however, theories attempting to explain the condition include the following:

• Hormonal factors—most likely androgenic hormones from either a maternal or fetal source, and possibly maternal progesterone or gonadotropic hormones from the maternal pituitary

• Inadequate testosterone levels

• Defect in the testes

• Defect in the gubernaculum

Signs and symptoms
Unilateral cryptorchidism
—Possible underdeveloped scrotum
—Nonpalpable testis on affected side
—Possible enlarged scrotum on unaffected side
Uncorrected bilateral crytorchidism
—Infertility

Diagnostic tests

Physical examination confirms cryptorchidism after laboratory tests determine sex.

• Buccal smear determines genetic sex by showing a male sex chromatin pattern.

• Serum gonadotropin measurement confirms the presence of testes by showing adequate circulating hormone.

Treatment

If the testes do not descend spontaneously by age 1, surgical correction is usually indicated. Orchiopexy secures the testes in the scrotum and is commonly performed before the boy reaches age 4 (optimum age is 1 to 2 years). Orchiopexy prevents sterility and excessive trauma from abnormal positioning. It also prevents harmful psychological effects. Rarely, human chorionic gonadotropin (HCG) I.M. may stimulate descent. However, hormonal therapy with HCG is ineffective if the testes are located in the abdomen.

Clinical implications

• Encourage parents of the child with undescended testes to express their concern about his condition. Provide information about causes, available treatments, and ultimate effect on reproduction. Emphasize that, especially in premature infants, the testes may descend spontaneously.

• If orchiopexy is necessary, explain the surgery to the child, using terms he understands. Tell him that a rubber band may be taped to his thigh for about 1 week after surgery to keep the testis in place. Explain that his scrotum may swell but should not be painful.

• After orchiopexy, monitor vital signs and intake and output. Check dressings. Encourage coughing and deep breathing. Watch for urinary retention.

• Keep the operative site clean. Tell the child to wipe from front to back after defecating. If a rubber band has been applied to keep the testis in place, maintain tension, but check that it is not too tight.

• Encourage parents to participate in postoperative care, such as bathing or feeding the child. Also urge the child to do as much for himself as possible.

Complications

If bilateral cryptorchidism persists untreated into adolescence, it may cause any of the following complications:

• Sterility

• Increased vulnerability to trauma

• Increased risk of testicular malignancy

Urinary tract infection

Description

Cystitis and urethritis, two forms of urinary tract infection (UTI), are nearly 10 times more common in women than in men and affect approximately 10% to 20% of all women at least once. Lower UTI is also a prevalent bacterial disease in children, with girls also most commonly affected. In men and children, lower UTI is frequently related to anatomic or physiologic abnormalities. UTIs often respond readily to treatment, but recurrence and resistant bacterial flareup during therapy are possible.

Causes

• Gram-negative enteric bacteria (typically *Escherichia coli*, *Klebsiella*, *Proteus*, *Enterobacter*, *Pseudomonas*, or *Seiratia*)

• Simultaneous infection with multiple pathogens in a patient with neurogenic bladder, an indwelling (Foley) catheter, or a fistula between the intestine and bladder

Signs and symptoms

Characteristic signs

—Urgency

—Frequency
—Dysuria
—Cramps or spasms of the bladder
—Itching
—Feeling of warmth during urination
—Nocturia
—Possible hematuria
—Possible fever
—Possible urethral discharge in males
Other common features
—Low back pain
—Malaise
—Nausea
—Vomiting
—Abdominal pain or tenderness over bladder
—Chills
—Flank pain

Diagnostic tests
• Microscopic urinalysis showing RBCs and WBCs greater than 10/high power field suggest UTI.
• Clean, midstream urine specimen revealing a bacterial count of more than 100,000/ml confirms the diagnosis.
• Sensitivity testing determines the appropriate therapeutic antimicrobial agent.
• Blood test or stained smear of the discharge rules out venereal disease.
• Voiding cystourethrography or intravenous pyelography may detect congenital anomalies.

Treatment
Appropriate antimicrobials are the treatment of choice for initial lower UTI in most cases. A 7- to 10-day course of antibiotic therapy is standard. After 3 days of antibiotic therapy, urine culture should show no organisms. If the urine is not sterile, bacterial resistance has probably occurred, making the use of a different antimicrobial necessary. Single-dose antibiotic therapy with amoxicillin or co-trimaxazole may be effective in women with acute noncomplicated UTI. A urine culture taken 1 to 2 weeks later indicates whether the infection has been eradicated.

Recurrent infections due to infected renal calculi, chronic prostatitis, or structural abnormality may necessitate surgery. Prostatitis also requires long-term antibiotic therapy. In patients without these predisposing conditions, long-term, low-dose antibiotic therapy is the treatment of choice.

Clinical implications
The care plan should include careful patient teaching, supportive measures, and proper specimen collection.
• Explain the nature and purpose of antimicrobial therapy. Emphasize the importance of completing the prescribed course of therapy or, with long-term prophylaxis, of adhering strictly to ordered dosage. Urge the patient to drink plenty of water (at least eight glasses a day). Stress the need to maintain a consistent fluid intake of about 2,000 ml/day. More or less than this amount may alter the effect of the prescribed antimicrobial. Fruit juices, especially cranberry juice, and oral doses of vitamin C may help acidify the urine and enhance the action of the medication.
• Watch for GI disturbances from antimicrobial therapy. Nitrofurantoin macrocrystals, taken with milk or a meal, prevent such distress. If therapy includes phenazopyridine, warn the patient that this drug may turn urine red-orange.
• Suggest warm sitz baths for relief of perineal discomfort. If baths are not effective, apply heat sparingly to the perineum, but be careful not to burn the patient. Apply topical antiseptics, such as povidone-iodine ointment, on the urethral meatus, as necessary.
• Collect all urine samples for culture and sensitivity testing carefully and promptly. Teach the female patient how to clean the perineum properly and keep the labia separated during voiding. A noncontaminated mid-

stream specimen is essential for accurate diagnosis.

• To prevent recurrent lower UTIs, teach the female patient to carefully wipe the perineum from front to back and to clean it thoroughly with soap and water after defecation. Advise an infection-prone woman to void immediately after sexual intercourse. Stress the need to drink plenty of fluids routinely and to avoid postponing urination. Recommend frequent comfort stops during long car trips. Also stress the need to empty the bladder completely. To prevent recurrent infections in men, urge prompt treatment of predisposing conditions such as chronic prostatitis.

Uterine cancer

Description

Uterine cancer (cancer of the endometrium) is the most common gynecologic cancer. Usually, it affects postmenopausal women between ages 50 and 60. It is uncommon between ages 30 and 40, and extremely rare before age 30. Most premenopausal women who develop uterine cancer have a history of anovulatory menstrual cycles or other hormonal imbalance. An average of 37,000 new cases of uterine cancer are reported annually; of these, 3,300 are eventually fatal.

Causes

• Adenocarcinoma (most common cause)
• Adenoacanthoma
• Endometrial stromal sarcoma
• Lymphosarcoma
• Mixed mesodermal tumors (including carcinosarcoma)
• Leiomyosarcoma

Risk factors

• Low fertility index and anovulation
• Abnormal uterine bleeding
• Obesity, hypertension, or diabetes

• Familial tendency
• History of uterine polyps or endometrial hyperplasia
• Estrogen therapy (still controversial)

Signs and symptoms

Early characteristic signs
—Uterine enlargement
—Unusual premenopausal or postmenopausal bleeding (discharge may be watery and blood-streaked at first but gradually becomes more bloody)
Late signs
Cancer is well advanced when these appear:
—Pain
—Weight loss

Diagnostic tests

Diagnosis of uterine cancer requires endometrial, cervical, and endocervical biopsies. (See *Staging Uterine Cancer*, p. 788.) Negative biopsies call for a fractional dilatation and curettage (D&C) to determine diagnosis. Positive diagnosis requires the following tests to provide baseline data and permit staging:

• Multiple cervical biopsies and endocervical curettage to pinpoint cervical involvement
• Schiller's test, staining the cervix and vagina with an iodine solution (healthy tissues turn brown; cancerous tissues resist the stain)
• Complete physical examination
• Chest X-ray or CT scan
• Intravenous pyelography and, possibly, cystoscopy
• Complete blood studies
• EKG
• Proctoscopy or barium enema studies (rarely used)

Treatment

Treatment varies, depending on the extent of the disease.
• Surgery usually involves total abdominal hysterectomy, bilateral sal-

Staging Uterine Cancer

Stage 0: Carcinoma in situ. Histologic findings are suspicious of malignancy; cases of Stage 0 should not be included in any therapeutic statistics.
Stage I: Carcinoma confined to the corpus
Stage Ia: Length of the uterine cavity 8 cm or less
Stage Ib: Length of the uterine cavity more than 8 cm
   Stage I cases should be subgrouped by histologic type of the adenocarcinoma as follows:
   • G1: Highly differentiated adenomatous carcinoma
   • G2: Moderately differentiated adenomatous carcinoma with partly solid areas
   • G3: Predominantly solid or entirely undifferentiated carcinoma
Stage II: Carcinoma has involved the corpus and the cervix but has not extended outside the uterus.
Stage III: Carcinoma has extended outside the uterus but not outside the true pelvis.
Stage IV: Carcinoma has extended outside the true pelvis or has obviously involved the mucosa of the bladder or rectum. A bullous edema as such does not permit a case to be allotted to Stage IV.
Stage IVa: Spread of the growth to adjacent organs
Stage IVb: Spread of the growth to distant organs

Reprinted from *Manual for Staging of Cancer* (Chicago: American Joint Committee for Cancer Staging and End Results Reporting, 1983). Used with permission.

pingo-oophorectomy, or possibly omentectomy with or without pelvic or paraaortic lymphadenectomy. Total exenteration removes all pelvic organs, including the vagina, and is done only when the disease is sufficiently contained to allow surgical removal of diseased parts. Partial exenteration may retain an unaffected colorectum or bladder.

• Radiation therapy (intracavitary or external radiation, or both, given 6 weeks before surgery) may inhibit recurrence and lengthen survival time when the tumor is not well differentiated.

• Hormonal therapy uses progesterone or chemotherapy with doxorubicin. Other combinations are useful for recurrence, especially vincristine, cyclophosphamide, and actinomycin D.

Clinical implications

The care plan for patients with uterine cancer should emphasize comprehensive patient teaching to help them cope with surgery, radiation, and chemotherapy. Provide good postoperative care and psychological support.

• Before surgery, reinforce what the physician has told the patient about the surgery, and explain the routine tests (e.g., repeated blood tests the morning after surgery) and postoperative care. If the patient is to have a lymphadenectomy *and* a total hysterectomy, explain that she will probably have a blood drainage system for about 5 days after surgery. Also explain indwelling (Foley) catheter care. Fit the patient with antiembolism stockings for use during and after surgery. Make sure the patient's blood has been typed and cross-matched. If the patient is premenopausal, inform her that removal of her ovaries will induce menopause.

• After surgery, measure fluid contents of the blood drainage system every shift. Notify the physician immediately if drainage exceeds 400 ml.

• If the patient has received subcutaneous heparin, continue administration, as ordered, until the patient is fully ambulatory again. Give prophylactic antibiotics, as ordered, and provide good Foley catheter care.

• Check vital signs every 4 hours. Watch for and immediately report any sign of complications, such as bleeding, abdominal distention, severe pain, wheezing, or other breathing difficulties. Provide analgesics, as ordered.

• Regularly encourage the patient to breathe deeply and cough to help prevent complications. Promote the use of an incentive spirometer once every waking hour to help keep lungs expanded.

• Find out if the patient is to have internal or external radiation or both. Usually, internal radiation therapy is done first. Check to see if the radioactive source will be inserted while the patient is in the operating room (preloaded) or at bedside (afterloaded). If the source is preloaded, the patient returns to her room "hot," and safety precautions begin immediately.

If the patient receives internal radiation, follow these guidelines:

• Explain the preloaded internal radiation procedure, and answer the patient's questions. Explain that internal radiation requires a 2- to 3-day hospital stay, bowel preparation, povidone-iodine vaginal douche, clear liquid diet, and nothing taken by mouth the night before the implantation; it also requires a Foley catheter.

• Tell the patient that the procedure is performed in the operating room under general anesthesia. She will be placed in a dorsal position, with knees and hips flexed, heels resting in footrests. The source is implanted in the vagina by the physician.

• Remember that safety precautions— time, distance, and shielding—must be imposed as soon as the patient's radioactive source is in place. Tell the patient that she will require a private room.

• Encourage the patient to limit movement while the source is in place. If she prefers, elevate the head of the bed slightly. Make sure the patient can reach everything she needs (call bell, telephone, water) without stretching or straining. Assist her in range-of-motion arm exercises (leg exercises and other body movements could dislodge the source). If ordered, administer a tranquilizer to help the patient relax and remain still. Organize the time you spend with the patient to minimize your exposure to radiation.

• Check the patient's vital signs every 4 hours. Watch for skin reaction, vaginal bleeding, abdominal discomfort, or evidence of dehydration.

• Inform visitors of safety precautions and hang a sign listing these precautions on the patient's door.

If the patient receives external radiation, follow these guidelines:

• Explain that a member of the radiation team will implant the source while the patient is in her room.

• Teach the patient and her family about the therapy before it begins. Tell the patient that treatment is usually given 5 days a week for 6 weeks. Warn her not to scrub body areas marked with indelible ink for treatment because it is important to direct treatment to exactly the same area each time.

• Instruct the patient to maintain a high-protein, high-carbohydrate, low-residue diet to reduce bulk and yet maintain calories. Administer diphenoxylate with atropine, as ordered, to minimize diarrhea, a possible side effect of pelvic radiation.

• To minimize skin breakdown and reduce the risk of skin infection, tell the patient to keep the treatment area dry, to avoid wearing clothes that rub against the area, and to avoid using heating pads, alcohol rubs, or irritating skin creams. Since radiation therapy increases susceptibility to infection (possibly by lowering WBC count), tell the patient to avoid persons with colds or other infections.

• Remember, a patient with uterine cancer needs special counseling and psychological support to help her cope with this disease and the necessary treatment measures. Fearful about her survival, she may also be concerned that treatment will alter her life-style and prevent sexual intimacy. Explain that except in total pelvic exenteration, the vagina remains intact and that once she recovers, sexual intercourse is possible. Your presence and interest alone will help the patient, even if you cannot answer every question she may ask.

Uterine leiomyomas
(Myomas, fibromyomas, fibroids)

Description
The most common benign tumors in women, uterine leiomyomas are smooth-muscle tumors. Usually, they are multiple and occur in the uterine corpus, although they may appear on the cervix or on the round or broad ligament. Uterine leiomyomas occur in approximately 20% of all women over age 35 and affect blacks three times more often than whites. Malignancy (leiomyosarcoma) develops in only 0.1% of patients.

Causes
The cause of uterine leiomyomas is unknown, but excessive levels of estrogen and human growth hormone (HGH) may influence tumor formation by stimulating susceptible fibromuscular elements. Large doses of estrogen and the later stages of pregnancy increase both tumor size and HGH levels. Conversely, uterine leiomyomas usually shrink or disappear after menopause, when estrogen production decreases.

Signs and symptoms
Common signs
—Submucosal hypermenorrhea (the cardinal sign)
—Possible other forms of abnormal endometrial bleeding, dysmenorrhea, and pain
Other features
If the tumor is large the following may occur:
—Feeling of heaviness in the abdomen
—Pain
—Intestinal obstruction
—Constipation
—Urinary frequency or urgency
—Possible irregular uterine enlargement

Diagnostic tests
• Blood studies showing anemia support the diagnosis.
• Dilatation and curettage or submucosal hysterosalpingography detect submucosal leiomyomas.
• Laparoscopy visualizes subserous leiomyomas on the uterine surface.

Treatment
Treatment depends on the severity of symptoms, size and location of the tumors, and the patient's age, parity, pregnancy status, desire to have children, and general health.

If they have caused problems in the past, or if they are likely to threaten a future pregnancy, small leiomyomas may be surgically removed. This is the treatment of choice for a young woman who wants to have children.

Tumors that twist or grow large enough to cause intestinal obstruction require a hysterectomy, with preservation of the ovaries, if possible.

If the patient is pregnant, but her uterus is no larger than a 6-month normal uterus by the 16th week of pregnancy, the outcome for the pregnancy is favorable, and surgery is usually unnecessary. However, if a pregnant woman has a leiomyomatous uterus the size of a 5- to 6-month normal uterus by the 9th week of pregnancy, spontaneous abortion will probably occur, especially with a cervical leiomyoma. If surgery is necessary, a hysterectomy is usually performed 5 to 6 months after delivery (when involution is complete), with preservation of the ovaries, if possible.

Clinical implications
• Tell the patient to report any abnormal bleeding or pelvic pain immediately.
• If a hysterectomy or oophorectomy is indicated, explain the effects of the operation on menstruation, menopause, and sexual activity to the patient.
• Reassure the patient that she will not experience premature menopause if her ovaries are left intact.
• If it is necessary for the patient to have a multiple myomectomy, make sure she understands pregnancy is still possible. However, if the uterine cavity is entered during surgery, explain that a cesarean delivery may be necessary.
• In a patient with severe anemia due to excessive bleeding, administer iron and blood transfusions, as ordered.

Uveitis

Description
Uveitis is inflammation of one uveal tract. It occurs as anterior uveitis, which affects the iris (iritis) or both the iris and the ciliary body (iridocyclitis); as posterior uveitis, which affects the choroid (choroiditis), or both the choroid and the retina (chorioretinitis); or as panuveitis, which affects the entire uveal tract. Although clinical distinction is not always possible, anterior uveitis occurs in two forms—granulomatous and nongranulomatous. (See *Granulomatous and Nongranulomatous Uveitis,* p. 792.) Untreated anterior uveitis progresses to posterior uveitis, causing scarring, cataracts, and glaucoma. With immediate treatment, anterior uveitis usually subsides after a few days to several weeks; however, recurrence is likely. Posterior uveitis generally produces some residual visual loss and marked blurring of vision.

Causes
• Typically, idiopathic
• Allergy
• Bacteria
• Viruses
• Fungi
• Chemicals
• Trauma
• Surgery
• Systemic diseases, such as rheumatoid arthritis, ankylosing spondylitis, and toxoplasmosis

Signs and symptoms
Anterior uveitis
—Moderate to severe eye pain
—Severe ciliary injection
—Photophobia
—Tearing
—Small, nonreactive pupil
—Blurred vision
—Possible deposits on the back of the cornea (seen in the anterior chamber)
Posterior uveitis
—Slightly decreased or blurred vision or floating spots
—Possible posterior synechia and photophobia

Diagnostic tests
• Slit-lamp examination shows a "flare and cell" pattern, which looks like light passing through smoke, and an increased number of cells over the inflamed area.
• Ophthalmoscopic examination or slit-lamp examination using a special

Granulomatous and Nongranulomatous Uveitis

FACTOR	GRANULOMATOUS	NONGRANULOMATOUS
Location	• Any part of uveal tract, but usually the posterior part	• Anterior portion: iris, ciliary body
Onset	• Insidious	• Acute
Pain	• None or slight	• Marked
Photophobia	• Slight	• Marked
Course	• Chronic	• Acute
Prognosis	• Fair to poor	• Good
Recurrence	• Occasional	• Common

Adapted with permission from Lillian S. Brunner and Doris S. Suddarth, *Textbook of Medical- Surgical Nursing*, 5th ed. (Philadelphia: J.B. Lippincott Co., 1984).

lens can identify active inflammatory fundus lesions involving the retina and/or choroid.
• Serologic tests can tell if toxoplasmosis is the cause of posterior uveitis.

Treatment
Uveitis includes treatment of any known underlying cause and application of a topical cycloplegic, such as 1% atropine sulfate, and of topical and subconjunctival corticosteroids. For severe uveitis, therapy includes oral systemic corticosteroids. However, because long-term steroid therapy can cause a rise in intraocular pressure (IOP) and/or cataracts, carefully monitor IOP during acute inflammation. If IOP rises, therapy should include an antiglaucoma medication, such as the beta blocker timolol, or a carbonic anhydrase inhibitor, such as acetazolamide (Diamox).

Clinical implications
• Encourage rest during the acute phase.
• Teach the patient the proper method of instilling eye drops.
• Suggest the use of dark glasses to ease the discomfort of photophobia.

• Instruct the patient to watch for and report side effects of systemic corticosteroid therapy (edema, muscle weakness).
• Stress the importance of follow-up care because of the strong likelihood of recurrence. Tell the patient to seek treatment immediately, at first signs of iritis.

V

Vaginal cancer

Description

Vaginal cancer varies in severity according to its location and effect on lymphatic drainage. It may progress from an intraepithelial tumor to an invasive cancer. A lesion in the upper third of the vagina (the most common site) usually metastasizes to the groin nodes. A lesion in the lower third (the second most common site) usually metastasizes to the hypogastric and iliac nodes. A lesion in the middle third metastasizes erratically. A posterior lesion displaces and distends the vaginal posterior wall before spreading to deep layers. By contrast, an anterior lesion spreads more rapidly into other structures and deep layers.

Vaginal cancer accounts for approximately 2% of all gynecologic malignancies. Incidence is increased in young women whose mothers took diethylstilbestrol. It usually occurs in women in their early to mid-50s, but some of the rarer types occur in younger women and children.

Causes

- Squamous cell carcinoma (most common)
- Melanoma
- Sarcoma
- Adenocarcinoma
- Rhabdomyosarcoma (in children)

Signs and symptoms

- Abnormal bleeding and discharge
- Possible vaginal lesions (large or small, often firm and ulcerated)
- Frequent voiding and bladder pain, with bladder involvement
- Rectal bleeding, with rectal involvement
- Vulvar lesion
- Pain, with involvement of pubic bone or other surrounding tissues

Diagnostic tests

- Vaginal Pap smear showing abnormal cells is the basis of diagnosis.
- Biopsy of any visible lesion permits histologic evaluation (see *Staging Vaginal Cancer*, p. 794).
- Colposcopy is done when lesions are not visible, to search out abnormalities.
- Painting the suspected vaginal area with Lugol's solution (strong iodine solution) also helps identify malignant areas by staining glycogen-containing normal tissue, while leaving abnormal tissue unstained.

Treatment

Early-stage treatment aims to treat the malignant area, while preserving the normal parts of the vagina. Radiation or surgery varies with the size, depth, and location of the lesion, and the patient's desire to maintain a functional vagina.

Surgery is usually recommended only when the tumor is so extensive that exenteration is needed, because close proximity to the bladder and rectum permits retention of only minimal tissue margins around resected vaginal tissue.

Staging Vaginal Cancer

Stage 0: Carcinoma in situ; intraepithelial carcinoma
Stage I: Carcinoma limited to vaginal wall
Stage II: Carcinoma involves subvaginal tissue but not the pelvic wall
Stage III: Carcinoma has extended to the pelvic wall
Stage IV: Carcinoma has extended beyond the true pelvis or has involved the mucosa of the bladder or rectum. Bullous edema as such does not permit assignment to Stage IV.
Stage IVa: Spread to adjacent organs
Stage IVb: Spread to distant organs

Reprinted from *Manual for Staging of Cancer* (Chicago: American Joint Committee for Cancer Staging and End Results Reporting, 1983). Used with permission.

Radiation therapy is the preferred treatment for advanced vaginal cancer. Most patients need preliminary external radiation treatment to shrink the tumor before internal radiation can begin. Then, if the tumor is localized to the vault and the cervix is present, radiation (radium or cesium) can be given with an intrauterine tandem or ovoids; if the cervix is absent, then a specially designed vaginal applicator is used instead. To minimize complications, radioactive sources and filters are carefully placed away from radiosensitive tissues such as the bladder and the rectum. Such treatment lasts 48 to 72 hours, depending on dosage.

Clinical implications

The patient receiving internal radiation needs special care.
• Before treatment begins, find out if the radiation source will be preloaded in the operating room or afterloaded while the patient is in her bed, so that you know how to plan patient care to minimize your exposure to radiation.
• Since the effects of radiation are cumulative, wear a radiosensitive badge and a lead shield (if available) when you enter the patient's room. Check with the radiation therapist concerning the maximum recommended time that you can safely spend with the patient when giving direct care.
• While the radiation source is in place, the patient must lie flat on her back. Insert an indwelling (Foley) catheter (usually done in the operating room), and do not change the patient's linens unless they are soiled. Give only partial bed baths, and make sure the patient has a call bell, telephone, water, or anything else she needs within easy reach. The physician will order a clear liquid or low-residue diet and an antidiarrheal drug to prevent bowel movements.
• To compensate for immobility, encourage the patient to do active range-of-motion exercises with both arms.
• Before radiation treatment, explain the necessity of immobilization, and tell the patient what it entails (such as no linen changes and the use of a Foley catheter). Throughout therapy, encourage her to express her anxieties and fears.
• Instruct the patient to use a stent or prescribed candle exercises to prevent vaginal stenosis. Coitus is also helpful in preventing such stenosis.

Valvular heart disease

Description

In valvular heart disease, two types of mechanical disruption can occur: stenosis, or narrowing, of the valve opening; or incomplete closure of the valve. Valvular heart disease occurs in varying forms and can affect any of the four valves of the heart: mitral, aortic, pulmonic, or tricuspid. Incidence varies depending on the form of valvular heart disease present. Mitral and tricuspid disease affects women more often than men. Aortic disease is more prevalent in men. Severe valvular heart disease can eventually lead to heart failure. Valvular heart disease occurs in varying forms:

• Mitral insufficiency: In this form, blood from the left ventricle flows back into the left atrium during systole, causing the atrium to enlarge to accommodate the backflow. As a result, the left ventricle also dilates to accommodate the increased volume of blood from the atrium and to compensate for diminishing cardiac output. Ventricular hypertrophy and increased end-diastolic pressure result in increased pulmonary artery pressure, eventually leading to left and right ventricular failure.

• Mitral stenosis: Narrowing of the valve by valvular abnormalities, fibrosis, or calcification obstructs blood flow from the left atrium to the left ventricle. Consequently, left atrial volume and pressure rise and the chamber dilates. Greater resistance to blood flow causes pulmonary hypertension, right ventricular hypertrophy, and eventually right ventricular failure. Also, inadequate filling of the left ventricle produces low cardiac output.

• Aortic insufficiency: Blood flows back into the left ventricle during diastole, causing a fluid overload in the ventricle, which, in turn, dilates and, ultimately, hypertrophies. The excess volume causes a fluid overload in the left atrium and finally in the pulmonary system. Left ventricular failure and pulmonary edema eventually result.

• Aortic stenosis: Increased left ventricular pressure attempts to overcome the resistance of the narrowed valvular opening. The added workload causes a greater demand for oxygen, while diminished cardiac output causes poor coronary artery perfusion, ischemia of the left ventricle, and eventually left ventricular failure.

• Pulmonic insufficiency: Blood ejected into the pulmonary artery during systole flows back into the right ventricle during diastole, causing a fluid overload in the ventricle, ventricular hypertrophy, and finally right ventricular failure.

• Pulmonic stenosis: Obstructed right ventricular outflow causes right ventricular hypertrophy in an attempt to overcome resistance to the narrow valvular opening. Right ventricular failure ultimately results.

• Tricuspid insufficiency: Blood flows back into the right atrium during systole, decreasing blood flow to the lungs and left side of the heart. Cardiac output also lessens. Fluid overload in the right side of the heart can eventually lead to right ventricular failure.

• Tricuspid stenosis: Obstructed blood flow from the right atrium to the right ventricle causes the right atrium to dilate and hypertrophy. Eventually, this leads to right ventricular failure and increases pressure in the vena cava.

Causes
Mitral stenosis
—Rheumatic fever (most common)
—Possibly associated with congenital anomalies
Mitral insufficiency
—Rheumatic fever
—Idiopathic hypertrophic subaortic stenosis (IHSS)
—Mitral valve prolapse
—Myocardial infarction
—Severe left ventricular failure
—Ruptured chordae tendineae
—Associated with congenital anomalies such as transposition of the great vessels
Tricuspid insufficiency
—Right ventricular failure
—Rheumatic fever
—Trauma (rare)
—Endocarditis (rare)
—Associated with congenital disorders

Tricuspid stenosis
—Rheumatic fever
—Congenital
—Associated with mitral or aortic valve disease

Pulmonic stenosis
—Congenital stenosis of valve cusps
—Rheumatic heart disease (infrequent)
—Associated with congenital heart defects such as tetralogy of Fallot

Pulmonic insufficiency
—Congenital
—Pulmonary hypertension
—Prolonged use of pressure monitoring catheter in the pulmonary artery (rare)

Aortic insufficiency
—Rheumatic fever
—Syphilis
—Hypertension
—Endocarditis
—Idiopathic
—Associated with Marfan's syndrome and ventricular septal defect, even after surgical closure

Aortic stenosis
—Congenital aortic bicuspid valve (associated with coarctation of the aorta)
—Congenital stenosis of valve cusps
—Rheumatic fever
—Atherosclerosis in the aged

Signs and symptoms

Mitral stenosis
—Dyspnea on exertion, paroxysmal nocturnal dyspnea, orthopnea, weakness, fatigue, palpitations
—Peripheral edema, jugular venous distention, ascites, hepatomegaly (right ventricular failure in severe pulmonary hypertension)
—Rales, cardiac dysrhythmias (atrial fibrillation), signs of systemic emboli
—On auscultation, a loud S_1 or opening snap, and a diastolic murmur at the apex

Mitral insufficiency
—Orthopnea, dyspnea, fatigue, angina, palpitations
—Peripheral edema, jugular vein distention, hepatomegaly (right ventricular failure)
—Tachycardia, rales, pulmonary edema
—On auscultation, a holosystolic murmur at the apex, possible split S_2, and an S_3

Tricuspid insufficiency
—Dyspnea and fatigue
—Possible peripheral edema, jugular venous distention, hepatomegaly, and ascites (right ventricular failure)
—On auscultation, possible S_3 and systolic murmur at the lower left sternal border that increases with inspiration

Tricuspid stenosis
—Possible dyspnea, fatigue, syncope
—Possible peripheral edema, jugular venous distention, hepatomegaly, and ascites (right ventricular failure)
—On auscultation, diastolic murmur at the lower left sternal border that increases with inspiration

Pulmonic stenosis
—Asymptomatic or symptomatic, with dyspnea on exertion, fatigue, chest pain, syncope
—Possible peripheral edema, jugular venous distention, hepatomegaly (right ventricular failure)
—On auscultation, a systolic murmur at the left sternal border, and a split S_2 with a delayed or absent pulmonic component

Pulmonic insufficiency
—Dyspnea, weakness, fatigue, chest pain
—Peripheral edema, jugular venous distention, hepatomegaly (right ventricular failure)
—On auscultation, diastolic murmur in pulmonic area

Aortic insufficiency
—Dyspnea, cough, fatigue, palpitations, angina, syncope
—Pulmonary vein congestion, congestive heart failure, pulmonary edema (left ventricular failure), "pulsating" nail beds (Quincke's sign)
—Rapidly rising and collapsing pulses (pulsus biferiens), cardiac dysrhythmias, wide pulse pressure in severe regurgitation

LAP Waveform: Picturing Mitral Insufficiency

If your patient has a left atrial catheter in place, you can identify mitral insufficiency by observing the waveform tracing during left atrial pressure (LAP) monitoring. On the waveform shown below, the heightened *v* wave indicates blood regurgitation through the mitral valve during ventricular contraction.

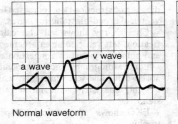

Normal waveform

Waveform of mitral insufficiency

—On auscultation, an S₃ and a diastolic blowing murmur at the left sternal border
—Palpation and visualization of apical impulse in chronic disease

Aortic stenosis
—Dyspnea on exertion, paroxysmal nocturnal dyspnea, fatigue, syncope, angina, palpitations
—Pulmonary venous congestion, congestive heart failure, pulmonary edema (left ventricular failure)
—Diminished carotid pulses, decreased cardiac output, cardiac dysrhythmias; possible pulsus alternans
—On auscultation, systolic murmur heard at the base or in carotids, and possibly an S₄

Diagnostic tests

Mitral stenosis
—Cardiac catheterization detects diastolic pressure gradient across the valve; elevated left atrial and pulmonary capillary wedge pressures (PCWP > 15) with severe pulmonary hypertension and pulmonary arterial pressures; elevated right heart pressure; decreased cardiac output; and abnormal contraction of the left ventricle. Catheterization may not be indicated in patients with isolated mitral stenosis

with mild symptoms.
—Chest X-ray shows left atrial and ventricular enlargement, enlarged pulmonary arteries, and mitral valve calcification.
—Echocardiography shows thickened mitral valve leaflets and left atrial enlargement.
—EKG detects left atrial hypertrophy, atrial fibrillation, right ventricular hypertrophy, and right axis deviation.

Mitral insufficiency
—Cardiac catheterization detects mitral regurgitation, with increased left ventricular end-diastolic volume and pressure; increased atrial and pulmonary capillary wedge pressures; and decreased cardiac output.
—Chest X-ray shows left atrial and ventricular enlargement and pulmonary venous congestion.
—Echocardiography detects abnormal valve leaflet motion and left atrial enlargement.
—EKG may show left atrial and ventricular hypertrophy, sinus tachycardia, and atrial fibrillation.

Tricuspid insufficiency
—Right heart catheterization detects high atrial pressure, tricuspid regurgitation, and decreased or normal cardiac output.

—Chest X-ray shows right atrial dilation and right ventricular enlargement.

—Echocardiography shows systolic prolapse of the tricuspid valve and right atrial enlargement.

—EKG shows right atrial or right ventricular hypertrophy and atrial fibrillation.

Tricuspid stenosis

—Cardiac catheterization detects increased pressure gradient across the valve, increased right atrial pressure, and decreased cardiac output.

—Chest X-ray shows right atrial enlargement.

—Echocardiography detects leaflet abnormality and right atrial enlargement.

—EKG shows right atrial hypertrophy, right or left ventricular hypertrophy, and atrial fibrillation.

Pulmonic stenosis

—Cardiac catheterization detects increased right ventricular pressure, decreased pulmonary artery pressure, and an abnormal valve orifice.

—EKG may show right ventricular hypertrophy, right axis deviation, right atrial hypertrophy, and atrial fibrillation.

Pulmonic insufficiency

—Cardiac catheterization detects pulmonary regurgitation, increased right ventricular pressure, and associated cardiac defects.

—Chest X-ray shows right ventricular and pulmonary arterial enlargement.

—EKG shows right ventricular or right atrial enlargement.

Aortic insufficiency

—Cardiac catheterization detects reduction in arterial diastolic pressures, aortic regurgitation, other valvular abnormalities, and increased left ventricular end-diastolic pressure.

—Chest X-ray shows left ventricular enlargement and pulmonary venous congestion.

—Echocardiography shows left ventricular enlargement, alterations in mitral valve movement (indirect indication of aortic valve disease), and mitral thickening.

—EKG shows sinus tachycardia, left ventricular hypertrophy, and left atrial hypertrophy in severe disease.

Aortic stenosis

—Cardiac catheterization detects pressure gradient across the valve (indicating obstruction) and increased left ventricular end-diastolic pressures.

—Chest X-ray shows valvular calcification, left ventricular enlargement, and pulmonary venous congestion.

—Echocardiography shows thickened aortic valve and left ventricular wall, possibly coexistent with mitral valve stenosis.

—EKG shows left ventricular hypertrophy.

Treatment and clinical implications

Treatment of valvular heart disease depends on the nature and severity of associated symptoms. For example, heart failure requires digoxin, diuretics, a sodium-restricted diet, and, in acute cases, oxygen. Other appropriate measures include anticoagulant therapy to prevent thrombus formation around diseased or replaced valves, and prophylactic antibiotics before and after surgery or dental care.

If the patient has severe signs and symptoms that cannot be managed medically, open heart surgery using cardiopulmonary bypass for valve replacement is indicated. (See *Prosthetic Heart Valves: Some Examples*.)

• Watch closely for signs of heart failure or pulmonary edema and side effects of drug therapy.

• Teach the patient about diet restrictions, medications, symptoms that should be reported, and the importance of consistent follow-up care.

• If the patient has surgery, watch for hypotension, dysrhythmias, and thrombus formation. Monitor vital signs, arterial blood gas measurements, intake and output, daily weights, blood chemistries, chest X-

Prosthetic Heart Valves: Some Examples

When choosing among prosthetic valves, the doctor weighs such factors as design, durability, and hemodynamic qualities. He also considers patient compliance for this reason: mechanical prostheses encourage thrombus formation, so the patient must undergo lifelong anticoagulant therapy and regular prothrombin time testing. For a patient unlikely to comply, the doctor may select a bioprosthesis instead because it doesn't require long-term anticoagulant therapy.

The following illustrations show several available prosthetic types.

Starr-Edwards ball cage mechanical valve

The *ball cage* mechanical valve (shown above), while durable, won't be used for tricuspid valve replacement because it's too large for the right ventricle.

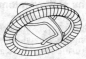

Bjork-Shiley tilting disk mechanical valve

Because of its flat design, the *tilting disk* mechanical valve (shown above) requires less space than the ball cage valve.

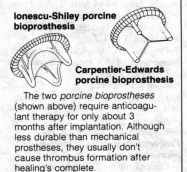

Ionescu-Shiley porcine bioprosthesis

Carpentier-Edwards porcine bioprosthesis

St. Jude's bileaflet mechanical valve

Among mechanical valve types, the *bileaflet* valve (shown above) creates the least resistance to blood flow, making it hemodynamically efficient.

The two *porcine bioprostheses* (shown above) require anticoagulant therapy for only about 3 months after implantation. Although less durable than mechanical prostheses, they usually don't cause thrombus formation after healing's complete.

---

rays, and pulmonary artery catheter readings.

Varicella
(Chicken pox)

Description
Varicella is a common, acute, and highly contagious infection. In its latent stage, it causes herpes zoster (shingles). Chicken pox can occur at any age, but it is most common in children ages 2 to 8. The incubation period lasts from 13 to 17 days. Chicken pox is probably communicable from 1 day before lesions erupt to 6 days after vesicles form. It is most contagious in the early stages of eruption of skin lesions.

Chicken pox occurs worldwide and is endemic in large cities. Outbreaks occur sporadically, usually in areas with large groups of susceptible children. It affects all races and both sexes equally. Seasonal distribution varies. In temperate areas, incidence is higher during late autumn, winter, and spring.

Causes
The herpesvirus varicella-zoster (V-Z)

Mode of transmission
Direct contact
—Respiratory secretions (most common)
—Skin lesions
—Acute maternal infection in the first or early second trimester (congenital varicella)
Indirect contact
—Air waves

Signs and symptoms
Childhood varicella
—Slight fever, malaise, and anorexia during prodromal phase
—Pruritic rash. Typically, rash begins as crops of small, erythematous macules on trunk or scalp that progress to papules and then clear vesicles on an erythematous base. Vesicles become cloudy, break, and form scabs. Rash spreads to face and rarely to extremities, with new vesicles continuing to appear for 3 to 4 days.
—Possible shallow ulcers on mucous membranes of the mouth, conjunctivae, and genitalia
Congenital varicella
—Hypoplastic deformity and scarring of a limb
—Retarded growth
—CNS and eye manifestations
Progressive varicella in immunocompromised person
—Lesions and high fever for more than 7 days

Treatment
Chicken pox calls for strict isolation until all the vesicles and most of the scabs disappear (usually for 1 week after the onset of the rash). Congenital chicken pox requires no isolation.

Usually, treatment consists of local or systemic antipruritics: cool bicarbonate of soda baths, calamine lotion, or diphenhydramine or another antihistamine. Antibiotics are unnecessary unless bacterial infection develops. Salicylates are contraindicated because of their link with Reye's syndrome.

Susceptible patients may need special treatment. Up to 72 hours after exposure to varicella-zoster, immune globulin may provide passive immunity. Vidarabine may slow vesicle formation, speed skin healing, and control the systemic spread of infection.

Clinical implications
Care is supportive and emphasizes patient and family teaching and preventive measures.
• Teach the child and his family how to apply topical antipruritic medications correctly. Stress the importance of good hygiene.
• Tell the patient not to scratch the lesions. However, because the need to scratch may be overwhelming, parents should trim the child's fingernails or tie mittens on his hands.
• Warn parents to watch for and immediately report signs of complications. Severe skin pain and burning may indicate a serious secondary infection and require prompt medical attention.
• To help prevent chicken pox, do not admit a child exposed to chicken pox to a unit that contains children who receive immunosuppressives or who have leukemia or immunodeficiency disorders. A vulnerable child who has been exposed to chicken pox should receive varicella-zoster immunoglobulin, to lessen severity.

Complications
Rare complications include pneumonia, myocarditis, fulminating encephalitis (Reye's syndrome), bleeding disorders, arthritis, nephritis, hepatitis, and acute myositis.

Variola
(Smallpox)

Description
Variola was an acute, highly contagious infectious disease. After a global eradication program, begun in 1967, the World Health Organization pronounced smallpox eradicated on Oc-

tober 26, 1979. Smallpox developed in three major forms: *variola major* (classic smallpox), which carried a high mortality; *variola minor*, a mild form that occurred in nonvaccinated persons and resulted from a less virulent strain; and *varioloid*, a mild variant of smallpox that occurred in previously vaccinated persons who had only partial immunity.

Causes
Poxvirus variola

Mode of transmission
Direct transmission
—Respiratory droplets
—Dried scales of virus-containing lesions
Indirect transmission
—Contact with contaminated linens or other objects

Signs and symptoms
Initial stage
—Chills
—High fever
—Headache
—Backache
—Severe malaise
—Vomiting (especially in children)
—Marked prostration
—Possible convulsive seizures (in children), violent delirium, stupor, or coma
Pustular stage
—Sore throat
—Cough
—Lesions on mucous membranes of mouth, throat, and respiratory tract
—Skin lesions (progress from macular to papular, vesicular, and pustular, then rupture and form scabs)
—Return of intial-stage symptoms
Final stage
—Intense pruritus
—Possible permanently disfiguring scars
—Diffuse dusky appearance on face and upper chest if fatal

Diagnostic tests
• Culture from an aspirate of vesicles and pustules was the most conclusive laboratory test.
• Microscopic examination of smears from lesion scrapings detected the virus or antibodies to the virus.
• Complement fixation detected the virus or antibodies to the virus.

Treatment and clinical implications
Treatment required hospitalization, with strict isolation, antimicrobial therapy to treat bacterial complications, vigorous supportive measures, and symptomatic treatment of lesions with antipruritics, starting during the pustular stage. Aspirin, codeine, or (as needed) morphine relieved pain; I.V. infusions and gastric tube feedings provided fluids, electrolytes, and calories, since pharyngeal lesions made swallowing difficult.

Complications
Fatal complications included the following:
• Encephalitic manifestations
• Extensive bleeding
• Secondary bacterial infections

Vasculitis

Description
Vasculitis includes a broad spectrum of disorders characterized by inflammation and necrosis of blood vessels. Its clinical effects depend on the vessels involved and reflect tissue ischemia caused by blood flow obstruction. Prognosis is also variable. For example, hypersensitivity vasculitis is usually a benign disorder limited to the skin, but more extensive polyarteritis nodosa can be rapidly fatal. Vasculitis can occur at any age, except for mucocutaneous lymph node syndrome, which occurs only during childhood. Vasculitis may be a primary disorder or secondary to other disorders such as rheumatoid arthritis or systemic lupus erythematosus.

Types of Vasculitis

TYPE	VESSELS INVOLVED
Polyarteritis nodosa	Small- to medium-sized arteries throughout body. Lesions tend to be segmental, occur at bifurcations and branchings of arteries, and spread distally to arterioles. In severe cases, lesions circumferentially involve adjacent veins.
Allergic angiitis and granulomatosis (Churg-Strauss syndrome)	Small- to medium-sized arteries and small vessels (arterioles, capillaries, and venules), mainly of the lung but also other organs
Polyangiitis overlap syndrome	Small- to medium-sized arteries and small vessels (arterioles, capillaries, venules) of lung and other organs
Wegener's granulomatosis	Small- to medium-sized vessels of the respiratory tract and kidney
Temporal arteritis	Medium- to large-sized arteries, most commonly branches of the carotid artery
Takayasu's arteritis (aortic arch syndrome)	Medium- to large-sized arteries, particularly the aortic arch and its branches and, possibly, the pulmonary artery
Hypersensitivity vasculitis	Small vessels, especially of the skin

SIGNS & SYMPTOMS	DIAGNOSIS
Hypertension, abdominal pain, myalgias, headache, joint pain, weakness	History of symptoms. Elevated ESR; leukocytosis; anemia; thrombocytosis; depressed C3 complement; rheumatoid factor titer >1:60; circulating immune complexes. Tissue biopsy shows necrotizing vasculitis.
Resembles polyarteritis nodosa with hallmark of severe pulmonary involvement	History of asthma. Eosinophilia; tissue biopsy shows granulomatous inflammation with eosinophilic infiltration.
Combines symptoms of polyarteritis nodosa and allergic angiitis and granulomatosis	Possible history of allergy. Eosinophilia; tissue biopsy shows granulomatous inflammation with eosinophilic infiltration.
Fever, pulmonary congestion, cough, malaise, anorexia, weight loss, mild to severe hematuria	Tissue biopsy shows necrotizing vasculitis with granulomatous inflammation. Leukocytosis; elevated ESR, IgA, and IgG; low titer rheumatoid factor; circulating immune complexes.
Fever, myalgia, jaw claudication, vision changes, headache (associated with polymyalgia rheumatica syndrome)	Decreased hemoglobin; elevated ESR; tissue biopsy shows panarteritis with infiltration of mononuclear cells, giant cells within vessel wall, fragmentation of internal elastic lamina, and proliferation of intima.
Malaise, pallor, nausea, night sweats, arthralgias, anorexia, weight loss, pain or paresthesia distal to affected area, bruits, loss of distal pulses, syncope, and, if carotid artery is involved, diplopia and transient blindness. May progress to congestive heart failure or cerebrovascular accident.	Decreased hemoglobin; leukocytosis; positive LE cell preparation and elevated ESR. Arteriography shows calcification and obstruction of affected vessels. Tissue biopsy shows inflammation of adventitia and intima of vessels, and thickening of vessel walls.
Palpable purpura, papules, nodules, vesicles, bullae, ulcers, or chronic or recurrent urticaria	History of exposure to antigen, such as a microorganism or drug. Tissue biopsy shows leukocytoblastic angiitis, usually in postcapillary venules, with infiltration of polymorphonuclear leukocytes, fibrinoid necrosis, and extravasation of erthyrocytes.

(continued)

Types of Vasculitis *(continued)*

TYPE	VESSELS INVOLVED
Mucocutaneous lymph node syndrome (Kawasaki disease)	Small- to medium-sized vessels, primarily of the lymph nodes; may progress to involve coronary arteries
Behçet's disease	Small vessels, primarily of the mouth and genitalia but also of the eyes, skin, joints, GI tract, and CNS

Causes

Exact cause is unknown; theories explaining how vasculitis develops include the following:

• Excessive antigen in the circulation, leading to vessel damage

• Cell-mediated (T cell) immune response, leading to release of intracellular enzymes, which cause vascular damage

Signs and symptoms/Diagnostic tests

(See *Types of Vasculitis,* pp. 802 to 805.)

Treatment

Treatment of vasculitis aims to minimize irreversible tissue damage associated with ischemia. In primary vasculitis, treatment may involve removal of an offending antigen or use of anti-inflammatory or immunosuppressive drugs. For example, antigenic drugs, food, and other environmental substances should be identified and eliminated, if possible. Drug therapy in primary vasculitis often involves low-dose cyclophosphamide (2 mg/kg P.O. daily) with daily corticosteroids. In rapidly fulminant vasculitis, cyclophosphamide dosage may be increased to 4 mg/kg daily for the first 2 to 3 days, followed by the regular dose.

Prednisone should be given in a dosage of 1 mg/kg daily in divided doses for 7 to 10 days, with consolidation to a single morning dose by 2 to 3 weeks. When the vasculitis appears to be in remission or when prescribed cytotoxic drugs take full effect, corticosteroids are tapered down to a single daily dose and then to an alternate-day schedule that may continue for 3 to 6 months before steroids are slowly discontinued.

In secondary vasculitis, treatment focuses on the underlying disorder.

Clinical implications

• Assess for dry nasal mucosa in patients with Wegener's granulomatosis. Instill nose drops to lubricate the mucosa and help diminish crusting, or irrigate the nasal passages with warm normal saline solution.

• Monitor vital signs. Use a Doppler ultrasonic flowmeter, if available, to auscultate blood pressure in the patient with Takayasu's arteritis, whose peripheral pulses are often difficult to palpate.

• Monitor intake and output. Check daily for edema. Keep the patient well

SIGNS & SYMPTOMS	DIAGNOSIS
Fever; nonsuppurative cervical adenitis; edema; congested conjunctivae; erythema of oral cavity, lips, and palms; and desquamation of fingertips. May progress to myocarditis, pericarditis, myocardial infarction, and cardiomegaly.	History of symptoms. Tissue biopsy shows intimal proliferation and infiltration of vessel walls with mononuclear cells.
Recurrent oral ulcers, eye lesions, genital lesions, and cutaneous lesions	History of symptoms.

hydrated (3 liters daily) to reduce the risk of hemorrhagic cystitis associated with cyclophosphamide therapy.

• Provide emotional support to help the patient and his family cope with an altered body image—the result of the disorder or its therapy. (For example, Wegener's granulomatosis may be associated with saddle nose, steroids may cause weight gain, and cyclophosphamide may cause alopecia.)

• Teach the patient how to recognize drug side effects. Monitor the patient's WBC count during cyclophosphamide therapy to prevent severe leukopenia.

Ventricular aneurysm

Description

Ventricular aneurysm is an outpouching, almost always of the left ventricle, that produces ventricular wall dysfunction in about 20% of patients. Untreated ventricular aneurysm can lead to dysrhythmias, systemic embolization, or congestive heart failure. It is potentially fatal. Resection improves prognosis in congestive heart failure or refractory disease with associated ventricular dysrhythmias.

Causes
Myocardial infarction

Signs and symptoms
• Dysrhythmias
• Palpitations
• Signs of cardiac dysfunction, such as weakness on exertion, fatigue, and angina
• Possible visible or palpable systolic precordial bulge
• Possible left ventricular dysfunction with chronic congestive heart failure
• Possible pulmonary edema, systemic embolization, or left ventricular failure with pulsus alternans

Diagnostic tests
Indicative tests include the following:
• Left ventriculography reveals left ventricular enlargement, with an area of akinesia or dyskinesia (during cineangiography) and diminished cardiac function.
• EKG may show persistent ST-T wave elevations 2 weeks after infarction.
• Chest X-ray may demonstrate an abnormal bulge distorting the heart's

contour if the aneurysm is large; the X-ray may be normal if the aneurysm is small.

• Noninvasive nuclear cardiology scan may indicate the site of infarction and suggest the area of aneurysm.

• Echocardiography shows abnormal motion in the left ventricular wall.

Treatment

Depending on the size of the aneurysm and the complications, treatment may necessitate only routine medical examination to follow the patient's condition or aggressive measures for intractable ventricular dysrhythmias, congestive heart failure, and emboli.

Emergency treatment of ventricular dysrhythmia includes antiarrhythmics I.V. or cardioversion. Preventive treatment continues with oral antiarrhythmics, such as procainamide, quinidine, or disopyramide.

Emergency treatment for congestive heart failure with pulmonary edema includes oxygen, digitalis I.V., furosemide I.V., morphine sulfate I.V., and, when necessary, nitroprusside I.V. and intubation. Maintenance therapy may include nitrates, prazosin, and hydralazine P.O. Systemic embolization requires anticoagulation therapy or embolectomy. Refractory ventricular tachycardia, heart failure, recurrent arterial embolization, and persistent angina with coronary artery occlusion may necessitate surgery, of which the most effective procedure is aneurysmectomy with myocardial revascularization.

Clinical Implications

• If ventricular tachycardia occurs, monitor blood pressure and heart rate. If cardiac arrest develops, initiate cardiopulmonary resuscitation (CPR) and call for assistance, resuscitative equipment, and medication.

• In a patient with congestive heart failure, closely monitor vital signs, heart sounds, intake and output, fluid and electrolyte balances, and BUN and creatinine levels. Because of the threat of systemic embolization, frequently check peripheral pulses and the color and temperature of extremities. Be alert for sudden changes in sensorium that indicate cerebral embolization and for any signs that suggest renal failure or progressive myocardial infarction.

• If dysrhythmias necessitate cardioversion, use a sufficient amount of conducting jelly to prevent chest burns. If the patient is conscious, give diazepam I.V., as ordered, before cardioversion. Explain that cardioversion is a lifesaving method using brief electroshock to the heart. If the patient is receiving antiarrhythmics, check appropriate laboratory tests. For instance, if the patient takes procainamide, check antinuclear antibodies because this drug may induce symptoms that mimic lupus erythematosus.

• If the patient is scheduled to undergo resection, explain expected postoperative care in the ICU (including use of endotracheal tube, ventilator, hemodynamic monitoring, chest tubes, and drainage bottle).

• After surgery, monitor vital signs, intake and output, heart sounds, and pulmonary artery catheter. Watch for signs of infection, such as fever and drainage.

• To prepare the patient for discharge, teach him how to check for pulse irregularity and rate changes. Encourage him to follow his prescribed medication regimen—even during the night—and to watch for side effects.

• Since dysrhythmias can cause sudden death, refer the family to a community-based CPR training program.

• Provide psychological support for the patient and family.

Ventricular septal defect

Description

In ventricular septal defect (VSD), the most common congenital heart disorder, an opening in the septum between the ventricles allows blood to shunt between the left and right ventricles. VSD accounts for up to 30% of all congenital heart defects. Prognosis is good for defects that close spontaneously or are correctable surgically, but poor for untreated defects, which are sometimes fatal by age 1, usually from secondary complications.

Causes

Failure of the ventricular septum to close completely by the 8th week of gestation

Risk factors

• Fetal alcohol syndrome
• Birth defects, especially Down's syndrome and other autosomal trisomies, renal anomalies, and such cardiac defects as patent ductus arteriosus and coarctation of the aorta

Signs and symptoms

Clinical features of VSD vary with the size of the defect, the effect of the shunting on the pulmonary vasculature, and the infant's age.

Small VSD
—Functional murmur or loud, harsh systolic murmur

Moderate-sized VSD
—Murmur (typically at least a grade 3, pansystolic, loudest at the fourth intercostal space)
—Possible thrill
—Loud pulmonic component of S_2
—Widely split S_2
—Displaced point of maximal impulse to the left on palpation

Large VSD
—Thin, small appearance of infant
—Slow weight gain
—Possible congestive heart failure with dusky skin; liver, heart, and spleen enlargement; diaphoresis; feeding difficulties; rapid, grunting respirations; and increased heart rate
—On auscultation and palpatation, murmur cannot be distinguished from that found in moderate-sized VSD

—In the presence of fixed pulmonary hypertension, diastolic murmur with systolic murmur becoming quieter and S_2 greatly accentuated

Diagnostic tests

• Chest X-ray is normal in small defects. In large VSDs, it shows cardiomegaly, left atrial and left ventricular enlargement, and prominent pulmonary vascular markings.
• EKG is normal in children with small VSDs. In large VSDs, it shows left and right ventricular hypertrophy, suggesting pulmonary hypertension.
• Echocardiography may detect a large VSD and its location in the septum, estimate the size of a left-to-right shunt, suggest pulmonary hypertension, and identify associated lesions and complications.
• Cardiac catheterization confirms VSD, determining its size and exact location; calculates the degree of shunting by comparing the blood oxygen saturation in each ventricle; determines the extent of pulmonary hypertension; and detects associated defects.

Treatment

Large defects usually require early surgical correction before irreversible pulmonary vascular disease develops. For small defects, surgery consists of simple suture closure. Moderate to large defects require insertion of a patch graft, using cardiopulmonary bypass.

If the child has other defects and will benefit from delaying surgery, pulmonary artery banding normalizes pressures and flow distal to the band and prevents pulmonary vascular disease, allowing postponement of surgery. (Pulmonary artery banding is done only when the child has other complications.)

Before surgery, treatment consists of the following:
• Digoxin, sodium restriction, and diuretics to prevent congestive heart failure
• Careful monitoring by physical examination, X-ray, and EKG to detect increased pulmonary hypertension, which indicates a need for early surgery
• Measures to prevent infection (prophylactic antibiotics, for example, to prevent infective endocarditis)

Usually, postoperative treatment includes a brief period of mechanical ventilation. The patient will need analgesics and may also require diuretics to increase urine output, continuous infusions of nitroprusside or adrenergic agents to regulate blood pressure and cardiac output, and, in rare cases, a temporary or permanent pacemaker if heart block occurs.

Clinical implications

Although the parents of an infant with VSD often suspect something is wrong with their child before diagnosis, they need psychological support to help them accept the reality of a serious cardiac disorder. Because surgery may take place months after diagnosis, parent teaching is vital to prevent complications until the child is scheduled for surgery or the defect closes. Thorough explanations of all tests are also essential.
• Instruct parents to watch for signs of congestive heart failure, such as poor feeding, sweating, and heavy breathing.
• If the child is receiving digoxin or other medications, tell the parents how to give it and how to recognize side effects. Caution them to keep medications out of the reach of all children.
• Teach parents to recognize and re-

port early signs of infection and to avoid exposing the child to persons with obvious infections.
• Encourage parents to let the child engage in normal activities.
• Stress the importance of prophylactic antibiotics before and after surgery.
• After surgery to correct VSD, monitor vital signs and intake and output. Maintain the infant's body temperature with an overbed warmer. Give catecholamines, nitroprusside, and diuretics, as ordered; analgesics, as needed.
• Monitor central venous pressure, intraarterial blood pressure, and left atrial or pulmonary artery pressure readings. Assess heart rate and rhythm for signs of conduction block.
• Check oxygenation, particularly in a child who requires mechanical ventilation. Suction as needed to maintain a patent airway and to prevent atelectasis and pneumonia.
• Monitor pacemaker effectiveness, if needed. Watch for signs of failure, such as bradycardia and hypotension.
• Reassure parents, and allow them to participate in their child's care.

Complications

A large VSD may cause a variety of complications.
• Cardiac hypertrophy
• Biventricular congestive heart failure
• Cyanosis
• Pneumonia
• Prominence of the anterior chest wall

Vitamin A deficiency

Description

Deficiency of vitamin A may result in night blindness, decreased color adjustment, keratinization of epithelial tissue, and poor bone growth. Each year, more than 80,000 persons worldwide—mostly children in underdeveloped countries—lose their sight from severe vitamin A deficiency. This condition is rare in the United States, but many disadvantaged children have substandard levels of vitamin A. With therapy, the chance of reversing symptoms of night blindness and milder conjunctival changes is excellent. When corneal damage is present, emergency treatment is necessary.

Causes
Inadequate diet
—Low intake of foods high in vitamin A (liver, kidney, butter, milk, cream, cheese, and fortified margarine)
—Low intake of carotene, a precursor of vitamin A (dark-green leafy vegetables and yellow or orange fruits and vegetables)
Malabsorption
—Celiac disease
—Sprue
—Obstructive jaundice
—Cystic fibrosis
—Giardiasis
—Habitual use of mineral oil as a laxative
Massive urinary excretion
—Cancer
—Tuberculosis
—Pneumonia
—Nephritis
—Urinary tract infection
Decreased storage and transport of vitamin A
—Hepatic disease

Signs and symptoms
• Visual change. Typical first symptom is night blindness, which may progress to xerophthalmia, or drying of the conjunctivae, with development of gray plaques (Biot's spots); perforation, scarring, and blindness may result.
• Keratinization of epithelial tissue (dry, scaly skin; follicular hyperkeratosis; and shrinking and hardening of mucous membranes)
• In an infant, failure to thrive and

apathy; dry skin; and corneal changes, which may lead to ulceration and rapid destruction of the cornea

Diagnostic tests
• Serum vitamin A levels less than 20 mcg/dl confirm vitamin A deficiency.
• Carotene levels less than 40 mcg/dl suggest vitamin A deficiency but fluctuate with seasonal ingestion of fruits and vegetables.

Treatment
Mild conjunctival changes or night blindness requires vitamin A replacement in the form of cod liver oil or halibut liver oil. Acute deficiency requires aqueous vitamin A solution I.M., especially when corneal changes have occurred. Therapy for underlying biliary obstruction consists of administration of bile salts; for pancreatic insufficiency, pancreatin. Dry skin responds well to cream- or petrolatum-based products.

In patients with chronic malabsorption of fat-soluble vitamins, and in those with low dietary intake, prevention of vitamin A deficiency requires aqueous I.V. supplements or a water-miscible preparation P.O.

Clinical implications
• Administer oral vitamin A supplements with or after meals or parenterally, as ordered. Watch for signs of hypercarotenemia (orange coloration of the skin and eyes) and hypervitaminosis A (rash, hair loss, anorexia, transient hydrocephalus, and vomiting in children; bone pain, hepatosplenomegaly, diplopia, and irritability in adults). If these signs occur, discontinue supplements, and notify the physician immediately. (Hypercarotenemia is relatively harmless; hypervitaminosis A may be toxic.)
• Since vitamin A deficiency usually results from dietary insufficiency, provide nutritional counseling and, if necessary, referral to an appropriate community agency.

Vitamin B deficiencies

Description
Vitamin B complex is a group of water-soluble vitamins essential to normal metabolism, cell growth, and blood formation. The most common deficiencies involve thiamine (B_1), riboflavin (B_2), niacin, pyridoxine (B_6), and cobalamin (B_{12}). (See *Incidence of Vitamin B Deficiencies*.)

Causes
Thiamine deficiency
—Malabsorption of vitamin B_1
—Inadequate dietary intake of vitamin B_1
Riboflavin deficiency
—Diet deficient in milk, meat, fish, green leafy vegetables, and legumes
—Prolonged diarrhea
—Exposure of milk to sunlight, which destroys riboflavin
—Treatment of legumes with baking soda, which destroys riboflavin
Niacin deficiency
—Inadequate dietary intake of niacin when diet is dominantly corn based
—Secondary to carcinoid syndrome or Hartnup disease
Pyridoxine deficiency
—Destruction of pyridoxine by autoclaving infant formulas
—Ingestion of pyridoxine antagonists, such as isoniazid and penicillamine
Cobalamin deficiency
—Absence of intrinsic factor in gastric secretions
—Absence of receptor sites after ileal resection
—Malabsorption syndromes associated with diverticulosis, sprue, intestinal infestation, regional ileitis, and gluten enteropathy
—Diet low in animal protein

Incidence of Vitamin B Deficiencies

Thiamine deficiency
Beriberi, a serious thiamine-deficiency disease, is most prevalent in Orientals who subsist mainly on diets of unenriched rice and wheat. Although uncommon in the United States, it most often occurs in alcoholics, malnourished young adults, and infants who are on low-protein diets or are being breast-fed by thiamine-deficient mothers. It also occurs in times of stress.

Riboflavin deficiency
Ariboflavinosis occurs in persons with chronic alcoholism or prolonged diarrhea.

Niacin deficiency
Pellagra, an advanced form of niacin deficiency, is now rarely found in the United States. Niacin deficiency is still common in parts of Egypt, Yugoslavia, Romania, and Africa, where corn is the dominant staple food.

Pyridoxine deficiency
A frank deficiency is uncommon in adults, except in persons taking pyridoxine antagonists, such as isoniazid and penicillamine.

Cobalamin deficiency
This type of deficiency is commonly found in persons with malabsorption syndromes associated with diverticulosis, sprue, intestinal infestation, regional ileitis, and gluten enteropathy.

Signs and symptoms
Thiamine deficiency
—General symptoms include polyneuritis, possibly Wenicke's encephalopathy and Korsakoff's psychosis, cardiomegaly, palpitations, tachycardia, dyspnea, circulatory collapse, constipation, indigestion, and possible ataxia, nystagmus, and ophthalmoplegia.

—Symptoms of wet beriberi include severe edema, starting in the legs and moving up through the body.

—Symptoms of dry beriberi include multiple neurologic effects and emaciated appearance.

—Symptoms of infantile beriberi include edema, irritability, abdominal pain, pallor, vomiting, loss of voice, and possible convulsions.

Riboflavin deficiency
—Early-stage symptoms include cheilosis (cracking of lips and corners of the mouth); sore throat; glossitis; seborrheic dermatitis in the nasolabial folds, scrotum, and vulva; possibly generalized dermatitis involving arms, legs, and trunk; and eye problems such as burning, itching, light sensitivity, tearing, and vascularization of the corneas.

—Late-stage symptoms include neuropathy, mild anemia, and growth retardation in children.

Niacin deficiency
—Early-stage symptoms include fatigue, anorexia, muscle weakness, headache, indigestion, mild skin eruptions, weight loss, and backache.

—Advanced-stage (pellagra) symptoms include dark scaly dermatitis, especially on exposed parts of the body; red and sore mouth, tongue, and lips; difficulty eating; nausea and vomiting; diarrhea; and associated CNS aberrations such as confusion, disorientation, neuritis, and possibly hallucinations and paranoia.

Pyridoxine deficiency
Infantile pyridoxine deficiency causes the following:
—Dermatitis

—Abdominal pain
—Vomiting
—Ataxia
—Convulsions
—Possible cheilosis, glossitis, and CNS disturbances

Cobalamin deficiency
—Pernicious anemia
—Peripheral neuropathy
—Possible spinal cord involvement (ataxia, spasticity, and hyperactive reflexes)

Diagnostic tests
Thiamine deficiency
—Serum thiamine levels are less than 2 mcg/dl.

—Serum pyruvate levels and alpha-ketoglutarate are elevated, especially after exercise and glucose administration.

—Urinary thiamine concentration is low.

Riboflavin deficiency
—Serum riboflavin levels are less than 15 mcg/dl.

Niacin deficiency
—Serum niacin levels are less than 30 mcg/dl.

—Urinary metabolites (N-methyl niacinamide and N-methylpyridone) are diminished or absent.

Pyridoxine deficiency
—24-hour urine collection after administration of 10 g of L-tryptophan shows xanthurenic acid more than 50 mg/day.

—Serum transaminase and RBC levels are decreased.

—Urinary excretion of pyridoxic acid is reduced.

Cobalamin deficiency
—Serum cobalamin levels are less than 150 pg/ml.

—Gastric analysis, Schilling test, hemoglobin studies, and gastric X-rays may be done to discover the cause of the deficiency.

Prevention and treatment
Appropriate dietary adjustments and supplementary vitamins can prevent or

correct vitamin B deficiencies.

• Thiamine deficiency requires a high-protein diet, with adequate calorie intake, possibly supplemented by B-complex vitamins for early symptoms. Thiamine-rich foods include pork, peas, wheat bran, oatmeal, and liver. Alcoholic beriberi may require thiamine supplements or administration of thiamine hydrochloride as part of a B-complex concentrate.

• Riboflavin deficiency requires supplemental riboflavin in patients with intractable diarrhea or increased demand for riboflavin as a result of growth, pregnancy, lactation, or wound healing. Good sources of riboflavin are meats, enriched flour, milk and dairy foods, green leafy vegetables, eggs, and cereal. Acute riboflavin deficiency requires daily oral doses of riboflavin alone or in combination with other B-complex vitamins. Riboflavin supplements can also be administered I.V. or I.M. as the sodium salt of riboflavin phosphate.

• Niacin deficiency requires supplemental B-complex vitamins and dietary enrichment in patients at risk due to marginal diets or alcoholism. Meats, fish, peanuts, brewer's yeast, enriched breads, and cereals are rich in niacin; milk and eggs, in tryptophan. Confirmed niacin deficiency requires daily doses of niacinamide P.O. or I.V.

• Pyridoxine deficiency requires prophylactic pyridoxine therapy in infants and epileptic children; supplemental B-complex vitamins in patients with anorexia or malabsorption, or in those taking isoniazid or penicillamine. Some women who take oral contraceptives may have to supplement their diets with pyridoxine. Confirmed pyridoxine deficiencies require oral or parenteral pyridoxine. Children with convulsive seizures stemming from metabolic dysfunction may require

daily doses of 200 to 600 mg pyridoxine.

• Cobalamin deficiency requires parenteral cyanocobalamin in patients with reduced gastric secretion of hydrochloric acid, lack of intrinsic factor, some malabsorption syndromes, or ileum resections. Strict vegetarians may have to supplement their diets with oral vitamin B_{12}. Depending on the severity of the deficiency, supplementary cyanocobalamin is usually given parenterally for 5 to 10 days, followed by monthly or daily vitamin B_{12} supplements.

Clinical implications

An accurate dietary history provides a baseline for effective dietary counseling.

• Identify and observe patients at risk for vitamin B deficiencies—alcoholics, the elderly, pregnant women, and persons on limited diets.

• Administer prescribed supplements. Make sure patients understand how important it is that they adhere strictly to their prescribed treatment for the rest of their lives. Watch for side effects from large doses of niacinamide, in patients with niacin deficiency. Remember, prolonged intake of niacin can cause hepatic dysfunction. Warn patients with Parkinson's disease that pyridoxine may impair response to levodopa therapy.

• Explain all tests and procedures. Reassure patients that, with treatment, prognosis is good. Refer patients to appropriate assistance agencies if their diets are inadequate due to socioeconomic conditions.

Vitamin C deficiency
(Scurvy)

Description

Vitamin C (ascorbic acid) deficiency leads to scurvy or inadequate production of collagen, an extracellular substance that binds the cells of the teeth, bones, and capillaries. Vitamin C deficiency is uncommon today in the United States, except in alcoholics, persons on restricted-residue diets, and infants weaned from breast milk to cow's milk without a vitamin C supplement.

Causes
• Diet lacking in foods rich in vitamin C, such as citrus fruits, tomatoes, cabbage, broccoli, spinach, and berries
• Destruction of vitamin C in foods by overexposure to air or by overcooking
• Excessive ingestion of vitamin C during pregnancy, which causes the newborn to require large amounts of the vitamin after birth
• Marginal intake of vitamin C during periods of physiologic stress—caused by infectious disease, for example—which can deplete tissue saturation of vitamin C

Signs and symptoms
Clinical features of vitamin C deficiency appear as capillaries become increasingly fragile.
Symptoms in adults
—Petechiae
—Ecchymoses
—Follicular hyperkeratosis, especially on buttocks and legs
—Anemia
—Anorexia
—Limb and joint pain, especially in knees
—Pallor
—Weakness
—Swollen or bleeding gums
—Loose teeth
—Lethargy
—Insomnia
—Poor wound healing
—Ocular hemorrhages in the bulbar conjunctivae
—Possible beading, fractures of the costochondral junction of the ribs or epiphysis, and psychological disturbances

Symptoms in children
—Tender, painful swelling in the legs, causing child to lie with legs partially flexed
—Fever
—Diarrhea
—Vomiting

Diagnostic tests
• Serum ascorbic acid levels less than 0.4 mg/dl help confirm the diagnosis.
• WBC ascorbic acid levels less than 25 mg/dl also help confirm it.

Treatment
Since scurvy is potentially fatal, treatment begins immediately to restore adequate vitamin C intake by daily doses of 100 to 200 mg vitamin C in synthetic form (or in orange juice in mild disease) and by doses as high as 500 mg/day in severe disease. Symptoms usually subside in 2 to 3 days; hemorrhages and bone disorders, in 2 to 3 weeks.

To prevent vitamin C deficiency, patients unable or unwilling to consume foods rich in vitamin C or those facing surgery should take daily supplements of ascorbic acid. Vitamin C supplements may also prevent this deficiency in recently weaned infants or those drinking formula not fortified with vitamin C.

Clinical implications
• Administer ascorbic acid P.O. or by slow I.V. infusion, as ordered. Avoid moving the patient unnecessarily to prevent irritation of painful joints and muscles. Encourage him to drink orange juice.
• Explain the importance of supplemental ascorbic acid. Counsel the patient and his family about good dietary sources of vitamin C.
• However, discourage the patient from taking too much vitamin C. Explain that excessive doses of ascorbic acid may cause nausea, diarrhea, and renal calculi formation and may also interfere with anticoagulant therapy.

Vitamin D deficiency
(Rickets)

Description
Vitamin D deficiency causes failure of normal bone calcification, which results in rickets in infants and young children, and osteomalacia in adults. With treatment, prognosis is good. In rickets, however, bone deformities usually persist. In osteomalacia, deformities may disappear.

Once a common childhood disease, rickets is now rare in the United States but occasionally appears in breast-fed infants who do not receive a vitamin D supplement or in infants receiving a formula with a nonfortified milk base. This deficiency may also occur in overcrowded, urban areas where smog limits sunlight penetration. Incidence is highest in black children who, because of their pigmentation, absorb less sunlight.

Osteomalacia, also uncommon in the United States, is most prevalent in the Orient, amoung young multiparas who eat a cereal diet and have minimal exposure to sunlight.

Causes
• Inadequate dietary intake of preformed vitamin D
• Malabsorption of vitamin D
• Conditions that lower absorption of vitamin D (typically, chronic pancreatitis, celiac disease, Crohn's disease, cystic fibrosis, gastric or small bowel resections, fistulas, colitis, and biliary obstruction)
• Too little exposure to sunlight
• Vitamin D-resistant rickets (refractory rickets, familial hypophosphatemia)
• Hepatic or renal disease that interferes with the formation of hydroxylated calciferol, necessary to initiate the formation of a calcium-binding protein in intestinal absorption sites
• Malfunctioning parathyroid gland, which contributes to calcium deficiency and interferes with activation of vitamin D in the kidneys

Signs and symptoms
Early symptoms
—Profuse sweating
—Restlessness
—Irritability
Chronic deficiency
—Numerous bone malformations (bowlegs, knock knees, rachitic rosary [beading of ends of ribs], enlargement of wrists and ankles, pigeon breast, delayed closing of fontanelles, skull softening and bulging of the forehead)
—Poorly developed muscles (potbelly)
—Infantile tetany
—Difficulty walking and climbing stairs
—Spontaneous multiple fractures
—Pain in legs and lower back

Diagnostic tests
• X-rays confirm diagnosis by showing characteristic bone deformities and abnormalities, such as Looser's zones.
• Plasma calcium levels are less than 7.5 mg/100 ml.
• Serum inorganic phosphorus levels are less than 3 mg/100 ml.
• Serum citrate levels are less than 2.5 mg/100 ml.
• Alkaline phosphatase is less than 4 Bodansky units/100 ml.

Treatment and clinical implications
For osteomalacia and rickets—except when due to malabsorption—treatment consists of massive P.O. doses of vitamin D or cod liver oil. For rickets refractory to vitamin D or in rickets accompanied by hepatic or renal disease, treatment includes 25-hydroxycholacalciferol, 1,25-dihydroxycholecalciferol, or a synthetic analog of active vitamin D.

• Obtain a dietary history to assess the patient's current vitamin D intake. Encourage him to eat foods high in vitamin D—fortified milk, fish liver oils, herring, liver, and egg yolks—and get sufficient sun exposure. If deficiency is due to socioeconomic conditions, refer the patient to an appropriate community agency.

• If the patient must take vitamin D for a prolonged period, tell him to watch for signs of vitamin D toxicity (headache, nausea, constipation, and, after prolonged use, renal calculi).

• To prevent rickets, administer supplementary aqueous preparations of vitamin D for chronic fat malabsorption, hydroxylated cholecalciferol for refractory rickets, and supplemental vitamin D for breast-fed infants.

Vitamin E deficiency

Description
In humans, vitamin E (tocopherol) appears to act primarily as an antioxidant, preventing intracellular oxidation of polyunsaturated fatty acids and other lipids. Deficiency of vitamin E usually manifests as hemolytic anemia in low-birth-weight or premature infants. With treatment, prognosis is good. Vitamin E deficiency is uncommon in adults.

Causes
• Vitamin E malabsorption
• Diet high in polyunsaturated fatty acids
• Formulas high in polyunsaturated fatty acids fortified with iron but not vitamin E
• Associated with fat malabsorption conditions such as kwashiorkor, celiac disease, or cystic fibrosis

Signs and symptoms
Premature infants
—Hemolytic anemia
—Thrombocythemia
—Erythematous papular skin eruption followed by desquamation
Infants
—Edema
—Skin lesions
Adults
—Muscle weakness
—Intermittent claudication

Diagnostic tests
• Serum alpha-tocopherol levels below 0.5 mg/dl in adults and below 0.2 mg/dl in infants confirm the diagnosis.
• Supporting studies include creatinuria, increased creatine phosphokinase, hemolytic anemia, and elevated platelet count.

Treatment and clinical implications
Replacement of vitamin E with a water-soluble supplement, either P.O. or parenteral, is the only appropriate treatment.

• As ordered, prevent deficiency by providing vitamin E supplements for low–birth-weight infants receiving formulas not fortified with vitamin E and for adults with vitamin E malabsorption. Many commercial multivitamin supplements are easily absorbed by patients with vitamin E malabsorption.
• Inform new mothers who plan to breast-feed that human milk provides adequate vitamin E.
• Encourage adult patients to eat foods high in vitamin E. Good sources include vegetable oils (corn, safflower, soybean, cottonseed), whole grains, dark-green leafy vegetables, nuts, and legumes. Tell them that heavy consumption of polyunsaturated fatty acids increases the need for vitamin E.
• If vitamin E deficiency is related to socioeconomic conditions, refer the patient to appropriate community agencies.

Vitamin K deficiency

Description
Deficiency of vitamin K, an element necessary for formation of prothrombin and other clotting factors in the liver, produces abnormal bleeding. If the deficiency is corrected, prognosis is excellent. Vitamin K deficiency is common among newborns in the first few days postpartum.

Causes
• Poor placental transfer of vitamin K and inadequate production of vitamin K (newborns)
• Prolonged use of drugs, such as the anticoagulant dicumarol and antibiotics
• Decreased flow of bile to the small intestine from obstruction of the bile duct or bile fistula
• Malabsorption of vitamin K (typically due to sprue, pellagra, bowel resection, ileitis, or ulcerative colitis)
• Improved response of hepatic ribosomes to vitamin K
• Cystic fibrosis, with fat malabsorption
• Insufficient dietary intake of vitamin K (rare)

Signs and symptoms
Abnormal bleeding tendency is the cardinal sign of vitamin K deficiency.

Diagnostic tests
Prothrombin time 25% greater than the normal range of 10 to 20 seconds, measured by the Quick method, confirms the diagnosis of vitamin K deficiency after other causes of prolonged prothrombin time (such as anticoagulant therapy or hepatic disease) have been ruled out. Repetition of this test in 24 hours (and regularly during treatment) monitors success of therapy.

Treatment and clinical implications
Administration of vitamin K corrects abnormal bleeding tendencies. To prevent vitamin K deficiency, follow these guidelines:
• Administer vitamin K to newborns and patients with fat malabsorption or with prolonged diarrhea resulting from colitis, ileitis, or long-term antibiotic drug therapy.
• Warn against self-medication with or overuse of antibiotics, because these drugs destroy the intestinal bacteria necessary to generate significant amounts of vitamin K.
• If the deficiency has a dietary cause, help the patient and family plan a diet that includes important sources of vitamin K, such as green leafy vegetables, cauliflower, tomatoes, cheese, egg yolks, and liver.

Vitiligo

Description
Marked by stark-white skin patches that may cause a serious cosmetic problem, this condition affects about 1% of the U.S. population, usually persons between ages 10 and 30, with peak incidence around age 20. It shows no racial preference, but the distinctive patches are most prominent in blacks. Vitiligo does not favor one sex; however, women tend to seek treatment more often than men. Repigmentation therapy, which is widely used in treating vitiligo, may necessitate several summers of exposure to sunlight. The effects of this treatment may not be permanent.

Causes
The causes of the destruction and loss of pigment cells are unknown. Possible theories include the following:
• Enzymatic self-destructing mechanisms
• Autoimmune mechanisms
• Abnormal neurogenic stimuli

Risk factors
- Inheritance
- Associated disorders (typically include thyroid dysfunction, pernicious anemia, Addison's disease, aseptic meningitis, diabetes mellitus, photophobia, hearing defects, alopecia areata, and halo nevi)

Signs and symptoms
- Depigmented or stark white patches on the skin (typically, this is bilaterally symmetrical, with sharp borders, which may be raised and hyperpigmented; appear over bony prominences around orifices [eyes, mouth], within body folds, and at sites of trauma)
- Possible whitening of hair within lesions
- Possible premature gray hair
- Possible ocular pigmentary changes

Diagnostic tests
- History of onset, associated illness, family history, and observation of charateristic lesions of vitiligo.
- Wood's light examination in a darkened room detects vitiliginous patches. Depigmented skin reflects the light; pigmented skin absorbs it.
- Other laboratory studies are done if autoimmune or endocrine disturbances are suspected.

Treatment
Repigmentation therapy combines systemic and topical psoralen compounds (methoxsalen and trioxsalen) with exposure to sunlight or artificial ultraviolet light, wavelength A (UVA). Body parts containing few hair follicles (such as the fingertips) may resist this therapy.

Depigmentation therapy is suggested for patients with vitiligo affecting more than 50% of the body surface. A cream containing 20% monobenzone permanently destroys pigment cells in unaffected areas of the skin and produces a uniform skin tone. This medication is applied initially to a small area of normal skin once daily to test for unfavorable reactions (contact dermatitis, for example). In the absence of adverse effects, the patient begins applying the cream twice daily to those areas he wishes to depigment first. (*Note:* Depigmentation is permanent and results in extreme sensitivity to sunlight.)

Commercial cosmetics may also help deemphasize vitiliginous skin. Some patients prefer dyes because these remain on the skin for several days, although the results are not always satisfactory. Although often impractical, complete avoidance of exposure to sunlight through the use of screening agents and protective clothing may minimize vitiliginous lesions in whites.

Clinical implications
- Instruct the patient to use psoralen medications three or four times weekly. (*Note:* Systemic psoralens should be taken 2 hours before exposure to sun; topical solutions should be applied 30 to 60 minutes before exposure.) Warn him to use a sunscreen (SPF 8 to 10) to protect both affected and normal skin during exposure and to wear sunglasses after taking the medication. If periorbital areas require exposure, tell the patient to keep his eyes closed during treatment.
- Suggest that the patient receiving depigmentation therapy wear protective clothing and use a sunscreen (SPF 15). Explain the therapy thoroughly, and allow the patient plenty of time to decide whether to undergo this treatment. Make sure he understands that the results of depigmentation are permanent and that he must thereafter protect his skin from the adverse effects of sunlight.
- Caution the patient about buying commercial cosmetics or dyes without trying them first, since some may not be suitable.

• For the child with vitiligo, modify repigmentation therapy to avoid unnecessary restrictions. Tell parents to give the initial dose of psoralen medication at 1 p.m. and then let the child go out to play as usual. After this, medication should be given 30 minutes earlier each day of treatment, provided the child's skin does not turn more than slightly pink from exposure. If marked erythema develops, parents should discontinue treatment and notify the physician. Eventually, the child should be able to take the medication at 9:30 a.m. and play outdoors the rest of the day without side effects. Tell the parents the child should wear clothing that permits maximum exposure of vitiliginous areas to the sun.

• Remind patients undergoing repigmentation therapy that exposure to sunlight also darkens normal skin. After being exposed to UVA for the prescribed amount of time, the patient should apply a sunscreen if he plans to be exposed to sunlight also. If sunburn occurs, advise the patient to discontinue therapy temporarily and to apply open wet dressings (using thin sheeting) to affected areas for 15 to 20 minutes, four or five times daily or as necessary for comfort. After application of wet dressings, allow the skin to air-dry. Suggest application of a soothing lubricating cream or lotion while the skin is still slightly moist.

• Reinforce patient teaching with written instructions.

• Be sensitive to the patient's emotional needs, but avoid promoting unrealistic hope for a total cure.

Vocal cord nodules and polyps

Description

Vocal cord nodules, which are hypertrophied fibrous tumors, form at the point where the cords come together forcibly. Vocal cord polyps are chronic, subepithelial, edematous masses. Both nodules and polyps have good prognoses, unless continued voice abuse causes recurrence, with subsequent scarring and permanent hoarseness. They are most common in teachers, singers, and sports fans, and in energetic children (ages 8 to 12) who continually shout while playing. Polyps are common in adults who smoke, live in dry climates, or have allergies.

Causes

Vocal cord nodules and polyps usually result from voice abuse, especially in the presence of infection.

Signs and symptoms

• Painless hoarseness
• Possible breathy or husky voice quality

Diagnostic tests

Indirect laryngoscopy confirms the diagnosis.

Treatment

Conservative management of small vocal cord nodules and polyps includes humidification, speech therapy (voice rest, training to reduce the intensity and duration of voice production), and treatment of any underlying allergies.

When conservative treatment fails to relieve hoarseness, nodules or polyps require removal under direct laryngoscopy. Microlaryngoscopy may be done for small lesions, to avoid injuring the vocal cord surface. If nodules or polyps are bilateral, excision may be performed in two stages: one cord is allowed to heal before excision of polyps on the other cord. Two-stage excision prevents laryngeal web, which occurs when epithelial tissue is removed from adjacent cord surfaces, and these surfaces grow together. For children, treatment consists of speech therapy. If possible, surgery should be delayed until the child is old enough to benefit from voice training, or until he can understand the need to abstain from voice abuse.

Clinical implications
• Postoperatively, stress the importance of resting the voice for 10 days to 2 weeks while the vocal cords heal. Provide an alternative means of communication—Magic Slate, pad and pencil, or alphabet board. Place a sign over the bed to remind visitors that the patient should not talk. Mark the intercom so other hospital personnel are aware the patient cannot answer. Minimize the need to speak by trying to anticipate the patient's needs.
• If the patient is a smoker, encourage him to stop smoking entirely or, at the very least, to refrain from smoking during recovery from surgery.
• Utilize a vaporizer to increase humidity and decrease throat irritation.
• Make sure the patient receives speech therapy after healing, if necessary, since continued voice abuse causes recurrence of growths.

Vocal cord paralysis

Description
Vocal cord paralysis results from disease of or injury to the superior or, most often, the recurrent laryngeal nerve. Vocal cord paralysis may be unilateral or bilateral. Unilateral paralysis is the most common form. However, bilateral paralysis is the most serious because it may cause incapacitating airway obstruction.

Causes
• Accidental severing of the recurrent laryngeal nerve, or one of its extralaryngeal branches, during thyroidectomy (most common)
• Pressure from aortic aneurysm or enlarged atrium (from mitral stenosis)
• Bronchial or esophageal carcinoma

• Trauma (neck injuries)
• Neuritis due to infections or metallic poisoning
• Hysteria
• CNS lesions (rare)

Signs and symptoms
Signs and symptoms of vocal cord paralysis depend on whether the paralysis is unilateral or bilateral, and on the position of the cord or cords when paralyzed.
Unilateral paralysis
—Vocal weakness
—Hoarseness
Bilateral paralysis
—Vocal weakness
—Possible incapacitating airway obstruction

Diagnostic tests
Indirect laryngoscopy shows one or both cords fixed in an adducted or partially abducted position, and confirms the diagnosis.

Treatment
Treatment of unilateral vocal cord paralysis consists of injection of Teflon into the paralyzed cord, under direct laryngoscopy. This procedure enlarges the cord and brings it closer to the other cord, which usually strengthens the voice and protects the airway from aspiration. Bilateral cord paralysis in an adducted position usually necessitates tracheotomy to restore a patent airway.

Alternative treatments for adult patients include arytenoidectomy to open the glottis, and lateral fixation of the arytenoid cartilage through an external neck incision. Excision or fixation of the arytenoid cartilage improves airway patency but produces residual voice impairment.

Treatment of hysterical aphonia may include psychotherapy and, for some patients, hypnosis.

Clinical implications
• If the patient chooses direct laryngoscopy and Teflon injection, explain

these procedures thoroughly. Tell him these measures will improve his voice but will not restore it to normal.

Many patients with bilateral cord paralysis prefer to keep a tracheostomy instead of having an arytenoidectomy; their voices are generally better with a tracheostomy alone than after corrective surgery.

• If the patient is scheduled to undergo a tracheotomy, explain the procedure thoroughly, and offer reassurance. Since the procedure is performed under a local anesthetic, the patient may be apprehensive.

• Teach the patient how to suction, clean, and change the tracheostomy tube.

• Reassure the patient that he can still speak by covering the lumen of the tracheostomy tube with his finger or a tracheostomy plug.

• If the patient elects to have an arytenoidectomy, explain the procedure thoroughly. Advise the patient that the tracheostomy will remain in place until the edema has subsided and the airway is patent.

Volvulus

Description

Volvulus is a twisting of the intestine at least 180° on its mesentery, which results in blood vessel compression. Volvulus usually occurs in a bowel segment with a mesentery long enough to twist. The most common area, particularly in adults, is the sigmoid. The small bowel is a common site in children. Other common sites include the stomach and cecum.

Causes

• Anomaly of rotation
• Ingested foreign body
• Adhesion
• Idiopathic
• Secondary to meconium ileus in patients with cystic fibrosis

Signs and symptoms

• Vomiting
• Rapid, marked abdominal distention
• Sudden onset of severe abdominal pain

Diagnostic tests

Sudden onset of severe abdominal pain and physical examination that may reveal a palpable mass suggest volvulus. Appropriate special tests include the following:

• Abdominal X-rays may show obstruction and abnormal air-fluid levels in the sigmoid and cecum; in midgut volvulus, abdominal X-rays may be normal.

• Barium enema fills the colon distal to the section of cecum in cecal volvulus. In sigmoid volvulus in children, barium may twist to a point, and in adults, barium may take on an "ace of spades" configuration.

• Upper GI series in midgut volvulus shows obstruction and possibly a twisted contour in a narrow area near the duodenojejunal junction, where the barium will not pass.

Treatment and clinical implications

Treatment varies according to the severity and location of the volvulus. For children with midgut volvulus, treatment is surgical. For adults with sigmoid volvulus, nonsurgical treatment includes proctoscopy to check for infarction, and reduction by careful insertion of a sigmoidoscope or a long rectal tube to deflate the bowel. Success of nonsurgical reduction is indicated by expulsion of gas and immediate relief of abdominal pain. If the bowel is distended but viable, surgery consists of detorsion (untwisting). If the bowel is necrotic, surgery includes resection and anastomosis. Prolonged hyperalimentation and I.V. antibiotics are usually necessary. Occasionally, sedatives are needed.

After surgical correction of volvulus, follow these guidelines:

• Monitor vital signs, watching for

temperature changes (a sign of sepsis), and a rapid pulse rate and falling blood pressure (signs of shock and peritonitis). Carefully monitor fluid intake and output (including stool), electrolytes, and CBC. Be sure to measure and record drainage from nasogastric tube and drains.

• Encourage frequent coughing and deep breathing. Reposition the patient often, and suction him, as needed.

• Keep dressings clean and dry. Record any excessive or unusual drainage. Later, check for incisional inflammation and separation of sutures.

• When bowel sounds and peristalsis return, begin oral feedings with clear liquids, as ordered. Before removing the nasogastric tube, clamp it for a trial period, and watch for abdominal distention. When solid food can be tolerated, gradually expand the diet. Reassure the patient and family, and explain all diagnostic procedures. If the patient is a child, encourage parents to participate in their child's care to minimize the stress of hospitalization.

Complications

Without immediate treatment, volvulus can lead to the following:

• Strangulation of the twisted bowel loop
• Ischemia
• Infarction
• Perforation
• Fatal peritonitis

Von Willebrand's disease

Description

Von Willebrand's disease is a hereditary bleeding disorder characterized by prolonged bleeding time, moderate deficiency of clotting Factor VIII_{AHF} (antihemophilic factor), and impaired platelet function. This disease commonly causes bleeding from the skin or mucosal surfaces and, in females, excessive uterine bleeding. Bleeding may range from mild and asymptomatic to severe, potentially fatal hemorrhage. Prognosis, however, is usually good. The disease occurs equally in males and females.

Causes

Inheritance of an autosomal dominant trait causes a mild to moderate deficiency of Factor VIII and defective platelet adhesion, which prolongs coagulation time.

Signs and symptoms

• Easy bruising
• Epistaxis
• Bleeding from the gums (severity may lessen with age)
• Possible hemorrhage after laceration or surgery, menorrhagia, and GI bleeding if severe form is present
• Possible massive soft-tissue hemorrhage and bleeding into joints (rare)

Diagnostic tests

Diagnosis is difficult, because symptoms are mild, laboratory values are borderline, and Factor VIII levels fluctuate. However, a positive family history and characteristic bleeding patterns and laboratory values help establish diagnosis. Typical laboratory data include the following:

• Prolonged bleeding time (more than 6 minutes)
• Slightly prolonged partial thromboplastin time (more than 45 seconds)
• Absent or reduced levels of Factor VIII-related antigens (VIII_{AGN}), and low Factor VIII activity level
• Defective in vitro platelet aggregation (using the ristocetin coagulation factor assay test)
• Normal platelet count and normal clot retraction

Treatment

The aims of treatment are to shorten bleeding time by local measures and to replace Factor VIII (and, consequently, Von Willebrand's factor (VWF) by infusion of cryoprecipitate or blood fractions that are rich in Factor VIII.

During bleeding episodes and before even minor surgery, I.V. infusion of cryoprecipitate or fresh-frozen plasma (in quantities sufficient to raise Factor VIII levels to 50% of normal) usually shortens bleeding time.

Clinical implications

The care plan should include local measures to control bleeding and patient teaching to prevent bleeding, unnecessary trauma, and complications.

• After surgery, monitor bleeding time for 24 to 48 hours, and watch for signs of new bleeding.

• During a bleeding episode, elevate and apply cold compresses and gentle pressure to the bleeding site.

• Refer parents of affected children for genetic counseling.

• Advise the patient to consult the physician after even minor trauma and before all surgery, to determine if replacement of blood components is necessary.

• Tell the patient to watch for signs of hepatitis within 6 weeks to 6 months after transfusion.

• Warn against using aspirin and other drugs that impair platelet function.

• If the patient has a severe form of this disease, instruct him to avoid contact sports.

Vulvar cancer

Description

Cancer of the vulva accounts for approximately 5% of all gynecologic malignancies. It can occur at any age, even in infants, but its peak incidence is in the mid-60s. The most common vulvar cancer is squamous cell carcinoma. Early diagnosis increases the chance of effective treatment and survival. Lymph node dissection allows 5-year survival in 85% of patients if it reveals no positive nodes; otherwise, the survival rate falls to less than 75%. (See *Staging Vulvar Cancer*.)

Causes

Unknown

Risk factors

• Leukoplakia (white epithelial hyperplasia)—reported in about 25% of patients

• Chronic vulvar granulomatous disease, including venereal disease

• Chronic pruritus of the vulva, with friction, swelling, and dryness

• Pigmented moles that are constantly irritated by clothing or perineal pads

• Irradiation of the skin, such as nonspecific treatment for pelvic cancer

• Obesity

• Hypertension

• Diabetes

• Nulliparity

Signs and symptoms

Characteristic

—Vulvar pruritus

—Vulvar bleeding

—Small vulvar mass (may start as a small ulcer on the surface, eventually becoming infected and painful)

Less common

—Mass in the groin

—Abnormal urination

—Abnormal defecation

—Cachexia

Diagnostic tests

• Pap smear revealing abnormal cells strongly suggests vulvar cancer.

• Biopsy of abnormal tissue identified by colposcopic examination with a histologic examination revealing abnormal skin changes and staining of diseased tissues confirms the diagnosis.

• Lymphangiography may pinpoint lymph node involvement.

• Other diagnostic tests include CBC,

Staging Vulvar Cancer

Stage 0: Carcinoma in situ
Stage I: Tumor confined to vulva—2 cm or less in diameter. Nodes are not palpable or are palpable in either groin, not enlarged, mobile (not clinically suspicious of neoplasm).
Stage II: Tumor confined to the vulva—more than 2 cm in diameter. Nodes are not palpable or are palpable in either groin, not enlarged, mobile (not clinically suspicious of neoplasm).
Stage III: Tumor of any size with (1) adjacent spread to the urethra and any or all of the vagina, the perineum, and the anus, and/or (2) nodes palpable in either or both groins (enlarged, firm, and mobile, not fixed but clinically suspicious of neoplasm).
Stage IV: Tumor of any size (1) infiltrating the bladder mucosa or the rectal mucosa or both, including the upper part of the urethral mucosa, and/or (2) fixed to the bone or other distant metastases. Fixed or ulcerated nodes in either or both groins.

Reprinted from *Manual for Staging of Cancer* (Chicago: American Joint Committee for Cancer Staging and End Results Reporting, 1983). Used with permission.

X-ray, EKG, and thorough physical (including pelvic) examination.

Treatment
Depending on the stage of the disease, cancer of the vulva usually calls for radical or simple vulvectomy (or laser therapy, for some small lesions). Radical vulvectomy requires bilateral dissection of superficial and deep inguinal lymph nodes. Depending on the extent of metastasis, resection may include the urethra, vagina, and bowel, leaving an open perineal wound until healing—about 2 to 3 months. Plastic surgery, including mucocutaneous graft to reconstruct pelvic structures, may be done later.

Small, confined lesions with no lymph node involvement may require a simple vulvectomy or hemivulvectomy (without pelvic node dissection). Personal considerations (young age of patient, active sexual life) may also mandate such conservative management. However, a simple vulvectomy requires careful postoperative surveillance, since it leaves the patient at higher risk of developing a new lesion.

If extensive metastasis, advanced age, or fragile health rules out surgery, irradiation of the primary lesion offers palliative treatment.

Clinical implications
Patient teaching, preoperative and postoperative care, and psychological support can help prevent complications and speed recovery.
• Before surgery, supplement and reinforce what the physician has told the patient about the surgery and postoperative procedures, such as the use of an indwelling (Foley) catheter, preventive respiratory care, and exercises to prevent venous stasis.
• Encourage the patient to ask questions, and answer them honestly.
• After surgery, provide scrupulous routine gynecologic care and special care to reduce pressure at the operative site, reduce tension on suture lines, and promote healing through better air circulation.
• Place the patient on an air mattress or egg-crate mattress, and use a cradle to support the top covers.
• Periodically reposition the patient with pillows. Make sure her bed has

a half-frame trapeze bar to help her move.

• For several days after surgery, the patient will be maintained on I.V. fluids or a clear liquid diet. As ordered, give her an antidiarrheal drug three times daily to reduce the discomfort and possible infection caused by defecation. Later, as ordered, give stool softeners and a low-residue diet to combat constipation.

• Teach the patient how to thoroughly cleanse the surgical site.

• Check the operative site regularly for bleeding, foul-smelling discharge, or other signs of infection. The wound area will look lumpy, bruised, and battered, making it difficult to detect occult bleeding. This situation calls for a physician or a primary nurse, who can more easily detect subtle changes in appearance.

• Within 5 to 10 days after surgery, as ordered, help the patient to walk. Encourage and assist her in coughing and range-of-motion exercises.

• To prevent urine contamination, the patient will have a Foley catheter in place for 2 weeks. Record fluid intake and output, and provide standard catheter care.

• Counsel the patient and her partner. Explain that sensation in the vulva will eventually return after the nerve endings heal, and they will probably be able to have sexual intercourse 6 to 8 weeks after surgery. Explain that they may want to try different sexual techniques, especially if surgery has removed the clitoris. Help the patient adjust to the drastic change in her body image.

Vulvovaginitis

Description
Vulvovaginitis is inflammation of the vulva (vulvitis) and vagina (vaginitis). Because of the proximity of these two structures, inflammation of one usually precipitates inflammation of the

other. Vulvovaginitis may occur at any age and affects most females at some time. Prognosis is good with treatment.

Causes
Vaginitis
With or without vulvitis, common causes include the following:
• Infection with *Trichomonas vaginalis,* a protozoan flagellate
• Infection with *Candida albicans (Monilia),* a fungus that requires glucose for growth
• Infection with *Hemophilus vaginalis,* a gram-negative bacillus
• Venereal infection with *Neisseria gonorrhoeae* (gonorrhea), a gram-negative diplococcus
• Viral infection with venereal warts (condylomata acuminata) or herpesvirus Type II
• Vaginal mucosa atrophy in menopausal women, which predisposes them to bacterial invasion

Vulvitis
Common causes include the following:
• Parasitic infection (*Phthirus pubis* [crab louse])
• Trauma (skin breakdown may lead to secondary infection)
• Poor personal hygiene, especially from contamination with urine, feces, or vaginal secretions
• Chemical irritations, or allergic reactions to feminine hygiene sprays, douches, detergents, clothing, or toilet paper
• Vulvar atrophy in menopausal women

Mode of transmission
Sexual intercourse is usually the mode of transmission for viral infections (condylomata acuminata, herpesvirus Type II), *Trichomonas vaginalis,* and venereal infection.

Signs and symptoms
Trichomonal vaginitis
—Vaginal discharge (thin, bubbly, green-tinged, and malodorous)
—Marked irritation

—Marked itching
—Burning on urination
—Frequent urination

Monilia vaginitis
—Vaginal discharge (thick, white, cottage-cheese–like in appearance)
—Red, edematous mucous membranes, with white flecks adhering to the vaginal wall
—Possible intense itching

Hemophilus vaginitis
—Gray, foul-smelling vaginal discharge

Gonorrhea
—Possible profuse, purulent vaginal discharge
—Dysuria

Acute vulvitis
—Edema
—Erythema
—Burning
—Pruritus
—Possible severe pain on urination and dyspareunia

Herpes infection
—Possible painful ulceration or vesicle formation

Chronic vulvitis
—Mild inflammation
—Possible severe edema that may involve the entire perineum

Diagnostic tests

• Microscopic examination of vaginal exudate identifying the infectious organism confirms the diagnosis.
• Biopsy of chronic lesions rules out malignancy.
• CBC, urinalysis, cytology screening and culture of exudate from acute lesions may diagnose vulvitis or suspected venereal disease.

Treatment

Common therapeutic measures include the following:
• Metronidazole P.O. for the patient with trichomonal vaginitis, and all sexual partners (if possible), since recurrence often results from reinfection by an asymptomatic male
• Vaginal ointments and suppositories, such as nystatin, for monilia vaginitis
• Local antibiotic therapy for hemophilus vaginitis
• Systemic antibiotic therapy (penicillin and probenicid) for the patient with gonorrhea, and all sexual partners

Cold compresses or cool sitz baths may provide relief from pruritus in acute vulvitis. Severe inflammation may require warm compresses. Other therapy includes avoiding drying soaps, wearing loose clothing to promote air circulation, and applying topical corticosteroids to reduce inflammation. Chronic vulvitis may respond to topical hydrocortisone or antipruritics and good hygiene (especially in elderly or incontinent patients). Topical estrogen ointments may be used to treat atrophic vulvovaginitis. No cure currently exists for herpesvirus infections; however, oral and topical acyclovir (Zovirax) decreases the duration and symptoms of active lesions.

Clinical implications

• Ask the patient if she has any drug allergies. Stress the importance of taking the medication for the length of time prescribed, even if symptoms subside.
• Teach the patient how to insert vaginal ointments and suppositories. Tell her to remain prone for at least 30 minutes after insertion to promote absorption (insertion at bedtime is ideal). Suggest she wear a pad to prevent staining her underclothing.
• Encourage good hygiene. Advise the patient with a history of recurrent vulvovaginitis to wear all-cotton underpants. Advise her to avoid wearing tight-fitting pants and pantyhose, which favor the growth of the infecting organisms.
• Report cases of venereal disease to the local public health authorities.
• Advise the patient of the correlation between sexual contact and the spread of vaginal infections.

W

Warts
(Verrucae)

Description
Warts are common, benign infections of the skin and adjacent mucous membranes. Although their incidence is highest in children and young adults, warts may occur at any age. Prognosis varies. Some warts disappear readily with treatment. Others necessitate more vigorous and prolonged treatment.

Causes
Human papillomavirus

Mode of transmission
- Direct contact
- Possible autoinoculation

Signs and symptoms
Clinical manifestations depend on the types of warts and location.
- Flat: multiple groupings of up to several hundred slightly raised lesions with smooth, flat, or slightly rounded tops; common on the face, neck, chest, knees, dorsa of hands, wrists, and flexor surfaces of the forearms; usually occur in children but can affect adults. Distribution is often linear, because these warts can spread from scratching or shaving.
- Plantar: slightly elevated or flat; occurs singly or in large clusters (mosaic warts), primarily at pressure points of the feet

- Digitate: fingerlike, horny projection arising from a pea-shaped base; occurs on the scalp or near the hairline
- Condyloma acuminatum (moist wart): usually small, pink to red, moist, and soft; may occur singly or in large cauliflowerlike clusters on the penis, scrotum, vulva, and anus. Although this type of wart may be transmitted through sexual contact, it is not always venereal in origin.
- Common (verruca vulgaris): rough, elevated, rounded surface; appears most frequently on extremities, particularly hands and fingers; most prevalent in children and young adults
- Filiform: single, thin, threadlike projection; commonly occurs around the face and neck
- Periungual: rough, irregularly shaped elevated surface; occurs around edges of finger- and toenails. When severe, the wart may extend under the nail and lift it off the nailbed, causing pain.

Diagnostic tests
- Visual examination usually confirms the diagnosis.
- Sigmoidoscopy may be done with recurrent anal warts to rule out internal involvement.

Treatment and clinical implications
Treatment of warts varies according to location, size, number, pain level (present and projected), history of therapy, the patient's age, and compliance with treatment. Most persons eventually develop an immune response that causes warts to disappear sponta-

neously and require no treatment.

Treatment may include the following:

• Electrodesiccation and curettage: High-frequency electric current destroys the wart and is followed by surgical removal of dead tissue at the base and application of an antibiotic ointment (such as polysporin), covered with a bandage, for 48 hours. This method is effective for common, filiform, and, occasionally, plantar warts.

• Cryotherapy: Liquid nitrogen or solid carbon dioxide kills the wart; the resulting dried blister is removed several days later. If initial treatment is not successful, it can be repeated at 2- to 4-week intervals. This method is useful for either periungual warts or for common warts on the face, extremities, penis, vagina, or anus.

• Acid therapy (primary or adjunctive): The patient applies plaster patches impregnated with acid (such as 40% salicylic acid plasters), or acid drops (such as 5% to 16.7% salicylic and lactic acid in flexible collodion) every 12 to 24 hours for 2 to 4 weeks. This method is not recommended for areas where perspiration is heavy or that are likely to get wet, or for exposed body parts where patches are cosmetically undesirable.

• 25% podophyllum in compound with tincture of benzoin (for venereal warts): For protection, cover adjacent unaffected skin with dimethicone or petrolatum before each treatment. The solution is then applied on moist warts. The patient must lie still while it dries, leave it on for 4 hours, and then wash it off with soap and water. Treatment may be repeated every 3 to 4 days and, in some cases, must be left on for a maximum of 24 hours, depending on the patient's tolerance. Apply trimacinolone cream 0.2% to relieve post-treatment inflammation.

The use of antiviral drugs is under investigation; suggestion and hypnosis are occasionally successful, especially with children. Conscientious adherence to prescribed therapy is essential. The patient's sexual partner may also require treatment.

Whiplash

Description

Acceleration-deceleration cervical injuries result from sharp hyperextension and flexion of the neck that damage muscles, ligaments, disks, and nerve tissue. Prognosis is excellent. Symptoms usually subside with symptomatic treatment.

Cause

Rear-end automobile accidents (most common)

Signs and symptoms

Symptoms may develop immediately although most often they are delayed 12 to 24 hours.

• Anterior and posterior neck pain (characteristic sign); initially moderate to severe, with anterior pain diminishing within a couple of days and posterior pain persisting or intensifying

• Possible dizziness, gait disturbances, vomiting, headache, nuchal rigidity, neck muscle asymmetry, and rigidity or numbness in the arms

Diagnostic tests

Full cervical spine X-rays rule out cervical fractures.

Treatment and clinical implications

In all suspected spinal injuries, assume the spine is injured until proven otherwise. Any patient with suspected whiplash or other injuries requires careful transportation from the accident scene. To do this, place him in a supine position on a spine board and immobilize his neck with tape and a hard cervical collar or sandbags. Until an X-ray rules out cervical fracture, move the patient as little as possible. Before the X-ray is taken, remove neck jewelry carefully. Do not undress the patient. Warn him against movements that could injure his spine.

Symptomatic treatment includes the following:

• Mild analgesic—such as aspirin with codeine or ibuprofen—and possibly a muscle relaxant—such as diazepam, cyclobenzaprine (Flexeril), or chlorzoxazone with acetaminophen

• Hot showers or warm compresses to the neck to relieve pain

• Immobilization with a soft, padded cervical collar for several days or weeks

• In severe muscle spasms, short-term cervical traction

Most whiplash patients are discharged immediately. Before discharge, teach patients to watch for possible drug side effects, to avoid alcohol if they are receiving diazepam or narcotics, and to rest for a few days and avoid lifting heavy objects. Warn them to return immediately if they experience persistent pain or if they develop numbness, tingling, or weakness on one side.

Whooping cough
(Pertussis)

Description

Whooping cough is a highly contagious respiratory infection. Characteristically, it produces an irritating cough that becomes paroxysmal and often ends in a high-pitched inspiratory whoop. Since the 1940s, immunization and aggressive diagnosis and treatment have significantly reduced mortality from whooping cough in the United States.

The disease is endemic throughout the world and usually occurs in early spring and late winter. About half the time, it strikes unimmunized children under the age of 2. Whooping cough

mortality in children under age 1 is usually a result of pneumonia and other complications. It is also dangerous in the elderly but tends to be less severe in older children and adults.

Causes

• Nonmotile, gram-negative coccobacillus *Bordetella pertussis* (most common)

• *Bordetella parapertussis*

• *Bordetella bronchiseptica*

Mode of transmission

• Direct inhalation of contaminated droplets from a patient in the acute stage

• Indirect contact with soiled linen and other articles contaminated by the phage

Signs and symptoms

Whooping cough follows a classic 6-week course that includes three stages, each of which lasts about 2 weeks.

Catarrhal stage (highly communicable)

—Irritating hacking, nocturnal cough

—Anorexia

—Sneezing

—Listlessness

—Infected conjunctivae

—Possible low-grade fever

Paroxysmal stage

—Spasmodic and recurrent coughing

—Loud, crowing inspiratory whoop at the end of each cough

—Possible tenacious mucus, choking on mucus, and vomiting

Convalescent stage

—Gradual subsidence of paroxysmal coughing

—Gradual subsidence of vomiting

—Possible return of paroxysmal coughing with any mild upper respiratory infection for months afterward

Diagnostic tests

• Nasopharyngeal and sputum culture showing *B. pertussis* in the early stages confirms the diagnosis.

• Fluorescent antibody screening of nasopharyngeal smears provides quicker results than cultures but is less reliable.

• WBC count is usually increased, especially in children older than 6 months and early in the paroxysmal stage. Sometimes the WBC count may reach 175,000 to 200,000/mm³ with 60% to 90% lymphocytes.

Treatment

Vigorous supportive therapy requires hospitalization of infants (often in the ICU), and fluid and electrolyte replacement. Other treatment includes adequate nutrition, codeine and mild sedation to decrease coughing, oxygen therapy in apnea, and antibiotics, such as erythromycin and, possibly, ampicillin, to shorten the period of communicability and prevent secondary infections.

Because very young infants are particularly susceptible to pertussis, immunization—usually with diphtheria and tetanus toxoids (DPT)—begins at 2, 4, and 6 months. Boosters follow at 18 months and at 4 to 6 years. The risk of pertussis is greater than the risk of vaccine complications, such as neurologic damage. However, if such vaccination causes convulsions or unusual and persistent crying, this may be a sign of severe neurologic reaction and the physician may not order the other doses. The vaccine is contraindicated in children over age 6, because it can cause a severe fever.

Clinical implications

Whooping cough calls for aggressive supportive care and respiratory isolation throughout the illness.

• Monitor acid-base, fluid, and electrolyte balances.

• Carefully suction secretions, and monitor oxygen therapy. Remember: Suctioning removes oxygen as well as secretions.

• Create a quiet environment to decrease coughing stimulation. Provide small, frequent meals, and treat constipation or nausea caused by codeine.

• Offer emotional support to parents of children with whooping cough.

• To decrease exposure to organisms, change soiled linen, empty the suction bottle, and change the trash bag at least once each shift.

Complications

• Paroxysmal coughing induces complications that include increased venous pressure, epistaxis, periorbital edema, conjunctival hemorrhage, hemorrhage of the anterior chamber of the eye, detached retina (and blindness), rectal prolapse, inguinal or umbilical hernia, convulsions, atelectasis, and pneumonitis.

• Choking spells in infants may produce apnea, anoxia, and disturbed acid-base balance.

• Paroxysmal stage complications include possible fatal bacterial infections and possible fatal viral infections.

Wilson's disease
(Hepatolenticular degeneration)

Description

Wilson's disease is a rare metabolic disorder characterized by retention of excessive amounts of copper in the liver, brain, kidneys, and corneas. These deposits produce the characteristic Kayser-Fleischer rings and eventually lead to tissue necrosis and fibrosis, causing a variety of clinical effects, especially hepatic disease and neurologic changes. Wilson's disease is progressive and, if untreated, leads to fatal hepatic failure. The disease occurs most often among eastern European Jews, Sicilians, and southern Italians, probably as a result of consanguineous marriages.

Causes

Wilson's disease is inherited as an autosomal recessive trait only when *both* parents carry the abnormal gene. There is a 25% chance that carrier parents will transmit Wilson's disease (and a 50% chance they will transmit the carrier state) to each of their offspring.

Signs and symptoms

Clinical manifestations usually appear between ages 6 and 20, but they may appear as late as age 40. They vary according to the patient and the state of his disease.

Common signs and symptoms

—Kayser-Fleischer ring (most characteristic symptom; appears as a rusty brown ring of pigment at the periphery of the corneas)

—Possible fever

Associated clinical features

—Liver and spleen: hepatomegaly, splenomegaly, ascites, jaundice, hematemesis, spider angiomas, and thrombocytopenia, eventually leading to cirrhosis or subacute necrosis of the liver

—Blood: anemia and leukopenia

—CNS: "wing-flapping" tremors in arms, "pill-rolling" tremors in hands, facial and muscular rigidity, dysarthria, unsteady gait, and emotional and behavioral changes

—Genitourinary tract: aminoaciduria, proteinuria, uricosuria, glycosuria, and phosphaturia

—Musculoskeletal system (in severe disease): muscle wasting, contractures, deformities, osteomalacia, and pathologic fractures

Diagnostic tests

• Serum ceruloplasmin is less than 20 mg/100 ml.

• Serum copper is less than 80 mcg/100 ml.

• Urine copper is more than 100 mcg/24 hours (may be as high as 1,000 mcg).

• Liver biopsy shows excessive copper deposits (250 mcg/g dry weight), tissue changes indicative of chronic active hepatitis, fatty liver, or cirrhosis.

• Slit-lamp ophthalmic examination revealing Kayser-Fleischer rings confirms the diagnosis; however, the rings are present only when the disease has progressed beyond the liver.

Treatment

Treatment aims to reduce the amount of copper in the tissues, prevent additional accumulation, and manage hepatic disease. The most effective treatment for Wilson's disease consists of lifetime therapy using pyridoxine (vitamin B_6) in conjunction with D-penicillamine, a copper-chelating agent that mobilizes copper from the tissues and promotes its excretion in the urine. However, about one third of patients are sensitive to penicillamine, necessitating dosage adjustment or discontinuation. If an adverse reaction recurs after penicillamine therapy is resumed, the patient may require treatment with corticosteroids, such as prednisone. Treatment also includes potassium and sodium supplements before meals, to prevent GI absorption of copper.

Clinical implications

• Since penicillamine is chemically related to penicillin, ask if the patient is allergic to penicillin before administering the first dose. Watch closely for allergic reactions such as fever, skin rash, adenopathy, severe leukopenia, and thrombocytopenia. Always give penicillamine on an empty stomach. If GI irritation develops, provide enteric-coated tablets.

• Tell the patient and his family what foods to avoid on a low-copper diet (mushrooms, nuts, chocolate, dried fruit, liver, and shellfish). Suggest the use of distilled water, since most tap water flows through copper pipes.

• Be sure to emphasize the necessity of lifetime therapy. Assist the patient and his family with arrangements for continuing education, physical or vocational rehabilitation, and community nursing services, as needed.

• Provide emotional support. The neurologic changes Wilson's disease produces often lead to its misdiagnosis as a psychiatric disorder. Reassure the patient that his condition has a treatable physical basis.

• For a patient in an advanced stage of the disease, encourage as much self-care as possible to prevent further mental and physical deterioration. Plan an exercise schedule. Avoid sensory deprivation or overload. Prevent accidents and injuries that could occur as a result of neurologic deficits.

• If the patient is in a terminal stage, support the family in their grief.

• Suggest genetic counseling for couples who are blood relatives or who have a relative with Wilson's disease. Explain that the chance of their having a child with Wilson's disease is 25% with *each* pregnancy. Teach parents the early symptoms, so they can seek prompt treatment for their child; stress regular pediatric examinations.

Wiskott-Aldrich syndrome

Description

Wiskott-Aldrich syndrome is an immunodeficiency disorder in which both B cell and T cell functions are defective. Its clinical features include thrombocytopenia with severe bleeding, eczema, recurrent infection, and an increased risk of lymphoid malignancy. Prognosis is poor. This syndrome causes early death (average life span is 4 years; rarely, affected children survive to their teens), usually from massive bleeding during infancy or from malignancy or severe infection in early childhood.

Causes

An inherited X-linked recessive trait causing immunodeficiency and thrombocytopenia

Signs and symptoms

Thrombocytopenic features in infancy
—Bloody stools
—Bleeding from a circumcision site
—Petechiae
—Purpura
—Possible hemorrhage

Immunodeficiency features in early childhood
—Recurrent systemic infections (typically, chronic pneumonia, sinusitis, otitis media, and herpes simplex of skin and eyes)
—Possible keratitis and vision loss
—Hepatosplenomegaly
—Eczema (becomes progressively more severe)
—Possible malignancy, especially leukemia and lymphoma

Diagnostic tests

• Platelet count is below 100,000/mm^3.
• Bleeding time is prolonged.
• IgE and IgA levels may be normal or elevated.
• IgM level is decreased.
• Isohemagglutinin levels are low or absent.

Treatment

Treatment aims to limit bleeding through the use of fresh, cross-matched platelet transfusions; to prevent or control infection with prophylactic or early and aggressive antibiotic therapy, as appropriate; to supply passive immunity with immune globulin infusion; and to control eczema with topical corticosteroids. (Systemic corticosteroids are contraindicated, since they further compromise immunity.) An antipruritic may relieve itching.

Treatment with transfer factor has had limited success. However, bone marrow transplantation has been remarkably successful in some patients.

Clinical implications

• Physical and psychological support and patient teaching can help these children and their families cope with this disorder. As soon as the child is old enough, begin teaching him about his disease and his limitations.

• Teach parents of an affected child to watch him for signs of bleeding, such as easy bruising, bloody stools, swollen joints, and tenderness in the trunk area. Help them plan their child's activity levels to ensure normal development. Although the child must avoid contact sports, he is allowed to ride a bike (while wearing protective football gear) and swim.

• Before giving platelet transfusions, establish the child's baseline platelet count. Be sure to check the platelet count often during therapy. Each platelet unit transfused should raise the count by 10,000/mm³.

• Instruct parents to observe the child for signs of infection and to report such signs promptly. Emphasize the importance of meticulous mouth and skin care (including careful cleansing of all skin wounds, no matter how superficial), good nutrition, and adequate hydration. Stress the need to avoid exposing the child to crowds or to persons who have active infections.

• Arrange for the parents to receive genetic counseling.

Wounds, open traumatic

Description

Open traumatic wounds are injuries that often result from home, work, or motor vehicle accidents and from acts of violence. Most open wounds require emergency treatment. In those with suspected nerve involvement, however, electromyography, nerve conduction, and electrical stimulation tests can provide more detailed information about possible peripheral nerve damage. (See *How to Manage Open Trauma*.)

How to Manage Open Trauma

ABRASION

Clinical action
Open surface wounds (scrapes) of epidermis and possibly the dermis, resulting from friction. Nerve endings exposed.

Diagnosis based on scratches, reddish welts, bruises, pain, and history of friction injury.

Type
• Obtain a history to distinguish injury from second-degree burn.
• Cleanse gently with topical germicide, and irrigate. Too vigorous scrubbing of abrasions will increase tissue damage.
• Remove all imbedded foreign objects. Apply local anesthetic if cleansing is very painful.
• Apply light, water-soluble antibiotic cream to prevent infection.
• If wound is severe, apply loose protective dressing that allows air to circulate.
• Administer tetanus prophylaxis, if necessary.

AVULSION

Clinical action
Complete tissue loss that prevents approximation of wound edges, resulting from cutting, gouging, or complete tearing of skin. Often affects nose tip, earlobe, fingertip, and penis.

Diagnosis based on full-thickness skin loss, hemorrhage, pain, history of trauma. X-ray required to rule out bone damage; CBC before surgery.

Type
• Check history for bleeding tendencies and use of anticoagulants.
• Record time of injury to help

How to Manage Open Trauma (continued)

determine if tissue is salvageable. Preserve tissue (if available) in cool saline solution for possible split-thickness graft or flap.
• Control hemorrhage with pressure, absorbable gelatin sponge, or topical thrombin.
• Cleanse gently, irrigate with saline solution, and debride, if necessary. Cover with a bulky dressing.
• Tell patient to leave dressing in place until return visit, to keep area dry, and to watch for signs of infection (pain, fever, redness, swelling).
• Administer analgesic and tetanus prophylaxis, if necessary.

CRUSH WOUND

Clinical action
Heavy falling object splits skin and causes necrosis along split margins and damages tissue underneath. May look like laceration.

Diagnosis based on history of trauma, edema, hemorrhage, massive hematomas, damage to surrounding tissues (fractures, nerve injuries, loss of tendon function), shock, pain, history of trauma. X-rays required to determine extent of injury to surrounding structures. CBC and differential, and electrolyte count also required.

Type
• Check history for bleeding tendencies and use of anticoagulants.
• Cleanse open areas gently with soap and water.
• Control hemorrhage with pressure and cold pack.
• Apply dry, sterile bulky dressing; wrap entire extremity in compression dressing.
• Immobilize injured extremity, and encourage patient to rest. Monitor vital signs, and check peripheral pulses and circulation often.
• Administer tetanus prophylaxis, if necessary.
• Severe injury may require I.V.

infusion of lactated Ringer's or saline solution with large-bore catheter, and surgical exploration, debridement, and repair.

PUNCTURE WOUND

Clinical action
Small-entry wounds that probably damage underlying structures, resulting from sharp, pointed objects.

Diagnosis based on hemorrhage (rare), deep hematomas (in chest or abdominal wounds), ragged wound edges (in bites), small-entry wound (in very sharp object), pain, and history of trauma. X-rays can detect retention of injuring object.

Type
• Check history for bleeding tendencies and use of anticoagulants.
• Obtain description of injury, including force of entry.
• Assess extent of injury.
• Do not remove impaling objects until injury is completely evaluated. (If the eye is injured, call ophthalmologist immediately.)
• Thoroughly cleanse injured area with soap and water. Irrigate all minor wounds with saline solution after removing foreign object.
• Leave human bite wounds open. Apply dry, sterile dressing to other minor puncture wounds.
• Tell patient to apply warm soaks daily.
• Administer tetanus prophylaxis and, if necessary, rabies vaccine.
• Deep wounds that damage underlying tissues may require exploratory surgery; retention of injuring object requires surgical removal.

LACERATION

Clinical action
Open wound, possibly extending into deep epithelium, resulting from penetration with knife or other
(continued)

How to Manage Open Trauma *(continued)*

sharp object or from a severe blow with a blunt object.

Diagnosis based on hemorrhage, torn or destroyed tissues, pain, and history of trauma.

Type

In laceration less than 8 hours old, and in all lacerations of face and areas of possible functional disability (such as the elbow):
• Apply pressure and elevate extremity to control hemorrhage.
• Cleanse wound gently; irrigate with normal saline solution (NSS).
• As necessary, debride necrotic margins, and close wound, using strips of tape or sutures.
• Severe laceration with underlying structural damage may require surgery.
In grossly contaminated laceration or laceration more than 8 hours old (except laceration of face and areas of possible functional disability):
• Administer broad-spectrum antibiotic, as ordered.
• *Do not* close wound immediately.
• Instruct patient to elevate injured extremity for 24 hours after injury to reduce swelling.
• Tell patient to keep dressing clean and dry and to watch for signs of infection.
• After 5 to 7 days, close wound with sutures or butterfly dressing if it appears uninfected and contains healthy granulated tissue.
• Apply sterile dressing and splint, as necessary.
In all lacerations:
• Check history for bleeding tendencies and anticoagulant use.
• Determine approximate time of injury, and estimate blood loss.
• Assess for neuromuscular, tendon, and circulatory damage.
• Administer tetanus prophylaxis, as necessary.
• Stress the need for follow-up and suture removal.
• If sutures become infected, culture the wound and scrub with

surgical soap preparation. Remove some or all sutures, and give broad-spectrum antibiotic, as ordered. Instruct patient to soak wound in warm, soapy water for 15 minutes, three times daily, and to return for follow-up every 2 to 3 days, until the wound heals.
• If injury is the result of suspected criminal activity, report it to police.

MISSILE INJURY

Clinical action

High velocity tissue penetration, such as a gunshot wound.

Diagnosis based on entry and possibly exit wounds, signs of hemorrhage, shock, pain, and history of trauma. X-ray, CBC, and differential and electrolyte levels required to assess extent of injury and estimate blood loss.

Type

• Check history for bleeding tendencies and use of anticoagulant.
• Control hemorrhage with pressure, if possible. Use large-bore catheters to start two I.V.s using lactated Ringer's or NSS for volume replacement and prepare for possible exploratory surgery.
• Maintain airway, and monitor for signs of hypovolemia, shock, and cardiac dysrhythmias. Check vital signs and neurovascular response often.
• Cover sucking chest wound during exhalation with petrolatum gauze and an occlusive dressing.
• Cleanse wound gently with soap and water; debride as necessary.
• If damage is minor, apply dry sterile dressing.
• Administer tetanus prophylaxis, if necessary.
• Obtain X-rays to detect retained fragments.
• If possible, determine caliber of weapon.
• Report to police.

X

X-linked infantile hypogammaglobulinemia
(Bruton's agammaglobulinemia)

Description
X-linked infantile hypogammaglobulinemia is a congenital disorder in which all five immunoglobulins—IgM, IgG, IgA, IgD, and IgE—and circulating B cells are absent or deficient. Affecting males almost exclusively, this disorder occurs in 1 in 50,000 to 100,000 births and causes severe, recurrent infections during infancy. Prognosis is good with early treatment, except in infants who develop polio or persistent viral infection. Infection usually causes some permanent damage, especially in the neurologic or respiratory system.

Causes
Unknown

Signs and symptoms
• Recurrent bacterial otitis media
• Pneumonia
• Dermatitis
• Bronchitis
• Meningitis
• Possible purulent conjunctivitis, dental caries, polyarthritis resembling rheumatoid arthritis, severe malabsorption, and retarded development

Diagnostic tests
• Immunoelectrophoresis reveals decreased or absence of IgM, IgA, and IgG; however, diagnosis by this method usually is not possible until the infant is 9 months old.
• Antigenic stimulation confirms an inability to produce specific antibodies.

Treatment and clinical implications
Treatment aims to prevent or control infections and to boost the patient's immune response. Injection of immune globulin helps maintain immune response. Since these injections are very painful, give them deep into a large muscle mass, and massage well. If the dose is more than 1.5 ml, divide it and inject it into more than one site; for frequent injections, rotate the injection sites. Because immune globulin is composed primarily of IgG, the patient may also need fresh frozen plasma infusions to provide IgA and IgM. Unfortunately, mucosal secretory IgA cannot be replaced by therapy, resulting in frequent crippling pulmonary disease.

Judicious use of antibiotics also helps combat infection. In some cases, chronic broad-spectrum antibiotics may be indicated. To help prevent severe infection, teach the patient and his family how to recognize its early signs and to report them promptly. Warn them to avoid crowds and persons who have active infections.

During acute infection, monitor the patient closely. Maintain adequate nutrition and hydration, and perform chest physiotherapy if required.

Suggest genetic counseling if parents have questions about vulnerability of future offspring.

Appendix A: Abbreviation List

A

ABGs — arterial blood gases
ACTH—adrenocorticotropic hormone
ADH—antidiuretic hormone
A/G ratio—albumin-globulin ratio
AHF—antihemophilia factor
AK — above the knee
ALT—alanine aminotransferase
ANA—antinuclear antibodies
AST—aspartate aminotransferase

B

BUN—blood urea nitrogen

C

C.—centigrade
CBC—complete blood count
CNS—central nervous system
CO—carbon monoxide
CO_2—carbon dioxide
COPD—chronic obstructive pulmonary disease
CPK—creatinine phosphokinase
CPR—cardiopulmonary resuscitation
CSF—cerebrospinal fluid
CT — computerized tomography
CVP—central venous pressure
CVS—cardiovascular system

D

D&C—dilatation and curretage
DLco—diffusing capacity for carbon monoxide
DNA—deoxyribonucleic acid
DPT—diphtheria, pertussis, tetanus (toxoids, vaccine)
DSM III—the American Psychiatric Association's Diagnostic and Statistical Manual of Mental Disorders, 3rd ed.

E

EEG—electroencephalogram
EKG/ECG—electrocardiogram
EMG—electromyogram
ENT—ear, nose, throat
ERV—expiratory reserve volume
ESR—erythrocyte sedimentation rate

F

F.—Fahrenheit
FDA—U.S. Food and Drug Administration
FEV—forced expiratory volume
FEV_1, FEV_2, FEV_3—forced expiratory volume measured in the 1st, 2nd, or 3rd second of the FVC maneuver
FHR—fetal heart rate
FIO_2—fraction of inspired oxygen

FRC—functional residual capacity
FSH—follicle-stimulating hormone
FUO—fever of undetermined origin
FVC—forced vital capacity

G

GFR—glomerular filtration rate
GI—gastrointestinal
GU—genitourinary

H

hCG—human chorionic gonadotropin
HCO_3—bicarbonate
Hct—hematocrit
Hgb—hemoglobin

I

IC—inspiratory capacity
ICP—increased intracranial pressure
IM—intramuscular
IOP—intraocular pressure
IPPB—intermittent positive pressure breathing
IRV—inspiratory reserve volume
IQ—intelligence quotient
I.V.—intravenous
IVP—intravenous pyelogram

L

LDH—lactic dehydrogenase
LE—lupus erythematosus
LH—luteinizing hormone

Abbreviation List (continued)

M

MCH—mean corpuscular hemoglobin
MCHC—mean corpuscular hemoglobin concentration
MCV—mean corpuscular volume
MI—myocardial infarction
MMEF—maximal midexpiratory flow
MVV—maximal voluntary ventilation

N

N—nitrogen
NG—nasogastric

O

O₂CT—oxygen content
O.D.—right eye
O.L.—left eye
O.S.—left eye
O₂Sat—oxygen saturation

P

PaCO₂—partial pressure of arterial carbon dioxide
PaO₂—partial pressure of arterial oxygen
PAP—pulmonary artery pressure
PAWP—pulmonary artery wedge pressure
PCWP—pulmonary capillary wedge pressure
PCG—phonocardiogram
PCO₂—partial pressure of carbon dioxide

PEEP—positive end expiratory pressure
pH—hyrogen-ion concentration
PID—pelvic inflammatory disease
PKU—phenylketonuria
PMI—point of maximum impulse
P.O.—by mouth, orally
PO₂—partial pressure of oxygen
PT—prothrombin time
PTH—parathyroid hormone
PTT—partial thromboplastin time
PWP—pulmonary wedge pressure

R

RBC—red blood cell
RES—reticulo-endothelial system
RF—rheumatoid factor
RNA—ribonucleic acid
RV—residual volume

S

SGOT—serum glutamic-oxaloacetic transaminase
SGPT—serum glutamic-pyruvic transaminase
STH—somatotropic hormone

T

TGV—throracic gas volume
TLC—total lung capacity
TSH—thyroid-stimulating hormone

V

VC—vital capacity
VCG—vectorcardiogram
VDRL—Venereal Disease Research Laboratory test

W

WBC—white blood cell

Appendix B: Additional Resources

ALCOHOLISM

Al-Anon Family Group Headquarters, 1372 Broadway, New York, N.Y. 10018; (212) 302-7240

Alateen World Service Headquarters, 1372 Broadway, New York, N.Y. 10018; (212) 302-7240

General Service Board of Alcoholics Anonymous (AA), 468 Park Ave., S., New York, N.Y., 10016; (212) 686-1100

ALLERGY AND ASTHMA

American Allergy Association (AAA), P.O. Box 7273, Menlo Park, Calif. 94025; (415) 322-1663

Asthma and Allergy Foundation of America (AAFA), 9604 Wisconsin Ave, Bethesda, Md. 20814; (301) 493-6552

ALZHEIMER'S DISEASE

Alzheimer's Disease and Related Disorders Association (ADRDA), 360 N. Michigan Ave., Chicago, Ill. 60601; (312) 853-3060

AMYOTROPHIC LATERAL SCLEROSIS

Amyotrophic Lateral Sclerosis Society of America, 15300 Ventura Blvd., Sherman Oaks, Calif. 91403; (213) 990-2151

National ALS Foundation, Inc., 185 Madison Ave., New York, N.Y. 10016; (212) 679-4016

ANOREXIA NERVOSA

American Anorexia Nervosa Association, 133 Cedar Lane, Teaneck, N.J. 07666; (201) 836-1800

Anorexia Nervosa and Associated Disorders (ANAD), Box 7, Highland Park, Ill. 60034; (312) 831-3438

ARTHRITIS

Arthritis Foundation (AF), 1314 Spring St., N.W., Atlanta, Ga. 30309; (404) 872-7100

American Rheumatism Association (ARA), c/o Arthritis Foundation

AUTISM

National Society for Autistic Children and Adults, 1234 Massachusetts Ave., N.W., Suite 1017, Washington, D.C. 20005; (202) 783-0125

BIRTH DEFECTS

March of Dimes Birth Defects Foundation (MDBDF), 1275 Mamaroneck Ave., White Plains, N.Y. 10605; (914) 428-7100

BLINDNESS

American Foundation for the Blind (AFB), 15 W. 16th St., New York, N.Y. 10011; (212) 620-2000

National Federation of the Blind, 1800 Johnson St., Baltimore, Md. 21230; (301) 659-9314

National Society to Prevent Blindness, 79 Madison Ave., New York, N.Y. 10016; (212) 684-3505

Additional Resources *(continued)*

CANCER

American Cancer Society (ACS), 90 Park Ave., New York, N.Y. 10016; (212) 599-8200

International Association of Laryngectomees (IAL), c/o American Cancer Society

Reach to Recovery Foundation, c/o American Cancer Society

United Ostomy Association (UOA), 2001 W. Beverly Blvd., Los Angeles, Calif. 90057; (213) 413-5510

CEREBRAL PALSY

United Cerebral Palsy Association, Inc., 66 E. 34th St., New York, N.Y. 10016; (212) 481-6300

CYSTIC FIBROSIS

Cystic Fibrosis Foundation (CFF), 6000 Executive Blvd., Suite 510, Rockville, Md. 20852; (800) 344-4823

DIABETES

American Association of Diabetes Educators (AADE), 500 N. Michigan Ave., Suite 1400, Chicago, Ill. 60611; (312) 661-1700

American Diabetes Association (ADA), National Service Center, 1600 Duke Street, Alexandria, Va. 22314; (800) 232-3472

Juvenile Diabetes Foundation International (JDFI), 60 Madison Ave., 4th Floor, New York, N.Y. 10010; (212) 889-7575

EPILEPSY

Epilepsy Foundation of America (EFA), 4351 Garden City Dr., Landover, Md. 20785; (301) 459-3700

HEART DISEASE

American Heart Association (AHA), 7320 Greenville Ave., Dallas, Tex. 75231; (214) 750-5300

HEMOPHILIA

National Hemophilia Foundation (NHF), 110 Green St., Room 406, New York, N.Y. 10012; (212) 219-8180

HUNTINGTON'S DISEASE

Huntington's Disease Foundation of America (HDFA), 140 W. 22nd St., 6th Floor, New York, N.Y. 10011; (212) 242-1968

National Huntington's Disease Association (NHDA), 1182 Broadway, Suite 402, New York, N.Y. 10001; (212) 684-2781

INFECTIOUS DISEASES

Centers for Disease Control, 1600 Clifton Rd., N.E., Atlanta, Ga. 30333; (404) 329-3311

KIDNEY DISEASE

National Kidney Foundation (NKF), 2 Park Ave., New York, N.Y. 10016; (212) 889-2210

(continued)

Additional Resources (continued)

LUPUS ERYTHEMATOSUS

American Lupus Society, 23751 Madison St., Torrance, Calif. 90505; (213) 373-1335

National Lupus Erythematosus Foundation (NLEF), 5430 Van Nuys Blvd., Suite 206, Van Nuys, Calif. 91401; (818) 885-8787

MENTAL HEALTH

National Mental Health Association, 1800 N. Kent St., Rosslyn, VA 22209; (703) 528-6405

MENTAL RETARDATION

Association for Children with Retarded Mental Development (ACRMD), 27 W. 23rd St., New York, N.Y. 10010; (212) 645-7000

President's Committee on Mental Retardation, 330 Independence Ave., S.W., Washington, D.C., 20201; (202) 245-7634

MIGRAINE HEADACHE

National Migraine Foundation, 5252 N. Western Ave., Chicago, Ill. 60625; (312) 878-7715

MULTIPLE SCLEROSIS

National Multiple Sclerosis Society (NMSS), 205 E. 42nd St., New York, N.Y. 10017; (212) 986-3240

MUSCULAR DYSTROPHY

Muscular Dystrophy Association, Inc., 810 7th Ave., New York, N.Y. 10019; (212) 586-0808

MYASTHENIA GRAVIS

Myasthenia Gravis Foundation, 7-11 South Broadway, Suite 304, White Plains, N.Y. 10601; (914) 328-1717

NEUROFIBROMATOSIS

The National Neurofibromatosis Foundation, Inc., 141 5th Ave., Suite 7-S, New York, N.Y. 10010; (212) 460-8980

PARKINSON'S DISEASE

American Parkinson Disease Association, 116 John St., New York, N.Y. 10038; (212) 732-9550

National Parkinson Foundation (NPF), 1501 N.W. 9th Ave., Miami, Fla. 33136; Fla.: (800) 433-7022; U.S.: (800) 327-4545

United Parkinson Foundation (UPF), 360 W. Superior St., Chicago, Ill. 60610; (312) 664-2344

PSORIASIS

National Psoriasis Foundation (NPF), 6443 S.W. Beaverton Hwy., Suite 210, Portland, Ore. 97221; (503) 297-1545

RAPE CRISIS SYNDROME

Pennsylvania Coalition Against Rape, 2200 N. 3rd St., Harrisburg, Pa. 17110; (800) 692-7445

REYE'S SYNDROME

National Reye's Syndrome Foundation (NRSF), 426 N. Lewis, Bryan, Ohio 43506; (419) 636-2679

Additional Resources *(continued)*

RETINITIS PIGMENTOSA

RP Foundation Fighting Blindness (RPFFB), 1401 Mount Royal Ave., Baltimore, Md. 21217; (301) 225-9400

SCOLIOSIS

Scoliosis Association, Inc., One Penn Plaza, New York, N.Y. 10119; (212) 845-1760

SEXUAL DYSFUNCTION

American Association of Sex Educators, Counselors and Therapists (AASECT), 11 Dupont Circle, Suite 220, Washington, D.C. 20036; (202) 462-1171

Herpes Resource Center (HRC), Box 100, Palo Alto, Calif. 94306; (415) 328-7710

SICKLE CELL DISEASE

National Association for Sickle Cell Disease, 3460 Wilshire Blvd., Suite 1012, Los Angeles, Calif. 90010; (213) 731-1166

SPEECH AND HEARING IMPAIRMENT

American Speech-Language-Hearing Association, 10801 Rockville Pike, Rockville, Md. 20852; (301) 897-5700

American Tinnitus Association, P.O. Box 5, Portland, Ore. 97207; (503) 248-9985

National Association of the Deaf, 814 Thayer Ave., Silver Spring, Md. 20910; (301) 587-1788

Self Help for Hard of Hearing People, Inc., P.O. Box 34889, Bethesda, Md. 20817; (301) 469-7222

SPINA BIFIDA

Spina Bifida Association of America (SBAA), 343 S. Dearborn Ave., Suite 310, Chicago, Ill. 60604; (312) 663-1562

SPINAL INJURY

American Spinal Injury Association, 250 E. Superior, Chicago, Ill. 60611; (312) 649-3425

SUDDEN INFANT DEATH SYNDROME

National Sudden Infant Death Syndrome Foundation (NSIDSF), 2 Metro Plaza, Suite 205, 8240 Professional Pl., Landover, Md. 20785; (800) 221-SIDS

TAY-SACHS DISEASE

National Tay-Sachs and Allied Diseases Association (NTSAD), 92 Washington Ave., Cedarhurst, N.Y. 11516; (516) 569-4300

MISCELLANEOUS

American Red Cross (ARC), 430 17th St., N.W., Washington, D.C. 20006; (202) 737-8300

Smokenders, 214 S. 42nd St., Philadelphia, Pa. 19104; (215) 386-1403

U.S. Committee for the World Health Organization (USC-WHO), 515 22nd St., N.W., Washington, D.C. 20037; (202) 861-4322

SELECTED REFERENCES

Adams, R.D., and Victor, M. *Principles of Neurology*, 3rd ed. New York: McGraw-Hill Book Co., 1981.

Arndt, Kenneth A. *Manual of Dermatologic Therapeutics*, 3rd ed. Boston: Little, Brown & Co., 1983.

Beck, Cornelia M., and Rawlins, Ruth Parmlee. *Mental Health in Psychiatric Nursing: A Holistic Life-Cycle Approach*. St. Louis: C.V. Mosby Co., 1984.

Bell, C. William. *Home Care and Rehabilitation in Respiratory Medicine*. Philadelphia: J.B. Lippincott Co., 1984.

Bobak, Irene M., and Jensen, Margaret D. *Essentials of Maternity Nursing*. St. Louis: C.V. Mosby Co., 1984.

Bockus, Henry, ed. *Gastroenterology*, 4th ed. Philadelphia: W.B. Saunders Co., 1984.

Boyda, Ellen K. *Respiratory Problems*, vol. 5. Oradell, N.J.: Medical Economics, 1983.

Braunwald, Eugene, M.D. *Heart Disease: A Textbook of Cardiovascular Medicine*, vol. 2. Philadelphia: W.B. Saunders Co., 1984.

Bricker, Neal S., and Kirschenbaum, Michael A. *The Kidney: Diagnosis and Management*. New York: John Wiley & Sons, 1984.

Brown, R.B. *Clinical Urology Illustrated*. Baltimore: Williams & Wilkins Co., 1982.

Brundage, Dorothy J. *Nursing Management of Renal Problems*, 2nd ed. St. Louis: C.V. Mosby Co., 1980.

Burgess, Ann W., and Baldwin, Bruce. *Crisis Intervention Theory and Pratice: A Clinical Handbook*. Englewood Cliffs, N.J.: Prentice Hall, 1981.

Burton, George G., and Hodgkin, John E., eds. *Respiratory Care: A Guide to Clinical Practice*, 2nd ed. Philadelphia: J.B. Lippincott Co., 1984.

Cadoret, Remi J., and King, L. *Psychiatry in Primary Care*, 2nd ed. St. Louis: C.V. Mosby Co., 1983.

Casciato, Dennis A., and Bennett, B.B. Lowitz. *Manual of Bedside Oncology*. Boston: Little, Brown & Co., 1983.

Cohen, Felissa L. *Clinical Genetics in Nursing Practice*. Philadelphia: J.B. Lippincott Co., 1984.

Cohn, Robert M., and Roth, Karl. *Metabolic Disease: A Guide to Early Recognition*. Philadelphia: W.B. Saunders Co., 1983.

Conn, Howard F., and Conn, Rex B., Jr. *Current Diagnosis*. Philadelphia: W.B. Saunders Co., 1980.

Conway-Rutkowski, Barbara L. *Carini and Owen's Neurological and Neurosurgical Nursing*, 8th ed. St. Louis: C.V. Mosby Co., 1982.

Coppleson, Malcom. *Gynecologic Oncology: Fundamental Principles and Clinical Practice*. New York: Churchill Livingstone, 1981.

Coventry, Mark B., ed. *Yearbook of Orthopedics, 1984*. Chicago: Year Book Medical Pubs., 1984.

Dalton, John R. *Basic Clinical Urology*. Philadelphia: J.B. Lippincott Co., 1982.

Dec, William G., Jr., et al. "Active Myocarditis in the Spectrum of Acute Dilated Cardiomyopathies," *New England Journal of Medicine* 312(14):885, April 4, 1985.

DeGroot, Leslie J., et al. *The Thyroid and Its Diseases*, 5th ed. New York: John Wiley & Sons, 1984.

DeVita, V.T., Jr., and Hellman, S. *Cancer: Principles and Practices of Oncology*. Philadelphia: J.B. Lippincott Co., 1982.

DeWeese, David D., and Saunders, William H. *Textbook of Otolaryngology*, 6th ed. St. Louis: C.V. Mosby Co., 1982.

DiSaia, Philip J., and Creasman, William T. *Clinical Gynecologic Oncology*. St. Louis: C.V. Mosby Co., 1981.

Donovan, M., and Pierce, S. *Cancer Care Nursing*. East Norwalk, Conn.: Appleton-Century-Crofts, 1984.

Duane, Thomas, ed. *Clinical Ophthalmology*. New York: Harper & Row Publishers, 1985.

English, Gerald, ed. "Otolaryngology," *Loose Leaf Reference Services*, vols. 1-5. Philadelphia: J.B. Lippincott Co., 1985.

First, Martin Roy. *Chronic Renal Failure: Pathophysiology, Clinical Manifestations, and Management.* New Hyde Park, N.Y.: Medical Examination Pub. Co., 1982.

Fitzpatrick, Thomas B., et al. *Dermatology in General Medicine: Update One.* New York: McGraw-Hill Book Co., 1982.

Flamenbaum, Walter. *Nephrology: An Approach to the Patient with Renal Disease.* Philadelphia: J.B. Lippincott Co., 1982.

Given, Barbara A., and Simmons, Sandra J. *Gastroenterology in Clinical Nursing,* 4th ed. St. Louis: C.V. Mosby Co., 1983.

Gilroy, John, and Holliday, Patti. *Basic Neurology.* New York: MacMillan Publishing Co., 1982.

Goldstein, William N. "DSM-III and the Diagnosis of Schizophrenia," *American Journal of Psychotherapy* 37(2):168-81, April 1983.

Gonick, Harvey C., ed. *Current Nephrology.* New York: John Wiley & Sons, 1983.

Green, Barth, et al. *Intensive Care for Neurologic Trauma and Disease.* Orlando, Fla.: Academic Press, 1982.

Guzzetta, C., and Dossey, B. *Cardiovascular Nursing: Bodymind Tapestry.* Philadelphia: J.B. Lippincott Co., 1983.

Haber, Judith, et al. *Comprehensive Psychiatric Nursing,* 2nd ed. New York: McGraw-Hill Book Co., 1982.

Hagerty, Bonnie K., and Packard, Karen L. *Psychiatric-Mental Health Assessment.* St. Louis: C.V. Mosby Co., 1984.

Hall, Ian S., and Colman, Bernard S. *Diseases of the Nose, Throat, and Ear,* 12th ed. New York: Churchill Livingstone, 1981.

Harley, Robinson D., ed. *Pediatric Ophthalmology.* Philadelphia: W.B. Saunders Co., 1983.

Hirsh, Jack, and Brain, Elizabeth A. *Hemostasis and Thrombosis: A Conceptual Approach,* 2nd ed. New York: Churchill Livingstone, 1983.

Holbrook, R.H., Jr., and Creasy, R.K. "Prevention of Preterm Delivery: The Important Role of Early Recognition," *Postgraduate Medicine* 75(8)177-85, June 1984.

Holland, J., and Frei, E. *Cancer Medicine.* Philadelphia: Lea & Febiger, 1982.

Hurst, J. Willis, et al. *The Heart.* New York: McGraw-Hill Book Co., 1982.

Hutchinson, Margaret McGahan. "Aplastic Anemia: Care of the Bone-Marrow-Failure Patient," *Nursing Clinics of North America* 18(3):543-51, September 1983.

Immunization Practices Advisory Committee. "Postexposure Prophylaxis of Hepatitis B," *Annals of Internal Medicine* 101(3):351-54, September 1984.

Jahss, Melvin H. *Disorders of the Foot,* vol. I. Philadelphia: W.B. Saunders Co., 1982.

JAMA. *Primer on Allergic and Immunologic Diseases.* November 26, 1982.

Kaplan, Helen S., et al. *The Evaluation of Sexual Disorders: Psychological and Medical Aspects.* New York: Brunner, Mazel, Inc., 1983.

Kaye, Donald, and Rose, Louis F. *Fundamentals of Internal Medicine.* St. Louis: C.V. Mosby Co., 1983.

Kelley, William N., et al. *Textbook of Rheumatology,* 2nd ed. Philadelphia: W.B. Saunders Co., 1985.

Kempe, C. Henry, et al., eds. *Current Pediatric Diagnosis and Treatment,* 8th ed. Los Altos, Calif.: Lange Medical Pubns., 1984.

Klenerman, L. *The Foot and Its Disorders,* 2nd ed. St. Louis: C.V. Mosby Co., 1982.

Krieger, Dorothy T., and Bardin, C. Wayne. *Current Therapy in Endocrinology, 1983-1984.* St. Louis: C.V. Mosby Co., 1983.

Lamb, H. Richard. "Deinstitutionalization and the Homeless Mentally Ill," *Hospital and Community Psychiatry* 35(9):899-907, September 1984.

Larson, Elaine. *Clinical Microbiology and Infection Control.* Boston: Blackwell Scientific Publications, 1984.

Lego, Suzanne. *The American Handbook of Psychiatric Nursing.* Philadelphia: J.B. Lippincott Co., 1984.

Lerner, Judith, and Khan, Zafar. *Mosby's Manual of Urologic Nursing.* St. Louis: C.V. Mosby Co, 1982.

Lichtenstein, Lawrence M., and Fauci, Anthony S. *Current Therapy in Allergy and Immunology 1983-1984.* St. Louis: C.V. Mosby Co., 1983.

(continued)

Loeb, J.M. "Cardiac Electrophysiology: Basic Concepts and Arrhythmogenesis," *Critical Care Quarterly* 7(2):9-19, September 1984.

McCarty, Daniel J. *Arthritis and Allied Conditions: A Textbook of Rheumatology,* 10th ed. Philadelphia: Lea & Febiger, 1985.

Magrinat, Gaston, et al. "A Reassessment of Catatonia," *Comprehensive Psychiatry* 24(3):218-28, May/June, 1983.

Menoascino, Frank J., and McCann, Brian. *Mental Health and Mental Retardation: Bridging the Gap.* Austin, Tex.: Pro-Ed, 1983.

Metheny, Norma, and Snively, W.D., Jr. *Nurses' Handbook of Fluid Balance,* 4th ed. Philadelphia: J.B. Lippincott Co., 1983.

Meyer, Jon K., and Schmidt, Chester M., Jr., eds. *Clinical Management of Sexual Disorders,* 2nd ed. Baltimore: Williams & Wilkins Co., 1983.

Milgrom, F., et al. *Principles of Immunological Diagnosis in Medicine.* Philadelphia: Lea & Febiger, 1981.

Moschella, Samuel L., et al. *Dermatology,* 2nd ed., vols 1 and 2. Philadelphia: W.B. Saunders Co., 1985.

Murray, Ruth B., and Huelskoetter, Marilyn W. *Psychiatric Mental Health Nursing: Giving Emotional Care.* Englewood Cliffs, N.J.: Prentice-Hall, 1983.

Nikas, Diana L. *Critically Ill Neurosurgical Patient.* New York: Churchill Livingstone, 1982.

Petersdorf, Robert G., et al. *Harrison's Principles of Internal Medicine,* 10th ed. New York: McGraw-Hill Book Co., 1983.

Plum, Fred, and Posner, Jerome. *The Diagnosis of Stupor and Coma,* 3rd ed. Philadelphia: F.A. Davis, 1983.

Platt-Koch, Lois M. "Borderline Personality Disorder: A Therapeutic Approach," *American Journal of Nursing* 83(12):1666-71, December 1983.

Potts, N.L. "Eating Disorders: The Secret Pattern of Binge/Purge," *American Journal of Nursing* 84(1):32-35, January 1984.

Rake, Robert F., ed. *Conn's Current Therapy.* Philadelphia: W.B. Saunders Co., 1984.

Rifkind, R.A., et al. *Fundamentals of Hematology.* Chicago: Year Book Medical Pubs., 1984.

Riggs, Gail K., and Gall, Eric P., eds. *Rheumatic Diseases: Rehabilitation and Management.* Boston: Butterworth Publishers, 1984.

Rodnan, Gerald P., et al., eds. *Primer on Rheumatic Diseases.* Atlanta: Arthritis Foundation, 1983.

Rosen, Peter, et al. *Emergency Medicine: Concepts and Clinical Practice,* vol. 1. St. Louis: C.V. Mosby Co., 1983.

Rudy, Ellen B., *Advanced Neurologic and Neurosurgical Nursing.* St. Louis: C.V. Mosby Co., 1984.

Sadler, Diane. *Nursing for Cardiovascular Health.* East Norwalk, Conn.: Appleton-Century-Crofts, 1984.

Salisbury, Roger E., and Newman, Nancy. *Manual of Burn Therapeutics.* Boston: Little, Brown & Co., 1983.

Schiff, Leon, ed. *Diseases of the Liver,* 5th ed. Philadelphia: J.B. Lippincott Co., 1982.

Schroeder, J.S., ed. *Invasive Cardiology.* Philadelphia: F.A. Davis Co., 1985.

Shortridge, L.A. "Using Ritodrine Hydrochloride to Inhibit Preterm Labor," *Journal of Maternal-Child Nursing* 8(1):58-61, January/February 1983.

Sleisinger, Marvin H., and Fordtran, John S. *Gastrointestinal Disease: Pathophysiology, Diagnosis, Management,* 3rd ed., vols. 1 and 2. Philadelphia: W.B. Saunders Co., 1983.

Smith, Donald R. *General Urology,* 11th ed. Los Altos, Calif.: Lange Medical Pubns., 1984.

Smith, J.B. *Pediatric Critical Care.* New York: John Wiley & Sons, 1983.

Spiro, Howard M. *Clinical Gastroenterology,* 2nd ed. New York: Macmillan Publishing Co., 1983.

Stanbury, John B., et al., eds. *The Metabolic Basis of Inherited Disease,* 5th ed. New York: McGraw-Hill Book Co., 1983.

Stites, Daniel P., et al, eds. *Basic and Clinical Immunology,* 5th ed. Los Altos, Calif.: Lange Medical Pubns., 1984.

Stone, William J., and Rabin, Pauline L., eds. *End-Stage Renal Disease*. Orlando, Fla.: Academic Press, 1983.

Stuart, Gail W., and Sundeen, Sandra J. *Principles and Practice of Psychiatric Nursing*, 2nd ed. St. Louis: C.V. Mosby Co., 1983.

"Symposium on Surgery of Stone Disease," *Urologic Clinics of North America* 10(1):583-766, November 1983.

Talal, N. "How to Recognize and Treat Sjögren's Syndrome," *Drug Therapy* 14:48-54, February 1984.

Thompson, Summer E., and Washington, A. Eugene. "Epidemiology of Sexually Transmitted Chlamydia Trachomatis Infections," *Epidemiologic Reviews* 5:96-123, 1983.

Twomey, Jeremiah J. *The Pathophysiology of Human Immunologic Disorders*. Baltimore: Urban & Schwarzenberg, 1982.

Underhill, Sandra, et al. *Cardiac Nursing*. Philadelphia: J.B. Lippincott Co., 1983.

Utsinger, Peter D., et al. *Rheumatoid Arthritis: Etiology, Diagnosis, Management*. Philadelphia: J.B. Lippincott Co., 1985.

Uyeda, Charles T., et al. "Rapid Diagnosis of Chlamydial Infections with the MicroTrak Direct Test," *Journal of Clinical Microbiology* 20(5):948-50, November 1984.

Vaughan, Daniel, and Asbury, Taylor. *General Ophthalmology*, 10th ed. Los Altos, Calif.: Lange Medical Pubs., 1983.

Vaughan, V., and McKay, R.J., eds. *Nelson Textbook of Pediatrics*, 12th ed. Philadelphia: W.B. Saunders Co., 1983.

Vogt, G. et al. *Manual of Neurosurgical Care*. St. Louis: C.V. Mosby Co., 1985.

Wachtel, Tom, et al. *Current Topics in Burn Care*. Rockville, Md.: Aspen Systems Corp., 1983.

Weir, D.M. *Immunology: An Outline for Students of Medicine and Biology*, 5th ed. New York: Churchill Livingstone, 1983.

Weisburg, Leon A., and Strub, Richard L. *Essentials of Clinical Neurology*. Baltimore: University Park Press, 1983.

Weller, R.O., et al. *Clinical Neuropathology*. New York: Springer-Verlag New York, 1983.

Whaley, L., and Wong, D. *Nursing Care of Infants and Children*, 2nd ed. St. Louis: C.V. Mosby Co., 1983.

Wilkins, Earle W., Jr. *MGH Textbook of Emergency Medicine*, 2nd ed. Baltimore: Williams & Wilkins Co., 1983.

Wilson, Holly S., and Kneisl, Carol Ren. *Psychiatric Nursing*, 2nd ed. Menlo Park, Calif.: Addison-Wesley Publishing Co., Medical/Nursing Division, 1983.

INDEX

i refers to an illustration; t to a table.

i refers to an illustration; t to a table.

i refers to an illustration; t to a table.

i refers to an illustration; t to a table.

i refers to an illustration; t to a table.

i refers to an illustration; t to a table.

i refers to an illustration; t to a table.

i refers to an illustration; t to a table.

N

O

i refers to an illustration; t to a table.

i refers to an illustration; t to a table.

i refers to an illustration; t to a table.

i refers to an illustration; t to a table.

i refers to an illustration; t to a table.